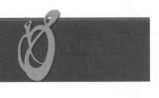

Preventive Cardiology

A Companion to Braunwald's Heart Disease

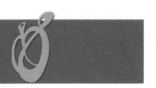

Preventive Cardiology

A Companion to Braunwald's Heart Disease

Roger S. Blumenthal, MD, FACC, FAHA
Professor of Medicine and Director
The Johns Hopkins Ciccarone Center for the Prevention of Heart Disease
Division of Cardiology, Johns Hopkins University
Baltimore, Maryland

JoAnne M. Foody, MD, FACC, FAHA
Associate Professor, Harvard Medical School
Director, Cardiovascular Wellness Center
Brigham and Women's/Faulkner Hospitals
Boston, Massachusetts

Nathan D. Wong, PhD, MPH, FACC, FAHA
Professor and Director
Heart Disease Prevention Program
Division of Cardiology, University of California, Irvine, California
Adjunct Professor, Department of Epidemiology
University of California, Irvine and Los Angeles, California
President, American Society for Preventive Cardiology

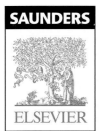

SAUNDERS

ELSEVIER

ELSEVIER
SAUNDERS

1600 John F. Kennedy Blvd.
Ste. 1800
Philadelphia, PA 19103-2899

Notices

Knowledge and best practice in this field are constantly changing. As new research and
experience broaden our understanding, changes in research methods, professional practices,
or medical treatment may become necessary.

Practitioners and researchers must always rely on their own experience and knowledge
in evaluating and using any information, methods, compounds, or experiments described
herein. In using such information or methods they should be mindful of their own safety
and the safety of others, including parties for whom they have a professional responsibility.

With respect to any drug or pharmaceutical products identified, readers are advised to
check the most current information provided (i) on procedures featured or (ii) by the
manufacturer of each product to be administered, to verify the recommended dose or
formula, the method and duration of administration, and contraindications. It is the
responsibility of practitioners, relying on their own experience and knowledge of their
patients, to make diagnoses, to determine dosages and the best treatment for each individual
patient, and to take all appropriate safety precautions.

To the fullest extent of the law, neither the Publisher nor the authors, contributors, or
editors, assume any liability for any injury and/or damage to persons or property as a matter
of products liability, negligence or otherwise, or from any use or operation of any methods,
products, instructions, or ideas contained in the material herein.

Library of Congress Cataloging-in-Publication Data
978-1-4377-1366-4

Executive Publisher: Natasha Andjelkovic
Developmental Editor: Bradley McIlwain
Publishing Services Manager: Patricia Tannian
Team Leader: Radhika Pallamparthy
Senior Project Manager: Sarah Wunderly
Project Manager: Joanna Dhanabalan
Design Direction: Steven Stave

Printed in the United States

Last digit is the print number: 9 8 7 6 5 4 3 2 1

This book is dedicated to the memory of Dr. Kenneth L. Baughman, who exemplified a tremendous commitment and personal passion for the principles and teachings of preventive cardiology during his entire life.

We would also like to thank our families for their support and encouragement during the development of this comprehensive textbook.

In addition, we extend special appreciation to those who inspired our careers in preventive cardiology, namely Drs. Eugene Braunwald, Peter Libby, Thomas Pearson, Adrian Ostfeld, William Kannel, William Castelli, Jeremiah Stamler, and Peter Kwiterovich.

Finally, we remember key colleagues and friends, including Dr. Stanley Blumenthal, Henry Ciccarone, David Kurtz, and John Yasuda, who made a difference in our lives and our commitment to preventive cardiology.

Ashkan Afshin, MD, MPH
Postdoctoral Research Fellow, Department of Epidemiology, Harvard School of Public Health, Boston, Massachusetts
Role of Ethnicity in Cardiovascular Disease: Lessons Learned from MESA and Other Population-Based Studies

George L. Bakris, MD
Professor of Medicine, Department of Medicine, University of Chicago Medical Center; Director, Hypertensive Disease Unit, Section of Endocrinology, Diabetes Metabolism and Hypertension, University of Chicago Medical Center, Chicago, Illinois
Advanced Risk Assessment in Patients with Kidney and Inflammatory Diseases

Christie M. Ballantyne, MD
Chief, Section of Cardiovascular Research; Interim Chief, Section of Cardiology, Department of Medicine, Baylor College of Medicine; Director, Center for Cardiovascular Disease Prevention, Methodist DeBakey Heart and Vascular Center, Houston, Texas
Novel Biomarkers and the Assessment of Cardiovascular Risk

Ronny A. Bell, PhD, MS
Professor of Epidemiology and Prevention, Division of Public Health Sciences, Wake Forest University School of Medicine, Winston-Salem, North Carolina
National and International Trends in Cardiovascular Disease: Incidence and Risk Factors

Jeffrey S. Berger, MD, MS, FACC
Assistant Professor of Medicine (Cardiology and Hematology); Assistant Professor of Surgery (Vascular Surgery); Director of Cardiovascular Thrombosis, New York University School of Medicine, New York, New York
Peripheral Arterial Disease Assessment and Management

Deepak L. Bhatt, MD, MPH, FACC, FAHA, FSCAI, FESC
Chief of Cardiology, VA Boston Healthcare System; Director, Integrated Interventional Cardiovascular Program, Brigham and Women's Hospital and VA Boston Healthcare System; Senior Investigator, TIMI Study Group; Associate Professor of Medicine, Harvard Medical School, Boston, Massachusetts
Antiplatelet Therapy

George L. Blackburn, MD, PhD
S. Daniel Abraham Associate Professor of Nutrition Medicine; Associate Director of Nutrition, Division of Nutrition, Harvard Medical School; Director of the Center for the Study of Nutrition and Medicine, Beth Israel Deaconess Medical Center, Boston, Massachusetts
Overweight, Obesity, and Cardiovascular Risk

Michael J. Blaha, MD, MPH
Johns Hopkins Ciccarone Center for the Prevention of Heart Disease, Baltimore, Maryland
Preventive Cardiology: Past, Present, and Future

Roger S. Blumenthal, MD, FACC
Professor of Medicine, The Johns Hopkins University School of Medicine; Director, Johns Hopkins Ciccarone Preventive Cardiology Center, Baltimore, Maryland
Preventive Cardiology: Past, Present, and Future; Role of Vascular Computed Tomography in Evaluation and Prevention of Cardiovascular Disease

Ariel Brautbar, MD
Assistant Professor, Section of Cardiovascular Research, Division of Atherosclerosis and Vascular Medicine, Department of Medicine, Department of Human and Molecular Genetics, Baylor College of Medicine, Houston, Texas
Novel Biomarkers and the Assessment of Cardiovascular Risk

Matthew J. Budoff, MD, FAHA, FACC
Professor of Medicine, David Geffen School of Medicine at UCLA, Los Angeles, California; Director, Cardiovascular Computed Tomography, Los Angeles Biomedical Research Institute, Torrance, California
Role of Vascular Computed Tomography in Evaluation and Prevention of Cardiovascular Disease

Gregory L. Burke, MD, MSc
Professor and Director, Division of Public Health Sciences, Wake Forest University School of Medicine, Winston-Salem, North Carolina
National and International Trends in Cardiovascular Disease: Incidence and Risk Factors

Javed Butler, MD, MPH
Professor of Medicine, Cardiology Division, Emory University; Deputy Chief Science Advisor, American Heart Association, Atlanta, Georgia
Heart Failure Prevention

Alison M. Coates, PhD
Senior Lecturer, Nutritional Physiology Research Centre, University of South Australia, Adelaide, Australia
Nutritional Approaches for Cardiovascular Disease Prevention

Mary C. Corretti, MD, FACC, FAHA, FASE
Associate Professor of Medicine; Director, Echocardiography Laboratory, The Johns Hopkins Hospital School of Medicine, Baltimore, Maryland
Endothelial Function and Dysfunction

Rebecca B. Costello, PhD, FACN
Office of Dietary Supplements, National Institutes of
Health, Bethesda, Maryland
*Integrative Medicine in the Prevention of Cardiovascular
Disease*

Michael H. Davidson, MD, FACC, FACP, FNLA
Clinical Professor and Director of Preventive Cardiology,
University of Chicago Pritzker School of Medicine;
Executive Medical Director, Radiant Research, Chicago,
Illinois
*Low-Density Lipoprotein Cholesterol: Role in
Atherosclerosis and Approaches to Therapeutic
Management*

Milind Y. Desai, MD
Staff Cardiologist, Cardiovascular Medicine, Heart and
Vascular Institute, Cleveland Clinic, Cleveland, Ohio
*Use of Cardiac Magnetic Resonance Imaging and
Positron Emission Tomography in Assessment of
Cardiovascular Disease Risk and Atherosclerosis
Progression*

William J. Elliott, MD, PhD
Professor of Preventive Medicine, Internal Medicine and
Pharmacology; Head, Division of Pharmacology, Pacific
Northwest University of Health Sciences, Yakima,
Washington
Hypertension: JNC 7 and Beyond

R. Curtis Ellison, MD
Professor of Medicine and Public Health; Director, Institute
on Lifestyle and Health, Boston University School of
Medicine, Boston, Massachusetts
Effects of Alcohol on Cardiovascular Disease Risk

Edward Fisher, MD, PhD
Leon H. Charney Professor of Cardiovascular Medicine;
Director, Center for the Prevention of Cardiovascular
Disease, Leon H. Charney Division of Cardiology, New
York University Langone Medical Center, New York,
New York
*Antihypertensive Drugs and Their Cardioprotective and
Renoprotective Roles in the Prevention and Management
of Cardiovascular Disease*

Puneet Gandotra, MD
Fellow in Cardiology, University of Maryland Hospital,
Baltimore, Maryland
*The Role of High-Density Lipoprotein Cholesterol in the
Development of Atherosclerotic Cardiovascular Disease*

Vasiliki V. Georgiopoulou, MD
Assistant Professor of Medicine, Emory University School
of Medicine, Division of Cardiology, Atlanta, Georgia
Heart Failure Prevention

Gary Gerstenblith, MD
Professor of Medicine, Division of Cardiology, Johns
Hopkins University, Baltimore, Maryland
*Cardiovascular Aging: The Next Frontier in
Cardiovascular Prevention*

Ty J. Gluckman, MD, FACC
Medical Director, Coronary Care Unit, Providence St.
Vincent Hospital, Portland, Oregon
Preventive Cardiology: Past, Present, and Future

M. Odette Gore, MD
Cardiology Fellow, Department of Internal Medicine,
Division of Cardiology, University of Texas Southwestern
Medical Center, Dallas, Texas
Diabetes and Cardiovascular Disease

Kristina A. Harris, BA, PhD candidate
Department of Nutritional Sciences, Pennsylvania State
University, University Park, Pennsylvania
*Nutritional Approaches for Cardiovascular Disease
Prevention*

Alison M. Hill, PhD
Postdoctoral Research Scholar, Department of Nutritional
Sciences, Pennsylvania State University, University Park,
Pennsylvania
*Nutritional Approaches for Cardiovascular Disease
Prevention*

P. Michael Ho, MD, PhD
Staff Cardiologist, Denver VA Medical Center; Associate
Professor of Medicine, University of Colorado Denver,
Denver, Colorado
*The Role of Treatment Adherence in Cardiac Risk Factor
Modification*

Paul N. Hopkins, MD, MSPH
Professor of Internal Medicine; Co-Director, Cardiovascular
Genetics, University of Utah School of Medicine, Salt
Lake City, Utah
Molecular Biology and Genetics of Atherosclerosis

Silvio E. Inzucchi, MD
Professor of Medicine; Clinical Director, Section of
Endocrinology; Program Director, Endocrinology &
Metabolism Fellowship, Yale University School of
Medicine; Director, Yale Diabetes Center, Yale-New Haven
Hospital, New Haven, Connecticut
Diabetes and Cardiovascular Disease

Heather M. Johnson, MD
Assistant Professor, University of Wisconsin School of
Medicine and Public Health, Madison, Wisconsin
*Carotid Intima-Media Thickness Measurement and
Plaque Detection for Cardiovascular Disease Risk
Prediction*

Steven R. Jones, MD, FACC, ABCL
Assistant Professor of Medicine, Cardiology, Johns Hopkins
University; Director, Inpatient Cardiology, The Johns
Hopkins Hospital School of Medicine, Baltimore,
Maryland
Endothelial Function and Dysfunction

Andreas P. Kalogeropoulos, MD
Assistant Professor of Medicine, Emory University School
Of Medicine, Division of Cardiology, Atlanta, Georgia
Heart Failure Prevention

Sekar Kathiresan, MD
Assistant Professor of Medicine, Harvard Medical School;
Director, Preventative Cardiology, Massachusetts
General Hospital; Associate Member, Broad Institute,
Massachusetts General Hospital, Boston, Massachusetts
*Genetics of Cardiovascular Disease and Its Role in Risk
Prediction*

Chad Kliger, MD
Fellow in Cardiovascular Disease, New York University
    Medical Center, New York, New York
    *Antihypertensive Drugs and Their Cardioprotective and
    Renoprotective Roles in the Prevention and Management
    of Cardiovascular Disease*

Penny M. Kris-Etherton, PhD, RD
Distinguished Professor of Nutrition, Department of
    Nutritional Sciences, Pennsylvania State University,
    University Park, Pennsylvania
    *Nutritional Approaches for Cardiovascular Disease
    Prevention*

Peter O. Kwiterovich, Jr., MD
Professor of Pediatrics and Medicine; Chief, Lipid Research
    Atherosclerosis Unit; Director, University Lipid Clinic,
    The Johns Hopkins Medical Institutions, Baltimore,
    Maryland
    *Evaluation and Management of Dyslipidemia in Children
    and Adolescents*

Edward G. Lakatta, MD
Director, Laboratory of Cardiovascular Science, National
    Institute on Aging, NIH; Professor of Medicine in
    Cardiology (part-time), The Johns Hopkins University
    School of Medicine; Adjunct Professor, Department of
    Physiology, University of Maryland School of Medicine,
    Baltimore, Maryland
    *Cardiovascular Aging: The Next Frontier in
    Cardiovascular Prevention*

Donald M. Lloyd-Jones, MD, ScM, FACC, FAHA
Chair, Department of Preventive Medicine; Associate
    Professor of Preventive Medicine and Medicine,
    Northwestern University Feinberg School of Medicine,
    Chicago, Illinois
    *Concepts of Screening for Cardiovascular Risk Factors
    and Disease*

John C. Longhurst, MD, PhD
Professor of Medicine; Professor, Departments of Physiology
    and Biophysics, Pharmacology and Biomedical
    Engineering; Director, Susan Samueli Center for
    Integrative Medicine, University of California, Irvine,
    California
    *Integrative Medicine in the Prevention of Cardiovascular
    Disease*

Russell V. Luepker, MD, MS
Mayo Professor, Division of Epidemiology, School of
    Public Health, University of Minnesota, Minneapolis,
    Minnesota
    *Tobacco Use, Passive Smoking, and Cardiovascular
    Disease: Research and Smoking Cessation Interventions*

Thomas M. Maddox, MD, Msc, FACC
Staff Cardiologist, Eastern Colorado Health Care System,
    U.S. Department of Veterans Affairs; Assistant Professor,
    Department of Medicine (Cardiology), University of
    Colorado Denver, Denver, Colorado
    *The Role of Treatment Adherence in Cardiac Risk Factor
    Modification*

Shaista Malik, MD, PhD, MPH
Assistant Professor, Division of Cardiology, University of
    California, Irvine, California
    Metabolic Syndrome and Cardiovascular Disease

Darren K. McGuire, MD, MHSc
Associate Professor of Medicine, Department of Internal
    Medicine, Division of Cardiology, University of Texas
    Southwestern Medical Center at Dallas, Dallas, Texas
    Diabetes and Cardiovascular Disease

C. Noel Bairey Merz, MD, FACC, FAHA
Director, Women's Heart Center; Director, Preventive and
    Rehabilitative Cardiac Center, Women's Guild Endowed
    Chair in Women's Health Heart Institute; Professor of
    Medicine, Cedars-Sinai Medical Center, Los Angeles,
    California
    Prevention of Ischemic Heart Disease in Women

Michael Miller, MD, FACC, FAHA
Professor of Medicine, Epidemiology and Public Health,
    University of Maryland School of Medicine; Director,
    Center for Preventive Cardiology, University of Maryland
    Medical Center, Baltimore, Maryland
    *The Role of High-Density Lipoprotein Cholesterol in the
    Development of Atherosclerotic Cardiovascular Disease*

Emile R. Mohler III, MD
Director of Vascular Medicine; Associate Professor of
    Medicine, University of Pennsylvania, Philadelphia,
    Pennsylvania
    Peripheral Arterial Disease Assessment and Management

Samia Mora, MD, MHS
Assistant Professor of Medicine, Harvard Medical School,
    Divisions of Cardiovascular Medicine, Preventive
    Medicine, Brigham and Women's Hospital, Boston,
    Massachusetts
    *Exercise Treadmill Stress Testing With and Without
    Imaging*

Kiran Musunuru, MD, PhD, MPH
Clinical and Research Fellow, Massachusetts General
    Hospital, Harvard Medical School, Broad Institute of MIT
    and Harvard, Johns Hopkins University School of
    Medicine, Boston, Massachusetts
    *Genetics of Cardiovascular Disease and Its Role in Risk
    Prediction*

Christian D. Nagy, MD
Adult and Pediatric Cardiology Fellow, The Johns Hopkins
    University School of Medicine, Ciccarone Center for the
    Prevention of Heart Disease, Baltimore, Maryland
    *Evaluation and Management of Dyslipidemia in Children
    and Adolescents*

Samer S. Najjar, MD
Medical Director, Heart Failure and Heart Transplantation,
    Washington Hospital Center, MedStar Health Research
    Institute, Washington, DC
    *Cardiovascular Aging: The Next Frontier in
    Cardiovascular Prevention*

Vijay Nambi, MD
Assistant Professor of Medicine, Baylor College of
    Medicine, Center for Cardiovascular Prevention,
    Methodist DeBakey Heart and Vascular Center, Ben Taub
    General Hospital, Houston, Texas
    *Novel Biomarkers and the Assessment of Cardiovascular
    Risk*

x **Khurram Nasir, MD, MPH**
Postdoctoral Fellow, Section of Cardiovascular Medicine, Yale School of Medicine, New Haven, Connecticut
Role of Vascular Computed Tomography in Evaluation and Prevention of Cardiovascular Disease

Raymond Oliva, MD
Fellow in Hypertensive Diseases, Department of Medicine, Hypertensive Disease Unit, Section of Endocrinology, Diabetes Metabolism and Hypertension, University of Chicago Medical Center, Chicago, Illinois
Advanced Risk Assessment in Patients with Kidney and Inflammatory Diseases

Raza H. Orakzai, MD
Fellow in Cardiovascular Disease, Cedars-Sinai Medical Center, Los Angeles, California
Prevention of Ischemic Heart Disease in Women

Gurusher S. Panjrath, MBBS
Clinical Fellow, The Johns Hopkins University School of Medicine, Baltimore, Maryland
Endothelial Function and Dysfunction

Jessica M. Peña, MD
Fellow in Cardiovascular Medicine, Cardiovascular Division, Brigham and Women's Hospital, Boston, Massachusetts
Antiplatelet Therapy

Tamar Polonsky, MD
Fellow, Cardiovascular Epidemiology and Prevention, Department of Preventive Medicine, Northwestern University, Chicago, Illinois
Advanced Risk Assessment in Patients with Kidney and Inflammatory Diseases

Prabhakar Rajiah, MBBS, MD, FRCR,
Clinical Fellow, Cardiovascular Imaging Laboratory, Imaging Institute, Cleveland Clinic, Cleveland, Ohio
Use of Cardiac Magnetic Resonance Imaging and Positron Emission Tomography in Assessment of Cardiovascular Disease Risk and Atherosclerosis Progression

Elizabeth V. Ratchford, MD, RVT/RPVI
Assistant Professor of Medicine; Director of the Johns Hopkins Center for Vascular Medicine, Division of Cardiology, The Johns Hopkins University School of Medicine, Baltimore, Maryland
Exercise for Restoring Health and Preventing Vascular Disease

Alan Rozanski, MD
Professor of Medicine, Division of Cardiology, Columbia University College of Physicians and Surgeons, St. Luke's-Roosevelt Hospital, New York, New York
Psychological Risk Factors and Coronary Artery Disease: Epidemiology, Pathophysiology, and Management

Arthur Schwartzbard, MD, FACC
Director, Clinical Lipid Research, NYU Center for Prevention of CV Disease; Assistant Professor of Medicine, Cardiology Section, NYUSOM; Director, Non Invasive Cardiology, Manhattan Campus of the NY Harbor Health Care System, New York, New York
Antihypertensive Drugs and Their Cardioprotective and Renoprotective Roles in the Prevention and Management of Cardiovascular Disease

Amil M. Shah, MD, MPH
Associate Physician, Divisions of Cardiovascular Medicine, Brigham and Women's Hospital, Instructor in Medicine, Harvard Medical School, Boston, Massachusetts
Exercise Treadmill Stress Testing With and Without Imaging

Leslee J. Shaw, PhD, FASNC, FACC, FAHA
Professor of Medicine; Co-Director, Emory Clinical Cardiovascular Research Institute, Emory University, Atlanta, Georgia
Prevention of Ischemic Heart Disease in Women

Chrisandra L. Shufelt, MD, MS, NCMP
Assistant Director, Women's Heart Center and Preventive and Rehabilitative Cardiac Center, Heart Institute, Cedars-Sinai Medical Center; Assistant Professor, Cedars-Sinai Medical Center; Assistant Clinical Professor, UCLA David Geffen School of Medicine, Los Angeles, California
Prevention of Ischemic Heart Disease in Women

Sidney C. Smith, Jr., MD, FACC, FAHA, FESC
Professor of Medicine; Director, Center for Cardiovascular Science and Medicine, University of North Carolina, Chapel Hill, North Carolina
Clinical Practice Guidelines and Performance Measures in the Treatment of Cardiovascular Disease

Kristina Spellman, RD, LD
Research Dietitian, Center for the Study of Nutrition Medicine, Beth Israel Deaconess Medical Center, Boston, Massachusetts
Overweight, Obesity, and Cardiovascular Risk

Laurence S. Sperling, MD, FACC, FACP, FAHA
Professor of Medicine (Cardiology); Director of Preventive Cardiology; Associate Director, Cardiology Fellowship Training Program, Emory University School of Medicine, Atlanta, Georgia
Heart Failure Prevention

James H. Stein, MD
Professor of Medicine, Cardiovascular Medicine Division; Director, Preventive Cardiology, University of Wisconsin School of Medicine and Public Health, Madison, Wisconsin
Carotid Intima-Media Thickness Measurement and Plaque Detection for Cardiovascular Disease Risk Prediction

Kerry J. Stewart, EdD, FAHA, MAACVPR, FACSM
Professor of Medicine; Director, Clinical and Research
  Exercise Physiology, The Johns Hopkins University
  School of Medicine, Johns Hopkins Bayview Medical
  Center, Baltimore, Maryland
  *Exercise for Restoring Health and Preventing Vascular
  Disease*

**Peter P. Toth, MD, PhD, FAAFP, FICA, FAHA,
FCCP, FACC**
Director of Preventive Cardiology, Sterling Rock Falls
  Clinic, Ltd., Sterling, Illinois; Clinical Professor,
  University of Illinois College of Medicine, Peoria, Illinois
  *Low-Density Lipoprotein Cholesterol: Role in
  Atherosclerosis and Approaches to Therapeutic
  Management*

Karol E. Watson, MD, PhD
Associate Professor of Medicine, Division of Cardiology,
  David Geffen School of Medicine at UCLA, Los Angeles,
  California
  *Role of Ethnicity in Cardiovascular Disease: Lessons
  Learned from MESA and Other Population-Based
  Studies*

Howard Weintraub, MD
Clinical Associate Professor, School of Medicine, Division
  of Cardiology, New York University Langone Medical
  Center, New York, New York
  *Antihypertensive Drugs and Their Cardioprotective and
  Renoprotective Roles in the Prevention and Management
  of Cardiovascular Disease*

Francine K. Welty, MD, PhD
Associate Professor of Medicine, Harvard Medical School;
  Director and Principal Investigator, NHLBI Specialized
  Center of Clinically Oriented Research in Vascular Injury,
  Repair and Remodeling, General and Preventative,
  Cardiologist, Division of Cardiology, Beth Israel
  Deaconess Medical Center, Boston, Massachusetts
  *The Contribution of Triglycerides and Triglyceride-Rich
  Lipoproteins to Atherosclerotic Cardiovascular Disease*

Mark A. Williams, PhD, FACSM, FAACVPR
Director, Cardiovascular Disease Prevention and
  Rehabilitation; Professor of Medicine, Division of
  Cardiology, Creighton University School of Medicine,
  Omaha, Nebraska
  *Exercise for Restoring Health and Preventing Vascular
  Disease*

Peter W. F. Wilson, MD
Professor of Medicine (Cardiology); Professor of Public
  Health (Epidemiology, Global Health), Emory University
  School of Medicine and Atlanta VAMC Epidemiology and
  Genetics Section, Atlanta, Georgia
  *Prediction of Cardiovascular Disease: Framingham Risk
  Estimation and Beyond*

Samuel Wollner, AB
Research Analyst, Center for the Study of Nutrition
  Medicine, Beth Israel Deaconess Medical Center, Boston,
  Massachusetts
  Overweight, Obesity, and Cardiovascular Risk

Nathan D. Wong, PhD, MPH, FACC, FAHA
Professor and Director, Heart Disease Prevention Program,
  Division of Cardiology, University of California,
  Irvine, California; Adjunct Professor, Department of
  Epidemiology, University of California, Irvine and
  Los Angeles, California; President, American Society
  for Preventive Cardiology
  *Metabolic Syndrome and Cardiovascular Disease; Role of
  Vascular Computed Tomography in Evaluation and
  Prevention of Cardiovascular Disease*

In the middle of the twentieth century, the development of an acute myocardial infarction was often totally unexpected and like the proverbial "bolt out of the blue." Frequently, *apparently* healthy persons were struck down during their most productive years, and at a time of large family responsibilities. These "heart attacks" often were either fatal or disabling. Medical attention was focused largely on the diagnosis and management of these catastrophic events. Forestalling or even better, preventing, myocardial infarction was rarely considered.

One notable exception, however, was Dr. Paul D. White, often called the "father of American cardiology." As early as the 1930s, White always included a section on prevention in his lectures on coronary artery disease, and he wrote about it in his famed textbook. The National Heart Institute (now the Heart, Lung and Blood Institute) was established in 1948 and was instrumental in furthering the concept of cardiac disease prevention. Two of the most important early actions by the Institute were the establishment of the Framingham Heart Study and of the Lipid Research Clinics. The former was (and continues to be) a long-term prospective study, with standardized examinations at intervals of adults who were initially without clinical manifestations of coronary artery disease. By 1961, it was evident that overtly healthy subjects with hypertension, hypercholesterolemia, and/or who were cigarette smokers were at higher risk to develop acute myocardial infarction than were their age- and sex-matched controls without these characteristics. Framingham investigators thus coined the term "coronary risk factors." These observations led to the important idea that the amelioration of risk factors would prevent, or at least delay, the development of clinical coronary artery disease. Considerable research has been done during the past half century that has supported this idea.

The institute's second major contribution was the Coronary Primary Prevention trial, which demonstrated that in subjects with hypercholesterolemia, but without overt coronary artery disease, the occurrence of coronary events could be reduced with a diet and cholestyramine, a resin that reduces elevated serum cholesterol. This confirmed, once and for all, the important role of cholesterol in atherogenesis. A breakthrough in coronary prevention occurred in the 1980s with the development of HMGCoA reductase inhibitors (statins), which caused a substantial lowering of LDL-cholesterol. Simultaneously, well tolerated blood pressure-reducing drugs and smoking cessation programs were developed.

At first, many cardiologists reacted sluggishly to these observations and often did not incorporate preventive measures into their practices. Both the glamour (and reimbursement) favored the diagnosis and management of acute illness over the more mundane (and poorly reimbursed) efforts required to maintain patients—particularly those who had no overt cardiovascular disease—on diet and other lifestyle measures as well as drugs, which often have some annoying side effects. However, during the 1990s, the evidence in favor of the clinical benefits of prevention became overwhelming, and in the first decade of this century, expert committees developed practice guidelines that provided strong support. Adherence to these guidelines became important measures of physician performance, a trend that only promises to increase in coming years.

Now, in the second decade of the current century, preventive cardiology has a robust and rapidly growing knowledge base. In addition to hypercholesterolemia, hypertension and cigarette smoking described a half century ago, we now recognize that diabetes, vascular inflammation, kidney disease, passive smoking, and a growing number of biomarkers and genetic variants may also be used in refining assessment of coronary risk.

Preventive Cardiology is very capably edited by Drs. Blumenthal, Foody, and Wong, and written by stellar authors, all experts in their subjects. It is a superb, well written and illustrated volume that elegantly weaves together the many separate strands of this critically important area of cardiology to provide a thorough understanding of the field. This volume should serve the needs of a broad audience. Prevention of cardiovascular disease is too important to leave to a relatively small group of experts, but instead must be carried out by all physicians, regardless of specialty, as well as by nurses and other health care professionals who care for patients with, or at risk of developing, cardiovascular disease. All of these groups and their trainees can profit enormously from this important book.

We are therefore very pleased to welcome *Preventive Cardiology* to the growing list of Companions to *Heart Disease*.

EUGENE BRAUNWALD

ROBERT BONOW

DOUGLAS MANN

DOUGLAS ZIPES

PETER LIBBY

For nearly a century, atherosclerotic cardiovascular disease has been the leading cause of death in industrialized countries. It often remains clinically silent for decades before resulting in an acute ischemic syndrome, myocardial infarction, stroke, or sudden cardiac death. Since atherosclerosis is a progressive disease that starts early in life, it challenges us to be more aggressive in our efforts regarding prevention.

Early identification of cardiovascular risk and modification of risk factors reduce the incidence of future cardiovascular events and improve peoples' quality of life. Unfortunately, rates of obesity and related conditions such as metabolic syndrome and diabetes are on the rise, in both developed and developing countries. Instead of prevention, significant health care dollars are spent on the end-stage complications of atherosclerotic vascular disease, such as drug-eluting stents, implantable cardioverter-defibrillators, and surgical revascularization.

Physicians, nurses, and other health care providers need to emphasize preventive strategies to slow or halt the progression of atherosclerosis. Health care providers need to understand how to optimize cardiovascular risk stratification. The Framingham and other global risk algorithms serve as an important starting point in risk assessment, but have limitations and often exclude key risk factors such as a family history of premature cardiovascular disease, glucose intolerance, triglycerides, waist size, and lifestyle habits. For example, although an adult with a glucose level of 126 mg/dL or higher is automatically placed into a very high risk category, a similar individual with a slightly lower glucose level but who may have additional risk factors or evidence of advanced subclinical atherosclerosis for their age may actually be at higher risk, but would not necessarily qualify for aspirin therapy, antihypertensive therapy, or lipid-lowering therapy.

A great need also exists for better understanding of the significance, clinical utility, and cost-effectiveness of more novel risk factors and screening for asymptomatic cardiovascular disease. Atherosclerosis imaging and measurement of biomarkers such as hs-CRP are now fairly widely performed, and there is a need for understanding how to incorporate into clinical practice the findings from large-scale epidemiologic studies (e.g., Cardiovascular Health Study and the Multi-Ethnic Study of Atherosclerosis) and clinical trials such as JUPITER. However, there are clear limitations to the data that we have so far on biomarkers such as hs-CRP and increasingly popular multimarker approaches, and imaging measures such as coronary artery calcium and carotid intima-media thickness. Experts are clearly split on how to incorporate emerging risk factors and subclinical disease into clinical practice.

The medical community needs to promote guideline adherence and reduce the gap in use of proven medical and lifestyle therapies. Moreover, federal, state, and local governments, education departments and schools, and the corporate sector need to play a greater role in ensuring environments conducive to promoting heart health. The cornerstone of prevention is based on therapeutic lifestyle changes, including regular brisk physical activity and a healthy diet, and strategies to better support these measures need to be developed and implemented at the health care and community level.

In this companion to *Braunwald's Heart Disease*, we approach cardiovascular disease prevention in a convenient ABCDE framework. In 2002 the AHA and ACC produced a guideline statement on the management of patients with chronic stable angina and arranged their recommendations into an ABCDE format. This approach has also been used as the basis for the training of fellows in preventive cardiology.[1] It has also been used in several evidence based reviews on primary and secondary prevention of CVD, management of non–ST-segment elevation myocardial infarction (NSTEMI) and management of metabolic syndrome.[2-4]

Prevention needs to be a central feature of a sustainable health care system, but implementation of preventive practices remains suboptimal. The ABCDE approach arranges prevention guidelines into an easy-to-remember framework that can be used by clinicians with each patient to ensure comprehensive care. The principal sections of this textbook include: (A) **a**ssessment of risk from a clinical and genetic perspective, **a**therothrombosis and **a**ntiplatelet therapy; (B) **b**lood pressure management; (C) **c**holesterol and dyslipidemia; (D) **d**iet and lifestyle issues (**d**iabetes mellitus ,metabolic syndrome; **d**isparities in care; **d**iagnostic testing to help improve risk prediction); and (E) **e**xercise prescriptions, cardiac rehabilitation and **e**motional aspects of preventive cardiology.

This text is meant to serve as a guide for those interested in prevention of cardiovascular disease. It provides an overview of the epidemiology and risk factors for cardiovascular disease, and the importance of risk stratification. It underscores the evidence base for the management of cardiovascular risk factors and provides recommendations for clinical care. It our hope that armed with the tools provided in this text we may achieve the promise of the prevention of most cardiovascular disease events in our lifetimes.

ROGER S. BLUMENTHAL, MD, FACC, FAHA

JOANNE FOODY, MD, FACC, FAHA

NATHAN D. WONG, PhD, MPH, FACC, FAHA

1. Blumenthal RS, et al. *J Am Coll Cardiol* 51:393, 2008.
2. Gluckman TJ, et al. *Arch Int Med* 164:1490, 2004.
3. Gluckman TJ, et al. *JAMA* 293:349, 2005.
4. Blaha MJ, et al. *Mayo Clin Proc* 83:932, 2008.

Contents

Look for These Other Titles in the Braunwald's Heart Disease Family

---

BRAUNWALD'S HEART DISEASE COMPANIONS

PIERRE THÉROUX
Acute Coronary Syndromes

ELLIOTT M. ANTMAN & MARC S. SABATINE
Cardiovascular Therapeutics

CHRISTIE M. BALLANTYNE
Clinical Lipidology

ZIAD ISSA, JOHN M. MILLER, & DOUGLAS P. ZIPES
Clinical Arrhythmology and Electrophysiology

DOUGLAS L. MANN
Heart Failure

HENRY R. BLACK & WILLIAM J. ELLIOTT
Hypertension

ROBERT L. KORMOS & LESLIE W. MILLER
Mechanical Circulatory Support

CATHERINE M. OTTO & ROBERT O. BONOW
Valvular Heart Disease

MARC A. CREAGER, JOSHUA A. BECKMAN, & JOSEPH LOSCALZO
Vascular Disease

BRAUNWALD'S HEART DISEASE IMAGING COMPANIONS

ALLEN J. TAYLOR
Atlas of Cardiac Computed Tomography

CHRISTOPHER M. KRAMER & **W. GREGORY HUNDLEY**
Atlas of Cardiovascular Magnetic Resonance

AMI E. ISKANDRIAN & **ERNEST V. GARCIA**
Atlas of Nuclear Imaging

JAMES D. THOMAS
Atlas of Echocardiography

SECTION 1

Assessment of Risk

CHAPTER **1**

Preventive Cardiology: Past, Present, and Future

Michael J. Blaha, Ty J. Gluckman, and Roger S. Blumenthal

KEY POINTS

- Atherosclerotic cardiovascular disease (CVD) is an ideal scenario for prevention efforts because (1) it is a common disease; (2) it is modifiable by behavior; (3) it has a long latency; (4) the time between symptom onset and severe disability or sudden cardiac death is short; and (5) no cure exists for systemic atherosclerosis once it is present.

- The Framingham Heart Study identified smoking, elevated blood pressure, and high cholesterol as the principal risk factors for CVD. More recently, the INTERHEART study has shown that 9 main CVD risk factors account for 90% of the population-attributable risk for a first myocardial infarction.

- The majority of improvement in rates of mortality from CVD since the 1960s is the result of prevention, not treatment, of acute CVD.

- Prevention occurs at three levels: primordial, primary, and secondary. However, there may be variable degrees of overlap as the cutoff points for risk factors change and as imaging modalities identify populations with disease burden that is not expected on the basis of traditional risk factors.

- There are two main approaches to prevention: a population-based approach, in which researchers seek to make small changes in risk factors across the entire population, and an individual-based approach, which emphasizes identifying individuals at high risk for CVD and aggressively lessening their risk factors.

- Guideline and scientific statements from the American Heart Association (AHA), American College of Cardiology (ACC), and other organizations direct population-based and individual-based preventive care.

- Despite guidelines, there is a wide gap between the burden of CVD and current preventive efforts. This gap can be narrowed with more simplified, comprehensive guidelines.

- This chapter offers an easy-to-remember memory tool that facilitates comprehensive preventive care: the "ABCDE" approach.

Since the early 1900s, atherosclerotic cardiovascular disease (CVD), including both coronary heart disease (CHD) and stroke, has been the leading cause of death in industrialized nations.[1] Atherosclerosis represents a unique public health challenge because it is a progressive, lifelong disease that is modified by behavior and yet produces few symptoms until late into its course. Unfortunately, when it does become clinically evident, there is often a short duration between symptom onset and disability, and sudden death is a common sentinel event.

In spite of numerous advances that have improved the treatment of acute CVD, many therapies remain costly, and their effectiveness depends on the prompt identification of the few individuals most likely to benefit. Both reperfusion and revascularization procedures are indicated in only a select group of patients with critical occlusive vascular disease; these treatments target localized areas of the vascular bed without addressing atherosclerosis throughout the rest of the body. As such, there remains no cure for atherosclerosis as a systemic disease.

Nonetheless, disproportionately large amounts of money are spent late in the disease course on relatively small numbers of patients with acute complications of CVD, rather than the far greater numbers in whom early preventive efforts might lead to markedly greater benefit. These factors underscore the true importance of CVD prediction and prevention, and they preface not only this chapter but the content of this entire text on preventive cardiology (Box 1-1).

With great foresight, the U.S. Public Health Service launched a publicly funded effort in the 1940s to identify modifiable CVD risk factors. Through modern clinical epidemiologic methods, the landmark Framingham Heart Study[2] helped define the field of preventive cardiology and led to the identification of smoking, hypertension,

BOX 1-1 Factors Making Atherosclerosis Ideal for Prevention

- High incidence
- Modifiable by behavior
- Long disease latency
- Short time between symptoms and disability
- Sudden death: a common manifestation
- Available treatments unable to cure underlying disease
- Treatment of acute disease associated with huge financial and societal cost

Risk Factor	Odds Ratio (99% CI) Multivariable Adjusted	Population-Attributable Risk Multivariable Adjusted
ApoB/ApoA-I	3.25 (2.82-3.76)	49%
Current smoking	2.87 (2.58-3.19)	36%
Diabetes	2.37 (2.07-2.71)	9.9%
Hypertension	1.91 (1.74-2.10)	18%
Abdominal obesity	1.62 (1.45-1.80)	20%
Psychosocial stress and depression	2.67 (2.21-3.22)	33%
Daily fruit and vegetable intake	0.70 (0.62-0.79)	14%
Exercise	0.86 (0.76-0.97)	12%
Alcohol intake	0.91 (0.82-1.02)	7%
Combined	129	90%

TABLE 1-1 Interheart: A Global Case-Control Study of Risk Factors for Acute Myocardial Infarction

Apo, apolipoprotein; CI, confidence interval.

and elevated cholesterol as the "principal risk factors" for CVD.[3] In the years that followed, the U.S. government launched several population-based educational campaigns and spent billions of dollars funding research aimed at controlling these risk factors. The Atherosclerosis Risk in Communities (ARIC) study, the Coronary Artery Risk Development in Young Adults (CARDIA) study, the Cardiovascular Health Study (CHS), and the Multi-Ethnic Study of Atherosclerosis (MESA) were instrumental in the effort to identify novel risk factors, to describe the determinants of early atherosclerosis, and to understand these factors and determinants in relation to younger, older, and multiple ethnic populations. Unfortunately, in spite of these efforts, smoking, hypertension, and hypercholesterolemia remain unacceptably common in the general population today.[1]

Risk factors for CVD begin accumulating at a young age, often while individuals are asymptomatic and unaware of the untoward consequences. Pathologic evidence of atherosclerosis can be identified soon after risk factor onset; persons with measurable risk demonstrate this evidence earliest.[4,5] Although risk factors are frequently present as early as the second and third decades of life, the presence of multiple risk factors is associated with an even higher prevalence of early atherosclerotic vascular disease.[6] Never has the risk for such individuals been more important than it is today, when a burgeoning global epidemic of childhood obesity further heightens the public health challenge.

Results from the global INTERHEART study suggest that nine modifiable risk factors—dyslipidemia, smoking, diabetes mellitus, hypertension, abdominal obesity, psychosocial stress, poor diet, physical inactivity, and alcohol consumption—account for more than 90% of the risk for a first myocardial infarction (Table 1-1).[7] The effects of these risk factors appear to be remarkably stable across gender, race, and geographic location. Such data have led the World Health Organization (WHO) to estimate that 80% of premature CHD can be prevented with comprehensive assessment and management of these risk factors.[8]

Because major CVD risk factors often co-occur, emerging risk factors probably account for disproportionately smaller numbers of CVD events.[9] In epidemiologic terms, biomarkers such as interleukin-6, adiponectin, and lipoprotein(a) are associated with a smaller incremental population-attributable risk. The value of measuring these factors, therefore, lies more in elucidating the pathophysiologic mechanisms of CVD and identifying novel therapeutic targets than in global risk prediction (Box 1-2).

Much research is still needed to better integrate existing risk variables into prediction models of short- and long-term global risk. This is important not only to ensure the cost-effective use of existing risk-reducing therapies (e.g., aspirin and statins) but to also determine who may benefit from measurement of biomarkers or detection of subclinical atherosclerosis through imaging techniques.[10] Improved treatment decisions—including delivery of existing options and the selective use of new modalities—remains the mainstay of

BOX 1-2 Modern Themes in Cardiovascular Disease Risk Prediction

- Novel risk factors: increasingly diminished population-attributable risk
- Novel risk factors: value is likely to be weighed in elucidating pathophysiologic mechanisms and guiding treatment
- Need for improved integration of existing risk factors into global risk prediction models
- Increased emphasis on delivery of care for existing risk factors

preventive cardiology. Only with improved risk prediction can treatment decisions be improved.

Success in preventive cardiology is defined by reduction in rates of mortality from CVD and the prevention of nonfatal CVD events. Since 1968, age-adjusted rates of mortality from CHD in the United States have been reduced by half, and similar trends have been noted in other industrialized countries around the world.[1,11,12] Concurrently, the prevalence of smoking, hypercholesterolemia, and high blood pressure has also decreased since 1968.[1] Public policy has played a tremendous role: Smoking bans have produced significant decreases in exposure to tobacco smoke,[13,14] dietary policies (including raising awareness of foods containing high amounts of saturated fats and bans on *trans*–fats in Europe[15]) have led to significant reductions in cholesterol levels,[16-18] and campaigns to decrease salt intake have resulted in significant reductions in systolic blood pressure.[19,20]

To explain the observed reduction in rates of mortality from CVD, researchers in several important studies have attempted to quantify the relative contribution of risk factor reduction versus treatment of acute CVD. Using IMPACT, a statistical model that incorporates risk factor and treatment data, researchers estimated that nearly half (44%) of the decline in U.S. CHD deaths from 1980 to 2000 resulted from population-wide risk factor reduction, and 47% resulted from evidence-based medical therapy directed at patients with known or suspected vascular disease.[21] Importantly, just 10% of the overall reduction was accounted for by acute therapy in acute coronary syndromes and 5% by revascularization in chronic stable angina. Similar results have been noted in other countries; in Finland, 76% of the cardiovascular disease mortality reduction was solely related to risk factor reduction.[22] The message from these studies is clear: the overwhelming majority of the reduction in rates of mortality from CVD is attributable to prevention, not to acute intervention.

Despite numerous successes in preventive cardiology, further innovation is urgently needed. Improvements in mortality rates are slowing, if not already at a plateau, and the increasing prevalence of obesity, diabetes mellitus, and the metabolic syndrome is probably responsible.[1] Increased caloric intake, greater consumption of refined carbohydrates, and decreased physical activity all have contributed to the emerging epidemic of abdominal obesity and insulin resistance. In fact, from 1980 to 2000, it is estimated that obesity and diabetes mellitus resulted in 8% and 10% increases in rates of mortality from CVD, respectively.[21]

Because of the broad range of topics within preventive cardiology, we have divided this chapter into four main parts. First, we discuss the three major levels of preventive cardiology: primordial prevention, primary prevention, and secondary prevention. Next, we review the current debate between population-based prevention strategies and strategies aimed at high-risk individuals, advocating for a mixture of the two. Then we highlight current prevention guideline statements, which serve as important references for health care providers. Last, we present the overarching theme for this text: The cardiovascular prevention community is desperately in need of simplified guidelines that are easy to implement. To that end, we present a concise "ABCDE" framework, which incorporates guidelines for most major modifiable risk factors into a simple memory tool for guiding comprehensive preventive care.

THE MAJOR LEVELS OF PREVENTION

Prevention of CVD occurs at three levels—primordial prevention, primary prevention, and secondary prevention—and each level has a different target population, a different setting in which care is provided, and different mechanisms of care delivery (Table 1-2).

Primordial Prevention

The term *primordial prevention,* first coined by Strasser[23] in 1978, describes efforts to *prevent the development* of CVD risk factors in a population. Primordial prevention occurs predominantly at the societal and community levels and includes policy decisions that influence dietary patterns, educational objectives, and the environment. One example of primordial prevention is policy-driven, population-wide reductions in intake of *trans*–fat and saturated fat in order to reduce total cholesterol levels.

The advantage of primordial prevention over other types of prevention is that intervention occurs before the onset of a given risk factor and its associated adverse effects. Primordial prevention also offers the possibility of sustainable gains in overall health and affordable care for a population, as the downstream need for subsequent acute CVD care is reduced or even eliminated. Also of importance is that primordial prevention can be applied to an entire population, without the need for screening to identify individuals at increased risk.

Primordial prevention measures usually produce only very small changes in risk factors at the individual patient level, inasmuch as these strategies are designed to reach larger numbers of individuals at a much earlier stage of life. As suggested by Rose, a leading epidemiologist, "A large number of people exposed to a small risk may generate many more cases than a small number exposed to a high risk."[24] In fact, according to some estimates, primordial prevention offers the possibility of much larger reductions in mortality rates than can be achieved with either primary or secondary prevention.[25]

The principal disadvantage of primordial prevention is that it is difficult to implement. Encouraging change in the behavior of an apparently "healthy" individual is challenging, partly because the relative risk reduction that occurs in such an individual over the near term is often small. In many cases, it is also difficult to predict the exact effect of such population-wide interventions until they are implemented. Finally, the up-front cost of initiating primordial prevention strategies is commonly enormous.

Primordial prevention frequently takes the form of policy change, educational programs, and environmental policy. These prevention plans are commonly implemented by politicians and are shaped by epidemiologic research. Clinicians, however, are becoming increasingly active in this area. This is particularly true in pediatrics and adolescent medicine, in which primordial prevention efforts are likely to have the greatest long-term benefit.

TABLE 1–2	Prevention of CVD		
		Level of Prevention	
Characteristic	**Primordial**	**Primary**	**Secondary**
Target patients	All patients, including children	Patients at increased risk for CVD	Patients with known CVD
Setting	Community, societal	Outpatient	Inpatient transitioning to outpatient
Delivery of care	Policy decisions Dietary patterns Education campaigns Environment	Education campaigns Behavioral intervention Medications	Behavioral intervention Medications Rehabilitation
Advantages	Intervention before risk factors develop Sustainable Does not require screening	Directed at higher risk individuals Tailored therapy Patients motivated to implement changes	Directed at highest risk individuals Tailored therapy Patients highly motivated to implement changes
Disadvantages	Difficult to implement Hard to quantify effect Up-front costs Individual risk reduction small	Requires screening of population May delay but not prevent disease "Medicalization" of asymptomatic individuals	Small segment of population eligible Attempts to attenuate loss of quality of life Not sustainable

CVD, cardiovascular disease.

Primary Prevention

Primary prevention consists of efforts to prevent adverse events, such as myocardial infarction and stroke, in individuals with known risk factors for CVD. Most frequently, such prevention takes the form of individualized lifestyle interventions, including diet and exercise, as well as pharmacotherapy aimed at risk factor improvement. Typically, primary prevention is initiated by primary care physicians and cardiologists in the outpatient setting and is guided by epidemiologic and clinical trial data. One example is the treatment of hypertensive patients with therapies to lower blood pressure in order to prevent subsequent CVD events.

The principal advantage of primary prevention is the ability to tailor therapy to individuals at higher risk before they develop clinically significant atherosclerotic disease. Because of this individualized approach, primary prevention strategies result in a larger relative risk reduction for the individual than does primordial prevention. Not surprisingly, patients receiving primary prevention are more receptive to risk factor modification, particularly if their individual CVD risk can be communicated appropriately.

In spite of this, there are several disadvantages to focusing solely on primary prevention. First, primary prevention requires screening of a large segment of the population to identify individuals with sufficient risk to warrant treatment. This can be an expensive process, and current risk prediction models are not perfect at identifying individuals for whom such therapy is appropriate. Second, primary prevention strategies probably delay rather than prevent the onset of overt disease. Finally, primary prevention strategies have been argued by some authorities to "medicalize" otherwise healthy people, potentially diverting attention away from persons who are acutely ill.

Despite these potential disadvantages, we believe that primary prevention strategies are crucial for lowering the burden of cardiovascular disease.

Secondary Prevention

Secondary prevention consists of efforts to prevent further CVD events and mortality among patients with clinically evident atherosclerotic CVD. Such efforts most commonly involve individualized lifestyle interventions, risk-reducing medications, and cardiac rehabilitation. Secondary prevention is usually guided by data from randomized clinical trials and is best initiated in the inpatient setting, with continuation in the outpatient setting to ensure long-term risk reduction. One example of secondary prevention is the use of aspirin, which reduces thrombotic events in patients with CVD.

The principal advantage of secondary prevention is the large relative risk reduction that can be achieved within a short period of time. In general, treatment of higher risk patients results in a smaller number-needed-to-treat (NNT) to prevent an adverse event. Such treatment is therefore usually more cost-effective for patients who qualify. Compliance with lifestyle changes and initiation of recommended therapies is also highest in patients who have experienced a previous CVD event, particularly if symptoms persist.

Focusing predominantly on secondary prevention, however, has several disadvantages. Even though a majority of adults in the United States eventually suffer a cardiovascular event, a proportionally smaller number are living with CVD at any one time. For example, in 2006, only 16.8 million individuals in the United States were living with CHD, and 6.5 million individuals in the United States were living with stroke; both groups represent only 7.8% of the total population.[1] Despite numerous available therapies, rates of recurrent events in secondary prevention also remain high. In fact, as many as 1 per 6 individuals with CHD and 1 per 7 individuals with stroke experience an adverse cardiovascular event within 1 year of follow-up.[26] Finally, isolated secondary prevention is costly. Without primordial and primary prevention to reduce the risk factor burden, the cost of secondary prevention in an increasingly obese, diabetic, and aging population is probably prohibitive. The financial burden is increased further when patients have become irreversibly disabled from an initial cardiovascular event.

Blurring of Prevention Types

Although each of the three levels of prevention is generally regarded as distinct, there can be variable degrees of overlap. This may be a source of potential confusion for patients, epidemiologists, and providers.

One such example is the case of a patient with a fasting blood glucose level of 132 mg/dL in the years 1996 and 1997. Between these two periods, the definition of diabetes mellitus was changed by the American Diabetes Association from a fasting blood glucose level of 140 mg/dL or higher to 126 mg/dL or higher.[27] From the perspective of the patient, despite no change in glycemic control, he or she was free of diabetes one month and then was considered to have the disease the next month. From the perspective of the epidemiologist, who views risk factors as continuous variables, changing thresholds simply reflects changing understanding of disease. This can be a common problem in clinical cardiology, inasmuch as continuous risk factor variables are commonly dichotomized as normal or abnormal on the basis of specific cutoff points. For the clinician, redefining the cutoff point for a given risk factor reclassifies patients from those needing primordial prevention to those needing primary prevention, and therapy is thus changed. This was illustrated again in 2002, when the National Cholesterol Education Program (NCEP) declared diabetes (as well as peripheral arterial disease, abdominal aortic aneurysm, and moderate carotid atherosclerosis) CHD risk equivalents[28]; patients with these conditions became classified as those requiring secondary prevention.

Another example is the case of a patient in whom significant subclinical atherosclerosis (e.g., increased coronary artery calcium score or increased carotid intima-media thickness) was identified on an imaging study. Should such an individual receive lipid-modifying therapy to an intensity recommended by primary prevention guidelines, or are even more aggressive secondary prevention goals warranted? The current management of advanced subclinical atherosclerosis occupies an uncertain middle ground between primary and secondary prevention, and in fact such an approach has been termed "primary and a half prevention."[29]

These reclassifications may appear to be a matter of semantics to the individual, but the implications are far greater at the public health level. By definition, lowering the cutoff point to define a given risk factor will decrease the numbers of individuals who qualify for primordial prevention and increase the numbers of those who qualify for primary prevention. Similarly, as technology improves the identification of subclinical atherosclerosis, there is the potential to decrease the numbers of individuals who qualify for primary prevention and increase the numbers of those who qualify for secondary prevention. These "rightward shifts" in the level of prevention invite a more aggressive treatment approach that is unfortunately also accompanied by increased up-front cost. Such is expected to be the case if future cholesterol guidelines adopt the results of the Justification for the Use of Statins in Primary Prevention: An Intervention Trial Evaluating Rosuvastatin (JUPITER).[30] In fact, it is estimated that 20% of middle-aged adults would be newly eligible for lipid-lowering therapy[31]; thus, approximately 6.5 million

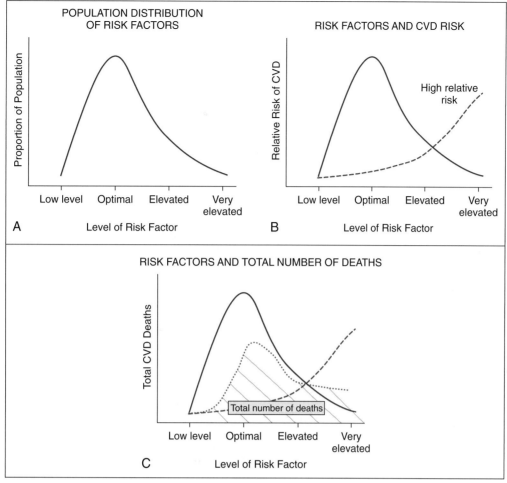

FIGURE 1-1 A, Population distribution of risk factors. **B,** Risk factors and risk for cardiovascular disease (CVD). **C,** Risk factors and total number of deaths.

additional middle-aged adults would be newly eligible for this therapy.[32]

POPULATION-BASED VERSUS INDIVIDUAL-BASED PREVENTION

Tremendous debate surrounds the question of which patients should be targeted for preventive therapy.[25,33] On opposite sides of the spectrum are two strategies: one founded on a population-based model, the other on an individual-based model. At the heart of each strategy are attempts to save the most lives, best increase quality of life, and be cost effective. Unfortunately, limited resources preclude complete delivery of both approaches, but a reasonable combination of the two is feasible.

Population-Based Prevention

The basic premise of a population-based prevention approach is that many CVD events occur in patients who are not considered a priori to be at high risk. This premise is driven by the distribution of risk factors within the population, which most commonly resembles a rightward skewed bell curve. Although individuals with the least well-controlled risk factors suffer the highest event rates, they represent a small fraction of the entire population. In contrast, although those with suboptimal control of mild risk factors have lower event rates, they represent a larger percentage of the population

and account for far greater numbers of adverse CVD events (Figure 1-1).

Proponents of a population-based strategy argue that small changes in the entire population can have a tremendous effect on CVD burden. One such example is a ban on *trans*–fats, which would be expected to result in a leftward-shift in the distribution of cholesterol levels and thus a substantial shift toward more optimal control of risk factors (Figure 1-2). This approach would have differing effects within the population, but the net effect would still be significant reduction in the population-wide rate of adverse CVD events.

Several advantages are associated with this approach. First, population-based strategies do not require broad screening efforts that rely on imperfect estimates of CVD risk. For example, taxing cigarettes or mandating reductions of salt in food affects broad numbers of individuals, even if not to the same degree. Second, like primordial prevention, population-based approaches have the potential to intervene early in the natural history of CVD, well before the development of CVD events. Third, population-based approaches to risk factor management produce numerous long-term benefits, not the least of which is a better quality of life. Last, this approach better accounts for behavioral and cultural differences between individual populations.

A population-based approach does, however, have several important drawbacks. Perhaps most important among these is the fact that such a strategy is likely to require broad-based governmental approval, which can be quite costly and whose implementation can be contentious. It is unlikely that

POPULATION-BASED APPROACH

INDIVIDUAL-BASED APPROACH

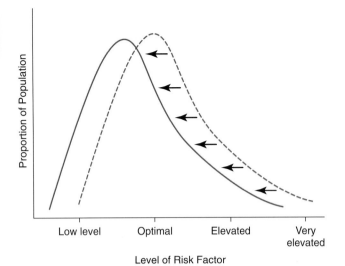

FIGURE 1-2 Population-based approach to control of risk factors.

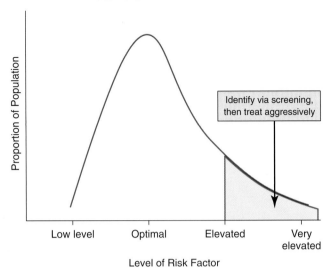

FIGURE 1-3 Individual-based approach to control of risk factors.

financial support will come from pharmaceutical and device companies, whose general focus is on the development of therapeutics that are applicable to a select portion of the population. In addition, public support for policy that encourages lifestyle change within a population that considers itself "healthy" may be difficult to achieve. In fact, people may believe in the "prevention paradox," a notion that broad-based interventions with large overall benefit produce modest, incremental benefits at the individual level.[34] Finally, population-based approaches are extraordinarily hard to implement, and even harder to assess in terms of benefit. For example, it is unclear to what extent U.S. educational programs about diets low in saturated fats from the 1960s and 1970s contributed to increased consumption of carbohydrates, which may underlie the current epidemics of obesity and diabetes mellitus. In spite of these challenges, the Osaka Declaration[35] serves as a good reference for population-based prevention by outlining economic and political barriers around the world.

Individual-Based Prevention

The basic premise of a targeted, patient-based strategy (commonly referred to as the *individual-based* or *high-risk approach*) is that the largest reductions in relative risk are achieved in patients with the highest event rates (Figure 1-3). These strategies are potentially cost saving, inasmuch as they can be applied to a smaller group of individuals guided by evidence from randomized-controlled trials. To be effective, however, an individual-based prevention strategy depends on effective risk-stratification tools to identify the portion of the population most likely to benefit. One such example is the cholesterol guidelines from the NCEP, in which the Framingham Risk Score is used.

First among the many advantages to this approach is its focused nature. Results of epidemiologic surveys suggest that as many as one third to half of all cardiovascular events occur in patients who have had a prior event, and nearly all of these patients have already sought medical attention.[36] Second, individualized approaches offer individualized care in a population in which there is often significant heterogeneity in the distribution of risk factors. Third, it is easier to quantify the long-term effects by directly comparing the findings with those from clinical trials (e.g., efficacy vs. effectiveness). Finally, patients at higher risk are usually more easily

motivated to achieve behavioral change and compliance with prescription medications.

The principal weakness of this approach is its reliance on currently imperfect risk assessment tools for screening and identification of patients at high risk. For example, although advanced age is a major factor that drives many risk prediction models, there is clear evidence that early prevention results in more favorable outcomes. Physicians' noncompliance also plays a significant role. The benefits obtained in clinical trials are rarely reproduced in the real-world setting, partly because risk assessment tools and available evidence-based therapies are used incompletely. Simplification of the guidelines represents one means that may help with compliance, but personalized risk assessment and the appropriate steps to reducing risk still must be communicated effectively to the individual patient.

CURRENT GUIDELINE STATEMENTS

To date, most guideline statements from the American Heart Association (AHA) and the American College of Cardiology (ACC) have focused on primary and secondary prevention of CVD at the individual level. However, increasing numbers of guidelines and consensus statements have advocated risk reduction at the community level. The most important of these documents, which serve as invaluable resources for this text, are listed as follows.

AHA Community-Level (Primordial) Prevention Guidelines

"American Heart Association Guide for Improving Cardiovascular Health at the Community Level: A Statement for Public Health Practitioners, Healthcare Providers, and Health Policy Makers from the American Heart Association Expert Panel on Population and Prevention Science"[37]

Primordial prevention begins in the community and encompasses recommendations for populations at the state, country, and even worldwide levels. Such a broad approach is important because of the remarkable regional variation in the incidence of CVD. To a large degree, behavioral and cultural differences probably account for a greater proportion of this

TABLE 1–3	Dimensions Encompassed by American Heart Association's Community Guidelines	
Behaviors	**Community Setting**	**Public Health Service**
Diet Physical activity level Tobacco use	Health care facilities and practitioners Schools Religious organizations Whole communities Food and tobacco industry Local/national government	Surveillance Education Mass media Policy and legislation

Adapted from Pearson TA, Bazzarre TL, Daniels SR, et al: American Heart Association guide for improving cardiovascular health at the community level: a statement for public health practitioners, healthcare providers, and health policy makers from the American Heart Association Expert Panel on Population and Prevention Science, *Circulation* 107:645-651, 2003.

variation than do genetic or other clinical variables, and there is ample evidence that community-level interventions can play a significant role in favorably changing behavior.

The AHA's community guidelines are organized around three dimensions: recognition of behaviors targeted for change, identification of community settings in which interventions can be implemented, and agreement on specific public health services that must be provided (Table 1-3). Specific risk-reducing recommendations are organized around six key strategies: assessment of CVD burden, education, community partnerships, access to screening and treatment, environmental change, and policy change at the governmental level (Table 1-4). Although these guidelines are extremely valuable, the most far-reaching contribution is probably the assistance of civic leaders in closing the significant gap between present-day community policies.

"Diet and Lifestyle Recommendations Revision 2006: A Scientific Statement from the American Heart Association Nutrition Committee"[38]

One principal feature that makes atherosclerotic CVD amenable to prevention is the ability of behavioral change to affect the disease course. Because of this, diet and lifestyle changes remain the foundation of CVD prevention. To this end, the AHA guidelines have identified seven diet and lifestyle goals: (1) consume an overall healthy diet; (2) aim for a healthy body weight; (3) aim for recommended levels of cholesterol subfractions and triglycerides; (4) aim for a normal blood pressure; (5) aim for a normal blood glucose level; (6) be physically active; and (7) avoid use of and exposure to tobacco products. To achieve these goals, the guidelines offer nine specific recommendations (Box 1-3).

"Understanding the Complexity of Trans Fatty Acid Reduction in the American Diet: American Heart Association Trans Fat Conference 2006"[39]

The process of partially hydrogenating fats (creation of *trans*–fatty acids) accelerated in the second half of the twentieth century as the demand for stable, cheap, and functional fats increased. These fats were subsequently found to increase levels of low-density lipoprotein (LDL) cholesterol, decrease levels of high-density lipoprotein (HDL) cholesterol, and contribute to an atherogenic lipid profile; therefore, the U.S. Food and Drug Administration (FDA) mandated on January 1, 2006, that all nutrition labels quantify the amount of *trans*–fat that is present in foods. Countries such as Denmark have taken significantly stronger steps by banning these fats completely.

TABLE 1–4	Improving Cardiovascular Health at the Community Level	
Strategy	**Goals**	**Example Recommendation**
Assessment	Informing community about incidence of CVD	Determining burden of CVD and risk factors at local level
Education	General health education School and youth education Worksite education Health care facility education	Mass media campaigns Early CVD curricula Promoting physical activity Availability of guidelines to all patients
Community organization and partnering	Community-specific action plan for CVD prevention	Identifying organizations in community that can provide services and resources
Ensuring personal health services	Increasing frequency of preventive care Providing adequate preventive training to clinicians	Increasing access to preventive services Requiring research-based curricula for behavior change
Environmental change	Ensuring access to healthy food Ensuring access to physical activities Ensuring tobacco-free environment	Promoting healthy food in school Increasing safety and infrastructure for walking, bicycling, etc. Banning smoking in public places and worksites
Policy change	Reducing initiation of tobacco use by young adults Providing adequate reimbursement for prevention	Tobacco taxes, reducing tobacco advertising Health insurance coverage of early prevention services

CVD, cardiovascular disease.
Adapted from Pearson TA, Bazzarre TL, Daniels SR, et al: American Heart Association guide for improving cardiovascular health at the community level: a statement for public health practitioners, healthcare providers, and health policy makers from the American Heart Association Expert Panel on Population and Prevention Science, *Circulation* 107:645-651, 2003.

BOX 1-3 Recommendations of the American Heart Association Nutrition Committee for Achieving Diet and Lifestyle Goals

- Balance calorie intake and physical activity to achieve healthy body weight
- Consume diet rich in vegetables and fruits
- Choose whole-grain, high-fiber foods
- Consume fish, especially oily fish, at least twice a week
- Limit intake of saturated fat to <7% of energy, *trans*–fat to <1%, and cholesterol to <300 mg
- Minimize intake of beverages and foods with added sugars
- Choose and prepare foods with little or no salt
- If you do consume alcohol, do so in moderation
- Follow AHA recommendations when eating outside of the home

Adapted from Lichtenstein AH, Appel LJ, Brands M, et al: Diet and lifestyle recommendations revision 2006: a scientific statement from the American Heart Association Nutrition Committee, *Circulation* 114:82-96, 2006.

This mandate[39] illustrates the complexity of population-based nutritional policy. Although there is strong interest in converting to healthier fats, such a change is limited by present-day agricultural practices, the lag time between agricultural policy and change in food supply, the need for new packaging and labeling, and issues of food stability and taste. The AHA advocates for increased awareness of *trans*–fats, agricultural-driven policies encouraging the production of healthier oils, exploration of new alternatives in food manufacturing, and rapid adoption of menus free of *trans*–fats by restaurants.

"Population-Based Prevention of Obesity: The Need for Comprehensive Promotion of Healthful Eating, Physical Activity, and Energy Balance"[40]

At current rates, 1 per every 2.5 adults and 1 per every 4 children in the United States will be obese by the year 2015.[41] Not surprisingly, the incidence of diabetes mellitus is concurrently rising. This trend extends well beyond the United States, unfortunately; major global epidemics for obesity and diabetes alike are expected.

Failure in most cases to achieve meaningful weight loss underscores the need for population-based prevention. This approach, however, entails challenges different from those of management of obesity on a clinical basis. The document from the AHA[40] raises awareness about the obesity epidemic, identifies high-risk subgroups, and, of most importance, highlights the difference between policy-driven environmental approaches to weight loss and clinical approaches by using an ecological model to identify targets for change. A number of potential strategies are outlined, including "big picture" architectural policies that reduce urban sprawl and increase navigability of neighborhoods.

"Air Pollution and Cardiovascular Disease: A Statement for Healthcare Professionals from the Expert Panel on Population and Prevention Science of the American Heart Association"[42]

The air is polluted with environmental gases such as nitrogen oxide, second-hand smoke from tobacco, and particulate matter small enough to reach the lower lungs. These air pollutants are associated with increases in rates of both short-term and long-term mortality from CVD. The National Mortality and Morbidity Air Pollution Study (NMMAPS) observed 50 million individuals in the 90 largest U.S. cities and demonstrated that for each $10\text{-}\mu\text{g/m}^3$ increase in thoracic particulate matter concentration, there is a 0.31% increase in rates of *daily* cardiopulmonary mortality.[43] An additional study of 500,000 adults monitored over a 16-year period similarly identified a 6% increase in rates of cardiopulmonary mortality for $10\text{-}\mu\text{g/m}^3$ increases in fine particulate matter.[44] In fact, it is speculated that a lifetime spent in one of the most polluted cities in the United States will reduce overall life expectancy (in 69% of cases, because of CVD) by 2 to 3 years.[45]

The mechanisms linking air pollution with CVD mortality include acute thrombosis, arrhythmias, acute arterial vasoconstriction, systemic inflammatory/oxidative responses, and chronic progression of atherosclerosis. At a minimum, the AHA supports expedited adoption of National Ambient Air Quality Standards, with a push for even more stringent policy. In addition, because the Air Quality Index is now calculated in more than 150 U.S. cities, the AHA supports guidelines for activity restriction among patients with known CVD when the Environmental Protection Agency activates the health alert system.

AHA Primary Prevention Guidelines

- "AHA Guidelines for Primary Prevention of Cardiovascular Disease and Stroke: 2002 Update"[46]
- "Primary Prevention of Ischemic Stroke"[47]
- "Evidence-Based Guidelines for Cardiovascular Disease Prevention in Women: 2007 Update"[48]

To implement primary prevention guidelines, which are based on an individual-based prevention model, physicians rely on accurate CVD risk assessment. Because of this, the strength of the intervention should match the degree of risk. Current AHA guidelines recommend the use of a global risk calculator for patients, beginning after age 40. Although this risk is calculated most commonly with the Framingham Risk Score to predict the 10-year risk of a devastating CHD event (myocardial infarction or CHD death),[49] the risk for other major CVD events (myocardial infarction, angina, stroke, peripheral artery disease, and heart failure) may be assessed as well.[50] Guidelines have not yet incorporated the new 30-year Framingham estimator,[51] but researchers will probably consider this in the near future.

The guidelines provide specific recommendations in nine areas (Table 1-5), drawing from documents produced by the Seventh Report of the Joint National Committee on Prevention (JNC7), the NCEP, the American Diabetes Association, and the U.S. Preventive Services Task Force (USPSTF). Although the recommendations are largely concordant in these documents, one exception is the recommendation to prescribe aspirin therapy: The AHA recommends it when the 10-year risk is 10% or higher, whereas the USPSTF's criterion is 6% or higher.[52]

Of importance is that the 2007 AHA statement "Treatment of Hypertension in the Prevention and Management of Ischemic Heart Disease"[53] advised physicians to lower the blood pressure goal even further, to <130/80 mm Hg in patients with a CHD risk equivalent (carotid artery disease, peripheral arterial disease, abdominal aortic aneurysm) or with a 10-year Framingham risk score of 10% or higher.

"American Heart Association Guidelines for Primary Prevention of Atherosclerotic Cardiovascular Disease Beginning in Childhood"[54]

It is now well-established that many behaviors associated with increased CVD risk are acquired during childhood. It is therefore crucial that prevention efforts begin while patients are young and receptive to change. Individual-based prevention programs in the pediatric population, like those for adults, rely on accurate assessment of risk. This can be more challenging, inasmuch as cutoff points for CVD risk factors are based on age, sex, and height.

In comparison to adults, lipid goals in the pediatric population are generally lower, and cutoff points for blood pressure and body mass index rely on percentiles established by a reference population (Table 1-6). Accordingly, physicians who treat individuals in these age groups should become familiar with these treatment goals.

In addition, the American Academy of Pediatrics issued an endorsed policy statement, "Cardiovascular Risk Reduction in High-Risk Pediatric Populations,"[55] and a clinical report, "Lipid Screening and Cardiovascular Health in Childhood,"[56] which replace their prior 1998 policy statement on this same subject. An emphasis is placed on risk stratification and treatment of elevated risk factors, including obesity, blood pressure, lipids, glucose, smoking, and lack of physical activity.

AHA Secondary Prevention Guidelines

"AHA/ACC Guidelines for Secondary Prevention for Patients with Coronary and Other Atherosclerotic Vascular Disease: 2006 Update"[57]

In the near future, the number of individuals qualifying for secondary prevention is expected to rise substantially. Numerous recommendations are provided in these guidelines

TABLE 1–5	Goals and Recommendations for CVD Risk Reduction: Primary Prevention	
Risk Factor	**Goal**	**Recommendation**
Smoking	Complete smoking cessation	Assessment, counseling, and pharmacotherapy
Blood pressure*	<140/90 mm Hg <130/85 mm Hg if patient has CRI or CHF <130/80 mm Hg if patient has diabetes	Lifestyle therapy, then individualized pharmacotherapy based on patient characteristics
Diet	Overall healthy eating pattern	Consistent with AHA Diet and Lifestyle Guidelines
Aspirin	Low-dose aspirin in patients with ≥10% 10-year risk	Doses 75-162 mg/day Contraindicated if patient has risk of GI or other hemorrhage
Lipid management	*Primary Goal* LDL-C level <160 mg/dL if ≤1 RF LDL-C level <130 mg/dL if ≥2 RFs LDL-C level <100 mg/dL if 10-year CHD risk >20% *Secondary Goal* If triglyceride levels ≥200 mg/dL, then 　Non–HDL-C level <190 mg/dL if ≤1 RF 　Non–HDL-C level <160 mg/dL if ≥2 RFs 　Non–HDL-C level <130 mg/dL if 10-year CHD risk >20% *Other Targets* Triglyceride levels <150 mg/dL HDL-C level >40 mg/dL in men HDL-C level >50 mg/dL in women *NCEP Optional Goals:* LDL-C level <100 mg/dL if ≥2 RFs LDL-C level <70 mg/dL if 10-year risk >20% Non–HDL-C level <130 mg/dL if ≥2 RFs Non–HDL-C level <100 mg/dL if 10-year CHD risk >20%	Lifestyle change, including dietary plant stanols/sterols, viscous fiber, and omega-3 fatty acids Then add statin therapy
Physical activity	≥30 min activity of moderate intensity per day most days of week	Additional benefits are obtained from vigorous intensity activity
Weight management	*Primary Goal* Achieve BMI of 18.5-24.9 kg/m² *Secondary Goal* Waist circumference: 　<40 inches in men 　<35 inches in women	Reduce body weight by 10% in first year of therapy
Diabetes	Normal fasting glucose HbA1c level < 7%	Lifestyle therapy Oral hypoglycemic agents Then insulin therapy
Chronic atrial fibrillation	Normal sinus rhythm or INR of 2.0-3.0	Aspirin, 325 mg, can be alternative if patient has high risk of bleeding

*The subsequent 2007 American Heart Association (AHA) statement "Treatment of Hypertension in the Prevention and Management of Ischemic Heart Disease" has advocated for a goal blood pressure of <130/80 mm Hg in patients with Framingham Risk Score ≥10%.[53]

BMI, body mass index; CHD, coronary heart disease; CHF, congestive heart failure; CRI, chronic renal insufficiency; CVD, cardiovascular disease; GI, gastrointestinal; HbA1c, glycated hemoglobin A1c; HDL-C, high-density lipoprotein cholesterol; INR, international normalized ratio; LDL-C, low-density lipoprotein cholesterol; NCEP, National Cholesterol Education Program; RF, risk factor.

TABLE 1–6	Thresholds for Risk Factors in Children
Risk Factor	**Level of Concern**
Lipid parameters	
Total cholesterol	≥170 mg/dL is borderline ≥200 mg/dL is elevated
LDL-C	≥110 mg/dL is borderline ≥130 mg/dL is elevated
Triglycerides	≥150 mg/dL
HDL-C	<35 mg/dL
Blood pressure	>90th percentile for age, sex, and height
Body size (BMI)	>85th percentile is at risk >95th percentile is overweight

BMI, body mass index; HDL-C, high-density lipoprotein cholesterol; LDL-C, low-density lipoprotein cholesterol.

(Table 1-7); the major differences from the primary prevention guidelines are more aggressive use of antiplatelet therapy; assessment of left ventricular ejection fraction; specific recommendations regarding angiotensin-converting enzyme (ACE) inhibitors, β-blockers, and aldosterone blockers; and administration of the influenza vaccine.

The 2007 AHA statement "Treatment of Hypertension in the Prevention and Management of Ischemic Heart Disease"[53] advocated further lowering of blood pressure goals to less than 130/80 mm Hg in patients with established CHD or a CHD risk equivalent (carotid artery disease, peripheral arterial disease, abdominal aortic aneurysm), particularly in patients with symptoms. This statement also encourages a goal of less than 120/80 mm Hg in patients with left ventricular dysfunction.

"Update to the AHA/ASA Recommendations for the Prevention of Stroke in Patients with Stroke and Transient Ischemic Attack"[58]

Stroke represents the third leading cause of death in the United States and is a major cause of disability.[1] In addition to specialized neurologic care, patients with ischemic stroke

Risk Factor	Goals	Recommendation
TABLE 1-7	**Goals and Recommendations for CVD Risk Reduction: Secondary Prevention**	
Smoking	Complete smoking cessation	Assessment, counseling, and pharmacotherapy
Blood pressure*	<140/90 mm Hg, <130/80 mm Hg if CKD or diabetes	Lifestyle therapy Prescribe β-blocker or ACE inhibitor or both
Lipid management	*Primary Goal* LDL-C level <100 mg/dL *Secondary Goal* If triglyceride levels ≥200 mg/dL, then non–HDL-C level <130 mg/dL *NCEP Optional Goals:* LDL-C level <70 mg/dL if 10-year risk >20% Non–HDL-C level <100 mg/dL	Lifestyle change Statin therapy
Physical activity	≥30 min activity of moderate intensity per day most days of week	Medically supervised programs for high-risk patients
Diabetes	HbA1c level <7%	Lifestyle therapy, then pharmacotherapy Coordinate with primary care
Antiplatelet agents		Aspirin, 75-162 mg/day, indefinitely Clopidogrel, 75 mg/day, for up to 12 months after acute coronary syndrome[†] Aspirin, 325 mg, for 1 month after stent
Renin-angiotensin-aldosterone system blockers		ACE inhibitor if LVEF ≤40% or if patient has hypertension, CKD, or diabetes ARBs in patients intolerant of ACE inhibitor Aldosterone blockers after MI if patient is taking ACE inhibitor and β-blocker and if LVEF ≤40%
β-Blockers		Continue indefinitely if after MI, acute coronary syndrome, or LV dysfunction unless contraindicated
Influenza vaccination		All patients

*The subsequent 2007 American Heart Association (AHA) statement "Treatment of Hypertension in the Prevention and Management of Ischemic Heart Disease" has advocated for a goal blood pressure of <130/80 mm Hg in patients with established coronary heart disease (CHD) and a goal of <120/80 mm Hg in patients with left ventricular dysfunction.[53]
[†]Duration of clopidogrel depends on stent type.
ACE, angiotensin-converting enzyme; ARB, angiotensin receptor blocker; CKD, chronic kidney disease; HbA1c, glycated hemoglobin A1c; HDL-C, high-density lipoprotein cholesterol; LDL-C, low-density lipoprotein cholesterol; LV, left ventricular; LVEF, left ventricular ejection fraction; MI, myocardial infarction; NCEP, National Cholesterol Education Program.

or transient ischemic attack benefit from many of the same recommendations outlined in the CHD secondary prevention guidelines. Three exceptions to these recommendations include those for blood pressure control, antiplatelet therapy, and lipid management (Table 1-8).

"Core Components of Cardiac Rehabilitation/Secondary Prevention Programs: 2007 Update"[59]

The goals of cardiac rehabilitation are to foster and increase compliance with healthy behaviors, to reduce disability, to promote an active lifestyle, and to alleviate or eliminate CVD risk factors. Cardiac rehabilitation involves significantly more than just exercise training. It provides a comprehensive, multidisciplinary framework for lifelong secondary prevention.

The AHA/ACC guidelines[57] have identified five components that are central to any cardiac rehabilitation program: individual patient assessment, nutritional counseling, risk factor management, psychosocial interventions, and physical activity counseling/exercise training. Beyond these components, the most recent guidelines[59] emphasize the increased role that rehabilitation programs should play in reinforcing compliance with evidence-based pharmacotherapy.

THE FUTURE OF PREVENTIVE CARDIOLOGY

Two trends within the field of medicine will almost certainly affect the direction of preventive cardiology. The first is a

Risk Factor/Intervention	Recommendation
TABLE 1-8	**Recommendations Specific for Secondary Prevention of Stroke[58]**
Blood pressure	All patients should begin taking an antihypertensive agent, even those without history of hypertension Absolute blood pressure target is uncertain and should be individualized
Antiplatelet therapy	Aspirin (50-325 mg/day) monotherapy, aspirin plus extended-release dipyridamole, and clopidogrel monotherapy are acceptable initial therapy choices The combination of aspirin with extended-release dipyridamole is preferred over aspirin alone
Lipid management	Treatment with statins is recommended for all patients, even when manifest CHD is not present Patients with hypercholesterolemia and CHD should be treated to achieve secondary prevention NCEP target

CHD, coronary heart disease; NCEP, National Cholesterol Education Program.

move toward more cost-effective health care, because only limited resources are available for an increasingly aged population. The second is a move toward "personalized medicine," which is based on recognition that disease manifestations can vary tremendously within a given population. Unfortunately, although both trends have substantial merit, they may not be easily compatible within the field of preventive cardiology.

Of the current prevention approaches, highly focused, individual-based prevention will probably remain the driving force. Because this type of prevention requires accurate tools for risk assessment at the individual patient level, risk prediction models must have better ways to integrate traditional risk factors. However, difficult ethical issues in terms of access to preventive services arise when risk algorithms are driven largely by chronologic age. A shift toward the concept of lifetime risk (and "biologic age") may be necessary to overcome the limitations of short-term risk prediction and improve communication of risk status with patients.

To account for further heterogeneity in patient risk, algorithms to stratify patients will probably need other means—including measurement of biomarkers or imaging—to assess for subclinical atherosclerosis. Imaging modalities enable direct visualization of the vascular system of individual patients, allowing identification of subgroups of at-risk individuals who have the largest burden of atherosclerosis. Resources could then be directed preferentially to those considered to be at highest risk. Clinical epidemiologic studies, however, have yet to define cost-effective strategies for using these exciting new technologies.

Missing from this approach, however, is the means to address the burgeoning epidemics of obesity, metabolic syndrome, and diabetes mellitus. Without tackling these problems, physicians run a risk of reversing all the gains in reduced rates of mortality from CVD that have been achieved since the 1960s. Solutions require a firm understanding of the behavioral, societal, and cultural forces underlying these epidemics and will probably borrow components from a population-based approach. In the interim, however, a multidisciplinary approach that includes cardiologists, diabetologists, internists, and nutritionists is sorely needed to close the "treatment gap" that currently exists between guidelines and practice.

RATIONALE FOR THE "ABCDE" APPROACH

There is now consensus among physicians and policymakers that CVD prevention is a crucial part of comprehensive care. Substantial data from clinical trials have demonstrated the safety and efficacy of preventive approaches and identified therapies that may halt or even reverse atherosclerosis. There is also a growing understanding that prevention needs to be a central feature of a sustainable, cost-effective health system. Despite this, however, implementation of preventive practices remains suboptimal.

Numerous reasons exist for the treatment gap in preventive cardiology. Some providers continue to believe that clinical trials, which are subject to strict inclusion criteria, may not be applicable to commonly encountered patient groups. Others have insufficient time to address preventive practices, especially when patients have active complaints. Still others believe that treatment guidelines are too complex and arduous to implement.

In early guideline statements, the AHA and ACC presented some of their recommendations in an "ABCDE" format. Since the early 2000s, the Johns Hopkins Ciccarone Center for the Prevention of Heart Disease has expanded this approach to be more broadly applied to the primary and secondary prevention of CVD,[60,61] the management of non–ST segment elevation acute coronary syndrome (NSTE-ACS),[62] and the metabolic syndrome.[63] Prevention guidelines are outlined in a memory tool that can be used by providers and patients alike. For any given patient, only select components of the approach may be applicable; however, the ABCDE approach ensures that no aspects of comprehensive preventive care are missed. Such an approach encourages patient and physician guideline compliance and can be helpful in closing the treatment gap.

The general ABCDE approach is shown below, including chapters in this text that address each component:

A

Assessment of Risk (see Chapters 3, 5, and 6)

- Cardiovascular risk stratification: Use of risk assessment tools, biomarkers, subclinical disease imaging, or other markers, or a combination of these, to identify patients at increased risk for CVD

Antiplatelet Therapy (see Chapter 7)

- Aspirin
- Adenosine diphosphate (ADP; P_2Y_{12}) receptor antagonists (e.g., clopidogrel)

Anticoagulant Therapy (see Chapter 7)

- Warfarin or related compounds

ACE Inhibitors, Angiotensin Receptor Blocker (ARB) Therapy, and Other Therapies That Modulate the Renin-Angiotensin-Aldosterone System (see Chapter 7)

- ACE inhibitors
- Angiotensin receptor blockers (ARB)
- Aldosterone blockers

B

Blood Pressure Control (see Chapter 9)

- Achievement of evidence-based blood pressure targets that are based on the Joint National Committee (JNC) guidelines[64]

β-Blocker Therapy (see Chapter 11)

- Role in primary and secondary prevention
- Role in atrial fibrillation

C

Cholesterol Management (see Chapters 13 and 14)

- Achievement of evidence-based lipid targets based on the NCEP[65] and American Diabetes Association/ACC[66] guidelines

Cigarette Smoking Cessation (see Chapter 20)

- Behavioral interventions
- Pharmacologic interventions

D

Diet and Weight Management (see Chapter 19)

- Macronutrient dietary composition recommendations
- Body composition goals
- Achievement of weight reduction through lifestyle modification and pharmacotherapy/surgery (in selected patients)

- Measurement of impaired fasting glucose level, impaired glucose tolerance, or both
- Metabolic syndrome: diagnosis, risk assessment, and management
- Achievement of tight glycemic control through lifestyle modification and pharmacotherapy

E

Exercise (see Chapter 33)

- Use of motivation tools (e.g., pedometers)
- Cardiac rehabilitation (in selected patients)

Ejection Fraction Assessment (see Chapter 10)

- Guide for pharmacotherapy and device implantation

CONCLUSION

Atherosclerotic CVD is an ideal scenario for prevention efforts because (1) it is a common disease; (2) it is modifiable by behavior; (3) the disease latency is long; (4) the time between symptom onset and severe disability or sudden cardiac death is short; and (5) no cure exists for systemic atherosclerosis once it is present.

The majority of improvement in rates of mortality from CVD since the 1960s is the result of prevention, not treatment, of acute CVD. Preventive cardiology must continue across all three levels (primordial, primary, and secondary) with a balance between the two main approaches to prevention (population-based and individual-based). Despite available guidelines, there is a wide gap between the burden of CVD and current preventive efforts. This gap can be narrowed partly by more simplified guidelines. The goal of this book is to provide a concise and yet comprehensive approach to preventive cardiology.

REFERENCES

1. Lloyd-Jones D, Adams R, Carnethon M, et al: Heart disease and stroke statistics—2009 update: a report from the American Heart Association Statistics Committee and Stroke Statistics Subcommittee. *Circulation* 119(3):480-486, 2009.
2. Dawber TR, Meadors GF, Moore FE Jr: Epidemiological approaches to heart disease: the Framingham Study. *Am J Public Health* 41:279-286, 1951.
3. Kannel WB, Dawber TR, Kagan A, et al: Factors of risk development of coronary heart disease—six year follow-up experience: the Framingham Study. *Ann Intern Med* 55:33-50, 1961.
4. Enos WF, Holmes RH, Beyer J: Coronary disease among United States soldiers killed in action in Korea: preliminary report. *JAMA* 552:1090-1093, 1953.
5. Relationship of atherosclerosis in young men to serum lipoprotein cholesterol concentrations and smoking: a preliminary report from the Pathobiological Determinants of Atherosclerosis in Youth (PDAY) Research Group. *JAMA* 264:3018-3024, 1990.
6. Berenson GS, Srinivasan SR, Bao W, et al: Association between multiple cardiovascular risk factors and atherosclerosis in children and young adults: the Bogalusa Heart Study. *N Engl J Med* 338:1650-1656, 1998.
7. Yusuf S, Hawken S, Ounpuu S, on behalf of the INTERHEART Study Investigators: Effect of potentially modifiable risk factors associated with myocardial infarction in 52 countries (the INTERHEART study): case-control study. *Lancet* 364:937-952, 2004.
8. World Health Organization: *Preventing chronic disease: a vital investment*, Geneva, Switzerland, 2005, World Health Organization.
9. Melander O, Newton-Cheh C, Almgren P, et al: Novel and conventional biomarkers for prediction of incident cardiovascular events in the community. *JAMA* 302:49-57, 2009.
10. Naghavi M, Falk E, Hecht HS, et al: The SHAPE Task Force. From vulnerable plaque to vulnerable patient—part III: executive summary of the Screening for Heart Attack Prevention and Education (SHAPE) Task Force report. *Am J Cardiol* 98(2A):2H-15H, 2006.
11. Unal B, Critchley JA, Capewell S: Explaining the decline in coronary heart disease mortality in England and Wales, 1981-2000. *Circulation* 109:1101-1107, 2004.
12. Laatikainen T, Critchley JA, Vartiainen E, et al: Explaining the decline in coronary heart disease mortality in Finland between 1982 and 1997. *Am J Epidemiol* 162:764-773, 2005.
13. Haw S, Gruer L: Changes in exposure of adult non-smokers to secondhand smoke after implementation of smoke-free legislation in Scotland: national cross sectional survey. *BMJ* 335:549, 2007.
14. Pell JP, Haw S, Cobbe S: Smoke-free legislation and hospitalizations for acute coronary syndrome. *N Engl J Med* 359:482-491, 2008.
15. Leth T, Jensen HG, Mikkelsen AA, et al: The effect of the regulation on *trans* fatty acid content in Danish food. *Atheroscler Suppl* 7:53-56, 2006.
16. Pekka P, Pirjo P, Ulla U: Influencing public nutrition for non-communicable disease prevention: from community intervention to national programme—experiences from Finland. *Public Health Nutr* 5:245-251, 2002.
17. Zatonski WA, Willett W: Changes in dietary fat and declining coronary heart disease in Poland: population based study. *BMJ* 331:187-188, 2005.
18. Hu FB: Diet and cardiovascular disease prevention: the need for a paradigm shift. *J Am Coll Cardiol* 50:22-24, 2007.
19. Sacks FM, Svetkey LP, Vollmer WM, et al: DASH-Sodium Collaborative Research Group. Effects on blood pressure of reduced dietary sodium and the Dietary Approaches to Stop Hypertension (DASH) diet. *N Engl J Med* 344:3-10, 2001.
20. Lichtenstein AH, Appeal LJ, Brands M, et al. Diet and lifestyle recommendations revision 2006: a scientific statement from the American Heart Association Nutrition Committee. *Circulation* 114:82-96, 2006.
21. Ford ES, Ajani UA, Croft JB, et al. Explaining the decrease in U.S. death from coronary disease, 1980-2000. *N Engl J Med* 356:2388-2398, 2007.
22. Vartiainen E, Puska P, Pekkanen J, et al: Changes in risk factors explain changes in mortality from ischaemic heart disease in Finland. *BMJ* 309:23-27, 1994.
23. Strasser T: Reflections on cardiovascular diseases. *Interdiscip Sci Rev* 3:225-230, 1978.
24. Rose G: *The strategy of preventive medicine*, Oxford, UK, 1992, Oxford University Press.
25. Capewell S: Will screening individuals at high risk of cardiovascular events deliver large benefits? No. *BMJ* 337:a1395, 2008.
26. Steg PG, Bhatt DL, Wilson PW, et al: REACH Registry Investigators. One-year cardiovascular event rates in outpatients with atherothrombosis. *JAMA* 297:1197-1206, 2007.
27. Expert Committee on the Diagnosis and Classification of Diabetes Mellitus: Report of the Expert Committee on the Diagnosis and Classification of Diabetes Mellitus. *Diabetes Care* 20:1183-1197, 1997.
28. Adult Treatment Panel III: Executive summary of the third report of the National Cholesterol Education Program (NCEP) Expert Panel on Detection, Evaluation, and Treatment of High Blood Cholesterol in Adults. *JAMA* 285:2486-2497, 2001.
29. Celermajer DS: Primary and a half prevention: can we identify asymptomatic subjects with high vascular risk? *J Am Coll Cardiol* 45:1994-1996, 2005.
30. Ridker PM, Danielson E, Fonseca FA, et al: JUPITER Study Group. Rosuvastatin to prevent vascular events in men and women with elevated C-reactive protein. *N Engl J Med* 359:2195-2207, 2008.
31. Spatz ES, Canavan ME, Desai MM: From here to JUPITER: identifying new patients for statin therapy using data from the 1999-2004 National Health and Nutrition Examination Survey. *Circ Cardiovasc Qual Outcomes* 2:41-48, 2009.
32. Michos ED, Blumenthal RS: Prevalence of low-density lipoprotein cholesterol with elevated high sensitivity C-reactive protein in the U.S.: implications of the JUPITER (Justification for the Use of Statins in Primary Prevention: An Intervention Trial Evaluating Rosuvastatin) study. *J Am Coll Cardiol* 53:931-935, 2009.
33. Jackson R, Wells S, Rodgers A: Will screening individuals at high risk of cardiovascular events deliver large benefits? Yes. *BMJ* 337:a1371, 2008.
34. Rose G: Strategy of prevention: lessons from cardiovascular disease. *BMJ* 282:1847-1851, 1981.
35. Advisory Board of the Fourth International Heart Health Conference: *The Osaka Declaration. Health, economics, and political action: stemming the global tide of cardiovascular disease*, Osaka, Japan, 2001, Osaka Prefectural Government. Available at http://www.med.mun.ca/chhdbc/pdf/Eng%20Osaka%20Declaration.pdf.
36. Kerr AJ, Broad J, Wells S, et al: Should the first priority in cardiovascular risk management be those with prior cardiovascular disease? *Heart* 95:125-129, 2009.
37. Pearson TA, Bazzarre TL, Daniels SR, et al: American Heart Association guide for improving cardiovascular health at the community level: a statement for public health practitioners, healthcare providers, and health policy makers from the American Heart Association Expert Panel on Population and Prevention Science. *Circulation* 107:645-651, 2003.
38. Lichtenstein AH, Appel LJ, Brands M, et al: Diet and lifestyle recommendations revision 2006: a scientific statement from the American Heart Association Nutrition Committee. *Circulation* 114:82-96, 2006.
39. Eckel RH, Borra S, Lichtenstein AH, et al: Understanding the complexity of *trans* fatty acid reduction in the American diet: American Heart Association *Trans* Fat Conference 2006: report of the *Trans* Fat Conference Planning Group. *Circulation* 115:2231-2246, 2007.
40. Kumanyika SK, Obarzanek E, Stettler N, et al: American Heart Association Council on Epidemiology and Prevention, Interdisciplinary Committee for Prevention. Population-based prevention of obesity: the need for comprehensive promotion of healthful eating, physical activity, and energy balance: a scientific statement from American Heart Association Council on Epidemiology and Prevention, Interdisciplinary Committee for Prevention (formerly the Expert Panel on Population and Prevention Science). *Circulation* 118:428-464, 2008.
41. Wang Y, Beydoun MA: The obesity epidemic in the United States—gender, age, socioeconomic, racial/ethnic, and geographic characteristics: a systematic review and meta-regression analysis. *Epidemiol Rev* 29:6-28, 2007.
42. Brook RD, Franklin B, Cascio W, et al: Expert Panel on Population and Prevention Science of the American Heart Association. Air pollution and cardiovascular disease: a statement for healthcare professionals from the Expert Panel on Population and Prevention Science of the American Heart Association. *Circulation* 109:2655-2671, 2004.
43. Dominici F, McDermott A, Daniels D, et al: Mortality among residents of 90 cities. In *Special report: revised analysis of time-series studies of air pollution and health*, Boston, 2003, Health Effects Institute, pp 9-24.
44. Pope CA, Burnett RT, Thun MJ, et al: Lung cancer, cardiopulmonary mortality, and long-term exposure to fine particulate air pollution. *JAMA* 287:1132-1141, 2002.

45. Pope CA: Epidemiology of fine particulate air pollution and human health: biologic mechanisms and who's at risk? *Environ Health Perspect* 108:713-723, 2000.

46. Pearson TA, Blair SN, Daniels SR, et al: AHA guidelines for primary prevention of cardiovascular disease and stroke: 2002 update: Consensus Panel Guide to Comprehensive Risk Reduction for Adult Patients Without Coronary or Other Atherosclerotic Vascular Diseases. American Heart Association Science Advisory and Coordinating Committee. *Circulation* 106:388-391, 2002.

47. Goldstein LB, Adams R, Alberts MJ, et al: American Heart Association/American Stroke Association Stroke Council. Primary prevention of ischemic stroke: a guideline from the American Heart Association/American Stroke Association Stroke Council. *Stroke* 37:1583-1633, 2006.

48. Mosca L, Banka CL, Benjamin EJ, et al: Evidence-based guidelines for cardiovascular disease prevention in women: 2007 update. *Circulation* 115:1481-1501, 2007.

49. Anderson KM, Wilson PW, Odell PM, et al: An updated coronary risk profile. A statement for health professionals. *Circulation* 83:356-362, 1991.

50. D'Agostino RB Sr, Vasan RS, Pencina MJ, et al: General cardiovascular risk profile for use in primary care: the Framingham Heart Study. *Circulation* 117:743-753, 2008.

51. Pencina MJ, D'Agostino RB Sr, Larson MG, et al: Predicting the 30-year risk of cardiovascular disease: the Framingham heart study. *Circulation* 119:3078-3084, 2009.

52. U.S. Preventive Services Task Force: Aspirin for the prevention of cardiovascular disease: U.S. Preventive Services Task Force recommendation statement. *Ann Intern Med* 150:396-404, 2009.

53. Rosendorff C, Black HR, Cannon CP, et al: Treatment of hypertension in the prevention and management of ischemic heart disease: a scientific statement from the American Heart Association Council for High Blood Pressure Research and the Councils on Clinical Cardiology and Epidemiology and Prevention. *Circulation* 115:2761-2788, 2007.

54. Kavey RE, Daniels SR, Lauer RM, et al: American Heart Association guidelines for primary prevention of atherosclerotic cardiovascular disease beginning in childhood. *Circulation* 107:1562-1566, 2003.

55. American Academy of Pediatrics: Cardiovascular risk reduction in high-risk pediatric populations. *Pediatrics* 119:618-621, 2007.

56. Daniels SR, Greer FR, Committee on Nutrition: Lipid screening and cardiovascular health in childhood. *Pediatrics* 122:198-208, 2008.

57. Smith SC Jr, Allen J, Blair SN, et al: AHA/ACC guidelines for secondary prevention for patients with coronary and other atherosclerotic vascular disease: 2006 update: endorsed by the National Heart, Lung and Blood Institute. *Circulation* 113:2363-2372, 2006.

58. Adams RJ, Albers G, Alberts MJ, et al: Update to the AHA/ASA recommendations for the prevention of stroke in patients with stroke and transient ischemic attack. *Stroke* 39:1647-1652, 2008.

59. Balady GJ, Williams MA, Ades PA, et al: Core components of cardiac rehabilitation/secondary prevention programs: 2007 update: a scientific statement from the American Heart Association Exercise, Cardiac Rehabilitation, and Prevention Committee, the Council on Clinical Cardiology; the Councils on Cardiovascular Nursing, Epidemiology and Prevention, and Nutrition, Physical Activity, and Metabolism; and the American Association of Cardiovascular and Pulmonary Rehabilitation. *Circulation* 115:2675-2682, 2007.

60. Braunstein JB, Cheng A, Fakhry C, et al: ABCs of cardiovascular disease risk management. *Cardiol Rev* 9(2):96-105, 2001.

61. Gluckman TJ, Baronowski B, Ashen MD, et al: A practical and evidence-based approach to cardiovascular disease risk reduction. *Arch Intern Med* 164:1490-1500, 2004.

62. Gluckman TJ, Sachdev M, Schulman SP, et al: A simplified approach to the management of non–ST-segment elevation acute coronary syndromes. *JAMA* 293:349-357, 2005.

63. Blaha MJ, Bansal S, Rouf R, et al: A practical "ABCDE" approach to the metabolic syndrome. *Mayo Clin Proc* 83:932-941, 2008.

64. Chobanian AV, Bakris GL, Black HR, et al: The seventh report of the Joint National Committee on Prevention, Detection, Evaluation, and Treatment of High Blood Pressure: the JNC 7 report. *JAMA* 289:2560-2572, 2003.

65. Adult Treatment Panel III: Executive summary of the third report of the National Cholesterol Education Program (NCEP) Expert Panel on Detection, Evaluation, and Treatment of High Blood Cholesterol in Adults. *JAMA* 285:2486-2497, 2001.

66. Brunzell JD, Davidson M, Furberg CD, et al: Lipoprotein management in patients with cardiometabolic risk: consensus conference report from the American Diabetes Association and the American College of Cardiology Foundation. *J Am Coll Cardiol* 51:1512-1524, 2008.

CHAPTER 2

National and International Trends in Cardiovascular Disease: Incidence and Risk Factors

Gregory L. Burke and Ronny A. Bell

KEY POINTS

- Cardiovascular disease (CVD) is the leading cause of death in the United States and other countries, accounting for more than half of all deaths. The burden of CVD is increasing among developing countries.

- About one third of U.S. residents have some form of CVD, and the economic cost of CVD in the United States exceeds $475 billion annually.

- CVD morbidity rates, mortality rates, and risk factors vary geographically in the United States and internationally, according to evidence from World Health Organization Multinational Monitoring of Trends and Determinants in Cardiovascular Disease (WHO-MONICA).

- CVD mortality rates have been declining substantially in most countries, whereas they have risen in Eastern European and Asian nations.

- CVD risk factors such as hypertension, hypercholesterolemia, cigarette smoking, obesity, and diabetes are very common in adult populations in the United States and around the world. Some of these risk factors are also increasing among children and adolescents.

- Many CVD risk factors have been declining, in accordance with improved awareness and medical care for these conditions, whereas other risk factors, such as physical inactivity, obesity, and diabetes, are rapidly increasing.

- Primary and secondary prevention strategies by the medical care system in the United States and other developed countries have

contributed to the decline in CVD mortality rates. A particular area of concern for the future is congestive heart failure.

- Future projections indicate that CVD will be the leading cause of death in both developed and developing regions of the world by the year 2020.

- In Western developed countries, specific steps should be taken to deal with the existing high burden of CVD. Primordial prevention should be emphasized, including increased physical activity, the promotion of a heart healthy diet, and a decreased prevalence of obesity.

Cardiovascular disease (CVD) continues to be the leading cause of death in the United States and other developed countries. The burden from CVD has been increasing in developing countries as well. According to current projections, overall CVD rates will continue to increase in the twenty-first century and will be the leading cause of death in both developed and the developing nations. The large global burden of CVD is occurring despite the availability of proven primary and secondary preventive strategies that have not been effectively disseminated. However, before a large-scale CVD prevention program is implemented, key decision-makers must be aware of the scope of the problem.

This chapter provides an overview of the data on differences between populations and secular trends in CVD risk factors, morbidity, and mortality. Specifically, we present data across age, gender, and geographic entities, and we provide a brief overview of time trends in CVD incidence and risk factors.

CARDIOVASCULAR DISEASE MORBIDITY AND MORTALITY: RATES AND TRENDS

The bulk of the U.S. data concerning the current burden from CVD and trends in CVD events were obtained from published reports of the National Center for Health Statistics (NCHS); the National Heart, Lung and Blood Institute (NHLBI); the American Heart Association (AHA); and region-specific surveillance studies. International data were extracted primarily from World Health

Organization (WHO) reports, as well as the World Health Organization Multinational Monitoring of Trends and Determinants in Cardiovascular Disease (WHO-MONICA) Project.[1-4]

International Comparisons of Morbidity and Mortality from Cardiovascular Disease

CVD (codes 390 to 459 in the ninth edition of the *International Classification of Diseases*[4a] and codes I00 to I99 in the tenth edition[4b]) is the leading cause of death in most countries, particularly in economically developed countries. Significant international variation in rates of mortality and morbidity from CVD has been documented from nation-specific data and in WHO-MONICA communities. Figure 2-1 shows rates of mortality from coronary heart disease (CHD) in 36 countries.[3] CHD death rates (per 100,000 population) among men aged 35 to 74 in these populations were highest in Eastern Europe and lowest in Asia, with more than a tenfold variation between the two regions. Among women aged 35 to 74, a similar pattern of CHD death rates was observed, with an approximately tenfold variation between the highest rates, also observed in Eastern Europe, and lowest rates, also observed in Asia. Of these 36 countries, the United States has the tenth highest rates of mortality from CHD among both men and women.

Figure 2-2 shows rates of mortality from stroke in 36 countries.[3] Rates of death from stroke (per 100,000 population) among men and women aged 35 to 74 in these populations were highest in the Russian

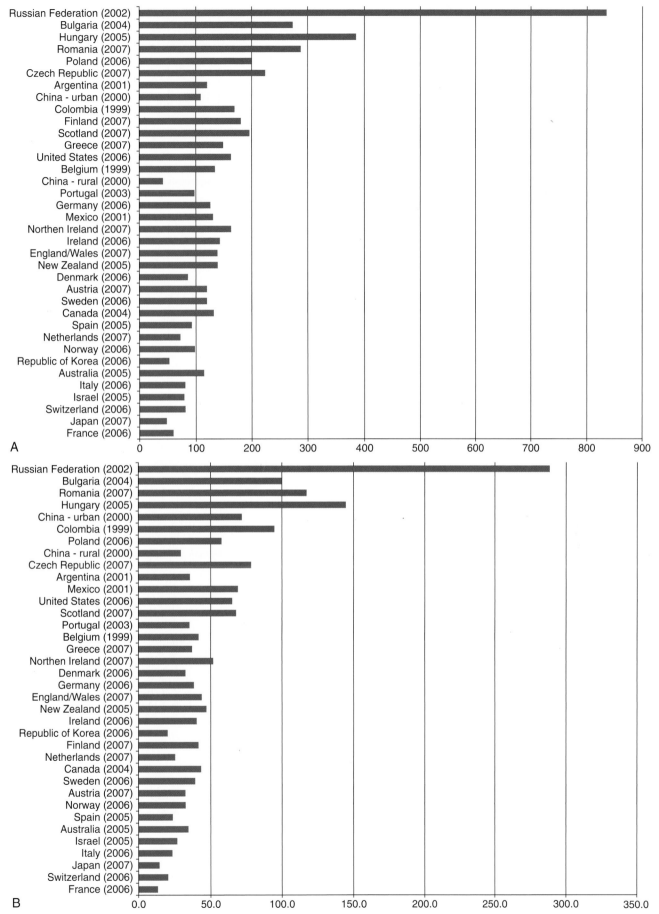

FIGURE 2-1 A, Age-adjusted rates of death from coronary heart disease (per 100,000 population) among men aged 35 to 74 in selected countries. **B,** Age-adjusted rates of death from coronary heart disease (per 100,000 population) among women aged 35 to 74 in selected countries. *(Adapted from American Heart Association:* Heart disease & stroke statistics—2010 update. A report from the American Heart Association, *Dallas, Tex, 2010, American Heart Association.)*

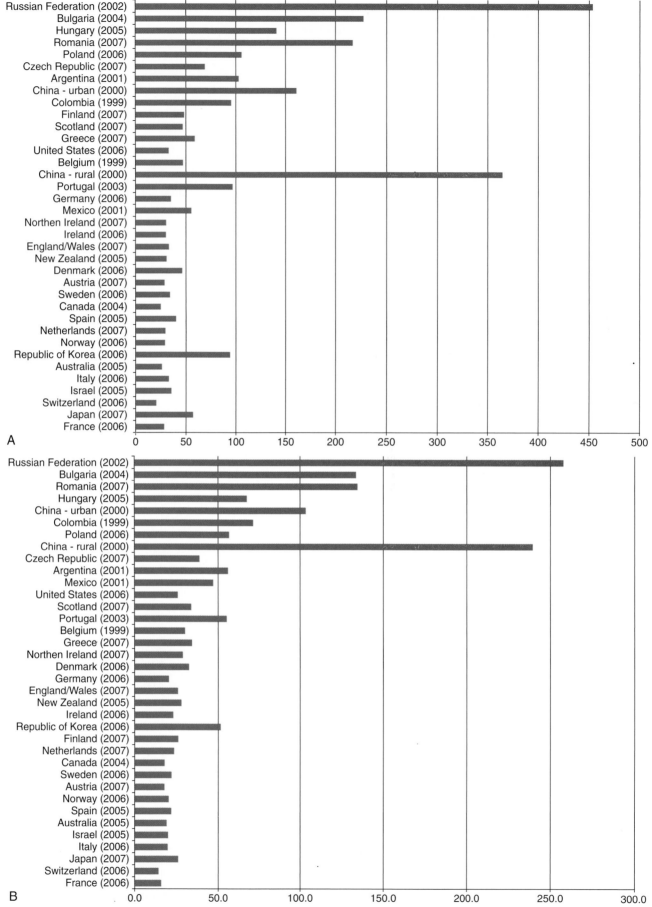

FIGURE 2-2 A, Age-adjusted rates of death from stroke (per 100,000 population) among men aged 35 to 74 in selected countries. **B,** Age-adjusted rates of death from stroke (per 100,000 population) among women aged 35 to 74 in selected countries. *(Adapted from American Heart Association:* Heart disease & stroke statistics—2010 update. A report from the American Heart Association, *Dallas, Tex, 2010, American Heart Association.)*

Federation, rural China, Bulgaria, and Romania and lowest in Switzerland, Canada, Australia, and France for men, with an approximately twenty-three–fold variation from lowest to highest. Of the 36 countries, the United States has the twelfth lowest rate of mortality from stroke among men. For women, rates of mortality from stroke range from 257.0 per 100,000 in the Russian Federation to 13.4 per 100,000 in Switzerland, a nearly twentyfold difference. Of the 36 countries, the United States has the sixteenth lowest rate of mortality from stroke among women.

Mortality from Cardiovascular Disease in the United States

In the United States, about 1.4 million people died from CVD in 2006; this number represents approximately 56% of all deaths. CVD was the underlying cause in about 830,000 deaths, or about 35% of all U.S. deaths.[3] CVD is the overall leading cause of death in the United States and is the leading cause of death in men older than 45 years and in women older than 65 years. In addition, CVD is the leading cause of death for all race/gender groups in the United States. Approximately 81 million Americans, or about one third of the population, have some form of CVD, which accounted for about 6.1 million hospital discharges in 2006. More than half of CVD deaths result from CHD, and about one per five result from stroke. The economic costs of CVD in the United States are enormous, estimated to be $475 billion in 2009.[3]

Table 2-1 presents 2005 U.S. data for rates of mortality from all causes and from CVD and years of potential life lost (YPLL) before the age of 75 by race/ethnicity group.[4] Overall, heart disease contributed to 211 deaths and 1110 YPLL before age 75 per 100,000 population, and stroke was associated with 47 deaths and 193 YPLL per 100,000 population. The highest CVD burden in the United States was found in the African American population: Rates of death from heart disease were approximately 30% higher among African Americans than among non-Hispanic white Americans. This gap was even wider for rates of death from stroke: Those rates

among African Americans were 41% higher than those among non-Hispanic white Americans. Rates of mortality from heart disease were lowest among Asian/Pacific Islanders (113 per 100,000). Rates of mortality from stroke were lowest among American Indian/Alaska Natives (35 per 100,000) and Hispanics (36 per 100,000) (NCHS). YPLL before age 75 for stroke were highest for African Americans and lowest for non-Hispanic white Americans; the difference in YPLL between these groups was nearly threefold. Thus, substantial differences in CVD burden in the United States were observed across race/ethnic groups.

There are also substantial differences in rates of mortality from CVD, ischemic heart disease, and stroke within the United States. Table 2-2 presents 2006 death rates by state, Puerto Rico, and Washington, D.C., and the rankings of incidence from the highest to lowest.[3] For CVD mortality, Mississippi had the highest rate (348.8 per 100,000), about 83% higher than the rate of the lowest ranked state, Minnesota (190.9 per 100,000). For CHD, Washington, D.C., had the highest rate (193.5 per 100,000), more than double the rate of the lowest ranked state, Utah (77.5 per 100,000). Arkansas had the highest rate of death from stroke (58.8 per 100,000), nearly double that of New York (29.7 per 100,000); of interest is that New York had the lowest rate of deaths from stroke but the second highest rate of death from CHD. Although the specific factors responsible for the great variation in ischemic heart disease and stroke rates are unclear, these data may suggest where statewide prevention programs are most needed.

Secular Trends in Mortality from Cardiovascular Disease

Mortality from CVD has been reduced substantially in most industrialized nations since the 1960s; this occurrence is congruent with changes in major CVD risk factors (discussed in the next section). Among 18 countries (Figure 2-3), rates of mortality from CHD in men and women aged 35 to 74 declined in all countries from 1999 to 2004; these declines included a nearly 5% reduction per year in the United States.[1]

Rates of mortality from stroke have also declined steadily.[1] In 18 countries, stroke-related mortality was reduced annually among men aged 35 to 74 from 1999 to 2004 (Figure 2-4). Reductions during this period were greatest among men in Australia and Norway and among women in Korea and Australia. In the United States, average annual reductions in stroke mortality during this period were 3% to 4%.[1]

Table 2-2 shows changes in total CVD, CHD, and stroke mortality in all 50 U.S. states, Washington, D.C., and Puerto Rico from 1996 to 2006.[3] In all states, CHD and stroke mortality declined substantially over the previous 10-year period, although there was a 7% increase in CHD in Washington, D.C. The percentage decreases were largest for CVD in Minnesota (–35.9%), for CHD in Utah and Nebraska (–44.0%) and for stroke in New Hampshire (–47.4%).

Table 2-3 shows the age-adjusted cause-specific mortality rates and the changes from 1972 to 2004 in the United States. Mortality from CHD overall was reduced 66% from 1972 (445.5 per 100,000 population) to 2004 (150.2 per 100,000 population).[1] Similar reductions were observed in mortality from stroke during these time periods (66.1% reduction).

Rosamond and colleagues[5] examined trends in heart disease incidence and mortality across four race/gender groups (white men and women, black men and women) in four U.S. communities (Forsyth County, N.C.; Jackson, Miss.; Minneapolis suburbs; and Washington County, Md.) from 1987 to 1994. Although CHD mortality was reduced in all four groups, the largest decreases in CHD mortality were observed among white men (average annual rate change,

TABLE 2–1	U.S. Mortality Rate and Years of Potential Life Lost Before Age 75 for Heart Disease and Stroke, 2005					
Race/ Gender Group	All Causes		Diseases of the Heart		Cerebrovascular Disease	
	Mortality Rate	YPLL	Mortality Rate	YPLL	Mortality Rate	YPLL
All persons	799	7300	211	1110	47	193
American Indian/ Alaska Native	663	8624	142	1010	35	209
Asian/ Pacific Islander	440	3533	113	514	39	163
Black	1017	11891	271	2046	65	442
Hispanic	591	5758	157	727	36	185
Non-Hispanic white	797	6853	210	1046	46	156

"Mortality Rate" refers to age-adjusted mortality rate per 100,000 population.
YPLL, years of potential life lost before age 75 per 100,000 population younger than 75 years.
Adapted from National Center for Health Statistics: *Health, United States, 2007,* Hyattsville, MD, 2008, National Center for Health Statistics.

TABLE 2–2 | **Age-Adjusted Death Rates for Total CVD, CHD, and Stroke by State in 2006 and Percentage Change from 1996**

State	Total CVD*			CHD†			Stroke‡		
	Rank	Death Rate	% Change 1996-2006	Rank	Death Rate	% Change 1996-2006	Rank	Death Rate	% Change 1996-2006
Alabama	51	330.9	−17.2	25	121.7	−32.4	51	55.5	−18.8
Alaska	11	227.5	−28.5	4	87.4	−38.2	34	46.8	−31.9
Arizona	5	215.4	−28.9	24	120.8	−31.1	3	34.5	−39.6
Arkansas	48	311.0	−23.8	47	160.1	−22.0	52	58.8	−35.1
California	29	257.3	−27.8	34	139.0	−36.3	29	44.9	−32.3
Colorado	4	212.8	−29.2	6	96.3	−35.9	13	38.7	−35.2
Connecticut	18	232.3	−35.1	13	110.0	−42.3	8	36.5	−37.7
Delaware	27	255.4	−26.1	37	140.8	−31.4	18	41.8	−24.0
District of Columbia (Washington, D.C.)	50	325.7	−19.1	52	193.5	7.0	10	37.6	−45.9
Florida	10	227.4	−30.1	28	129.2	−37.2	4	35.3	−33.3
Georgia	41	288.8	−28.2	12	108.7	−41.5	43	51.4	−33.6
Hawaii	2	206.2	−30.9	3	85.2	−40.2	22	43.2	−32.9
Idaho	20	238.5	−25.3	14	110.2	−34.0	44	51.6	−27.3
Illinois	33	268.2	−29.8	31	134.8	−39.4	31	45.4	−33.0
Indiana	40	288.7	−27.7	35	139.7	−36.0	39	49.1	−34.8
Iowa	22	246.7	−29.6	39	141.6	−36.2	20	42.9	−31.6
Kansas	28	255.4	−26.1	17	114.1	−35.0	33	46.7	−28.0
Kentucky	44	307.7	−25.6	42	148.6	−32.2	42	50.5	−30.4
Louisiana	46	308.4	−22.4	33	138.3	−32.4	46	52.1	−24.7
Maine	17	232.2	−33.1	15	112.2	−43.3	17	41.3	−28.6
Maryland	32	266.6	−25.4	40	141.7	−29.7	23	43.6	−31.6
Massachusetts	8	224.0	−31.3	9	105.6	−39.9	11	37.7	−28.2
Michigan	42	291.7	−27.8	45	156.6	−35.2	28	44.5	−34.5
Minnesota	1	190.9	−35.9	2	79.7	−45.5	14	39.3	−40.1
Mississippi	52	348.8	−23.4	41	146.8	−38.1	49	53.7	−25.7
Missouri	43	293.2	−27.4	44	155.2	−34.2	41	49.4	−27.3
Montana	7	223.3	−30.2	7	99.0	−36.1	16	41.2	−33.9
Nebraska	13	228.8	−34.5	5	89.9	−44.0	25	43.9	−29.5
Nevada	39	287.7	−22.0	23	119.5	−38.5	15	39.7	−33.8
New Hampshire	16	230.1	−34.4	21	116.3	−42.7	5	35.4	−47.4
New Jersey	26	254.1	−30.1	38	141.2	−36.1	6	35.9	−33.8
New Mexico	9	224.0	−24.4	18	114.6	−30.8	9	37.5	−35.9
New York	37	278.6	−30.9	51	181.2	−32.9	1	29.7	−37.2
North Carolina	34	268.2	−30.4	27	126.1	−39.3	47	52.4	−36.0
North Dakota	23	246.7	−28.8	30	133.7	−26.6	40	49.2	−29.8
Ohio	38	283.8	−28.0	43	154.0	−32.6	30	45.2	−28.1
Oklahoma	49	322.0	−21.2	50	177.4	−23.2	48	53.3	−23.0
Oregon	14	228.8	−29.6	8	99.2	−40.2	36	48.0	−38.8
Pennsylvania	35	268.8	−29.9	32	136.0	−37.4	24	43.6	−30.0
Puerto Rico	6	219.4	−27.5	10	106.6	−23.7	26	43.9	−25.0

| TABLE 2–2 | Age-Adjusted Death Rates for Total CVD, CHD, and Stroke by State in 2006 and Percentage Change from 1996—cont'd | | | | | | | | |

| | Total CVD* | | | CHD† | | | Stroke‡ | | |
State	Rank	Death Rate	% Change 1996-2006	Rank	Death Rate	% Change 1996-2006	Rank	Death Rate	% Change 1996-2006
Rhode Island	24	249.8	−25.7	48	162.4	−27.3	2	31.4	−38.4
South Carolina	36	270.5	−33.1	22	119.2	−43.0	45	51.6	−41.8
South Dakota	19	235.6	−30.0	36	140.0	−27.7	19	42.4	−30.9
Tennessee	45	307.7	−25.1	49	167.8	−30.0	50	54.6	−31.2
Texas	31	262.8	−28.6	29	132.2	−37.4	37	48.3	−30.5
Utah	3	208.2	−28.0	1	77.5	−44.0	7	36.2	−40.7
Vermont	15	229.3	−33.0	26	124.5	−37.8	12	37.8	−39.7
Virginia	30	258.1	−31.1	20	115.6	−36.8	38	49.0	−33.5
Washington	12	228.0	−28.7	19	114.7	−31.7	21	42.9	−39.0
West Virginia	47	309.2	−27.4	46	158.7	−35.8	35	47.6	−21.7
Wisconsin	21	241.8	−30.9	16	113.9	−39.2	27	44.3	−38.9
Wyoming	25	250.1	−26.6	11	107.1	−36.5	32	45.4	−37.2
Total United States		262.5	−29.5		135.0	−35.9		43.6	−32.7

*Total cardiovascular disease (CVD) is defined by the 10th edition of the *International Classification of Diseases* (ICD-10) codes I00 to I99.
†Coronary heart disease (CHD) is defined here by the ICD-10 codes I20 to I25.
‡Stroke is defined here by the ICD-10 codes I60 to I69.
Rank is from lowest to highest. Percent change based on log linear slope of rates each year.
From American Heart Association: *Heart disease & stroke statistics—2010 update. A report from the American Heart Association,* Dallas, Tex, 2010, American Heart Association.

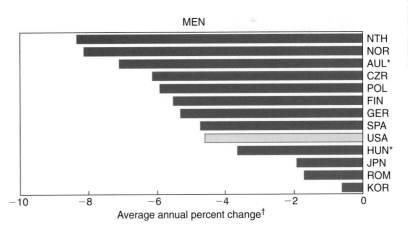

FIGURE 2-3 Change in age-adjusted rates of death from coronary heart disease by country and sex, ages 35 to 74, 1999 to 2004. *Age adjusted to European standard; †Data for 1998-2003. *(From National Heart, Lung and Blood Institute:* Morbidity and mortality: 2007 chart book on cardiovascular, lung, and blood diseases, *Bethesda, Md, 2007, National Institutes of Health.)*

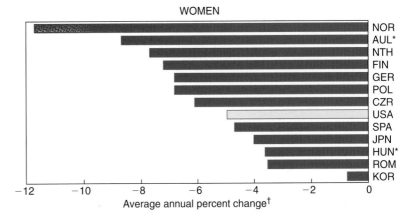

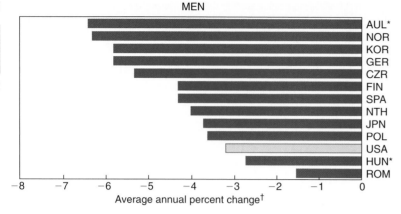

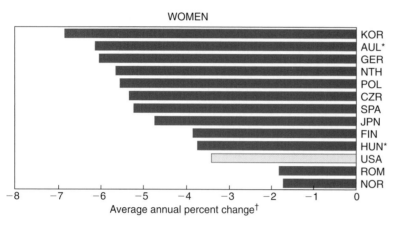

FIGURE 2-4 Change in age-adjusted rates of death from stroke by country and sex, ages 35 to 74, 1999 to 2004. *Age adjusted to European standard; †Data for 1998-2003. *(From National Heart, Lung and Blood Institute:* Morbidity and mortality: 2007 chart book on cardiovascular, lung, and blood diseases, *Bethesda, Md, 2007, National Institutes of Health.)*

TABLE 2–3	Age-Adjusted Death Rates and Percentage Change for All Causes and Cardiovascular Diseases, United States, 1972 and 2004			
	Deaths/100,000 Population			
Cause of Death	**1972**	**2004**	**1972-2004 Difference**	**Percentage Change**
All causes	1214.8	800.8	−414.0	−34.1
CVD*	695.4	289.5	−405.9	−58.4
CHD	445.5	150.2	−295.3	−66.3
Heart failure	9.3	18.9	9.6	103.2
Stroke	147.3	50.0	−97.3	−66.1
Other CVD	93.3	70.4	−22.9	−24.5
Non-CVD	519.4	511.3	−8.1	−1.6

*Excluding congenital malformations of the circulatory system.
CHD, coronary heart disease; CVD, cardiovascular disease.
From National Heart, Lung and Blood Institute: *Morbidity and mortality: 2007 chart book on cardiovascular, lung and blood diseases,* Bethesda, Md, 2007, National Institutes of Health.

−4.7%), and the smallest decline in CHD mortality was observed for black men (average annual rate change, −2.5%). Average annual rates of hospitalization for a first myocardial infarction actually increased during this time period among black women (7.4%) and black men (2.9%) but remained essentially unchanged among white men (−0.3%) and decreased among white women (−2.5%). There was also evidence of an overall decrease in rates of recurrent myocardial infarction and improvement in survival after myocardial infarction.[5]

In summary, although CVD mortality and morbidity were reduced significantly in most economically developed nations after the 1950s, CVD rates and the rates of reduction of CVD mortality were substantially heterogeneous between nations. In the United States, rates of CVD mortality and morbidity continue to decline, although there is still significant variation among regions (states) and among race/ethnic groups in the burden of CVD; African Americans bear the greatest burden from CVD. These data suggest which high-risk groups or regions have the greatest need for preventive efforts and programs.

CARDIOVASCULAR DISEASE RISK FACTORS: NATIONAL AND INTERNATIONAL RATES AND TRENDS

Data on the prevalence and trends in selected CVD risk factors (i.e., high blood pressure, high cholesterol, cigarette smoking, obesity, and diabetes) in the United States and other countries are described as follows. These data are potential mediating factors for the previously discussed trends for CVD morbidity and mortality.

High Blood Pressure

Elevated systolic (≥140 mm Hg) and diastolic (≥90 mm Hg) blood pressure, or hypertension, greatly increases the risk of heart disease and stroke. In the *Seventh Report of the Joint National Committee on Prevention, Detection, Evaluation, and Treatment of High Blood Pressure,*[6] an additional category of "pre-hypertension" (systolic blood pressure of 120 to 139 mm Hg or diastolic blood pressure of 80 to 89 mm Hg) was recognized in order to emphasize the role of increased risk of CVD associated with elevated blood pressure above 115/75 mm Hg.

International data indicate a great deal of geographic variation in blood pressure.[7] Among adults aged 35 to 64 from WHO MONICA communities in the final wave of the survey, systolic blood pressure ranged, on average, from 121 mm Hg (Catalonia, Spain) to 142 mm Hg (North Karelia, Finland) among men and from 117 mm Hg (Toulouse, France) to 138.5 mm Hg (Kuopio Province, Finland) among women (Table 2-4). During the approximately 10-year period from the initial to the final WHO MONICA surveys, systolic blood pressure was reduced in most participating communities. The downward trends were greater for women than for men: Nearly 75% of the communities demonstrated significant reductions for women (see Table 2-4). Only one of these communities (Halifax [Nova Scotia], Canada) demonstrated a significant increase in systolic blood pressure.[8]

In the United States, approximately 74.5 million individuals have hypertension (Table 2-5).[3] Hypertension affects approximately one third of the adult population and was responsible for more than 56,500 deaths in 2006 and 514,000 hospitalizations in 2006. The estimated burden of hypertension is approximately $76.6 billion. Hypertension is much more prominent in African Americans than in other racial/ethnic groups, among both men and women.

The prevalence of hypertension among adults increased to approximately 29% in the period 1999 to 2000; this was an increase of about 4.0% from the period 1988 to 1994.[9] The prevalence of hypertension was also 29% in the 2005-2006 wave of the National Health and Nutrition Examination Survey (NHANES), with an additional 28% having prehypertension.[10] Across the United States, there is significant variation in the prevalence of self-reported hypertension, ranging from 19.7% in Utah to 33.3% in West Virginia (Table 2-6).[11]

Awareness, treatment, and control of hypertension have improved significantly in the United States since the mid-1970s.[6] Seventy percent of adults aged 18 to 74 were aware of hypertension in 1999 to 2000, up from 51% in 1976 to 1980. During the same later period, treatment for hypertension increased from 31% to 59%, and control of hypertension increased from 10% to 64% (albeit much lower than the Healthy People 2010 goal of 50% of persons with hypertension being in control).[11a] More recent data from the 2005-2006 NHANES[10] showed that 78% of adults aged 18 or older with hypertension were aware of their condition, 68% were receiving antihypertension treatment, and 64% were controlling their hypertension adequately (Figure 2-5). Improvements in treatment, however, have been exclusively those in men; treatment in women has not improved significantly during the past decade. Also, control of hypertension has improved exclusively in non-Hispanic white men.[9,10]

Cholesterol

Elevation in serum cholesterol is an established risk factor for CVD among middle-aged adults. International data from WHO MONICA indicates significant geographic variation in mean cholesterol values, ranging from 4.5 mmol/L (173 mg/dL) among men and women in Beijing, China, to 6.4 mmol/L (246 mg/dL) and 6.2 mmol/L (239 mg/dL) among men and women in Ticino, Switzerland. The difference between the centers with highest and lowest mean cholesterol values is approximately 40% to 45% (see Table 2-4).[7] The prevalence of diagnosed hypercholesterolemia ranges from 1% and 2.1% among men and women in Kaunus, Lithuania, to 42.4% and 35.0% in North Karelia, Finland.

Population cholesterol levels have declined consistently in the WHO MONICA populations. From the initial to the final survey periods, mean cholesterol values declined significantly in about half the centers for both men and women; the greatest of these differences were observed in Lille, France, for men, a reduction of 0.7 mmol/L (27 mg/dL), and in Gothenburg, Sweden, for women, a reduction of 0.8 mmol/L (31 mg/dL). The greatest increases during this period for both men and women were observed in Ticino, Switzerland (0.97 mmol/L, or 37 mg/dL, for men; 0.76 mmol/L, or 29 mg/dL, for women).[8]

In the United States, approximately 102 million adults aged 20 years and older have high cholesterol levels (total cholesterol, ≥200 mg/dL) (Table 2-7). The mean serum cholesterol value in the United States is approximately 199 mg/dL.[3] The prevalence of elevated levels of serum cholesterol is slightly higher among women (47.9%) than among men (45.2%), and rates are higher among Hispanic and non-Hispanic white Americans. About 10% of U.S. adolescents have elevated levels of serum cholesterol. The incidence of self-reported hypercholesterolemia in the adult population ranges in the United States from 33.5% in Colorado to 42.4% in West Virginia (see Table 2-6).[11] The mean level of low-density lipoprotein (LDL) cholesterol in the United States is 115.0 mg/dL, and approximately 25.3% of American adults have elevated (≥160 mg/dL) levels of LDL cholesterol. The mean level of high-density lipoprotein (HDL) cholesterol among U.S. adults is 54.3 mg/dL, and approximately 16.2% of U.S. adults have low levels (<40 mg/dL) of HDL cholesterol. The mean level of triglycerides among U.S. adults is 144.2 mg/dL.[3]

Despite increased awareness of the effects of hypercholesterolemia on cardiovascular disease and the availability of medications to treat this condition, evidence suggests that much work is needed in this area. Less than half of patients who qualify for lipid therapy are receiving it, and only about one third of patients treated for high LDL cholesterol are achieving their goals.[3]

Cigarette Smoking

Data from WHO MONICA populations indicate very high rates of cigarette smoking across the world[8] (see Table 2-4). Population percentages of regular smokers (those reporting smoking cigarettes every day) among men aged 35 to 64 ranged from 17.0% in Auckland, New Zealand, to 63.5% in Beijing, China, and among women, the percentages ranged from 3.0% in Beijing, China, to 44.7% in Glostrup, Denmark. An additional 20% to 35% of the populations in most of these sites were identified as occasional smokers and ex-smokers.

International data about secular trends in smoking prevalence in the WHO MONICA populations indicate significant declines in most areas.[8] In more than half the communities, smoking prevalence was reduced significantly among men in more than half the communities and reduced nonsignificantly in another third. In only one community, Beijing, China, did rates increase significantly among men from baseline to final survey periods. Among women, smoking prevalence declined significantly in only about one third of the communities, whereas some degree of increase occurred in more than half. Among both men and women, the greatest declines were observed in the Stanford, California (U.S.), community: absolute decreases of 13.4% among men and 15.3% among women.

In the United States, approximately 49 million adults (25.7% of men and 21.0% of women) are considered current smokers.[3] Cigarette use is more common among men and women of lower socioeconomic status across all race/ethnic groups. Between states, there is an nearly threefold variation in adult smoking prevalence, ranging from 9.2% in Utah to 26.4% in West Virginia (see Table 2-6).[11] California, having an active tobacco prevention program funded by tobacco tax

TABLE 2–4 | **Prevalence of Risk Factors for Cardiovascular Disease Across Selected Countries**

Country	% Daily Smokers		Systolic Blood Pressure (mm Hg)		Total Cholesterol (mmol)		Mean BMI (kg/m²)	
	Men	Women	Men	Women	Men	Women	Men	Women
Australia: Newcastle (New South Wales)	21.8	16.5	130.9	127.1	5.76	5.58	27.9	27.3
Australia: Perth (Western Australia)	24.2	12.5	134.0	125.4	5.53	5.36	26.4	26.1
Belgium: Charleroi	48.3	29.3	130.7	124.9	6.18	6.10	27.1	26.8
Belgium: Ghent	42.9	26.8	129.0	121.5	6.03	5.96	26.4	26.1
Canada: Halifax (Nova Scotia)	31.7	24.9	129.5	125.7	5.64	5.77	27.5	27.6
China: Beijing	63.5	9.0	131.5	130.2	4.52	4.49	24.1	24.5
Czech Republic	38.7	23.0	137.2	133.8	6.17	6.14	27.6	27.8
Denmark: Glostrup	43.5	44.7	125.8	121.1	5.96	5.82	26.0	24.7
Finland: Kuopio Province	30.4	13.4	140.2	138.5	6.01	5.75	27.3	27.1
Finland: North Karelia	27.0	11.5	142.2	137.2	6.03	5.75	27.5	27.1
Finland: Turku/Loimaa	29.4	18.7	139.5	135.1	5.88	5.72	27.1	26.2
France: Lille	32.8	16.7	134.8	128.7	5.84	5.82	26.4	26.4
France: Strasbourg	23.3	14.9	135.3	127.0	6.03	5.91	27.3	26.2
France: Toulouse	24.2	21.6	124.9	117.0	5.82	5.65	26.1	24.5
Germany: Augsburg (Rural)	24.3	15.7	135.6	128.8	6.09	5.93	27.8	26.8
Germany: Augsburg (Urban)	35.4	24.9	136.8	130.7	6.19	5.92	27.1	26.5
Germany: Breman	44.8	30.0	132.3	128.3	6.05	5.85	26.8	26.3
Germany: East Germany	31.7	16.8	140.3	138.0	6.16	6.03	26.7	26.4
Iceland: Reykjavik	20.9	30.8	125.9	121.6	6.22	5.99	26.9	26.5
Italy: Area Brianza	34.0	22.8	130.6	126.8	5.93	5.89	26.4	25.5
Italy: Fruili	29.0	22.2	139.5	134.3	5.87	5.66	26.9	25.8
Lithuania: Kaunas	34.9	4.4	137.4	134.2	5.96	6.19	27.1	28.0
New Zealand: Auckland	17.0	14.2	126.1	122.4	5.70	5.56	26.7	25.6
Poland: Tarnobrzeg Voivodship	54.4	20.7	133.8	133.9	5.58	5.51	25.9	28.5
Poland: Warsaw	51.5	33.9	132.4	128.1	5.75	5.65	27.1	27.5
Russia: Moscow (Control)	47.1	13.6	130.0	132.7	5.26	5.55	25.2	26.5
Russia: Moscow (Intervention)	41.8	14.2	133.4	132.9	5.38	5.51	25.6	26.3
Spain: Catalonia	41.2	15.0	121.1	118.3	N/A	N/A	N/A	N/A
Sweden: Gothenburg	25.5	28.6	133.9	129.5	5.57	5.44	26.2	24.9
Sweden: Northern Sweden	21.0	28.2	130.0	125.9	6.28	6.12	26.4	25.7
Switzerland: Ticino	35.5	26.2	131.7	124.0	6.54	6.19	26.5	25.3
Switzerland: Vaud/Fribourg	26.7	24.8	132.4	124.4	6.31	6.06	26.5	24.7
United Kingdom: Belfast	28.8	24.6	134.9	129.5	5.90	5.91	26.3	25.6
United Kingdom: Glasgow	41.1	41.0	132.6	126.2	6.05	6.08	26.8	26.9
United States: Stanford	23.0	18.7	128.6	119.4	5.40	5.31	26.9	26.6
Yugoslavia: Novi Sad	48.6	29.8	136.1	137.0	6.37	6.19	27.3	27.8

BMI, body mass index; N/A, not available.

TABLE 2–5	Prevalence, Mortality, Hospital Discharges, and Estimated Costs of Hypertension in the United States, 2006: Overall, by Sex, and by Race/Ethnicity			
Population Group	Prevalence, 2006, Age ≥20 Years	Mortality,* 2006, All Ages	Hospital Discharges, 2006, All Ages	Estimated Cost, 2010
Both sexes	74,500,000 (33.6%)	56,561	514,000	$76.6 billion
Men	35,700,000 (34.4%)	24,382 (43.1%)†	204,000	—
Women	38,800,000 (32.6%)	32,179 (56.9%)†	309,000	—
NH white men	34.3%	17,581	—	—
NH white women	31.1%	24,888	—	—
NH black men	43.04%	6089	—	—
NH black women	44.8%	6480	—	—
Mexican American men	25.9%	—	—	—
Mexican American women	31.6%	—	—	—
Hispanic or Latino‡ ≥18 years	21.0%	—	—	—
Asian‡ ≥18 years	21.0%	—	—	—
American Indians/ Alaska Natives‡ ≥18 years	25.4%	—	—	—

*Mortality data are for whites and blacks and include Hispanics.

†These percentages represent the portion of total HBP mortality that is for males vs. females.

‡NHIS (2008), NCHS: data are weighted percentages for Americans ≥18 years of age. NH, non-Hispanic.

Data from American Heart Association: Heart disease & stroke statistics—2010 update. A report from the American Heart Association, *Circ* 121:e46, 2010.

monies, reported a smoking prevalence of 14%, which is consistent with the declines observed in the Stanford cohort participating in the WHO MONICA survey.

Cigarette smoking has been declining in the United States since 1980. According to data from the National Health Interview Survey (Figure 2-6),[12] the prevalence of current cigarette smoking among adults older than 25 years of age was 37% in 1974, a rate that is 82% higher than the 2006 estimate of 20.3%. Declines were greatest among African American men; 53.4% of adult African American men smoked in 1974, in comparison with 25.4% in 2006, a decrease of almost 50%.

Rates of exposure to second-hand smoke are also declining. The percentage of nonsmokers with detectable serum levels of cotinine decreased dramatically, from 83.9% in the period 1988 to 1994 to 46.4% in the period 1999 to 2004. Significant variation exists in that African Americans have much higher rates of exposure (70.5%) than do non-Hispanic white Americans (43.0%) and Mexican Americans (40.0%).[3]

Obesity

Obesity is a well-established risk factor for CVD and contributes to an increased prevalence of other CVD risk factors, such as hypertension, hypercholesterolemia, and diabetes mellitus. In the final wave of WHO MONICA surveys, the mean body mass index (BMI) for men and women ranged from a low of 25.2 and 23.5 for men and women, respectively, in Moscow and Gothenburg, Sweden, to a high of 27.9 and 28.5 for men and women, respectively, in Newcastle (New South Wales), Australia, and Tarnobrzeg Voivodship, Poland.[7]

Unlike some other CVD risk factors, BMI has been increasing in most communities across the world. Only three WHO MONICA communities demonstrated reductions in BMI among men from initial to final survey periods, and about half the communities demonstrated significant increases. Among women, about half of the communities demonstrated increases and half demonstrated decreases, and in both cases, about half of these changes were significant.[8] The greatest increases for men and women were observed in Newcastle (New South Wales), Australia, and in Halifax (Nova Scotia), Canada, respectively (1.8 kg/m² in both communities).

In the United States, approximately 144 million adults are overweight (BMI, 25.0 to 29.9) or obese (BMI, ≥30) (Table 2-8).[3] This represents about two thirds of the adult population. Also, about one third of youth aged 2 to 19 years are overweight or obese, and this percentage has increased dramatically since 1980. The estimated costs associated with obesity are approximately $147 billion. Obesity is most common among persons of lower socioeconomic status and among some ethnic minority groups. According to NHANES data from 2007 to 2008, the prevalence of overweight varied across race/gender groups from 45.5% (white women) to 67.6% (Mexican American women). The prevalence of obesity ranged from 31.9% (non-Hispanic white men) to 49.6% (African American women). Rates of overweight or obesity ranged from 61.2% (non-Hispanic white women) to 79.3% (Hispanic men; Figure 2-7).[13] Among states, the prevalence of obesity ranges from 19.1% in Colorado to 33.4% in Mississippi (see Table 2-6). Similarly, there are great variations in the prevalence of the lack of physical activity (during the past month), ranging from 39.2% in Alaska to 61.4% in Louisiana (see Table 2-6).[11]

Although the prevalence of overweight and obesity is much greater than in past decades, evidence suggests that the trend may be leveling off. In an analysis of NHANES data from 1999 to 2008, Flegal and colleagues[13] showed that the prevalence of obesity did not change significantly for women and that the rates for men did not differ across the most recent time periods (2003 to 2008).

Abdominal obesity, a key component of the CVD risk associated with obesity, is also highly prevalent in the United States. According to NHANES data from 2003 to 2004, 42.4% of men and 61.3% of women had abdominal obesity.[14] Rates have increased significantly among both men and women since the period 1999 to 2000.

Diabetes Mellitus

Diabetes is now recognized as an established risk factor for CVD. Diabetes is now considered a CHD "risk equivalent," which means that for persons with diabetes, the risk of developing CHD is equivalent to that for persons with a history of CHD, and it also means that such persons should be treated in accordance with secondary prevention guidelines.[15] Diabetes increases the risk of CVD by two to four times, and CVD accounts for 60% to 70% of deaths among persons with diabetes.[16] Risk factors for type 2 diabetes (the most common form of diabetes) include increasing age; family history of

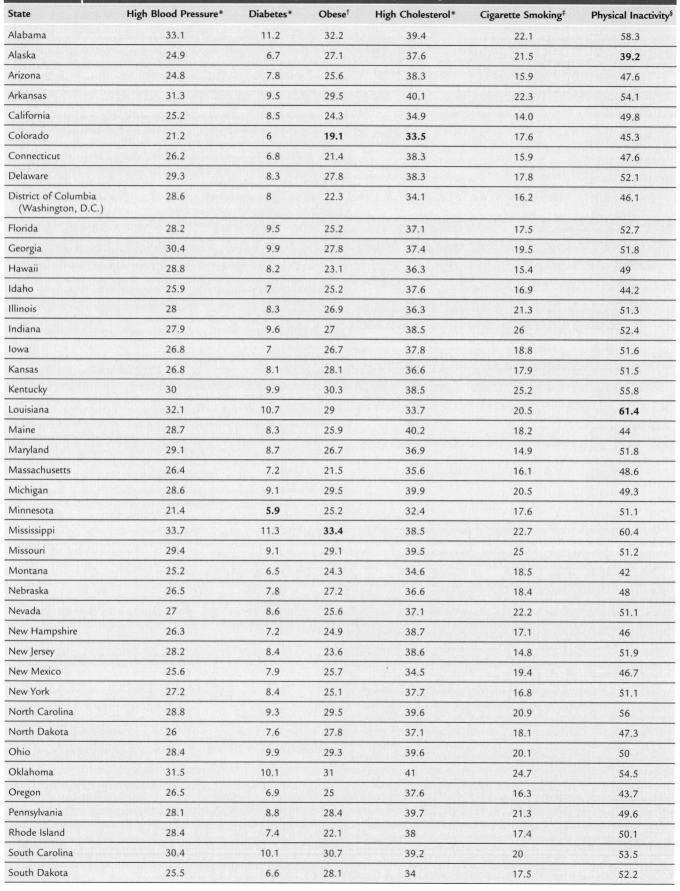

State	High Blood Pressure*	Diabetes*	Obese†	High Cholesterol*	Cigarette Smoking‡	Physical Inactivity§
Alabama	33.1	11.2	32.2	39.4	22.1	58.3
Alaska	24.9	6.7	27.1	37.6	21.5	**39.2**
Arizona	24.8	7.8	25.6	38.3	15.9	47.6
Arkansas	31.3	9.5	29.5	40.1	22.3	54.1
California	25.2	8.5	24.3	34.9	14.0	49.8
Colorado	21.2	6	**19.1**	**33.5**	17.6	45.3
Connecticut	26.2	6.8	21.4	38.3	15.9	47.6
Delaware	29.3	8.3	27.8	38.3	17.8	52.1
District of Columbia (Washington, D.C.)	28.6	8	22.3	34.1	16.2	46.1
Florida	28.2	9.5	25.2	37.1	17.5	52.7
Georgia	30.4	9.9	27.8	37.4	19.5	51.8
Hawaii	28.8	8.2	23.1	36.3	15.4	49
Idaho	25.9	7	25.2	37.6	16.9	44.2
Illinois	28	8.3	26.9	36.3	21.3	51.3
Indiana	27.9	9.6	27	38.5	26	52.4
Iowa	26.8	7	26.7	37.8	18.8	51.6
Kansas	26.8	8.1	28.1	36.6	17.9	51.5
Kentucky	30	9.9	30.3	38.5	25.2	55.8
Louisiana	32.1	10.7	29	33.7	20.5	**61.4**
Maine	28.7	8.3	25.9	40.2	18.2	44
Maryland	29.1	8.7	26.7	36.9	14.9	51.8
Massachusetts	26.4	7.2	21.5	35.6	16.1	48.6
Michigan	28.6	9.1	29.5	39.9	20.5	49.3
Minnesota	21.4	**5.9**	25.2	32.4	17.6	51.1
Mississippi	33.7	11.3	**33.4**	38.5	22.7	60.4
Missouri	29.4	9.1	29.1	39.5	25	51.2
Montana	25.2	6.5	24.3	34.6	18.5	42
Nebraska	26.5	7.8	27.2	36.6	18.4	48
Nevada	27	8.6	25.6	37.1	22.2	51.1
New Hampshire	26.3	7.2	24.9	38.7	17.1	46
New Jersey	28.2	8.4	23.6	38.6	14.8	51.9
New Mexico	25.6	7.9	25.7	34.5	19.4	46.7
New York	27.2	8.4	25.1	37.7	16.8	51.1
North Carolina	28.8	9.3	29.5	39.6	20.9	56
North Dakota	26	7.6	27.8	37.1	18.1	47.3
Ohio	28.4	9.9	29.3	39.6	20.1	50
Oklahoma	31.5	10.1	31	41	24.7	54.5
Oregon	26.5	6.9	25	37.6	16.3	43.7
Pennsylvania	28.1	8.8	28.4	39.7	21.3	49.6
Rhode Island	28.4	7.4	22.1	38	17.4	50.1
South Carolina	30.4	10.1	30.7	39.2	20	53.5
South Dakota	25.5	6.6	28.1	34	17.5	52.2

TABLE 2–6 State-Specific Prevalence of Risk Factors for Cardiovascular Disease (High Blood Pressure, Overweight, High Cholesterol, Diabetes, Cigarette Smoking, Physical Inactivity) Among Adults

State	High Blood Pressure*	Diabetes*	Obese†	High Cholesterol*	Cigarette Smoking‡	Physical Inactivity§
TABLE 2–6 State-Specific Prevalence of Risk Factors for Cardiovascular Disease (High Blood Pressure, Overweight, High Cholesterol, Diabetes, Cigarette Smoking, Physical Inactivity) Among Adults—cont'd						
Tennessee	33.8	10.4	31.2	34.2	23.1	61.2
Texas	27.8	9.7	28.9	38.5	18.5	53.5
Utah	**19.7**	6.1	23.1	32.6	**9.3**	43.8
Vermont	24.8	6.4	23.3	35.1	16.8	42.4
Virginia	27.1	7.9	25.8	37.4	16.4	50.5
Washington	25.4	6.9	26	36.7	15.7	46.3
West Virginia	**33.3**	**11.9**	31.9	**42.4**	**26.5**	54.1
Wisconsin	26.3	7.2	26.1	34.9	19.9	44.9
Wyoming	25.1	7.4	25.2	38.1	19.4	43.3

Boldfaced entries represent the highest and lowest rates for each risk factor category.
*Diagnosed by physician.
†Obesity defined as body mass index (BMI) ≥ 30 kg/m².
‡Current smokers.
§Percentage reporting less than the recommended level of physical activity (≥30 minutes of moderate physical activity 5 or more days per week, or vigorous physical activity for ≥20 minutes 3 or more days per week).
Data for Hypertension, High Cholesterol, and Physical Inactivity from *Behavioral Risk Factor Surveillance System*, Atlanta, 2007, Centers for Disease Control and Prevention; and for Obesity, Current Smoking, and Diabetes from *Behavioral Risk Factor Surveillance System*, Atlanta, 2008, Centers for Disease Control and Prevention.

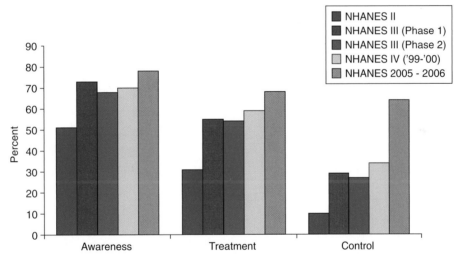

FIGURE 2-5 Trends in awareness, treatment, and control of high blood pressure in adults aged 18 to 74. *(Chobanian AV, Bakris GL, Black HR, et al; National Heart, Lung and Blood Institute Joint National Committee on Prevention, Detection, Evaluation, and Treatment of High Blood Pressure; National High Blood Pressure Education Program Coordinating Committee: The seventh report of the Joint National Committee on prevention, detection, evaluation, and treatment of high blood pressure.* JAMA *289:2560-2571, 2003; and Ostchega Y, Yoon SS, Hughes J, Tatiana L: Hypertension awareness, treatment, and control—continued disparities in adults: United States, 2005-2006,* NCHS Data Brief No. 3, Hyattsville, Md: National Center for Health Statistics; 2008. Available at http://www.cdc.gov/nchs/data/databriefs/db03.pdf.)*

diabetes; overweight/obesity, particularly central adiposity; being a member of certain ethnic minority groups, especially African Americans, Native Americans, and Hispanic Americans; and a history of gestational diabetes.[17]

Approximately 24 million Americans, or 7.8% of the population, have diabetes (fasting glucose level ≥126 mg/dL, or taking hypoglycemic medication), the majority of whom have type 2 diabetes.[17] About the same number have "pre-diabetes," which is defined as impaired fasting glucose level, based on fasting glucose values of 110 to 125 mg/dL, or impaired glucose tolerance, based on glucose values of 140 to 199 mg/dL after a 2-hour oral glucose tolerance test.[18] The

incidence of diabetes in the United States ranges from 5.9% in Minnesota to 11.9% in West Virginia (see Table 2-6).[11] Diabetes is diagnosed in about 1.6 million people aged 20 and older each year.[17] Data from the SEARCH for Diabetes in Youth Study estimate that diabetes has been diagnosed in approximately 154,000 youth younger than 20 years, or about 1 of every 523 children and youth in the United States.[19] This study also showed that the incidence of diagnosed diabetes in youth is approximately 24.3 per 100,000.[20] Type 1 diabetes is more common, but type 2 diabetes is also common, particularly among African American, Hispanic, Asian/Pacific Islander, and American Indian adolescents.

	Prevalence of Total Cholesterol ≥200 mg/dL, 2006, Age ≥20 Years	Prevalence of Total Cholesterol ≥240 mg/dL, 2006, Age ≥20 Years	Prevalence of LDL Cholesterol ≥130 mg/dL, 2006, Age ≥20 Years	Prevalence of HDL Cholesterol <40 mg/dL, 2006, Age ≥20 Years
Population Group				
Both sexes*	102,200,000 (46.8%)	35,700,000 (16.2%)	71,200,000 (32.6%)	35,100,000 (16.2%)
Men*	47,700,000 (45.2%)	15,900,000 (15.0%)	34,900,000 (33.1%)	26,400,000 (25.0%)
Women*	54,500,000 (47.9%)	19,700,000 (17.2%)	36,300,000 (32.0%)	8,700,000 (7.9%)
NH white men (%)	45.0	15.3	31.5	25.4
NH white women (%)	48.7	18.1	33.8	7.9
NH black men (%)	40.2	10.9	34.4	14.7
NH black women (%)	41.8	13.1	28.6	6.5
Mexican American men (%)	51.1	16.8	42.7	29.3
Mexican American women (%)	49.0	14.3	30.4	11.7
Total Hispanics† ≥20 years of age (%)	—	29.9	—	—
Total Asian/Pacific Islanders† ≥20 years of age (%)	—	29.2	—	—
Total American Indians/Alaska Natives† ≥20 years of age (%)	—	31.2	—	—

TABLE 2–7 Prevalence of Elevated Total, Elevated LDL, and Low HDL Cholesterol in the United States, Overall and by Sex and Race/Ethnicity, 2006

*Total data for total cholesterol are for Americans ≥20 years of age. Data for LDL cholesterol, HDL cholesterol, and all racial/ethnic groups are age adjusted for age ≥20 years.
†BRFSS (1991-2003, CDC), *MMWR;* data are self-reported data for Americans ≥20 years of age.
HDL, high-density lipoprotein; LDL, low-density lipoprotein; NH, non-Hispanic.
Data from American Heart Association: Heart disease & stroke statistics—2010 update. A report from the American Heart Association, *Circ* 121:e46, 2010.

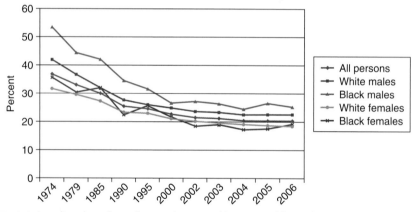

FIGURE 2-6 Age-adjusted prevalence of current cigarette smoking among adults aged 25 years and older, by race and sex, 1974 to 2000. *(Data from the National Health Interview Survey. Adapted from National Center for Health Statistics:* Health, United States, 2008 with special feature on the health of young adults, *Hyattsville, Md, 2008, National Center for Health Statistics.)*

The number of adults with diabetes increased dramatically in the 1990s, which is consistent with increases in obesity and physical inactivity during that period. Diabetes prevalence increased 33% from 1990 to 1998 and 61% from 1990 to 2001. More recent data, from 2003 to 2006, indicates that prevalence rates have leveled off since the increases in the 1990s (Figure 2-8).[21-23] Internationally, it was estimated that 285 million adults would have diabetes in 2010, and this number would increase to 439 million people by 2030. A 69% increase is projected in the numbers of persons with diabetes in developing countries, and a 20% increase is projected in developed countries.[24] One analysis in the United States indicated that by 2034, the prevalence of diabetes would nearly double to 44.1 million, and the estimated diabetes-related spending would triple to $336 billion.[25]

Metabolic Syndrome

Some CVD risk factors (including abdominal obesity, impaired fasting glucose, low HDL cholesterol, elevated triglyceride levels, and elevated blood pressure) occur in conjunction with each other in a condition referred to as the *metabolic syndrome.* This clustering greatly increases the risk of CVD. Commonly used definitions of the metabolic syndrome

TABLE 2–8	Prevalence of Overweight and Obesity among U.S. Adults and Children (2006), Overall and By Gender and Race/Ethnicity, and Estimated Costs (2008)				
Population Group	Prevalence of Overweight and Obesity in Adults, 2006, Age ≥20 Years	Prevalence of Obesity in Adults, 2006, Age ≥20 Years	Prevalence of Overweight and Obesity in Children, 2006, Ages 2-19 Years	Prevalence of Obesity in Children, 2006, Ages 2-19 Years	Cost, 2008*
Both sexes					$147 billion
n	144,100,000	71,600,000	23,500,000	12,000,000	
%	66.3	32.9	31.9	16.3	
Men					—
n	75,500,000	33,600,000	12,300,000	6,400,000	
%	71.7	31.8	32.7	17.1	
Women					—
n	68,600,000	38,000,000	11,200,000	5,600,000	
%	61.0	34.0	31.0	15.5	
NH white men (%)	71.4	31.6	31.9	15.6	—
NH white women (%)	57.5	31.3	29.5	13.6	—
NH black men (%)	71.4	35.2	30.8	17.4	—
NH black women (%)	79.6	53.2	39.2	24.1	—
Mexican American men (%)	75.1	29.1	40.8	23.2	—
Mexican American women (%)	74.1	41.8	35.0	18.5	—
Hispanic or Latino, aged ≥18 years[†] (%)	70.3	31.3	—	—	—
Asian-only, aged ≥18 years[†] (%)	40.7	9.4	—	—	—
American Indian/Alaska Native, aged ≥18 years[†] (%)	69.6	42.1	—	—	—

*Data *Health Affairs (Millwood)* 28:w822, 2009.
[†]NIHS (2008), NCHS (provisional); data are based on self-reported height and weight and are age adjusted for Americans ≥18 years old. Overweight is BMI ≥25 kg/m² and <30 kg/m². Obese is BMI ≥30 kg/m².
Data from American Heart Association: Heart disease & stroke statistics—2010 update. A report from the American Heart Association, *Circ* 121:e46, 2010.

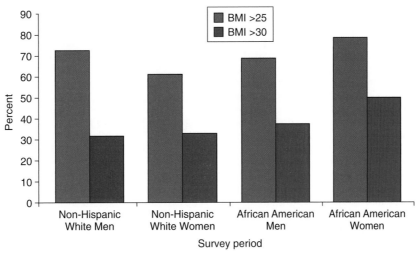

FIGURE 2-7 Prevalence of overweight and obesity among U.S. adults, by gender and race or ethnicity, 2007 to 2008. *(From Flegal KM, Carroll MD, Ogden CL, et al: Prevalence and trends in obesity among US adults, 1999-2008. JAMA 303:235-241, 2010.)*

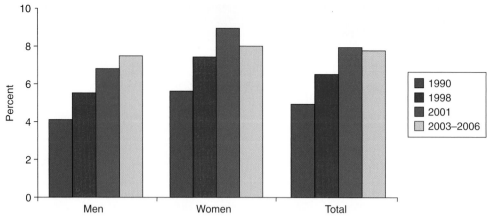

FIGURE 2-8 Time trends for diagnosed diabetes in the United States, overall and by sex, 1990, 1998, 2001, and 2003 to 2006. *(Adapted from Mokad AH, Ford ES, Bowman BA, et al: Diabetes trends in the U.S.: 1990-1998, Diabetes Care, 23:1278, 2000; Mokad AH, Ford ES, Bowman BA, et al: Prevalence of obesity, diabetes, and obesity-related health risk factors, 2001, JAMA, 289:76, 2003; Cowie CC, Rust KF, Byrd-Holt DD, et al: Prevalence of diabetes and high risk for diabetes using A1C criteria in the U.S. population in 1988-2006, Diabetes Care 33:562, 2010.)*

include that provided by the World Health Organization (WHO), the European Group for Study of Insulin Resistance (EGIR), the AHA/NHLBI (revised Third Adult Treatment Panel definition), the American Association of Clinical Endocrinologists (AACE), and the International Diabetes Federation (IDF) (Table 2-9).[26] It is estimated that 22% of the U.S. population have the metabolic syndrome.[27] The prevalence of the metabolic syndrome increases with age, from approximately 6.7% among adults aged 20 to 29 years to about 40% to 45% among adults older than 60 years. Mexican Americans have the highest likelihood of developing the metabolic syndrome; rates are 28.3% among men and 35.6% among women.[27]

MEDICAL CARE TRENDS

The medical care of CVD changed substantially from the 1980s into the early twenty-first century. These changes occurred both in CVD risk factor reduction in high-risk groups and in the treatment administered during and after acute CVD events. Since the 1980s, awareness, treatment, and control of hypertension and elevated serum cholesterol levels have improved dramatically in the United States; these improvements are linked to more aggressive treatment thresholds and treatment goals. It is thought that the increased use of both pharmacologic and nonpharmacologic modalities to reduce risk factors for CVD has contributed to up to 50% of the observed decline in CHD mortality, and changes in medical care have been suggested to contribute the remaining 50% of the decline. There continue to be substantial opportunities for significant improvement in the identification, management, and control of elevated cholesterol levels[28,29] or hypertension.[30] The need for improvements in treatment of high-risk groups is compounded by the effects of the ongoing obesity epidemic on risk factors and diabetes.

The overall burden of CVD is illustrated by the increasing number of CVD-related hospitalizations (Figure 2-9). The number of discharges increased from slightly more than 3 million per year in 1970 to more than 6 million per year in 2006. In addition, CVD procedures have been used increasingly in the United States since 1970 (Figure 2-10).[3] Specifically, the number of cardiac catheterizations has increased from approximately 300,000 per year in 1979 to more than 1.3 million in 2000. Increases in the number of procedures

from the 1980s into the mid-1990s, followed by a leveling off through 2006, were observed for coronary artery bypass graft procedures, pacemaker implantations and carotid endarterectomies. Technologic advances during this period have resulted in a nearly fourfold increase in the number of percutaneous coronary interventions (PCIs), from fewer than 300,000 in 1990 to more than 1.2 million per year by 2006.

The total number of discharges after hospitalizations for congestive heart failure in the United States (Figure 2-11) have increased from 200,000 discharges in 1979 to nearly 500,000 in 2006.[3] This shift is probably attributable both to the increased numbers of individuals who survive acute coronary events and to the aging of the U.S. population.

It is not surprising that these trends in CVD medical care have resulted in increased health expenditures in the United States. It was estimated that in 2009, more than $160 billion in costs (direct and indirect) would be incurred for CHD, about $70 billion for both stroke and hypertension, and nearly $40 billion for heart failure. Because the total expenditures for U.S. health care exceed 16% of gross domestic product, cardiovascular care has been a major factor associated with the increase in costs (Figure 2-12).

MIGRANT STUDIES

As mentioned, CVD burden is substantially different among different countries. These differences may be attributable to many factors, including country or regional differences in genotypes, gene-environment interactions, differences in health behaviors, and differences in the awareness and diagnosis of CVD. Studies of individuals who migrate from areas of low CVD prevalence to areas of higher CVD prevalence provide valuable evidence that corroborates the observed ecological comparisons of countries.

In the Ni-Hon-San Study, Japanese individuals who remained in Japan were compared with those who immigrated to Hawaii and with those who immigrated to the San Francisco Bay area (Figure 2-13). The data showed that risk factor–related behaviors of the immigrants become more similar to those observed in their newly adopted country.[31] Likewise, rates of morbidity and mortality from CVD among immigrants to the U.S. mainland were observed to approach levels observed in U.S. white populations, rather than

| TABLE 2–9 | Definitions of the Metabolic Syndrome |

Feature	WHO (1998)*	EGIR†	ATP III (2001)‡	AACE (2003)§	IDF (2005)‖	AHA/NHLBI (2006)¶
Insulin resistance	IGT, IFG, or lowered insulin sensitivity	Plasma insulin level >75th percentile	None	IGT or IFG (also includes family history, polycystic ovarian syndrome, sedentary lifestyle, advancing age, and ethnic groups susceptible to type 2 diabetes)	None	
Central adiposity	Waist-to-hip ratio >0.90 in men or >0.85 in women, or BMI >30 kg/m²	Waist circumference ≥94 cm in men and ≥80 cm in women	Waist circumference ≥102 cm in men and ≥88 cm in women	BMI ≥25 kg/m²	Increased waist circumference (population specific)	Waist circumference ≥102 cm in men and ≥88 cm in women
Lipid levels	Triglyceride levels ≥150 mg/dL; HDL cholesterol level <35 mg/dL in men and <39 mg/dL in women; or both	Triglyceride levels ≥150 mg/dL; HDL cholesterol level <39 mg/dL in men or women; or both	Triglyceride levels ≥150 mg/dL, or taking medication for elevated triglyceride levels; HDL cholesterol level <40 mg/dL in men and <50 mg/dL in women, or taking medication for low HDL level	Triglyceride levels ≥150 mg/dL, or receiving triglyceride therapy; HDL cholesterol level <40 mg/dL in men or <50 mg/dL in women	Triglyceride levels ≥150 mg/dL, or receiving triglyceride therapy; HDL cholesterol level <40 mg/dL in men or <50 mg/dL in women or taking medication for low HDL level	Triglyceride levels ≥150 mg/dL, or taking medication for elevated triglyceride levels; HDL cholesterol level <40 mg/dL in men and <50 mg/dL in women, or taking medication for low HDL level
Blood pressure	≥140/90 mm Hg	≥140/90 mm Hg, or medication taken for hypertension	≥130/85 mm Hg, or medication taken for hypertension	≥130/85 mg/dL	≥130 mm Hg systolic or ≥85 mm Hg diastolic, or medication taken for hypertension	≥130 mg/dL systolic or >85 mm Hg diastolic, or medication taken for hypertension
Glucose level	IFG, IGT, or type 2 diabetes	IFG or IGT (but not diabetes)	≥110 mg/dL (or diabetes), or hypoglycemic therapy received (updated to ≥100 mg/dL in 2004)	IFG or IGT (but not diabetes)	≥100 mg/dL (includes diabetes)	≥100 mg/dL (includes diabetes), or drug treatment received for elevated glucose level
Microalbuminuria	Urinary albumin excretion rate >20 µg/min or an albumin-to-creatinine ratio >20 mg/g	N/A	N/A	N/A	N/A	N/A

*The World Health Organization (WHO) defines metabolic syndrome as diabetes, impaired glucose tolerance, impaired fasting glucose, or insulin resistance plus two or more risk factors.

†The European Group for the Study of Insulin Resistance (EGIR) defines metabolic syndrome as plasma insulin levels >75th percentile plus two or more risk factors.

‡The Adult Treatment Panel III (ATP III) defines metabolic syndrome as three or more of the risk factors. Hypertriglyceridemia and low high-density lipoprotein (HDL) cholesterol count as separate risk factors. Microalbuminuria is not included in ATP III.

§The American Association of Clinical Endocrinologists (AACE) defines metabolic syndrome as IGT or IFG or any of the risk factors on the basis of clinical judgment.

‖The International Diabetes Foundation (IDF) defined metabolic syndrome as increased waist circumference (population specific) plus two or more risk factors.

¶The American Heart Association/National Heart, Lung and Blood Institute (AHA/NHLBI) defines metabolic syndrome as three or more of the risk factors.

BMI, body mass index; IFG, impaired fasting glucose; IGT, impaired glucose tolerance.

Adapted from Grundy SM, Cleeman JI, Daniels SR, et al: Diagnosis and management of the metabolic syndrome: an American Heart Association/National Heart, Lung and Blood Institute Scientific Statement. *Circulation* 112:2735-2752, 2005.

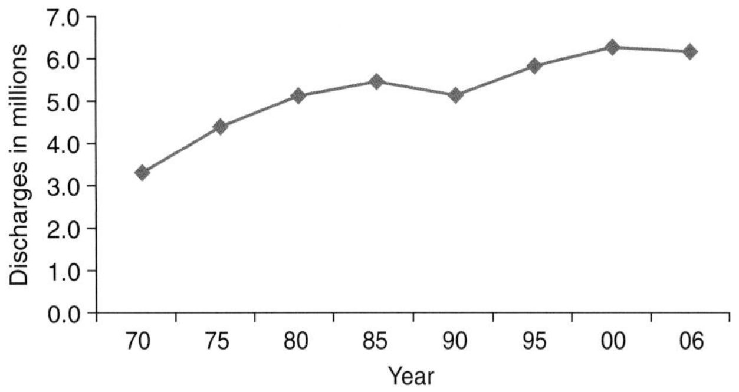

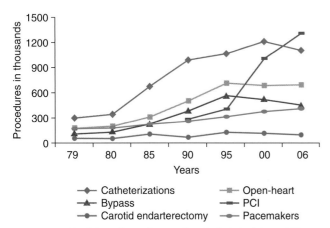

FIGURE 2-9 Trends in the overall burden of cardiovascular disease, 1970 to 2006. *(From American Heart Association:* Heart disease & stroke statistics: 2009, *Dallas, Tex, 2010, American Heart Association.)*

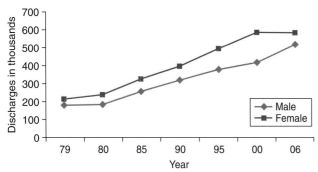

FIGURE 2-10 Trends in cardiovascular procedures in the United States, 1979 to 2006. *(From American Heart Association:* Heart disease & stroke statistics: 2009, *Dallas, Tex, 2010, American Heart Association.)*

FIGURE 2-11 Discharges after hospitalization for congestive heart failure in the United States, 1979 to 2006. *(From American Heart Association:* Heart disease & stroke statistics: 2009, *Dallas, Tex, 2010, American Heart Association.)*

remaining at the lower rates observed in individuals remaining in Japan (Figure 2-14).

This information suggests that environmental factors probably play a key role in mediating some of the large differences observed between countries. It is unlikely that individuals genetically predisposed toward a more abnormal CVD risk profile and higher rates of CVD morbidity and mortality are more likely to emigrate from their homelands. Therefore, the adoption of new health behaviors by immigrants probably mediates the majority of the increase in CVD burden. This possibility is extremely important in the context of international CVD prevention. It suggests that current and future expected increases in rates of CVD in countries with previously low rates of CVD are probably mediated to a great extent by the adoption of a more Westernized lifestyle.

FUTURE TRENDS IN CARDIOVASCULAR DISEASE

Using currently observed trends in CVD to predict subsequent trends and global disease burden is a challenging task. A number of key points can, however, be elucidated with some confidence: (1) A continued unacceptably high burden of CVD is observed in developed countries; (2) the CVD burden is rapidly increasing in countries with emerging economies; and (3) a large number of modifiable risk factors are identifiable, and their modification is known to prevent CVD.

Projections by Murray and Lopez[32] indicate that CVD will be the leading cause of death in both developed and developing regions of the world by the year 2020. These projections are shown in Figure 2-14, in which the leading causes of death projected for 2020 are contrasted for developed and developing countries. In developed countries, ischemic heart disease and cerebral vascular disease are projected to account for nearly 37% of all-cause mortality and for more than 25% of all-cause mortality in developing countries. Of importance is that both the endemically high rates of CVD in developed countries and the rapidly increasing rates of CVD in developing countries are linked to population levels of CVD risk factors.

The remarkable declines in cardiovascular mortality observed in Western countries since 1980 are attributable largely to successful primary and secondary prevention of CVD disease. Despite these dramatic improvements in developed countries, substantial opportunities remain to further reduce CVD burden. For example, cigarette smoking continues to be a habit of more than 20% to 40% of adults in many of these countries. Further opportunities remain for identification and treatment of elevated blood pressure, dyslipidemia, and obesity. Prognosis after myocardial infarction and stroke has improved dramatically, but further advances in the early detection and early treatment of these conditions would certainly be of great benefit. Therefore, despite huge

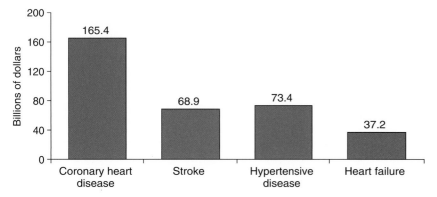

FIGURE 2-12 Costs of major cardiovascular diseases and stroke in the U.S., 2009. *(Data from the National Heart, Lung and Blood Institute.)*

improvements in CVD burden in developed countries, large subgroups of the population remain at unacceptably high risk for CVD events.

Conversely, in developing countries, less emphasis has been placed on prevention of chronic disease; this is because of economic pressures and the historically lower rates of CVD burden in these societies. Unless these societies are able to learn from the unfortunate lessons associated with the epidemic of CVD in developed countries, they will probably repeat the history of increasing CVD burden in the developed countries during much of the twentieth century.

Many developing countries currently have high rates of cigarette smoking, increasing rates of obesity, and increasing rates of other CVD risk factors. Ironically, what puts individuals in the developing world at risk for CVD is the ongoing adoption of Western lifestyles. Active efforts are required even to maintain current levels of physical activity and healthy components of traditional diets in these countries. In addition, the development of effective strategies for prevention of CVD—such as risk factor screening and treatment and appropriate medical intervention for acute events— is necessary to reverse the current path toward increasing CVD burden.

Important steps should be taken to reduce the future burden of CVD in both developing and developed countries and the existing high burden of CVD in developed nations. Prevention of the development of risk factors in the first place should be emphasized, including increased physical activity, the promotion of a heart healthy diet, and a decrease in the prevalence of obesity. Interventions that focus on reducing the prevalence of traditional risk factors should continue to be an important part of primary and secondary prevention efforts. Specific efforts should include the identification and treatment of hypertension, the identification and treatment of dyslipidemia, and enhanced efforts to prevent smoking initiation and to encourage smoking cessation. Because of the large number of individuals at high risk with existing CVD in developed countries, secondary prevention efforts are an important strategy to reduce subsequent CVD morbidity and mortality.

Although the strategy for CVD interventions in developing countries is similar, it should be tailored to the specific needs of each country. In many of these settings, the current burden of CVD is relatively low, but the potential for a substantial burden is high. In these countries, primordial prevention for CVD will be a key part of these prevention efforts. It is of paramount importance to encourage the maintenance of existing heart healthy habits such as physical activity, a traditional (and healthier) diet, and low rates of obesity.

A secondary strategy should be the identification and treatment of traditional risk factors. One very important risk factor in developing countries is a cigarette smoking rate that is often higher than that in developed countries. Because of the lower prevalence of CVD in these countries, secondary prevention efforts in these emerging countries are often poorer than in developed countries. However, secondary prevention programs need to be initiated. It is hoped that the emerging economies will learn from the mistakes of developed countries and hence avoid the epidemic of CVD.

CONCLUSION

Despite the fact that the overall prevalence of CVD risk factors has been reduced in most countries, the prevalence of major CVD risk factors, as well as incidence of CVD, varies tremendously around the world. The exception to the pattern of an improving CVD risk profile is the increasing rates of obesity and diabetes, particularly in the more developed countries, which may have a deleterious effect on future trends in CVD

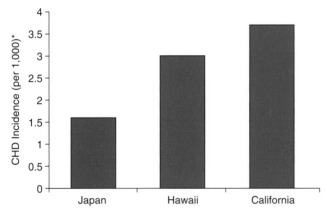

FIGURE 2-13 Incidence of coronary heart disease in middle-aged Japanese men residing in Japan, Hawaii, and California. *Age-adjusted with Hawaii sample as standard. (Adapted from Robertson TL, Kato H, Rhoads GG, et al: Epidemiologic studies of coronary heart disease and stroke in Japanese men living in Japan, Hawaii and California, Am J Cardiol 39:239-243, 1977.)

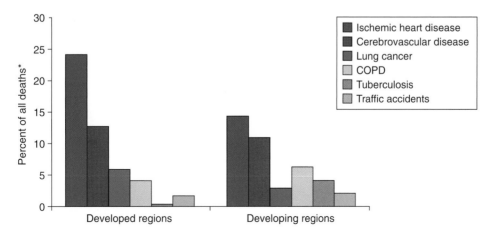

FIGURE 2-14 Projected leading causes of death in 2020 by region of the world. (Adapted from Murray CJL, Lopez AD: The global burden of disease: a comprehensive assessment of global mortality and disability from diseases, injuries and risk factors in 1990 and projected to 2020, Cambridge, Mass, 1996, Harvard University Press on behalf of the World Health Organization and the World Bank.)

incidence. The overall reductions in CVD risk factors may explain, in part, the concordant reductions in rates of mortality and morbidity from CVD in the United States and in other developed countries.

This chapter has focused on describing trends in CVD in the United States and in other countries. Substantial heterogeneity exists in CVD mortality among countries. Encouraging improvements have been observed since the 1970s in some of the countries with the highest rates of CVD mortality, but less encouraging developments have occurred in regions of the world with lower rates of CVD, such as Eastern Europe. In addition, projections suggest that in developing countries in South Asia and in the Pacific Rim, the burden of CVD will increase rapidly. As would be expected, international trends in CVD morbidity and mortality are highly correlated with the presence or absence of health-oriented behaviors and traditional CVD risk factors.

Substantial opportunities exist to further reduce the burden in developed countries and prevent further increases in CVD in developing countries. Subsequent chapters in this book focus on effective strategies for CVD prevention both in clinical and community settings. Substantial allocation of human and monetary resources is needed to implement these prevention and treatment strategies; however, in view of the potential payoffs in reduction of death and disability, this effort is essential.

REFERENCES

1. National Heart, Lung and Blood Institute: *Morbidity and mortality: 2007 chart book on cardiovascular, lung, and blood diseases*, Bethesda, Md, 2007, National Institutes of Health.
2. The WHO MONICA Project: Myocardial infarction and coronary deaths in the World Health Organization MONICA Project. *Circulation* 90:583-612, 1994.
3. American Heart Association: *Heart disease & stroke statistics—2010 update. A report from the American Heart Association*, Dallas, Tex, 2010, American Heart Association.
4. U.S. Department of Health and Human Services: *Chart book on trends in the health of Americans. Health, United States, 2008*, Hyattsville, Md, 2008, National Center for Health Statistics.
4a. *International classification of diseases and related health problems*, ed 9, Geneva, Switzerland, 1977, World Health Organization.
4b. *International classification of diseases and related health problems*, ed 10, Geneva, Switzerland, 1992, World Health Organization.
5. Rosamond WD, Chambless LE, Folsom AR, et al: Trends in the incidence of myocardial infarction and in mortality due to coronary heart disease, 1987 to 1994. *N Engl J Med* 339:861-867, 1998.
6. Chobanian AV, Bakris GL, Black HR, et al; National Heart, Lung, and Blood Institute Joint National Committee on Prevention, Detection, Evaluation, and Treatment of High Blood Pressure; National High Blood Pressure Education Program Coordinating Committee: The seventh report of the Joint National Committee on prevention, detection, evaluation, and treatment of high blood pressure. *JAMA* 289:2560-2571, 2003.
7. The WHO MONICA Project: *WWW-Publications from the WHO MONICA Project* (online database): www.ktl.fi/publications/monica. Accessed July 18, 2010.
8. Evans A, Tolonen H, Hense H-W, et al, for the WHO MONICA Project: Trends in coronary risk factors in the WHO MONICA project. *Int J Epidemiol* 30:S35-S40, 2001.
9. Hajjar I, Kotchen TA: Trends in prevalence, awareness, treatment, and control of hypertension in the United States, 1988-2000. *JAMA* 290:199-206, 2003.
10. Ostchega Y, Yoon SS, Hughes J, Tatiana L: *Hypertension awareness, treatment, and control—continued disparities in adults: United States, 2005-2006*, NCHS Data Brief No. 3, Hyattsville, Md, 2008, National Center for Health Statistics. Available at http://www.cdc.gov/nchs/data/databriefs/db03.pdf.
11. Centers for Disease Control and Prevention: *Behavioral risk factor surveillance system* (online database): www.cdc.gov/brfss. Accessed July 19, 2010.
11a. U.S. Department of Health and Human Services: *Healthy people 2010* (website): http://www.healthypeople.gov/Document/HTML/Volume1/12Heart.htm#_Toc490544222.
12. National Center for Health Statistics: *Health, United States, 2008 with socioeconomic status and health chartbook*, Hyattsville, Md, 2008, National Center for Health Statistics.
13. Flegal KM, Carroll MD, Ogden CL, et al: Prevalence and trends in obesity among US adults, 1999-2008. *JAMA* 303:235-241, 2010.
14. Chaoyang L, Ford ES, McGuire LC, et al: Increasing trends in waist circumference and abdominal obesity among U.S. adults. *Obesity (Silver Spring)* 15:216-224, 2007.
15. Executive Summary of the Third Report of the National Cholesterol Education Program (NCEP). Expert Panel on Detection, Evaluation, and Treatment of High Blood Cholesterol in Adults (Adult Treatment Panel III). *JAMA* 285:2486-2497, 2001.
16. National Diabetes Data Group, editors: *Diabetes in America*, ed 2, NIH Publication No. 95-1468, Washington, D.C., 1995, U.S. Department of Health and Human Services, National Institutes of Health, National Institute of Diabetes and Digestive and Kidney Diseases.
17. Centers for Disease Control and Prevention: *National diabetes fact sheet: general information and national estimates on diabetes in the United States, 2007*, Atlanta, GA, 2008, U.S. Department of Health and Human Services, Centers for Disease Control and Prevention.
18. Benjamin SM, Valdez R, Geiss LS, et al: Estimated number of adults with prediabetes in the U.S. in 2000: opportunities for prevention. *Diabetes Care* 26(3):645-649, 2003.
19. The SEARCH for Diabetes in Youth Study Group: The burden of diabetes among U.S. youth: prevalence estimates from the SEARCH for Diabetes in Youth Study. *Pediatrics* 118:1510-1518, 2006.
20. The SEARCH for Diabetes in Youth Study Group: Incidence of diabetes in youth in the United States: the SEARCH for Diabetes in Youth Study. *JAMA* 297:2716-2724, 2007.
21. Mokdad AH, Ford ES, Bowman BA, et al: Diabetes trends in the U.S.: 1990-1998. *Diabetes Care* 23:1278-1283, 2000.
22. Mokdad AH, Ford ES, Bowman BA, et al: Prevalence of obesity, diabetes, and obesity-related health risk factors, 2001. *JAMA* 289:76-79, 2003.
23. Cowie CC, Rust KF, Byrd-Holt DD, et al: Prevalence of diabetes and high risk for diabetes using A1c criteria in the U.S. population in 1988-2006. *Diabetes Care* 33:562-568, 2010.
24. Shaw JE, Sicree RA, Zimmet PZ: Global estimates of the prevalence of diabetes for 2010 and 2030. *Diabetes Res Clin Pract* 87:4-14, 2010.
25. Huang ES, Basu A, O'Grady M, et al: Projecting the future diabetes population size and related costs for the U.S. *Diabetes Care* 32:2225-2229, 2009.
26. Grundy SM, Cleeman JI, Daniels SR, et al: Diagnosis and management of the metabolic syndrome: an American Heart Association/National Heart, Lung and Blood Institute Scientific Statement. *Circulation* 112:2735-2752, 2005.
27. Ford ES, Giles WH, Dietz WH: Prevalence of the metabolic syndrome among U.S. adults: findings from the Third National Health and Nutrition Examination Survey. *JAMA* 287:356-359, 2002.
28. Stafford RS, Blumenthal D, Pasternak RC: Variations in cholesterol management practices by U.S physicians. *J Am Coll Cardiol* 29:139-146, 1997.
29. Danias PG, O'Mahony S, Radford M, et al: Serum cholesterol levels are underevaluated and undertreated. *Am J Cardiol* 81:1353-1356, 1998.
30. The sixth report of the Joint National Committee on Prevention, Detection, Evaluation, and Treatment of High Blood Pressure. *Arch Intern Med* 157:2413-2446, 1997 [Erratum in *Arch Intern Med* 158:573, 1998].
31. Robertson TL, Kato H, Rhoads GG, et al: Epidemiologic studies of coronary heart disease and stroke in Japanese men living in Japan, Hawaii and California. *Am J Cardiol* 39:239-243, 1977.
32. Murray CJL, Lopez AD: *The global burden of disease: a comprehensive assessment of global mortality and disability from diseases, injuries and risk factors in 1990 and projected to 2020*, Cambridge, Mass, 1996, Harvard University Press on behalf of the World Health Organization and the World Bank.

CHAPTER 3

Prediction of Cardiovascular Disease: Framingham Risk Estimation and Beyond

Peter W. F. Wilson

KEY POINTS

- Risk estimation usually originates with observational studies of the incidence of coronary heart disease events over time.

- Prediction of risk is dependent on accurate and precise baseline measurements in persons without coronary disease at the time of measurement.

- Follow-up of 10 years is a typical interval of interest for the prediction of coronary disease events in adults who are asymptomatic at baseline.

- Performance criteria for risk estimation include discrimination, calibration, and reclassification.

- Newer risk factors and biomarkers for heart disease can be evaluated in the context of existing risk estimation approaches.

Prediction of heart disease has become possible because of the long-term experience in observational studies that included detailed information on elements of risk before the development of clinical disease. Storage of information, computerization, and exportability of risk prediction tools have facilitated this process. The origins of coronary heart disease (CHD) risk estimation, the role of baseline measurements, determination of outcomes, statistical programming, algorithm development, and performance evaluation are the key concepts that underlie this discipline.

Many factors contribute to the risk for CHD and to the risk for cardiovascular disease (CVD) in general. The primary focus of this chapter is estimation of risk for CHD over a 10-year interval. There is considerable agreement about the key factors that are effective predictors of initial CHD events.[1-4] Although there are differences between the predictions of CVD and of its constituent events (peripheral arterial disease,[5] stroke,[6] and heart failure[7]), there are many similarities, and information on the prediction of CVD is also provided.

ORIGINS OF ESTIMATION OF RISK FOR CORONARY HEART DISEASE

The prediction of CVD outcomes has evolved considerably over recent years. Initial efforts were related to the development of logistic regression data analysis and its adaptation to the prediction of CHD events. The Framingham Heart Study began in 1948, and the researchers initially evaluated the role of factors such as age, sex, high blood pressure, high blood levels of cholesterol, diabetes mellitus, and smoking as risk factors for the onset of first CHD events. Logistic regression methods became available on large-frame computers in the 1950s and 1960s.[8,9] This process involved assembling data for a population sample that had been monitored prospectively for the occurrence of a dichotomous event such as clinical CHD.

The initial approach involved identifying persons free of the vascular event of interest, obtaining baseline data on factors that might affect risk for the outcome, and monitoring the participants prospectively for the development of the clinical outcome under investigation.[1] The original participants in the Framingham study returned for new examinations and assessment of new cardiovascular events every 2 years, and the researchers, using logistic regression in the data from the original Framingham cohort, developed cross-sectional pooling methods to assess risk over time.

BASELINE MEASUREMENTS AS PREDICTORS OF RISK FOR CORONARY HEART DISEASE

To develop reliable estimations of CHD risk, it is important to have a longitudinal study, standardized measurements at baseline, and adjudicated outcomes that are consistent over the follow-up interval. It is possible to undertake multivariate analyses of factors that might be associated with a vascular disease outcome in a cross-sectional study,[10] but it is preferable to have a prospective design to fully understand the role of factors that might increase risk for developing a vascular disease event.

A prospective design is necessary because critical risk factors may change after the occurrence of CHD, and such a design allows the inclusion of fatal events as outcomes. The literature related to tobacco use and risk of CHD is informative with regard to this issue. After experiencing a myocardial infarction, a person may stop smoking or may underreport the amount of smoking that occurred before the occurrence of a myocardial infarction, which could lead to analyses in which the effect of smoking on risk for myocardial infarction would be underestimated.

Standardized measurements are important to use in assessing the role of factors that might increase risk for vascular disease outcomes. For example, blood pressure levels are typically measured in the arm

3

with a cuff that is of appropriate size and is inflated and deflated according to a protocol; the level of the arm is maintained near the level of heart; measurements are taken in patients who have been sitting in a room at ambient temperature for a specified number of minutes; a sphygmomanometer that has been standardized is used; and determinations are made by properly trained personnel. Blood pressure can be measured inaccurately for many reasons, including inconsistent positioning of the patient, varying the time the subject is at rest before measurement, varying credentials of the examiner (e.g., nurses vs. doctors), and rounding errors when the measurements are recorded.[11]

Lipid standardization has been helpful in ensuring accuracy and precision of lipid measurements, which are used to help assess risk for cardiovascular events, and measurements are typically obtained in the fasting state. The Lipid Research Clinics Program, initiated in the 1970s, led to the development of a Lipid Standardization Program at the Centers for Disease Control and Prevention, with monitoring of research laboratories that measure cholesterol, high-density lipoprotein (HDL) cholesterol, and triglyceride levels.[12-14] This program updated the laboratory methods and techniques over time to accommodate newer methods of measurement.[15-17]

Laboratory determinations have several potential sources of variability, including preanalytic, analytic, and biologic sources.[18,19] Preanalytic sources of error include fasting status, appropriate use of tourniquets during phlebotomy, room temperature, and sample transport conditions. Laboratory variability is minimized through the use of high-quality instruments, use of reliable assays, performance of replicate assays, and use of algorithms to repeat assays if the difference between results of replicate assays exceeds specified thresholds. Other methods to ensure accuracy and precision with laboratory determinations include the use of external standards, using batching samples, and minimizing the number of lots for calibration. Sources of biologic variability include fasting status, time of day, season of the year, and intervening illnesses.[18]

Another key risk factor is diabetes status. In many of the older studies, subjects did not fast for each clinical visit, and an expert-derived diagnosis of diabetes mellitus was used on the basis of available glucose information, medication use, and chart reviews. The American Diabetes Association has changed the criteria for diabetes since the 1970s. For example, diabetes was considered present in 1979 if fasting glucose level was 140 mg/dL or higher or if a nonfasting glucose level was higher than 200 mg/dL.[20] These criteria were revised in 1997 so that a fasting glucose level of 126 mg/dL or higher was considered to be diagnostic for diabetes mellitus.[21]

CORONARY HEART DISEASE OUTCOMES

Total CHD (angina pectoris, myocardial infarction, and death from CHD) and "hard" CHD (myocardial infarction and death from CHD) are the outcomes that have been studied most frequently, but other investigators have reported on the risk of "hard" CHD; their studies included persons with a baseline history of angina pectoris,[2] and the European CHD risk estimates have focused on the occurrence of death from CHD.[4]

HISTORY OF ESTIMATION OF RISK FOR CORONARY HEART DISEASE

In the early 1970s, CHD risk was estimated with the use of logistic regression methods and cross-sectional pooling with the variables age, sex, blood pressure, cholesterol level, smoking, and diabetes.[22] In initial research on CHD

prediction, investigators used logistic regression analyses, and the relative risk effects for each of the predictor variables were provided. Time-dependent regression methods and the addition of HDL cholesterol levels as an important predictor led to improved prediction models for CHD,[23] in which score sheets and regression equation information with intercepts were used to estimate absolute risk for CHD over an interval that typically spanned 8 to 12 years of follow-up.

Score sheets to estimate CHD risk were highlighted in a 1991 Framingham study–related publication about CHD risk in which total CHD was predicted,[24] as were various first cardiovascular events.[25] The outcome of interest was prediction of a first CHD event on the basis of the independent variables age, sex, high blood pressure, high blood cholesterol, diabetes mellitus, smoking, and left ventricular hypertrophy detected on the electrocardiogram (ECG-LVH). Risk equations with coefficients were provided to allow estimation of CHD risk by means of score sheets, pocket calculators, and computer programs.[24]

A 1998 Framingham study–related article on CHD risk estimation[1] showed little difference in the overall predictive capability for total CHD when total cholesterol level was replaced in the calculations by low-density lipoprotein (LDL) cholesterol, which suggested that an initial lipid screening with total cholesterol, HDL cholesterol, age, sex, systolic blood pressure, diabetes mellitus, and smoking had good overall predictive capabilities without lipid subgroup measurements. The 1998 CHD risk analyses did not include information on ECG-LVH as a risk predictor because the Joint National Committee on Prevention, Detection, Evaluation, and Treatment of High Blood Pressure had not recommended that electrocardiography be performed on asymptomatic middle-aged persons.[26] Also, the prevalence of ECG-LVH was very low (a small percentage) in middle-aged white populations. In contrast, among African Americans, ECG-LVH has been much more common. It is thought that including electrocardiography might be particularly helpful for estimating CHD risk in African Americans and in other racial and ethnic groups in which ECG-LVH is more common and in which the population burden of hypertension is greater.[27]

A workshop was convened by the National Heart, Lung and Blood Institute in 2001 to assess the ability to estimate risk of first CHD events in middle-aged Americans. In summaries of the workshop proceedings, D'Agostino and colleagues[28] and Grundy and associates[29] compared the predictive results for CHD in several studies by using equations used in the Framingham study or equations in which the variables were the same as those in the Framingham risk-estimation equations but with study-specific predictions. Participants in the workshop evaluated the role of calibration and used statistical adjustments for differences in risk factor levels and incidence rates.[28] The summary findings included the following: (1) Relative risks for the individual variables were similar to those in the Framingham experience; (2) the Framingham equations predicted CHD quite well when applied to other populations, and the C-statistic for the Framingham prediction was usually very similar to the C-statistic from the study-specific predictor equation; and (3) in African Americans and Japanese American men from the Honolulu Heart Study, the Framingham equation had much less capability for discrimination.[28]

CORONARY HEART DISEASE RISK ALGORITHM DEVELOPMENT

It is helpful to understand how CHD risk algorithms are currently developed and how performance criteria are used to evaluate prediction algorithms. The key starting point is the experience of a well-characterized prospective study cohort that is generally representative of a larger population group. That initial stipulation can help to ensure the generalizability of the results. Only data from subjects with complete outcome and covariate information for a given endpoint are used in the analyses.

Risk estimates for CHD are usually derived from proportional hazards regression models according to methods developed by Cox.[30] The variables that are significant in the individual analyses are then considered for inclusion in multivariable prediction models according to a fixed design or a stepwise model in which an iterative approach is used to select the variables for inclusion. Pairwise interactions can be considered for inclusion in the model, but it may be difficult to interpret those results, and interactions may be less generalizable when tested in other population groups.

Traditional candidate variables considered for these analyses in American and European formulations have typically included systolic or diastolic blood pressure, blood pressure treatment, cholesterol level, diabetes mellitus, current smoking, and body mass index.[1,4] Information related to treatment, such as blood pressure medication, should be included with caution in this situation because the risk algorithm is typically being developed from an observational study with a prospective design, not from a clinical trial in which treatments are randomly assigned. Some prediction equations have included data from persons with diabetes mellitus,[1] but the Adult Treatment Panel guidelines reflected the opinion that persons with diabetes mellitus were already at high risk for CHD and that risk assessment was therefore not needed for these individuals.[31] Reports and reviews published since 2001 have called into question whether diabetes mellitus is a "CHD risk equivalent," and data have shown that the risk of a subsequent CHD event is approximately twofold for persons known to have diabetes mellitus and fourfold for those who have already experienced CHD.[32]

A validation group is used to test the usefulness of the risk prediction algorithm. One approach is to use an internal validation sample within the study. By this method, a fraction of the data are used for model development, and the other fraction of the data are used for validation. An alternative to this approach is to take a very large fraction of the persons in the study and successively develop models from near-complete data sets. External validation of a risk prediction model—testing the use of the model in other population samples—is especially useful and provides the first indication of whether it is possible to generalize the risk prediction model to other scenarios.

PERFORMANCE CRITERIA FOR CORONARY HEART DISEASE RISK ALGORITHMS

A variety of statistical evaluations are now available to evaluate the usefulness of CHD risk prediction and they are discussed successively as follows.

Relative Risk

For each risk factor, proportional hazards modeling yields regression coefficients for a study cohort. The relative risk of a variable is computed by exponentiating the regression coefficient in the multivariate regression models. This measure estimates the difference in risk between someone with a given risk factor such as cigarette smoking and someone who does not smoke. An analogous approach can be undertaken to estimate effects for continuous variables by showing effects for a specific number of units for the variable or by identifying differences in risk that are associated with a difference in

the number of units that, in turn, are associated with a standard deviation for the factor.

Discrimination

Discrimination is the ability of a statistical model to distinguish patients who experience clinical CHD events from those who do not. The C-statistic is the typical performance measure used, which is analogous to the area under a receiver operator characteristic curve; it is a composite of the overall sensitivity and specificity of the prediction equation (Figure 3-1).[33] The C-statistic represents an estimate of the probability that a model will assign a higher risk to patients who develop CHD within a specified follow-up period than to patients who do not. The error associated with C-statistic estimates can itself be estimated.[33,34]

Values for the C-statistic range from 0.00 to 1.00, and a value of 0.50 reflects discrimination by chance. Higher values generally indicate agreement between observed and predicted risks. The average C-statistic for the prediction of CHD is approximately 0.70.[1,28] Using a large number of independent predictor variables can lead to better discrimination but can also "overfit" the model, whereby the statistical model can work very well for the derivation data set but have much lower discriminatory capability and limited accuracy in predicting the occurrence of outcomes with other data.

Calibration

Calibration is a measure of how closely predicted estimates correspond with actual outcomes. To present calibration analyses, the data are separated into deciles of risk, and observed rates are tested for differences from the expected rates across the deciles; they are tested with a version of the Hosmer-Lemeshow chi-square statistic.[28] Smaller chi-square values indicate good calibration, and values higher than 20 generally indicate significant lack of calibration.

Recalibration

An existing CHD prediction model can be recalibrated if it provides relatively useful ranking of risk for the population being studied, but the model systematically overestimates or

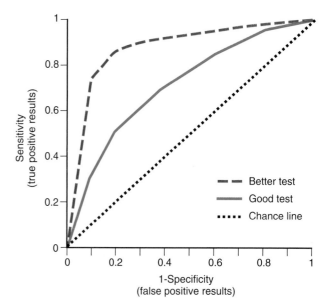

FIGURE 3-1 Schematic for receiver operator characteristic curves and disease prediction, based on sensitivity and specificity of multivariate prediction models.

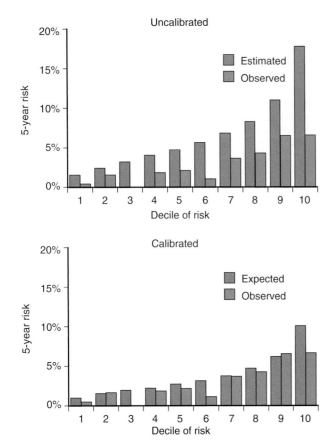

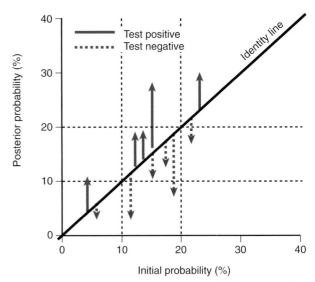

FIGURE 3-3 Example of reclassification strategy and risk of disease according to initial and posterior probabilities. Gridlines represent potential levels that are associated with reclassification of risk.

FIGURE 3-2 Hypothetical example of uncalibrated and calibrated estimated and observed risk for coronary heart disease (CHD), according to deciles of CHD risk.

underestimates CHD risk in the new population. For example, recalibrating the Framingham risk-prediction equation would involve inserting the mean risk factor values and average incidence rate for the new population into the equation. Kaplan-Meier estimates can be used to determine average incidence rates.[35] This approach was undertaken for Framingham risk-prediction equations that were applied to the CHD experience of Japanese-American men in the Honolulu Heart Study and for Chinese men and women.[28,35] In each of these scenarios, the Framingham risk-prediction equation provided relatively good discrimination but did not provide reliable estimates of absolute risk. A schematic of such an approach is shown in Figure 3-2, where the left panel shows CHD risk is systematically overestimated when the Framingham equation is applied to another population. After calibration, the estimation fits the observed experience much more closely, and the Hosmer-Lemeshow chi-square value is much lower.

Reclassification

Specialized testing in subgroups has been used to reclassify risk for vascular disease. An example of such an approach is the use of exercise testing to upgrade, downgrade, or confirm estimates of vascular disease risk in patients being evaluated for angina pectoris.[36] CHD algorithms may do a reasonably good job in prediction of CHD risk, and the inclusion of a new variable may have minimal effects on C-statistic estimates.[37-40] Methods developed to assess this approach have used a multivariate estimation procedure and tested the utility of a new test to increase, decrease, or confirm risk estimates.[36] Pencina and coworkers[41] published an updated method to assess reclassification that takes into account the potential reclassification of both cases and noncases.

Reclassification has practical applications, as shown in Figure 3-3, in which an initial probability of CHD is estimated from a multivariate prediction equation, and additional information then provides an updated estimation of risk, which is commonly called the *posterior estimate.* If the new information did not provide any added value, the risk estimate would be the same as for the initial calculation, and the risk estimate would lie close to the identity line. The schematic shows the hypothetical effects for a small number of patients. For some individuals, the test result was positive, increasing the posterior risk estimates. On the other hand, negative tests moved the risk estimates downward for some individuals.

The magnitude of effects can be shown graphically by the length of the vertical lines and how they differ from the identity line. It is important to evaluate a posterior risk estimate that would reclassify the individual to a lower or higher risk category. For example, Figure 3-3 shows seven persons with an initial probability of developing disease in the 10% to 20% range. At the intermediate level the risk was increased in three persons and decreased in four persons with new variable information, but some of the risk differences did not differ appreciably from the initial estimates. Risk was reclassified into a higher category for only one person and to a lower category for two persons. Some authors have used performance measures such as the Bayes Information Criteria as another method to interpret potential effects of reclassification.[38]

CURRENT ESTIMATION OF RISK FOR CORONARY HEART DISEASE

The current starting point for using a CHD risk-prediction equation in a person being screened for CHD is a medical history and a clinical examination with standardized collection of key predictor (independent) risk factors: age, sex, fasting lipids (total, LDL, and HDL cholesterol; ratio of total cholesterol to HDL cholesterol), systolic blood pressure, history of diabetes mellitus treatment, fasting and postprandial glucose levels, and use of tobacco and other substances (Table 3-1).[1,2] This information can be used to estimate risk of CHD over a 10-year interval through the use of score sheets or computer programs, as described at the website for

| TABLE 3–1 | Examples of Algorithms for Predicting CHD and Other CVD Events |

Variable	Wilson et al (1998)[1]	ATP III ("Executive Summary," 2001)[31]	Assmann et al (2002)[2]	Reference euroSCORE (Conroy et al, 2003)[4]	Wolf et al (1991)[6]	Murabito et al (1997)[5]	Butler et al (2008)[46]	D'Agostino et al (2008)[54]
Source	Framingham study	Framingham study	PROCAM	Europe	Framingham study	Framingham study	Health ABC study	Framingham study
Outcome*	Total CHD	Hard CHD	Hard CHD	CHD mortality	Stroke	Intermittent claudication	Cardiac failure	Total CVD
Age interval	5 years	5 years	5 years	5 years	Intervals vary	5 years	5 years	5 years
Inclusion criteria	No CHD	No CHD	Possible CHD	No CHD	Possible CHD	Possible CHD	Possible CHD	No CVD
Sex	Men, women	Men, women	Men	Men, women	Men, women	Men, women	Men, women	Men, women
BP levels	JNC category	Systolic BP	Systolic BP	Systolic BP	Systolic BP	JNC category	Systolic BP	Systolic BP
BP therapy	No	Yes	No	No	Yes	No	No	Yes
Cholesterol	Yes	Yes	No	Yes	No	Yes	No	Yes
HDL cholesterol	Yes	Yes	Yes	No	No	No	No	Yes
LDL cholesterol	Optional	No	Yes	No	No	No	No	No
Cigarette smokers	Yes	Yes	Yes	Yes	Yes	Yes, number/day	No	Yes
Glycemia	Patients with DM included	Patients with DM excluded	Diabetes status	Diabetes status	Diabetes status	Diabetes status	Glucose level	Diabetes status
Other factors	—	—	—	—	ECG-LVH, atrial fibrillation	—	Heart rate ECG-LVH, serum albumin, creatinine	—
Baseline CVD included	ECG-LVH	No	MI history	No	CHD	No	CHD	No

*"Total CHD" refers to angina pectoris, myocardial infarction, and death from CHD; "hard CHD" refers to myocardial infarction and death from CHD.
ATP III, Adult Treatment Panel, third report; BP, blood pressure; CHD, coronary heart disease; CVD, cardiovascular disease; DM, diabetes mellitus; ECG-LVH, left ventricular hypertrophy detected on electrocardiogram; Health ABC, Health, Aging, and Body Composition; euroSCORE, European System for Cardiac Operative Risk Evaluation; HDL, high-density lipoprotein; JNC, Joint National Committee on Prevention, Detection, Evaluation, and Treatment of High Blood Pressure; LDL, low-density lipoprotein; MI, myocardial infarction; PROCAM, Prospective Cardiovascular Munster (study).

the Framingham Heart Study (http://www.framinghamheart study.org). Risk estimation over 10 years with a score sheet based on the Framingham experience was used by the National Cholesterol Education Program in the Adult Treatment Panel III Guidelines (Figure 3-4), and an interactive calculator is also available on the Internet (http://hp2010. nhlbihin.net/atpiii/calculator.asp?usertype=prof).

Specialized models have been developed for persons with type 2 diabetes in which additional potential predictor variables are considered. The experience of diabetic patients who participated in the United Kingdom Prospective Diabetes Study has been used to develop this prediction algorithm, which can be accessed on the Internet (www.dtu.ox.ac.uk/ riskengine). Stevens and colleagues,[42] the authors of the algorithm, reported that the key predictor variables for initial CHD events were age, diabetes duration, presence of atrial fibrillation, glycosylated hemoglobin level, systolic blood pressure level, total cholesterol concentration, HDL cholesterol concentration, race, and smoking status.

European groups have developed strategies to estimate risk of CHD with European data. Investigators from the Prospective Cardiovascular Munster (PROCAM) in Germany[2] monitored a cohort for the development of CHD, and their results were generally similar to what has been estimated from Framingham data (see Table 3-1).[2] Their analyses were restricted to men. The factors significantly associated with the development of a next CHD event included age, LDL cholesterol concentration, smoking, HDL cholesterol concentration, systolic blood pressure, family history of premature myocardial infarction, diabetes mellitus, and triglyceride levels. The investigators in the Operative Urban Centers for Economic Requalification (CUORE) cohort study in Italy[3] undertook prediction analyses in middle-aged men who were monitored for 10 years for CHD events. They found that age, total cholesterol concentration, systolic blood pressure, cigarette smoking, HDL cholesterol concentration, diabetes mellitus, hypertension drug treatment, and family history of CHD were associated with initial CHD events.

The CUORE investigators also tested the utility of Framingham and PROCAM estimating equations in Italy. They found that, in general, both Framingham and PROCAM overestimated CHD risk in Italian men, and after calibration of the Framingham equations, it was possible to reliably predict CHD events in their study cohort.[3] Risk scores have also been developed in the United Kingdom (the QRISK calculator) and Scotland (the ASSIGN calculator) with consideration of the effects of social deprivation.[43,44] The QRISK algorithm predicts total CVD according to age, sex, smoking status, systolic blood pressure, ratio of total serum cholesterol to high-density lipoprotein level, body mass index, family

A

Age y	Points
20-34	−9
35-39	−4
40-44	0
45-49	3
50-54	6
55-59	8
60-64	10
65-69	11
70-74	12
75-79	13

Total Cholesterol (mg/dL)	Points				
	Age 20-39 y	Age 40-49 y	Age 50-59 y	Age 60-69 y	Age 70-79 y
<160	0	0	0	0	0
160-199	4	3	2	1	0
200-239	7	5	3	1	0
240-279	9	6	4	2	1
>280	11	8	5	3	1

	Points				
	Age 20-39 y	Age 40-49 y	Age 50-59 y	Age 60-69 y	Age 70-79 y
Nonsmoker	0	0	0	0	0
Smoker	8	5	3	1	1

HDL, mg/dL	Points
<60	−1
50-59	0
40-49	1
>40	2

Systolic BP (mm Hg)	Number untreated	Number treated
<120	0	0
120-129	0	1
130-139	1	2
140-159	1	2
>160	2	3

Point total	10-year risk (%)
<0	<1
0	1
1	1
2	1
3	1
4	1
5	2
6	2
7	3
8	4
9	5
10	6
11	8
12	10
13	12
14	16
15	20
16	25
>17	>30

B

Age y	Points
20-34	−7
35-39	−3
40-44	0
45-49	3
50-54	6
55-59	8
60-64	10
65-69	12
70-74	14
75-79	16

Total Cholesterol (mg/dL)	Points				
	Age 20-39 y	Age 40-49 y	Age 50-59 y	Age 60-69 y	Age 70-79 y
<160	0	0	0	0	0
160-199	4	3	2	1	1
200-239	8	6	4	2	1
240-279	11	8	5	3	2
>280	13	10	7	4	2

	Points				
	Age 20-39 y	Age 40-49 y	Age 50-59 y	Age 60-69 y	Age 70-79 y
Nonsmoker	0	0	0	0	0
Smoker	9	7	4	2	1

HDL, mg/dL	Points
<60	−1
50-59	0
40-49	1
>40	2

Systolic BP (mm Hg)	Number untreated	Number treated
<120	0	0
120-129	1	3
130-139	2	4
140-159	3	5
>160	4	6

Point total	10-year risk (%)
<9	<1
9	1
10	1
11	1
12	1
13	2
14	2
15	3
16	4
17	5
18	6
19	8
20	11
21	14
22	19
23	22
24	27
>25	>30

FIGURE 3-4 Risk of hard coronary heart disease (CHD) events according to the National Cholesterol Education Program, Adult Treatment Program III Guidelines. **A,** Men. **B,** Women. BP, blood pressure; HDL, high-density lipoprotein. *(From Executive Summary of the third report of the National Cholesterol Education Program (NCEP) Expert Panel on Detection, Evaluation, and Treatment of High Blood Cholesterol in Adults (Adult Treatment Panel III). JAMA 285:2486-2497, 2001.)*

Risk factor points									
Risk factor	0	+1	+2	+3	+4	+5	+6	+7	Line score
Age, yr	45-49	50-54	55-59	60-64	65-69	70-74	75-79	80-84	
Sex	Female			Male					
Cholesterol, mg/dL	<170	170-209	210-249	250-289	>289				
Blood pressure	Normal	High normal	Stage 1		Stage 2+				
Cigarettes/d, n	0	1-5	6-10	11-20	>20				
Diabetes	No					Yes			
CHD	No					Yes			
								Point total	

Points	4-year probability		Points	4-year probability
<10	<1%		23	10%
10-12	1%		24	11%
13-15	2%		25	13%
16-17	3%		26	16%
18	4%		27	18%
19	5%		28	21%
20	6%		29	24%
21	7%		30	28%
22	8%			

FIGURE 3-5 Risk of intermittent claudication over 4 years in Framingham Heart Study participants aged 45 to 84 years. *(From Murabito JM, D'Agostino RB, Silbershatz H, et al: Intermittent claudication: a risk profile from the Framingham Heart Study.* Circulation 96:44-49, 1997.)

history of CHD (in a first-degree relative younger than 60), area measure of deprivation, and existing treatment with antihypertensive agent.

The European System for Cardiac Operative Risk Evaluation (euroSCORE)[4] algorithm is currently the most popular CHD prediction algorithm in Europe (see Table 3-1). It predicts CHD mortality and includes data from a large number of studies across Europe to generate the risk-prediction algorithms. The factors used in the prediction included age, sex, smoking, systolic blood pressure, and the ratio of total cholesterol concentration to HDL cholesterol concentration. Slightly different versions of the risk-scoring algorithm are used in regions of higher risk (generally more Northern latitudes) than in regions of lower risk (more Southern regions of Europe). Unfortunately, not enough of the participating centers had data on CHD morbidity, and a prediction algorithm for total CHD that is based on experience across Europe is still in development.

Prediction of First Cardiovascular Disease Events

Approximately two thirds of CVD events represent CHD (myocardial infarction, angina pectoris, CHD death). There is considerable interest in the prediction of CVD in general and in the vascular disease events that do *not* represent CHD, such as intermittent claudication, stroke, and cardiac failure.[5-7,45] For example, the determinants of intermittent claudication in the Framingham study were shown to be age, male sex, blood pressure, diabetes mellitus, cigarette smoking, cholesterol level, and HDL cholesterol level (Figure 3-5; see also Table 3-1).[5] A slightly different approach[6] was

undertaken in the prediction of first stroke events, and data from persons with heart disease at baseline were included in the analyses undertaken by Framingham investigators. They reported that age, male sex, blood pressure level, diabetes mellitus, and CHD were predictive of the incidence of stroke during follow-up (Figures 3-6 and 3-7; see also Table 3-1). Similarly, the prediction of cardiac failure has often included data from persons known to have experienced CHD as at-risk individuals.[7] For example, predictors of cardiac failure in the Health, Aging, and Body Composition (Health ABC) cohort included age, sex, coronary artery disease at baseline, systolic blood pressure, heart rate, left ventricular hypertrophy, cigarette smoking, fasting glucose level, serum creatinine concentration, and serum albumin concentration (see Table 3-1 and Figure 3-8).[45,46]

Prediction of Secondary Cardiovascular Disease Events in Persons with Preexisting Cardiovascular Disease

Persons with established CVD, or a CVD risk equivalent, are at increased risk for cardiovascular events. The absolute risk of a "hard" CHD event in these patients often exceeds 2% per year,[1] and such patients may have a wide range of absolute risks (typically 2% to 5% per year). Risk assessment may be useful in this setting. In evaluating a patient with preexisting coronary artery disease, physicians should consider obtaining the medical history and performing a physical examination, 12-lead electrocardiography, and selected laboratory tests. The Framingham Heart Study researchers have developed algorithms for estimating the 2-year risk for CHD events,

Risk factor	0	1	2	3	4	5	6	7	8	9	10
						Points					
Age (yr)	54-56	57-59	60-62	63-65	66-68	69-71	72-74	75-77	78-80	81-83	84-86
SBP (mm Hg)	95-105	106-116	117-126	127-137	138-148	149-159	160-170	171-181	182-191	192-202	203-213
Hyp Rx	No		Yes								
DM	No		Yes								
Cigs	No			Yes							
CVD	No			Yes							
AF	No				Yes						
LVH	No										

Points	10-year probability	Points	10-year probability	Points	10-year probability
1	2.6%	11	11.2%	21	41.7%
2	3.0%	12	12.9%	22	46.6%
3	3.5%	13	14.8%	23	51.8%
4	4.0%	14	17.0%	24	57.3%
5	4.7%	15	19.5%	25	62.8%
6	5.4%	16	22.4%	26	68.4%
7	6.3%	17	25.5%	27	73.8%
8	7.3%	18	29.0%	28	79.0%
9	8.4%	19	32.9%	29	83.7%
10	9.7%	20	37.1%	30	87.9%

FIGURE 3-6 Risk of stroke over 10 years in men aged 55 to 84 years in the Framingham Heart Study. AF, atrial fibrillation; Cigs, number of cigarettes smoked per day; CVD, cardiovascular disease; DM, diabetes mellitus; Hyp Rx, medication for hypertension; LVH, left ventricular hypertrophy; SBP, systolic blood pressure. *(From Wolf PA, D'Agostino RB, Belanger AJ, et al: Probability of stroke: a risk profile from the Framingham study. Stroke 3:312-318, 1991.)*

stroke, or death from cerebrovascular disease in women (Table 3-2) and men (Table 3-3) with existing CHD.[47,48] Tables such as those in the publication by Califf and colleagues[48] may be useful for initial risk stratification, but clinical manifestation, including the type of chest pain present and the presence of any associated comorbid conditions, should also be considered in the determination of prognosis (Table 3-4).

Measurement of risk factors that arise in particular patients, proinflammatory markers after a CVD event, or both can further enhance risk stratification. For example, increased levels of C-reactive protein confer a worse prognosis, especially levels higher than 10 mg/dL after myocardial infarction.[49] Moreover, higher coronary calcium scores determined by electron beam computed tomography and reduced vascular endothelial function are predictive of worse outcomes in patients with known CVD.[50,51] Measurement of these factors is not currently recommended in this setting, primarily because such patients are already regarded as being at extremely high risk.

The individual major CVD risk factors are important predictors of long-term prognosis in persons with established CHD. Over an average of nearly 10 years of follow-up, systolic blood pressure, total cholesterol, and diabetes remained significant predictors for the risk of repeated myocardial infarction or death from CHD among subjects who had sustained a previous myocardial infarction in the Framingham Heart Study.[52] Other studies have also confirmed the role of key risk factors in promoting the recurrence of CVD events and mortality, and their importance as therapeutic targets is suggested.[53]

FUTURE OF PREDICTION OF VASCULAR DISEASE RISK

The prediction of CHD has helped guide clinical decisions for persons free of clinical CVD at baseline. It is especially helpful in identifying middle-aged individuals who should be treated aggressively with management of cholesterol level and blood pressure. As blood pressure and lipid treatment strategies become more widespread, more efficacious, and achievable at lower cost, it makes sense to try to prevent total cardiovascular events. Furthermore, clinicians and patients alike are interested not only in their risk of CHD but also their risk of stroke, peripheral arterial disease, and cardiac failure. For the preceding reasons, it is likely that first CVD events (including total CHD, peripheral arterial disease, cerebrovascular disease, and cardiac failure) may become the clinical outcome of greatest interest and significance in the future.[25,54] Some investigations, especially those with large cardiovascular registries, have also been involved with the prediction of subsequent cardiovascular events and bedside risk estimation of 6-month mortality in patients who survive admission for an acute coronary syndrome.[48,55]

Coronary disease risk can be estimated by several methods, and simple prediction tools can potentially be self-administered. For example, analyses undertaken by Mainous and associates[56] for participants in the Atherosclerosis Risk in Communities Study revealed that the variables age, diabetes, hypertension, hypercholesterolemia, smoking, physical activity, and family history were predictive of initial CHD events in men, and similar results were available for women.

Risk factor	Points										
	0	1	2	3	4	5	6	7	8	9	10
Age (yr)	54-56	57-59	60-62	63-65	66-68	69-71	72-74	75-77	78-80	81-83	84-86
SBP (mm Hg)	95-104	105-114	115-124	125-134	135-144	145-154	155-164	165-174	175-184	185-194	195-204
Hyp Rx	No; if yes, see below		*								
DM	No		*	Yes							
Cigs	No			Yes							
CVD	No										
AF	No						Yes				
LVH	No		Yes		Yes						

*If currently under antihypertensive therapy, add points depending on SBP:

	SBP (mm Hg)										
	95-104	105-114	115-124	125-134	135-144	145-154	155-164	165-174	175-184	185-194	195-204
Points	6	5	5	4	3	3	2	1	1	0	0

Points	10-year probability	Points	10-year probability	Points	10-year probability
1	1.1%	10	6.3%	19	31.9%
2	1.3%	11	7.6%	20	37.3%
3	1.6%	12	9.2%	21	43.4%
4	2.0%	13	11.1%	22	50.0%
5	2.4%	14	13.3%	23	57.0%
6	2.9%	15	16.0%	24	64.2%
7	3.5%	16	19.1%	25	71.4%
8	4.3%	17	22.8%	26	78.2%
9	5.2%	18	27.0%	27	84.4%

FIGURE 3-7 Risk of stroke over 10 years in women aged 55 to 84 years in the Framingham Heart Study. AF, atrial fibrillation; Cigs, number of cigarettes smoked per day; CVD, cardiovascular disease; DM, diabetes mellitus; Hyp Rx, medication for hypertension; LVH, left ventricular hypertrophy; SBP, systolic blood pressure. *(From Wolf PA, D'Agostino RB, Belanger AJ, et al: Probability of stroke: a risk profile from the Framingham study. Stroke 3:312-318, 1991.)*

Similarly, Gaziano and colleagues[57] used data from the National Health and Nutrition Examination Survey to demonstrate that a simple set of variables, including age, systolic blood pressure, smoking status, body mass index, reported diabetes status, and current treatment for hypertension were predictive of CHD risk. Such approaches may be useful in developing parts of the world, where lower cost estimates of CHD risk would be particularly useful. Much of the research in the prediction of vascular disease events since 1990 has focused on CHD, but there is considerable interest to enlarge this category to total CVD, and more complete details are included in the report by D'Agostino and colleagues.[54]

Imaging information related to atherosclerotic burden can be particularly helpful in predicting risk for CHD events, but the cost of such procedures is high in comparison with the low cost of health risk screening.[58] Atherosclerotic imaging may be particularly successful when coupled with reclassification: Persons at intermediate risk are first identified by low-cost screening methods and then undergo an imaging test of an arterial bed (coronary arteries, aorta, or carotid arteries), and risk is then reclassified, depending on the results of the imaging test. As the result of such a combined imaging-global risk assessment approach, some persons would be reassigned to a higher risk group; however, it is unknown whether more aggressive risk factor modification in such persons will ultimately result in reduced morbidity or mortality from CVD.

Reclassification strategies may have their greatest utility as a follow-up to sensitive, lower cost, but not highly specific screening strategies such as CHD risk algorithms that are currently in place. Such strategies have not yet been worked out but are likely to be considered in the next round of recommendations for screening and follow-up, especially in situations for which risk algorithms are already in place and atherosclerotic imaging or other specialized laboratory testing is available. Genetic information can potentially be used to develop an estimate of CHD risk, and some investigators have undertaken analyses with this approach.[58] It is likely that this method will achieve greater efficacy when the genetic information is coupled with clinically useful information such as blood pressure and lipid levels.

SUMMARY

Observational studies have provided the richest source of information to develop estimation of CHD and CVD risk. Most risk estimation has been derived from an era when aggressive treatment of risk factors was not common. Treatment of risk factors with lipid and blood pressure medications will complicate risk estimation in the future. Follow-up intervals of 5 to 15 years are typical in the development of CHD and CVD risk-estimating equations, and a 10-year interval is commonly used for reporting. Future strategies may incorporate longer term and lifetime risk estimates.

Age	
Years	**Points**
≤ 71	-1
72-75	0
76-78	1
≥ 79	2

Coronary Artery Disease	
Status	**Points**
No	0
Possible	2
Definite	5

LV Hypertrophy	
Status	**Points**
No	0
Yes	2

Systolic Blood Pressure	
mm Hg	**Points**
≤ 90	-4
95–100	-3
105–115	-2
120–125	-1
130–140	0
145–150	1
155–165	2
170–175	3
180–190	4
195–200	5
> 200	6

Heart Rate	
Bpm	**Points**
≤ 50	-2
55–60	-1
65–70	0
75–80	1
85–90	2
≥ 95	3

Smoking	
Status	**Points**
Never	0
Past	1
Current	4

Albumin	
g/dL	**Points**
≥ 4.8	-3
4.5–4.7	-2
4.2–4.4	-1
3.9–4.1	0
3.6–3.8	1
3.3–3.5	2
≤ 3.2	3

Fasting Glucose	
Mg/dL	**Points**
≤ 80	-1
85–125	0
130–170	1
175–220	2
225–265	3
≥ 270	5

Creatinine	
mg/dL	**Points**
≤ 0.7	-2
0.8–0.9	-1
1.0–1.1	0
1.2–1.4	1
1.5–1.8	2
1.9–2.3	3
> 2.3	6

Key:
Systolic BP to nearest 5 mm Hg
Heart Rate to nearest 5 bpm
Albumin to nearest 0.1 g/dL
Glucose to nearest 5 mg/dL
Creatinin to nearest 0.1 mg/dL

Health ABC HF Risk Score	HF Risk Group	5-yr HF Risk
≤ 2 Points	Low	< 5%
3-5 Points	Average	5-10%
6-9 Points	High	10-20%
≥ 10 Points	Very high	> 20%

FIGURE 3-8 Risk of heart failure (HF) over 5 years in Health, Aging, and Body Composition (Health ABC) participants. BP, blood pressure; bpm, beats per minute; LV, left ventricular. *(From Butler J, Kalogeropoulos A, Georgiopoulou V, et al: Incident heart failure prediction in the elderly: the Health ABC Heart Failure score.* Circ Heart Fail *1:125-133, 2008.)*

| TABLE 3–2 | Risk of Coronary Artery Disease Event, Stroke, or Cerebrovascular Disease Death in Women with Existing Coronary Artery Disease |

Age*	Points	Total-C (mg/dL)*	Points by HDL-C (mg/dL)									SBP (mm Hg)	Points
			25	30	35	40	45	50	60	70	80		
35	0	160	4	3	3	2	2	1	1	0	0	100	0
40	1	170	4	3	3	2	2	2	1	1	0	110	0
45	2	180	4	3	3	2	2	2	1	1	0	120	1
50	3	190	4	4	3	3	2	2	1	1	1	130	1
55	4	200	4	4	3	3	2	2	2	1	1	140	2
60	5	210	4	4	3	3	3	2	2	1	1	150	2
65	6	220	5	4	4	3	3	2	2	1	1	160	2
70	7	230	5	4	4	3	3	3	2	2	1	170	3
75	7	240	5	4	4	3	3	3	2	2	1	180	3
		250	5	4	4	4	3	3	2	2	1	190	3
		260	5	5	4	4	3	3	2	2	1	200	3
		270	5	5	4	4	3	3	2	2	2	210	4
Other		280	5	5	4	4	3	3	3	2	2	220	4
Diabetes	3	290	5	5	4	4	4	3	3	2	2	230	4
Smoking	3	300	6	5	4	4	4	3	3	2	2	240	4
												250	4

TABLE 3–2	Risk of Coronary Artery Disease Event, Stroke, or Cerebrovascular Disease Death in Women with Existing Coronary Artery Disease—cont'd

		Average 2-Year Risk in Women with CVD	
Total Points	2-Year Probability (%)	Age (Years)	Probability (%)
0	0	35-39	<1
2	1	40-44	<1
4	1	45-49	<1
6	1	50-54	4
8	2	55-59	6
10	4	60-64	8
12	6	65-69	12
14	10	70-74	12
16	15		
18	23		
20	35		
22	51		
24	68		
26	85		

*The points assigned to specific ages are to the right of the Age column. The points assigned to Total-C are to the left of the Total-C column.

CVD, cardiovascular disease; HDL-C, high-density lipoprotein cholesterol; SBP, systolic blood pressure; Total-C, total cholesterol.

From Califf RM, Armstrong PW, Carver JR, et al: 27th Bethesda Conference: matching the intensity of risk factor management with the hazard for coronary disease events. Task Force 5. Stratification of patients into high, medium and low risk subgroups for purposes of risk factor management. *J Am Coll Cardiol* 27:1007-1019, 1996, with permission.

TABLE 3–3	Risk of Coronary Artery Disease Event, Stroke, or Cerebrovascular Disease Death in Men with Existing Coronary Artery Disease

						Points by HDL-C (mg/dL)							
Age*	Points	Total-C (mg/dL)*	25	30	35	40	45	50	60	70	80	SBP (mm Hg)	Points
35	0	160	6	5	4	4	3	2	1	1	0	100	0
40	1	170	6	5	5	4	3	3	2	1	0	110	1
45	1	180	7	6	5	4	4	3	2	1	1	120	1
50	2	190	7	6	5	4	4	3	2	2	1	130	2
55	2	200	7	6	5	5	4	4	3	2	1	140	2
60	3	210	7	6	6	5	4	4	3	2	1	150	3
65	3	220	8	7	6	5	5	4	3	2	2	160	3
70	4	230	8	7	6	5	5	4	3	3	2	170	4
75	4	240	8	7	6	6	5	4	4	3	2	180	4
		250	8	7	6	6	5	5	4	3	2	190	4
		260	8	7	7	6	5	5	4	3	2	200	5
		270	9	8	7	6	6	5	4	3	3	210	5
Other points		280	9	8	7	6	6	5	4	4	3	220	5
Diabetes	1	290	9	8	7	7	6	5	4	4	3	230	6
		300	9	8	7	7	6	6	5	4	3	240	6
												250	6

Continued

TABLE 3–3	Risk of Coronary Artery Disease Event, Stroke, or Cerebrovascular Disease Death in Men with Existing Coronary Artery Disease—cont'd

Total Points	2-Year Probability (%)	Average 2-Year Risk in Men with CVD	
		Age (Years)	Probability (%)
0	2	35-39	<1
2	2	40-44	8
4	3	45-49	10
6	5	50-54	11
8	7	55-59	12
10	10	60-64	12
12	14	65-69	14
14	20	70-74	14
16	28		
18	37		
20	49		
22	63		
24	77		

*The points assigned to specific ages are to the right of the Age column. The points assigned to Total-C are to the left of the Total-C column.

CVD, cardiovascular disease; HDL-C, high-density-lipoprotein cholesterol; SBP, systolic blood pressure; Total-C, total cholesterol.

From Califf RM, Armstrong PW, Carver JR, et al: 27th Bethesda Conference: matching the intensity of risk factor management with the hazard for coronary disease events. Task Force 5. Stratification of patients into high, medium and low risk subgroups for purposes of risk factor management. *J Am Coll Cardiol* 27:1007-1019, 1996, with permission.

TABLE 3–4	Risk of Mortality at 1 Year: Clinical History Variables

1. Find points for each risk factor:

Age (Years)	Points	Angina: Pain Type	Points	Comorbid Factor	Points*
20	0	Nonanginal pain	3	Cerebrovascular disease	20
30	13	Atypical angina	25	PVD	23
40	25	Typical angina		Diabetes	20
50	38	Stable	41	Prior MI	17
60	50	Progressive	46	Hypertension	8
70	62	Unstable	51	Mitral regurgitation	
80	75			Mild	19
90	88			Severe	38
100	100				

2. Sum points for all risk factors:

Age + pain score + comorbidity = point total

3. Look up risk corresponding to point total:

Total Points	Probability of 1-Year Death	Total Points	Probability of 1-Year Death
84	1%	184	20%
106	2%	199	30%
120	3%	211	40%
136	5%	220	50%
160	10%	229	60%

*Zero points for each "no."

MI, myocardial infarction; PVD, peripheral vascular disease.

From Califf RM, Armstrong PW, Carver JR, et al: 27th Bethesda Conference: matching the intensity of risk factor management with the hazard for coronary disease events. Task Force 5. Stratification of patients into high, medium and low risk subgroups for purposes of risk factor management. *J Am Coll Cardiol* 27:1007-1019, 1996, with permission.

Performance criteria for risk estimation include discrimination, calibration, and reclassification. These methods provide information concerning the usefulness of the prediction equation to distinguish future cases from noncases, allows evaluation on how well the risk-estimating equation might work in other regions, and can help to provide a context for the evaluation of risk factors that arise in particular people.

REFERENCES

1. Wilson PW, D'Agostino RB, Levy D, et al: Prediction of coronary heart disease using risk factor categories. *Circulation* 97:1837-1847, 1998.
2. Assmann G, Cullen P, Schulte H: Simple scoring scheme for calculating the risk of acute coronary events based on the 10-year follow-up of the Prospective Cardiovascular Munster (PROCAM) study. *Circulation* 105(3):310-315, 2002.
3. Ferrario M, Chiodini P, Chambless LE, et al: Prediction of coronary events in a low incidence population. Assessing accuracy of the CUORE Cohort Study prediction equation. *Int J Epidemiol* 34:413-421, 2005.
4. Conroy RM, Pyorala K, Fitzgerald AP, et al: Estimation of ten-year risk of fatal cardiovascular disease in Europe: the SCORE project. *Eur Heart J* 24:987-1003, 2003.
5. Murabito JM, D'Agostino RB, Silbershatz H, et al: Intermittent claudication: a risk profile from the Framingham Heart Study. *Circulation* 96:44-449, 1997.
6. Wolf PA, D'Agostino RB, Belanger AJ, et al: Probability of stroke: a risk profile from the Framingham study. *Stroke* 3:312-318, 1991.
7. Kannel WB, D'Agostino RB, Silbershatz H, et al: Profile for estimating risk of heart failure. *Arch Intern Med* 159:1197-1204, 1999.
8. Walker SH, Duncan DB: Estimation of the probability of an event as a function of several independent variables. *Biometrika* 54:167-179, 1967.
9. Truett J, Cornfield J, Kannel WB: A multivariate analysis of risk of coronary heart disease in Framingham. *J Chron Dis* 20:511-524, 1967.
10. Schlesselman JJ: *Case-control studies*, ed 1, New York, 1982, Oxford University Press.
11. Chobanian AV, Bakris GL, Black HR, et al: The seventh report of the Joint National Committee on Prevention, Detection, Evaluation, and Treatment of High Blood Pressure: the JNC 7 report. *JAMA* 289:2560-2572, 2003.
12. Lipid Research Clinics Population Studies: *Data book: volume 1. The prevalence study 1980 (NIH Publication No. 80-1527)*. Bethesda, Md, 1990, National Institutes of Health.
13. Lipid Research Clinics Program. *Manual of laboratory operation*, ed 1, Bethesda, Md, 1974, National Institutes of Health.
14. Rifkind BM, Segal P: Lipid Research Clinics Program reference values for hyperlipidemia and hypolipidemia. *JAMA* 250:1869-1872, 1983.
15. Warnick GR, Myers GL, Cooper GR, et al: Impact of the third cholesterol report from the Adult Treatment Panel of the National Cholesterol Education Program on the Clinical Laboratory. *Clin Chem* 48(1):11-17, 2002.
16. McNamara JR, Leary ET, Ceriotti F, et al: Point: status of lipid and lipoprotein standardization. *Clin Chem* 43(8 Pt 1):1306-1310, 1997.
17. Myers GL, Cooper GR, Sampson EJ: Traditional lipoprotein profile: clinical utility, performance requirement, and standardization. *Atherosclerosis* 108(Suppl):S157-S169, 1994.
18. Cooper GR, Myers GL, Smith J, et al: Blood lipid measurements: variations and practical utility. *JAMA* 267:1652-1660, 1992.
19. Cooper GR, Smith SJ, Myers GL, et al: Estimating and minimizing effects of biologic sources of variation by relative range when measuring the mean of serum lipids and lipoproteins. *Clin Chem* 40:227-232, 1994.
20. National Diabetes Data Group: Classification and diagnosis of diabetes mellitus and other categories of glucose intolerance. *Diabetes* 28:1039-1057, 1979.
21. Report of the Expert Committee on the Diagnosis and Classification of Diabetes Mellitus. *Diabetes Care* 20:1183-1197, 1997.
22. Kannel WB, Castelli WP, Gordon T, et al: Serum cholesterol, lipoproteins, and the risk of coronary heart disease: the Framingham study. *Ann Intern Med* 74:1-12, 1971.
23. Wilson PWF, Castelli WP, Kannel WB: Coronary risk prediction in adults: the Framingham Heart Study. *Am J Cardiol* 59(G):91-94, 1987.
24. Anderson KM, Wilson PWF, Odell PM, et al: An updated coronary risk profile. A statement for health professionals. *Circulation* 83:357-363, 1991.
25. Anderson KM, Odell PM, Wilson PWF, et al: Cardiovascular disease risk profiles. *Am Heart J* 121:293-298, 1991.
26. National High Blood Pressure Education Program: The 1988 report of the Joint National Committee on Detection, Evaluation, and Treatment of High Blood Pressure. *Arch Intern Med* 148:1023-1038, 1988.
27. Joint National Committee: The fifth report of the Joint National Committee on Detection, Evaluation, and Treatment of High Blood Pressure (JNC V). *Arch Intern Med* 153:154-183, 1993.
28. D'Agostino RB Sr, Grundy S, Sullivan LM, et al: Validation of the Framingham coronary heart disease prediction scores: results of a multiple ethnic groups investigation. *JAMA* 286:180-187, 2001.
29. Grundy SM, D'Agostino RB Sr, Mosca L, et al: Cardiovascular risk assessment based on US cohort studies: findings from a National Heart, Lung and Blood Institute workshop. *Circulation* 104:491-496, 2001.
30. Cox DR: Regression models and life tables. *J R Stat Soc Ser B* 34:187-220, 1972.
31. Executive summary of the third report of the National Cholesterol Education Program (NCEP) Expert Panel on Detection, Evaluation, and Treatment of High Blood Cholesterol in Adults (Adult Treatment Panel III). *JAMA* 285:2486-2497, 2001.
32. Bulugahapitiya U, Siyambalapitiya S, Sithole J, et al: Is diabetes a coronary risk equivalent? Systematic review and meta-analysis. *Diabet Med* 26:142-148, 2009.
33. Pencina MJ, D'Agostino RB: Overall C as a measure of discrimination in survival analysis: model specific population value and confidence interval estimation. *Stat Med* 23:2109-2123, 2004.
34. D'Agostino RB Sr, Nam BH: Evaluation of the performance of survival analysis models: discrimination and calibration measures. In Balakrishnan N, Rao CR, editors: *Handbook of statistics, volume 23: advances in survival analysis*, ed 1, Amsterdam, 2004, Elsevier, pp 1-26.
35. Liu J, Hong Y, D'Agostino RB Sr, et al: Predictive value for the Chinese population of the Framingham CHD risk assessment tool compared with the Chinese Multi-Provincial Cohort Study. *JAMA* 291(21):2591-2599, 2004.
36. Diamond GA, Hirsch M, Forrester JS, et al: Application of information theory to clinical diagnostic testing. The electrocardiographic stress test. *Circulation* 63:915-921, 1981.
37. Wilson PW, Nam BH, Pencina M, et al: C-reactive protein and risk of cardiovascular disease in men and women from the Framingham Heart Study. *Arch Intern Med* 165:2473-2478, 2005.
38. Cook NR, Buring JE, Ridker PM: The effect of including C-reactive protein in cardiovascular risk prediction models for women. *Ann Intern Med* 145:21-29, 2006.
39. Pepe MS, Thompson ML: Combining diagnostic test results to increase accuracy. *Biostatistics* 1:123-140, 2000.
40. Pepe MS, Janes H, Longton G, et al: Limitations of the odds ratio in gauging the performance of a diagnostic, prognostic, or screening marker. *Am J Epidemiol* 159:882-890, 2004.
41. Pencina MJ, D'Agostino RB Sr, D'Agostino RB Jr, et al: Evaluating the added predictive ability of a new marker: from area under the ROC curve to reclassification and beyond. *Stat Med* 27:157-172, 2008.
42. Stevens RJ, Kothari V, Adler AI, et al: The UKPDS risk engine: a model for the risk of coronary heart disease in type II diabetes (UKPDS 56). *Clin Sci (Lond)* 101:671-679, 2001.
43. Hippisley-Cox J, Coupland C, Vinogradova Y, et al: Derivation and validation of QRISK, a new cardiovascular disease risk score for the United Kingdom: prospective open cohort study. *BMJ* 335:136, 2007.
44. Woodward M, Brindle P, Tunstall-Pedoe H: Adding social deprivation and family history to cardiovascular risk assessment: the ASSIGN score from the Scottish Heart Health Extended Cohort (SHHEC). *Heart* 93:172-176, 2007.
45. Kalogeropoulos A, Georgiopoulou V, Kritchevsky SB, et al: Epidemiology of incident heart failure in a contemporary elderly cohort: the Health, Aging, and Body Composition study. *Arch Intern Med* 169:708-715, 2009.
46. Butler J, Kalogeropoulos A, Georgiopoulou V, et al: Incident heart failure prediction in the elderly: the Health ABC Heart Failure score. *Circ Heart Fail* 1:125-133, 2008.
47. D'Agostino RB, Russell MW, Huse DM, et al: Primary and subsequent coronary risk appraisal: new results from the Framingham study. *Am Heart J* 139:272-281, 2000.
48. Califf RM, Armstrong PW, Carver JR, et al: 27th Bethesda Conference: matching the intensity of risk factor management with the hazard for coronary disease events. Task Force 5. Stratification of patients into high, medium and low risk subgroups for purposes of risk factor management. *J Am Coll Cardiol* 27:1007-1019, 1996.
49. Pearson TA, Mensah GA, Alexander RW, et al: Markers of inflammation and cardiovascular disease: application to clinical and public health practice: a statement for healthcare professionals from the Centers for Disease Control and Prevention and the American Heart Association. *Circulation* 107:499-511, 2003.
50. Salazar HP, Raggi P: Usefulness of electron-beam computed tomography. *Am J Cardiol* 89(4A):17B-22B, 2002.
51. Quyyumi AA: Prognostic value of endothelial function. *Am J Cardiol* 91(12A):19H-24H, 2003.
52. Wong ND, Cupples LA, Ostfeld AM, et al: Risk factors for long-term coronary prognosis after initial myocardial infarction: the Framingham study. *Am J Epidemiol* 130:469-480, 1989.
53. Dankner R, Goldbourt U, Boyko V, et al: Predictors of cardiac and noncardiac mortality among 14,697 patients with coronary heart disease. *Am J Cardiol* 91:121-127, 2003.
54. D'Agostino RB Sr, Vasan RS, Pencina MJ, et al: General cardiovascular risk profile for use in primary care: the Framingham Heart Study. *Circulation* 117:743-753, 2008.
55. Eagle KA, Lim MJ, Dabbous OH, et al: A validated prediction model for all forms of acute coronary syndrome: estimating the risk of 6-month postdischarge death in an international registry. *JAMA* 291:2727-2733, 2004.
56. Mainous AG III, Koopman RJ, Diaz VA, et al: A coronary heart disease risk score based on patient-reported information. *Am J Cardiol* 99:1236-1241, 2007.
57. Gaziano TA, Young CR, Fitzmaurice G, et al: Laboratory-based versus non–laboratory-based method for assessment of cardiovascular disease risk: the NHANES I Follow-up Study cohort. *Lancet* 371:923-931, 2008.
58. Detrano R, Guerci AD, Carr JJ, et al: Coronary calcium as a predictor of coronary events in four racial or ethnic groups. *N Engl J Med* 358:1336-1345, 2008.
59. Humphries SE, Yiannakouris N, Talmud PJ: Cardiovascular disease risk prediction using genetic information (gene scores): is it really informative? *Curr Opin Lipidol* 19:128-132, 2008.

CHAPTER 4

Genetics of Cardiovascular Disease and Its Role in Risk Prediction

Kiran Musunuru and Sekar Kathiresan

HERITABILITY OF CARDIOVASCULAR DISEASE

Coronary heart disease (CHD) and myocardial infarction (MI) are among the leading causes of death and infirmity worldwide. Traditional risk factors for MI include age, blood lipid concentrations, blood pressure, diabetes mellitus, and tobacco use. Family history is also an important risk factor for MI; individuals in the offspring cohort of the Framingham Heart Study who had at least one parent with early-onset cardiovascular disease (age at onset <55 in men and <65 in women) had a more than twofold increase in age-adjusted risk of suffering a cardiovascular event in comparison with individuals with no such family history.[1] This increase in risk persisted even after adjustment for multiple traditional risk factors, which implies a genetic basis for the increased risk. Early-onset MI appears to be particularly heritable,[2] which is suggestive of the importance of inherited risk factors for early manifestation of the disease, as opposed to "acquired" risk factors, such as age and tobacco use, that predispose to MI later in life.

Some of the heritability of MI can be attributed to heritability of various MI risk factors. As much as half of the interindividual variability in blood lipid concentrations—low-density lipoprotein cholesterol (LDL-C), high-density lipoprotein cholesterol (HDL-C), and triglycerides—appears to result from inherited factors.[3-6] Blood pressure[7,8] and type 2 diabetes mellitus[9] also appear to have substantial heritability.

The evidence for strong heritable components of MI and some of its risk factors has motivated the search for genetic loci that account for this heritability. In principle, investigation of all of the underlying genetic loci enable researchers to quantify the level of inherited risk for each individual, which should greatly improve cardiovascular risk prediction. With the completion of the Human Genome Project and International Haplotype Map Project,[10,11] it has become possible to perform large-scale genome-wide screens of common DNA sequence variants for association with phenotypes of interest; this approach is termed *genome-wide association* (GWA).[12] Successful GWA studies have been performed for many clinical traits and diseases, including cardiovascular disease.[13]

This chapter focuses primarily on GWA studies and the clinical implications of their results. A large body of work on the genetics of myocardial infarction and cardiovascular risk factors—which preceded the advent of the GWA approach and in which approaches such as linkage analyses and candidate gene studies were used—is summarized in Chapter 8.

GENOME-WIDE ASSOCIATION STUDIES

GWA studies are designed to detect common DNA variants—those distributed widely in a given population, in contrast to rare mutations that exist in only a few individuals—that are associated with traits or diseases. For each of the traits and diseases that have been shown to be at least partly heritable, it is presumed that there are specific "causal" DNA variants that affect gene function and thereby contribute to the phenotype. Other common DNA variants that are noncausal but are located very close to a causal DNA variant "mark" the latter; variants that are in close proximity on a chromosome often remain linked to one another through many human generations, rather than becoming uncorrelated by the effects of homologous recombination that occurs during meiosis. In principle, in European populations, it is possible to cover the entire genome and detect any common causal DNA variants with about 500,000 "marker" DNA variants.[14] (This number varies among ethnic groups because of differences in correlation structure among DNA variants in distinct ancestral populations.)

Thus, GWA studies have been made possible by the cataloging of more than 3 million single-nucleotide polymorphisms (SNPs) in the human genome.[11] In GWA studies, hundreds of thousands of SNPs are interrogated by genotyping arrays, and the variants at these SNPs are determined (a typical SNP has two possible variant alleles). This genome-wide genotyping is performed for thousands of individuals. For diseases, the study includes individuals with the disease and healthy control individuals; for quantitative traits such as blood lipid concentrations, the study cohort comprises people representing the full range of values for the trait.

Statistical analyses are performed to determine whether variants at any of the SNPs are associated with disease status or changes (higher or lower) in the quantitative trait. Because hundreds of thousands of SNPs are being used, each of which can be regarded as a unique statistical experiment, a corrected P value threshold of 5×10^{-8} (rather than the usual 0.05) is used to determine statistical significance. Any SNP meeting this stringent criterion (an "index" SNP on a chromosomal locus) is considered to be associated with the phenotype, although causality cannot be inferred because the SNP may simply be a marker for a nearby causal DNA variant.

Genome-wide Association Studies of Blood Lipid Concentrations

In the first reported GWA study for blood lipid concentrations, the investigators used data from nearly 3000 individuals in the Diabetes Genetics Initiative. This initial study identified SNPs in three loci at genome-wide significance ($P < 5 \times 10^{-8}$), one for each of the three lipid traits: LDL-C, HDL-C, and triglyceride levels.[15] The index SNP for LDL-C was near the *APOE* gene (which encodes the apolipoprotein E protein, a component responsible for cellular uptake of large lipoprotein particles such as chylomicrons and very low-density lipoproteins), and the index SNP for HDL-C was near the *CETP* gene (which encodes the cholesteryl ester transfer protein, a component responsible for facilitating the transfer of cholesteryl esters from HDL to other lipoproteins). Thus, this first GWA study provided internal validation of the technique by mapping common DNA variants in known lipid regulators.

In addition, the GWA study identified a triglyceride level–associated locus that harbored no genes previously known to be involved in lipoprotein metabolism. The index SNP for triglycerides was in an intron of *GCKR* (which encodes glucokinase regulatory protein), and results of subsequent analyses suggested that a coding missense variant (i.e., an alteration of a single amino acid) is responsible for the association with triglyceride levels.[16,17]

Data from a second set of lipid GWA studies built upon data from the first; the Finland–United States Investigation of NIDDM Genetics (FUSION) study and the SardiNIA Project, added to the Diabetes Genetics Initiative, included a total of almost 9000 individuals.[18,19] In order to increase the power to detect statistically significant ($P < 5 \times 10^{-8}$) associations, the top-scoring SNPs in the initial 9000 participants were genotyped in more than 18,000 additional individuals from other cohorts. This staged approach revealed a total of 19 loci associated with one or more of the three lipid traits. In addition to the three loci already identified, these studies revealed loci containing well-characterized lipid regulators, including *APOB* (apolipoprotein B), *APOAI* (apolipoprotein A-I), *LDLR* (LDL receptor), *PCSK9* (proprotein convertase subtilisin/kexin type 9), *LPL* (lipoprotein lipase), and *HMGCR* (3-hydroxy-3-methylglutaryl–coenzyme A reductase). The last is of particular note because it is the drug target of the widely used statin class of LDL-C–lowering medications. These studies also identified six novel loci whose causal genes have yet to be characterized. Two of these novel loci were confirmed in simultaneously published, independent GWA studies on LDL-C (on chromosome 1p13) and triglyceride levels (on chromosome 7q11).[20-22]

In a third wave of even larger GWA studies, genotyping was performed in up to 40,000 individuals from various prospective cohort studies, case-control studies (for conditions

such as diabetes and coronary disease), and family-based studies. These studies identified more than 30 lipid-associated loci, of which about half harbor established lipid regulators (Table 4-1).[23-25] A notable finding of these studies is that genes in 11 of the loci are known to harbor rare mutations that cause monogenic (mendelian) lipid disorders, such as familial hypercholesterolemia (see Table 4-1). These rare mutations have large effects on gene function, which leads to a phenotype (such as premature MI) that comes to clinical attention.

One lesson from the GWA studies is that the same genes that cause mendelian disorders also have common variants that have more subtle effects on gene function and lead to small changes in lipid levels. GWA studies have been criticized for the ability only to discover common variants that have little clinical importance; however, a GWA-identified gene can prove to be highly clinically relevant if the gene's activity is modulated by a large degree, either by virtue of a naturally occurring rare mutation in an individual or in a family or by deliberate targeting of the gene by a pharmacologic agent. A case in point is *HMGCR:* If statins had not been discovered before the GWA era, the finding that common variants in *HMGCR* lead to modest changes in LDL-C would have suggested inhibition of 3-hydroxy-3-methylglutaryl–coenzyme A reductase as a potential new therapeutic strategy. By this reasoning, some of the more than 15 novel GWA loci discovered to date may harbor clinically useful drug targets and, thus, merit functional investigation.

Increasingly larger GWA studies with more than 100,000 participants of European descent (e.g., by the Global Lipids Genetics Consortium), as well as GWA studies in other ethnic groups (e.g., African Americans in the National Heart, Lung, and Blood Institute Candidate Gene Association Resource [NHLBI CARe]), are expected to uncover dozens more novel loci for which functional investigation will show numerous causal genes that will greatly enhance the understanding of lipoprotein metabolism and perhaps eventually lead to the development of new lipid-modifying medications.

Genome-wide Association Studies of Other Risk Factors for Myocardial Infarction

GWA studies have been performed for a number of cardiovascular risk factors besides blood lipid concentrations. Studies on blood pressure have identified more than a dozen loci with common DNA variants that are associated significantly ($P < 5 \times 10^{-8}$) with systolic blood pressure or diastolic blood pressure (Table 4-2).[26,27] However, the effects of each SNP on blood pressure are quite small, in no case exceeding 1–mm Hg change per allele (see Table 4-2), and in most cases, potential functional links between the genes in each locus and the phenotype remain obscure.

One interesting exception is the chromosome 1p36 locus, which harbors five different genes with credible connections to blood pressure and cardiovascular disease: *MHFTR,* which encodes methylenetetrahydrofolate reductase, a catalyst in a critical step in homocysteine metabolism; *CLCN6,* which encodes a chloride channel; *NPPA* and *NPPB,* which encode atrial natriuretic peptide and B-type natriuretic peptide, respectively, which have vasodilatory effects; and *AGTRAP,* which encodes angiotensin II receptor–associated protein, a modulator of the renin-angiotensin-aldosterone axis. Although common DNA variants directly within the *NPPA* and *NPPB* genes have also been demonstrated to be highly associated with blood pressure,[28] it is difficult to know which of the five 1p36 genes (or combination of genes) exerts the effect on blood pressure detected by the GWA study; this lack of information highlights the general challenge that will be faced repeatedly by investigators seeking

TABLE 4–1 | **Loci Associated with Blood Lipid Concentrations**

Unique Locus	Trait	Chr	SNP	Sample Size	P Value	Gene(s) of Interest within or near Associated Interval	Associated Mendelian Lipid Disorder
1	LDL	1p13	rs12740374	19,648	2×10^{-42}	CELSR2-PSRC1-SORT1	—
2	LDL	2p24	rs515135	19,648	5×10^{-29}	APOB	Familial hypercholesterolemia
3	LDL	19q13	rs4420638	11,881	4×10^{-27}	APOE-APOC1-APOC4-APOC2	Type III hyperlipoproteinemia
4	LDL	19p13	rs6511720	19,648	2×10^{-26}	LDLR	Familial hypercholesterolemia
5	LDL	2p21	rs6544713	23,456	2×10^{-20}	ABCG5-ABCG8	Sitosterolemia
6	LDL	5q13	rs3846663	19,648	8×10^{-12}	HMGCR	—
7	LDL	5q23	rs1501908	27,280	1×10^{-11}	TIMD4-HAVCR1	—
8	LDL	20q12	rs6102059	28,895	4×10^{-9}	MAFB	—
9	LDL	7p15	rs12670798	17,797	6×10^{-9}	DNAH11	—
10	LDL	12q24	rs2650000	39,340	2×10^{-8}	HNF1A	—
11	LDL	1p32	rs11206510	19,629	4×10^{-8}	PCSK9	Familial hypercholesterolemia
12	HDL	16q13	rs1532624	21,412	9×10^{-94}	CETP	CETP deficiency
13	HDL	15q22	rs1532085	21,412	1×10^{-35}	LIPC	Hepatic lipase deficiency
14	HDL	16q22	rs2271293	21,412	8×10^{-16}	CTCF-PRMT8-LCAT	LCAT deficiency
15	HDL	18q21	rs4939883	19,785	7×10^{-15}	LIPG	—
16	HDL	9q31	rs3905000	21,412	9×10^{-13}	ABCA1	Tangier disease
17	HDL	11p11	rs7395662	21,412	6×10^{-11}	MADD-FOLH1	—
18	HDL	9p22	rs471364	40,414	3×10^{-10}	TTC39B	—
19	HDL	20q13	rs1800961	30,714	8×10^{-10}	HNF4A	—
20	HDL	12q24	rs2338104	19,793	1×10^{-10}	MMAB-MVK	—
21	HDL	19p13	rs2967605	35,151	1×10^{-8}	ANGPTL4	—
22	HDL	1q42	rs4846914	19,794	4×10^{-8}	GALNT2	—
23	TG	11q23	rs964184	19,840	4×10^{-62}	APOA1-APOC3-APOA4-APOA5	Primary hypoalphalipoproteinemia
24	TG	8p21	rs12678919	19,840	2×10^{-41}	LPL	Familial hyperchylomicronemia
25	TG	2p23	rs1260326	19,840	2×10^{-31}	GCKR	—
26	TG	8q24	rs2954029	19,840	3×10^{-19}	TRIB1	—
27	TG	7q11	rs714052	19,840	3×10^{-15}	MLXIPL	—
28	TG	11q12	rs174547	38,846	2×10^{-14}	FADS1-FADS2-FADS3	—
29	TG	1p31	rs1167998	17,815	2×10^{-12}	DOCK7-ANGPTL3	—
30	TG	19p13	rs17216525	19,840	4×10^{-11}	NCAN-CILP2-PBX4	—
31	TG	20q13	rs7679	38,561	7×10^{-11}	PLTP	—
32	TG	8p23	rs7819412	33,336	3×10^{-8}	XKR6-AMAC1L2	—

CETP, cholesteryl ester transfer protein; Chr, chromosome locus; HDL, high-density lipoprotein; LCAT, lecithin-cholesterol acyltransferase; LDL, low-density lipoprotein; SNP, single-nucleotide polymorphism; TG, triglycerides.

Data from Kathiresan S, Willer CJ, Peloso GM, et al: Common variants at 30 loci contribute to polygenic dyslipidemia, *Nat Genet* 41:56-65, 2009; and from Aulchenko YS, Ripatti S, Lindqvist I, et al: Loci influencing lipid levels and coronary heart disease risk in 16 European population cohorts, *Nat Genet* 41:47-55, 2009.

to understand the functional effects of GWA loci with multiple genes.

Type 2 diabetes mellitus is one of the most exhaustively studied phenotypes, having been analyzed in several successive phases of GWA studies of increasingly large size; to date, more than 20 genome-wide significantly associated loci have been identified.[29-34] Many of these loci harbor genes that appear to alter insulin processing and secretion by the pancreatic beta cell. For example, *TCF7L2* (transcription factor 7–like 2), the gene in the GWA locus most strongly associated with type 2 diabetes, encodes a transcription factor that interacts with the Wnt signaling pathway and regulates proglucagon gene expression in gut endocrine cells[35]; patients with diabetes risk–conferring variants in the *TCF7L2* gene exhibit decreased levels of insulin secretion from beta cells.[36] Despite the fact that diabetes is a strong risk factor for cardiovascular disease, it remains unclear whether genes such as *TCF7L2* that have been identified in diabetes GWA studies will prove to significantly contribute to cardiovascular disease.

TABLE 4–2	Loci Associated with Blood Pressure						
Unique Locus	Chr	SNP	P Value	Change in Blood Pressure (mm Hg) per Allele (SE)	Gene(s) of Interest within or near Associated Interval	Trait
1	10q24	rs11191548	7×10^{-24}	1.16 (0.12)	CYP17A1-NT5C2	SBP
2	15q24	rs1378942	1×10^{-23}	0.43 (0.04)	CSK-ULK3	DBP
3	4q21	rs16998073	1×10^{-21}	0.50 (0.05)	FGF5	DBP
4	12q24	rs653178	3×10^{-18}	0.46 (0.05)	SH2B3-ATXN2	DBP
5	1p36	rs17367504	2×10^{-13}	0.85 (0.11)	MTHFR-CLCN6-NPPA-NPPB-AGTRAP	SBP
6	12q21	rs2681492	4×10^{-11}	0.85 (0.13)	ATP2B1	SBP
7	10q21	rs1530440	1×10^{-9}	0.39 (0.06)	C10orf107	DBP
8	11p15	rs381815	2×10^{-9}	0.65 (0.11)	PLEKHA7	SBP
9	3p22	rs9815354	3×10^{-9}	0.49 (0.08)	ULK4	DBP
10	17q21	rs16948048	5×10^{-9}	0.31 (0.05)	ZNF652	DBP
11	17q21	rs12946454	1×10^{-8}	0.57 (0.10)	PLCD3	SBP
12	10p12	rs11014166	1×10^{-8}	0.37 (0.06)	CACNB2	DBP
13	12q24	rs2384550	4×10^{-8}	0.35 (0.06)	TBX3-TBX5	DBP

Chr, chromosome locus; DBP, diastolic blood pressure; SE, standard error; SBP, systolic blood pressure; SNP, single-nucleotide polymorphism.
Data from Newton-Cheh C, Johnson T, Gateva V, et al: Genome-wide association study identifies eight loci associated with blood pressure, Nat Genet 41:666-676, 2009; and from Levy D, Ehret GB, Rice K, et al: Genome-wide association study of blood pressure and hypertension, Nat Genet 41:677-687, 2009.

Several nontraditional risk factors for cardiovascular disease have also been studied with GWA investigations. For example, C-reactive protein (CRP) and fibrinogen, two inflammatory biomarkers that are predictive of disease in prospective cohort studies, each have several loci that are significantly associated with the biomarker's blood concentration.[37-40] Not surprisingly, among the associated SNPs are variants in the CRP gene (for CRP) and in the FGB gene, which encodes fibrinogen beta chain (for fibrinogen). Also found to be associated with either of the two biomarkers were SNPs near a variety of metabolic, inflammatory, and immunity genes, which suggests that the blood biomarker levels integrate signals from multiple metabolic, inflammatory, and immune pathways.

Every clinical trait demonstrated to be associated with cardiovascular risk will probably be subjected ultimately to the GWA approach.

Genome-wide Association Studies of Myocardial Infarction and Coronary Artery Disease

Three GWA studies for coronary artery disease were published simultaneously in 2007: one from the Ottawa Heart Study,[41] one from the Icelandic company deCODE genetics,[42] and one from the Wellcome Trust Case-Control Consortium.[43] Despite using independent cohorts and different genotyping arrays, all three studies demonstrated the same novel locus on chromosome 9p21 to be associated with disease. Of particular note was the finding that genotypes of index SNPs in the 9p21 locus were not associated with any of the traditional risk factors for cardiovascular disease; this suggests that the genetic mechanism encoded in this locus operates through a previously unknown risk pathway. Furthermore, the minimally defined locus (≈58 kilobases in individuals of European descent) harbors no known genes, and so it is unclear how the causal DNA variant or variants in the locus influence phenotype. In subsequent studies, the association of the 9p21 locus with coronary artery disease and, specifically, MI has been replicated, as have a variety of other vascular phenotypes such as abdominal aortic aneurysm, intracranial aneurysm, and peripheral arterial disease; these findings are suggestive of a pathogenetic mechanism in vascular tissue.[44-46]

Besides the 9p21 locus, the study from the Wellcome Trust Case Control Consortium[43] identified SNPs in several additional loci associated with coronary artery disease at or near the statistical significance threshold of $P < 5 \times 10^{-8}$. A second set of GWA studies for either coronary artery disease or MI, each with several thousand disease cases, confirmed some of these loci and characterized several more associated loci.[45,47-49] To date, strong statistical evidence links more than a dozen loci to disease development (Table 4-3), and future GWA studies of larger size, such as those by the Coronary ARtery DIsease Genome-wide Replication And Meta-analysis (CARDIoGRAM) consortium, are likely to identify more. Several of these loci are linked to blood lipid concentrations (see Table 4-3), but the remainder are not clearly associated with any of the traditional cardiovascular risk factors or even emerging biomarkers such as CRP. Functional characterization of these loci may reveal multiple risk pathways, previously unknown, that represent new therapeutic opportunities for the prevention of MI.

IMPLICATIONS OF GENETICS FOR CAUSALITY OF RISK FACTORS

The ability to perform genetic analyses in large cohorts of individuals being monitored for incident cardiovascular events now makes it possible to probe the relationships between cardiovascular risk factors and disease. Mendelian randomization is a technique in which DNA variants are used to address the question of whether an epidemiologic association between a given risk factor and disease signifies a causal relationship between the two.[50] If a DNA variant is known to directly influence an intermediate phenotype, and the intermediate phenotype is causal for disease, then the DNA variant should be associated with the disease to the extent predicted

TABLE 4–3 | **Loci Associated with Myocardial Infarction or Coronary Artery Disease**

Unique Locus	Chr	SNP	P Value	Odds Ratio (95% CI) per Risk Allele	Gene(s) of Interest within or near Associated Interval	Associated With Lipids?
1	9p21	rs4977574	3×10^{-44}	1.29 (1.25-1.34)	CDKN2A-CDKN2B-ANRIL	No
2	1p13	rs646776	8×10^{-12}	1.19 (1.13-1.26)	CELSR2-PSRC1-SORT1	Yes
3	21q22	rs9982601	6×10^{-11}	1.20 (1.14-1.27)	SLC5A3-MRPS6-KCNE2	No
4	1q41	rs17465637	1×10^{-9}	1.14 (1.10-1.19)	MIA3	No
5	10q11	rs1746048	7×10^{-9}	1.17 (1.11-1.24)	CXCL12	No
6	6p24	rs12526453	1×10^{-9}	1.12 (1.08-1.17)	PHACTR1	No
7	19p13	rs1122608	2×10^{-9}	1.15 (1.10-1.20)	LDLR	Yes
8	2q33	rs6725887	1×10^{-8}	1.17 (1.11-1.23)	WDR12	No
9	1p32	rs11206510	1×10^{-8}	1.15 (1.10-1.21)	PCSK9	Yes
10	12q24	rs2259816	4×10^{-8}	1.08 (1.05-1.11)	HNF1A	Yes
11	12q24	rs3184504	9×10^{-8}	1.13 (1.08-1.18)	SH2B3	No
12	3q22	rs9818870	5×10^{-7}	1.15 (1.11-1.19)	MRAS	No
13	6q26-6q27	rs2048327-rs3127599-rs7767084-rs10755578 (haplotype)	4×10^{-15}	1.82 (1.57-2.12)	LPA	Yes

Chr, chromosome locus; CI, confidence interval; SNP, single-nucleotide polymorphism.

Data from Myocardial Infarction Genetics Consortium, Kathiresan S, Voight BF, et al: Genome-wide association of early-onset myocardial infarction with single nucleotide polymorphisms and copy number variants, *Nat Genet* 41:334-341, 2009; from Erdmann J, Grosshennig A, Braund PS, et al: New susceptibility locus for coronary artery disease on chromosome 3q22.3, *Nat Genet* 41:280-282, 2009; and from Tregouet DA, Konig IR, Erdmann J, et al: Genome-wide haplotype association study identifies the SLC22A3-LPAL2-LPA gene cluster as a risk locus for coronary artery disease, *Nat Genet* 41:283-285, 2009.

by (1) the effect of the DNA variant on the phenotype and (2) the effect of the phenotype on the risk of developing disease. Lack of the predicted association between the DNA variant and disease in an adequately powered sample would argue against a purely causal role for the intermediate phenotype in the pathogenesis of the disease.

This study design mimics a prospective randomized clinical trial, wherein the randomization of each individual occurs at the moment of conception: genotypes of DNA variants are "assigned" to gametes in a random manner during meiosis, a process that is assumed not to be influenced by the typical confounders observed in observational epidemiologic studies; for example, a parent's disease status or socioeconomic status should not affect which of his or her two alleles of an SNP is passed to a child, each allele having an equal (50%) chance of being transmitted via the gamete to the zygote. In other words, mendelian randomization should be unaffected by confounding or reverse causation. This technique has potential shortcomings: for example, it is only as reliable as the robustness of the estimates of the variant's effects on phenotype and effects of phenotype on disease, and the DNA variant is assumed not to influence the disease by means other than the intermediate phenotype being studied (pleiotropy), which in many cases may not be true. However, when this technique is carefully executed, the results can be as informative as those of a well-conducted randomized clinical trial.

Although no formal mendelian randomization studies of LDL-C and other lipid traits have yet been reported, studies in this vein have confirmed a causal relationship between LDL-C and cardiovascular disease. For example, nonsense coding variants in the *PCSK9* gene that were discovered in African Americans result in significantly reduced blood LDL-C concentrations; these reduced concentrations were, in turn, observed to be associated with the reduced incidence of CHD in a large African American cohort.[51,52] Similarly, a common missense coding variant in *PCSK9* in European Americans associated with lower LDL-C levels was also found to be associated with a lower risk of CHD and MI.[52,53] More recently, 11 SNPs found to be associated with LDL-C in a GWA study were reported to be associated with CHD.[54]

In contrast, three independent mendelian randomization studies of variants in the *CRP* gene that affect blood CRP concentrations, performed in thousands of individuals, did not show an association between these variants and either ischemic vascular disease or CHD.[38,55,56] Although these findings cannot definitively rule out some causal role of CRP in MI, they suggest that any such causal role is minor in comparison with the role of LDL-C. They also suggest that the cardiovascular risk reduction obtained with rosuvastatin therapy in the Justification for the Use of Statins in Primary Prevention: an Intervention Trial Evaluating Rosuvastatin (JUPITER),[57] in which patients with baseline normal LDL-C levels and elevated CRP levels were studied, resulted more from the lipid-lowering effects of the statin rather than its CRP-lowering effects.

A parallel line of evidence similarly casts doubt on the notion that inflammatory molecules such as CRP are critical mediators of cardiovascular disease. Of the 13 loci most highly associated with MI and coronary artery disease (see Table 4-3), 5 are related to blood lipid concentrations, which is strongly indicative of a causal relationship between lipid levels and disease. In contrast, none of the other 8 loci are clearly related to inflammation, which suggests that inflammatory molecules are of less pathobiologic importance to MI than are lipid levels or, for that matter, to the as-of-yet-uncharacterized risk mechanisms represented by the 8 non–lipid-related loci. This observation cannot be attributed to a bias of GWA studies against inflammatory gene SNPs, inasmuch as classical inflammatory diseases such as rheumatoid arthritis and Crohn disease have been found to be associated with numerous inflammatory gene SNPs at genome-wide significance.[58,59]

Thus, although inflammation may contribute to the pathogenesis of MI, results of research with the currently available genetic techniques suggest that, on a population-wide basis, inflammation is of modest causal importance in comparison with other risk factors such as LDL-C.

UTILITY OF GENETIC RISK SCORES FOR DISEASE PREDICTION

Conventional cardiovascular risk algorithms such as the Framingham risk score, which includes several traditional risk factors and is generally limited to 10-year predictions, do not yield accurate predictions about many cardiovascular events. Much energy in the field of preventive cardiology has been directed toward identification of novel risk factors that, when combined with conventional risk algorithms, will enable more accurate predictions of who will develop disease. In view of the partial heritability of cardiovascular disease, there is considerable interest in determining whether the use of genetic data will improve risk prediction.

A genetic risk score (ranging from 0 to 18) that accounts for nine SNPs associated with either LDL-C or HDL-C was found to be correlated with incidental cardiovascular disease in a prospective cohort study[60]; each unfavorable allele (a single point in the score) conferred a 15% increase in risk after adjustment for traditional risk factors, including blood lipid concentrations. When stratified into groups with a high risk score or a low risk score, individuals with a high risk score were found to have an actual 63% increase in risk in comparison with those with a low risk score.

The association of the lipid genetic risk score with disease that was independent of blood lipid concentrations was attributed to the genetic risk score reflecting lifetime exposure to higher or lower lipid levels, whereas a single fasting lipid profile represents a snapshot of a patient's condition at the time the profile is measured. It is also possible that some of the lipid-associated SNPs have pleiotropic effects that contribute to cardiovascular disease but are not reflected in traditional risk factor measurements.

Addition of the genotype score to traditional risk factors did not significantly improve risk discrimination; no change was found in the C-statistic (area under the receiver operator characteristic curve). Nonetheless, modest numbers of individuals at intermediate cardiovascular risk, as judged by the Adult Treatment Panel III criteria, were correctly reclassified into a higher or lower risk category. Of note was that all of the lipid SNPs used in this genetic risk score predated the GWA studies reported since 2007; thus, the genetic risk score does not include dozens of SNPs now known to be associated with lipid levels. Those SNPs may be expected to significantly improve the predictive value of the risk score.

A comprehensive genetic risk score would include SNPs that are not associated with traditional risk factors—such as index SNPs in the chromosome 9p21 locus identified in GWA studies to be most highly associated with coronary artery disease and MI—and thereby have more independent predictive value than a lipid level–only genetic risk score. The 9p21 genotype by itself confers up to a 60% increase in risk in individuals with two unfavorable alleles.[41,45,61] A risk score that includes nine SNPs identified in GWA studies as being associated with early-onset MI, including an SNP at locus 9p21 and three SNPs associated with LDL-C, is even more highly associated with disease, with a 2.2-fold difference in risk for MI between extreme quintiles of risk score.[45]

Nevertheless, attempts to incorporate SNPs at locus 9p21 into risk-prediction models have yielded disappointing results to date. As with the lipid genetic risk score, adding the 9p21 genotype to traditional risk factors in prospective cohort studies with men[61] and women[62] yielded no improvement in risk discrimination (as judged by C-statistic) and reclassified only small proportions of individuals to more accurate risk categories. However, investigators do await the evaluation of a comprehensive genotype score that includes many or all of the SNPs discovered to be strongly associated with cardiovascular disease.

Finally, as noted at the start of this chapter, a personal family history of early-onset MI in at least one parent more than doubles the risk of a cardiovascular event. As more genetic variants associated with disease are discovered, it will be important to assess whether a comprehensive genetic risk score will add any predictive value above and beyond simply asking about a patient's family history. For this reason, determining a genetic risk score may ultimately prove to be most useful in infants and children (whose parents may not be old enough to have developed coronary artery disease) for the purpose of determining lifetime cardiovascular risk and engaging in more stringent primordial prevention practices.

UTILITY OF GENETICS FOR PERSONALIZED MEDICINE

Another potential use of genetics information is its application to pharmacogenetics: determining which individuals are more likely to benefit from (or to suffer an adverse effect from) the use of a particular medication. The design of pharmacogenetic studies is similar to that of traditional genetic studies except that the phenotype of interest, instead of being a disease or clinical trait, is the outcome upon receiving a therapy.

At least three examples of pharmacogenetic findings are relevant to the prevention or treatment of cardiovascular disease. First, the statin drugs are the most widely used medications used to lower lipid levels because of their consistent efficacy in reducing cardiovascular endpoints in numerous clinical trials. These trials have documented wide variability in individuals' response to statin therapy in the degree of LDL-C lowering. Pharmacogenetic studies in some of these trials, as well as in other cohorts, have reproducibly demonstrated that variants of SNPs in lipid level–related genes, *HMGCR* and *APOE,* are associated with the percentage decrease in blood LDL-C concentration experienced by statin users.[63-68] Thus, in principle, genotyping before initiation of lipid-lowering therapy could help predict response to statin drugs and guide practitioners in choosing among the statins (low- vs. high-potency) or choosing the starting dose for an individual patient—so-called personalized medicine.

A second, converse finding is that statin use occasionally causes myopathy that in extreme cases is life-threatening. A GWA study for statin-induced myopathy identified an SNP in the *SLCO1B1* gene as highly associated with this adverse effect.[69] In individuals with two unfavorable alleles at this SNP, the risk of developing myopathy while they take statin therapy is 17 times higher than that in individuals with no unfavorable alleles. Thus, a genetic test for this SNP could be useful in screening patients before initiation of therapy, particularly if there is already concern that the patient is at risk for myopathy because of family history or has a personal history of muscle symptoms while receiving statin therapy. Patients with the risk-conferring genotype may wish to avoid statins and choose alternative therapies for lowering lipid levels.

The third example involves the antiplatelet agent clopidogrel, which is widely used in patients after acute coronary syndrome, percutaneous coronary intervention, or both. Clopidogrel is converted into its active metabolite by the CYP2C19 enzyme of hepatic cytochrome P-450. In three large

52 studies of patients receiving clopidogrel after acute coronary syndromes, individuals with reduced-function alleles of the *CYP2C19* gene experienced significantly higher rates of cardiovascular death, myocardial infarction, and stroke.[70-72] This is consistent with the finding in one of the studies that reduced-function allele carriers harbored lower plasma levels of the active metabolite of clopidogrel.[70] In principle, patients with reduced-function *CYP2C19* alleles would benefit from higher doses of clopidogrel or alternative antiplatelet medications such as prasugrel, although this remains to be tested in prospective clinical trials.

CONCLUSION

The development of the GWA technique has elucidated the genetics of cardiovascular disease and cardiovascular risk factors; studies with this technique have revealed numerous loci that represent previously unknown biologic mechanisms and, ultimately, potential new therapeutic opportunities. Future studies from groups such as the Global Lipids Genetics Consortium and CARDIoGRAM will extend these findings even further by screening very large populations and identifying even more loci associated with blood lipid concentrations and coronary artery disease, and the NHLBI CARe and other studies will yield fresh insights into human genetics by applying GWA to non-European populations. Although it remains unclear whether genetics will be useful for cardiovascular risk prediction in adults, it may eventually be useful in other applications such as primordial prevention and personalized medicine.

REFERENCES

1. Lloyd-Jones DM, Nam BH, D'Agostino RB Sr, et al: Parental cardiovascular disease as a risk factor for cardiovascular disease in middle-aged adults: a prospective study of parents and offspring. *JAMA* 291:2204-2211, 2004.
2. Nora JJ, Lortscher RH, Spangler RD, et al: Genetic-epidemiologic study of early-onset ischemic heart disease. *Circulation* 61:503-508, 1980.
3. Rao DC, Laskarzewski PM, Morrison JA, et al: The Cincinnati Lipid Research Clinic Family Study: cultural and biological determinants of lipids and lipoprotein concentrations. *Am J Hum Genet* 34:888-903, 1982.
4. Namboodiri KK, Kaplan EB, Heuch I, et al: The Collaborative Lipid Research Clinic Family Study: biological and cultural determinants of familial resemblance for plasma lipids and lipoproteins. *Genet Epidemiol* 2:227-254, 1985.
5. Heller DA, de Faire U, Pedersen NL, et al: Genetic and environmental influences on serum lipid levels in twins. *N Engl J Med* 328:1150-1156, 1993.
6. Pilia G, Chen WM, Scuteri A, et al: Heritability of cardiovascular and personality traits in 6,148 Sardinians. *PLoS Genet* 2(8):e132, 2006.
7. Havlik RJ, Garrison RJ, Feinleib M, et al: Blood pressure aggregation in families. *Am J Epidemiol* 110:304-312, 1979.
8. Levy D, DeStefano AL, Larson MG, et al: Evidence for a gene influencing blood pressure on chromosome 17. Genome scan linkage results for longitudinal blood pressure phenotypes in subjects from the Framingham Heart Study. *Hypertension* 36:477-483, 2000.
9. Barroso I: Genetics of type 2 diabetes. *Diabet Med* 22:517-535, 2005.
10. Lander ES, Linton LM, Birren B, et al: Initial sequencing and analysis of the human genome. *Nature* 409:860-921, 2001.
11. International HapMap Consortium, Frazer KA, Ballinger DG, et al: A second generation human haplotype map of over 3.1 million SNPs. *Nature* 449:851-861, 2007.
12. Musunuru K, Kathiresan S: HapMap and mapping genes for cardiovascular disease. *Circ Cardiovasc Genet* 1:66-71, 2008.
13. Donnelly P: Progress and challenges in genome-wide association studies in humans. *Nature* 456:728-731, 2008.
14. Dudbridge F, Gusnanto A: Estimation of significance thresholds for genomewide association scans. *Genet Epidemiol* 32:227-234, 2008.
15. Diabetes Genetics Initiative of Broad Institute of Harvard and MIT, Lund University, Novartis Institutes of BioMedical Research, et al: Genome-wide association analysis identifies loci for type 2 diabetes and triglyceride levels. *Science* 316:1331-1336, 2007.
16. Orho-Melander M, Melander O, Guiducci C, et al: Common missense variant in the glucokinase regulatory protein gene is associated with increased plasma triglyceride and C-reactive protein but lower fasting glucose concentrations. *Diabetes* 57:3112-3121, 2008.
17. Beer NL, Tribble ND, McCulloch LJ, et al: The *P446L* variant in *GCKR* associated with fasting plasma glucose and triglyceride levels exerts its effect through increased glucokinase activity in liver. *Hum Mol Genet* 18:4081-4088, 2009.
18. Willer CJ, Sanna S, Jackson AU, et al: Newly identified loci that influence lipid concentrations and risk of coronary artery disease. *Nat Genet* 40:161-169, 2008.
19. Kathiresan S, Melander O, Guiducci C, et al: Six new loci associated with blood low-density lipoprotein cholesterol, high-density lipoprotein cholesterol or triglycerides in humans. *Nat Genet* 40:189-197, 2008.
20. Sandhu MS, Waterworth DM, Debenham SL, et al: LDL-cholesterol concentrations: a genome-wide association study. *Lancet* 371:483-491, 2008.
21. Wallace C, Newhouse SJ, Braund P, et al: Genome-wide association study identifies genes for biomarkers of cardiovascular disease: serum urate and dyslipidemia. *Am J Hum Genet* 82:139-149, 2008.
22. Kooner JS, Chambers JC, Aguilar-Salinas CA, et al: Genome-wide scan identifies variation in *MLXIPL* associated with plasma triglycerides. *Nat Genet* 40:149-151, 2008.
23. Kathiresan S, Willer CJ, Peloso GM, et al: Common variants at 30 loci contribute to polygenic dyslipidemia. *Nat Genet* 41:56-65, 2009.
24. Aulchenko YS, Ripatti S, Lindqvist I, et al: Loci influencing lipid levels and coronary heart disease risk in 16 European population cohorts. *Nat Genet* 41:47-55, 2009.
25. Sabatti C, Service SK, Hartikainen AL, et al: Genome-wide association analysis of metabolic traits in a birth cohort from a founder population. *Nat Genet* 41:35-46, 2009.
26. Newton-Cheh C, Johnson T, Gateva V, et al: Genome-wide association study identifies eight loci associated with blood pressure. *Nat Genet* 41:666-676, 2009.
27. Levy D, Ehret GB, Rice K, et al: Genome-wide association study of blood pressure and hypertension. *Nat Genet* 41:677-687, 2009.
28. Newton-Cheh C, Larson MG, Vasan RS, et al: Association of common variants in *NPPA* and *NPPB* with circulating natriuretic peptides and blood pressure. *Nat Genet* 41:348-353, 2009.
29. Frayling TM: Genome-wide association studies provide new insights into type 2 diabetes aetiology. *Nat Rev Genet* 8:657-662, 2007.
30. Zeggini E, Scott LJ, Saxena R, et al: Meta-analysis of genome-wide association data and large-scale replication identifies additional susceptibility loci for type 2 diabetes. *Nat Genet* 40:638-645, 2008.
31. Yasuda K, Miyake K, Horikawa Y, et al: Variants in *KCNQ1* are associated with susceptibility to type 2 diabetes mellitus. *Nat Genet* 40:1092-1097, 2008.
32. Unoki H, Takahashi A, Kawaguchi T, et al: SNPs in *KCNQ1* are associated with susceptibility to type 2 diabetes in East Asian and European populations. *Nat Genet* 40:1098-1102, 2008.
33. Lyssenko V, Nagorny CL, Erdos MR, et al: Common variant in *MTNR1B* associated with increased risk of type 2 diabetes and impaired early insulin secretion. *Nat Genet* 41:82-88, 2009.
34. Bouatia-Naji N, Bonnefond A, Cavalcanti-Proenca C, et al: A variant near *MTNR1B* is associated with increased fasting plasma glucose levels and type 2 diabetes risk. *Nat Genet* 41:89-94, 2009.
35. Yi F, Brubaker PL, Jin T: TCF-4 mediates cell type–specific regulation of proglucagon gene expression by beta-catenin and glycogen synthase kinase-3beta. *J Biol Chem* 280:1457-1464, 2005.
36. Florez JC, Jablonski KA, Bayley N, et al: *TCF7L2* polymorphisms and progression to diabetes in the Diabetes Prevention Program. *N Engl J Med* 355:241-250, 2006.
37. Ridker PM, Pare G, Parker A, et al: Loci related to metabolic-syndrome pathways including *LEPR, HNF1A, IL6R,* and *GCKR* associate with plasma C-reactive protein: the Women's Genome Health Study. *Am J Hum Genet* 82:1185-1192, 2008.
38. Elliott P, Chambers JC, Zhang W, et al: Genetic loci associated with C-reactive protein levels and risk of coronary heart disease. *JAMA* 302:37-48, 2009.
39. Danik JS, Pare G, Chasman DI, et al: Novel loci, including those related to Crohn disease, psoriasis, and inflammation, identified in a genome-wide association study of fibrinogen in 17,686 women: the Women's Genome Health Study. *Circ Cardiovasc Genet* 2:134-141, 2009.
40. Dehghan A, Yang Q, Peters A, et al: Association of novel genetic loci with circulating fibrinogen levels: a genome-wide association study in 6 population-based cohorts. *Circ Cardiovasc Genet* 2:125-133, 2009.
41. McPherson R, Pertsemlidis A, Kavaslar N, et al: A common allele on chromosome 9 associated with coronary heart disease. *Science* 316:1488-1491, 2007.
42. Helgadottir A, Thorleifsson G, Manolescu A, et al: A common variant on chromosome 9p21 affects the risk of myocardial infarction. *Science* 316:1491-1493, 2007.
43. Samani NJ, Erdmann J, Hall AS, et al: Genomewide association analysis of coronary artery disease. *N Engl J Med* 357:443-453, 2007.
44. Schunkert H, Gotz A, Braund P, et al: Repeated replication and a prospective meta-analysis of the association between chromosome 9p21.3 and coronary artery disease. *Circulation* 117:1675-1684, 2008.
45. Myocardial Infarction Genetics Consortium, Kathiresan S, Voight BF, et al: Genome-wide association of early-onset myocardial infarction with single nucleotide polymorphisms and copy number variants. *Nat Genet* 41:334-341, 2009.
46. Helgadottir A, Thorleifsson G, Magnusson KP, et al: The same sequence variant on 9p21 associates with myocardial infarction, abdominal aortic aneurysm and intracranial aneurysm. *Nat Genet* 40:217-224, 2008.
47. Erdmann J, Grosshennig A, Braund PS, et al: New susceptibility locus for coronary artery disease on chromosome 3q22.3. *Nat Genet* 41:280-282, 2009.
48. Tregouet DA, Konig IR, Erdmann J, et al: Genome-wide haplotype association study identifies the SLC22A3-LPAL2-LPA gene cluster as a risk locus for coronary artery disease. *Nat Genet* 41:283-285, 2009.
49. Gudbjartsson DF, Bjornsdottir US, Halapi E, et al: Sequence variants affecting eosinophil numbers associate with asthma and myocardial infarction. *Nat Genet* 41:342-347, 2009.
50. Davey Smith G, Ebrahim S: "Mendelian randomization": can genetic epidemiology contribute to understanding environmental determinants of disease? *Int J Epidemiol* 32:1-22, 2003.
51. Cohen J, Pertsemlidis A, Kotowski IK, et al: Low LDL cholesterol in individuals of African descent resulting from frequent nonsense mutations in PCSK9. *Nat Genet* 37:161-165, 2005.
52. Cohen JC, Boerwinkle E, Mosley TH Jr, et al: Sequence variations in PCSK9, low LDL, and protection against coronary heart disease. *N Engl J Med* 354:1264-1272, 2006.
53. Kathiresan S, Myocardial Infarction Genetics Consortium: A PCSK9 missense variant associated with a reduced risk of early-onset myocardial infarction. *N Engl J Med* 358:2299-2300, 2008.
54. Willer CJ, Sanna S, Jackson AU, et al: Newly identified loci that influence lipid concentrations and risk of coronary artery disease. *Nat Genet* 40:161-169, 2008.

55. Zacho J, Tybjaerg-Hansen A, Jensen JS, et al: Genetically elevated C-reactive protein and ischemic vascular disease. *N Engl J Med* 359:1897-1908, 2008.

56. Lawlor DA, Harbord RM, Timpson NJ, et al: The association of C-reactive protein and CRP genotype with coronary heart disease: findings from five studies with 4,610 cases amongst 18,637 participants. *PLoS One* 3(8):e3011, 2008.

57. Ridker PM, Danielson E, Fonseca FA, et al: Rosuvastatin to prevent vascular events in men and women with elevated C-reactive protein. *N Engl J Med* 359:2195-2207, 2008.

58. Raychaudhuri S, Remmers EF, Lee AT, et al: Common variants at CD40 and other loci confer risk of rheumatoid arthritis. *Nat Genet* 40:1216-1223, 2008.

59. Barrett JC, Hansoul S, Nicolae DL, et al: Genome-wide association defines more than 30 distinct susceptibility loci for Crohn's disease. *Nat Genet* 40:955-962, 2008.

60. Kathiresan S, Melander O, Anevski D, et al: Polymorphisms associated with cholesterol and risk of cardiovascular events. *N Engl J Med* 358:1240-1249, 2008.

61. Talmud PJ, Cooper JA, Palmen J, et al: Chromosome 9p21.3 coronary heart disease locus genotype and prospective risk of CHD in healthy middle-aged men. *Clin Chem* 54:467-474, 2008.

62. Paynter NP, Chasman DI, Buring JE, et al: Cardiovascular disease risk prediction with and without knowledge of genetic variation at chromosome 9p21.3. *Ann Intern Med* 150:65-72, 2009.

63. Ballantyne CM, Herd JA, Stein EA, et al: Apolipoprotein E genotypes and response of plasma lipids and progression-regression of coronary atherosclerosis to lipid-lowering drug therapy. *J Am Coll Cardiol* 36:1572-1578, 2000.

64. Chasman DI, Posada D, Subrahmanyan L, et al: Pharmacogenetic study of statin therapy and cholesterol reduction. *JAMA* 291:2821-2827, 2004.

65. Krauss RM, Mangravite LM, Smith JD, et al: Variation in the 3-hydroxyl-3-methylglutaryl coenzyme A reductase gene is associated with racial differences in low-density lipoprotein cholesterol response to simvastatin treatment. *Circulation* 117:1537-1544, 2008.

66. Voora D, Shah SH, Reed CR, et al: Pharmacogenetic predictors of statin-mediated low-density lipoprotein cholesterol reduction and dose response. *Circ Cardiovasc Genet* 1:100-106, 2008.

67. Mega JL, Morrow DA, Brown A, et al: Identification of genetic variants associated with response to statin therapy. *Arterioscler Thromb Vasc Biol* 29:1310-1315, 2009.

68. Thompson JF, Hyde CL, Wood LS, et al: Comprehensive whole-genome and candidate gene analysis for response to statin therapy in the Treating to New Targets (TNT) cohort. *Circ Cardiovasc Genet* 2:173-181, 2009.

69. SEARCH Collaborative Group, Link E, Parish S, et al: SLCO1B1 variants and statin-induced myopathy—a genomewide study. *N Engl J Med* 359:789-799, 2008.

70. Mega JL, Close SL, Wiviott SD, et al: Cytochrome P-450 polymorphisms and response to clopidogrel. *N Engl J Med* 360:354-362, 2009.

71. Simon T, Verstuyft C, Mary-Krause M, et al: Genetic determinants of response to clopidogrel and cardiovascular events. *N Engl J Med* 360:363-375, 2009.

72. Collet JP, Hulot JS, Pena A, et al: Cytochrome P450 *2C19* polymorphism in young patients treated with clopidogrel after myocardial infarction: a cohort study. *Lancet* 373:309-317, 2009.

CHAPTER 5

Novel Biomarkers and the Assessment of Cardiovascular Risk

Vijay Nambi, Ariel Brautbar, and Christie M. Ballantyne

KEY POINTS

- Cardiovascular risk stratification must be improved, and biomarkers, genetic markers, and imaging provide the best avenue toward this improvement.

- All currently available markers (biomarkers and genetic markers) provide only limited to modest improvements in the ability to predict cardiovascular risk.

- In the future, the combination of genetic markers, imaging markers, and biomarkers will probably be used in an attempt to identify at-risk individuals while investigators continue to refine risk prediction with traditional risk factors.

The limitations of traditional coronary heart disease (CHD) risk stratification through the use of scores such as the Framingham Risk Score have been well documented and discussed.[1-3] The majority of individuals who have CHD events would have been classified as having low or intermediate risk by traditional risk stratification schemes, because most of the general population has low to intermediate 10-year (short-term) risk. Furthermore, although the risk factors for CHD and stroke are similar, the risk prediction algorithms are different[4-9]; therefore, an individual may have low risk for CHD and yet high risk for stroke, and vice versa.[10] In addition, although risk prediction tools are available, many clinicians do not use them, and those who do typically estimate only CHD risk and do not estimate risk for stroke, peripheral arterial disease, or heart failure. Newer tools that estimate total cardiovascular disease (CVD) risk are available[10a] and would be preferred to those that are limited to estimating CHD risk; however, the newer tools still focus on traditional risk factors and do not address longer term risk. Finally, most risk scores have been derived in populations with a predominance of one ethnicity, and the applicability of those scores to other ethnicities is therefore not known. Hence, improved CVD risk assessment tools are needed. Strategies to improve risk prediction have focused on identifying individuals who have an increased long-term risk (i.e., lifetime risk)[11] and in identifying novel markers. These additional markers include those identified on imaging, genetic markers, and biomarkers measured in plasma or urine.

CRITERIA FOR EVALUATING A NEW MARKER IN RISK PREDICTION

On average, more than 1100 reports of investigations of independent predictors or risk factors for various clinical outcomes are published every year, and CHD is one of the outcomes more frequently assessed.[12] Some of the newly discovered markers have been reported to improve CHD risk prediction in comparison with traditional risk factors.

Tzoulaki and colleagues[13] assessed studies reporting improved CHD risk prediction beyond the Framingham risk score and found that the majority of the studies had design, analytical, or reporting flaws. A scientific statement from the American Heart Association[14] therefore recommended that certain important parameters be evaluated and reported to determine whether a marker adequately improves CHD risk prediction (Box 5-1).

Among the first things to consider is whether the marker is tested in an appropriate population. A cohort from a population-based epidemiologic study is ideal because the participants are representative of the population at large. Even in this cohort, however, there are limitations: for example, whether findings are generalizable to other ethnicities not studied. After basic analyses, including whether the marker is associated with the outcome of interest, odds ratio, risk ratio, and hazards ratio, the marker should be tested for (1) its ability to discriminate between persons who have the disease of interest (e.g., CHD) and those who do not, (2) its accuracy in risk prediction, and (3) its effect on reclassifying individuals in the low- and intermediate-risk groups.

The ability of a marker to "discriminate" between persons with and those without a particular outcome is generally tested by describing the C-statistic, or the area under the receiver operating characteristic (ROC) curve, which essentially plots sensitivity against $1 -$ specificity, or true-positive findings against true-negative findings. A value of 0.50 indicates that the marker has no more value than chance. However, the use of the C-statistic in model selection (i.e., to decide what variables to include in a model) has limitations.[15] Other tests based on likelihood, such as the likelihood ratio statistic or the Bayes information criterion, which adjusts for the number of variables in the model, are more sensitive[15,16] and may be better for use in model selection and as a measure of model fit. Another marker used in discrimination is the integrated discrimination improvement, which tests whether the novel marker correctly increases the predicted risk (i.e., reclassification to a higher risk category) of persons who

BOX 5-1 Recommendations for Reporting of Novel Risk Markers

1. Report the basic study design and outcomes in accord with accepted standards for observational studies
2. Report levels of standard risk factors and the results of risk model, using these established factors
3. Evaluate the novel marker in the population, and report:
   a. Relative risk, odds ratio, or hazard ratio conveyed by the novel marker alone, with the associated confidence limits and P value
   b. Relative risk, odds ratio, or hazard ratio for novel marker after statistical adjustment for established risk factors, with the associated confidence limits and P value
   c. P value for addition of the novel marker to a model that contains the standard risk markers
4. Report the discrimination of the new marker:
   a. C-index and its confidence limits for model with established risk markers
   b. C-index and its confidence limits for model, including novel marker and established risk markers
   c. Integrated discrimination index, discrimination slope, or binary R^2 for the model with and without the novel risk marker
   d. Graphic or tabular display of predicted risk in cases and noncases separately, before and after inclusion of the new marker
5. Report the accuracy of the new marker:
   a. Display observed vs. expected event rates across the range of predicted risk for models without and with the novel marker
   b. Using generally recognized risk thresholds, report the number of subjects reclassified and the event rates in the reclassified groups

From Hlatky MA, Greenland P, Arnett DK, et al: Criteria for evaluation of novel markers of cardiovascular risk: a scientific statement from the American Heart Association, *Circulation* 119:2408-2416, 2009.

TABLE 5–1	Calculation of Net Reclassification Index (NRI)			
Risk Category by Traditional Risk Factors	Risk Category by Traditional Risk Factors + Biomarker X			
	<5%	5% to 20%	>20%	Total
Individuals Who Have a Clinical Event (n)				
<5%	37	14	0	51
5% to 20%	5	85	16	106
>20%	0	4	24	28
Total	40	104	41	185
Individuals Who Do Not Have a Clinical Event (n)				
<5%	1650	145	0	1795
5% to 20%	150	680	33	863
>20%	2	32	69	103
Total	1802	857	102	2761

NRI = [(number of individuals with events among those who were reclassified to a higher risk group/total number of individuals with events) − (number of individuals with events among those who were reclassified to a lower risk group/total number of individuals with events)] − [(number of individuals without events among those who were reclassified to a higher risk group/total number of individuals without events) − (number of individuals without events among those who were reclassified to a lower risk group/total number of individuals without events)].

For the data in this table:

1. Number of individuals *with* events among those who were reclassified to a *higher* risk group/total number of individuals with events = (14 + 16)/185 = 30/185 = 0.162
2. Number of individuals *with* events among those who were reclassified to a *lower* risk group/total number of individuals with events = (5 + 4)/185 = 9/185 = 0.049
3. Number of individuals *without* events among those who were reclassified to a *higher* risk group/total number of individuals without events = (145 + 33)/2761 = 188/2761 = 0.064
4. Number of individuals *without* events among those who were reclassified to a *lower* risk group/total number of individuals without events = (150 + 2 + 32)/2761 = 174/2761 = 0.066

Therefore, NRI = (0.162 − 0.049) − (0.064 − 0.066) = 0.113 − 0.005 = 0.115, or 11.5%.

have the event and decreases the predicted risk of those who do not.[17]

Although these tests of discrimination are important, they do not assess whether risk prediction is accurate. For this, a goodness-of-fit test is necessary to evaluate whether there is any difference between the predicted and observed risk. The number of individuals who are reclassified (i.e., will change risk groups) by the inclusion of the risk marker of interest and the net effect of the reclassification (net reclassification index [NRI]) then need to be determined.[17] The NRI, a statistical test designed to study the net effect of reclassification, determines whether reclassifications were appropriate; for example, if an individual was reclassified to a higher risk group and then had an event, the reclassification would be considered appropriate ("good"), whereas if the individual was reclassified to a lower risk group and then had an event, the reclassification would be considered inappropriate ("bad"). The net effect of the "good" and "bad" reclassification determines the NRI, and the clinical NRI is determined by the effect in the intermediate-risk group (in general, persons who have a 5% to 20% estimated 10-year risk for CHD), in which the test might be used to refine risk assessment and need for treatment (Table 5-1).

It would be useful to show that a clinical strategy that used the novel marker in risk prediction and in treating individuals can decrease the incidence of CHD. In this chapter, we discuss the use of biomarkers and genetic markers that have been studied for their use in the improvement of CVD risk prediction.

BIOMARKERS ASSESSED IN CARDIOVASCULAR DISEASE RISK PREDICTION

Several markers have been associated with CHD, stroke, or both, but only a very few have been tested for their influence on risk prediction. The marker that has been best studied is high-sensitivity C-reactive protein (hsCRP) level. Other markers that appear promising include lipoprotein-associated phospholipase A_2 (LpPLA$_2$) level and amino-terminal pro–B-type (or brain) natriuretic peptide (NT-proBNP) level.

C-Reactive Protein

C-reactive protein is a nonspecific marker of inflammation. C-reactive protein was initially tested for association with CVD as investigators increasingly appreciated the role played by inflammation in the pathogenesis of atherosclerosis.[18] In several studies, researchers have reported associations between hsCRP level and incidental CHD, stroke, or both.[19-28]

In view of the consistent association, Ridker and associates[29] evaluated the value of hsCRP in risk prediction in a number of analyses. They first examined the value of hsCRP level when added to variables used in the Framingham risk score (age, total cholesterol level, high-density lipoprotein cholesterol [HDL-C] level, smoking, and blood pressure) in the Women's Health Study.[29] In a cohort of 15,048 women aged 45 and older, 390 women had incident CVD events (116 myocardial infarctions, 217 coronary revascularization procedures, 65 deaths from cardiovascular causes, and 100 ischemic strokes) in an average follow-up period of 10 years. Although adding hsCRP level to a risk prediction model based on Framingham variables only marginally improved the area under the ROC curve (to 0.815, in comparison with 0.813 for the model without hsCRP level), other tests of discrimination, such as the Bayes information criterion, suggested that a model that included hsCRP level would be better. According to model calibration tested with the Hosmer-Lemeshow goodness-of-fit test, the model with hsCRP level was a better fit when expected and observed events were compared. Of the individuals predicted to have a 5% to 20% risk over 10 years, about 20% were reclassified after the addition of hsCRP level.

Ridker and colleagues[30] then investigated whether risk prediction could be improved with the inclusion of several novel markers (e.g., levels of hsCRP, hemoglobin A1c, homocysteine, soluble intercellular adhesion molecule–1, apolipoproteins) that had been identified since the Framingham risk score had been described. They divided the Women's Health Study cohort into a model derivation cohort ($n = 16,400$) and a model validation cohort ($n = 8158$). The variables that resulted in the best fitting model included age, hemoglobin A1c in subjects with diabetes, current smoking, lipoprotein(a) levels (if apolipoprotein B level $\geq$ 100 mg/dL), apolipoprotein B level, apolipoprotein A-I level, parental history of myocardial infarction (at age <60 years), and natural logarithms of systolic blood pressure and hsCRP level. Ridker and colleagues then simplified this model for clinical use by substituting levels of total cholesterol and HDL-C for levels of apolipoproteins B-100 and A-I and eliminating the measurement of lipoprotein(a) level (Table 5-2). This Reynolds risk score,[31] which differed from the Framingham risk score mainly in its use of hsCRP level and parental history of myocardial infarction, was found to have better model discrimination and calibration and reclassified 40% to 50% of individuals in the intermediate-risk group into higher risk or lower risk categories. However, no patient was reclassified from the low-risk group (<5% CHD risk over 10 years) to the high-risk group (>20% CHD risk over 10 years) or vice versa; this suggests that prior probability of disease should be considered in determining for whom additional testing is recommended.

The Reynolds risk score was subsequently described in men as well: in comparison with a traditional model, the Reynolds risk score reclassified 18% of subjects in the Physicians Health Study II, including 20% of subjects at intermediate risk, and was associated with a better model fit and discrimination.[32] In addition, the Reynolds risk score was associated with an NRI of 5.3% and a clinical NRI of 14.2%. Other analyses have also suggested that the NRI for adding hsCRP level is approximately 5% to 7%.[33,34] However, in a case-control study of individuals in the European Prospective Investigation into Cancer and Nutrition (EPIC)–Norfolk study, the NRI for adding hsCRP level was 12.0%.[35]

More recently, a strategy of treating individuals with elevated hsCRP levels was studied in the Justification for the Use of Statins in Primary Prevention: an Intervention Trial Evaluating Rosuvastatin (JUPITER). Individuals with low-density lipoprotein cholesterol (LDL-C) levels lower than 130 mg/dL and hsCRP levels of 2 mg/L or higher were treated with rosuvastatin; treatment with this drug was associated with a 44% relative risk reduction in major adverse cardiovascular events, and the trial was discontinued early because of clear benefit.[36] Yang and coworkers[37] analyzed data on participants in the Atherosclerosis Risk in Communities (ARIC) study according to the entry criteria for JUPITER; their findings suggested that elevated hsCRP level confers high risk regardless of LDL-C levels (either <130 mg/dL or $\geq$130 mg/dL) and after various traditional risk factors are taken into account.

The 2009 evaluation of hsCRP level by the United States Preventive Services Task Force (USPSTF)[38] concluded that there is strong evidence that hsCRP level is associated with incident CHD, moderate evidence that hsCRP level can help in risk stratification of the intermediate-risk group, but insufficient evidence that reducing hsCRP level can prevent CHD events. However, in its systematic review of nine "emerging" CHD risk factors, including hsCRP level, the USPSTF concluded that current evidence does not support the use of any of these factors in further risk stratification.[39] Similarly, other investigators have questioned whether adding hsCRP level has any additional value in risk stratification.[40] Part of the reason that these questions have been raised is the significant correlation of hsCRP level with traditional risk factors and its minimal effect on the area under the ROC curve.

In an analysis of National Health and Nutrition Examination Survey (NHANES) data, Miller and associates reported that hsCRP levels were rarely high (>3 mg/L) in the absence of traditional risk factors associated with CHD, occurring in 4.4% of men and 10.3% of women, and that elevations in hsCRP levels that were attributable to a borderline or abnormal CHD risk factor occurred in 78% of men and 67% of women.[41] Epidemiologic studies such as the Framingham Heart Study and the ARIC study have also demonstrated that the effect of hsCRP level on improving the area under the ROC curve is minimal and not statistically significant.[42,43] However, using area under the ROC curve as the only metric to evaluate value in risk stratification can be suboptimal, because the C-statistic is based solely on ranks and is not as sensitive as measures based on likelihood. In fact, several well-established risk factors such as LDL-C and HDL-C may add little to the area under the ROC curve when added to other traditional risk factors.[15]

Our own impression of the available data is that hsCRP level can help identify higher risk individuals among those classified as having intermediate short-term (10-year) risk for CHD by traditional risk prediction algorithms. However, it is unclear whether hsCRP level is a risk marker or a risk factor; that is, it is unclear whether hsCRP level plays a role in the pathogenesis of atherosclerosis or adverse cardiovascular events, or whether it is merely a bystander marking other changes that lead to atherogenesis and adverse cardiovascular

TABLE 5–2	Reynolds Risk Score	
Best-Fitting Model	**Clinically Simplified Model: Reynolds Risk Score**
Age	Age
Systolic blood pressure	Systolic blood pressure
Current smoking	Current smoking
hsCRP	hsCRP
Parental history of MI < age 60	Parental history of MI < age 60
Hemoglobin A1c (if diabetic)	Hemoglobin A1c (if diabetic)
Apo B-100	Total cholesterol
Apo A-I	HDL-C
Lp(a) [if apo B-100 ≥ 100]	

Note: The Reynolds Risk Score was originally described in women and has since been described in men by means of the same clinically simplified model.[32]

Apo A-I, apolipoprotein A-I; apo B-100, apolipoprotein B-100; HDL-C, high-density lipoprotein cholesterol; hsCRP, high-sensitivity C-reactive protein; Lp(a), lipoprotein(a); MI, myocardial infarction.

From Ridker PM, Buring JE, Rifai N, et al: Development and validation of improved algorithms for the assessment of global cardiovascular risk in women: the Reynolds Risk Score, *JAMA* 297:611-619, 2007.

events. Genetic studies have identified several loci associated with hsCRP levels but not with CVD,[44,45] which suggests that hsCRP level may be a risk marker. However, whether it is a risk marker or a risk factor should not affect the ability of hsCRP level to predict risk.

In summary, there is consensus that elevation in hsCRP level is associated with increased risk for CHD and stroke. In our opinion, a clinically relevant number of individuals are reclassified, and a prospective trial has shown that treatment of individuals who have elevated hsCRP levels, "normal" LDL-C levels, and intermediate CHD risk can reduce both CHD and stroke. In addition, an expert panel convened by the National Academy of Clinical Biochemistry concluded, on the basis of a thorough literature review for a number of emerging risk factors, that only hsCRP level met all the criteria for acceptance for risk assessment in primary prevention.[46]

Lipoprotein-Associated Phospholipase A₂

LpPLA$_2$ level is another biomarker that has consistently been shown to be associated with both CHD and stroke.[22,47-51] LpPLA$_2$, which is predominantly associated with LDL in the circulation, is thought to mediate its inflammatory effects through its action on oxidized phospholipids, releasing lysophosphatidylcholine and oxidized nonesterified fatty acids, both of which are capable of attracting monocytes to an atherosclerotic lesion and further induce the expression of adhesion molecules.[52]

LpPLA$_2$ level has been evaluated as a marker for improving risk prediction. In the ARIC study, LpPLA$_2$ level was the only marker (of 19 markers studied, including hsCRP level) that significantly increased the area under the ROC curve (by 0.006) when added to traditional risk factors that included age, race, sex, total cholesterol level, HDL-C level, systolic blood pressure, antihypertensive medication use, smoking status, and diabetes.[43] However, in a more recent report from the EPIC-Norfolk study in which several markers were examined for their ability to improve risk prediction when added to a Framingham risk score–based model, only hsCRP level improved the C-statistic significantly; LpPLA$_2$ level had no significant effect.[35] Addition of LpPLA$_2$ level in this study resulted in an NRI of 1.7% and a clinical NRI of 8.8%, whereas adding hsCRP level was associated with an NRI of 12.0% and a clinical NRI of 28.4%. However, the model fit was better with LpPLA$_2$ level than with hsCRP level.

In view of the strong association of LpPLA$_2$ level with stroke (ischemic), Nambi and colleagues, using an analysis of a case–cohort random sample ($n = 949$, of whom 183 had incident ischemic stroke) from the ARIC study, evaluated whether LpPLA$_2$ level could improve stroke risk prediction.[10] Nambi and colleagues classified individuals' 5-year risk for stroke as low (<2%), intermediate (2% to 5%), or high (>5%) on the basis of a traditional risk factor model that included age, sex, race, current smoking, systolic blood pressure, LDL-C level, HDL-C level, diabetes, antihypertensive medication, and body mass index and then added hsCRP and LpPLA$_2$ levels separately and together to the analysis. Overall, adding LpPLA$_2$ level significantly improved the area under the ROC curve (from 0.732 to 0.752; 95% confidence interval [CI] for change in area under the ROC curve, 0.0028 to 0.0310), whereas adding hsCRP level did not significantly increase the area under the ROC curve (from 0.732 to 0.743; 95% CI for change in area under the ROC curve, −0.0005 to 0.0183). However, adding both LpPLA$_2$ and hsCRP levels, as well as their interaction, resulted in the best improvement in the area under the ROC curve, which increased to 0.774 (95% CI for change in area under the ROC curve, 0.0182 to 0.0607). The addition of hsCRP level, LpPLA$_2$ level, and

their interaction reclassified 4%, 39%, and 34% of the individuals originally classified as being at low, intermediate, and high risk, respectively.

In summary, LpPLA$_2$ level has not been as well studied as hsCRP level, especially with regard to improving risk prediction. Available data suggest that its ability to improve CHD risk prediction may be modest, but its ability to improve ischemic stroke risk prediction may be better. Additional studies are needed to examine whether pharmacologic treatment of patients who have elevated LpPLA$_2$ levels can reduce CVD events. LpPLA$_2$ level may be a risk factor, not only a risk marker, and a large outcomes trial is examining whether inhibition of LpPLA$_2$ in patients at high risk can reduce CVD events.[52a] Further studies will be needed to evaluate and identify the role for LpPLA$_2$ level in CVD risk stratification.

Amino-Terminal Pro–B-Type Natriuretic Peptide

B-type (or brain) natriuretic peptide (BNP) is a cardiac hormone secreted by cardiomyocytes in response to pressure and ventricular volume overload. The amino-terminal fragment of its prohormone (NT-proBNP), which has traditionally been thought of as a marker for congestive heart failure, has also been associated with both CHD and stroke.[53] The contribution of NT-proBNP level in risk stratification was examined in the Rotterdam study,[54] in which NT-proBNP level was analyzed with traditional risk factors to investigate its ability to predict 10-year risk of CVD. For a group of 5063 individuals older than 55 years and free of CHD, addition of NT-proBNP level to traditional risk factors significantly improved the C-statistic both in men (0.661 to 0.694; change in C-statistic, 0.033; 95% CI, 0.012 to 0.052) and in women (0.729 to 0.761; change in C-statistic, 0.032; 95% CI, 0.016 to 0.047) and resulted in an NRI of 9.2% (95% CI, 3.5% to 14.9%; $P = 0.001$) in men and 13.3% (95% CI 5.9% to 20.8%; $P < 0.001$) in women. In the Rancho Bernardo Study,[54a] increased NT-proBNP levels or detectable troponin T levels in asymptomatic elderly participants were associated with increased risk for CVD death and total mortality rate, and participants with elevations of both markers had even higher risk.

Other Markers

Several other markers also have associations with CVD; however, information regarding their use in CVD risk stratification is limited. In the analysis from the ARIC study noted previously, in which researchers examined the effect of adding various markers ($n = 19$) to traditional risk factors, only LpPLA$_2$ level improved the area under the ROC curve.[43] Rana and associates[35] investigated the effect of adding levels of hsCRP, myeloperoxidase, LpPLA$_2$, secretory phospholipase A$_2$ group IIA (sPLA$_2$), fibrinogen, paraoxonase, macrophage chemoattractant protein–1 (MCP-1), and adiponectin to analyses of CHD risk stratification. Overall, hsCRP level was the only marker that significantly improved the area under the ROC curve (to 0.65, from 0.59 for a Framingham risk score–based model; $P = 0.005$). Level of hsCRP was also associated with the best NRI and clinical NRI (12% and 28.4%, respectively), and sPLA$_2$ level was the next best (6.4% and 16.3%, respectively). However, when model fit was examined, adding hsCRP or paraoxonase or MCP-1 level to the Framingham risk score was associated with lack of model fit, whereas the addition of the other markers was associated with a good model fit. In the intermediate-risk group, the greatest numbers of individuals were accurately reclassified with the addition of sPLA$_2$ level, followed by levels of fibrinogen, LpPLA$_2$, adiponectin, and myeloperoxidase. In separate case-control analyses from the

EPIC-Norfolk study,[54b] CHD risk was noted to increase across increasing quartiles of myeloperoxidase level.

Multiple Markers

Because many of these markers improve risk prediction marginally, efforts have been made to evaluate the value of a multimarker approach by combining several biomarkers. With many of these multimarker approaches, the researchers examined primarily the association of markers (in concert) with CHD/CVD but not their use in risk stratification (reviewed by Koenig[55]).

Wang and coworkers[56] assessed 10 biomarkers (levels of hsCRP, BNP, N-terminal pro–atrial natriuretic peptide, aldosterone, renin, fibrinogen, D-dimer, plasminogen-activator inhibitor type 1, and homocysteine, and the urinary albumin-to-creatinine ratio) in the Framingham Heart Study ($n = 3209$) for their ability to predict major adverse cardiovascular events. BNP level (hazard ratio = 1.25) and urinary albumin-to-creatinine ratio (hazard ratio = 1.20) had the strongest association with major adverse cardiovascular events, and BNP level (hazard ratio = 1.40), hsCRP level (hazard ratio = 1.39), and urinary albumin-to-creatinine ratio (hazard ratio = 1.22) had the strongest association with death, but none of the markers affected the C-statistic significantly. The C-statistic for major cardiovascular events was 0.70 in a model that included age, sex, and the multimarker score; 0.76 in a model with age, sex, and conventional risk factors; and 0.77 in a model with all predictors.

Melander and associates[57] evaluated the additional value of 6 biomarkers (levels of hsCRP, cystatin C, LpPLA$_2$, midregional proadrenomedullin [MR-proADM], midregional pro–atrial natriuretic peptide, and NT-proBNP) in 5067 participants without CVD from Malmö, Sweden (mean age, 58 years). After using a backwards elimination model to identify the best markers for prediction of CVD events ($n = 418$) and CHD events ($n = 230$) (median follow-up, 12.8 years), they reported that hsCRP and NT-proBNP levels best improved the C-statistic for prediction of CHD events (increase in C-statistic, 0.007; $P = 0.04$), whereas NT-BNP and MR-proADM levels best improved prediction of CVD events, although the improvement was not statistically significant (increase in C-statistic, 0.009; $P = 0.08$). Very few individuals were reclassified: 8% of the study population was reclassified for CVD risk prediction and 5% for CHD risk prediction. Similarly, improvements in NRI for CVD and CHD were nonsignificant, although improvements in clinical NRI were significant (7% and 15%, respectively, largely through reclassification to a lower risk category).

Multiple markers have also been studied in older individuals. In one study in individuals older than 85 years, traditional risk factors were poor predictors of cardiovascular mortality, and of the markers studied (levels of hsCRP, homocysteine, folic acid, and interleukin-6), homocysteine level was the best predictor of cardiovascular mortality (area under the ROC curve, 0.65; 95% CI, 0.55 to 0.75). On the other hand, Zethelius and associates[58] reported significant improvement in prediction of CHD death in individuals older than 75 years with the use of biomarkers (levels of troponin I, NT-proBNP, cystatin C, and hsCRP); the C-statistic improved from 0.664 for traditional risk factors alone to 0.766 (difference, 0.102; 95% CI, 0.056 to 0.147) in the whole cohort and from 0.688 to 0.748 (difference, 0.059; 95% CI, 0.007 to 0.112) in subjects without CVD. The NRI for adding all the biomarkers was significant (26%, $P = 0.005$). Overall, this study was limited by the fact that only 136 subjects died from CVD.

Hence, even with the use of multiple markers, a consistent reliable set of markers has not been identified for CVD risk prediction. Of the novel markers studied, the addition of BNP level to hsCRP level appears the most reliable.

Advanced Lipoprotein Testing

Assessment of apolipoprotein B concentration and measurement of lipoprotein particle sizes with nuclear magnetic resonance (NMR) have been suggested as tests that may refine and improve risk prediction in comparison with cholesterol measures currently used clinically. Mora and colleagues[59] examined the association of these tests with CVD and their ability to improve risk prediction in the Women's Health Study, a study of healthy female health care professionals aged 45 years or older. Although both NMR lipid profile and apolipoprotein B concentration were associated with CVD after adjustment for nonlipid risk factors, the hazard ratios were similar to those for traditional lipid measures. The C-index was 0.784 for the model with nonlipid risk factors and ratio of total cholesterol to HDL-C levels, and it was not significantly different with the addition of LDL level measured by NMR (0.785) or apolipoprotein B level (0.786). NRI also did not show net improvement; in comparison with nonlipid risk factors and the total cholesterol–to–HDL-C ratio, NRI was 0% with NMR-measured LDL level and 1.9% with apolipoprotein B. This finding suggests that these novel lipid measures do not significantly enhance risk prediction in comparison with the traditional lipid measure of total cholesterol–to–HDL-C ratio. However, other studies in populations with higher baseline triglyceride values have demonstrated that apolipoprotein B level and other measures of LDL particle number provided additive prognostic value over LDL-C level.[59a]

GENETIC MARKERS AND ASSESSMENT OF RISK FOR CORONARY HEART DISEASE

Numerous new discoveries have helped investigators link genetic variants to human disease processes. Genetic and epidemiologic studies of cardiovascular genetics and CHD in particular have identified genetic variants directly associated with CHD and CHD risk factors. However, the practical clinical implementation of this information for management and prevention of CHD continues to be evaluated. The major studies in which researchers have evaluated the application of genetic variants associated with CHD in risk prediction and preventive cardiovascular management (Table 5-3) are described in this section.

Genetic Variation in the Human Genome

The human genome comprises millions of DNA base pairs that constitute either coding regions, which code for proteins that are essential for cell function, or noncoding regions of unknown significance. One of the major characteristics of the human genome is its interindividual variation. This variation in genomic content and structure between individuals is large, and its importance in normal function varies. There are rare variants with a large effect on disease risk, common variants that usually have a small effect on disease susceptibility, and variants with no apparent influence on known disease.

The most frequent type of genomic sequence variation in the human genome is the single nucleotide polymorphism (SNP). A SNP is a change in a single base pair at a specific genomic locus, so that the same single base pair is not in that locus for everyone; there may be a different base pair in a subgroup of the population. It is estimated that there is 1 SNP every 1000 base pairs and about 3 million base pair differences between any given two human genomes. Some of these SNPs are inherited together as part of a block of DNA called a *haplotype*. This phenomenon is useful in research because it enables a single SNP (a "tag" SNP) to be tested as a marker

TABLE 5–3	Statistical Metrics for Examining the Clinical Utility of Genetic Variants to Improve CHD Risk Prediction						
Subjects, n	Gender	Variant(s)	Traditional Risk Factor Model	Improvement in Area under the ROC Curve	NRI	CNRI	Reference
2742	Men	9p21	FRS	0.02	≈4.3%*		Talmud et al[72]
22,000	Women	9p21	FRS	0	2.70%	≈7%*	Paynter et al[70]
9998	Both	9p21	ACRS	0.004	0.80%	6.20%	Brautbar et al[71]
5414	Both	GRS	FRS	0	≈6.1%*		Kathiresan et al[74]

*Estimated on the basis of the published reclassification table.

ACRS, ARIC [Atherosclerosis Risk in Communities] Risk Score; CHD, coronary heart disease; CNRI, clinical net reclassification index; FRS, Framingham risk score; NRI, net reclassification index.

for multiple SNPs. The less frequent SNP or allele usually has a frequency of greater than 5%, which is defined as the minor allele frequency.

Because of the relatively large numbers of SNPs in the human genome and their interindividual variation, they are natural candidates for research on differences in disease susceptibility between individuals. According to the "common disease–common variant" hypothesis,[59b] complex diseases such as atherosclerosis and CHD are caused by not one gene but rather multiple genes, each of which contributes a small additive effect toward a certain threshold that results in the overall condition. SNPs are the ideal tool with which to examine and discover genes or noncoding areas that participate in diseases such as CHD.

To identify SNPs that may be associated with disease processes, different approaches have been applied, including the candidate-gene approach, which had limited success, and genome-wide association (GWA) studies, which have successfully identified multiple loci associated with various disease conditions and traits. GWA studies are based on the testing of thousands and up to a million SNPs at once to identify loci associated with a disease, such as CHD, and traits, such as LDL-C level. Important considerations for both candidate-gene and GWA approaches are the need to correct the statistical metrics used for discovery for multiple testing, replication of the results in a study population that is similar to the original discovery cohort, and examining the association in other populations and ethnicities.

The 9p21 Chromosomal Region and Coronary Heart Disease

In 2007, two independent GWA studies reported a number of SNPs in a 58-kilobase interval on the 9p21 chromosomal region that demonstrated a strong association with CHD in white persons.[60,61] These SNPs defined a single haplotype (i.e., they were closely linked together and inherited together) and were found to be associated with increases in CHD risk of approximately 20% in heterozygotes and approximately 40% in homozygotes. After the initial report, multiple studies replicated and validated this association in the white population[62-64] and demonstrated the association in additional populations, including Han Chinese,[65] East Asian,[66] South Korean,[67] Hispanic,[66] and Italian.[68] However, this association was not demonstrated in African American populations.[60,66] Interestingly, there are no known genes in this 58-kilobase interval in the 9p21 chromosomal region, although two genes, CDKN2A and CDKN2B, are located adjacent to it. Results of one study suggested that the 9p21 risk allele has a major role in the cardiac expression of CDKN2A and CDKN2B, which directly affect the proliferation properties of vascular cells.[69]

The importance of the 9p21 chromosomal region was not only its association with CHD but was also the high frequency of the risk allele in the white population: 45% to 55% in

various studies.[62,63,70-72] The combination of a large effect size with high population frequency made the 9p21 risk allele an attractive marker with which to enhance CHD risk prediction.

Talmud and associates[72] were the first investigators to evaluate whether the addition of the 9p21 risk allele to traditional risk factors improves CHD risk prediction. To examine their hypothesis, they used the Northwick Park Heart Study II (NPHS-II), a prospective study of 2742 white men monitored for 14 years, during which this population sustained 270 CHD events. The hazard ratio after adjustment for traditional risk factors (including age, smoking, systolic blood pressure, cholesterol, and HDL-C level) was 1.70 (95% CI, 1.19 to 2.41) for individuals who are homozygous for the risk allele. Adjustment for family history modestly decreased the hazard ratio, which was suggestive of some correlation between the 9p21 risk allele and family history. However, there was no statistically significant association between the two (P = 0.48).

Discrimination was examined by adding the 9p21 risk allele to a model with age and clinical practice (site of patient recruitment) only. Although the area under the ROC curve increased from 0.62 to 0.64, the increase was not statistically significant. Calibration, examined with the Hosmer-Lemeshow metrics, revealed a nonsignificant P value, indicating a good fit for the models with and without the 9p21 risk allele. After the addition of the 9p21 risk allele, approximately 22% of individuals were reclassified. NRI and clinical NRI were not calculated, but 63% of patients reclassified were assigned to a more accurate risk as reflected by a more appropriate event rate in their new category. Additional metrics assessing model fit—the likelihood ratio and the Bayes information criterion—were improved by the addition of the 9p21 risk allele.

Because of the lack of improvement in discrimination, Talmud and associates[72] suggested a potential approach to enhance the use of the 9p21 risk allele to improve risk prediction. Incremental addition of 1 to 10 hypothetical variants (with similar effect sizes and frequency as the 9p21 risk allele) to a traditional risk factor–based model significantly improved the area under the ROC curve after the addition of the first variant. These findings suggested that SNPs may be combined to construct a genetic risk score that may improve risk prediction; this concept is developed later in this section.

Following the analysis by Talmud and associates,[72] who used a cohort comprising only men, Paynter and colleagues[70] examined the clinical utility of the 9p21 risk allele added to traditional risk factors in a cohort of 22,129 white women who were prospectively monitored for a period of approximately 10 years; in this cohort, 715 total incident CVD events (CHD and stroke) were sustained. The hazard ratio was 1.15 per 9p21 risk allele for CVD events, and when tested for association with traditional risk factors, the 9p21 risk allele had a modest association with family history and diabetes. The addition of the 9p21 risk allele did not significantly increase the C-index in comparison with models based on the Framingham risk score and Reynolds risk score. Only 2.7% of the women were reclassified, most of whom (approximately 86%) were reclassified correctly. The NRI and integrated discrimination improvement was 2.7% and 0.001, respectively; clinical NRI was not calculated. Goodness of fit was tested with the Hosmer-Lemeshow metrics, which demonstrated a good fit for both models, with and without the 9p21 risk allele. The conclusion of Paynter and colleagues was that the addition of the 9p21 risk allele to traditional risk factors in analysis was not useful clinically. However, because this large cohort had a relatively low number of incident events (715 CVD events for 22,129 subjects), the statistical power of the study was substantially limited.

Brautbar and coworkers[71] examined whether the addition of the 9p21 risk allele to traditional risk factors improves CHD risk prediction in the ARIC study. The ARIC population examined included 9998 white middle-aged men and women who were monitored for approximately 14 years, of whom 13.5% had 1349 incident CHD events. The calculated hazard ratio was 1.2 per allele for the 9p21 risk allele after adjustment for traditional risk factors. The ARIC Cardiovascular Risk Score (ACRS), a model based on traditional risk factors that was created and tested in the ARIC study, was used to evaluate the utility of adding the 9p21 risk allele to traditional risk factors along with the Framingham risk score. The ACRS is based on age, gender, smoking, diabetes, systolic blood pressure, antihypertensive medication use, total cholesterol level, and HDL-C level. The frequency of the risk allele was 49% in the entire cohort and, as expected, significantly higher among subjects with CHD events. Discrimination was evaluated by calculation of the area under the ROC curve, which was modestly but significantly improved for the model with the 9p21 risk allele over the model without it (0.780 and 0.776, respectively). Goodness of fit examined with the Grønnesby-Borgan metrics was better for the model with the 9p21 risk allele, although both models did not demonstrate a good fit.

When the 9p21 risk allele was added to traditional risk factors, approximately 13% in the intermediate-low category (5% to 10% risk over 10 years) and intermediate-high category (10% to 20% risk over 10 years) were reclassified in both the ACRS and Framingham risk score models. The NRI and clinical NRI after the addition of the 9p21 risk allele were 0.8% and 6.2%, respectively, for the ACRS model. The clinical NRI for the Framingham risk score model was 6.8%. To evaluate the clinical utility of reclassification, Brautbar and coworkers measured the baseline LDL-C distribution in the categories for 5% to 10% and 10% to 20% CHD risk over 10 years before reclassification. In both risk groups, approximately 90% had LDL-C levels higher than 100 mg/dL, and thus reclassification to a higher risk category would have practical implications for many individuals by changing LDL-C target goal and initiation level for lipid-modifying therapy based on National Cholesterol Education Program Adult Treatment Panel III guidelines. In summary, the largest effect on reclassification in this analysis was on the intermediate-risk categories, 90% of whom had LDL-C levels above the recommended goals after reclassification.

Genetic Risk Score

Before the discovery of the 9p21 chromosomal region, extensive efforts were made to identify a panel of SNPs that would enable better estimation of CHD risk. The first study to examine this question included approximately 15,000 individuals from the ARIC study who developed approximately 1400 CHD events.[73] SNPs to be examined were chosen on the basis of prior GWA and candidate-gene studies. After extensive effort to genotype the SNPs in ARIC,

frequency and association with CHD were tested in both African American and white subjects. Within each race, SNPs associated with P values higher than 0.10 were excluded, which left 11 SNPs for each race. The SNPs were then modeled for an additive effect of the risk-raising allele and were individually evaluated by Cox proportional-hazards models. The genetic risk score, comprising these 11 SNPs, was added to traditional risk factors on the basis of the ACRS model. Calculation of the area under the ROC curve demonstrated modest improvement for African American subjects (0.758 to 0.769) and marginal improvement for white subjects (0.764 to 0.766). Reclassification was not examined in this study. The study's conclusion was that the improvement in discrimination was modest and probably not clinically applicable. However, the additive approach taken in this study was widely adopted in subsequent genetic studies of CHD risk prediction.

An interesting approach to a constructing a genetic risk score for CHD prediction was presented by Kathiresan and associates,[74] who examined the additive effect of SNPs that were already known to be associated with LDL-C and HDL-C. The main hypothesis was that although these SNPs were associated with an intermediate phenotype that is already well established for CHD risk assessment, they represent a measurement of lifelong exposure to that particular intermediate phenotype. This exposure has an additional predictive value beyond that of the intermediate phenotype itself, and these SNPs capture that value.

To examine this hypothesis, the investigators used a cohort of 5414 subjects who developed 238 CHD events. When discrimination was examined, the C-statistic was the same for the models with and without the genetic risk score. After reclassification, the NRI was modestly improved. However, reclassification was poor, especially for the 10% to 20% CHD risk category. In our opinion, both discrimination and reclassification in this study did not show a substantial improvement, which suggests that it would be more beneficial to use SNPs that are associated directly with CHD and not through a known intermediate phenotype.

Paynter and colleagues[75] examined the hypothesis suggested by Kathiresan and associates[74] in the Women's Genome Health Study. SNPs were included in a genetic risk score based on a literature search for GWA studies. The genetic risk score was based on 101 SNPs known to be associated with an intermediate phenotype of CHD. A model based on Adult Treatment Panel III variables with and without the genetic risk score showed no improvement in the C-statistic and no significant increase in the NRI (0.5). These results further suggest that genetic risk score models based on SNPs that are not associated with an intermediate phenotype may have better clinical utility for CHD risk prediction.

Summary on the Use of Genetic Markers in Assessment of Risk for Cardiovascular Disease

The use of genetic information for CHD risk prediction is an attractive possibility and has made considerable progress. However, no clinical guidelines currently exist for either the conduct of GWA studies or the assessment of SNPs to refine assessment of CVD risk. Multiple examinations of genetic risk scores as means to improve risk prediction have demonstrated only limited clinical utility. However, the discovery of the 9p21 risk allele has demonstrated that certain genetic markers with large effect size and high population frequency may help improve risk prediction models in the future. As the area of discovery of genetic markers develops, better genetic risk prediction models are possible and may lead to the use of genetic markers to improve risk prediction and prevention of CHD.

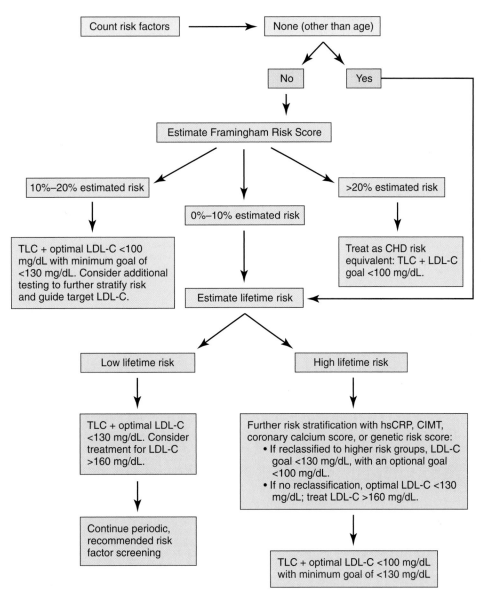

FIGURE 5-1 Risk assessment algorithm. CHD, coronary heart disease; CIMT, carotid intima–media thickness (measured by ultrasound); hsCRP, high-sensitivity C-reactive protein; LDL-C, low-density lipoprotein cholesterol; TLC, therapeutic lifestyle change. *(From Nambi V, Ballantyne CM: "Risky business": ten years is not a lifetime,* Circulation *119:362-364, 2009.)*

CONCLUSION

Cardiovascular risk stratification must be improved, and biomarkers, genetic markers, and imaging provide the best avenue toward this improvement (Figure 5-1).[76] However, all currently available markers (biomarkers and genetic markers) confer only limited to modest improvements in the ability to predict risk. The combination of genetic markers, imaging markers, and biomarkers will probably be used in concert in an attempt to identify at-risk individuals while investigators continue to refine risk prediction with traditional risk factors. However, both the clinical utility and cost-effectiveness of such approaches need to be determined. On the other hand, risk stratification will be of clinical use (for disease management) primarily when treatment plans change with assessed risk or when therapies are available to target novel risk factors. Currently, the only risk factors whose goals vary according to estimated risk are LDL-C level and blood pressure. With the price of statins decreasing, the cost- and risk-benefit ratios may allow a single cut point, as for other risk

factors, in determining the need for statin therapy in the future. Hence, while risk stratification needs continued improvement, simultaneous advances in therapeutics are also crucial for attaining the eventual goals of personalized cardiovascular risk stratification and primary prevention.

REFERENCES

1. Pasternak RC, Abrams J, Greenland P, et al: 34th Bethesda Conference: Task Force #1—identification of coronary heart disease risk: is there a detection gap? *J Am Coll Cardiol* 41:1863-1874, 2003.
2. Grundy SM, Pasternak R, Greenland P, et al: Assessment of cardiovascular risk by use of multiple–risk-factor assessment equations: a statement for healthcare professionals from the American Heart Association and the American College of Cardiology. *Circulation* 100:1481-1492, 1999.
3. Wilson PW, D'Agostino RB, Levy D, et al: Prediction of coronary heart disease using risk factor categories. *Circulation* 97:1837-1847, 1998.
4. Expert Panel on Detection, Evaluation, and Treatment of High Blood Cholesterol in Adults: Executive summary of the third report of the National Cholesterol Education Program (NCEP) Expert Panel on Detection, Evaluation, and Treatment of High Blood Cholesterol in Adults (Adult Treatment Panel III). *JAMA* 285:2486-2497, 2001.

5. Chambless LE, Folsom AR, Sharrett AR, et al: Coronary heart disease risk prediction in the Atherosclerosis Risk in Communities (ARIC) study. *J Clin Epidemiol* 56:880-890, 2003.
6. Wolf PA, D'Agostino RB, Belanger AJ, et al: Probability of stroke: a risk profile from the Framingham study. *Stroke* 22:312-318, 1991.
7. D'Agostino RB, Wolf PA, Belanger AJ, et al: Stroke risk profile: adjustment for antihypertensive medication. The Framingham study. *Stroke* 25:40-43, 1994.
8. Wang TJ, Massaro JM, Levy D, et al: A risk score for predicting stroke or death in individuals with new-onset atrial fibrillation in the community: the Framingham Heart Study. *JAMA* 290:1049-1056, 2003.
9. Chambless LE, Heiss G, Shahar E, et al: Prediction of ischemic stroke risk in the Atherosclerosis Risk in Communities Study. *Am J Epidemiol* 160:259-269, 2004.
10. Nambi V, Hoogeveen RC, Chambless L, et al: Lipoprotein-associated phospholipase A_2 and high-sensitivity C-reactive protein improve the stratification of ischemic stroke risk in the Atherosclerosis Risk in Communities (ARIC) study. *Stroke* 40:376-381, 2009.
10a. D'Agostino RB Sr, Vasan RS, Pencina MJ, et al: General cardiovascular risk profile for use in primary care: the Framingham Heart Study. *Circ* 117:743-753, 2008.
11. Lloyd-Jones DM, Leip EP, Larson MG, et al: Prediction of lifetime risk for cardiovascular disease by risk factor burden at 50 years of age. *Circulation* 113:791-798, 2006.
12. Brotman DJ, Walker E, Lauer MS, et al: In search of fewer independent risk factors. *Arch Intern Med* 165:138-145, 2005.
13. Tzoulaki I, Liberopoulos G, Ioannidis JP: Assessment of claims of improved prediction beyond the Framingham risk score. *JAMA* 302:2345-2352, 2009.
14. Hlatky MA, Greenland P, Arnett DK, et al: Criteria for evaluation of novel markers of cardiovascular risk: a scientific statement from the American Heart Association. *Circulation* 119:2408-2416, 2009.
15. Cook NR: Use and misuse of the receiver operating characteristic curve in risk prediction. *Circulation* 115:928-935, 2007.
16. Harrell FE Jr: *Regression modeling strategies*, New York, 2001, Springer.
17. Pencina MJ, D'Agostino RB Sr, D'Agostino RB Jr, et al: Evaluating the added predictive ability of a new marker: from area under the ROC curve to reclassification and beyond. *Stat Med* 27:157-172, 2008.
18. Ross R: Atherosclerosis—an inflammatory disease. *N Engl J Med* 340:115-126, 1999.
19. Ridker PM, Cushman M, Stampfer MJ, et al: Inflammation, aspirin, and the risk of cardiovascular disease in apparently healthy men. *N Engl J Med* 336:973-979, 1997.
20. Ridker PM, Rifai N, Rose L, et al: Comparison of C-reactive protein and low-density lipoprotein cholesterol levels in the prediction of first cardiovascular events. *N Engl J Med* 347:1557-1565, 2002.
21. Koenig W, Lowel H, Baumert J, et al: C-reactive protein modulates risk prediction based on the Framingham score: implications for future risk assessment: results from a large cohort study in southern Germany. *Circulation* 109:1349-1353, 2004.
22. Ballantyne CM, Hoogeveen RC, Bang H, et al: Lipoprotein-associated phospholipase A_2, high-sensitivity C-reactive protein, and risk for incident coronary heart disease in middle-aged men and women in the Atherosclerosis Risk in Communities (ARIC) study. *Circulation* 109:837-842, 2004.
23. Danesh J, Wheeler JG, Hirschfield GM, et al: C-reactive protein and other circulating markers of inflammation in the prediction of coronary heart disease. *N Engl J Med* 350:1387-1397, 2004.
24. Pai JK, Pischon T, Ma J, et al: Inflammatory markers and the risk of coronary heart disease in men and women. *N Engl J Med* 351:2599-2610, 2004.
25. Ridker PM, Wilson PW, Grundy SM: Should C-reactive protein be added to metabolic syndrome and to assessment of global cardiovascular risk? *Circulation* 109:2818-2825, 2004.
26. Cushman M, Arnold AM, Psaty BM, et al: C-reactive protein and the 10-year incidence of coronary heart disease in older men and women: the Cardiovascular Health Study. *Circulation* 112:25-31, 2005.
27. Ridker PM, Rifai N, Cook NR, et al: Non-HDL cholesterol, apolipoproteins A-I and B_{100}, standard lipid measures, lipid ratios, and CRP as risk factors for cardiovascular disease in women. *JAMA* 294:326-333, 2005.
28. Laaksonen DE, Niskanen L, Nyyssonen K, et al: C-reactive protein in the prediction of cardiovascular and overall mortality in middle-aged men: a population-based cohort study. *Eur Heart J* 26:1783-1789, 2005.
29. Cook NR, Buring JE, Ridker PM: The effect of including C-reactive protein in cardiovascular risk prediction models for women. *Ann Intern Med* 145:21-29, 2006.
30. Ridker PM, Buring JE, Rifai N, et al: Development and validation of improved algorithms for the assessment of global cardiovascular risk in women: the Reynolds risk score. *JAMA* 297:611-619, 2007.
31. Reynolds risk score: calculating heart and stroke risk for women and men (online calculator): http://www.reynoldsriskscore.org. Accessed July 28, 2010.
32. Ridker PM, Paynter NP, Rifai N, et al: C-reactive protein and parental history improve global cardiovascular risk prediction: the Reynolds risk score for men. *Circulation* 118:2243-2251, 4 pp following 2251, 2008.
33. Wilson PW, Pencina M, Jacques P, et al: C-reactive protein and reclassification of cardiovascular risk in the Framingham Heart Study. *Circ Cardiovasc Qual Outcomes* 1:92-97, 2008.
34. Cook NR: Comments on "Evaluating the added predictive ability of a new marker: From area under the ROC curve to reclassification and beyond" by M. J. Pencina et al., *Statistics in Medicine* (DOI: 10.1002/sim.2929). *Stat Med* 27:191-195, 2008.
35. Rana JS, Cote M, Despres JP, et al: Inflammatory biomarkers and the prediction of coronary events among people at intermediate risk: the EPIC-Norfolk prospective population study. *Heart* 95:1682-1687, 2009.
36. Ridker PM, Danielson E, Fonseca FA, et al: Rosuvastatin to prevent vascular events in men and women with elevated C-reactive protein. *N Engl J Med* 359:2195-2207, 2008.
37. Yang EY, Nambi V, Tang Z, et al: Clinical implications of JUPITER (Justification for the Use of statins in Prevention: an Intervention Trial Evaluating Rosuvastatin) in a U.S. population insights from the ARIC (Atherosclerosis Risk in Communities) study. *J Am Coll Cardiol* 54:2388-2395, 2009.
38. Buckley DI, Fu R, Freeman M, et al: C-reactive protein as a risk factor for coronary heart disease: a systematic review and meta-analyses for the U.S. Preventive Services Task Force. *Ann Intern Med* 151:483-495, 2009.
39. Helfand M, Buckley DI, Freeman M, et al: Emerging risk factors for coronary heart disease: a summary of systematic reviews conducted for the U.S. Preventive Services Task Force. *Ann Intern Med* 151:496-507, 2009.
40. Farkouh ME, Bansilal S, Mathew V: CRP has little incremental value over traditional cardiovascular risk factors in risk stratification. *Nat Clin Pract Cardiovasc Med* 4:290-291, 2007.
41. Miller M, Zhan M, Havas S: High attributable risk of elevated C-reactive protein level to conventional coronary heart disease risk factors: the Third National Health and Nutrition Examination Survey. *Arch Intern Med* 165:2063-2068, 2005.
42. Wilson PW, Nam BH, Pencina M, et al: C-reactive protein and risk of cardiovascular disease in men and women from the Framingham Heart Study. *Arch Intern Med* 165:2473-2478, 2005.
43. Folsom AR, Chambless LE, Ballantyne CM, et al: An assessment of incremental coronary risk prediction using C-reactive protein and other novel risk markers: the Atherosclerosis Risk in Communities study. *Arch Intern Med* 166:1368-1373, 2006.
44. Elliott P, Chambers JC, Zhang W, et al: Genetic loci associated with C-reactive protein levels and risk of coronary heart disease. *JAMA* 302:37-48, 2009.
45. Zacho J, Tybjaerg-Hansen A, Jensen JS, et al: Genetically elevated C-reactive protein and ischemic vascular disease. *N Engl J Med* 359:1897-1908, 2008.
46. Myers GL, Christenson RH, Cushman M, et al: National Academy of Clinical Biochemistry Laboratory Medicine Practice guidelines: emerging biomarkers for primary prevention of cardiovascular disease. *Clin Chem* 55:378-384, 2009.
47. Packard CJ, O'Reilly DS, Caslake MJ, et al, for the West of Scotland Coronary Prevention Study Group: Lipoprotein-associated phospholipase A_2 as an independent predictor of coronary heart disease. *N Engl J Med* 343:1148-1155, 2000.
48. Blake GJ, Dada N, Fox JC, et al: A prospective evaluation of lipoprotein-associated phospholipase A_2 levels and the risk of future cardiovascular events in women. *J Am Coll Cardiol* 38:1302-1306, 2001.
49. Blankenberg S, Stengel D, Rupprecht HJ, et al: Plasma PAF-acetylhydrolase in patients with coronary artery disease: results of a cross-sectional analysis. *J Lipid Res* 44:1381-1386, 2003.
50. Koenig W, Khuseyinova N, Lowel H, et al: Lipoprotein-associated phospholipase A_2 adds to risk prediction of incident coronary events by C-reactive protein in apparently healthy middle-aged men from the general population: results from the 14-year follow-up of a large cohort from southern Germany. *Circulation* 110:1903-1908, 2004.
51. Oei HH, van der Meer IM, Hofman A, et al: Lipoprotein-associated phospholipase A_2 activity is associated with risk of coronary heart disease and ischemic stroke: the Rotterdam Study. *Circulation* 111:570-575, 2005.
52. Caslake MJ, Packard CJ: Lipoprotein-associated phospholipase A_2 as a biomarker for coronary disease and stroke. *Nat Clin Pract Cardiovasc Med* 2:529-535, 2005.
52a. The Stabilization of Atherosclerotic Plaque by Initiation of Darapladib Therapy Trial (STABILITY). Available at: http://clinicaltrials.gov/ct2/show/NCT00799903. Accessed September 15, 2010.
53. Di Angelantonio E, Chowdhury R, Sarwar N, et al: B-type natriuretic peptides and cardiovascular risk: systematic review and meta-analysis of 40 prospective studies. *Circulation* 120:2177-2187, 2009.
54. Rutten JH, Mattace-Raso FU, Steyerberg EW, et al: Amino-terminal pro–B-type natriuretic peptide improves cardiovascular and cerebrovascular risk prediction in the population: the Rotterdam study. *Hypertension* 55:785-791, 2010.
54a. Daniels LB, Laughlin GA, Clopton P, et al: Minimally elevated cardiac troponin T and elevated N-terminal pro-B-type natriuretic peptide predict mortality in older adults: results from the Rancho Bernardo Study. *J Am Coll Cardiol* 52:450-459, 2008.
54b. Meuwese MC, Stroes ES, Hazen SL, et al: Serum myeloperoxidase levels are associated with the future risk of coronary artery disease in apparently healthy individuals: the EPIC-Norfolk Prospective Population Study. *J Am Coll Cardiol* 50:159-165, 2007.
55. Koenig W: Update on integrated biomarkers for assessment of long-term risk of cardiovascular complications in initially healthy subjects and patients with manifest atherosclerosis. *Ann Med* 41:332-343, 2009.
56. Wang TJ, Gona P, Larson MG, et al: Multiple biomarkers for the prediction of first major cardiovascular events and death. *N Engl J Med* 355:2631-2639, 2006.
57. Melander O, Newton-Cheh C, Almgren P, et al: Novel and conventional biomarkers for prediction of incident cardiovascular events in the community. *JAMA* 302:49-57, 2009.
58. Zethelius B, Berglund L, Sundstrom J, et al: Use of multiple biomarkers to improve the prediction of death from cardiovascular causes. *N Engl J Med* 358:2107-2116, 2008.
59. Mora S, Otvos JD, Rifai N, et al: Lipoprotein particle profiles by nuclear magnetic resonance compared with standard lipids and apolipoproteins in predicting incident cardiovascular disease in women. *Circulation* 119:931-939, 2009.
59a. Sniderman AD: Applying apoB to the diagnosis and therapy of the atherogenic dyslipoproteinemias: a clinical diagnostic algorithm. *Curr Opin Lipidol* 15:433-438, 2004.
59b. Schork NJ, Murray SS, Frazer KA, Topol EJ: Common vs. rare allele hypotheses for complex diseases. *Curr Opin Genet Dev* 19:212-219, 2009.
60. McPherson R, Pertsemlidis A, Kavaslar N, et al: A common allele on chromosome 9 associated with coronary heart disease. *Science* 316:1488-1491, 2007.
61. Helgadottir A, Thorleifsson G, Manolescu A, et al: A common variant on chromosome 9p21 affects the risk of myocardial infarction. *Science* 316:1491-1493, 2007.
62. Samani NJ, Erdmann J, Hall AS, et al: Genomewide association analysis of coronary artery disease. *N Engl J Med* 357:443-453, 2007.
63. Schunkert H, Gotz A, Braund P, et al: Repeated replication and a prospective meta-analysis of the association between chromosome 9p21.3 and coronary artery disease. *Circulation* 117:1675-1684, 2008.

64. Wellcome Trust Case Control Consortium: Genome-wide association study of 14,000 cases of seven common diseases and 3,000 shared controls. *Nature* 447:661-678, 2007.

65. Zhou L, Zhang X, He M, et al: Associations between single nucleotide polymorphisms on chromosome 9p21 and risk of coronary heart disease in Chinese Han population. *Arterioscler Thromb Vasc Biol* 28:2085-2089, 2008.

66. Assimes TL, Knowles JW, Basu A, et al: Susceptibility locus for clinical and subclinical coronary artery disease at chromosome 9p21 in the multi-ethnic ADVANCE study. *Hum Mol Genet* 17:2320-2328, 2008.

67. Shen GQ, Li L, Rao S, et al: Four SNPs on chromosome 9p21 in a South Korean population implicate a genetic locus that confers high cross-race risk for development of coronary artery disease. *Arterioscler Thromb Vasc Biol* 28:360-365, 2008.

68. Shen GQ, Rao S, Martinelli N, et al: Association between four SNPs on chromosome 9p21 and myocardial infarction is replicated in an Italian population. *J Hum Genet* 53:144-150, 2008.

69. Visel A, Zhu Y, May D, et al: Targeted deletion of the 9p21 non-coding coronary artery disease risk interval in mice. *Nature* 464:409-412, 2010.

70. Paynter NP, Chasman DI, Buring JE, et al: Cardiovascular disease risk prediction with and without knowledge of genetic variation at chromosome 9p21.3. *Ann Intern Med* 150:65-72, 2009.

71. Brautbar A, Ballantyne CM, Lawson K, et al: Impact of adding a single allele in the 9p21 locus to traditional risk factors on reclassification of coronary heart disease risk and implications for lipid-modifying therapy in the Atherosclerosis Risk in Communities (ARIC) study. *Circ Cardiovasc Genet* 2:279-285, 2009.

72. Talmud PJ, Cooper JA, Palmen J, et al: Chromosome 9p21.3 coronary heart disease locus genotype and prospective risk of CHD in healthy middle-aged men. *Clin Chem* 54:467-474, 2008.

73. Morrison AC, Bare LA, Chambless LE, et al: Prediction of coronary heart disease risk using a genetic risk score: the Atherosclerosis Risk in Communities study. *Am J Epidemiol* 166:28-35, 2007.

74. Kathiresan S, Melander O, Anevski D, et al: Polymorphisms associated with cholesterol and risk of cardiovascular events. *N Engl J Med* 358:1240-1249, 2008.

75. Paynter NP, Chasman DI, Pare G, et al: Association between a literature-based genetic risk score and cardiovascular events in women. *JAMA* 303:631-637, 2010.

76. Nambi V, Ballantyne CM: "Risky business": ten years is not a lifetime. *Circulation* 119:362-364, 2009.

Advanced Risk Assessment in Patients with Kidney and Inflammatory Diseases

Raymond Oliva, Tamar Polonsky, and George L. Bakris

KEY POINTS

- The number of patients around the world with chronic kidney disease (CKD) has increased alarmingly.

- Even mild to moderate worsening of kidney function has become an independent risk factor for cardiovascular morbidity and mortality.

- In the future, novel risk markers—such as cystatin C, adiponectin, and possibly new inflammatory markers other than C-reactive protein (CRP) and microalbuminuria—may be used to assess risk for cardiovascular events.

- Management of patients with CKD is important for protection against both progression of kidney disease and progression of cardiovascular disease.

- Close monitoring and follow-up are key in the therapeutic management of patients with CKD.

Chronic kidney disease (CKD), defined as persistent kidney damage reflected by a glomerular filtration rate (GFR) of less than 60 mL/min/1.73 m^2 for 3 months,[1] is a major public health problem worldwide. More than 8 million people in the United States have stage 3 CKD, and the number is rising. This trend in CKD is reflected around the world, not just in the United States.[2]

Patients with stage 3 or higher CKD have higher rates of cardiovascular morbidity, manifested by higher incidences of heart failure, arrhythmias, and myocardial infarctions. Progression of CKD in these patients to end-stage kidney disease—defined as a GFR of less than 10 mL/min/1.73 m^2—further increases the risk for cardiovascular events; the annual mortality rate has improved since 2000 but remains approximately 19% per year.[3] In earlier stage nephropathy (i.e., GFR >60 and <90 mL/min/1.73 m^2), less is known regarding cardiovascular risk.[4-6] Investigators increasingly appreciate, however, the fact that risk markers such as microalbuminuria that are associated with vascular inflammation are indicative of higher cardiovascular risk (Table 6-1).[7]

PATHOPHYSIOLOGY

Various abnormalities are commonly observed in patients with CKD that may enhance their risk for cardiovascular disease (CVD) events. Although the precise mechanism by which CKD increases CVD risk is not fully elucidated, most cases of CKD are clearly associated with increased oxidative stress and magnified inflammatory responses at the level of the vasculature. Endothelial dysfunction is an early event in people with CKD, and microalbuminuria is associated with the presence of endothelial dysfunction.[7] In most patients with advanced CKD, atherosclerosis is accelerated and characterized by more advanced, heavily calcified plaques that extend to both the intima and medial layers of the coronary vessels.[8,9] Increased expression of several cytokines, as well as of macrophages, plays a role in the evolution of the plaque development.

Several inflammatory markers have been implicated as potential triggers of atherosclerotic complications. High-sensitivity C-reactive protein (hs-CRP) is considered a biomarker of chronic systemic inflammation, as well as a mediator of atherosclerosis. Of patients with end-stage kidney disease, 20% to 50% have been shown to have elevated CRP levels.[10,11] Hyperhomocysteinemia is also a predictor of future CVD events in patients with established coronary artery disease and in patients with type 2 diabetes, as well as those undergoing dialysis.[12,13] Adiponectin level also plays an important role in modulating atherosclerosis and is decreased in people with impaired glucose homeostasis or diabetes. In the Mild and Moderate Kidney Disease (MMKD) study group, patients with low adiponectin levels experienced significant cardiovascular events.[14]

The amount of nitric oxide present is reflective of how well the endothelium is functioning. It has a protective role in that it inhibits vascular muscle cell proliferation, platelet aggregability, and the adhesion of monocytes to the endothelium. The enzyme responsible for the genesis of nitric oxide can be inhibited by endogenous methyl arginine production such as asymmetric dimethylarginine (ADMA). Levels of ADMA are postulated to be increased in patients with advanced nephropathy, and such elevation is recognized as a putative biomarker in cardiovascular and kidney disease.[15] Two large clinical trials, the Coronary Artery Risk Determination investigating the Influence of ADMA Concentration (CARDIAC) and the AtheroGene Study, demonstrated that ADMA is an independent risk factor for cardiovascular disease. In these studies, baseline ADMA levels were independently predictive of cardiovascular events.[16,17]

Hypertension is a complex phenotype because neurohumoral factors such as angiotensin II, norepinephrine, and other cytokines, as well as chronic volume overload, exert inflammatory and growth-promoting effects in the cardiovascular system.[18] Angiotensin II is a proinflammatory substance and a recognized growth

TABLE 6–1	Risk Factors and Novel Risk Markers of Chronic Kidney Disease in Predicting Cardiovascular Morbidity and Mortality
Risk Factors for Cardiovascular Disease	**Novel Risk Markers for Cardiovascular Disease**
Older age	Cystatin C level
Race	C-reactive protein level
Smoking history	Microalbuminuria
Hypertension	Adiponectin level
Diabetes	Albumin level
Dyslipidemia	Asymmetric dimethylarginine
Anemia	
Chronic kidney disease	

promoter. The sympathetic system not only is a major regulator of cardiovascular function but also affects immune response, as does angiotensin II. It is interesting to note that in patients with CKD, circulating levels of norepinephrine are directly related to the muscular component of the left ventricle. Norepinephrine levels are also a strong and independent predictor of death from cardiovascular causes. Chronic volume overload is a major stressor, and in the long run, the deleterious effects of volume overload depend on the fact that hemodynamic burden activates a series of adaptive processes that modify the very structure of the myocardium.[18]

The aforementioned factors—together with retention of toxins, increased calcium intake, and decreased phosphate excretion; abnormalities in bone mineral metabolism; and poor nutrition state—all increase inflammatory markers and potentiate vascular disease.[14,19-21]

RISK IN COMMUNITY-BASED POPULATIONS

CKD itself is a major risk factor for cardiovascular events. In many cohort studies, risk for coronary heart disease (CHD) has been assessed in relation to changes in CKD stage. The findings of these studies have led to the formation of recommendations from both The National Kidney Foundation and the American College of Cardiology/American Heart Association that CKD be considered as a CHD risk equivalent. Many physicians may not be aware that increases in risk for CHD parallel reductions in GFR, highest risk being at GFR values lower than 45 mL/min.[4]

The Framingham Heart Study[22] is one prospective, community-based study of the burden of CVD in patients with kidney disease. The study has revealed that the majority of patients with mild to moderate CKD are older, are more likely to be obese, have lower levels of high-density lipoprotein (HDL), and higher triglyceride levels. They also have a high prevalence of hypertension, diabetes, and elevated levels of low-density lipoprotein (LDL). The CKD population is less likely to achieve optimal control of blood pressure and controlled hemoglobin A1c concentrations of less than 7%.

Another large cohort study involved the Kaiser Permanente Renal Registry. Among 1,120,295 adults within a large, integrated system of health care delivery, the GFR was estimated.[4] After adjustment, the risk of death increased as the estimated GFR decreased below 60 mL/min/1.73 m². The adjusted hazard ratio for cardiovascular events also increased inversely with the estimated GFR. The adjusted risk of hospitalization with a reduced estimated GFR followed a similar pattern. The findings highlighted the clinical and public health importance of CKD. In the Atherosclerosis Risk in Communities (ARIC) study,[23] participants with a GFR of 15 to 59 mL/min/1.73 m² (hazard ratio, 1.38; 95% confidence interval, 1.02 to 1.87) and 60 to 89 mL/min/1.73 m² (hazard ratio, 1.16; 95% confidence interval, 1.00 to 1.34) had an increased adjusted risk for atherosclerotic CVD events, in comparison with subjects with normal GFR levels, after a mean follow-up of 6.2 years.

In the National Health and Nutrition Examination Survey (NHANES), rates of CVD-related mortality were 4.1, 8.6, and 20.5 deaths per 1000 person-years among participants with estimated GFRs of higher than 90, 70 to 89, and lower than 70 mL/min/1.73 m², respectively. Those with an estimated GFR lower than 70 mL/min/1.73 m² had significantly higher relatively risks of death from cardiovascular disease (1.7; 95% confidence interval, 1.3 to 2.1) and from all causes.[24]

CARDIOVASCULAR RISK FACTORS IN PATIENTS WITH CHRONIC KIDNEY DISEASE

CVD is the major cause of morbidity and mortality among patients with CKD. Most patients share risk factors, including diabetes, hypertension, obesity, lipid abnormalities, and smoking (see Table 6-1). Even people with early stage 3 nephropathy (i.e., estimated GFR < 60 mL/min/1.73 m²) have a higher risk of mortality than those with a GFR above 60 mL/min/1.73 m².

Diabetes is the most common cause of CKD, accounting for nearly 50% of all new cases of renal replacement therapy. In a cohort of Chinese patients with type 2 diabetes who did not have macrovascular disease or end-stage renal disease, all-cause mortality increased from 1.2% to 18.3% as kidney function deteriorated from stage 1 to stage 4.[25] Hypertension is another modifiable risk for CVD. The degree and duration of hypertension strongly influence outcomes and also accelerate CKD progression.[26] Most patients with CKD have both hypertension and diabetes as comorbid conditions, and the effect on CVD risk is more than additive.

Obesity is a major global health concern and may precede the development of many CVD risk factors, including diabetes, hypertension, and dyslipidemia. In the Framingham Heart Study,[27] obesity was noted to be associated with increased risk of developing stage 3 CKD during nearly 20 years of follow-up. This finding suggests that the association of obesity with stage 3 CKD may be mediated by vascular disease risk factors.

Patients with CKD are at high risk for insulin resistance and other features of the classical metabolic syndrome. The association of higher body mass index (BMI), insulin resistance, hyperglycemia, and hypertriglyceridemia supports the notion that early in the disease state, other well-known CVD risk factors are present and may be magnified by the presence of advanced CKD.[9]

Overweight and obesity are also associated with increased risk of proteinuria and risk of worsening kidney function, inasmuch as increased levels of proteinuria are associated with faster CKD progression.[28] Conversely, in patients undergoing dialysis, the relationship is different: The greater the BMI with better nutrition, the lower the incidence of CVD events. In short, survival is higher in patients with end-stage kidney disease who have higher BMIs.

The sequelae of CKD, such as anemia and low active vitamin D levels, may also contribute to the increased risk for CVD.[29,30] In a registry cohort study of 5549 adults hospitalized with acute myocardial infarction or unstable angina, profound anemia was independently associated with increased mortality rate (hazard ratio, 1.8 for hemoglobin levels of <9 vs. >12 g/dL) among patients with an estimated GFR of 30 to 59.[31]

TABLE 6–2 | **Clinical Trials of Lipid-Lowering Therapy in Patients with Chronic Kidney Disease**

Trial	Design	Population	Sample Size	Intervention	Duration	Outcome
Pravastatin Pooling Project (PPP)	Post hoc subanalysis of West of Scotland Coronary Prevention Study (WOSCOPS), Cholesterol and Recurrent Events (CARE), and Long-term Intervention with Pravastatin in Ischaemic Disease (LIPID)	Moderate CKD (CG-GFR, 30-59 mL/min/1.73 min^2	4491	Pravastatin, 40 mg/day	≈5 years	Decile risk (HR, 0.77) of adjusted incidence of primary outcome
Heart Protection Study (HPS)	Post hoc subanalysis	CKD (serum creatinine clearance >110 µmol/L for women and >130 µmol/L for men but <200 µmol/L)	1329	Simvastatin, 40 mg/day	5 years	Decile risk (HR, 0.72) of major vascular events
Anglo-Scandinavian Cardiac Outcomes Trial–Lipid Lowering Arm (ASCOT-LLA)	Post hoc subanalysis	Renal dysfunction (microalbuminuria, proteinuria)	6571	Atorvastatin, 10 mg/day	3.3 years	Decile risk (HR, 0.61) of primary endpoint
Veterans' Affairs High Density Lipoprotein Intervention Trial (VA-HIT)	Post hoc, subanalysis	Predialysis CKD	1046	Gemfibrozil, 1200 mg/day	5.3	Decile risk (HR, 0.73) of primary outcome and decile risk (HR, 0.74) of combined outcome of coronary death, nonfatal MI, or stroke
Study of Heart and Renal Protection (SHARP)	Prospective double-blind RCT	Predialysis status Hemodialysis Peritoneal dialysis	9000 (6000 before dialysis and 3000 undergoing dialysis)	Simvastatin, 20 mg, and ezetimibe, 10 mg	4 years	Major vascular events, rates of progression to ESR in patients before dialysis

CG-GFR, glomerular filtration rate calculated with Cockcroft-Gault equation; CKD, chronic kidney disease; ESR, end-stage renal disease; HR, hazard ratio; MI, myocardial infarction; RCT, randomized controlled trial.

Elevated cholesterol levels are very prevalent among people with estimated GFR values lower than 60 mL/min/1.73 m^2. Lowering cholesterol levels in people who have diabetes and an estimated GFR higher than 60 mL/min/1.73 m^2 is beneficial, as observed in the Scandinavian Simvastatin Survival Study (4S), in which patients with type 2 diabetes had a 2.5-fold greater risk for coronary artery disease than did nondiabetic patients.[32,33] Ongoing trials are currently being conducted to examine the benefit of lowering cholesterol levels in early- to moderate-stage CKD[34]; however, it is clear that lowering cholesterol levels in patients with advanced-stage CKD who are undergoing dialysis does not alter CVD outcomes.[35,36] Thus, early use of statins slows nephropathy progression and reduces CVD risk, whereas late use once dialysis has been instituted fails to alter CVD risk (Table 6-2).

There is also a relationship between cardiovascular disease and microalbuminuria.[37] In a secondary analysis of the Multiple Risk Factor Interventional Trial, the presence of minimal proteinuria conferred nearly a 2.5-fold greater risk for cardiovascular morbidity events.[38] The presence of microalbuminuria in patients with diabetes is a useful marker for patients at greatest risk for the development of macrovascular disease.[7] In addition, post hoc analyses from the Losartan Intervention For Endpoint reduction in hypertension (LIFE) trial clearly demonstrated that reduction in albuminuria progression over time is associated with a lower incidence of CVD outcomes.[39]

ASSOCIATION OF CHRONIC KIDNEY DISEASE AFTER MYOCARDIAL INFARCTION

There is a significant rise in mortality among CKD patients after an acute coronary event. The prognosis of patients after acute myocardial infarction may be poor partly because of a relatively increased number of presentations, resulting from underdiagnosis and undertreatment.[40,41] For example, the presence of dyspnea in a patient with end-stage renal disease may be mistakenly attributed to volume overload. In a survey, 44% of patients undergoing dialysis present with chest pains, in comparison with 68% of patients with CKD who are not undergoing dialysis.[40] Medications are underused, and aggressive therapy such as thrombolysis and angiography is not prescribed because of further increase of creatinine levels, which leads to acute renal failure. As a result, the rate of 1-year mortality after an acute myocardial infarction in patients with CKD is approximately 50%.[42] The Cooperative Cardiovascular Project performed a cohort study with 130,099 elderly patients with mild to moderate CKD who had myocardial infarctions.[43] The rates of 1-year mortality were 46% among patients with stage 3 CKD (creatinine level, 1.5 to 2.4 mg/dL) and 66% among patients with stage 4 CKD (creatinine level, 2.5 to 3.9 mg/dL). Problems with the management of these types of patients arose because they received less therapy—whether aspirin, beta blockers, thrombolytic therapy, angiography, or angioplasty—during hospitalization.

In another retrospective cohort study, outcomes after an acute myocardial infarction were compared between patients with varying levels of CKD and patients without CKD. In-hospital mortality rates were 2% among patients with normal kidney function, 6% among those with CKD, 14% among those with advanced CKD, 21% among those with severe kidney failure, and 30% among those with end-stage kidney disease. Postdischarge death was less likely in patients who received acute reperfusion therapy (odds ratio, 0.7), aspirin (odds ratio, 0.7), and beta blocker therapy (odds ratio, 0.7).[44]

MEASURES TO PREVENT CARDIOVASCULAR EVENTS IN PATIENTS WITH CHRONIC KIDNEY DISEASE

Risk modification and lifestyle changes can decrease cardiac events in patients with CKD. In general, similar conditions apply to patients who have CKD and those who do not with regard to smoking cessation, maintaining ideal body weight, active lifestyle, and glycemic control in diabetes.

The treatment of hypertension is important in patients with CKD to protect against both progressive kidney disease and cardiovascular disease. As stated in the guidelines of the Joint National Committee on Prevention, Detection, Evaluation, and Treatment of High Blood Pressure,[45] the goal for blood pressure in proteinuric CKD is lower than 130/80 mm Hg to slow the rate of progression of kidney disease. Angiotensin-converting enzyme inhibitors and angiotensin receptor blockers have been shown to significantly reduce cardiovascular morbidity and mortality in multiple, large, prospective randomized trials.[46] They have a dose-dependent beneficial effect on atherosclerosis progression and may prevent the development and recurrence of atrial fibrillation. The Perindopril Protection against Recurrent Stroke Study (PROGRESS) had a post hoc analysis in which 29% of patients with creatinine clearance of less than 60 mL/min were evaluated; the use of perindopril, an antihypertensive therapy, reduced the risk of all cardiovascular events in patients with CKD.[47]

The use of lipid-lowering agents such as statins, as previously discussed, is very useful in slowing nephropathy and reducing CVD risk among patients with an estimated GFR above 30 mL/min, but these agents were not useful in altering CVD events in patients undergoing dialysis (see Table 6-2). The 2003 Kidney Disease Outcomes Quality Initiative (K/DOQI) guidelines recommend a goal LDL cholesterol level of less than 100 mg/dL.[48] Hypertriglyceridemia and low HDL concentrations are common lipoprotein abnormalities in patients with CKD. Fibrates effectively lower triglycerides and elevate HDL-cholesterol concentrations, which could complement the effectiveness of statins. The Veterans' Affairs High Density Lipoprotein Interventional Trial (VA-HIT) demonstrated lower cardiovascular events with gemfibrozil in patients with creatinine clearance of less than 75 mL/min.[49]

Data on the use of aspirin in patients with chronic kidney disease is sparse. Three studies have shown the benefit of giving aspirin to patients with CKD. A retrospective observational analysis from the Dialysis Outcomes and Practice Patterns Study (DOPPS) revealed that aspirin resulted in a decreased risk of stroke (relative risk, 0.82) in all patients undergoing dialysis.[50] A secondary subgroup analysis of the Hypertension Optimal Treatment (HOT) study found that in patients with serum creatinine levels higher than 1.3 mg/dL, low-dose aspirin (75 mg/day) significantly reduced the numbers of cardiovascular events and myocardial

infarctions.[51] The safety of aspirin was evaluated in the first United Kingdom Heart and Renal Protection (UK-HARP I) study.[52] It was not associated with an increased risk of major bleeding in comparison with placebo. The National Kidney Foundation suggests that the prescription of low-dose aspirin is probably safe in most patients with CKD.[1]

CONCLUSION

The number of CKD patients around the world has increased alarmingly. Even mild to moderate worsening of kidney function has become an independent risk factor for cardiovascular morbidity and mortality. In the future, novel risk markers such as cystatin C, adiponectin, and possibly new inflammatory markers other than hs-CRP and microalbuminuria may be used to assess risk for cardiovascular events. Management of patients with CKD is important for protection against both progression of kidney disease and progression of cardiovascular disease. Close monitoring and follow-up are key in the therapeutic management of patients with CKD.

REFERENCES

1. Goolsby MJ: National Kidney Foundation Guidelines for chronic kidney disease: evaluation, classification, and stratification. *J Am Acad Nurse Pract* 14:238-242, 2002.
2. Bakris GL, Ritz E: The message for World Kidney Day 2009. Hypertension and kidney disease: a marriage that should be prevented. *Am J Nephrol* 30:95-98, 2009.
3. Coresh J, Astor B, Sarnak MJ: Evidence for increased cardiovascular disease risk in patients with chronic kidney disease. *Curr Opin Nephrol Hypertens* 13:73-81, 2004.
4. Go AS, Chertow GM, Fan D, et al: Chronic kidney disease and the risks of death, cardiovascular events, and hospitalization. *N Engl J Med* 351:1296-1305, 2004.
5. Ruilope LM, Salvetti A, Jamerson K, et al: Renal function and intensive lowering of blood pressure in hypertensive participants of the hypertension optimal treatment (HOT) study. *J Am Soc Nephrol* 12:218-225, 2001.
6. Boos CJ: Cardiovascular protection with ACE inhibitors—more HOPE for EUROPA? *Med Sci Monit* 10:SR23-SR28, 2004.
7. Khosla N, Sarafidis PA, Bakris GL: Microalbuminuria. *Clin Lab Med* 26:635-653, vi-vii, 2006.
8. Schwarz U, Buzello M, Ritz E, et al: Morphology of coronary atherosclerotic lesions in patients with end-stage renal failure. *Nephrol Dial Transplant* 15:218-223, 2000.
9. Chan DT, Irish AB, Dogra GK, et al: Dyslipidaemia and cardiorenal disease: mechanisms, therapeutic opportunities and clinical trials. *Atherosclerosis* 196:823-834, 2008.
10. Grootendorst DC, de Jager DJ, Brandenburg VM, et al: Excellent agreement between C-reactive protein measurement methods in end-stage renal disease patients—no additional power for mortality prediction with high-sensitivity CRP. *Nephrol Dial Transplant* 22:3277-3284, 2007.
11. Lacson E Jr, Levin NW: C-reactive protein and end-stage renal disease. *Semin Dial* 17:438-448, 2004.
12. Heinz J, Kropf S, Luley C, et al: Homocysteine as a risk factor for cardiovascular disease in patients treated by dialysis: a meta-analysis. *Am J Kidney Dis* 54:478-489, 2009.
13. Menon V, Sarnak MJ, Greene T, et al: Relationship between homocysteine and mortality in chronic kidney disease. *Circulation* 113:1572-1577, 2006.
14. Becker B, Kronenberg F, Kielstein JT, et al: Renal insulin resistance syndrome, adiponectin and cardiovascular events in patients with kidney disease: the Mild and Moderate Kidney Disease Study. *J Am Soc Nephrol* 16:1091-1098, 2005.
15. Jacobi J, Tsao PS: Asymmetrical dimethylarginine in renal disease: limits of variation or variation limits? A systematic review. *Am J Nephrol* 28:224-237, 2008.
16. Schulze F, Lenzen H, Hanefeld C, et al: Asymmetric dimethylarginine is an independent risk factor for coronary heart disease: results from the multicenter Coronary Artery Risk Determination investigating the Influence of ADMA Concentration (CARDIAC) study. *Am Heart J* 152:493-498, 2006.
17. Schnabel R, Blankenberg S, Lubos E, et al: Asymmetric dimethylarginine and the risk of cardiovascular events and death in patients with coronary artery disease: results from the AtheroGene Study. *Circ Res* 97:e53-e59, 2005.
18. Zoccali C, Mallamaci F, Tripepi G: Novel cardiovascular risk factors in end-stage renal disease. *J Am Soc Nephrol* 15(suppl 1):S77-S80, 2004.
19. Horl WH, Cohen JJ, Harrington JT, et al: Atherosclerosis and uremic retention solutes. *Kidney Int* 66:1719-1731, 2004.
20. Cooper BA, Penne EL, Bartlett LH, et al: Protein malnutrition and hypoalbuminemia as predictors of vascular events and mortality in ESRD, *Am J Kidney Dis* 43:61-66, 2004.
21. Becker BN, Himmelfarb J, Henrich WL, et al: Reassessing the cardiac risk profile in chronic hemodialysis patients: a hypothesis on the role of oxidant stress and other non-traditional cardiac risk factors. *J Am Soc Nephrol* 8:475-486, 1997.
22. Parikh NI, Hwang SJ, Larson MG, et al: Cardiovascular disease risk factors in chronic kidney disease: overall burden and rates of treatment and control. *Arch Intern Med* 166:1884-1891, 2006.
23. Manjunath G, Tighiouart H, Ibrahim H, et al: Level of kidney function as a risk factor for atherosclerotic cardiovascular outcomes in the community. *J Am Coll Cardiol* 41:47-55, 2003.
24. Muntner P, He J, Hamm L, et al: Renal insufficiency and subsequent death resulting from cardiovascular disease in the United States. *J Am Soc Nephrol* 13:745-753, 2002.

25. So WY, Kong AP, Ma RC, et al: Glomerular filtration rate, cardiorenal end points, and all-cause mortality in type 2 diabetic patients. *Diabetes Care* 29:2046-2052, 2006.

26. Norris K, Bourgoigne J, Gassman J, et al: Cardiovascular outcomes in the African American Study of Kidney Disease and Hypertension (AASK) trial. *Am J Kidney Dis* 48:739-751, 2006.

27. Foster MC, Hwang SJ, Larson MG, et al: Overweight, obesity, and the development of stage 3 CKD: the Framingham Heart Study. *Am J Kidney Dis* 52:39-48, 2008.

28. Kalaitzidis RG, Bakris GL: Should proteinuria reduction be the criterion for antihypertensive drug selection for patients with kidney disease? *Curr Opin Nephrol Hypertens* 18:386-391, 2009.

29. Astor BC, Coresh J, Heiss G, et al: Kidney function and anemia as risk factors for coronary heart disease and mortality: the Atherosclerosis Risk in Communities (ARIC) study. *Am Heart J* 151:492-500, 2006.

30. Levin A, Li YC: Vitamin D and its analogues: do they protect against cardiovascular disease in patients with kidney disease? *Kidney Int* 68:1973-1981, 2005.

31. Keough-Ryan TM, Kiberd BA, Dipchand CS, et al: Outcomes of acute coronary syndrome in a large Canadian cohort: impact of chronic renal insufficiency, cardiac interventions, and anemia. *Am J Kidney Dis* 46:845-855, 2005.

32. Huskey J, Lindenfeld J, Cook T, et al: Effect of simvastatin on kidney function loss in patients with coronary heart disease: findings from the Scandinavian Simvastatin Survival Study (4S). *Atherosclerosis* 205:202-206, 2009.

33. Pyorala K, Ballantyne CM, Gumbiner B, et al: Reduction of cardiovascular events by simvastatin in nondiabetic coronary heart disease patients with and without the metabolic syndrome: subgroup analyses of the Scandinavian Simvastatin Survival Study (4S). *Diabetes Care* 27:1735-1740, 2004.

34. Landray M, Baigent C, Leaper C, et al: The second United Kingdom Heart and Renal Protection (UK-HARP-II) study: a randomized controlled study of the biochemical safety and efficacy of adding ezetimibe to simvastatin as initial therapy among patients with CKD. *Am J Kidney Dis* 47:385-395, 2006.

35. Wanner C, Krane V, Marz W, et al: Atorvastatin in patients with type 2 diabetes mellitus undergoing hemodialysis. *N Engl J Med* 353:238-248, 2005.

36. Fellstrom BC, Jardine AG, Schmieder RE, et al: Rosuvastatin and cardiovascular events in patients undergoing hemodialysis. *N Engl J Med* 360:1395-1407, 2009.

37. Keane WF: Proteinuria: its clinical importance and role in progressive renal disease. *Am J Kidney Dis* 35:S97-S105, 2000.

38. Grimm RH Jr, Svendsen KH, Kasiske B, et al: Proteinuria is a risk factor for mortality over 10 years of follow-up. MRFIT Research Group. Multiple Risk Factor Intervention Trial. *Kidney Int Suppl* 63:S10-S14, 1997.

39. Ibsen H, Olsen MH, Wachtell K, et al: Does albuminuria predict cardiovascular outcomes on treatment with losartan versus atenolol in patients with diabetes, hypertension, and left ventricular hypertrophy? The LIFE study. *Diabetes Care* 29:595-600, 2006.

40. Herzog CA: How to manage the renal patient with coronary heart disease: the agony and the ecstasy of opinion-based medicine. *J Am Soc Nephrol* 14:2556-2572, 2003.

41. Collins AJ, Li S, Gilbertson DT, et al: Chronic kidney disease and cardiovascular disease in the Medicare population. *Kidney Int Suppl* (87):S24-S31, 2003.

42. Shik J, Parfrey PS: The clinical epidemiology of cardiovascular disease in chronic kidney disease. *Curr Opin Nephrol Hypertens* 14:550-557, 2005.

43. Shlipak MG, Heidenreich PA, Noguchi H, et al: Association of renal insufficiency with treatment and outcomes after myocardial infarction in elderly patients. *Ann Intern Med* 137:555-562, 2002.

44. Wright RS, Reeder GS, Herzog CA, et al: Acute myocardial infarction and renal dysfunction: a high-risk combination. *Ann Intern Med* 137:563-570, 2002.

45. Chobanian AV, Bakris GL, Black HR, et al: The Seventh Report of the Joint National Committee on Prevention, Detection, Evaluation, and Treatment of High Blood Pressure: the JNC 7 report. *JAMA* 289:2560-2572, 2003.

46. Ryan MJ, Tuttle KR: Elevations in serum creatinine with RAAS blockade: why isn't it a sign of kidney injury? *Curr Opin Nephrol Hypertens* 17:443-449, 2008.

47. Perkovic V, Ninomiya T, Arima H, et al: Chronic kidney disease, cardiovascular events, and the effects of perindopril-based blood pressure lowering: data from the PROGRESS study. *J Am Soc Nephrol* 18:2766-2772, 2007.

48. Kidney Disease Outcomes Quality Initiative (K/DOQI) Group: K/DOQI clinical practice guidelines for management of dyslipidemias in patients with kidney disease. *Am J Kidney Dis* 41(4 suppl 3):I-IV, S1-S91, 2003.

49. Tonelli M, Collins D, Robins S, et al: Gemfibrozil for secondary prevention of cardiovascular events in mild to moderate chronic renal insufficiency. *Kidney Int* 66:1123-1130, 2004.

50. Ethier J, Bragg-Gresham JL, Piera L, et al: Aspirin prescription and outcomes in hemodialysis patients: the Dialysis Outcomes and Practice Patterns Study (DOPPS), *Am J Kidney Dis* 50:602-611, 2007.

51. Hansson L, Zanchetti A, Carruthers SG, et al: Effects of intensive blood-pressure lowering and low-dose aspirin in patients with hypertension: principal results of the Hypertension Optimal Treatment (HOT) randomised trial. HOT Study Group. *Lancet* 351:1755-1762, 1998.

52. Baigent C, Landray M, Leaper C, et al: First United Kingdom Heart and Renal Protection (UK-HARP-I) study: biochemical efficacy and safety of simvastatin and safety of low-dose aspirin in chronic kidney disease. *Am J Kidney Dis* 45:473-484, 2005.

Atherothrombosis and Antiplatelet Therapy

CHAPTER 7

Antiplatelet Therapy

Jessica M. Peña and Deepak L. Bhatt

KEY POINTS

- Six randomized trials of aspirin therapy for the primary prevention of cardiovascular disease have demonstrated a 12% relative reduction in the risk of major adverse cardiovascular events.

- In large randomized trials of secondary prevention, aspirin has resulted in a 25% reduction in serious vascular events.

- For a decision of whether to initiate aspirin in a primary prevention setting, current U.S. Preventive Services Task Force guidelines recommend incorporating an estimation of an individual patient's risk of hemorrhage.

- Dual-antiplatelet therapy with clopidogrel and aspirin is the mainstay of treatment after acute coronary syndromes and percutaneous coronary intervention.

- Clopidogrel resistance is an increasingly recognized phenomenon that underscores the importance of newer antiplatelet agents such as prasugrel and the oral $P2Y_{12}$ receptor antagonist ticagrelor.

- Novel agents targeting the platelet $P2Y_{12}$ and thrombin receptors are currently being studied in phase II and III trials and hold promise for the future.

Platelet activation plays a central role in the development of atherothrombosis, and antiplatelet therapy is thus a cornerstone of prevention and treatment of cardiovascular disease. Initial platelet activation and rapid platelet amplification occurs in response to potent agonists such as thromboxane A_2, adenosine diphosphate (ADP), and thrombin.[1] Investigators' understanding of these pathways has led to the development of pivotal pharmacotherapies for treating cardiovascular disease. For example, the thromboxane inhibitor aspirin has resulted in substantial reductions in cardiovascular morbidity, and some authors have estimated that it could avert 100,000 vascular deaths per year.[2] In this chapter, we review the mechanism of action, data from primary and secondary prevention trials, and guidelines for antiplatelet agents currently in widespread use. We also discuss ongoing trials of novel antiplatelet agents directed at platelet targets such as the ADP receptor and the less exploited thrombin receptor.

ASPIRIN

Mechanism of Action

Acetylsalicylic acid, or aspirin, is the most widely used antiplatelet agent in the treatment of cardiovascular disease. Aspirin exerts its principal antiplatelet effect by acetylating a serine residue on the cyclooxygenase (COX) or prostaglandin H synthase enzyme and thus irreversibly inhibiting the action of this enzyme.[3] After exposure to aspirin, the anucleate platelet is largely unable to synthesize COX during its 7- to 10-day lifespan.[4] COX enzymes, which exist in at least two isoforms, are responsible for production of

prostaglandins and thromboxane from arachidonic acid. Preferential inhibition of COX-1 results in decreased production of thromboxane A_2, a potent mediator of platelet aggregation.[5] Other potential mechanisms of action include inhibition of intrinsic nitric oxide synthase[6] and inhibition of transcription factors involved in inflammation[7] (Figure 7-1).

Secondary Prevention

The salutary effect of aspirin for the secondary prevention of cardiovascular disease is well established. In the first small studies to examine this relationship in patients with a history of myocardial infarction, the results were suggestive of a mortality benefit but were statistically inconclusive.[8-10] More convincing evidence arose from the Antiplatelet Trialists' Collaboration (ATC), a meta-analysis of 31 randomized trials of antiplatelet therapy primarily with aspirin in patients who had sustained prior myocardial infarction, stroke, transient ischemic attack (TIA), or unstable angina.[11] Of 29,000 patients, those treated with antiplatelet therapy demonstrated a 25% reduction in the odds of suffering a recurrent vascular event.[11] In a second study, the ATC demonstrated an 18% reduction in the odds of vascular death among patients at high risk, as defined by history of myocardial infarction, stroke, TIA, or unstable angina.[12]

Although intuited from smaller randomized studies,[13] the benefit of aspirin in the setting of an acute myocardial infarction was persuasively demonstrated in the Second International Study of Infarct Survival (ISIS-2).[14] In this trial of 17,187 patients with a suspected acute myocardial infarction, a 162.5-mg daily dose of aspirin administered for 1 month significantly

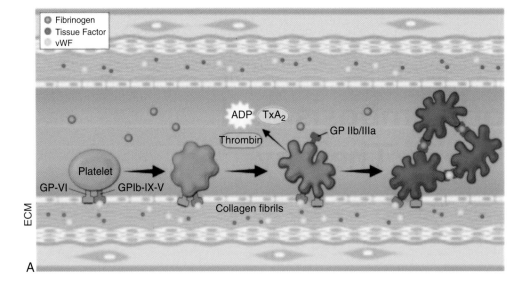

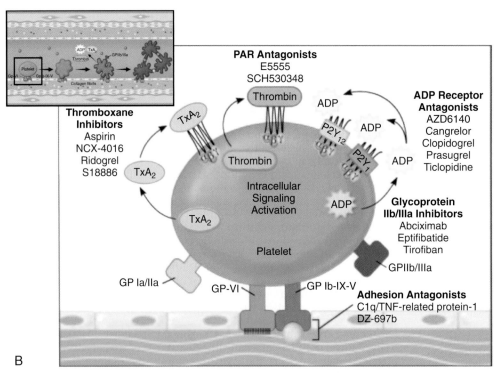

FIGURE 7-1 Platelet activation and the mechanism of thrombus formation. **A,** Endothelial injury exposes components of the extracellular environment such as collagen and von Willebrand factor (vWF). After binding to these components by means of glycoprotein receptors, platelets adhere to the subendothelium and become activated. Activation of the platelet causes a conformational change in the shape of the platelet, release of adenosine diphosphate (ADP) and thromboxane A₂ (TxA₂), and formation of thrombin on the platelet surface. The release of factors such as ADP and TxA₂ causes activation of circulating platelets and amplifies the platelet response. These responses cause the platelet glycoprotein (GP) IIb/IIIa receptor to change shape and increase its affinity for adhesive proteins such as vWF and fibrinogen. Platelet aggregation ensues, and the additional interaction of the platelet aggregate with thrombin and fibrin results in thrombus formation. **B,** The agonists ADP, TxA₂, and thrombin bind to G protein–coupled receptors and trigger an intracellular signaling cascade. Several antiplatelet therapies are directed at inhibiting the interaction between these agonists and their respective receptors such as the ADP receptor antagonists, thromboxane inhibitors, and emerging protease activating receptor (PAR) antagonists. C1q/TNF, C1q complex/tumor necrosis factor; P2Y₁ and P2Y₁₂, G protein–coupled purinergic receptors. *(From Meadows TA, Bhatt DL: Clinical aspects of platelet inhibitors and thrombus formation,* Circ Research *100:1261-1275, 2007.)*

reduced early vascular mortality in comparison with placebo (9.4% versus 11.8%, respectively).[14] The protection afforded by aspirin extended to patients with unstable angina in a study of 1266 male veterans.[15] In this randomized, placebo-controlled trial, a daily 324-mg buffered aspirin administered for 12 weeks resulted in a 51% reduction in myocardial infarction or death.[15] Similar results emerged from the study by the Research Group on Instability in Coronary Artery Disease (RISC), which demonstrated a 57% to 69% reduction in the rate of the combined endpoint of myocardial infarction

| TABLE 7-1 | Primary Prevention Trials of Aspirin |

Trial	Year of Publication	Population	Aspirin Dose	Stroke	Relative Risk Myocardial Infarction	All-Cause Mortality
British Doctors' Trial	1988	5139 male physicians	500 mg or 300 mg daily	1.13	0.97	0.89
Physicians' Health Study	1989	22,071 male physicians	325 mg every other day	1.22	0.59	0.96
Thrombosis Prevention Trial	1998	5085 men	75 mg daily	0.98	0.68	1.06
Hypertension Optimal Treatment Study	1998	18,790 men and women	75 mg daily	0.98	0.64	0.93
Primary Prevention Project	2001	4495 men and women	100 mg daily	0.67	0.69	0.81
Women's Health Study	2005	39,876 female health professionals	100 mg every other day	0.83	1.02	0.95

Adapted from Meadows T, Bhatt DL: Clinical aspects of platelet inhibitors and thrombus formation, *Circ Res* 100:1261-1275, 2007.

or death among 796 men with unstable angina or non–Q-wave myocardial infarction who were treated with low-dose aspirin.[16]

The benefits of early aspirin therapy after an ischemic stroke were elucidated in two contemporaneous large, randomized trials of patients with acute stroke: the Chinese Acute Stroke Trial (CAST)[17] and the Ischemic Stroke Trial (IST).[18] In more than 20,000 patients enrolled in CAST, 160 mg of aspirin given within 48 hours of an ischemic stroke prevented 6.8 deaths or recurrent nonfatal strokes per 1000 patients treated.[17] In a 2 × 2 factorial open-label design, IST investigators examined the effects of subcutaneous heparin, 300 mg of aspirin, or both administered within 48 hours of an ischemic stroke. Aspirin was associated with 11 fewer deaths or recurrent stroke per 1000 patients treated.[18] The results of these trials, analyzed together, revealed that this benefit was offset slightly by an excess of 2 cases of intracranial hemorrhage per 1000 patients treated.[19]

Treatment with aspirin has also been an essential adjunct in patients undergoing coronary revascularization. Among patients undergoing coronary artery bypass grafting (CABG), aspirin administration both before and soon after surgery has been demonstrated to improve both early and 1-year patency of the saphenous vein graft.[20,21] Aspirin administered after coronary angioplasty has been associated with a decreased risk of the composite endpoint of death, restenosis, or myocardial infarction in comparison with placebo (30% versus 41%, respectively).[22] As might be expected, the addition of aspirin to thrombolytic therapy also reduces rates of recurrent ischemia and infarct-related reocclusion of arteries.[23]

The ATC provided irrefutable evidence in favor of aspirin for secondary prevention with a more recent meta-analysis of 195 trials that included more than 135,000 patients.[24] This meta-analysis revealed similar risk reduction with antiplatelet therapy among patients at high risk, and this reduction also extended to patients with stable angina, atrial fibrillation, and peripheral artery disease.[24]

Primary Prevention

To date, six large, randomized trials have been undertaken to study aspirin for the primary prevention of cardiovascular disease (Table 7-1). The British Doctors' Trial was conducted to evaluate the effect of a daily 500-mg dose of aspirin in healthy male physicians.[25] Of the 5139 subjects studied, a majority of participants were older than 60 years and were either current or ex-smokers. After 6 years of follow-up, there were no statistically significant differences in the rates of fatal or nonfatal myocardial infarction, stroke, or all-cause

mortality between patients assigned to receive aspirin therapy and those assigned to receive no aspirin. There was, however, an approximate 50% reduction in TIA among physicians treated with aspirin. This trial was not blinded and did not have a placebo control group. Over the course of the study, 44.3% of physicians assigned to receive aspirin therapy discontinued the drug.[25]

The Physicians' Health Study, a larger trial designed to assess the efficacy of aspirin in reducing cardiovascular events, enrolled 22,071 male physicians in the United States.[26] In a double-blind, placebo-controlled design, healthy physicians were randomly assigned to receive 325 mg of aspirin every other day or beta-carotene in a 2 × 2 factorial design. The study, which was terminated early, demonstrated a significant (44%) risk reduction in the rate of total myocardial infarction. Similarly, there was an 18% risk reduction in the composite outcome of nonfatal myocardial infarction, nonfatal stroke and cardiovascular death. Despite this robust finding, aspirin therapy did not confer a cardiovascular mortality benefit in this study.[26]

The effect of aspirin and warfarin in reducing cardiovascular events in 5085 men was evaluated in the Thrombosis Prevention Trial, a randomized, double-blind, placebo-controlled trial.[27] In a 2 × 2 factorial design, men who did not have established cardiovascular disease but were deemed to be at high risk for vascular disease were randomly assigned to receive treatment with aspirin, 75 mg daily, and warfarin with a target international normalized ratio (INR) of 1.5. Aspirin therapy, either alone or in combination with warfarin, conferred a 20% reduction in the primary endpoint of cardiovascular death and fatal and nonfatal myocardial infarction. This reduction was driven primarily by a 32% reduction in the risk of nonfatal myocardial infarction. In a result concordant with those of the large studies preceding the Thrombosis Prevention Trial, no mortality benefit with aspirin therapy was demonstrated.[27]

In the Hypertension Optimal Treatment study, the effect of low-dose aspirin was investigated in an international cohort of 18,790 men and women, aged 50 to 80, with hypertension.[28] A separate arm of the study was concerned with the effect of antihypertensive therapy directed at diastolic blood pressure and cardiovascular outcomes. In this randomized, placebo-controlled, double-blind study, a daily dose of 75 mg of aspirin was associated with a 15% relative risk reduction in major cardiovascular events, defined as both fatal and nonfatal stroke, fatal and nonfatal myocardial infarction, or cardiovascular death.[28]

Another trial designed to examine the efficacy of aspirin among men and women at risk for cardiovascular disease was the Primary Prevention Project.[29] In an open-label 2 × 2 factorial design, 4495 patients were randomly assigned to receive a 100-mg daily dose of aspirin, as well as vitamin E. Patients were eligible for inclusion in the trial if they had a history of hypertension, hypercholesterolemia, diabetes, family history of premature coronary artery disease, were obese, or were older than 65. A majority of patients included in the study had at least two or more of these risk factors. The mean age of participants was more than 60 years, and 57.7% were women. The trial was terminated prematurely in part because data from the Hypertension Optimal Treatment and Thrombosis Prevention Trial provided evidence in favor of aspirin for primary prevention. After a mean follow-up period of 3.6 years, investigators demonstrated a 44% relative risk reduction in cardiovascular death among patients assigned to treatment with aspirin. Similarly, they demonstrated a 22% relative risk reduction in the primary endpoint of cardiovascular death, nonfatal myocardial infarction, or stroke.[29]

The Women's Health Study was designed to address the role of aspirin in the primary prevention of cardiovascular disease in women. A total of 39,876 female health professionals were randomly assigned to receive 100 mg of aspirin every other day.[30] After a mean follow-up period of 10 years, this treatment was found to confer 17% and 22% reductions in the risk of stroke and TIAs, respectively, but no significant reduction in the risk of myocardial infarction or cardiovascular death. In the subgroup of women aged 65 and older, however, aspirin was associated with a significant (26%) reduction in the risk of the primary endpoint of cardiovascular death, nonfatal myocardial infarction, or stroke.[30]

A large meta-analysis[31] of the six aforementioned primary prevention trials concluded that aspirin reduces composite cardiovascular events by 12% and 14% in women and men, respectively. Overall, aspirin was not associated with a lower risk of cardiovascular death.

In an update, the ATC performed another meta-analysis[32] of the six major primary prevention trials, which was strengthened by the availability of individual participant data. In primary prevention studies, aspirin was associated with a 12% reduction in the risk ratio of a major adverse cardiovascular event in comparison with no aspirin (0.51% versus 0.57% per year, respectively). The magnitude of this effect was similar in both men and women and was independent of age. Moreover, the small absolute benefit was counterbalanced by an increase in major extracranial hemorrhage in comparison to no aspirin (0.10% versus 0.07% per year, respectively). For secondary prevention, aspirin conferred an absolute reduction of 1.5% per year in the rate of occurrence of a serious vascular event.[32]

Although previous primary prevention trials of aspirin included analyses of data from subgroups of patients with diabetes, these provided insufficient information with regard to efficacy in this important patient population. In the Japanese Primary Prevention of Atherosclerosis with Aspirin for Diabetes (JPAD) trial, 2539 men and women with well-controlled type 2 diabetes, with a mean age of 65 and without known cardiovascular disease, were randomly assigned to receive 81 or 100 mg daily of aspirin versus no aspirin.[33] The overall event rate was low in this population, and a significant reduction in major cardiovascular events was not observed in the subjects taking aspirin. However, a reduction in the secondary composite endpoint of fatal stroke or myocardial infarction was observed. In a prespecified subgroup analysis of diabetic patients older than 65, a benefit was derived from low-dose aspirin in comparison with the control condition in the primary endpoint (6.3% versus 9.2% respectively).[33]

In the Prevention of Progression of Arterial Disease and Diabetes (POPADAD) trial, which was contemporaneous with the JPAD trial, the efficacy of low-dose (100 mg) daily aspirin and antioxidant therapy in preventing cardiovascular events

was evaluated in 1276 patients with diabetes and asymptomatic peripheral artery disease.[34] The investigators did not observe a statistically significant benefit of aspirin over placebo in this randomized, controlled, double-blind study. In another trial, Aspirin for Asymptomatic Atherosclerosis, 3350 healthy men and women with asymptomatic peripheral artery disease (as defined by an ankle-brachial index <0.95) were randomly assigned to receive aspirin, 100 mg daily, or placebo. After a mean follow-up period of 8.2 years, no difference in major cardiovascular events or all-cause mortality was observed between participants randomly assigned to receive aspirin or placebo.[35]

Several ongoing trials have been designed to address remaining questions regarding the efficacy of aspirin in primary prevention. The plan of A Study of Cardiovascular Events in Diabetes (ASCEND) is to assess the effectiveness of low-dose daily aspirin in 10,000 patients with diabetes.[36] Similarly, the Aspirin and Simvastatin Combination for Cardiovascular Events Prevention Trial in Diabetes (ACCEPT-D) is designed to assess the efficacy of open-label daily aspirin, either alone or in combination with simvastatin, in reducing cardiovascular events in approximately 5000 patients with diabetes.[37] Because researchers in most primary prevention studies have examined the benefit of aspirin in populations at relatively low risk, the ongoing Aspirin to Reduce Risk of Vascular Events (ARRIVE) trial will address the role of aspirin in an international cohort of approximately 12,000 patients deemed to be at moderate risk (20% to 30%) of developing a cardiovascular event over 10 years.[38] The role of aspirin in the primary prevention of cardiovascular disease in elderly patients is being studied in the Aspirin in Reducing Events in the Elderly (ASPREE) trial.[39] The aim of the Japanese Primary Prevention Project with Aspirin is to evaluate cardiovascular outcomes in 10,000 Japanese patients older than 60 with at least one additional traditional cardiovascular risk factor who are treated with 100 mg of aspirin daily.[40]

Dosing

Daily aspirin doses of only 30 mg have been demonstrated to completely inhibit synthesis of platelet thromboxane.[41] Despite this observation, the optimal dose of aspirin for an individual patient is not known. Some investigators have speculated that higher dosages of aspirin may paradoxically attenuate the antithrombotic effect of thromboxane inhibition by causing inhibition of the vasodilator prostacyclin.[42] However, a wide variety of aspirin dosages (ranging from 50 to 1500 mg) have been demonstrated to be efficacious for prevention of cardiovascular events, and a formal comparison of several different doses has never been performed in the context of a randomized, controlled, prospective trial in coronary artery disease.[24]

Results of one ATC meta-analysis suggested similar reduction in vascular events across a wide range of aspirin dosages.[24] In a post hoc analysis of the Clopidogrel in Unstable Angina to prevent Recurrent Events (CURE) study, increasing dosages of aspirin (<100 mg, 101 to 199 mg, and >200 mg daily) administered with either placebo or clopidogrel were not associated with greater clinical benefit.[43] Moreover, higher rates of major bleeding were observed with escalating dosages of aspirin compared with placebo (1.9%, 2.8%, and 3.7%, respectively).[43] A meta-analysis of 31 randomized trials that included more than 192,000 patients reached a similar conclusion; the risk of major bleeding events was lowest in patients who took the lowest aspirin dosage.[44] This finding was confirmed in an observational study of participants in the Clopidogrel for High Atherothrombotic Risk and Ischemic Stabilization (CHARISMA) trial.[45] In this large prospective study of patients at high risk of cardiovascular events, patients were randomly assigned to receive clopidogrel or placebo in addition to background aspirin therapy (at daily doses of 162 mg or lower). A post hoc analysis demonstrated no significant reduction in the composite outcome of myocardial infarction, death, or stroke with increasing doses of aspirin. In fact, there was a suggestion of harm to patients treated with higher doses of aspirin in addition to clopidogrel, with increased rates of cardiovascular events and a greater incidence of bleeding, although this was not statistically significant.[45]

Results of the Clopidogrel Optimal Loading Dose Usage to Reduce Recurrent Events/Optimal Antiplatelet Strategy for Interventions (CURRENT-OASIS 7) trial have enhanced the understanding of both aspirin and clopidogrel dosing in acute coronary syndromes (ACS).[46] In a double-blind 2×2 factorial design, approximately 25,000 patients with ACS treated with an early invasive strategy were randomly assigned to receive conventional clopidogrel dosages (300-mg loading dose, followed by 75 mg daily) versus high-dose clopidogrel (600-mg loading dose, followed by 150 mg daily for 6 days and subsequent maintenance dosing of 75 mg daily).[47] Subjects in each of these groups were further randomly assigned, in an open-label manner, to receive high-dose aspirin (300 to 325 mg) or low-dose aspirin (75 to 100 mg) after an initial 300-mg dose of aspirin. High-dose clopidogrel was associated with a significant reduction in the composite of death, myocardial infarction, or stroke at 30 days in patients undergoing percutaneous coronary intervention (PCI).[46] No difference in efficacy or hemorrhagic risk was observed between patients who received low-dose aspirin and those who received high-dose aspirin.[46] A prespecified substudy will also be conducted to examine the effects of aspirin dosing on urinary metabolites of thromboxane and prostacyclin among patients who experience adverse cardiac events and those who do not.[47]

Formulations

Aspirin exists in a "regular" form, as well as in buffered and enteric-coated preparations. Aspirin is rapidly absorbed in the stomach and small intestine after ingestion; inhibition of portal platelet COX enzyme occurs before complete systemic absorption.[48] Levels of aspirin in the systemic circulation peak within 40 minutes after ingestion of regular aspirin and 3 to 4 hours after ingestion of an enteric-coated preparation.[49] A pharmacodynamic study in 12 healthy volunteers demonstrated that near-maximal platelet thromboxane inhibition, occurring over a mean of 13.6 minutes, is achieved most efficiently when a 325-mg aspirin tablet is chewed.[50] Swallowing a whole buffered tablet doubles the time necessary to achieve maximal platelet inhibition.[50] Although enteric-coated preparations may have theoretical benefit in reducing gastric irritation and bleeding, the risk of gastrointestinal bleeding observed with aspirin is also increased because of its systemic effect. Enteric-coated aspirin does not seem to confer protection against gastrointestinal bleeding in comparison with buffered or regular preparations of the same dose.[51]

Hemorrhagic Complications

The most feared complications of antiplatelet therapy are sequelae from hemorrhage. The majority of bleeding complications arise from the gastrointestinal tract; the estimated relative risk was 2.1 in one meta-analysis of 22 randomized primary or secondary prevention studies in which 75- to 325-mg dosages of aspirin were compared with placebo.[52] The relative risk of intracranial hemorrhage was 1.7; no differences between major bleeding and dosages of aspirin were observed. This translated to an annual absolute increase in major bleeding of 0.12%.[52] In a prospective, observational study of 991 patients with coronary artery disease who

were treated with 75- to 300-mg of aspirin, the incidence of upper gastrointestinal hemorrhage was 1.5% over 2 years of follow-up.[53] It has been estimated that aspirin contributes to an excess of 5 cases of gastrointestinal hemorrhage per 1000 patients treated.[54] Gastric toxicity, as measured by inhibition of gastric prostaglandin synthesis, is thought to be dose dependent, and a 50% reduction in gastric prostaglandin is observed at dosages as low as 30 mg/day.[55] Therefore, all dosages currently prescribed in clinical practice can be expected to heighten the risk of gastrointestinal hemorrhage.[56]

The extent to which this risk can be attenuated by proton pump inhibition has been examined in both asymptomatic patients and those with prior gastroduodenal ulcers. In a prospective, double-blind study of more than 900 asymptomatic patients requiring low-dose aspirin therapy, use of a proton pump inhibitor (PPI) for 26 weeks was associated with a lower rate of endoscopic ulcers than was placebo (1.6% versus 5.4%, respectively).[57] In another study of 123 patients with recently healed gastroduodenal ulcers and treated *Helicobacter pylori* infection, the combination of 100 mg of aspirin and 30 mg of lansoprazole was associated with fewer recurrent ulcer complications was the combination of aspirin and placebo over 1 year (1.6% versus 14.8%, respectively).[58] In a similar randomized, placebo-controlled trial of 320 patients with a recent bleeding ulcer, investigators studied the combination of clopidogrel 75 mg daily plus esomeprazole placebo twice daily versus 80 mg aspirin plus esomeprazole 20 mg twice daily.[59] Clopidogrel was associated with a higher rate of recurrent bleeding over 1 year than was the combination of aspirin and PPI (0.7% versus 8.6%, respectively).[59] During 12 weeks of follow-up, the histamine H2 receptor antagonist famotidine was demonstrated to decrease the risk of endoscopic esophagitis and peptic ulcers in comparison with placebo in patients who received 75 to 325 mg of daily aspirin therapy.[60]

By consensus, the American College of Cardiology Foundation (ACCF), American College of Gastroenterology (ACG), and American Heart Association (AHA) recommend reducing chronic aspirin dosages to 81 mg daily with the addition of a daily dose of a PPI in patients with a history of gastrointestinal hemorrhage or ulcer or in patients at risk of these complications, such as those who take maintenance steroid medication, elderly patients, or patients with a history of dyspepsia.[61]

In addition, testing and treatment of *H. pylori* is advocated initiation of chronic antiplatelet therapy in patients with a history of peptic ulcer disease. Replacing aspirin with clopidogrel is not recommended as a strategy for reducing the risk of recurrent gastrointestinal complications.[61]

Drug Interactions

Other nonsteroidal anti-inflammatory drugs (NSAIDs) can interact in deleterious ways with aspirin. The addition of NSAIDs to aspirin potentiates the risk of gastrointestinal events. However, concomitant NSAID use may also mitigate the protective effect of aspirin. MacDonald and Wei[62] reported on trends in mortality among more than 7000 patients with cardiovascular disease discharged from the hospital with prescriptions for aspirin or for the combination of aspirin and ibuprofen. The latter combination was associated with an excess risk of both all-cause mortality and cardiovascular death (hazard ratios, 1.9 and 1.7, respectively). The potential mechanism of this interaction was evaluated in healthy volunteers who were administered ibuprofen, followed by 81 mg of aspirin.[63] Ibuprofen administered before aspirin or several times daily blocked normal aspirin-induced platelet inhibition. However, the administration of aspirin 2 hours before a single dose of ibuprofen resulted in expected irreversible COX-1 inhibition.[63] Naproxen has also been demonstrated

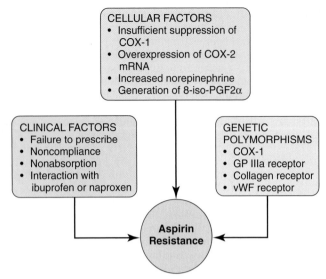

FIGURE 7-2 Possible mechanisms of aspirin resistance. COX, cyclooxygenase; GP, glycoprotein; mRNA, messenger ribonucleic acid; PGF$_{2\alpha}$, prostaglandin factor 2α; vWF, von Willebrand factor. *(From Bhatt DL: Aspirin resistance: more than just a laboratory curiosity,* J Am Coll Cardiol *43:1127-1129, 2004.)*

to antagonize the COX-1 inhibition of aspirin in vitro, presumably by functioning as a competitive inhibitor of the COX enzyme.[64] Amplifying concerns about NSAIDs as a class, a large Finnish case-control study demonstrated a significant increase in the risk of first myocardial infarction with use of either conventional or selective COX-2 inhibitor NSAIDs.[65,66]

Aspirin Resistance

Despite appropriate doses of aspirin, many patients develop recurrent ischemic events. This clinical dilemma has often been attributed to *aspirin resistance,* a broad term that encompasses the wide variety of factors thought to contribute to this phenomenon (Figure 7-2). At the simplest level, patients' nonadherence to aspirin therapy, underprescription by physicians, drug interaction with ibuprofen or naproxen, and malabsorption may all play a role.[67] It is also known that platelet activation can occur via thromboxane-independent pathways.[68] One such mechanism may involve COX independent production of the arachidonic acid derivative 8-iso-prostaglandin factor F$_{2\alpha}$ PGF$_{2\alpha}$, a potent vasoconstrictor and platelet aggregant, released in response to oxidative stress.[69] Because aspirin is a relatively weak inhibitor of COX-2, it has also been postulated that platelet COX-2, normally expressed in response to inflammatory stimuli, may result in sufficient synthesis of thromboxane A$_2$ to contribute to aspirin resistance.[70] Other genetic factors may also contribute to observed differences in platelet responsiveness. The platelet polymorphism PI^{A2} has been associated with aspirin resistance.[68] Aspirin resistance has been observed in patients with acute myocardial infarction[71] and elicited by exercise in patients with stable coronary artery disease.[72] One systematic review of 15 studies revealed a wide range in estimates of the prevalence of laboratory aspirin resistance (5% to 65%).[73] The lack of a uniform definition of aspirin resistance and its measurement has limited the understanding of this entity. The "gold standard" test of platelet function, light transmission aggregometry, is the most precise; however, it is time consuming and cannot be performed at the patient's bedside.[74]

The implications of inadequate aspirin-induced platelet inhibition were assessed in a nested case-control study of participants in the Heart Outcomes Prevention Evaluation (HOPE). Eikelboom and colleagues[75] found an independent association between increasing urinary thromboxane levels, a marker of aspirin resistance, and major cardiovascular events. In another prospective study of 326 patients with stable cardiovascular disease, aspirin resistance, as measured by a one-time optical platelet aggregation test, was present in 5.2% of patients and associated with a significant increase in the rate of the combined endpoint of myocardial infarction, stroke, or death in comparison with patients not deemed resistant (24% versus 10%, respectively).[76] In data congruent with these findings, Chen and colleagues[77] demonstrated an almost threefold increase in the risk of periprocedural myocardial infarction in patients undergoing nonurgent PCI who were deemed aspirin resistant according to a commercial point-of-care assay. More recently, a prespecified analysis of the CHARISMA trial confirmed the findings of the HOPE substudy and revealed an increased risk of stroke, myocardial infarction, or death in patients whose urinary 11-dehydrothromboxane B$_2$ levels were in the highest quartile.[78] Moreover, clopidogrel (in subjects who received it) did not appear to attenuate this relationship. Interestingly, female sex, increasing age, peripheral artery disease, tobacco use, and use of angiotensin-converting enzyme inhibitors or oral hypoglycemic agents were independently associated with incomplete thromboxane inhibition.[78]

Guidelines

The U.S. Preventive Services Task Force (USPSTF) recommends the use of aspirin in men aged 45 to 79 and women aged 55 to 79 for the primary prevention of a cardiovascular event if the perceived benefit of aspirin outweighs the potential harm caused by an increased risk of gastrointestinal hemorrhage (Figure 7-3).[79] For patients at moderate risk for cardiovascular events, the American College of Chest Physicians (ACCP) recommends 75 to 100 mg of aspirin daily.[80] The American Diabetes Association advocates the use of 75 to 162 mg of aspirin daily in patients with diabetes who are older than 40 or for those who have other traditional risk factors for cardiovascular disease.[81] For patients with peripheral artery disease, the American College of Cardiology (ACC)/AHA recommends 75 to 325 mg of aspirin daily for the prevention of stroke, myocardial infarction, or cardiovascular death.[82]

After an ST-elevation myocardial infarction (STEMI), the ACCP recommends initiation of aspirin at a dose of 160 to 325 mg, with subsequent reduction to 75 to 100 mg, to be continued indefinitely.[80] The ACCP also recommends indefinite low-dose aspirin (75 to 100 mg daily) after PCI, CABG, carotid endarterectomy, and peripheral revascularization.[80] A focused update of the 2004 STEMI guidelines recommends aspirin initiation at a dose of 162 to 325 mg for 1, 3, and 6 months after bare-metal, sirolimus, and paclitaxel drug-eluting stents, respectively, with reduction to 75 to 162 mg daily thereafter (ACC/AHA Class 1, level of evidence B).[83] The AHA/American Stroke Association (ASA) recommends administration of 325 mg of aspirin within 24 to 48 hours of an acute ischemic stroke, except for patients receiving thrombolytic therapy, for whom aspirin should be deferred 24 hours.[84]

THIENOPYRIDINES

Mechanism of Action

The thienopyridines, of which ticlopidine and clopidogrel are the prototypes, irreversibly inhibit platelets by binding to P2Y$_{12}$, the G protein–coupled receptor that is normally activated by ADP released from injured endothelium and red blood cells.[85] Through interaction with the P2Y$_{12}$ and P2Y$_1$ platelet receptors, ADP triggers a cascade of events that result in platelet aggregation and in further release of ADP from the activated platelet, thus potentiating the initial response.[86,87]

ASPIRIN FOR THE PREVENTION OF CARDIOVASCULAR DISEASE
CLINICAL SUMMARY OF U.S. PREVENTIVE SERVICES TASK FORCE RECOMMENDATIONS

75

Population	Men Age 45–79 Years	Women Age 55–79 Years	Men Age <45 Years	Women Age <55 Years	Men and Women Age ≥80 Years
Recommendation	Encourage aspirin use when potential CVD benefit (MIs prevented) outweighs potential harm of GI hemorrhage	Encourage aspirin use when potential CVD benefit (strokes prevented) outweighs potential harm of GI hemorrhage	Do not encourage aspirin use for MI prevention	Do not encourage aspirin use for stroke prevention	No recommendation
	Grade: A		Grade: D		Grade: I (insufficient evidence)

| How to Use This Recommendation | Shared decision making is strongly encouraged with individuals whose risk is close to (either above or below) the estimates of 10-year risk levels indicated below. As the potential CVD benefit increases above harms, the recommendation to take aspirin should become stronger.

To determine whether the potential benefit of MI's prevented (men) and strokes prevented (women) outweighs the potential harm of increased GI hemorrhage, both 10-year CVD risk and age must be considered. |
|---|---|

Risk Level at Which CVD Events Prevented (Benefit) Exceeds GI Harm

Men		Women	
Age	10-Year CHD Risk	Age	10-Year Stroke Risk
45–59 years	≥4%	55–59 years	≥3%
60–69 years	≥9%	60–69 years	≥8%
70–79 years	≥12%	70–79 years	≥11%

The table above applies to adults who are not taking NSAIDs and who do not have upper GI pain or a history of GI ulcers.

NSAID use and history of GI ulcers increase the risk for serious GI bleeding events considerably and should be considered in determining the balance of benefits and harm.

NSAID use combined with aspirin use approximately quadruples the risk for serious GI bleeding events compared with the risk with aspirin use alone. The rate of serious bleeding in aspirin users is approximately 2 to 3 times greater in patients with a history of GI ulcers

| Risk Assessment | **For men:** Risk factors for CHD include age, diabetes, total cholesterol level, HDL cholesterol level, blood pressure, and smoking.
CHD risk estimation tool: http://healthlink.mcw.edu/article/923521437.html

For women: Risk factors for ischemic stroke include age, high blood pressure, diabetes, smoking, history of CVD, atrial fibrillation, and left ventricular hypertrophy.
Stroke risk estimation tool: www.silentstroke.org/PersonalStrokeRisk1.xls |
|---|---|
| Relevant Recommendations from USP-STF | The USPSTF has made recommendations on screening for abdominal aortic aneurysm, carotid artery stenosis, CHD, high blood pressure, lipid disorders, and peripheral arterial disease. These recommendations are available at www.preventiveservices.ahrq.gov. |

FIGURE 7-3 U.S. Preventive Services Task Force (USPSTF) recommendations for aspirin use in primary prevention. CHD, coronary heart disease; CVD, cardiovascular disease; GI, gastrointestinal; HDL, high-density lipoprotein; MI, myocardial infarction; NSAID, nonsteroidal anti-inflammatory drug. *(From U.S. Preventive Services Task Force:* Aspirin for the prevention of cardiovascular disease: clinical summary of U.S. Preventive Services Task Force Recommendation, *AHRQ Publication No. 09-05129-EF-3, Rockville, MD, March 2009, Agency for Healthcare Research and Quality. Available at: http://www.ahrq.gov/clinic/uspstf09/aspirincvd/aspcvdsum.htm.)*

Ticlopidine

Ticlopidine, first studied in humans in 1975, inhibits ADP-induced platelet aggregation in a dose-dependent manner, with an onset of action of 24 to 48 hours.[88] Like clopidogrel, ticlopidine is a prodrug and must be metabolized by the cytochrome P-450 system to an active metabolite.[89] Although many early trials provided evidence to support the use of ticlopidine in patients with established cardiovascular disease, adverse hematologic side effects and rather slow onset of action in comparison with clopidogrel have curtailed its widespread subsequent use. Among patients taking ticlopidine, serious neutropenia has been reported in fewer than

1% to as high as 3.4%,[90-94] and thrombotic thrombocytopenic purpura has been reported in 0.02%.[95]

Two such early trials were the Canadian American Ticlopidine Study (CATS)[90] and the Ticlopidine Aspirin Stroke Study (TASS).[92] In the CATS trial, more than 1000 patients with recent thromboembolic stroke were randomly assigned to receive treatment with ticlopidine or placebo; a nearly 25% relative risk reduction was demonstrated in the rate of the combined endpoint of vascular death, myocardial infarction, or death.[90] In TASS, ticlopidine was compared with high-dose aspirin in more than 3000 patients who had sustained a recent neurologic event; a 21% relative risk reduction was demonstrated in the rate of recurrent fatal and nonfatal stroke in favor of ticlopidine.[92] Incongruent with this result were the findings of the African-American Antiplatelet Stroke Prevention Study (AAASPS), which did not show a reduction in the composite endpoint of stroke, myocardial infarction, or vascular death in African American patients treated with ticlopidine after an ischemic stroke.[91]

The Swedish Ticlopidine Multicentre Study demonstrated a 29% reduction in all-cause mortality among 687 patients with established peripheral artery disease treated with ticlopidine, in comparison with placebo.[93] This mortality benefit was explained entirely by a reduction in fatal myocardial infarction. The early use of ticlopidine was further supported by a study that demonstrated a nearly 47% relative risk reduction in vascular death among 653 patients with unstable angina treated with ticlopidine in an open-label trial.[96] The additional antiplatelet benefit of ticlopidine was later demonstrated to extend to PCIs, previously complicated by stent thrombosis in the era of single antiplatelet therapy and oral anticoagulation.[94,97,98] Soon after, the results of the Clopidogrel Aspirin Stent International Cooperative Study (CLASSICS) suggested superiority of the combination of aspirin and clopidogrel over that of aspirin and ticlopidine in patients undergoing placement of coronary stents.[99] Although this study was not statistically powered to compare the efficacy of these two antiplatelet regimens, the combination of aspirin and clopidogrel was associated with significantly fewer noncardiac adverse effects than was the combination of ticlopidine and aspirin (4.6% versus 9.1%, respectively).[99] More conclusive evidence arose from a meta-analysis of both registry and randomized trial data in which clopidogrel and ticlopidine were compared: The rate of major adverse cardiac events was reduced 50% with combination clopidogrel and aspirin in comparison with ticlopidine and aspirin.[100]

Clopidogrel

Secondary Prevention

Clopidogrel has been tested in the secondary prevention of cardiovascular disease in several trials (Table 7-2). The Clopidogrel versus Aspirin in Patients at Risk of Ischemic Events (CAPRIE) study was the first large, randomized, placebo-controlled trial to test the efficacy of clopidogrel in preventing cardiovascular events.[101] This international, multicenter study included 19,185 patients, predominately male, with a mean age of 63 who had sustained a recent myocardial infarction, stroke, or symptomatic peripheral artery disease. The subjects were monitored for a mean of almost 2 years. Clopidogrel (75 mg daily) conferred an 8.7% relative risk reduction in the rate of the composite endpoint of myocardial infarction, stroke, or vascular death in comparison with a daily 325-mg dose of aspirin.[101] In subgroup analyses of patients with diabetes and prior CABG in the CAPRIE trial, clopidogrel was also more efficacious than aspirin in reducing the rate of the combined endpoint of vascular death, myocardial infarction, or stroke.[102,103]

The salutary effect of dual-antiplatelet therapy with clopidogrel and aspirin in patients with ACS was established in the CURE trial.[104] Among 12,562 men and women with unstable angina or non–ST-elevation myocardial infarction, a 300-mg loading dose of clopidogrel followed by a dose of 75 mg of clopidogrel daily with open-label aspirin therapy (75 to 325 mg) was associated with a lower rate of the combined endpoint of cardiovascular death, myocardial infarction, or stroke than was placebo (9.6% versus 11.4%, respectively). The protective effect of clopidogrel was evident within the first 24 hours after randomization, and clopidogrel also reduced the risk of in-hospital ischemia, recurrent angina, revascularization, and heart failure.[104] The additional early benefit of clopidogrel in comparison with placebo was

also shown to extend to patients in the CURE study who subsequently underwent CABG[105] and PCI.[106] Another CURE substudy demonstrated the consistent benefit of clopidogrel across various risk groups, as defined by the Thrombolysis In Myocardial Infarction (TIMI) risk score.[107]

The use of dual-antiplatelet therapy with clopidogrel and aspirin before PCI was supported by evidence from the Clopidogrel for the Reduction of Events During Observation (CREDO) trial.[108] In 2116 patients undergoing elective PCI, pretreatment with a 300-mg loading dose of clopidogrel followed by 1 year of dual-antiplatelet therapy (clopidogrel 75 mg daily and aspirin 81-325 mg daily) was associated with a nearly 27% relative risk reduction in the composite endpoint of myocardial infarction, death, or need for target vessel revascularization in comparison with placebo.[108]

On the basis of the premise that combination therapy with clopidogrel and aspirin might attenuate cardiovascular risk beyond that observed with clopidogrel alone, the CHARISMA trial was conducted to evaluate the efficacy of clopidogrel and low-dose aspirin for the prevention of major cardiovascular events.[109] The 15,603 patients with established cardiovascular disease or multiple cardiovascular risk factors were monitored for a median of 28 months. Clopidogrel and aspirin did not result in significant benefit with regard to the composite endpoint of stroke, myocardial infarction, or cardiovascular death in comparison with placebo plus aspirin.[109] However, in a subsequent analysis of patients with prior myocardial infarction, symptomatic peripheral artery disease, or stroke, the combination of clopidogrel and aspirin afforded a 1.5% absolute risk reduction in the composite endpoint of stroke, myocardial infarction, or cardiovascular death.[110]

The additional benefit of clopidogrel among patients with STEMI has been demonstrated in two large-scale randomized, placebo-controlled trials.[111,112] The Clopidogrel and Metoprolol in Myocardial Infarction Trial (COMMIT) enrolled 45,852 Chinese patients with an acute myocardial infarction to receive clopidogrel, 75 mg daily, or placebo in addition to aspirin, 162 mg daily.[111] Also in this 2×2 factorial design, the effect of metoprolol (intravenous followed by oral preparations) was evaluated. Clopidogrel treatment for a mean of approximately 2 weeks was associated with a 9% odds reduction in the composite of myocardial infarction, stroke, or death, as well as a 7% odds reduction in all-cause mortality.[111] Similarly, the Clopidogrel as Adjunctive Reperfusion Therapy–Thrombolysis In Myocardial Infarction 28 (CLARITY-TIMI 28) study demonstrated a 36% odds reduction in the composite endpoint of death, myocardial infarction, or infarct-related artery occlusion, demonstrated angiographically, in 3491 patients with STEMI who were treated with clopidogrel and fibrinolytics.[112] This reduction was achieved without a significant increase in the risk of major bleeding in both trials. In a prespecified analysis of patients who underwent PCI in the CLARITY-TIMI 28 study, random assignment to pretreatment with a 300-mg loading dose of clopidogrel was associated with a 46% odds reduction at 30 days in the composite endpoint of stroke, myocardial infarction, or death.[113]

The role of clopidogrel in the prevention of cerebrovascular events has been addressed in a prospective manner. Diener and colleagues[114] studied the addition of low-dose aspirin to background clopidogrel therapy among patients with recent stroke or TIA and at least one additional cardiovascular risk factor in the Management of Atherothrombosis with Clopidogrel in High-Risk Patients (MATCH) study. After 18 months of treatment, there was no statistically significant benefit of dual-antiplatelet therapy with regard to stroke, myocardial infarction, or vascular death, and an important increase in major bleeding was observed in comparison with clopidogrel and placebo.[114] With this background, the Prevention Regimen

TABLE 7–2 | **Major Randomized Trials of Clopidogrel Therapy**

Trial	No. of Patients	Population	Follow-Up	Treatment	Primary Endpoint	Relative Risk Reduction	P
Clopidogrel versus Aspirin in Patients at Risk of Ischemic Events (CAPRIE)	19,185	Patients with established vascular disease	Mean: 1.9 years	Clopidogrel versus aspirin	Stroke, vascular death, or MI	8.7%	0.043
Clopidogrel in Unstable Angina to prevent Recurrent Events (CURE)	12,562	Patients with ACS	3-12 months	Clopidogrel + aspirin versus aspirin alone	CV death, nonfatal MI, or stroke	20%	<0.001
PCI-CURE	2658	Patients with NSTEMI and undergoing PCI	30 days	Clopidogrel + aspirin versus aspirin alone	CV death, MI, urgent TLR	30%	0.03
Clopidogrel and Metoprolol in Myocardial Infarction Trial (COMMIT)	45,852	Patients with acute MI	Mean: 15 days	Clopidogrel + aspirin versus aspirin alone	Death, stroke, or reinfarction	9%	0.002
Clopidogrel as Adjunctive Reperfusion Therapy–Thombolysis In Myocardial Infarction (CLARITY-TIMI 28)	3491	Patients with STEMI and receiving fibrinolytics	Angiography after median of 84 hours	Clopidogrel + aspirin versus aspirin alone	Death, MI, or infarct-related occlusion of artery	31%	<0.001
Clopidogrel for the Reduction of Events During Observation (CREDO)	2116	Patients undergoing elective PCI or with high likelihood of needing PCI	1 year	Clopidogrel + aspirin versus aspirin alone	Death, stroke, or MI	26.9%	0.02
PCI-CLARITY	1863	Patients with STEMI and receiving fibrinolytics and PCI	30 days after PCI	Clopidogrel + aspirin versus aspirin alone	Death, recurrent MI, or stroke	42%	0.008
Clopidogrel for High Atherothrombotic Risk and Ischemic Stabilization (CHARISMA)	15,603	Patients with known CV disease or multiple risk factors for CV disease	Median: 28 months	Clopidogrel + aspirin versus aspirin alone	CV death, stroke, or MI	7%	0.22
Management of Atherothrombosis with Clopidogrel in High-Risk Patients (MATCH)	7599	Patients with recent TIA or stroke and risk factor for stroke	18 months	Clopidogrel + aspirin versus clopidogrel alone	Ischemic stroke, vascular death, MI, or rehospitalization for ischemia	6.4%	0.244
Atrial Fibrillation Clopidogrel Trial with Irbesartan for Prevention of Vascular Events (ACTIVE)–W	6706	Patients with AF and risk factors for stroke	Median: 1.28 years	Clopidogrel + aspirin versus warfarin	Stroke, MI, vascular death, or non-CNS systemic embolus	−44%	<0.001
ACTIVE-A	7554	Patients with AF and risk factors for stroke but ineligible for VKA	Median: 3.6 years	Clopidogrel + aspirin versus aspirin alone	Stroke, MI, vascular death, or non-CNS systemic embolus	11%	0.01

ACS, acute coronary syndrome; AF, atrial fibrillation; CNS, central nervous system; CV, cardiovascular; MI, myocardial infarction, NSTEMI, non–ST-elevation myocardial infarction; PCI, percutaneous coronary intervention; STEMI, ST-elevation myocardial infarction; TIA, transient ischemic attack; TLR, target lesion revascularization; VKA, vitamin K antagonists.

Adapted from Meadows T, Bhatt DL: Clinical aspects of platelet inhibitors and thrombus formation, *Circ Res* 100:1261-1275, 2007.

for Effectively Avoiding Second Strokes (PRoFESS) investigators randomly assigned more than 20,000 men and women with a mean age of 66 who had suffered a recent ischemic stroke to receive either fixed-dose aspirin, 25 mg, and extended-release dipyridamole, 250 mg, twice daily or clopidogrel, 75 mg daily.[115] The effect of telmisartan was also studied in a 2 × 2 factorial design. After a mean follow-up period of 2.5 years, there was no statistical difference in either the rate of the primary endpoint of recurrent stroke or the secondary composite endpoint of vascular death, stroke, or myocardial infarction.[115]

The first prospective investigation of the role of dual-antiplatelet therapy in preventing cardiovascular events in patients with atrial fibrillation was part of the Atrial Fibrillation Clopidogrel Trial with Irbesartan for Prevention of Vascular Events (ACTIVE) family of studies.[116,117] The ACTIVE-W trial enrolled 6706 patients with atrial fibrillation and additional risk factors for stroke, with a mean CHADS$_2$ (congestive heart failure, hypertension, age >75 years, diabetes mellitus, and either stroke or TIA) score of 2, to test the hypothesis that combination clopidogrel and low-dose aspirin would be noninferior to oral anticoagulation with vitamin K antagonists targeted to an INR goal of 2 to 3.[116] The trial was halted prematurely because the combination of clopidogrel and aspirin was associated with an excess risk of the composite endpoint of stroke, myocardial infarction, vascular death, or systemic embolus in comparison with oral anticoagulation (5.6% versus 3.9%, respectively). The superiority of oral anticoagulation was driven largely by a significant reduction in the risk of stroke and systemic embolism.[116] As expected, maintenance of a therapeutic INR is an important proviso.[118]

The superiority of oral anticoagulation over dual-antiplatelet therapy in stroke prevention has also been demonstrated in subgroups of ACTIVE-W participants who were at relatively lower risk.[119] Despite the clear superiority of oral anticoagulation over antiplatelet therapy in patients at high risk with atrial fibrillation, it is not appropriate for certain patients. The ACTIVE-A trial, in which 7554 such patients were randomly assigned to receive either clopidogrel or placebo with the background of aspirin, demonstrated a 28% reduction in the risk of stroke with clopidogrel and aspirin.[117] However, dual-antiplatelet therapy resulted in a 51% increase in the risk of major extracranial hemorrhage.[117] In the ongoing Secondary Prevention of Small Subcortical Strokes (SPS3) trial, researchers will examine the efficacy of dual-antiplatelet therapy with aspirin and clopidogrel in comparison with aspirin and placebo in the prevention of recurrent stroke in patients with lacunar strokes.[120]

Although dual-antiplatelet therapy with a thienopyridine and aspirin has become the standard of care after PCI and stent placement, the optimal duration of this therapy, particularly after drug-eluting stent placement, remains a subject of great debate. The most feared complication after stent placement is stent thrombosis, an uncommon but highly morbid event. An early meta-analysis focused on data from 6675 patients enrolled in randomized trials in which first-generation drug-eluting stents were compared with bare-metal stents; the data revealed a significant increase in the risk of late stent thrombosis in patients treated with drug-eluting stents and less than 6 months of dual-antiplatelet therapy.[121] Although the risk of early stent thrombosis (<30 days) appeared similar, the risk of stent thrombosis after 1 year was almost five times higher in patients treated with drug-eluting stents.[121] Elaborating on these findings, a registry analysis of more than 4000 patients receiving drug-eluting or bare-metal stents demonstrated a significantly lower rate of the combined endpoint of death or myocardial infarction in patients with drug-eluting stents who were treated with extended clopidogrel than in those treated with 6 or 12 months of clopidogrel.[122] In another observational study of patients treated with drug-eluting stents, the overall rate of stent thrombosis was 1.9% during 18 months of follow-up, and the major predictor of stent thrombosis within 6 months of placement of a drug-eluting stent was discontinuation of clopidogrel.[123]

The possibility of rebound phenomena after cessation of clopidogrel was raised in a retrospective study of more than 3000 patients treated with clopidogrel after ACS.[124] In this Veterans Affairs cohort of patients treated with treated with either medical therapy or PCI, increased rates of the combined endpoint of all-cause mortality or acute myocardial infarction were observed in both medically treated and post-PCI patients after cessation of clopidogrel. Interestingly, there was a grouping of events in the first 90 days after clopidogrel cessation, which raised the specter of a rebound effect.[124] This possibility was supported by in vitro

upregulation of proinflammatory markers and increased platelet aggregation after clopidogrel withdrawal in a small study of patients with diabetes.[125] On the other hand, biologic rebound is less likely with an irreversible antiplatelet agent.

Clopidogrel Resistance

An important clinical conundrum arises from the great variability observed in platelet responsiveness to clopidogrel.[126] A growing body of evidence suggests that clopidogrel resistance is associated with poorer cardiovascular outcomes. In a small study of 60 patients with STEMI, hyporesponsiveness to clopidogrel was observed in up to 25% of patients and associated with greater risk of a recurrent cardiovascular event over a 6-month follow-up period.[127] The pharmacogenetic factors underlying this observation have been further elucidated: Approximately 80% of the prodrug clopidogrel is metabolized to inactive metabolites.[128] The remainder must undergo hepatic metabolism through a two-step cytochrome P-450–dependent process. Among healthy volunteers, Mega and colleagues[129] demonstrated a 30% prevalence of the CYP2C19 allele, a genetic polymorphism that confers loss of function and hence a reduction of the active metabolite of clopidogrel. These investigators also examined the relationship between presence of the CYP2C19 polymorphism and clinical outcomes among 1477 participants assigned to receive clopidogrel in the Trial to Assess Improvement in Therapeutic Outcomes by Optimizing Platelet Inhibition with Prasugrel–Thrombolysis In Myocardial Infarction 38 (TRITON-TIMI 38). In this retrospective analysis, there was a 54% increase in the risk of the composite endpoint of myocardial infarction, cardiovascular death, or stroke among carriers of at least one CYP2C19 allele over that of noncarriers. Presence of the CYP2C19 allele was also associated with a threefold increase in the risk of stent thrombosis.[129] These findings were supported by a contemporaneous report from the French registry of Acute ST Elevation Myocardial Infarction and Non–ST-Elevation Myocardial Infarction (FAST-MI).[130] In patients with an acute myocardial infarction who underwent PCI, the presence of two copies of the CYP2C19 allele was associated with more than a threefold increase in the risk of adverse cardiovascular events.[130] A genome-wide association study confirmed that this allele may affect clopidogrel response.[131,132]

Despite these data, the optimal management strategy for patients with apparent clopidogrel resistance is not known. In a small case series of 7 patients with stent thrombosis and clopidogrel resistance measured by platelet reactivity, escalation of clopidogrel maintenance doses did not result in improved platelet responsiveness.[128] The ongoing Gauging Responsiveness with a VerifyNow Assay–Impact on Thrombosis and Safety (GRAVITAS) trial is a randomized, placebo-controlled study that should add important information in this regard.[133] With the use of a point-of-care assay, approximately 2200 patients with high platelet reactivity will be randomly assigned to receive conventional dosages of clopidogrel (75 mg daily) versus 150 mg daily after placement of a drug-eluting stent for 6 months and will be monitored for the occurrence of nonfatal myocardial infarction, cardiovascular death, or stent thrombosis.[133]

Drug-drug interactions may also contribute to clinically observed clopidogrel resistance. Because clopidogrel must be hepatically metabolized through a cytochrome P-450–dependent process, coadministration with CYP450 substrates has also been implicated in reducing the efficacy of clopidogrel. Although results of a small early study of 44 patients undergoing elective stent implantation suggested such an interaction with atorvastatin,[134] later reports have refuted this.[135-137] In a small study of 45 patients randomly assigned to receive either atorvastatin or pravastatin in the background of clopidogrel after ACS, neither statin attenuated clopidogrel-induced platelet aggregation after 5 weeks of treatment.[135]

A prospective study of 75 patients undergoing coronary stenting also confirmed the absence of an early interaction between clopidogrel and atorvastatin, according to several measures of platelet function.[136] In fact, patients treated with statins alone had decreased platelet activity and decreased expression of the thrombin receptor protease-activating receptor 1, which support the notion of an independent statin antiplatelet effect.[136]

The drug interaction between clopidogrel and the widely used PPIs has also raised concerns. The mechanism of this interaction is not certain, but it may stem from impaired intestinal absorption of clopidogrel and PPI-induced inhibition of CYP2C19, the major enzyme involved in the activation of clopidogrel.[138] An early report highlighted this interaction, demonstrating greater levels of platelet reactivity as measured by vasodilator-stimulated phosphoprotein (VASP) phosphorylation in patients treated with clopidogrel and PPIs.[139] In the Omeprazole Clopidogrel Aspirin Study (OCLA), 124 patients receiving coronary stents were randomly assigned in a double-blind manner to receive omeprazole, 20 mg daily, or placebo in addition to standard clopidogrel and aspirin therapy.[36] With the use of a VASP assay, a marker of clopidogrel-induced platelet inhibition, the investigators demonstrated greater mean platelet reactivity in patients treated with omeprazole. However, the attenuation of platelet inhibition by PPIs may not be a class effect. In another study of platelet activity in patients treated with clopidogrel and pantoprazole or esomeprazole, neither PPI was associated with a change in the mean platelet reactivity index in comparison to patients taking clopidogrel without PPIs.[140] In a retrospective analysis of more than 8000 veterans treated with clopidogrel after ACS, use of PPIs was associated with a greater risk of rehospitalization for ACS or death after adjustment for multiple potential confounders (adjusted odds ratio 1.25).[141] Among patients treated with clopidogrel and PPIs, 14.6% had a recurrent hospitalization for ACS, in comparison with 6.9% treated with clopidogrel alone.[141] A more recent observational study from a randomized clinical trial did not demonstrate any clinical interaction, despite ex vivo evidence of a blunting of the antiplatelet effect of clopidogrel.[142] The clinical significance of this interaction and its contribution to adverse cardiac events was not addressed in the context of a randomized controlled trial until as recently as 2009. In the results of the Clopidogrel and the Optimization of Gastrointestinal Events (COGENT) trial, there was no evidence of cardiovascular harm from the combination of clopidogrel with proton pump inhibitors.[143]

Prasugrel

Prasugrel is a newer member of the thienopyridine family with several theoretical advantages over its predecessors ticlopidine and clopidogrel. Although it is also a prodrug, its onset of action occurs in less than 30 minutes, and it has been demonstrated to be 10 times more potent than clopidogrel in animal models.[144] Furthermore, common genetic variants of CYP450 polymorphisms do not appear to be associated with a reduction in the antiplatelet effect of prasugrel.[145,146] In the TRITON-TIMI 38 study, more than 13,000 patients at moderate to high risk with ACS who were undergoing PCI were randomly assigned to receive either prasugrel (a 60-mg loading dose, followed by 10 mg daily) or clopidogrel (a 300-mg loading dose, followed by 75 mg daily) for up to 15 months.[147] Prasugrel was associated with a 19% relative rate reduction in the composite endpoint of cardiovascular death, nonfatal myocardial infarction, or stroke. This finding was counterbalanced by a 32% increase in the rate of major bleeding in subjects who took prasugrel.[147] A post hoc analysis by the investigators concluded that there was either no net clinical benefit or net harm in three particular subgroups: elderly subjects, patients with prior stroke or TIA, and those weighing less than 60 kg. In a prespecified analysis of patients with and without diabetes in the TRITON-TIMI 38 study, a 30% reduction in major cardiovascular events was observed in patients with diabetes treated with prasugrel, in comparison with a 14% reduction in those without diabetes.[148] There was also no significant difference in the rate of major bleeding in patients with diabetes who took prasugrel or clopidogrel, which represented a greater net clinical benefit than in patients without diabetes.[148]

Prasugrel has also been shown to confer benefit after stent placement with regard to ischemic complications and stent thrombosis. In a subgroup analysis of patients receiving stents in TRITON-TIMI 38, prasugrel conferred 20% and 18% relative reductions in the rate of the primary endpoint among patients receiving bare-metal and drug-eluting stents, respectively.[149] In patients with stents, prasugrel was also associated with a 58% relative reduction in stent thrombosis.[149] According to an analysis of STEMI patients in TRITON-TIMI 38, prasugrel was also more efficacious than clopidogrel with a 3% absolute risk reduction in the primary endpoint at 30 days.[150,151]

Guidelines

In a focused update of the STEMI guidelines, the ACC/AHA gave a Class 1 recommendation to the addition of a 300- to 600-mg loading dose of clopidogrel or 60 mg loading dose of prasugrel in all patients with STEMI who were undergoing PCI.[152] In patients receiving fibrinolytic therapy and nonprimary PCI, clopidogrel is favored as the thienopyridine of choice, because of the lack of data for prasugrel in the setting of fibrinolytic therapy.[152] Similarly, for patients with a history of stroke or TIA, prasugrel is not recommended. Clopidogrel (75 mg daily) or prasugrel (10 mg daily) is recommended for 12 months after placement of a bare-metal or drug-eluting stent. In patients scheduled to undergo elective CABG, discontinuation of clopidogrel and prasugrel for a minimum of 5 and 7 days, respectively, is recommended.[152] The ACCP recommended the addition of clopidogrel, 75 mg daily, to aspirin for patients with symptomatic coronary artery disease.[80] With regard to secondary prevention of stroke, the AHA/ASA suggested that aspirin, combination aspirin and dipyridamole, and clopidogrel alone are all reasonable antiplatelet strategies.[153] Combination aspirin and dipyridamole is preferred over aspirin alone, however.[153]

NOVEL AGENTS

Although a full discussion of glycoprotein IIb/IIIA (GP IIb/IIIA) inhibition is not within the scope of this chapter, the historical experience with oral GP IIb/IIIA inhibition is noteworthy. A meta-analysis of the four large, randomized trials of oral GP IIb/IIIa inhibitors that included more than 33,000 patients conclusively demonstrated the deleterious effects of this class of antiplatelet agents.[154] According to aggregate data, oral GP IIb/IIIa inhibitors were associated with a 31% increase in mortality.[154] Hence, these agents are no longer used for antiplatelet therapy.

Several ongoing trials of novel platelet inhibitors may add to the current therapies for cardiovascular disease. The oral reversible P2Y$_{12}$ receptor antagonist, AZD 6140 (ticagrelor), was studied in the Platelet Inhibition and Patient Outcomes (PLATO) trial.[155] Unlike the thienopyridines, it is not a prodrug, and thus hepatic metabolism is not needed to produce an active metabolite.[156] Additional theoretical benefits are rapid onset and offset of action, as well as greater platelet inhibition than with clopidogrel.[157] In a randomized, double-blind study of 18,624 patients with ACS, the PLATO trial demonstrated a decreased risk of the composite endpoint of vascular death, stroke, or myocardial infarction in patients who received ticagrelor, 90 mg twice daily, in comparison with clopidogrel, 75 mg daily (9.8% versus 11.8% respectively).[155] This benefit was achieved without an increase in major bleeding. The results of a phase II study evaluating the efficacy of ticagrelor in patients identified as clopidogrel nonresponders are also awaited.[158] Another reversible P2Y$_{12}$ receptor antagonist available in both intravenous and oral forms, PRT060128, is also being compared with clopidogrel in phase II trials of patients undergoing elective PCI (INtraveNous and Oral administration of elinogrel, a selective and reversible P2Y$_{12}$-receptor inhibitor, versus clopidogrel to eVAluate Tolerability and Efficacy in nonurgent Percutaneous Coronary Interventions patients [INNOVATE-PCI])[159] and STEMI (Early Rapid ReversAl of platelet thromboSis with intravenous Elinogrel before PCI to optimize reperfusion in acute Myocardial Infarction [ERASE MI]).[160]

Yet another target of platelet inhibition is thrombin-mediated platelet aggregation. Thrombin is a potent agonist of platelet aggregation through its interaction with the protease-activating receptor 1.[161] The potential incremental clinical benefit of the thrombin receptor antagonist SCH 53038 is being evaluated in two large phase III trials. In the Thrombin Receptor Antagonist for Clinical Event Reduction in Acute Coronary Syndrome (TRA*CER) study, approximately 12,500 patients with ACS will be randomly assigned to receive SCH 53038 or placebo for 1 year, in addition to standard medical therapy.[160] The Thrombin Receptor Antagonist in Secondary Prevention of Atherothrombotic Ischemic Events–Thrombolysis In Myocardial Infarction 50 (TRA 2°P-TIMI 50) trial is a large, randomized, double-blind, placebo-controlled trial designed to evaluate the efficacy of a 2.5-mg daily dose of SCH 53038 in comparison with placebo in patients with a history of myocardial infarction, stroke, or peripheral artery disease who were being treated with aspirin, clopidogrel, or both.[162] Another novel platelet-activating receptor antagonist, E5555, is being investigated in phase II trials in the Lessons from Antagonizing the Cellular Effects of Thrombin (LANCELOT) study.[163] In vitro, E5555 also appears to possess biologic activity beyond protease-activating receptor 1 blockade.[164]

Cilostazol

Although first approved in the United States in 1999 for the treatment of intermittent claudication, cilostazol has been used as an antiplatelet agent in Asia since 1988.[165] Cilostazol exerts its principal antiplatelet effect through selective inhibition of phosphodiesterase 3 in platelets and vascular smooth muscle cells.[165] This leads to increased levels of platelet cyclic adenosine monophosphate (cAMP) and ultimately results in inhibition of platelet aggregation and arteriolar vasodilation.[166] Antimitogenic effects and inhibition of cAMP uptake may also play a role in the mechanism of action of cilostazol.[166] The efficacy of cilostazol in the symptomatic management of patients with intermittent claudication has been demonstrated in several trials. In one randomized, placebo-controlled trial that included more than 600 patients with intermittent claudication, cilostazol, either 50 mg or 100 mg twice daily, significantly improved pain-free walking distance in comparison with placebo.[167] In a meta-analysis of eight randomized, placebo-controlled trials that included 2702 patients with moderate to severe claudication, cilostazol resulted in a 67% increase in pain-free walking distance and a 50% increase in maximal walking distance.[168] Furthermore, this benefit was maintained in stratification by gender, age, and diabetes.

With its pleiotropic effects, cilostazol may be added to the armamentarium of antiplatelet therapy after PCI. In early studies of cilostazol, researchers reported a reduction in intimal proliferation and restenosis after directional coronary atherectomy and balloon angioplasty.[169,170] In a pooled analysis of 23 trials that included more than 5000 patients, cilostazol was found to be associated with a reduction in the risk of both restenosis and the need for repeat revascularization after PCI.[171] More recently, a prospective, randomized trial of triple-antiplatelet therapy—in which diabetic patients who had received drug-eluting stents were given aspirin, clopidogrel, and cilostazol—demonstrated reduced angiographic restenosis, as well as target lesion revascularization, in comparison with standard dual-antiplatelet therapy.[172] The protective effect of cilostazol may be attributable partly to attenuation of endothelial senescence induced by drug-eluting stents.[173] As might be expected, triple-antiplatelet therapy results in more potent inhibition of ADP-induced platelet aggregation than does conventional dual-antiplatelet therapy.[174,175] Despite these data, the role of triple-antiplatelet therapy in current clinical practice remains uncertain. A retrospective study from a Korean registry provided important insight in this area. In this study of 4203 patients with STEMI who underwent PCI, triple-antiplatelet therapy was associated with fewer major cardiac events, cardiac death, and total mortality than was dual-antiplatelet therapy.[176] The incremental benefit of cilostazol may prove to be particularly useful in patients with clopidogrel resistance. This hypothesis was tested in the Adjunctive Cilostazol Versus High Maintenance Dose Clopidogrel in Patients with Clopidogrel Resistance (ACCEL-RESISTANCE) study.[177] In this small study of 60 patients undergoing PCI, patients with high post-treatment platelet reactivity more than 12 hours after a 300-mg dose of clopidogrel were randomized to receive either 100 mg of cilostazol twice daily or 150 mg of clopidogrel daily. Adjunctive cilostazol was associated with greater platelet inhibition after 30 days than were high maintenance doses of clopidogrel.[177]

Dipyridamole

Dipyridamole has a variety of vascular effects that may contribute to its efficacy in cerebrovascular disease, for which it has been widely studied. Dipyridamole inhibits adenosine uptake by red blood cells, which in turn stimulates adenylyl cyclase and subsequent platelet formation of cAMP, an inhibitor of platelet aggregation.[178] An additional antithrombotic effect arises from inhibition of endothelium phosphodiesterase 5, and stimulation of nitric oxide/cyclic guanosine monophosphate (cGMP) signaling.[179] Dipyridamole has also been shown to exhibit antioxidant and direct anti-inflammatory effects.[178] Although results of an early randomized trial of high-dose aspirin and dipyridamole versus aspirin or placebo were not suggestive of an additional benefit with regard to recurrent stroke,[180] subsequent large-scale studies have provided an evidence base to support its use. The first European Stroke Prevention Study (ESPS) revealed a 33.5% reduction in stroke or all-cause death among 2500 patients with a recent stroke or TIA who were treated with 75 mg of dipyridamole and 330 mg of aspirin three times daily, in comparison with placebo.[181] In a 2 × 2 factorial design, the European Stroke Prevention Study 2 (ESPS 2) randomly assigned 6602 patients with prior stroke or TIA to receive aspirin alone (25 mg twice daily), fixed-dose aspirin (25 mg) plus dipyridamole (200 mg) twice daily, dipyridamole alone (200 mg twice daily), or placebo.[182] In comparison with placebo, combination therapy produced a 37% relative risk reduction in stroke, aspirin alone produced an 18% reduction, and dipyridamole alone produced a 16% reduction.[182] In an open-label design in the European/Australasian Stroke Prevention in Reversible Ischaemia Trial (ESPRIT), 2764 patients with recent minor stroke or TIA were randomly assigned to receive aspirin (30 to 325 mg daily) alone or aspirin plus dipyridamole (200 mg twice daily).[183] Over a mean follow-up period of 3.5 years,

TABLE 7–3	Antiplatelet Agents and Supporting Trials

Antiplatelet Agent	Dose	Major Supporting Trials and Endpoint Reductions
Aspirin	75-325 mg daily	**Primary Prevention** Antithrombotic Trialists (ATT): 12% RRR in MI, stroke, or vascular death per year **Secondary Prevention** ATT: 19% RRR in MI, stroke, or vascular death per year, 20% RRR in major coronary event per year
Ticlopidine	250 mg twice daily	**Stroke** Canadian American Ticlopidine Study (CATS): 23.3% RRR in recurrent stroke, MI, or vascular death in comparison to placebo Ticlopidine Aspirin Stroke Study (TASS): 12% RRR in all-cause mortality or nonfatal stroke **Peripheral Artery Disease** Swedish Ticlopidine Multicentre Study (STIMS): 29.1% RRR in all-cause mortality; no significant difference in primary endpoint of MI, stroke, or TIA **Percutaneous Coronary Intervention** **Stent Anticoagulation Restenosis Study (STARS): 80%-85% RRR in death, TLR, stent thrombosis, or nonfatal MI in comparison to aspirin alone or aspirin plus warfarin**
Clopidogrel	75 mg daily	**ACS/Coronary Disease** Clopidogrel versus Aspirin in Patients at Risk of Ischemic Events (CAPRIE): 8.7% RRR in ischemic stroke, vascular death, or MI in comparison to aspirin alone Clopidogrel in Unstable Angina to prevent Recurrent Events (CURE): 20% RRR in CV death, nonfatal MI, or stroke after NSTEMI/ACS in comparison to placebo Clopidogrel for the Reduction of Events During Observation (CREDO): 26.9% RRR in MI, death, or stroke for early and sustained treatment with clopidogrel after PCI in comparison with placebo Clopidogrel for High Atherothrombotic Risk and Ischemic Stabilization (CHARISMA): No significant difference in CV death, MI, or stroke in population at high risk with DAT, in comparison to aspirin alone Clopidogrel and Metoprolol in Myocardial Infarction Trial (COMMIT): 9% RRR in death, stroke or reinfarction after MI in comparison to placebo Clopidogrel as Adjunctive Reperfusion Therapy–Thrombolysis In Myocardial Infarction (CLARITY-TIMI 28): 36% odds reduction in death, recurrent MI, or infarct-related occlusion of artery after STEMI in comparison to placebo **Stroke** Management of Atherothrombosis with Clopidogrel in High-Risk Patients (MATCH): No significant reduction in ischemic stroke, MI, vascular death, or rehospitalization for ischemia with DAT in comparison to clopidogrel alone after stroke or TIA Prevention Regimen for Effectively Avoiding Second Strokes (PRoFESS): No significant difference in rate of recurrent stroke in comparison to ASA-ERDP after ischemic stroke Atrial Fibrillation Clopidogrel Trial with Irbesartan for Prevention of Vascular Events (ACTIVE)-W: DAT inferior to oral anticoagulation in patients with AF with RR of 1.44 for stroke, embolic event, MI, or vascular death ACTIVE-A: 11% RRR in major vascular events in patients with AF in comparison to placebo plus background aspirin
Prasugrel	10 mg daily*	**ACS** Trial to Assess Improvement in Therapeutic Outcomes by Optimizing Platelet Inhibition with Prasugrel-Thrombolysis in Myocardial Infarction (TRITON-TIMI 38): 19% RRR in CV death, nonfatal MI, or nonfatal stroke in comparison to clopidogrel
Aspirin-Dipyridamole	25 mg/200 mg twice daily	**Stroke** European Stroke Prevention Study (ESPS): 33.5% RRR in all-cause mortality or stroke in comparison to placebo European Stroke Prevention Study 2 (ESPS 2): 24% RRR in stroke or death in comparison to aspirin alone or dipyridamole alone European/Australasian Stroke Prevention in Reversible Ischaemia Trial (ESPRIT): 20% RRR in vascular death, nonfatal MI, nonfatal stroke, or nonfatal major bleeding in comparison to aspirin alone
Cilostazol	50-100 mg twice daily	**Peripheral Artery Disease** Improves maximal walking distance by 50%, pain-free walking distance by 67%

*Consider 5 mg if patient weighs <60 kg.

ACS, acute coronary syndrome; AF, atrial fibrillation; ASA-ERDP; aspirin-extended release dipyridamole; CV, cardiovascular; DAT, dual-antiplatelet therapy; MI, myocardial infarction; NSTEMI, non–ST-elevation myocardial infarction; RR, relative risk; RRR, relative risk reduction; STEMI, ST-elevation myocardial infarction; TIA, transient ischemic attack; TLR, target lesion revascularization.

the rate of the primary composite endpoint of cardiovascular death, nonfatal myocardial infarction, nonfatal stroke, or major bleeding was 13% among subjects who took aspirin plus dipyridamole and 16% among patients who took only aspirin. After 5 years of follow-up, 34% of patients discontinued the combination of aspirin and dipyridamole, many because of headache.[183] The awaited Japanese Aggrenox Stroke Prevention vs. Aspirin Programme (JASAP) is comparing fixed-dose dipyridamole plus aspirin with aspirin, 81 mg daily, for the secondary prevention of stroke.[184]

CONCLUSION

Platelets play a fundamental role in thrombosis and inflammation, processes germane to the development of cardiovascular disease. Inhibition of thromboxane synthesis through aspirin has formed the basis of modern cardiovascular disease prevention. Similarly, ADP inhibition by thienopyridines has proved an essential adjunct in the treatment of patients with ACS, cerebrovascular disease, and peripheral artery disease (Table 7-3). However, despite these therapies, a significant number of patients experience vascular events because of the multiple pathways available for platelet activation. New strategies for platelet inhibition must be developed to achieve greater successes in the treatment of cardiovascular disease.

REFERENCES

1. Davi G, Patrono C: Platelet activation and atherothrombosis. *N Engl J Med* 357:2482-2494, 2007.
2. Peto R, Collins R, Gray R: Large-scale randomized evidence: large, simple trials and overviews of trials. *J Clin Epidemiol* 48:23-40, 1995.
3. Roth GJ, Majerus P: The mechanism of the effect of aspirin on human platelets. *J Clin Invest* 56:624-632, 1975.
4. Patrono C: Aspirin as an antiplatelet drug. *N Engl J Med* 330:1287-1294, 1994.
5. Schror K: Aspirin and platelets: the antiplatelet action of aspirin and its role in thrombosis treatment and prophylaxis. *Semin Thromb Hemost* 23:349-356, 1997.
6. Amin AR, Vyas P, Attur M, et al: The mode of action of aspirin-like drugs: effect on inducible nitric oxide synthase. *Proc Natl Acad Sci* 92:7926-7930, 1995.
7. Kopp E, Sankar G: Inihibition of NF-kappa B by sodium salicylate and aspirin. *Science* 265:956-959, 1994.
8. Coronary Drug Project Research Group: Aspirin in coronary heart disease. *J Chronic Dis* 29:625-642, 1976.
9. Elwood PC, Cochrane AL, Burr ML, et al: A randomized controlled trial of acetyl salicylic acid in the secondary prevention of mortality from myocardial infarction. *BMJ* 1:436-440, 1974.
10. Persantine and aspirin in coronary heart disease. The Persantine-Aspirin Reinfarction Study Research Group. *Circulation* 62:449-461, 1980.
11. Antiplatelet Trialists' Collaboration: Secondary prevention of vascular disease by prolonged antiplatelet treatment. *BMJ* 296:320-331, 1988.
12. Antiplatelet Trialists' Collaboration: Collaborative overview of randomized trials of antiplatelet therapy–I: prevention of death, myocardial infarction, and stroke by prolonged antiplatelet therapy in various categories of patients. *BMJ* 308:81-106, 1994.
13. Elwood PC, Sweetnam PM: Aspirin and secondary mortality after myocardial infarction. *Lancet* 314:1313-1315, 1979.
14. ISIS-2 (Second International Study of Infarct Survival) Collaborative Group: Randomised trial of intravenous streptokinase, oral aspirin, both, or neither among 17,187 cases of suspected myocardial infarction. *Lancet* 2:349-360, 1988.
15. Lewis HD, Davis JW, Archibald DG, et al: Protective effects of aspirin against acute myocardial infarction and death in men with unstable angina. Results of a Veterans Administration cooperative study. *N Engl J Med* 309:396-403, 1983.
16. Research Group on Instability in Coronary Artery Disease (RISC) Investigators: Risk of myocardial infarction and death during treatment with low dose aspirin and intravenous heparin in men with unstable coronary artery disease. *Lancet* 336:827-830, 1990.
17. Chen ZM and CAST (Chinese Acute Stroke Trial) Investigators: CAST: randomised placebo-controlled trial of early aspirin use in 20,000 patients with acute ischaemic stroke. *Lancet* 349:1641-1649, 1997.
18. International Stroke Trial Collaborative Group: The International Stroke Trial (IST): a randomised trial of aspirin, subcutaneous heparin, both, or neither among 19,435 patients with acute ischaemic stroke. *Lancet* 349:1569-1581, 1997.
19. Chen Z, Sandercock P, Pan H, et al: Indications for early aspirin use in acute ischemic stroke: a combined analysis of 40,000 randomized patients from the Chinese Acute Stroke Trial and the International Stroke Trial. *Stroke* 31:1240-1249, 2000.
20. Gavaghan TP, Gebski V, Baron DW: Immediate postoperative aspirin improves vein graft patency early and late after coronary artery bypass graft surgery. A placebo-controlled, randomized study. *Circulation* 83:1526-1533, 1991.
21. Goldman S, Copeland J, Moritz T, et al: Saphenous vein graft patency 1 year after coronary artery bypass surgery and effects of antiplatelet therapy. Results of a Veterans Administration cooperative study. *Circulation* 80:1190-1197, 1989.
22. Savage MP, Goldberg S, Bove AA, et al: Effect of thromboxane A_2 blockade on clinical outcome and restenosis after successful coronary angioplasty: Multi-Hospital Eastern Atlantic Restenosis Trial (M-Heart II). *Circulation* 92:3194-3200, 1995.
23. Roux S, Christeller S, Ludin E: Effects of aspirin on coronary reocclusion and recurrent ischemia after thrombolysis: a meta-analysis. *J Am Coll Cardiol* 19:671-677, 1992.
24. Antithrombotic Trialists' Collaboration: Collaborative meta-analysis of randomized trials of antiplatelet therapy for prevention of death, myocardial infarction, and stroke in high risk patients. *BMJ* 324:71-86, 2002.
25. Peto R, Gray R, Collins R, et al: Randomised trial of prophylactic daily aspirin in British male doctors. *BMJ* 296:313-316, 1988.
26. Steering Committee of the Physicians' Health Study Group: Final report on the aspirin component of the ongoing Physicians' Health Study. *N Engl J Med* 321:129-135, 1989.
27. Medical Research Council's General Practice Research Framework: Thrombosis Prevention Trial: randomised trial of low-intensity oral anticoagulation with warfarin and low-aspirin in the primary prevention of ischaemic heart disease in men at increased risk. *Lancet* 351:233-241, 1998.
28. Hansson L, Zanchetti A, Carruthers S, et al: Effects of intensive blood-pressure lowering and low-dose aspirin in patients with hyertension: principal results of the Hypertension Optimal Treatment (HOT) randomised trial. *Lancet* 351:1755-1762, 1998.
29. Collaborative Group of the Primary Prevention Project: Low-dose aspirin and vitamin E in people at cardiovascular risk: a randomised trial in general practice. *Lancet* 357:89-95, 2001.
30. Ridker P, Cook N, Lee I, et al: A randomized trial of low-dose aspirin in the primary prevention of cardiovascular disease in women. *N Engl J Med* 352:1293-1304, 2005.
31. Berger JS, Roncaglioni MC, Avanzini F, et al: Aspirin for the primary prevention of cardiovascular events in women and men. *JAMA* 295:306-313, 2006.
32. Antithrombotic Trialists' Collaboration: Aspirin in the primary and secondary prevention of vascular disease: collaborative meta-analysis of individual participant data from randomised trials. *Lancet* 373:1849-1860, 2009.
33. Ogawa H, Nakayama M, Morimoto T, et al: Low-dose aspirin for primary prevention of atherosclerotic events in patients with type 2 diabetes: a randomized controlled trial. *JAMA* 300:2134-2141, 2008.
34. Belch J, MacCuish A, Campbell I, et al: The Prevention of Progression of Arterial Disease and Diabetes (POPADAD) trial: factorial randomised placebo controlled trial of aspirin and antioxidants in patients with diabetes and asymptomatic peripheral arterial disease. *BMJ* 337:a1840, 2008.
35. Fowkes G, Patrono C: AAA: randomized controlled trial of low dose aspirin in the prevention of cardiovascular events and death in subjects with asymptomatic atherosclerosis, presented at the European Society of Cardiology Congress, Barcelona, Spain, August 30, 2009. Available at: http://www.escardio.org/congresses/esc-2009/congress-reports/Pages/706001-706002-fowkes-patrono.aspx. Accessed August 3, 2010.
36. Gilard M, Arnaud B, Cornily JC, et al: Influence of omeprazole on the antiplatelet action of clopidogrel associated with aspirin: the randomized, double-blind OCLA (Omeprazole CLopidogrel Aspirin) study. *J Am Coll Cardiol* 51:256-260, 2008.
37. De Berardis G, Sacco M, Evangelista V: Aspirin and Simvastatin Combination for Cardiovascular Events Prevention Trial in Diabetes (ACCEPT-D): design of a randomized study of the efficacy of low-dose aspirin in the prevention of cardiovascular events in subjects with diabetes mellitus treated with statins. *Trials* 8:21, 2007 (online journal article): http://www.trialsjournal.com/content/8/1/21. Accessed August 3, 2010.
38. *A study to assess the efficacy and safety of enteric-coated acetylsalicylic acid in patients at moderate risk of cardiovascular disease (ARRIVE)*, (online U.S. government report): http://clinicaltrials.gov/ct2/show/NCT00501059. Accessed August 3, 2010.
39. Nelson M, Reid C, Beilin L, et al: Rationale for a trial of low-dose aspirin for the primary prevention of major adverse cardiovascular events and vascular dementia in the elderly: ASPirin in Reducing Events in the Elderly (ASPREE). *Drugs Aging* 20:897-903, 2003.
40. *Japanese Primary Prevention Project with Aspirin* (online U.S. government report): http://clinicaltrials.gov/ct2/show/NCT00225849. Accessed August 3, 2010.
41. Patrono C: Aspirin as an antiplatelet drug. *N Engl J Med* 330:1287-1294, 1994.
42. Clarke RJ, Mayo G, Price P, et al: Suppression of thromboxane A_2 but not of systemic prostacyclin by controlled-release aspirin. *N Engl J Med* 325:1137-1141, 1991.
43. Peters RJG, Mehta SR, Fox KAA, et al: Effects of aspirin dose when used alone or in combination with clopidogrel in patients with acute coronary syndromes: observations from the Clopidogrel in Unstable Angina to Prevent Recurrent Events (CURE) study. *Circulation* 108:1682-1687, 2003.
44. Serebruany VL, Steinhubl SR, Berger PB, et al: Analysis of risk of bleeding complications after different doses of aspirin in 192,036 patients enrolled in 31 randomized controlled trials. *Am J Cardiol* 95:1218-1222, 2005.
45. Steinhubl SR, Bhatt DL, Brennan DM, et al: Aspirin to prevent cardiovascular disease: the association of aspirin dose and clopidogrel with thrombosis and bleeding. *Ann Intern Med* 150:379-386, 2009.
46. Mehta SR: *A randomized comparison of a clopidogrel high loading and maintenance dose regimen versus standard dose and high versus low dose aspirin in 25,000 patients with acute coronary syndromes: results of the CURRENT-OASIS 7 trial,* presented at the European Society of Cardiology Congress 2009, Barcelona, Spain, August 30, 2009.
47. Mehta SR, Bassand JP, Chrolavicius S, et al: Design and rationale of CURRENT-OASIS 7: a randomized, 2 × 2 factorial trial evaluating optimal dosing strategies for clopidogrel and aspirin in patients with ST and non–ST-elevation acute coronary syndromes managed with an early invasive strategy. *Am Heart J* 156:1080-1088.e1, 2008.
48. Campbell CL, Smyth S, Montalescot G, et al: Aspirin dose for the prevention of cardiovascular disease: a systematic review. *JAMA* 297:2018-2024, 2007.
49. Patrono C, Coller B, Fitzgerald G, et al: Platelet-active drugs: the relationships among dose, effectiveness, and side effects. *Chest* 126:234S-264S, 2004.
50. Feldman M, Cryer B: Aspirin absorption rates and platelet inhibition times with 325-mg buffered aspirin tablets (chewed or swallowed intact) and with buffered aspirin solution. *Am J Cardiol* 84:404-409, 1999.
51. Kelly JP, Kaufman DW, Jurgelon JM, et al: Risk of aspirin-associated major upper-gastrointestinal bleeding with enteric-coated or buffered product. *Lancet* 348:1413-1416, 1996.
52. McQuaid KR, Laine L: Systematic review and meta-analysis of adverse events of low-dose aspirin and clopidogrel in randomized controlled trials. *Am J Med* 119:624-638, 2006.
53. Ng W, Wong W, Chen W, et al: Incidence and predictors of upper gastrointestinal bleeding in patients receiving low dose aspirin for secondary prevention of cardiovascular events in patients with coronary artery disease. *World J Gastroenterol* 12:2923-2927, 2006.
54. Hernández-Díaz S, García Rodríguez LA: Cardioprotective aspirin users and their excess risk of upper gastrointestinal complications. *BMC Med* 4:22, 2006.
55. Lee M, Cryer B, Feldman M: Dose effects of aspirin on gastric prostaglandins and stomach mucosal injury. *Ann Intern Med* 120:184-189, 1994.
56. Cryer B: Reducing the risks of gastrointestinal bleeding with antiplatelet therapies. *N Engl J Med* 352:287-289, 2005.
57. Yeomans N, Lanas A, Labenz J, et al: Efficacy of esomeprazole (20 mg once daily) for reducing the risk of gastroduodenal ulcers associated with continuous use of low-dose aspirin. *Am J Gastroenterol* 103:2465-2473, 2008.
58. Lai KC, Lam SK, Chu KM, et al: Lansoprazole for the prevention of recurrences of ulcer complications from long-term low-dose aspirin use. *N Engl J Med* 346:2033-2038, 2002.

59. Chan FKL, Ching JYL, Hung LCT, et al: Clopidogrel versus aspirin and esomeprazole to prevent recurrent ulcer bleeding. *N Engl J Med* 352:238-244, 2005.
60. Taha AS, McCloskey C, Prasad R, et al: Famotidine for the prevention of peptic ulcers and oesophagitis in patients taking low-dose aspirin (FAMOUS): a phase III, randomised, double-blind, placebo-controlled trial. *Lancet* 374:119-125, 2009.
61. Bhatt DL, Scheiman J, Abraham NS, et al: ACCF/ACG/AHA 2008 expert consensus document on reducing the gastrointestinal risks of antiplatelet therapy and NSAID use: a report of the American College of Cardiology Foundation Task Force on Clinical Expert Consensus Documents. *Circulation* 118:1894-1909, 2008.
62. Macdonald TM, Wei L: Effect of ibuprofen on cardioprotective effect of aspirin. *Lancet* 361:573-574, 2003.
63. Catella-Lawson F, Reilly MP, Kapoor SC, et al: Cyclooxygenase inhibitors and the antiplatelet effects of aspirin. *N Engl J Med* 345:1809-1817, 2001.
64. Capone ML, Sciulli MG, Tacconelli S, et al: Pharmacodynamic interaction of naproxen with low-dose aspirin in healthy subjects. *J Am Coll Cardiol* 45:1295-1301, 2005.
65. Bhatt DL: NSAIDS and the risk of myocardial infarction: do they help or harm? *Eur Heart J* 27:1635-1636, 2006.
66. Helin-Salmivaara A, Virtanen A, Vesalainen R, et al: NSAID use and the risk of hospitalization for first myocardial infarction in the general population: a nationwide case-control study from Finland. *Eur Heart J* 27:1657-1663, 2006.
67. Bhatt DL: Aspirin resistance: more than just a laboratory curiosity. *J Am Coll Cardiol* 43:1127-1129, 2004.
68. Quinn MJ, Topol EJ: Common variations in platelet glycoproteins: pharmacogenomic implications. *Pharmacogenomics* 2:341-352, 2001.
69. Csiszar A, Stef G, Pacher P, et al: Oxidative stress–induced isoprostane formation may contribute to aspirin resistance in platelets. *Prostaglandins Leukot Essent Fatty Acids* 66:557-558, 2002.
70. Weber AA, Zimmermann KC, Meyer-Kirchrath J, et al: Cyclooxygenase-2 in human platelets as a possible factor in aspirin resistance. *Lancet* 353:900, 1999.
71. Poulsen TS, Jorgensen B, Korsholm L, et al: Prevalence of aspirin resistance in patients with an evolving acute myocardial infarction. *Thromb Res* 119:555-562, 2007.
72. Christiaens L, Macchi L, Herpin D, et al: Resistance to aspirin in vitro at rest and during exercise in patients with angiographically proven coronary artery disease. *Thromb Res* 108:115-119, 2002.
73. Snoep JD, Hovens MMC, Eikenboom JCJ, et al: Association of laboratory-defined aspirin resistance with a higher risk of recurrent cardiovascular events: a systematic review and meta-analysis. *Arch Intern Med* 167:1593-1599, 2007.
74. Dalen JE: Aspirin resistance: is it real? Is it clinically significant? *Am J Med* 120:1-4, 2007.
75. Eikelboom JW, Hirsh J, Weitz JI, et al: Aspirin-resistant thromboxane biosynthesis and the risk of myocardial infarction, stroke, or cardiovascular death in patients at high risk for cardiovascular events. *Circulation* 105:1650-1655, 2002.
76. Gum PA, Kottke-Marchant K, Welsh PA, et al: A prospective, blinded determination of the natural history of aspirin resistance among stable patients with cardiovascular disease. *J Am Coll Cardiol* 41:961-965, 2003.
77. Chen WH, Lee PY, Ng W, et al: Aspirin resistance is associated with a high incidence of myonecrosis after non-urgent percutaneous coronary intervention despite clopidogrel pretreatment. *J Am Coll Cardiol* 43:1122-1126, 2004.
78. Eikelboom JW, Hankey GJ, Thom J, et al: Incomplete inhibition of thromboxane biosynthesis by acetylsalicylic acid: determinants and effect on cardiovascular risk. *Circulation* 118:1705-1712, 2008.
79. U.S. Preventive Services Task Force: Aspirin for the prevention of cardiovascular disease: U.S. Preventive Services Task Force Recommendation Statement. *Ann Intern Med* 150:396-404, 2009.
80. Hirsh J, Guyatt G, Albers GW, et al: Executive summary: American College of Chest Physicians Evidence-Based Clinical Practice Guidelines (8th edition). *Chest* 133(6 suppl):71S-109S, 2008.
81. American Diabetes Association: Standards of medical care in diabetes. *Diabetes Care* 32:S13-S61, 2009.
82. Hirsch AT, Haskal ZJ, Hertzer NR, et al: ACC/AHA 2005 guidelines for the management of patients with peripheral arterial disease (lower extremity, renal, mesenteric, and abdominal aortic): executive summary a collaborative report from the American Association for Vascular Surgery/Society for Vascular Surgery, Society for Cardiovascular Angiography and Interventions, Society for Vascular Medicine and Biology, Society of Interventional Radiology, and the ACC/AHA Task Force on Practice Guidelines (Writing Committee to Develop Guidelines for the Management of Patients with Peripheral Arterial Disease): endorsed by the American Association of Cardiovascular and Pulmonary Rehabilitation; National Heart, Lung and Blood Institute; Society for Vascular Nursing; Transatlantic Inter-Society Consensus; and Vascular Disease Foundation. *J Am Coll Cardiol* 47:1239-1312, 2006.
83. Antman EM, Hand M, Armstrong PW, et al: 2007 Focused update of the ACC/AHA 2004 Guidelines for the Management of Patients with ST-Elevation Myocardial Infarction: a report of the American College of Cardiology/American Heart Association Task Force on Practice Guidelines: developed in collaboration with the Canadian Cardiovascular Society endorsed by the American Academy of Family Physicians: 2007 Writing Group to Review New Evidence and Update the ACC/AHA 2004 Guidelines for the Management of Patients with ST-Elevation Myocardial Infarction, Writing on Behalf of the 2004 Writing Committee. *Circulation* 117:296-329, 2008.
84. Adams HP, Jr, del Zoppo G, Alberts MJ, et al: Guidelines for the early management of adults with ischemic stroke: a guideline from the American Heart Association/American Stroke Association Stroke Council, Clinical Cardiology Council, Cardiovascular Radiology and Intervention council, and the Atherosclerotic Peripheral Vascular Disease and Quality of Care Outcomes in Research Interdisciplinary Working Groups: the American Academy of Neurology affirms the value of this guideline as an educational tool for neurologists. *Stroke* 38:1655-1711, 2007.
85. Hollopeter G, Jantzen HM, Vincent D, et al: Identification of the platelet ADP receptor targeted by antithrombotic drugs. *Nature* 409:202-207, 2001.
86. Meadows TA, Bhatt DL: Clinical aspects of platelet inhibitors and thrombus formation. *Circ Res* 100:1261-1275, 2007.
87. Storey RF, Sanderson HM, White AE, et al: The central role of the P2T receptor in amplification of human platelet activation, aggregation, secretion and procoagulant activity. *Br J Haematol* 110:925-934, 2000.
88. Thebault JJ, Blatrix C, Blanchard JF, et al: Effects of ticlopidine, a new platelet aggregation inhibitor in man. *Clin Pharmacol Ther* 18:485-490, 1975.
89. Savi P, Herbert JM: Clopidogrel and ticlopidine: $P2Y_{12}$ adenosine diphosphate–receptor antagonists for the prevention of atherothrombosis. *Semin Thromb Hemost* 31:174-183, 2005.
90. Gent M, Donald Easton J, Hachinski VC, et al: The Canadian American Ticlopidine Study (CATS) in thromboembolic stroke. *Lancet* 333:1215-1220, 1989.
91. Gorelick PB, Richardson D, Kelly M, et al: Aspirin and ticlopidine for prevention of recurrent stroke in black patients: a randomized trial. *JAMA* 289:2947-2957, 2003.
92. Hass WK, Easton JD, Adams HP, et al: A randomized trial comparing ticlopidine hydrochloride with aspirin for the prevention of stroke in high-risk patients. Ticlopidine Aspirin Stroke Study Group. *N Engl J Med* 321:501-507, 1989.
93. Janzon L, Bergqvist J, Bober J, et al: Prevention of myocardial infarction and stroke in patients with intermittent claudication; effects of ticlopidine. Results from STIMS, the Swedish Ticlopidine Multicentre Study. *J Intern Med* 227:301-308, 1990.
94. Leon MB, Baim DS, Popma JJ, et al: A clinical trial comparing three antithrombotic-drug regimens after coronary-artery stenting. *N Engl J Med* 339:1665-1671, 1998.
95. Steinhubl SR, Tan WA, Foody JM, et al: Incidence and clinical course of thrombotic thrombocytopenic purpura due to ticlopidine following coronary stenting. *JAMA* 281:806-810, 1999.
96. Balsano F, Rizzon P, Violi F, et al: Antiplatelet treatment with ticlopidine in unstable angina. A controlled multicenter clinical trial. The Studio della Ticlopidina nell'Angina Instabile Group. *Circulation* 82:17-26, 1990.
97. Bertrand ME, Legrand V, Boland J, et al: Randomized multicenter comparison of conventional anticoagulation versus antiplatelet therapy in unplanned and elective coronary stenting: the Full Anticoagulation Versus Aspirin and Ticlopidine (FANTASTIC) study. *Circulation* 98:1597-1603, 1998.
98. Urban P, Macaya C, Rupprecht HJ, et al: Randomized evaluation of anticoagulation versus antiplatelet therapy after coronary stent implantation in high-risk patients: the Multicenter Aspirin and Ticlopidine Trial after Intracoronary Stenting (MATTIS). *Circulation* 98:2126-2132, 1998.
99. Bertrand ME, Rupprecht HJ, Urban P, et al: Double-blind study of the safety of clopidogrel with and without a loading dose in combination with aspirin compared with ticlopidine in combination with aspirin after coronary stenting: the Clopidogrel Aspirin Stent International Cooperative Study (CLASSICS). *Circulation* 102:624-629, 2000.
100. Bhatt DL, Bertrand ME, Berger PB, et al: Meta-analysis of randomized and registry comparisons of ticlopidine with clopidogrel after stenting. *J Am Coll Cardiol* 39:9-14, 2002.
101. CAPRIE Steering Committee: A randomised, blinded, trial of clopidogrel versus aspirin in patients at risk of ischaemic events (CAPRIE). *Lancet* 348:1329-1339, 1996.
102. Bhatt DL, Marso SP, Hirsch AT, et al: Amplified benefit of clopidogrel versus aspirin in patients with diabetes mellitus. *Am J Cardiol* 90:625-628, 2002.
103. Bhatt DL, Chew DP, Hirsch AT, et al: Superiority of clopidogrel versus aspirin in patients with prior cardiac surgery. *Circulation* 103:363-368, 2001.
104. Clopidogrel in Unstable Angina to Prevent Recurrent Events Trial Investigators: Effects of clopidogrel in addition to aspirin in patients with acute coronary syndromes without ST-segment elevation. *N Engl J Med* 345:494-502, 2001.
105. Fox KAA, Mehta SR, Peters R, et al: Benefits and risks of the combination of clopidogrel and aspirin in patients undergoing surgical revascularization for non–ST-elevation acute coronary syndrome: the Clopidogrel in Unstable Angina to prevent Recurrent ischemic Events (CURE) trial. *Circulation* 110:1202-1208, 2004.
106. Mehta SR, Yusuf S, Peters RJG, et al: Effects of pretreatment with clopidogrel and aspirin followed by long-term therapy in patients undergoing percutaneous coronary intervention: the PCI-CURE study. *Lancet* 358:527-533, 2001.
107. Budaj A, Yusuf S, Mehta SR, et al: Benefit of clopidogrel in patients with acute coronary syndromes without ST-segment elevation in various risk groups. *Circulation* 106:1622-1626, 2002.
108. Steinhubl SR, Berger PB, Mann JT III, et al: Early and sustained dual oral antiplatelet therapy following percutaneous coronary intervention: a randomized controlled trial. *JAMA* 288:2411-2420, 2002.
109. Bhatt DL, Fox KAA, Hacke W, et al: Clopidogrel and aspirin versus aspirin alone for the prevention of atherothrombotic events. *N Engl J Med* 354:1706-1717, 2006.
110. Bhatt DL, Flather MD, Hacke W, et al: Patients with prior myocardial infarction, stroke, or symptomatic peripheral arterial disease in the CHARISMA trial. *J Am Coll Cardiol* 49:1982-1988, 2007.
111. Chen ZM, Jiang LX, Chen YP, et al: Addition of clopidogrel to aspirin in 45,852 patients with acute myocardial infarction: randomised placebo-controlled trial. *Lancet* 366:1607-1621, 2005.
112. Sabatine MS, Cannon CP, Gibson CM, et al: Addition of clopidogrel to aspirin and fibrinolytic therapy for myocardial infarction with ST-segment elevation. *N Engl J Med* 352:1179-1189, 2005.
113. Sabatine MS, Cannon CP, Gibson CM, et al: Effect of clopidogrel pretreatment before percutaneous coronary intervention in patients with ST-elevation myocardial infarction treated with fibrinolytics: the PCI-CLARITY study. *JAMA* 294:1224-1232, 2005.
114. Diener HC, Bogousslavsky J, Brass LM, et al: Aspirin and clopidogrel compared with clopidogrel alone after recent ischaemic stroke or transient ischaemic attack in high-risk patients (MATCH): randomised, double-blind, placebo-controlled trial. *Lancet* 364:331-337, 2004.

115. Sacco RL, Diener HC, Yusuf S, et al: Aspirin and extended-release dipyridamole versus clopidogrel for recurrent stroke. *N Engl J Med* 359:1238-1251, 2008.
116. ACTIVE Writing Group on Behalf of the ACTIVE Investigators: Clopidogrel plus aspirin versus oral anticoagulation for atrial fibrillation in the Atrial fibrillation Clopidogrel Trial with Irbesartan for Prevention of Vascular Events (ACTIVE W): a randomised controlled trial. *Lancet* 367:1903-1912, 2006.
117. ACTIVE Investigators: Effect of clopidogrel added to aspirin in patients with atrial fibrillation. *N Engl J Med* 360:2066-2078, 2009.
118. Connolly SJ, Pogue J, Eikelboom J, et al: Benefit of oral anticoagulant over antiplatelet therapy in atrial fibrillation depends on the quality of international normalized ratio control achieved by centers and countries as measured by time in therapeutic range. *Circulation* 118:2029-2037, 2008.
119. Healey JS, Hart RG, Pogue J, et al: Risks and benefits of oral anticoagulation compared with clopidogrel plus aspirin in patients with atrial fibrillation according to stroke risk: the Atrial Fibrillation Clopidogrel Trial with Irbesartan for Prevention of Vascular Events (ACTIVE-W). *Stroke* 39:1482-1486, 2008.
120. *Secondary Prevention of Small Subcortical Strokes Trial (SPS3)* (online U.S. government report): http://clinicaltrials.gov/ct2/show/NCT00059306. Accessed August 3, 2010.
121. Bavry AA, Kumbhani DJ, Helton TJ, et al: Late thrombosis of drug-eluting stents: a meta-analysis of randomized clinical trials. *Am J Med* 119:1056-1061, 2006.
122. Eisenstein EL, Anstrom KJ, Kong DF, et al: Clopidogrel use and long-term clinical outcomes after drug-eluting stent implantation. *JAMA* 297:159-168, 2007.
123. Airoldi F, Colombo A, Morici N, et al: Incidence and predictors of drug-eluting stent thrombosis during and after discontinuation of thienopyridine treatment. *Circulation* 116:745-754, 2007.
124. Ho PM, Peterson ED, Wang L, et al: Incidence of death and acute myocardial infarction associated with stopping clopidogrel after acute coronary syndrome. *JAMA* 299:532-539, 2008.
125. Angiolillo DJ, Fernandez-Ortiz A, Bernardo E, et al: Clopidogrel withdrawal is associated with proinflammatory and prothrombotic effects in patients with diabetes and coronary artery disease. *Diabetes* 55:780-784, 2006.
126. Serebruany VL, Steinhubl SR, Berger PB, et al: Variability in platelet responsiveness to clopidogrel among 544 individuals. *J Am Coll Cardiol* 45:246-251, 2005.
127. Matetzky S, Shenkman B, Guetta V, et al: Clopidogrel resistance is associated with increased risk of recurrent atherothrombotic events in patients with acute myocardial infarction. *Circulation* 109:3171-3175, 2004.
128. Pena A, Collet JP, Hulot JS, et al: Can we override clopidogrel resistance? *Circulation* 119:2854-2857, 2009.
129. Mega JL, Close SL, Wiviott SD, et al: Cytochrome P-450 polymorphisms and response to clopidogrel. *N Engl J Med* 360:354-362, 2009.
130. Simon T, Verstuyft C, Mary-Krause M, et al: Genetic determinants of response to clopidogrel and cardiovascular events. *N Engl J Med* 360:363-375, 2009.
131. Bhatt DL: Tailoring antiplatelet therapy based on pharmacogenomics: how well do the data fit? *JAMA* 302:896-897, 2009.
132. Shuldiner AR, O'Connell JR, Bliden KP, et al: Association of cytochrome P450 2C19 genotype with the antiplatelet effect and clinical efficacy of clopidogrel therapy. *JAMA* 302:849-857, 2009.
133. Price MJ, Berger PB, Angiolillo DJ, et al: Evaluation of individualized clopidogrel therapy after drug-eluting stent implantation in patients with high residual platelet reactivity: design and rationale of the GRAVITAS trial. *Am Heart J* 157:818-824, 824.e1, 2009.
134. Lau WC, Waskell LA, Watkins PB, et al: Atorvastatin reduces the ability of clopidogrel to inhibit platelet aggregation: a new drug-drug interaction. *Circulation* 107:32-37, 2003.
135. Mitsios JV, Papathanasiou AI, Rodis FI, et al: Atorvastatin does not affect the antiplatelet potency of clopidogrel when it is administered concomitantly for 5 weeks in patients with acute coronary syndromes. *Circulation* 109:1335-1338, 2004.
136. Serebruany VL, Midei MG, Malinin AI, et al: Absence of interaction between atorvastatin or other statins and clopidogrel: results from the Interaction Study. *Arch Intern Med* 164:2051-2057, 2004.
137. Wenaweser P, Windecker S, Billinger M, et al: Effect of atorvastatin and pravastatin on platelet inhibition by aspirin and clopidogrel treatment in patients with coronary stent thrombosis. *Am J Cardiol* 99:353-356, 2007.
138. Norgard NB, Mathews KD, Wall GC: Drug-drug interaction between clopidogrel and the proton pump inhibitors. *Ann Pharmacother* 43:1266-1274, 2009.
139. Gilard M, Arnaud B, Gal GL, et al: Influence of omeprazol on the antiplatelet action of clopidogrel associated to aspirin. *J Thromb Haemost* 4:2508-2509, 2006.
140. Siller-Matula JM, Spiel AO, Lang IM, et al: Effects of pantoprazole and esomeprazole on platelet inhibition by clopidogrel. *Am Heart J* 157:148.e1-148.e5, 2009.
141. Ho PM, Maddox TM, Wang L, et al: Risk of adverse outcomes associated with concomitant use of clopidogrel and proton pump inhibitors following acute coronary syndrome. *JAMA* 301:937-944, 2009.
142. O'Donoghue ML, Braunwald E, Antman EM, et al: Pharmacodynamic effect and clinical efficacy of clopidogrel and prasugrel with or without a proton-pump inhibitor: an analysis of two randomised trials. *Lancet* 374:989-997, 2009.
143. Bhatt DL, Cryer B, Contant CF: *COGENT: a prospective, randomized, placebo-controlled trial of omeprazole in patients receiving aspirin and clopidogrel,* presented at the 21st Annual Transcatheter Cardiovascular Therapeutics Meeting, San Francisco, CA, September 24, 2009.
144. Sugidachi A, Asai F, Ogawa T, et al: The in vivo pharmacologic profile of CS-747, a novel antiplatelet agent with platelet ADP receptor antagonist properties. *Br J Pharmacol* 129:1439-1446, 2000.
145. Mega JL, Close SL, Wiviott SD, et al: Cytochrome P450 genetic polymorphisms and the response to prasugrel: relationship to pharmacokinetic, pharmacodynamic, and clinical outcomes. *Circulation* 119:2553-2560, 2009.
146. Varenhorst C, James S, Erlinge D, et al: Genetic variation of CYP2C19 affects both pharmacokinetic and pharmacodynamic responses to clopidogrel but not prasugrel in aspirin-treated patients with coronary artery disease. *Eur Heart J* 30:1744-1752, 2009.
147. Wiviott SD, Braunwald E, McCabe CH, et al: Prasugrel versus clopidogrel in patients with acute coronary syndromes. *N Engl J Med* 357:2001-2015, 2007.
148. Wiviott SD, Braunwald E, Angiolillo DJ, et al: Greater clinical benefit of more intensive oral antiplatelet therapy with prasugrel in patients with diabetes mellitus in the Trial to Assess Improvement in Therapeutic Outcomes by Optimizing Platelet Inhibition with Prasugrel–Thrombolysis In Myocardial Infarction 38. *Circulation* 118:1626-1636, 2008.
149. Wiviott SD, Braunwald E, McCabe CH, et al: Intensive oral antiplatelet therapy for reduction of ischaemic events including stent thrombosis in patients with acute coronary syndromes treated with percutaneous coronary intervention and stenting in the TRITON-TIMI 38 trial: a subanalysis of a randomised trial. *Lancet* 371:1353-1363, 2008.
150. Bhatt DL: Prasugrel in clinical practice. *N Engl J Med* 361:940-942, 2009.
151. Montalescot G, Wiviott SD, Braunwald E, et al: Prasugrel compared with clopidogrel in patients undergoing percutaneous coronary intervention for ST-elevation myocardial infarction (TRITON-TIMI 38): double-blind, randomised controlled trial. *Lancet* 373:723-731, 2009.
152. Kushner FG, Hand M, Smith Jr SC, et al: 2009 Focused updates: ACC/AHA guidelines for the management of patients with ST-elevation myocardial infarction (updating the 2004 guideline and 2007 focused update) and ACC/AHA/SCAI guidelines on percutaneous coronary intervention (updating the 2005 guideline and 2007 focused update): a report of the American College of Cardiology Foundation/American Heart Association Task Force on Practice Guidelines. *J Am Coll Cardiol* 54:2205-2241, 2009.
153. Sacco RL, Adams R, Albers G, et al: Guidelines for prevention of stroke in patients with ischemic stroke or transient ischemic attack: a statement for healthcare professionals from the American Heart Association/American Stroke Association Council on Stroke: co-sponsored by the Council on Cardiovascular Radiology and Intervention: the American Academy of Neurology affirms the value of this guideline. *Stroke* 37:577-617, 2006.
154. Chew DP, Bhatt DL, Sapp S, et al: Increased mortality with oral platelet glycoprotein IIb/IIIa antagonists: a meta-analysis of phase III multicenter randomized trials. *Circulation* 103:201-206, 2001.
155. Wallentin L, Becker RC, Budaj A, et al: Ticagrelor versus clopidogrel in patients with acute coronary syndromes. *N Engl J Med* 361:1045-1057, 2009.
156. James S, Akerblom A, Cannon CP, et al: Comparison of ticagrelor, the first reversible oral $P2Y_{12}$ receptor antagonist, with clopidogrel in patients with acute coronary syndromes: rationale, design, and baseline characteristics of the PLATelet inhibition and patient Outcomes (PLATO) trial. *Am Heart J* 157:599-605, 2009.
157. Husted S, Emanuelsson H, Heptinstall S, et al: Pharmacodynamics, pharmacokinetics, and safety of the oral reversible $P2Y_{12}$ antagonist AZD6140 with aspirin in patients with atherosclerosis: a double-blind comparison to clopidogrel with aspirin. *Eur Heart J* 27:1038-1047, 2006.
158. A study of the antiplatelet effects comparing AZD6140 with clopidogrel responder and non-responders (RESPOND) (online U.S. government report): http://clinicaltrials.gov/ct2/show/NCT00642811. Accessed August 3, 2010.
159. *A phase 2 safety and efficacy study of PRT060128, a novel intravenous and oral $P2Y_{12}$ inhibitor, in non-urgent PCI (INNOVATE-PCI)* (online U.S. government report): http://clinicaltrials.gov/ct2/show/NCT00751231. Accessed August 3, 2010.
160. Safety and efficacy of adjunctive antiplatelet therapy prior to primary PCI in patients with STEMI (ERASE-MI) (online U.S. government report): http://clinicaltrials.gov/ct2/show/NCT00546260. Accessed August 3, 2010.
161. Chackalamannil S, Wang Y, Greenlee WJ, et al: Discovery of a novel, orally active himbacine-based thrombin receptor antagonist (SCH 530348) with potent antiplatelet activity. *J Med Chem* 51:3061-3064, 2008.
162. Trial to assess the effects of SCH 530348 in preventing heart attack and stroke in patients with atherosclerosis (TRA 2°P–TIMI 50) (online U.S. government report): http://clinicaltrials.gov/ct2/show/NCT00526474. Accessed August 3, 2010.
163. Angiolillo DJ, Capranzano P: Pharmacology of emerging novel platelet inhibitors. *Am Heart J* 156:10S-15S, 2008.
164. Serebruany VL, Kogushi M, Dastros-Pitei D, et al: The in-vitro effects of E5555, a protease-activated receptor (PAR)–1 antagonist, on platelet biomarkers in healthy volunteers and patients with coronary artery disease. *Thromb Haemost* 102:111-119, 2009.
165. Ikeda Y: Antiplatelet therapy using cilostazol, a specific PDE 3 inhibitor. *Thromb Haemost* 82:435-438, 1999.
166. Schror K: The pharmacology of cilostazol. *Diabetes Obes Metab* 4:S14-S19, 2002.
167. Beebe HG, Dawson DL, Cutler BS, et al: A new pharmacological treatment for intermittent claudication: results of a randomized, multicenter trial. *Arch Intern Med* 159:2041-2050, 1999.
168. Thompson PD, Zimet R, Forbes WP, et al: Meta-analysis of results from eight randomized, placebo-controlled trials on the effect of cilostazol on patients with intermittent claudication. *Am J Cardiol* 90:1314-1319, 2002.
169. Tsuchikane E, Katoh O, Sumitsuji S, et al: Impact of cilostazol on intimal proliferation after directional coronary atherectomy. *Am Heart J* 135:495-502, 1998.
170. Tsuchikane E, Fukuhara A, Kobayashi T, et al: Impact of cilostazol on restenosis after percutaneous coronary balloon angioplasty. *Circulation* 100:21-26, 1999.
171. Biondi-Zoccai GGL, Lotrionte M, Anselmino M, et al: Systematic review and meta-analysis of randomized clinical trials appraising the impact of cilostazol after percutaneous coronary intervention. *Am Heart J* 155:1081-1089, 2008.
172. Lee SW, Park SW, Kim YH, et al: Drug-eluting stenting followed by cilostazol treatment reduces late restenosis in patients with diabetes mellitus: The DECLARE-DIABETES trial (A Randomized Comparison of Triple Antiplatelet Therapy with Dual Antiplatelet Therapy After Drug-Eluting Stent Implantation in Diabetic Patients). *J Am Coll Cardiol* 51:1181-1187, 2008.

173. Ota H, Eto M, Ako J, et al: Sirolimus and everolimus induce endothelial cellular senescence via sirtuin 1 down-regulation: therapeutic implication of cilostazol after drug-eluting stent implantation. *J Am Coll Cardiol* 53:2298-2305, 2009.

174. Kim JY, Lee K, Shin M, et al: Cilostazol could ameliorate platelet responsiveness to clopidogrel in patients undergoing primary percutaneous coronary intervention. *Circ J* 71:1867-1872, 2007.

175. Lee BK, Lee SW, Park SW, et al: Effects of triple antiplatelet therapy (aspirin, clopidogrel, and cilostazol) on platelet aggregation and P-selectin expression in patients undergoing coronary artery stent implantation. *Am J Cardiol* 100:610-614, 2007.

176. Chen KY, Rha SW, Li YJ, et al: Triple versus dual antiplatelet therapy in patients with acute ST-segment elevation myocardial infarction undergoing primary percutaneous coronary intervention. *Circulation* 119:3207-3214, 2009.

177. Jeong YH, Lee SW, Choi BR, et al: Randomized comparison of adjunctive cilostazol versus high maintenance dose clopidogrel in patients with high post-treatment platelet reactivity: Results of the ACCEL-RESISTANCE (Adjunctive Cilostazol versus High Maintenance Dose Clopidogrel in Patients with Clopidogrel Resistance) randomized study. *J Am Coll Cardiol* 53:1101-1109, 2009.

178. Kim HH, Liao JK: Translational therapeutics of dipyridamole. *Arterioscler Thromb Vasc Biol* 28:S39-S42, 2008.

179. Aktas B, Utz A, Hoenig-Liedl P, et al: Dipyridamole enhances NO/cGMP-mediated vasodilator-stimulated phosphoprotein phosphorylation and signaling in human platelets: in vitro and in vivo/ex vivo studies. *Stroke* 34:764-769, 2003.

180. Bousser MG, Eschwege E, Haguenau M, et al: "AICLA" controlled trial of aspirin and dipyridamole in the secondary prevention of athero-thrombotic cerebral ischemia. *Stroke* 14:5-14, 1983.

181. ESPS Group: European Stroke Prevention Study. *Stroke* 21:1122-1130, 1990.

182. Diener HC, Cunha L, Forbes C, et al: European Stroke Prevention Study 2. Dipyridamole and acetylsalicylic acid in the secondary prevention of stroke. *J Neurol Sci* 143:1-13, 1996.

183. Esprit Study Group: Aspirin plus dipyridamole versus aspirin alone after cerebral ischaemia of arterial origin (ESPRIT): randomised controlled trial. *Lancet* 367:1665-1673, 2006.

184. JASAP: Japanese Aggrenox Stroke Prevention vs. Aspirin Programme (online U.S. government report): http://clinicaltrials.gov/ct2/show/NCT00311402. Accessed August 3, 2010.

7

Antiplatelet Therapy

CHAPTER 8

Molecular Biology and Genetics of Atherosclerosis

Paul N. Hopkins

KEY POINTS

- Atherogenesis and contributing factors may be conceptualized in steps, including *initiation* of endothelial activation and inflammation, *promotion* of foam cell formation, *progression* of complex plaques, and *precipitation* of acute events.

- Redundant signaling pathways lead to endothelial activation in areas of slow flow (especially with flow reversal) and a quiescent endothelial phenotype in areas of higher, unidirectional flow, providing an explanation for predictable locations of atherosclerosis-prone sites.

- Dyslipidemia can lead to endothelial activation through several redundant pathways including LOX-1, TLR4, RAGE, and possibly inadequate protection from HDL.

- Numerous cytokines and chemokines binding to their cognate receptors (many with redundant or overlapping roles) direct accumulation of subendothelial macrophages and other leukocytes.

- Multiple lipoprotein modifications, including nonoxidative, are likely to contribute to foam cell formation in atherosclerotic lesions.

- Knockout studies in mice usually have modest effects on atherosclerosis, perhaps because of redundancy in the pathways.

- The difficulty of demonstrating human genetic associations and their modest effects documented to date (other than the few genes that strongly affect major risk factors) may be explained, in part, by the redundant nature of pathways involved in atherogenesis.

During the past 10 to 15 years, there has been an explosion of knowledge regarding the molecular basis of many diseases, including atherosclerosis. Indeed, the various aspects of atherogenesis illustrate most of the major themes of contemporary molecular biology and cell signaling. Whereas some reluctance to delve into the complexities of these pathways is natural, it is reassuring that many of these signaling pathways and their oddly named members are becoming canonical. Indeed, knowledge of at least some of this newer information will become ever more necessary. This chapter emphasizes the molecular biology and genetics of atherosclerosis, with little discussion of the arguably equally important genetic determinants of the major risk factors.

Perhaps one of the major insights to be gleaned from consideration of the various pathways involved in atherogenesis is their sheer number and complexity. Advances in the science of intracellular signaling[1] and a growing appreciation for the number of cytokines, chemokines, and receptors involved in cellular communication during atherogenesis led this reviewer to recognize one remarkable feature of such systems—*redundancy*. Redundancy is seen as a means to ensure the operation of critically important pathways even when one or more elements may be dysfunctional. Thus, a similar element may take over the function of another element or provide a slightly different but overlapping utility. Redundancy is particularly evident in pathways important for survival, on both a cellular and an organismal level. In this regard, atherosclerosis shares numerous pathways involved in defenses against pathogens, inflammation, and cell survival. As it turns out, these pathways are characterized by redundancy (see Table 8-1).

The question then arises: What will be the expected impact of redundancy on our efforts to find genes related to atherosclerosis risk? Whereas the effects on atherosclerosis of many genes may be clearly evident in highly controlled experiments during the short term, their apparent effects may become lost over time if other mechanisms can substitute for or duplicate their action. If this is the case, redundancy of complex systems may help explain the remarkable difficulty in identifying genes for such complex, common diseases as atherosclerosis and hypertension. Redundancy of the various activation and transduction pathways will be a recurrent theme throughout this chapter.

A GENERAL OVERVIEW OF ATHEROGENESIS

Atherogenesis and its clinical expression may be divided into four major steps. Terminology for this model borrows from the cancer literature and was fairly complete in general outline fully 30 years ago.[2] The steps include *initiation* of endothelial activation and inflammation; *promotion* of intimal lipoprotein deposition, retention, modification, and foam cell formation; *progression* of complex plaques by plaque growth, enlargement of the necrotic core, fibrosis, thrombosis, and remodeling; and *precipitation* of acute events, primarily through plaque destabilization and acute thrombosis. Note that acute events may be precipitated by factors unrelated to atherogenesis, for example, through mismatch of arterial oxygen supply and myocardial demand (as with heavy exercise in the setting of uncompensated subtotal coronary occlusion and vulnerable myocardium, leading to ischemia and ventricular fibrillation).

In this scheme, factors frequently act at more than one step of atherogenesis, particularly the major risk factors. For example, elevated lipids can contribute to endothelial activation (with or without oxidation),[3-5] impair nitric oxide (NO) synthesis by endothelium or its availability,[6,7] lead to foam cell formation (after a variety of possible modifications),[8] increase platelet activation and thrombotic potential,[9] and promote reversible plaque destabilization.[10,11] Obviously, factors that increase thrombotic potential may also help precipitate an acute event if an occluding thrombus ensues.

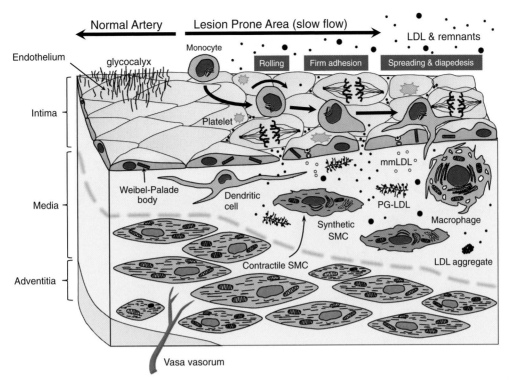

FIGURE 8-1 Initiation of atherosclerosis.

Factors that initiate inflammation also are likely to lead to an unstable plaque.[12]

During initiation, several key events occur as illustrated in Figure 8-1. In areas predisposed by hemodynamic factors, atherogenic lipoproteins, including low-density lipoproteins (LDL) and smaller very low-density lipoproteins (VLDL) as well as other remnants of triglyceride-rich lipoproteins (TGRL), infiltrate the intima and are modified by several potential mechanisms. The modified lipoproteins appear to release inflammatory signals to endothelial cells, causing them to become activated. Activated endothelial cells elaborate various chemoattractant and adhesion molecules, such as monocyte chemoattractant protein 1 (MCP-1) and vascular cell adhesion molecule 1 (VCAM-1) recognized by cognate receptors on passing monocytes (and, to a lesser extent, other white cells and platelets) that lead to a sequence of rolling, firm adhesion with spreading and diapedesis or transmigration into the subendothelial layer of the intima. Slow or disrupted flow is a major determinant of endothelium activation.

Once in the intima, monocytes transform into activated macrophages capable of ingesting the modified lipoproteins and further amplifying the inflammatory response. Concomitantly, inflammatory cytokines, such as platelet-derived growth factor (PDGF) from adherent platelets and other cells, summon smooth muscle cells to move into the intima, where they change from a contractile to a synthetic phenotype capable of ingesting modified lipoproteins, synthesizing and secreting collagen, and producing various cytokines. Note that platelets can adhere directly to activated endothelial cells, much as white cells do[13]; desquamation of the endothelium is not a prerequisite. T cells and mast cells also participate importantly in immune signaling and amplification. Thus, during initiation, the intima becomes populated with inflammatory cells poised to do battle with the modified lipoproteins, which are seen as foreign invaders in unauthorized territory.

During the promotion phase (Fig. 8-2), insudation of lipoproteins and their modification continue in proportion to their plasma levels, endothelial permeability, and transarterial pressure gradient that drives fluid convection. Unchecked uptake of remnants or modified lipoproteins by several scavenger receptors on macrophages and smooth muscle cells leads to formation of foam cells, the hallmark of the growing atherosclerotic lesion. Macrophage foam cells remain capable of relatively rapid egress from the lesion if conditions are favorable (such as a marked reduction in serum lipoprotein concentration) but seem to be retained when lipid levels are high.[14] Thus, if the balance between lipoprotein entry, foam cell formation, reverse cholesterol transport, and foam cell egress favors cholesterol accumulation, the lesion grows. If excess free cholesterol accumulates within foam cells (particularly with cholesterol monohydrate crystal formation), both apoptosis and necrosis can occur.[15,16] This marks the beginning of the formation of the necrotic core as illustrated in Figure 8-2.

As the lipid-rich plaque progresses (Fig. 8-3), accumulating macrophages secrete a host of cytokines and matrix metalloproteinases (MMPs). All migrating cells secrete MMPs to facilitate their diapedesis through extracellular matrix. Thus, highly cellular plaques would be expected to be more friable. MMPs also undermine the stability of the overlying fibrous cap and contribute to plaque rupture with exposure of the blood to the thrombogenic underlying matrix. In addition, interferon-γ (IFN-γ), secreted by activated T cells, acts to strongly inhibit collagen formation by smooth muscle cells, further weakening the plaque and fibrous cap.[12] The result can be catastrophic thrombosis and downstream tissue infarction; but more often, there is limited mural thrombosis with subsequent organization leading to saltatory growth of lesions. Other precipitating changes in the plaque include erosions and, importantly, eruption through the endothelium of underlying cholesterol crystals.[17] Before such episodes of thrombosis, there may be little if any encroachment of the plaque into the arterial lumen because of outward remodeling of the arterial wall to accommodate the growing plaque. Hemodynamic factors and other risk factors seem to influence remodeling and the percentage of the plaque filled with

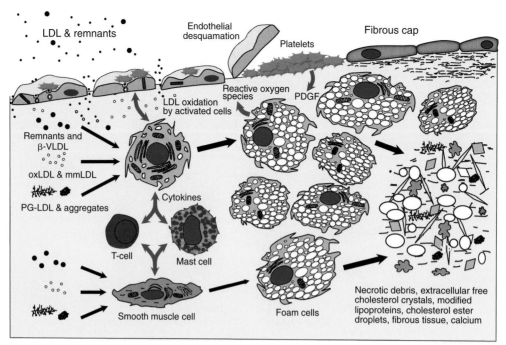

FIGURE 8-2 Promotion of atherosclerosis and foam cell formation.

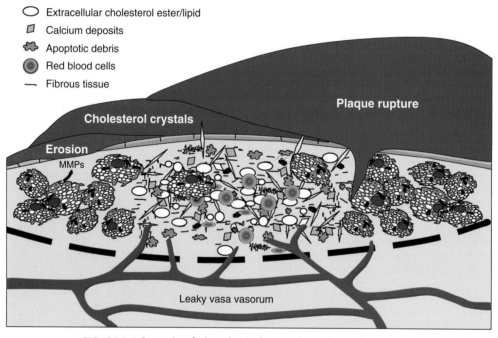

FIGURE 8-3 Progression of atherosclerotic plaques and precipitation of acute events.

fibrous tissue versus lipid.[18] Calcification appears to be associated with healing or more fibrous plaques, although the overall coronary calcium score remains a powerful predictor of overall atherosclerosis and subsequent risk for coronary events.

When the intimal thickness increases beyond just 0.5 mm, hypoxia induces ingrowth of vasa vasorum.[19] In recent years, there has been growing appreciation for the potentially major destabilizing effects of these leaky, friable vessels. Vasa vasorum invading lipid-rich plaques remain highly permeable because of constant exposure to inflammatory factors,

possibly in a large measure from mast cells. Rather than sudden hemorrhage, a constant leak of red blood cells leads to progressively larger amounts of red cell markers found in unstable plaques. Thus, red cell membranes may greatly exacerbate the accumulation of free cholesterol and promote formation of toxic cholesterol crystals. Furthermore, the red cells are a source of strongly pro-oxidant heme iron, which would favor inflammation and lesion progression generally. Such a scenario may favor progression of lesions for some time even after plasma lipoprotein levels are reduced.

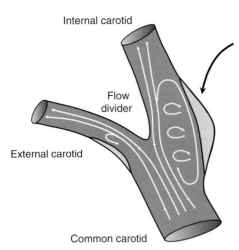

Internal carotid

Flow divider

External carotid

Common carotid

SLOW, mildly oscillatory flow with LOW shear stress results in:
• increased cell adhesion molecules
• increased inflammatory markers
• decreased NO production
• more white cell adherence
• disordered endothelial actin fibers
• less elongated endothelial cells
• shorter glycocalyx
• increased lipoprotein permeability
• altered subendothelial extracellular matrix (e.g., increased fibronectin)
• negative artery remodeling and increased intima-medial thickness
• **PREDISPOSITION TO ATHEROSCLEROSIS**

FIGURE 8-4 Location and features of atherosclerosis-prone sites.

INITIATION OF ATHEROSCLEROSIS

Disturbed Flow and the Atherosclerosis-Prone Endothelial Phenotype

In recent years, endothelial response to flow has been the subject of intense investigation. Sites of atherosclerosis predilection occur in areas of low shear or eddy currents (Fig. 8-4) characterized by slow, oscillating (back-and-forth) flow. Such a pattern is referred to as disturbed flow even though the pattern is stable over time in specific areas of the arterial tree. This observation has been confirmed in many observational and experimental studies and is supported by extensive mathematical modeling.[20-22] Progression of plaque is predictable in individual human subjects at such locations in the arterial tree.[23-25] Turbulence is virtually never a feature of flow in these sites.[26] Experimentally, atherosclerotic lesions accumulate exclusively in areas of low shear just beyond stenoses created by carotid casts in hyperlipidemic mice.[18] The unique hemodynamics of the coronary circulation, with near cessation of flow or flow reversal during systole, together with the high pressures generated at the aortic root may explain the marked predilection of coronary arteries to atherosclerosis. Interestingly, rabbit coronary artery endothelial cells expressed only one fifth the endothelial nitric oxide synthase (eNOS) and greater endothelin-1 (ET-1) compared with aortic endothelial cells.[27] As heart rate increases, relatively more time is spent in systole, when flow is essentially nil. This may help explain the fourfold increase in coronary artery disease (CAD) risk as resting heart rate increased from below 60 to above 100 beats per minute.[28]

Multiple, redundant transduction mechanisms endow endothelial cells with exquisite sensitivity to abrupt changes in shear stress. These mechanisms include ion channels, G protein–coupled receptors (GPCRs), the lipid bilayer itself, and the endothelial glycocalyx, with stress transmitted throughout the cell by microfibers and sensed by integrins and at cell junctions.[20,29] In general, more rapid flow induces remodeling, which results in larger vessels. Conversely, slow flow results in diminution in the size of the vessel. In this way, flow becomes a fundamental stimulus for blood vessel development during embryogenesis.[21] In addition, flow strongly affects numerous endothelial responses, including endothelial cell migration, mitosis, apoptosis, endothelial layer permeability, inflammation (including white cell adhesion), NO release, and thrombosis.[20,21,30]

The pattern of flow is critical in determining the endothelial phenotype. Direct measurement of flow patterns by ultrasound and magnetic resonance imaging techniques in atherosclerosis-resistant compared with atherosclerosis-prone areas revealed marked differences as shown in Figure 8-5.[31] Endothelial cells exposed to the atherosclerosis-prone flow pattern, characterized by slow flow that reversed direction slightly during the course of a cardiac cycle (referred to as oscillatory or disturbed flow), developed a proatherosclerotic phenotype, whereas cells exposed to higher flow rates (higher shear stress or laminar flow) that remained unidirectional although pulsatile had an antiatherosclerotic phenotype. The time course of phenotypic changes and some of the molecular signaling events in the endothelial cells exposed to the respective flow patterns are also shown in Figure 8-5. Platelets and white cells are also much more likely to attach to areas of slow flow, either to endothelium or even when measured for attachment to artificial surfaces such as one coated with E-selectin.[29]

Of great importance is the relatively recent recognition that proinflammatory endothelial responses occur only transiently with onset of flow, after a sudden stepped increase in flow, or with directional change in flow.[29] However, after several hours of continued unidirectional, laminar high shear stress or pulsatile flow (suggesting undulation in the rate of flow but always unidirectional and faster than disturbed, oscillatory flow), these proinflammatory responses are suppressed to below initial (no flow) conditions (see Fig. 8-5). After prolonged exposure (10 to 12 hours) to unidirectional flow, the cells thus display an anti-inflammatory, antioxidant, antiproliferative phenotype, remaining in a relatively quiescent state but active in production of protective NO and prostacyclin (PGI$_2$). In contrast, when endothelial cells are exposed to slow oscillatory flow, where direction of flow actually reverses however slightly during the cycle, they never suppress their proinflammatory responses, do not align with the flow, have disorganized cytoskeletons, and develop other features characteristic of lesion-prone areas including increased apoptosis, frequent mitoses, greater permeability (particularly at sites of mitosis), shorter glycocalyx, elaboration of cell adhesion molecules, secretion of MCP-1 and endothelin, decreased bioavailability of NO, and increased production of superoxide by NADPH oxidase and heme oxidase. In addition, these endothelial cells increase production of subendothelial matrix components, such as fibronectin, which results in enhanced inflammatory responses and a thickening of the basement membrane that may be seen as an increase of intima-medial thickness on ultrasound.[20,21,31] The classic inflammatory markers nuclear factor κB (NF-κB)[32] and protein kinase Cβ (PKCβ)[33] as well as other markers of

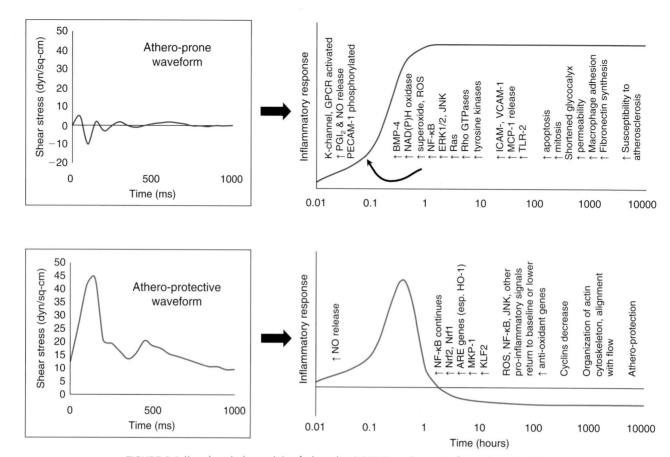

FIGURE 8-5 Hemodynamic characteristics of atherosclerosis-initiating and protective flow and resulting effects.

inflammation have been used to track the increased inflammatory signal seen with early exposure to rapid flow or prolonged exposure to slow flow as well as its suppression with longer term exposure to high shear.

Redundant Mechanotransduction and Cell Signaling Mechanisms

A number of generally proinflammatory signaling pathways are activated immediately or soon after abrupt onset of flow (Fig. 8-6). If disrupted flow continues (either low shear stress or back-and-forth flow), the proinflammatory, proatherogenic state described earlier becomes more fully established. A number of genes in these pathways have been subject to knockout or overexpression in atherosclerosis-prone mice. Although a thorough review of each of the affected signaling pathways cannot be undertaken here, an attempt is made to orient the reader to the location and general function of the specific signaling pathway in the endothelial cell to appreciate the general stage of atherogenesis in which a particular gene may function. Note that whereas a number of the following pathways may be considered canonical and dealt with in general reviews of signaling or in textbooks, they may subserve rather different purposes in specific tissues. Emphasis in the following paragraphs is on such signaling in endothelial cells and in the context of disturbed flow.

The endothelial glycocalyx is important in mechanotransduction, particularly in mediating responses seen in the first few minutes after flow change. The glycocalyx is also involved in inflammatory cell adhesion, thrombosis, migration, and endothelial permeability. The endothelial glycocalyx can be thicker (up to 500 nm or more) than the endothelial cell itself

(300 to 400 nm). The glycocalyx is composed primarily of the proteoglycan syndecan 1 (which consists of a core protein and three or more glycosaminoglycan chains attached). Syndecan 1 is arranged in a highly structured hexagonal lattice spread over the luminal surface of the endothelial cell with interconnections to the actin cortical web, part of the cytoskeleton.[34,35] The stiffness of the proteoglycans and their ability to transmit torque to the endothelial cytoskeleton make for an "exquisitely designed transducer of fluid shearing stresses."[34] Treatment of endothelial cells with heparinase selectively removes heparan sulfate but not the syndecan 1 core protein[36] and markedly disrupts the glycocalyx layer, reducing many but not all flow-induced responses in endothelial cells, such as NO release in response to shear stress.[37]

In the following paragraphs, several pathways of endothelial mechanotransduction are reviewed roughly in the order in which they are activated by onset of shear stress. They include (1) PKC activation through calcium channels and a GPCR; (2) bone morphogenic protein 4 (BMP4) activation with subsequent generation of reactive oxygen species (ROS) and activation of NF-κB; (3) platelet and endothelial cell adhesion molecule 1 (PECAM-1) and integrin activation; (4) activation of MAPK pathways, particularly JNK; and (5) activation of heat shock proteins.

Within a few seconds after onset of blood flow, there is an influx of calcium (e.g., through the polycystin-2 channel), potassium, and chloride through respective ion channels and activation of GPCRs (such as the bradykinin B2 receptor, which is activated without binding of agonists). The resultant G protein signaling activates phospholipase C with production of diacylglycerol and subsequent activation of PKCβ. In addition, there is a sudden initial burst of NO production that is

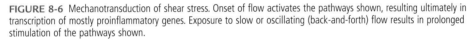

FIGURE 8-6 Mechanotransduction of shear stress. Onset of flow activates the pathways shown, resulting ultimately in transcription of mostly proinflammatory genes. Exposure to slow or oscillating (back-and-forth) flow results in prolonged stimulation of the pathways shown.

calcium, calmodulin, PKC, and G protein dependent.[38] There may also be a mechanical effect from glypican and CD44 to assist in caveolin-1 phosphorylation and removal of its suppressive effect on eNOS.[39] This stimulation of NO production is generally considered anti-inflammatory and antiatherosclerotic. However, PKC signaling can activate proinflammatory signaling through several MAPK pathways, and knockout of PKCβ resulted in marked reduction in atherosclerosis.[40]

BMP4 activation with subsequent activation of NADPH oxidase and heme oxygenase 1 activity together with accumulation of superoxide and other ROS can lead to NF-κB activation.[41] NADPH oxidase may also be upregulated directly in response to onset of shear stress.

Abrupt onset of flow results in torsional forces transmitted by the glycocalyx to the actin cortical web. This force is thought to be transmitted through actin stress fibers to the dense peripheral actin band and to syndecan 4 and integrins that anchor the endothelial cell to the extracellular matrix. Tractional forces may also be transmitted to lamins on the nuclear envelope.[30] The dense peripheral actin band surrounds the endothelial cell much like a rubber bumper encircles a bumper car.[35] It has been proposed that the tractional forces on this band disrupt the weak links between vascular endothelial cadherin (VE-cadherin) proteins of adjoining cells, resulting in the transmission of a signal that is dependent on PECAM-1, VE-cadherin, and vascular endothelial growth factor receptor 2 (VEGFR-2, also called Flk-1).[42] In this process, PECAM-1 appears to act as the true mechanical transducer that directly activates a Src family kinase and also results in release of bound Gαqr.[43] VE-cadherin functions as an adapter protein allowing Src to activate VEGFR-2, which then activates phosphatidylinositol 3-kinase (PI3K), which in turn activates integrins as indicated in Figure 8-6. The

activated integrins then form new bonds to the extracellular matrix, which triggers activation of Rho, Rac, and Cdc42. In endothelial cells, these work in a coordinated fashion to modify actin polymerization and to mediate cell alignment to flow and other responses. Early changes lead to contraction and increased intercellular permeability. The adapter protein Shc is phosphorylated in response to integrin activation, enabling signaling through other adapters, Grb and Sos, to Ras and Raf with subsequent signaling to the MAPK pathway. Integrin binding and activation also lead to phosphorylation of focal adhesion kinase (FAK), which in turn binds and activates Src, followed by phosphorylation of paxillin and p130[cas], which then activate Ras. Alternatively, FAK may first bind Shc with subsequent activation of Src; a third pathway results in activation of Rho. The kinase Src may also directly transmit signals to the MAPK pathway.[21,30,44]

Yet another result of integrin activation is activation of p21-activated kinase (PAK), which may be one of the most important activators of the MAPK pathway resulting from shear stress. This activation appears to depend on PI3K signaling from the PECAM-1, VE-cadherin, VEGFR-2 complex.[45] Not only does PAK activation lead to activated JNK (a terminal MAPK), but it may also directly affect various cell junctional adhesion molecules, resulting in increased endothelial permeability.[46] Importantly, the activation of PAK appears to depend on integrin binding to fibronectin in the extracellular matrix. The protein ZO-1, associated with tight junctions, is also involved in the increase in endothelial permeability after onset of flow or prolonged oscillatory slow flow. Connexin43 (Cx43), unlike other connexins, relocates to cell junctions in response to onset of shear stress and is increased in atherosclerosis-prone areas of the endothelium.[47]

8

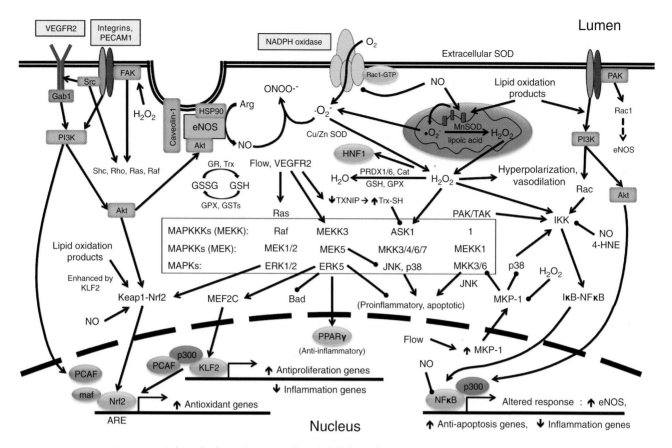

FIGURE 8-7 Pathways leading to the transition from the initial proinflammatory, pro-oxidant state to the quiescent, anti-inflammatory, antioxidant state after prolonged exposure to more rapid flow (high shear stress). Lipid oxidation products include 4-hydroxy-2-nonenal (4-HNE) and others.

Importantly, there is greater inflammatory response to onset of shear stress when integrins are bound to fibronectin or fibrinogen (characteristically found in extracellular matrix underlying previously injured endothelium) compared with components of the normal extracellular matrix unexposed to prior injury. This difference in inflammatory response seems to be mediated by the binding specificity of different integrins, but activation of Akt also seems to play a role.[45] The alteration of the extracellular matrix, with increase in fibronectin, occurs early in atherosclerosis-prone areas as part of the cellular response to disrupted flow, whereas deposition of fibrinogen may occur later.[21]

As noted before, several of the signals activated on abrupt onset of flow converge on the MAPK/ERK (mitogen-activated protein kinase/extracellular signal-regulated kinase) or simply MAPK pathway, which results, ultimately, in activation of a variety of transcription factors, including Egr-1 (early growth factor 1) and AP-1 (activator protein 1, which contains c-fos and c-Jun). NF-κB may also be activated by crosstalk with MAP kinases.

The canonical MAPK pathway represents a generic designation for a series of three kinases, often held in juxtaposition by a scaffolding protein (with other regulatory proteins sometimes attached, such as IMP or "impedes mitogenic signal propagation"). MAPK designates the terminal kinase. It is activated by a MAPK kinase (MAPKK), also called a MAPK/ERK kinase (MEK). This intermediate kinase is phosphorylated by an upstream MAPKK kinase (MAPKKK or MAP3K) also known as a MEK kinase (MEKK). The MAPK pathway or complex is activated by upstream kinases often in response to tyrosine receptor kinases (classically worked out for EGFR, the endothelial growth factor receptor) or kinases interacting

with integrins or other flow sensors. In the canonical EGFR pathway, after binding endothelial growth factor, the receptor self-phosphorylates its cytoplasmic domains, allowing binding of one or more adaptor proteins (e.g., Grb2, which binds directly to the receptor or through another adaptor, Shc). Grb2 interacts with the guanine nucleotide exchange factor Sos (son of sevenless), which then activates membrane-bound Ras by promoting exchange of GDP for GTP. Once bound by GTP, Ras is active. In this example (for EGFR), active Ras leads to activation of the protein tyrosine kinase RAF1. RAF1 is actually a MAP3K, the first of a series of three kinases leading to activation of the MAPK ERK. A variety of potential kinases may serve as the initial kinase, MAP3K or MEKK (such as RAF1), as well as multiple potential intermediate kinases and terminal kinases. Mammalian terminal kinases include ERK(1-7), JNK(1-3), and p38(α, β, δ, and γ). Traditionally, ERKs are the terminal kinases for mitogens; p38 and JNK result from stress or cytokine activation. Once activated, terminal kinases can phosphorylate membrane proteins, transcriptional factors in the nucleus, proteins associated with the actin cytoskeleton, various additional signaling molecules, and MAP kinase–activated kinases (MK), which in turn have a series of substrates (such as transcription factors, cell survival, and other signaling proteins). Some examples are given in Figure 8-7. Their control and signal termination are also complex. In endothelial cells, terminal kinases in MAPK/ERK signaling pathways can phosphorylate eNOS and may have diverse other effects on cell function. Whereas p38 and JNK are generally proinflammatory, ERK5 appears to have multiple anti-inflammatory effects.

Another consequence of early-onset shear stress is activation of heat shock proteins (HSPs).[48] These are generally considered protective proteins,[49] and recent evidence suggests that an increase in HSP-90, which can act to stimulate eNOS, is brought about not only by prolonged rapid flow but also by statins as a beneficial, pleiotropic effect.[50] HSPs can act as protein chaperones to promote proper folding (especially HSP-70) and other protective functions. HSP-60 may act to chaperone certain cytosolic proteins into the mitochondria. When cells are not under stress, HSPs are bound to heat shock transcription factor 1 (HSF1) in the cytoplasm. When misfolded proteins are present or the cell is stressed by a number of factors, including ROS,[51] oxidized lipids, or cytokines, the HSP binds to the misfolded protein (or is otherwise used in the cell), thus becoming separated from HSF1. HSF1 then forms a trimer, moves to the nucleus, and stimulates transcription of HSPs. In the case of HSP-60, levels are clearly upregulated in endothelial cells in atherosclerosis-prone areas of slow flow, with increased expression on the luminal membrane. Cell surface HSP-60 may be important in triggering an autoimmune response that may be important in promoting atherosclerosis (see later).[52]

Transition to an Atherosclerosis-Resistant Endothelial Phenotype

After several hours of exposure to laminar flow, the quiescent state described earlier is induced, the actin cytoskeleton organizes itself into a pattern such that the cells align themselves to be elongated in the direction of the flow with tight cellular junctions, and most cells are found in an arrested state of growth (G_0 or G_1). Not only are shear-stressed endothelial cells relatively quiescent, but they become frankly resistant to even potent inflammatory cytokines such as tumor necrosis factor-α (TNF-α).[53,54] The molecular mechanisms that mediate this transition have been the subject of intensive investigation.

Some of the complex intracellular events that appear to underlie the transition from an activated to a quiescent state are depicted in Figure 8-7. Of great importance is the recent recognition that the organized sequence of protective events is at least in part dependent on an initial burst of ROS produced together with increased NO. At the onset of flow, there is a marked increase in production of superoxide anion ($\cdot O_2^-$) by NADPH oxidase, mediated possibly by increased activation of the small GTPase Rac (produced by mechanotransduction mechanisms reviewed earlier) or direct effects transmitted through the cell membrane. At the same time, there is a surge in NO production by eNOS due to calmodulin binding and phosphorylation by PKCβ. Surprisingly, Rac appears to be required for normal expression of eNOS as well.[55] Continued and enhanced production of NO is one of the features of the atheroprotective state. This seems to be mediated by a gradual increase in eNOS mRNA as well as by multiple post-transcription changes in the eNOS enzyme (such as binding to HSP-90, calcineurin, and certain phosphorylations) that decrease the dependence of eNOS on calcium and calmodulin and increase overall activity.[43]

Because $\cdot O_2^-$ reacts rapidly with NO to form peroxynitrite (ONOO$\cdot^-$), there is a balance between NO and $\cdot O_2^-$ production that may be significant for signaling events.[56] Excess or prolonged $\cdot O_2^-$ clearly has detrimental effects and can promote cellular damage and apoptosis.[57,58] Nevertheless, more controlled release of ROS may be an important signaling mechanism that is key to subsequent protective adaptations by the cell. Early after onset of laminar flow, or with prolonged slow, oscillatory flow, the balance favors $\cdot O_2^-$ production with neutralization of vasodilating effects of NO; after several hours of laminar flow, NO is favored through multiple mechanisms.[59] However, some of the vasodilation seen immediately after initiation of flow is mediated by hydrogen peroxide

(H_2O_2), which acts as an "endothelial derived hyperpolarizing factor."[60] In addition, NO can inhibit mitochondrial electron transport chain complex I and IV and thereby at least transiently increase mitochondrial production of superoxide anion.[58,61] Lipid oxidation products, such as 4-hydroxy-nonenal, potentially produced during the $\cdot O_2^-$ spike, are taken up actively into mitochondria, where they also promote $\cdot O_2^-$ production.[58,61] In the cytosol, $\cdot O_2^-$ is rapidly converted to H_2O_2 by copper/zinc superoxide dismutase (Cu/Zn SOD); in the mitochondria, this function is performed by manganese superoxide dismutase (MnSOD). Much of the subsequent "redox signaling" is likely to be mediated by H_2O_2, as it is more stable and freely membrane permeable, unlike $\cdot O_2^-$ or other free radicals.[61,62] Nevertheless, H_2O_2, $\cdot O_2^-$, ONOO$\cdot^-$, and hydroxyl radical ($\cdot OH$) can all contribute to a pro-oxidant environment sensed, in part, through effects on free -SH groups on cysteine residues in various signaling proteins.

Cellular antioxidant defenses depicted in Figure 8-7 include not only the SOD enzymes but catalase, various glutathione peroxidase enzymes, and glutathione-S-transferases (GSTs, which not only convert superoxide to water but reduce a number of other toxic, oxidized molecules by coupling with the GSH to GSSG reaction) as well as glutathione reductase, peroxiredoxins (PRDXs), and thioredoxin (Trx), which regenerate reduced glutathione. Trx also acts as a signaling "gate" by binding (when Trx is in the reduced form) to the MEKK ASK1 (apoptosis signal-regulating kinase 1). Thus, ASK1 is a redox-responsive MEKK. ASK1 appears to be the major mediator of TNF-induced JNK activation in endothelial cells.[63] JNK, as noted before, has major proinflammatory and apoptotic effects. When ASK1 is bound by Trx, it is unresponsive to upstream signals, such as those generated from the binding of TNF-α to its receptor. Trx-bound ASK1 is also targeted for ubiquitination and degradation.[64] Trx is highly responsive to ROS and is released from ASK1 on early exposure to the onset of flow or oxidative stress or during prolonged slow or disturbed flow. In addition, Trx is bound by thioredoxin-interacting protein (TXNIP), which inactivates Trx. Importantly, TXNIP is downregulated by prolonged laminar flow through an unknown pathway.[53] Finally, NO can bind to Trx and increase its binding to and inactivation of ASK1.[63]

A key, critically protective pathway that is stimulated by flow in endothelial cells and the early ROS burst involves the induction of numerous antioxidant genes. Many of these genes (which include most of the antioxidant enzymes depicted in Figure 8-7) share an antioxidant responsive element (ARE) in their promoters and are activated by the transcription factor Nrf2 (nuclear factor erythroid 2–like related factor 2). Importantly, Nrf2 is activated by both disturbed and laminar flow, but only laminar flow results in increased expression of the antioxidant genes. This was thought to be mediated in part by the oxidized lipid d15-PGJ$_2$ generated through cyclooxygenase 2 (COX-2).[65] Nrf2 is bound in cytoplasm by an inhibitor, Keap1 (Kelch-like erythroid-derived cap'n'collar homology–associated protein 1). Keap1 binding targets Nrf2 for proteosomal degradation. Recently, a mechanism was proposed that is dependent on early stimulation of superoxide and hydrogen peroxide by mitochondria, increased early production of NO, and activation of Akt, which all converge to inactivate Keap1 and to release Nrf2 for transport to the nucleus. Effects of oxidized lipids also seem to accelerate the pathway.[61] Direct binding of NO to Keap1 and phosphorylation by Akt appeared particularly important. Critically important for the Nrf2 pathway is the recently discovered effect of KLF2 to prime Nrf2 for greater upregulation of ARE-responsive genes (see later). This interaction, affecting dozens of genes, is one of several major effects promoted by shear stress and KLF2.[66]

The early post-flow, pro-oxidant state promotes signaling through ASK1 and promotes activation of inhibitor of κB

(IκB) kinase (IKK). IKK phosphorylates IκB, thereby releasing IκB from NF-κB, targeting IκB for proteosomal degradation, and freeing NF-κB to be transported to the nucleus, where it acts as a transcription factor for numerous proinflammatory genes. As noted before, NF-κB expression is frequently found to be increased in atherosclerosis-prone regions (see Fig. 8-6). Nevertheless, NF-κB also acts early to support an increase in eNOS synthesis and has antiapoptotic effects.[67] This yin-yang behavior is modified in the setting of prolonged laminar flow, in which the proinflammatory actions of NF-κB are almost entirely abrogated or "uncoupled" (as seen by a marked suppression of VCAM-1, E-selectin, and IL-8 production in response to TNF-α), leaving the cytoprotective effects of NF-κB (such as an induction of MnSOD and eNOS) intact.[54] Recent insights into the mechanism of this transition suggest activation by Akt (also activated early after the initiation of flow) of a histone acetylator, p300 (generally referred to as p300/CBP; CBP refers to the p300 homologue CREB-binding protein). p300/CBP may also be activated by a short burst of oxidant stress. The activated p300 acts as a coactivator with NF-κB and greatly affects NF-κB activation of genes, especially seen as a marked increase in eNOS transcription.[68] In addition, there is negative feedback exerted by NO at several steps of the NF-κB pathway. Thus, nitrosylation inhibits IKK, stabilizes IκB, induces IκB mRNA, decreases NF-κB transport to the nucleus, and inhibits NF-κB binding to DNA.[69]

Not only does NO provide feedback inhibition to NF-κB, but it also appears to be critical for downregulation of NADPH oxidase subunits after prolonged exposure to laminar flow. Thus, when endothelial cells were subjected to shear forces in a cone-and-plate viscometer, NO and $\cdot O_2^-$ production were upregulated 6-fold and 2.5-fold, respectively, by 2 hours. There was no change in NADPH oxidase subunit number at this point. It is possible that a higher earlier peak for $\cdot O_2^-$ was missed. Thereafter, $\cdot O_2^-$ declined until it was about 50% of the initial level after 24 hours of laminar shear stress while NO production had increased markedly. The investigators found that there was an approximate 50% decrease in the expression of the activity-limiting gp91^{phox} subunit of NADPH oxidase while eNOS protein expression was increased 3.5-fold. The reduction in gp91^{phox} expression was shown to be NO dependent, although the specific signal transduction pathway was not demonstrated.[70] Interestingly, endothelial expression of the angiotensin type 1 receptor (AT1R) is also downregulated by shear stress and NO signaling.[71]

Crosstalk between different MAPK pathway kinases appears to be another important mechanism whereby the protective endothelial phenotype is brought on by laminar flow. As depicted in Figure 8-7, activation of MEK5 by flow inhibits activation of the proapoptotic, inflammatory MAPK JNK.[63,72] Furthermore, MEK5 activates ERK5, which interferes with signaling downstream of JNK.[63] Perhaps even more important is the induction of KLF2 (Kruppel-like factor 2) by the transcription factor MEF2C (myocyte enhancer factor 2C), which is activated by ERK5. ERK5 also phosphorylates and thereby inactivates the proapoptotic factor Bad.

Numerous studies have pointed to the induction of KLF2 as a critical step in the conversion to and maintenance of an atheroprotective state.[73-77] KLF2 is expressed almost exclusively in areas of the vasculature protected from atherosclerosis, whereas it is nearly absent in atherosclerosis-prone areas and is clearly upregulated by laminar flow. It is also important in embryonic vascular development. The molecular effects of KLF2 are protean and include: inhibition of activating transcription factor 2 (ATF2), which can be one of the heterodimeric components of AP-1, the key product of the MAPK p38 and a required activating factor for many proinflammatory effects of NF-κB[78]; induction of inhibitory Smad7, which blocks transmission of proatherosclerotic signals through the transforming growth factor-β (TGF-β)

receptor, together with reduction of nuclear c-Jun, a second component of AP-1, thereby further blocking many inflammatory signals[79]; enhanced transcription of eNOS and the enzyme dimethylarginine dimethylaminohydrolase, which degrades the eNOS inhibitor ADMA (asymmetric dimethylarginine); increased transcription of protective thrombomodulin (TM); inhibition of ET-1 and MCP-1; and other major effects. In one study, KLF2 decreased the expression of the following genes by 80% to 90% after exposure of cells to IL-1β: IL-1α, IL-1β, IL-6, IL-8, IL-15, MCP-1, E-selectin, TNF-α, CXCL10, CXCL11, IFN-γ, COX-2, and CCL5.[75]

An important mechanism to upregulate KLF2 involves activation of p300/CBP-associated factor (PCAF) by a PI3K-dependent but Akt-independent mechanism.[80] Activated PCAF acts together with p300 to acetylate histones and greatly increase transcription of KLF2-regulated genes. Increased PCAF activity is also related to induction of COX-2 independent of KLF2. Thus, PCAF activation appears to be yet another critical mechanism linking early signaling events to the onset of flow. Interestingly, statin drugs are potent inducers of KLF2, possibly by way of Akt activation, a finding that lends credibility to the potential importance of so-called pleiotropic effects of these drugs.[75]

MAPK phosphatase 1 (MKP-1) is another gene found to be expressed exclusively in arterial regions protected by high laminar flow.[81] As MKP-1 deactivates p38 and JNK by dephosphorylating these terminal MAP kinases, it also has the potential for major anti-inflammatory effects. The precise mechanism whereby MKP-1 is induced by flow is currently unknown.

In summary, prolonged flow establishes a quiescent endothelial phenotype by the following redundant and somewhat interacting mechanisms: (1) use of the initial pro-oxidant burst as a trigger for the induction of cellular antioxidant defenses; (2) capitalizing on the reduction of ROS to downregulate JNK (through decreased TXNIP and increased Trx) and NF-κB signaling; (3) activation of Akt/PKB, resulting in strong eNOS upregulation and antiapoptotic signals as well as diversion of NF-κB to a largely anti-inflammatory role with further support of eNOS induction; (4) greatly upregulated NO production, resulting in inhibition of NF-κB inflammatory signaling, downregulation of NADPH oxidase activity, and decreased expression of the AT1R as well as other protective activities; and (5) MAPK pathway crosstalk and induction of MKP-1, leading to inhibition of p38 and JNK signaling while promoting signaling by protective MEK5, ERK5, and, most important, KLF2.

GENOMIC STUDIES OF FLOW-MEDIATED CHANGE IN ENDOTHELIAL PHENOTYPE

Several groups have examined RNA expression profiles of endothelial cells exposed to the atherosclerosis-prone versus protective flow patterns.[31,66,73,78,82-86] In these studies, expression of up to 10,000 or more genes could be assessed simultaneously by examining differences in the levels of mRNA found in harvested endothelial cells exposed in vitro to the different flow patterns. Although there were a number of differences in technical approaches used in these studies and differences in specific findings of which genes were significantly upregulated or downregulated, this genome-wide approach generally confirmed the findings of candidate gene and molecular studies in which genes associated with inflammation and susceptibility to atherosclerosis tended to be increased in cells exposed to the slow-flow, oscillatory pattern, whereas such genes were suppressed in the cells exposed to rapid, unidirectional pulsatile flow.

In one of the studies, endothelial cells were harvested from atherosclerosis-prone and atherosclerosis-protected areas of aorta from normal pigs.[85,87] This in vivo approach suggested that whereas proinflammatory genes were frequently increased in the atherosclerosis-prone areas, some potentially compensating genes were also upregulated, including several antioxidant genes, such as glutathione peroxidase. Also, there seemed to be little evidence of frank inflammation in these arteries. Thus, active NF-κB was not found in greater levels in nuclei, nor were several key adhesion receptors found to be expressed at higher levels on the cell surface. The authors interpreted these results to suggest that disrupted or slow flow primes the endothelium to respond with an enhanced inflammatory response if it is exposed to additional risk factors. Thus, "a delicate balance of pro- and antiatherosclerotic mechanisms may exist simultaneously in endothelium of lesion-prone sites of the aorta to create a setting of net vulnerability to atherogenesis, but with protective measures also present. A shift from athero-susceptibility to atherogenesis may occur by inhibition of the protection."[87]

This concept of predisposition is supported by the finding of an increase in both bound NF-κB and its inhibitor IκB in the cytoplasm of endothelial cells from atherosclerosis-prone areas of the aorta in mice but with no increase of NF-κB in the nucleus. Nevertheless, there was much greater activation of NF-κB and its inducible gene products in these same hemodynamically prone areas after the mice were treated with lipopolysaccharide or after feeding LDL receptor (LDLR)–deficient mice a high-fat diet to induce hyperlipidemia.[88]

Further Endothelial Activation by Dyslipidemia

The well-known observation of monocyte adherence to endothelium in atherosclerosis-prone areas just days after induction of severe hypercholesterolemia by cholesterol feeding in animals can be better appreciated in light of the above molecular mechanisms.[89,90] Factors that even modestly activate endothelial cells would be expected to initiate substantially greater effects in the already "primed" cells found in atherosclerosis-prone areas.[88] Hyperlipidemia clearly provides one or more signals for such activation,[91] whereas lowering of serum cholesterol, even if only by dietary means, clearly decreases endothelial activation.[7,92] As early as 2 hours after injection of human LDL into rabbits, grapelike clusters of aggregated LDL could be seen enmeshed in focal areas of the subendothelial matrix.[93] VCAM-1 and MCP-1 are expressed by endothelial cells within at least 3 weeks of starting of a high-cholesterol diet in rabbits.[92] Not only do lipoproteins preferentially accumulate in atherosclerosis-prone areas, but hyperlipidemia itself clearly increases the permeability of the endothelium and total area of susceptibility, suggesting direct activation.[89,90] Both activation of endothelium with increased cell turnover and diminished glycocalyx height appear to mediate this increased permeability due to hyperlipidemia.[94] This appeared true with even modest hyperlipidemia as newly synthesized, radiolabeled thymidine (an index of cell turnover) in aortic endothelial cells tripled in just 3 days after starting of a high-cholesterol diet in pigs when serum cholesterol levels had increased to only 187 mg/dL (normal, 74 mg/dL).[95] Thus, hyperlipidemia clearly activates endothelium, but the precise signals mediating this effect have been less easily identified.[96,97] Given the current evidence, it would appear that multiple mechanisms linking hyperlipidemia to endothelial activation are likely, further illustrating the principle of redundancy. Several of these possible mechanisms are presented briefly here.

LDL Oxidation

Much evidence has been forwarded in support of the LDL oxidation hypothesis for endothelial activation (and still

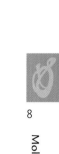

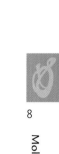

FIGURE 8-8 Staining for elements of early plaque in aortas from 82 spontaneously aborted fetuses, aged 5.0 to 7.3 months. *(Modified from Napoli C, D'Armiento FP, Mancini FP, et al: Fatty streak formation occurs in human fetal aortas and is greatly enhanced by maternal hypercholesterolemia. Intimal accumulation of low density lipoprotein and its oxidation precede monocyte recruitment into early atherosclerotic lesions,* J Clin Invest 100:2680, 1997.*)*

more for foam cell formation, to be discussed later).[96,98] Native LDL appears to accumulate in the intima of human fetuses before macrophages are found. Appearance of oxidized LDL seems to follow native LDL, and the oxidized LDL are frequently present without macrophages nearby. However, the most common finding was the presence of intimal macrophages together with oxidized LDL (Fig. 8-8).[99] Severely oxidized LDL (oxLDL) have been shown to stimulate adhesion of both macrophages and T cells to endothelial cells, to promote diapedesis into the subendothelium, and to lead to the arrest of egress.[96] Whereas LDL bearing oxidation-related epitopes were seen frequently when macrophages were present, even in fetal aorta (see Fig. 8-8), the more severely oxidized oxLDL are generally found in advanced lesions primarily in association with macrophages. Such oxLDL are thought to be more likely formed by exposure to myeloperoxidase-produced hypochlorous acid from activated macrophages.[57,100] This consideration raises the question of whether oxLDL help summon the macrophages initially or whether oxLDL are formed only after activated macrophages have arrived. Nevertheless, even if formation of oxLDL or chlorinated and nitrosylated forms of LDL require preexisting macrophages, such modified LDL could subsequently perpetuate endothelial activation and otherwise promote atherosclerosis.[101] One important issue to note in this regard is the near absence of myeloperoxidase in experimental mouse atherosclerotic lesions, suggesting a major species difference with humans and providing a likely explanation for the lack of effect on murine atherosclerosis after knockout of myeloperoxidase, whereas humans with myeloperoxidase deficiency appear to be protected from atherosclerosis.[98] Perhaps the strongest evidence in favor of the oxidized LDL hypothesis comes from the decrease in atherosclerosis seen after immunization of animals with various forms of oxidized LDL or malondialdehyde-treated LDL.[102-104] Still, the immunization appeared to be most effective at later stages of atherosclerosis.[103] Given these considerations, there remains the need to explain how the endothelium is activated to attract the monocytes in the first place.

Aside from oxLDL (usually produced in vitro with nonphysiologic exposure to copper or iron ions), endothelial and smooth muscle cells can mildly oxidize LDL in culture, and

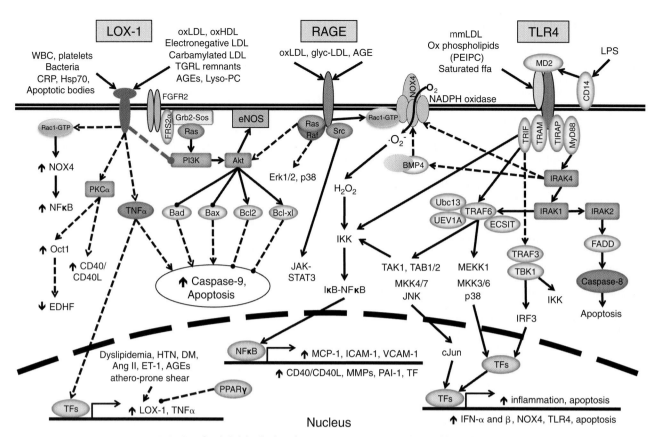

FIGURE 8-9 Activation of endothelial cells through LOX-1, RAGE, or TLR4 signaling. Highly parallel pathways are present in macrophages that can lead to activation and foam cell formation.

such "minimally modified" LDL (mmLDL) can also activate endothelial cells and initiate monocyte adherence and transmigration. These events were prevented by the presence of high-density lipoproteins (HDL) or antioxidants.[105] In these studies, only monocyte, not neutrophil, adhesion and migration was stimulated, much as might be expected for atherosclerosis-related endothelial activation. Presumably, LDL trapped in the subendothelial space would be exposed to sufficient ROS from activated endothelial cells to result in such minimally oxidized LDL. Formation of mmLDL or oxLDL in the plasma is thought to be unlikely because of potent antioxidant factors there. Some have questioned whether even mmLDL are formed in vivo in the surprisingly antioxidant-rich intima.[57] However, the observations in human fetuses cited before would suggest that at least some oxidation is possible and occurs before the arrival of macrophages.

mmLDL and Toll-Like Receptor 4 (TLR4)

Perhaps the strongest evidence for a pathway mediating endothelial activation by mmLDL is by way of toll-like receptor 4 (TLR4).[106-108] TLR4 is a major mediator of innate immunity and the main response receptor for bacterial lipopolysaccharide. A number of pathogen-associated molecular patterns (PAMPs) appear to trigger inflammatory responses through TLRs. Oxidized or otherwise altered phospholipids protrude abnormally (much like whiskers) from the cell membrane and trigger innate immune receptors and natural antibodies that act to clear the damaged phospholipids.[109,110] These considerations may be most relevant to macrophage activation and foam cell formation, considered later. Nevertheless, endothelial cells from C3H/HeJ mice, which have an inbred mutation in TLR4, are essentially unresponsive to mmLDL and are protected from diet-induced atherosclero-

sis.[111] Furthermore, mmLDL as well as associated oxidized phospholipids were shown to transmit signals to activate NF-κB through TLR4.[106] Knockout of TLR4 or its downstream adapter protein MyD88 (myeloid differentiation factor 88) resulted in unresponsiveness to mmLDL in endothelial cells and decreased atherosclerosis.[108] As noted later, TLR4 may also be involved in other mechanisms of endothelial activation in relation to atherosclerosis. Several features of TLR4 signaling are shown in Figure 8-9. TLR2 may also be involved in endothelial activation.[112]

Role of the Oxidized LDL Receptor 1 (LOX-1)

Early studies with oxLDL demonstrated powerful proinflammatory and apoptotic effects on incubation with endothelial cells. Subsequent studies identified LOX-1 (lectin-like oxidized LDL receptor 1), coded by the *OLR1* gene (oxidized LDL receptor 1), as a scavenger-type receptor expressed on the surface of endothelial cells that likely mediated these effects. LOX-1 is also expressed on monocyte-macrophages and platelets, but unlike macrophages, LOX-1 is the only scavenger-type receptor expressed highly on endothelial cells. LOX-1 may be considered another PAMP-recognizing receptor with a key role in innate immunity.[109] Importantly, LOX-1 is not expressed constitutively but is induced by most of its ligands, including oxLDL, as well as by factors that upregulate NADPH oxidase, such as angiotensin II. Besides oxLDL, LOX-1 is bound and activated by gram-positive and gram-negative bacteria, apoptotic bodies, senescent red blood cells, activated white blood cells and platelets, advanced glycation end products (AGEs), lysolecithin, and, recently recognized, C-reactive protein.[113,114] LOX-1 is expressed particularly in atherosclerosis-prone areas or over atherosclerotic plaque and has been reported to be increased by hyperlipidemia, diabetes, and hypertension and after exposure to various cytokines.[115-117]

Details of LOX-1–mediated intracellular signaling continue to be worked out. Some of the identified pathways are depicted in Figure 8-9. Intracellular signaling pathways activated by LOX-1 include RhoA (resulting in eNOS downregulation); a Rac1-mediated burst in NADPH oxidase activity[118]; the Ras, Raf, ERK1/2 cascade, leading to increased PAI-1 expression[119]; and increased expression of CD40 and CD40L (CD40 ligand) through PKCα signaling, which may act in an autocrine fashion through CD40L signaling to further upregulate several inflammatory genes including TNF-α and P-selectin.[120] Importantly, activation of LOX-1 leads to inactivation of PI3K. In endothelial cells, PI3K is strongly protective as it normally upregulates eNOS and inhibits apoptosis. Upregulation of PI3K is key to the protective autoregulation by fibroblast growth factor 2 (FGF2) through its own receptor, FGFR2, as shown in Figure 8-9. Therefore, by blocking of PI3K and through increased TNF-α production, apoptosis is greatly accelerated.[121,122]

If oxLDL were the only lipoprotein to bind to the LOX-1 receptor, its relevance to early endothelial activation would not be so readily apparent for reasons noted before. However, studies note that in addition to oxLDL, LOX-1 is bound and strongly activated by electronegative LDL.[121] This finding is consistent with a substantial literature demonstrating the endothelial activating and apoptotic potential of electronegative LDL. These particles can be formed by a number of nonoxidative mechanisms as well as by oxidation, including glycation, enrichment with nonesterified fatty acids, treatment with cholesteryl esterases, phospholipase A_2, platelet-activating factor acyl hydrolase (PAF-AH, also called LpPLA$_2$), and, importantly, sphingomyelinase.[123,124] Electronegative LDL are found in a much higher proportion of plasma LDL than are oxidized LDL (up to 10% of normolipidemic LDL). Recently, evidence was presented that LDL themselves carry a sphingomyelinase activity that promotes formation of electronegative LDL and that promotes LDL aggregation as seen in subendothelial, trapped LDL.[125] Further, sphingomyelinase and other enzymes capable of modifying LDL and promoting aggregation are present in the artery wall and likely promote aggregation of LDL.[124] Importantly, other studies identify LOX-1 as a receptor that can mediate inflammatory responses to TGRL (triglyceride-rich lipoprotein) remnants.[126]

Particles that bind to LOX-1 appear to be relevant in vivo because overexpression of LOX-1 in the liver to remove such particles from plasma led to virtual arrest of atherosclerosis progression.[127] Knockout of LOX-1 reduced atherosclerosis approximately 50% in a high-cholesterol/fat–fed LDLR knockout model and preserved endothelial function.[128] Overexpression of LOX-1 in coronary arteries in apo E knockout mice leads to an atherosclerosis-like vasculopathy.[129]

TGRL remnants may be particularly atherogenic. In one study, TGRL appeared to activate endothelial cells without any need for modification.[5] In another study, apo C-III, which accumulates on TGRL, appeared to activate PKCß and thereby inhibit protective Akt signaling in endothelial cells.[130] In a gene expression study comparing VLDL with oxidized VLDL (oxVLDL), different endothelial pathways were activated.[131] Thus, native VLDL upregulated ERK1/2 and NF-κB modestly with little effect on ROS generation, whereas oxVLDL resulted in substantial stimulation of the MAPK p38, NF-κB, and marked increase in ROS production as well as evidence for decreased viability. Later studies by this same group showed much greater endothelial activation by postprandial TGRL after a cream meal compared with fasting TGRL from hypertriglyceridemic patients. In addition, flow-mediated dilation of the brachial artery was impaired by the fatty meal. Postprandial TGRL resulted in upregulation of p38 MAPK, CREB, NF-AT, NF-κB, VCAM-1, PECAM-1, ELAM-1, ICAM-1,

P-selectin, MCP-1, IL-6, TLR4, CD40, ADAMTS1, and PAI-1.[132] The receptors or other mechanisms mediating these responses were not identified.

RAGE

The receptor for advanced glycation end products (RAGE) is present on endothelial cells and, like TLR4 and LOX-1, can activate endothelial cells by overlapping intracellular signaling pathways (see Fig. 8-9). JNK activation seems to be particularly important in this regard, but RAGE also activates the JAK-STAT3 pathway.[133] RAGE is generally considered in the context of diabetes-related modifications to proteins or LDL. Indeed, it recognizes a ligand generated by nonenzymatic reactions between glucose and protein lysine residues (carboxy-methyl lysine). Certainly, ligation of RAGE by this ligand, generated in proportion to degree of hyperglycemia, is one means whereby diabetes contributes to endothelial activation and atherosclerosis, as demonstrated by use of soluble RAGE competition[134] as well as diabetic RAGE knockout models.[135] However, hyperlipidemia without diabetes also generates a substantial load of ligands for the RAGE. Indeed, 52% reduction in atherosclerosis was seen in nondiabetic, apo E knockout mice that were also deficient in RAGE, whereas those expressing endothelial cell–specific dominant-negative RAGE mutations had more than 70% reduction.[136] Ligands for RAGE present in oxLDL identified in this model included proinflammatory S100/calgranulins and HMGB1 (high-mobility group box 1). Incubation with S100 activated JNK with elaboration of VCAM-1 in cultured wild-type endothelial cells, whereas activation was substantially reduced in the RAGE knockout or dominant-negative cells.[136] Thus, RAGE represents yet another pathway for endothelial cell activation.

REFLECTIONS ON ENDOTHELIAL ACTIVATION

One of the major messages in these discussions is the redundancy of pathways potentially leading to endothelial cell activation. For modified lipoproteins alone, activation may occur by way of TLR4, LOX-1, or RAGE. The TLR4 and RAGE responses may require oxidative changes, as found in mmLDL or oxidized phospholipids, but may also be triggered by saturated fatty acids (for TLR4); the LOX-1 response appears to include a broader array of triggers. Other potential pathways resulting in endothelial activation from various lipoprotein moieties are also likely. Thus, an intervention that focuses on only one of these pathways, such as oral antioxidants (even acknowledging the limitations of the antioxidants tested thus far), might be expected to be ineffectual in reducing coronary events. This can be expected even if oxidation is causally related to disease because of the redundancy of lipoprotein modifications that can lead to endothelial activation. For the same reason, effects from single genes in these pathways may be difficult to detect. Indeed, not shown in Figure 8-9 are the numerous cytokine-mediated pathways that lead to activation. Additional pathways are illustrated by numerous knockout models reviewed in Tables 8-1 and 8-2.

Redundancy seems to be the rule for pathways vital to the survival of the organism. In the case of endothelial activation, the key role such activation plays in defense from microorganisms as well as in clearing the bloodstream of senescent or apoptotic debris seems evident. In this sense, it may be disingenuous to describe the state of endothelial activation associated with various risk factors as "dysfunction." Indeed, the cells seem to be performing admirably and as expected in response to perceived threats.

8

Molecular Biology and Genetics of Atherosclerosis

TABLE 8–1		Effects on Atherosclerosis of Gene Knockout, Transgenic Expression, or Other Genetic Manipulations Involving Endothelial Cell Activation and Other Early Steps in Initiation*
Gene	**Effect†**	**Gene Function**
PKCβ1/2	↓↓	A proinflammatory conventional PKC
Egr-1	↓↓	Proinflammatory transcription factor activated by JNK
PECAM-1	↓ to ↓↓	Flow sensor, involved in intercellular junction
Fibronectin, EIIIA	↓↓	Extracellular matrix component, proinflammatory
Cx37 (BMT)	↑	Regulates macrophage adhesion to endothelium
Cx43	↓↓	Promotes leukocyte accumulation
eNOS	↑	Synthesis of NO
p47^{phox}	↓↓	Critical component of NADPH oxidase
Renin	↓↓	Produces angiotensin I from angiotensinogen
AT1R	↓↓	Angiotensin receptor 1 (can activate NADPH oxidase)
HO-1	↑↑	Important cellular enzymatic antioxidant
MnSOD	↑↑	Important cellular enzymatic antioxidant
PRDX1	↑	Important cellular enzymatic antioxidant
LIAS	↑	Synthesis of lipoic acid, a mitochondrial antioxidant
NEMO	↓	Component of IKK that phosphorylates IκB
IκB (DN)	↓↓	Sequesters NF-κB in cytoplasm until phosphorylated
TLR2	↓	A toll-like receptor—normally recognizes PAMPs
TLR4	↓↓	A toll-like receptor, binds modified lipoproteins
MyD88	↓↓	Adaptor protein critical for TLR signaling
LOX-1, OLR1	↓↓	Activation of endothelial cells by modified lipoproteins
RAGE	↓↓	Activation of endothelial cells by modified lipoproteins
PARP-1	↓↓	DNA repair and stress enzyme–activated DNA damage
ROCK1	↓↓	Transmits contraction signals from Rho
PI3Kγ, p110γ	↓↓	Regulates macrophage chemotaxis
5-LO	↓↓↓	Rate-limiting enzyme for leukotriene synthesis

*In this and the following tables, studies were whole-body knockout of the gene unless otherwise indicated, performed in either apo E–deficient or LDL receptor knockout mice.

†Effects on atherosclerosis (for all tables): ↓, <50% reduction; ↓↓, 50%-80% reduction; ↓↓↓, >80% reduction; ↑, <100% increase; ↑↑, 100% or greater increase.

BMT, bone marrow transplantation; DN, dominant negative.

TABLE 8–2			Genetic Studies Involving Ligands and Corresponding Cognate Receptors in Endothelial Cell–Leukocyte Interactions*
Endothelium	**Effect**	**Leukocyte**	**Effect**
Tethering or Rolling			
E-selectin	↓	ESL-1, CD44	↓↓
P-selectin	↓	PSGL-1	↓
PSGL-1, CD24, CD34	↓	L-selectin	—
Activation by Chemokines/Chemoattractants			
M-CSF	↓↓↓	CSF1R	↓↓
MCP-1 (CCL2)	↓↓ to ↓↓↓	CCR2	↓↓ to ↓↓↓
CCL5 (RANTES)	↓ to ↓↓	CCR1 CCR5	↑↑↓
CXCL1 (GROα)	↓	CXCR2 (BMT)	↓↓
CXCL2 (GROβ) CXCL3 (GROγ) CXCL5-7	—	CXCR2	↓↓
CXCL4 (PF 4)	↓↓	CXCR3B	—
CXCL8 (IL-8)	—	CXCR2	↓↓
CXCL9, 10, 11	↓	CXCR3	NS
CXCL12 (SDF-1)	—	CXCR4	↑
CXCL16	↑	CXCR6	↓
CX3CL1 (fractalkine)	↓↓	CX3CR1	↓↓
CD40	NS	CD40L (CD154)	↓↓↓
Slow Rolling and Firm Adhesion			
VCAM-1	↓	α$_4$β$_1$ integrin (VLA4)	—
Fibronectin	↓↓	α$_4$β$_1$, α$_5$β$_1$	—
ICAM-1	NS to ↓↓	α$_L$β$_2$ integrin (LFA1)	↓
E-selectin	↓	α$_M$β$_2$ integrin	—
vWF	—	α$_{IIb}$β$_3$ integrin	—
Thrombospondin-1 (VN)	—	α$_V$β$_3$ integrin	↑↑
MADCAM1	—	α$_4$β$_7$ integrin	—
CD137	—	CD137L	—
Transmigration			
JAM-A	—	LFA1, JAM-A	—
JAM-B	—	VLA4, JAM-C	—
JAM-C (also in smooth muscle cells)	—	MAC1, JAM-B	—
CD99	↓	CD99	—
PECAM-1	↓ to ↓↓	PECAM-1	↓ to ↓↓
ICAM-2	—	MAC1, LFA1	—

*In most cases, monocyte interactions are shown. Interactions with other leukocytes and platelets may follow similar steps. Cells other than endothelial cells may produce the chemokines shown.

BMT, bone marrow transplantation; NS, not significant; —, not tested.

Molecular Biology of Leukocyte Transmigration into Intima

The first step of capturing passing leukocytes has generally been considered to be mediated by endothelial cells expressing on their surface the adhesion molecules P-selectin and E-selectin. Binding of these selectins to their cognate receptors on leukocytes is relatively loose, with breaking and reforming of the bonds, thereby leading to partial tethering and rolling of leukocytes under the shear forces of the blood circulation. L-selectin on virtually all leukocytes can recognize several markers on activated endothelial cells as well.

Tethering and rolling bring the leukocyte into intimate contact with the endothelial surface, where the leukocyte encounters chemotactic cytokines or chemokines such as MCP-1 (also referred to as CCL2) and monocyte colony-stimulating factor (M-CSF) as well as other surface-immobilized chemokines that are held close to the endothelial surface by proteoglycans in the glycocalyx. More than 40 chemokines are known, again illustrating the redundancy of key systems.[137]

The current terminology for the chemokines refers to characteristic conserved cysteine residues in the N terminus. These cysteines can have no intervening amino acids (CC chemokines), one separating amino acid (CXC chemokines), or three intervening amino acids (CXXXC or CX3C chemokines); L refers to the chemokine ligand and R to the receptor. For example, some of surface-immobilized chemokines noted before include CXCL1, CXCL2, CXCL4, and CCL5 in addition to MCP-1 (CCL2). Chemokines presented by activated endothelial cells bind to cognate receptors that are all GPCRs (such as CCR2, the receptor for MCP-1) located on the surface of the leukocyte. This binding leads to further activation. At least 20 such receptors are known. Even before this step, rolling appears to promote movement of these GPCRs from intracellular sites to the cell surface in association with cholesterol-rich rafts. One study demonstrated the presence of MCP-1, GROα, and IL-8 on the endothelium of human atherosclerotic plaque that was capable of inducing attachment and spreading of test monocytes, suggesting the relevance of prior, mostly mouse-based models and further illustrating redundancy in this early step of atherogenesis.[138]

Binding of chemokines to their cognate GPCRs initiates "inside-out signaling," with the result being an alteration in the extracellular configuration of leukocyte integrins leading to enhanced binding affinity to endothelial VCAM-1 and ICAM-1 (or other ligands). This enhanced interaction then leads to slow rolling, adhesion strengthening, spreading, and firm adhesion. The firm binding of leukocyte integrins with their ligands then initiates "outside-in signaling" and clustering of the integrins into focal adhesions. Outside-in signaling refers to a host of integrated signals initiated by the bound integrins that result in intraluminal crawling as the leukocyte seeks an opportune site for penetration and finally diapedesis or transmigration of the leukocyte into the subendothelium. This may occur by passage of the leukocyte between endothelial cells by interactions with various gap junction proteins (paracellular migration) or directly through thinned segments of endothelial cells (transcellular migration). For monocytes, this is followed by transformation into tissue macrophages or dendritic cells. There are at least 24 different integrin heterodimers that mediate this signaling on various leukocytes.[139]

Each progressive step of this process is associated with greater activation of the leukocyte and coordinated intracellular and intercellular signaling with endothelial cells. Whereas monocyte transmigration has been considered to predominate in atherosclerotic lesion formation, the participation of other leukocytes and subsets of monocytes and T cells has recently been more fully recognized.[140] Platelets can also adhere to activated endothelial cells and may aid in binding of other white cells. T cells, mast cells, and even a few B cells and neutrophils also find their way into the incipient lesion. Once they are in the subendothelial space, there is an exchange of cytokines between the various activated cells that further amplifies the inflammatory response. The molecular biology of these steps in relation to atherosclerosis has been extensively studied and is the focus of several recent, excellent reviews.[13,140-144] Some of the ligands and receptors mediating these endothelial cell–leukocyte interactions are listed in Table 8-2. However, virtually any presentation of leukocyte activation and interaction with the endothelium must be considered a simplification. One review

listed 47 proteins that were thought to be regulatory for at least 900 total proteins and 6000 protein-protein interactions.[145] Gene expression profiling identified 400 genes that were upregulated or downregulated by at least twofold after exposure of endothelial cells to IL-1β, IFN-γ, and TNF-α.[146] About 600 to 1000 genes were similarly regulated during the transition of monocytes to macrophages.[147,148] Only a few additional details of some of the key processes are provided here.

As noted before, initial tethering and rolling of leukocytes are mediated, in part, by P-selectin and E-selectin on activated endothelial cells and L-selectin on leukocytes. PSGL1 (P-selectin glycoprotein ligand 1) can bind all these selectins. Other ligands can also bind E-selectin. Nonactivated integrins can bind weakly to VCAM-1 and ICAM-1 and can also mediate rolling. However, activated integrins are generally considered more important in leukocyte firm adhesion and spreading. P-selectin is also expressed on activated platelets. P-selectin is presynthesized and stored in Weibel-Palade bodies and can be expressed on the cell surface rapidly by fusion of the Weibel-Palade body with the cell membrane. In contrast, E-selectin is not stored and must be synthesized de novo; thus, levels rise more slowly on activation.

The early recognition of the predominance of macrophages in human and experimental plaques focused most attention on the early entrance of these cells into the intimal space. However, the importance of other cells has been increasingly recognized. Further stimulation of macrophages or dendritic cells by Th1 cells as well as mutual stimulation by macrophages and dendritic cells seems to establish inflammatory cells within the intima as long as any inciting risk factors (such as hyperlipidemia) are present. Neutrophils may become particularly important in destabilizing advanced lesions.[140,143]

In a startling set of experiments, an extensive network of dendritic cells were found to be the earliest inhabitants of this space, concentrated clearly in atherosclerosis-prone areas of disturbed flow. This network was established in all specimens examined even in infancy or early childhood in the absence of any risk factors, well before the presence of any evidence of macrophage accumulation or lipid-filled cells, and was universally present in normolipidemic animals as well.[149] The participation of these cells in addition to early appearance of proinflammatory Th1 lymphocytes, which may respond to the self antigen HSP-60, together with the observation that patients with CAD were found to have increased plasma titers of anti–HSP-60 antibodies that strongly cross-reacted to certain *Cytomegalovirus* antigens has raised considerable interest.[150] Evidence has been presented that immunization of LDLR knockout mice with the bacterial homologue HSP-65, HSP-60, or desensitizing peptide fragments shifts lymphocyte counts to greater numbers of regulatory Th2 (anti-inflammatory) in relation to Th1 cells with increased IL-10 production and substantially reduces atherosclerosis by 50% to as much as 80%.[151,152] Whether such desensitization therapy may be effective to prevent progression of human atherosclerosis is unknown.

Because movement of leukocytes has been so extensively studied in the context of many diseases, the elegant mechanisms controlling their movement and chemotaxis will not be discussed in detail. It is recommended that the interested reader consult recent textbooks for the elegant coordination of these events, in which GTPase molecules Cdc42 and Rac serve as both controlling "switches" and membrane attachment points for growing and branching actin microfibers that provide a pushing force to propel the cell forward, while Rho works at the back of the cell to promote uropod retraction. Kinesin motors serve to recycle integrins and other key cell machinery forward while other signaling mechanisms maintain cell polarity.

TABLE 8–3	Genetic Effects on Atherosclerosis—Cytokine Signaling
Gene	**Effect**
Secreted by Macrophages in response to Toll Receptor and Scavenger Receptor Binding	
IL-1α	↓↓
IL-1β	↓
IL-6	NS
gp130 (IL6ST, in humans)	↓
IL-12	↓↓
IL-18	↓
TNF-α	↓↓
MIF	↓↓
Secreted primarily by Th1 cells after Activation by Antigen Presentation (Dendritic Cell or Macrophage), Reinforced by CD40-CD40L Costimulation	
IL-2	↓
IFN-γ	↓ to ↓↓
Secreted primarily by Th2 cells after Activation by Antigen Presentation (Primarily Anti-Inflammatory)	
IL-4	NS
IL-5	↑
IL-10	↑
Secreted primarily by T Regulatory Cells	
TGF-β	↑↑
Secreted by Mast Cells	
GM-CSF	↓ to ↑
Miscellaneous	
IL-1Ra (TG)	↓
IL-1R	↓↓↓
TNFR1 (p55)	↑↑
IFN-γR	↓↓

NS, not significant; TG, transgenic with overexpression.

Once early inflammatory changes have been established, particularly with recruitment of the various leukocytes to the subendothelial space, numerous cytokines are secreted by activated cells that reinforce the inflammatory response and further activate endothelial cells as well as surrounding leukocytes. This exchange of cytokines acts as a positive feedback loop to ensure a vigorous response to perceived threats. In Table 8-3, a list is provided of some of these cytokines as well as other genes affecting early stages of endothelial activation and inflammation and effects on atherosclerosis of genetic manipulation. The receptors and intracellular signaling in response to these cytokines have been the subject of much study, and many illustrations of these pathways are available for free download from commercial sources on the Internet (e.g., *http://www.sabiosciences.com/pathwaycentral. php* and *http://www.cellsignal.com/reference/pathway/ index.html*) as well as a recent on-line textbook of cell signaling pathways (*http://www.cellsignallingbiology.org/*). They will not be discussed further here.

While reviewing Tables 8-1 through 8-3, the reader should keep in mind that the apparent impact on atherosclerosis of manipulating a given gene can change over time. Most of these models are double knockouts; the first knockout (of the apo E gene or the LDL receptor) results in hyperlipidemia, and the second knockout is of the test gene under study. Short-term studies generally report a greater percentage reduction in atherosclerosis due to test gene knockout than longer term studies do. For example, in one study, at 5 weeks there was a clear effect of even heterozygous CCR2 (the receptor for MCP-1) knockout, with atherosclerosis clearly increasing progressively from CCR2$^{-/-}$ (strongly protected) to CCR2$^{+/-}$ to CCR2$^{+/+}$ (wild type). By 9 weeks, however, the heterozygous knockout had caught up to the wild type. By 13 weeks, even the homozygous knockout mice had atherosclerosis extent similar to that for wild type at 9 weeks, although the trajectories for atherosclerosis remained different between CCR2$^{-/-}$ and CCR2$^{+/-}$ mice.[153]

What do such observations imply for gene effects in human atherosclerosis, a disease that develops over decades? Even with powerful (but presumably rare) effects on a clearly important gene, there may be no observable effect in the long run in a redundant system. This principle may help explain the extreme difficulty that human gene hunters have had in identifying consistently replicable genetic associations with atherosclerosis, particularly involving initiating pathways (endothelial activation and inflammation). A corollary may be that interventions that have global impact on such pathways (such as control of hyperlipidemia or a reduction in blood pressure) will likely have more success than efforts to affect a single genetic element. An additional consideration with regard to inflammatory pathways is that a focused intervention such as that noted for CCR2 knockout that resulted in marked reductions in monocytes may be associated with unacceptable increases in susceptibility to infection.

Effects of Selected Risk Factors on Initiation of Atherosclerosis

Blood Pressure

Pressure, stretch, and flow are the first risk factors to which the endothelium is exposed. Blood pressure in the arterial range is an essential requirement for the development of atherosclerosis. Venous atherosclerosis does not occur even in patients with homozygous familial hypercholesterolemia.[154] The relatively rapid progression of atherosclerosis in saphenous veins used in coronary artery bypass suggests that there is nothing uniquely resistant about veins themselves. Normally, the pulmonary arterial circulation with its systolic pressures of 12 to 22 mm Hg is another entirely protected site. Nevertheless, with pulmonary hypertension, atherosclerotic plaques are commonly seen.[155]

The major mechanism whereby pressure promotes atherosclerosis appears to be through increased pressure-driven convection of LDL and other lipoproteins into the intima.[156] For example, LDL accumulation in the intima of pressurized rabbit aorta increased 44-fold when pressure was raised from 70 to 160 mm Hg.[157] Stretch may also play a role.[158] Approximately 90% of the convection of LDL into the subendothelial space appears to be through gaps created between mitotic endothelial cells in areas of low shear stress, whereas only 10% was estimated to enter by way of transcellular vesicular traffic.[159] A thinner glycocalyx, also associated with atherosclerosis-prone areas with low shear stress, also appears to contribute to greater LDL permeability.[160]

Exercise

Even modest exercise serves as a potent stimulus to improved endothelial function as measured by vasodilation in response to acetylcholine, particularly in older animals and humans.[161-163] Aged mice had much higher levels of nitrotyrosine (a marker of chronic oxidative stress) in their aortas compared with younger mice, and this was markedly reduced by modest amounts of voluntary running on an exercise wheel.[161] Exercise acutely increases flow and hence shear stress experienced by endothelial cells in many vascular beds, not just the exercising limb. This increased flow is sensed by multiple transduction mechanisms, several of which acutely stimulate NO production as well as pro-oxidant systems. NO can acutely block several pro-oxidant pathways and inflammatory pathways, including direct inhibition of NADPH oxidase and IKK. Further, NO alters transcription of eNOS and leads to increased expression of eNOS protein. Thus, inhibition of eNOS activity abrogates the exercise-induced increase in eNOS protein expression.[164]

Stimulation of flow has a number of additional effects. An acute increase in flow with exercise results in a transient increase in endothelial superoxide anion generation by mitochondria and NADPH oxidase.[165] This superoxide is converted rapidly to hydrogen peroxide. The modest, controlled burst of hydrogen peroxide, in turn, also acts to promote increased expression and activity of eNOS, possibly (as noted before) through altered expression of NF-κB as well as stimulation of HSP-90 (which strongly supports eNOS activity) through stimulation of HNF1. Importantly, when high levels of human catalase were expressed in endothelial cells of exercising mice, blocking signaling by hydrogen peroxide, the expected increase in eNOS expression in response to exercise was entirely blocked.[166]

Endothelial cells also adapt to chronic laminar flow by stimulation of a number of antioxidant defenses (at least in part through Nrf2 signaling), resulting in increased expression of extracellular superoxide dismutase and Cu/Zn SOD as well as a decrease in NADPH oxidase.[165] Similar adaptive changes occur with exercise training, explaining the longer term antioxidant effects of exercise despite acute modest stimulation of superoxide and hydrogen peroxide production during acute bouts of exercise.[161,166] Parallel benefits from exercise on insulin signaling pathways in skeletal muscle appear to be blocked by large doses of oral antioxidants, suggesting potential deleterious effects of such interventions.[167] Finally, exercise was shown to clearly reduce atherosclerosis in apo E–deficient mice together with marked reduction of macrophage and Th1 cell accumulation in the intima. This effect of exercise was entirely blocked by inhibition of eNOS.[164] Other effects of exercise on endothelial function, including increased PGI$_2$, thrombomodulin, and plasmin, have also been reviewed.[168]

Hyperlipidemia

Extensive effects of hyperlipidemia to initiate atherosclerosis are reviewed earlier. Not only does hyperlipidemia activate the endothelium and otherwise promote atherosclerosis, but effects on circulating white cells are also apparent. Thus, expression of CCR2, the cognate receptor on monocytes for MCP-1, was approximately twofold higher in hypercholesterolemic patients with average LDL of 167 mg/dL compared with persons with LDL of 80 mg/dL. Incubation of monocytes in hypercholesterolemic serum, without LDL oxidation, led to similar marked increases of CCR2, apparently through uptake by the LDL receptor. Additional unexpected effects of hypercholesterolemia include suppression of the inward rectifying potassium current in endothelial cells (which might be expected to lead to diminished NO response to acute changes in flow).[169] Hypercholesterolemia affects phosphatidylinositol 4,5-bisphosphate (PIP$_2$)–sensing amino acids in inwardly rectifying K (Kir2) channels, not by altering membrane physical properties.[170] Interestingly, patients with

familial hypercholesterolemia were shown to have reduced glycocalyx volume, which could be partially restored by treatment with rosuvastatin.[171]

Hypercholesterolemia and particularly hypertriglyceridemia appear to increase activity of xanthine oxidoreductase (XOR).[172] There may be both greater conversion in the liver of the enzyme from the dehydrogenase form to the oxidase form (accompanied by greater production of superoxide) and increased release of the oxidase from the liver. Xanthine oxidase is then thought to adhere to the glycocalyx of endothelial cells, where it can contribute to endothelial oxidative stress and promote endothelial dysfunction that may be ameliorated by XOR inhibitors such as allopurinol.[173] XOR knockout studies are not feasible in mice as the pups are stunted and live only 4 to 6 weeks, presumably because of renal failure.[174] Nevertheless, tungsten administration (a relatively specific inhibitor of XOR) to apo E–deficient mice fed a Western-type diet for 6 months resulted in 83% reduction of aortic atherosclerosis.[175]

HDL Effects

Besides reverse cholesterol transport, HDL has been shown to mediate a number of protective effects on the endothelium. HDL protects endothelial cells from apoptosis induced by oxLDL, TGRL, TNF-α, and activated complement. HDL stimulates NO production by eNOS and increases prostacyclin (PGI$_2$) production through COX-2. Finally, HDL suppresses expression of VCAM-1, ICAM-1, and E-selectin by endothelial cells as well as other signs of endothelial activation after exposure to oxLDL or cytokines.[176] These effects are mediated by both apo A-I and lipid components carried in HDL, particularly sphingosine 1-phosphate (S1P) and related lysosphingolipids.[177,178]

There are five known S1P receptors, S1P1 through 5. These are G protein–coupled receptors (GPCR) with the potential to be coupled to a variety of heterotrimeric G proteins with diverse and frequently divergent functions. The atheroprotective functions of HDL on endothelial cells appear to be mediated by S1P signaling primarily through the S1P1 receptor and to a lesser extent through S1P3.[177,178] HDL carries more than 50% of the S1P in plasma.[179,180] Activation of the S1P1 receptor recapitulates a number of the protective features of prolonged exposure to laminar flow (see Fig. 8-7). These effects appear to be mediated by ERK1/2, PI3K, Akt, and Rac1 activation, with resulting increased barrier integrity, increased NO production, suppression of inflammatory responses, promotion of cellular antioxidants, and increased cell survival (by suppression of caspases). Activation of these pathways is supported by and possibly dependent on the binding of apo A-I to endothelial SR-B1. Binding to SR-B1 not only brings the HDL into proximity with S1P1 receptors but also supports cytosolic signaling to activate Src. Src can then activate MEK1/2 followed by ERK1/2 as well as PI3K. PDZK1 is an adaptor or scaffolding protein that binds to the cytosolic side of SR-B1. PDZK1 is required for Src activation by HDL. Indeed, PDZK1 knockout completely blocked HDL-mediated increases in eNOS and promotion of endothelial repair after injury.[181] HDL may also inhibit monocyte activation after interactions with T cells.[177]

Another mechanism whereby HDL protects endothelial cells and promotes NO production is by removal of the oxysterol 7-keto cholesterol by way of the ABCG1 transporter.[182] This oxidized sterol built up when mice were fed a Western-type diet. HDL also helps prevent LDL oxidation or detoxifies oxidized phospholipids in LDL through the HDL-associated enzyme PON1. PON1 knockout mice express increased atherosclerosis, whereas overexpression of PON1 was protective.[183] These findings contrast with the much more variable outcomes associated with milder effects on PON1 caused by common human variants.[184]

Whereas other risk factors may recapitulate a form of endothelial activation that in some settings would be advantageous (such as in infection or physical injury), the endothelial response in diabetes is truly maladaptive and finds few if any parallels in normal physiology. Therefore, the term *endothelial dysfunction* applies most aptly in diabetes. Unlike other risk factors, hyperglycemia leads to endothelial dysfunction that is systemic, resulting in both aggravation of atherosclerosis and a microvascular disease that is unique to diabetes. In type 2 diabetes, excess free fatty acid exposure and insulin resistance appear to further exacerbate this response.

An elegant, unified model to explain the seemingly disparate aspects of endothelial dysfunction in diabetes has been forwarded.[185,186] The endothelial cell is one of a handful of cell types that are unable to regulate entry of glucose into their cytoplasm. Thus, hyperglycemia leads to unregulated uptake of glucose through GLUT1 transporters and elevated intracellular glucose in endothelial cells. Rapid flux of substrate through the glycolytic pathway then ensues, leading to an abundance of pyruvate for transfer into mitochondria, synthesis of acetyl coenzyme A, and generation of reducing equivalents (NADH, FADH$_2$) by the citric acid cycle. The transfer of high-energy electrons from NADH and FADH$_2$ to complexes of the electron transport chain provides energy to pump hydrogen ions from the matrix into the mitochondrial intermembrane space, thereby generating the hydrogen ion gradient that subsequently drives ATP synthesis through F$_0$F$_1$ complexes. With an overabundance of energy substrate, the hydrogen gradient increases to a critical level, at which point the final electron transport to complex IV is impaired (where water is normally formed from controlled electron transport to oxygen). The "backed up" electrons then begin to be transported from coenzyme Q$_{10}$ (ubiquinone) to oxygen directly, forming superoxide anion. (Paradoxically, a similar phenomenon occurs with hypoxia.) This formation of superoxide anion can be blocked by dissipating the hydrogen ion gradient (e.g., by overexpression of uncoupling proteins) or by preventing transfer of electrons into the transport chain. In larger arteries, uncontrolled endothelial uptake and oxidation of free fatty acids, which are excessively abundant in type 2 diabetes, further exacerbate the energy surfeit and excess generation of superoxide anion.

Although superoxide anion does not penetrate membranes, a substantial amount of the excess superoxide is formed on the outer side of the mitochondrial inner membrane and can be transferred to the cytosol through the voltage-dependent anion channel in the outer mitochondrial membrane.[58] A modest or transient increase in superoxide production might be expected to produce primarily a transient rise in hydrogen peroxide and potentially stimulate an antioxidant response through Nrf2 signaling, as apparently occurs with exercise. Such a response is seen with short-term incubation of endothelial cells in high glucose. However, prolonged incubation, as in diabetes or with frequently repeated although transient exposures to high glucose, appears to result in sufficient superoxide production to overwhelm SOD antioxidant defenses and results in nuclear (as well as mitochondrial) DNA damage, such as single-strand breaks. In response, a DNA repair enzyme, poly(ADP-ribose) polymerase 1 (PARP-1), is activated. PARP-1 uses NAD$^+$ as a substrate and adds long ADP-ribose chains to various proteins and transcription factors, to itself, and, importantly, to histones. ADP-ribosylation of histones alters their conformation and allows greater access to the damaged DNA for other repair enzymes. Hydrogen peroxide, although less reactive than other ROS, can also activate PARP-1 (perhaps through formation of highly reactive hydroxyl radical), but to a lesser extent than superoxide and peroxynitrite.[187] PARP-1 can signal for apoptosis or extensive inflammation in the setting of extensive DNA repair, and pharmacologic inhibition or genetic deletion of PARP-1 decreased inflammation and reduced atherosclerosis in hyperlipidemic mice.[188] Activated PARP-1 leads to inhibition of glyceraldehyde-3-phosphate dehydrogenase with accumulation of the 3-carbon substrates, with subsequent promotion of AGE synthesis as well as diacylglycerol production with stimulation of PKC.

Stimulation of the expression of Nrf2 (by inactivation of Keap1 with sulforaphane, a naturally occurring substance in broccoli) upregulated antioxidant defenses and led to a marked reduction in the adverse effects of hyperglycemia, further supporting the role of ROS in mediating endothelial dysfunction in diabetes.[189] Lipoic acid is an important mitochondrial antioxidant, and supplementation was shown to decrease atherosclerosis in hyperlipidemic, diabetic mice.[190] Heterozygous deficiency of lipoic acid synthase in such mice resulted in a 48% increase in atherosclerosis extent.[191]

There is growing evidence for selective endothelial insulin resistance for the vasodilating Akt pathway while the vasoconstricting ERK1/2 pathway (through Shc, Grb2-Sos, Ras, Raf, and MEK1/2) is left intact. The vasoconstriction seems to be particularly promoted through the activation of PKCθ by fatty acids, such as palmitate. PKCθ both inhibits insulin signaling through IRS-1 and Akt and promotes signaling through the ERK1/2 pathway.[192,193] Perhaps more relevant are increases in adhesion molecule expression in endothelial cells after exposure to insulin. Insulin-induced expression of VCAM-1 in endothelial cells was recently shown to be mediated through the insulin-like growth factor 1 receptor and could be completely abrogated by inhibiting the MAPK p38. Interestingly, insulin also stimulated expression of ICAM-1 by way of the insulin receptor. In both cases, MEK1 appeared to be involved but primarily by activating p38 rather than ERK1/2.[194] Endothelial dysfunction (including impaired eNOS phosphorylation and production of NO) was clearly induced recently by exposure to saturated free fatty acid (particularly palmitate) regardless of insulin signaling (with use of mice lacking insulin receptors in all the vasculature or knockout of Akt).[195] These mice also developed hypertension.

Autoimmune and Inflammatory Disease

Increased risk of atherosclerotic disease has been documented for several autoimmune diseases, including systemic lupus erythematosus,[196-201] rheumatoid arthritis or elevated rheumatoid factor,[202,203] systemic sclerosis,[204] and psoriasis.[205-207] It would be reasonable to expect that the elevated plasma cytokines, including TNF-α and IL-6,[208,209] seen particularly in systemic lupus erythematosus, would activate endothelial cells and thereby initiate atherosclerotic processes, particularly at atherosclerosis-prone sites. Other mechanisms have recently been forwarded. Mice that lack functional Fas ligand or Fas have impaired ability to clear apoptotic debris and have features of autoimmune disease. When crossed with apo E–deficient mice, these mice have increased atherosclerosis.[210,211] Apoptotic debris may present autoantigens to dendritic cells and thereby lead to autoantibody production and increased circulation of immune complexes, which could cause immune injury and promote inflammation. Alternatively, apoptotic debris itself could directly promote inflammation in atherosclerotic plaques.

Several older studies illustrated a potential synergism between immune injury and hyperlipidemia. Rabbits made only mildly hypercholesterolemic (200 to 250 mg/dL) and subjected to repeated injection of horse serum (a form of immunologic assault with antigen-antibody deposition on lesion-prone areas of endothelium) developed atherosclerosis that was more similar to human atherosclerosis than the usual severe hypercholesterolemia-induced lesions in rabbits. The rabbits appeared to be protected by antihistamines in this setting.[212] A counterpart in humans was suggested to be the finding of increased levels of serum antibodies to heat-dried cow's milk and boiled egg in patients with coronary heart disease.[213] The display of HSP-60 on endothelial cells in association with activation of endothelial cells from a variety of initiating factors could lead to autoimmune reactions, endothelial damage, and increased atherosclerosis, especially coupled with hyperlipidemia and other risk factors.[52]

A large literature has accumulated relating to immune activation by repeated or latent infections, which suggests another potential mechanism for endothelial activation and atherosclerosis initiation.[214] Macrophage activation may be involved as well. Infection of apo E–deficient mice with *Chlamydia pneumoniae*[215] or herpesvirus[216] accelerated atherosclerosis. Indeed, so did nonspecific activation of TLR2 receptors.[112] However, treatment of coronary patients with macrolide antibiotics failed to alter subsequent event rates.[217-219] Thus, causality for the infectious disease hypothesis remains to be proved. Furthermore, if the relationship to infectious disease requires only exposure resulting in an immune response, not continued infection, then the hypothesis may not be provable by any antimicrobial intervention.

Cigarette Smoking

Smoking has long been considered an endothelial cell stressor and activator. A genome-wide analysis of expression changes in 35,000 genes was recently reported after exposure of cultured endothelial cells to cigarette smoke extract.[220] There was massive upregulation of genes related to the unfolded protein response, thought to be due to immense oxidative stress. Generation of free radicals was apparently mediated by metals as well as by reactive species in the extract. This was accompanied by mitochondrial dysfunction, upregulation of HSF1 and heat shock proteins (including HSP-60), and cell cycle arrest. These observations are consistent with prior reports of the pro-oxidant effects of smoking leading to activation of endothelial cells.[221] The rapid reversibility of cardiovascular risk after smoking cessation suggests that this activation affects not only early endothelial activation but precipitating factors such as clotting and stability of advanced plaques as well (probably also through inflammatory effects).[222] Nevertheless, some evidence suggests that persistent inflammatory effects can last for years after smoking cessation.[223]

PROMOTION OF ATHEROSCLEROSIS

The promotion of atherosclerosis centers on the development of foam cells, their retention in or egress from the intima, their apoptosis or necrosis, and formation of the necrotic core. Insudation of lipoproteins into the subendothelial space and lipoprotein retention and modification are thought to be the major drivers of this stage of atherogenesis. The risk of coronary events is clearly proportional to the exponent of LDL plasma concentrations (hence the frequently replicated log-linear relationship, with a 30% increase in risk associated with a 30 mg/dL linear rise in plasma LDL).[224] Other apo B–containing lipoproteins are also proatherogenic; the order of atherogenicity, as demonstrated by matching cholesterol levels in apo E and LDLR knockout mice,[225] is roughly as follows: smaller LDL > larger LDL > β-VLDL > IDL > smaller VLDL > larger VLDL.

These findings are concordant with findings in humans. Patients with homozygous familial hypercholesterolemia (LDLR mutations) have the highest risk for CAD, followed by LDLR heterozygotes, type III patients, then type IV and possibly type V patients. Interestingly, human subjects with heterozygous LDLR mutations and either heterozygous or homozygous for apo E2-2 (and who clearly manifest type

III hyperlipidemia in addition to high LDL) do not have a higher risk than that of other persons with familial hypercholesterolemia.[226-228] This may be due to a reduction in conversion of remnants to LDL and somewhat reduced LDL levels in this combined lipid disorder. In contrast, mice with combined LDLR and apo E deficiency suffer extremely accelerated atherosclerosis and experience spontaneous myocardial infarction, which seems also to be related to endothelin signaling as a precipitating event.[229] Low levels of HDL are clearly associated with elevated atherosclerosis risk. The association of low HDL with elevated triglycerides can be associated with remarkably elevated risk.[230,231] The remainder of this section focuses on mechanisms whereby lipoproteins promote foam cell formation. Genetic determinants of lipoprotein levels are treated elsewhere in this volume.

As reviewed earlier, endothelial cells are activated by several different forms of modified lipoproteins. Macrophages share with endothelial cells many common receptors and activating mechanisms. In general, macrophages will be activated once they reach the subendothelial space through signaling with activated endothelial cells. However, they become more fully activated, expressing various scavenger receptors with increased secretion of various cytokines as well as activation of myeloperoxidase, after they encounter proinflammatory, modified lipoproteins. These changes generally occur concomitantly during foam cell formation.

Lipoprotein Retention and Modification

The level of LDL found in the interstitial fluid of the intima is approximately double the plasma concentration.[232] As demonstrated recently in human autopsy specimens, lipoprotein entry and retention in the intima precede macrophage infiltration into this space.[233] Once partially activated macrophages enter the subendothelial space, they encounter trapped lipoproteins. As shown by the classic experiments of Brown and Goldstein, unmodified LDL cannot lead to foam cell formation as the uptake of native, unmodified LDL is by way of the LDLR, which is downregulated once cellular cholesterol stores are replete.[234] β-VLDL was the only native lipoprotein that was taken up into macrophages and that led to foam cell formation without modification in those pioneering studies. These earlier observations have been amply verified.[235]

A number of LDL modifications have now been shown to also suffice in formation of foam cells. Many of these modifications are not by way of oxidation.[236] Clearly, the LDL and other lipoproteins must remain trapped in the intima long enough for modification to occur and for macrophages to take them up for atherosclerosis to progress. The importance of retention of LDL by binding to proteoglycans in the intimal extracellular matrix (particularly to those bearing chondroitin sulfate) was clearly demonstrated by the decrease in atherosclerosis seen in mice whose apo B lacked a proteoglycan binding determinant.[237] Other proteoglycan binding sequences appear to be present in apo B48 as well.[8] Lipoprotein lipase (LPL), when expressed by macrophages, can provide a nonenzymatic bridge between lipoproteins and proteoglycans and promote retention in the arterial wall and increased atherosclerosis (as shown by bone marrow transplantation studies with LPL-deficient macrophages).[238] Conversely, when LPL is playing its more commonly considered role on endothelial cells, it promotes lipoprotein delipidation of TGRL and is protective, especially when it is overexpressed in LDLR knockout mice.[239]

One of the most important mechanisms for both retention and modification of trapped lipoproteins appears to be mediated by secreted phospholipases (sPLA$_2$), particularly groups III and V sPLA$_2$.[240] Apo E knockout mice fed an atherogenic diet and overexpressing human group III sPLA$_2$ had a more than twofold increase in atherosclerosis.[240] LDL modified by group V sPLA$_2$ aggregates and binds proteoglycans more avidly and is taken up into macrophages, leading to foam cell formation. Accelerated atherosclerosis was seen in LDLR knockout mice when group V sPLA$_2$ was overexpressed; reduced atherosclerosis was seen in mice with bone marrow transplants from mice deficient in group V sPLA$_2$.[241] Group IIa sPLA$_2$ may also contribute but is less active than the group V enzyme.[242] Group V sPLA$_2$ is the major sPLA$_2$ enzyme released by activated endothelial cells.[243,244]

8   Sphingomyelinase is another enzyme released by activated endothelial cells and other lesional cells that has been implicated in LDL modification. Importantly, sphingomyelinase produces ceramide in the lipoprotein and promotes greater retention by proteoglycans and greatly promotes uptake and foam cell formation for several lipoprotein types. Deficiency of acid sphingomyelinase in LDLR knockout mice resulted in a 55% decrease in atherosclerosis.[245] Not only might sphingomyelinase be important within the subendothelial space, but a fraction of plasma LDL appears to carry substantial sphingomyelinase activity. These LDL were also electronegative. Electronegative LDL can also carry substantial PAF-AH (also referred to as Lp-PLA$_2$). Electronegative LDL, when incubated in vitro, were shown to degrade their own phospholipids in vitro, rendering them highly subject to aggregation and macrophage uptake. This activity was not blocked by antioxidants and could represent an important means of LDL modification. However, the source of the activity was apparently not secreted sphingomyelinase.[125] It would be of great interest to assess the effect of knocking out both group V sPLA$_2$ and sphingomyelinase in hyperlipidemic animals as these two enzymes appear to work synergistically to modify LDL.

Much has been written about oxidative modification of lipoproteins. Certainly, when oxidized by various methods, including incubation with cultured endothelial cells (which are generally at least partially activated in most in vitro settings), LDL and other lipoproteins are taken up avidly by macrophages with resultant macrophage activation, proliferation, and foam cell formation.[97] Some of these effects are likely to be mediated by oxidation of phospholipids[246]; oxidized cholesteryl esters[247] and changes to apo B characterized by chlorination of tyrosine and nitrations by myeloperoxidase are important as well.[101] Furthermore, oxidation of HDL clearly impairs its antiatherosclerotic activity.[101] These and many other observations make a persuasive argument that oxidation of lipoproteins contributes to atherosclerosis.[97,248] However, human clinical trials with antioxidants have been resoundingly negative (particularly the larger and more recent ones).

A potential explanation to resolve this apparent discrepancy may be, once again, redundancy. Here, the redundancy involves multiple possible lipoprotein modifications that could all lead to foam cell formation. One additional consideration may be important. The chemical oxidative footprint found predominantly on LDL from human atherosclerotic plaque clearly points to myeloperoxidase as the source of pro-oxidant acitvity.[249] This would suggest that activated macrophages and possibly (in more advanced lesions) neutrophils are the main cause of such oxidized LDL. This brings into question the primacy of oxLDL (or possibly even mmLDL) in foam cell formation because activated macrophages would have to already be present in the lesion to initiate such oxidation. Whereas oxLDL generated by myeloperoxidase would undoubtedly be atherogenic and promote further foam cell formation as well as inflammation and apoptosis, it would seem unlikely to be an initial cause of macrophage activation (and perhaps not even a necessary one). Furthermore, the LDL could be oxidized after it was taken up into the macrophage.

Unfortunately, standard mouse models of atherosclerosis are not of much help in resolving this issue as mice express much lower levels of myeloperoxidase in their macrophages than is seen in human lesions. Furthermore, knockout of mouse myeloperoxidase does not decrease atherosclerosis. However, when human myeloperoxidase is expressed in the mouse macrophages, which results in increased levels, atherosclerosis is increased.[101] These considerations support the notion that myeloperoxidase is potentially proatherogenic but redundant, as mouse atherosclerosis can progress extensively in its absence.

Carbamylation is a recently recognized form of LDL modification that may be particularly important in renal disease and smoking. A small fraction of urea can spontaneously and reversibly form highly reactive cyanate, which can then bind to lysine residues in proteins, forming homocitrulline. Many proteins in uremia have been noted to be altered, but carbamylated LDL from uremic patients or prepared in vitro activated endothelial cells primarily by way of LOX-1 on endothelial cells.[250] Furthermore, carbamylated LDL binds to macrophage SR-AI receptor and causes foam cell formation.[251] Importantly, thiocyanate, which is markedly increased in the plasma of cigarette smokers, can be converted to cyanate by myeloperoxidase, which might mediate a substantial portion of carbamylation in vivo. Protein homocitrulline levels were found to be strongly related to cardiovascular risk with an odds ratio of 7 to 8 in the top versus bottom quartile.[251]

Uptake of Modified Lipoproteins to Form Foam Cells

Traditionally, scavenger receptors have been considered the primary mechanism whereby modified lipoproteins are taken up relentlessly by macrophages, leading to foam cell formation and promotion of atherosclerosis. However, recent evidence points to non–scavenger receptor uptake as a quantitatively more important pathway. LDL treated with group V sPLA$_2$ is taken up by macropinocytosis, which is mediated by syndecan 4. This process is accelerated by macrophage activation and can lead to foam cell formation. Unlike uptake of oxLDL through scavenger receptors, macropinocytosis is blocked by inhibition of PI3K.[252] Thus, foam cells can clearly be formed independent of scavenger receptors. In a sense, then, scavenger receptors and uptake of oxidized LDL may be considered yet another example of redundant pathways.

Oxidatively modified LDL as well as some other modified LDL and β-VLDL are taken up by a variety of scavenger receptors.[253] These include the class A (AI, AII, MARCO, SRCL, SCARA5), class B (CD36, SR-B1), class C (dSR-C1, in *Drosophila* only), class D (CD68, an endosomal receptor), class E (LOX-1), class F (SREC-I, SREC-II), class G (SR-PSOX = CXCL16), class H (FEEL-1, FEEL-2, primarily bacterial binding), and class I (CD163, may help clear hemoglobin) receptors. A number of these receptors bind acetylated LDL and especially oxLDL (SR-AI/II, MARCO, SRCL, SR-B1, LOX-1, SREC-I, FEEL-1/2). CD36 also binds VLDL and TGRL remnants. However, only SR-A and CD36 have been subject to extensive studies.

Importantly, all these scavenger receptors bind alternative ligands, which may reflect their physiologic roles. Thus, scavenger receptors bind various bacteria, bacterial lipopolysaccharide, lipoteichoic acid, microbial diglycerides, apoptotic debris, amyloid, and AGEs. Macrophages from mice deficient in SR-AI/II bound AGEs much less avidly. Also, the mice were more prone to death from infection with *Listeria* and particularly with HSV-1 infections.[254] Thus, macrophage scavenger receptors play a major role in recognizing PAMPs and hence participating in innate immunity. Later it was shown that SR-A is the main scavenger receptor for group B streptococcus and *Streptococcus pyogenes* but could also bind *Neisseria meningitidis*, *Staphylococcus aureus*, and *Escherichia coli*.[253] Binding of CD36 can trigger inflammatory activation of NF-κB and MAPK cascade signaling by interactions with Src kinases and toll-like receptors or certain integrins as coreceptors with CD36.[255] Nevertheless, scavenger receptors can also play an important anti-inflammatory role in clearing apoptotic debris.

The history of scavenger receptor knockouts has been controversial. Thus, a recent knockout study of both SR-A (coded by the *MSR* gene) and CD36 showed no alteration in extent of atherosclerotic lesions in apo E knockout mice.[256] Importantly, however, these MSR/CD36/apo E triple knockout mice did have much less apoptosis and necrosis and fewer inflammatory markers in their lesions. The transcription factor STAT1 was also recently shown to be critical for apoptosis in this setting.[257] Thus, scavenger receptors may be more important for later progression of atherosclerosis, including formation of the necrotic core and plaque instability.

Cholesterol Homeostasis in Macrophages

As macrophages indulge, atherosclerotic lesions bulge.[258]

As macrophages take up modified LDL and TGRL remnants, cholesteryl ester in lysosomes is hydrolyzed by acid cholesteryl ester hydrolase (CEH). The released free cholesterol is then esterified by ACAT1 and stored in intracellular lipid droplets. These droplets are surrounded by several proteins including perilipin, ADRP (adipose differentiation-related protein), TIP47 (tail-interacting protein of 47 kDa), and S3-12.[259] Cholesteryl ester stored in these droplets can be hydrolyzed by neutral CEH. Free cholesterol released in this manner appears to be targeted for efflux from the macrophage through the ABCA1 receptor, which interacts primarily with lipid-free apo A-I or very small pre-β HDL; the AGCG1 or AGCG4 receptors, which release cholesterol to larger HDL; or the SR-B1, also to HDL. Macrophages also constitutively secrete apo E, which can act, with phospholipid, as a free cholesterol acceptor, forming discs, much like nascent HDL.[260]

Some intracellular free cholesterol is spontaneously or enzymatically (by CYP27A) oxidized to oxysterols (such as 25- or 27-hydroxycholesterol), which bind to and activate the liver X receptor (LXR). When thus bound, LXR dimerizes with the retinol X receptor (RXR) and affects transcription of genes involved with cellular cholesterol balance. Thus, activated LXR increases transcription of Niemann-Pick type C 1 and 2 proteins (which are involved in cholesterol intracellular trafficking), ABCA1, ABCG1, apo E, and PLTP (phospholipid transfer protein). Activated LXR can also be sumoylated and, as such, strongly suppresses transcription of a number of proinflammatory genes. Pharmacologic activation of LXR inhibits atherosclerosis, whereas knockout results in increased atherosclerosis.[261,262] Activation of PPARγ also upregulates LXR expression but induces CD36 expression as well.[263] Interestingly, the fatty acid–binding protein aP2 appears to bind natural ligands of PPARγ, and knockout of aP2 leads to greater stimulation of PPARγ and suppression of atherosclerosis.[264]

In considering effects of various genes on cholesterol homeostasis in macrophages, one key fact must be recognized. Excess free or unesterified cholesterol (FC) is toxic to cells.[15,265] Foam cells can accumulate large amounts of cholesteryl ester with relative impunity. However, in the process of cholesteryl ester hydrolysis in lysosomes, free cholesterol can rise to high levels. This is the location of most free cholesterol in foam cells found in advanced plaques; yet it is excess FC transported to endoplasmic reticulum that

may lead to the earliest cellular dysfunction, possibly by precipitating release of endoplasmic reticulum calcium and triggering the unfolded protein response, leading to apoptosis.[265]

Necrosis can follow more severe elevations of FC. In this situation, it may be cholesterol crystals that induce damage to intracellular organelles to cause necrosis. One response of cells to mitigate the potential toxicity of FC is stimulation of phosphatidylcholine (PC) synthesis and the formation of cellular whorls consisting of FC and PC. If the molar ratio of FC:PC remains above 0.4, necrosis ensues.[266] Limitation of PC synthesis therefore aggravates FC toxicity. In addition, incubation of cholesterol-loaded foam cells with HDL helped prevent necrosis. Deficiency in macrophage-specific ACAT1 in LDLR-deficient mice led to increased free cholesterol and plaque size,[267] possibly due to an excessive increase in FC:PC.[266] In contrast, overexpression of neutral CEH resulted in increased cholesterol efflux from macrophages and decreased atherosclerosis.[268] A key difference appeared to be the lack of upregulated efflux of free cholesterol in the case of ACAT1 deficiency, resulting in toxic accumulation of free cholesterol. These observations suggest different intracellular trafficking of FC and release after inhibition of ACAT1 compared with CEH.

The Niemann-Pick C1 (NPC1) protein appears to act as a shuttle for FC between cell organelles. Apo E–deficient mice with NPC1 knockout have worse atherosclerosis and, interestingly, severe, spontaneous thrombosis. The cause of the prothrombotic state was not clear.[269]

Other genetic models with impaired cholesterol unloading of foam cells show accelerated atherosclerosis. One such model is clearly apo A-I deficiency (with protection shown by overexpression of apo A-I).[270,271] Severe, fulminant atherosclerosis and coronary lesions with appearance similar to human lesions develop in apo E–deficient mice lacking the SR-B1 receptor.[272] Macrophage-specific knockout of SR-B1 had a much lesser effect on atherosclerosis, suggesting overall reverse cholesterol transport (or uptake of HDL-cholesterol into the liver through SR-B1) as perhaps more important than macrophage-specific transport through SR-B1.[273] Other studies also question the importance of macrophage SR-B1 in reverse cholesterol transport, whereas ABCA1 and ABCG1 do facilitate such transport from cholesterol-filled macrophages (Table 8-4).[274]

ABCA1 (the gene found deficient in Tangier disease) facilitates free cholesterol efflux to lipid-poor apo A-I discs; the more recently identified ABCG1 can promote efflux to larger, spherical HDL_2 and HDL_3 particles. In addition, ABCG1 promotes efflux of oxysterols. Both receptors appear to be important for macrophage cholesterol efflux and reverse cholesterol transport.[270,271] Strangely, whole-body knockout of ABCA1 in either apo E– or LDLR-deficient mice did not affect atherosclerosis, but serum cholesterol levels were much lower in these mice. On the other hand, macrophage-specific knockout of ABCA1 in apo E–deficient mice did not affect lipoprotein levels but did result in a modest increase in atherosclerosis.[275] In contrast, either whole-body or macrophage-specific knockout of ABCG1 did not consistently increase atherosclerosis (some studies even showed a decrease), possibly because of upregulation through LXR of both ABCA1 and apo E–mediated adequate efflux. LXR may also have been stimulated by increased exposure to oxysterols in these ABCG1 knockout mice. However, macrophage-specific knockout of both ABCG1 and ABCA1 resulted in much more atherosclerosis than either ABCA1 or AGCG1 deficiency alone did.[276] These results strongly suggest that both ABCA1 and ABCG1 are important for cholesterol efflux from macrophages in vivo but again demonstrate redundant pathways.

Studies generally support the concept that reverse cholesterol transport is atheroprotective. An assay to document

TABLE 8–4	Genes Related to Promotion of Atherosclerosis*	
Gene	**Effect**	**Gene Function**
apo B	↓↓	Proteoglycan binding–defective apo B tested
LPL (BMT)	↓	Macrophage LPL can bind lipoproteins
LRP1	↑	LRP1 internalization defective knock-in; triglyceride-rich remnant receptor
ASM	↓↓	Acid sphingomyelinase cleaves sphingomyelin to ceramide
sPLA₂, group III	↑↑	Produces lysophosphatidyl choline in LDL
sPLA₂ ,group V	↓	Produces lysophosphatidyl choline in LDL; BMT study
EP4	↓↓	Macrophage PGE₂ receptor
5-LO (BMT)	↓	Global heterozygote had much lower levels of atherosclerosis
iNOS (BMT)	↓	Produced both excess NO and superoxide in lesions
MSR	NS to ↓↓	Macrophage scavenger receptor; variable subsequent studies
CD36	NS to ↓	A class B scavenger receptor
Grb2 (BMT)	↓	Adapter protein coupling receptor signals to the MAPK pathway
NF-κB, p50 (BMT)	↓	More macrophages in lesions but absence of foam cells
JNK1	NS	Strongly proinflammatory MAPK
JNK2	↓↓	Important in macrophages; less foam cell formation in knockout
LXRαβ (BMT)	↑↑	Multiple effects on macrophage cholesterol homeostasis
PPARγ (BMT)	↑	PPARγ/RXR dimer upregulates LXR as well as CD36 transcription
aP2 (BMT)	↓	Fatty acid–binding protein found in macrophages and adipocytes
ADFP (BMT)	↓	Promotes lipid storage
ACAT1 (BMT)	↑↑	Catalyzes cholesterol esterification in macrophages
CEH (TG)	↓↓	Macrophage-specific cholesteryl ester hydrolase transgenic
NPC1	↑↑	Intracellular FC trafficking
SR-B1	↑↑	An HDL receptor; whole-body knockout showed severe disease
ABCA1 (BMT)	↑	Cellular cholesterol exporter
ABCG1 (BMT)	NS to ↑↑	Increased atherosclerosis when combined with ABCA1 knockout

*Note: many of these studies were performed as bone marrow transplantation (BMT) of the knockout to show that it affected macrophage function specifically.
NS, not significant; TG, transgenic with overexpression.

reverse cholesterol transport in vivo was developed in which macrophages loaded with radiolabeled cholesterol are injected intraperitoneally into mice. Appearance of the labeled cholesterol in the blood and feces is tracked.[271,277] Several examples of counterintuitive findings are consistent with the general concept of reverse cholesterol transport as measured by this in vivo assay. Perhaps most clearly illustrated is the seemingly paradoxical finding of increased HDL seen with whole-body or hepatic SR-B1 deficiency. Reverse cholesterol transport through HDL to the liver is clearly impaired in this model. Conversely, overexpression of hepatic SR-B1 lowers HDL but increases reverse cholesterol transport as well as inhibits atherosclerosis.[277]

Surprising findings regarding lecithin-cholesterol acyltransferase (LCAT) knockout or overexpression models may also be reconciled by the same technique. Thus, LCAT overexpression may actually increase atherosclerosis and seems to impair whole-body reverse cholesterol transport by decreasing availability of very small, lipid-poor HDL, which are the most active cholesterol acceptors. Conversely, LCAT knockout has been reported to decrease atherosclerosis in some mouse models. Furthermore, in LCAT-overexpressing mice, transgenic expression of cholesteryl ester transport protein appears to facilitate reverse cholesterol transport and to decrease atherosclerosis.[271]

PROGRESSION OF ATHEROSCLEROSIS AND PRECIPITATION OF EVENTS

As noted in the introduction, this phase of atherogenesis has to do with growth of complicated plaques, thrombosis, plaque instability, and precipitation of acute events. Animal models of these more advanced stages of atherosclerosis are relatively few and may be less comparable to the human condition. Indeed, only a few genetic models of atherosclerosis clearly progress to atherothrombotic complications such as myocardial infarction. For example, one model required placing apo E–deficient mice on a high-fat diet after placement of a cast around the carotid artery, giving intraperitoneal injections of lipopolysaccharide to cause immune activation, and producing a hyperdynamic circulation and stress with noise and foot shocks. More than 60% of such animals had carotid plaque ruptures, but thrombosis was still rare because of the vigorous fibrinolytic activity of mice.[278,279] In another model, stable transgenic overexpression of human PAI-1 resulted in frequent coronary artery thrombi and myocardial infarction in normolipidemic mice, but this occurred without atherosclerosis.[280] The relevance of this model to the human situation is clearly questionable.

Despite difficulties, advances in this area continue to be made rapidly through direct study of human plaque and pathophysiologic studies. Of major importance was recognition of the vulnerable plaque, whose thin fibrous cap, decreased collagen content, and greater inflammatory activity including MMP expression lead to rupture or fissuring in the fibrous cap, exposure of the highly thrombogenic plaque substance to blood, and precipitation of acute thrombotic events.[281-283] Other prominent features of vulnerable plaques include a high free cholesterol content, markers of red blood cell infiltration, and increased vasa vasorum.[283-285]

Recently, hypoxia within advanced human atherosclerotic plaques, with release of hypoxia-inducible factors and plaque penetration with vasa vasorum, has been related to enlargement of lesions.[286,287] Red cells appear to be major contributors of free cholesterol in advanced plaques as well as a source of strongly proinflammatory and pro-oxidant material. Degree of instability has been correlated with degree of neovascularization of plaques. Whereas the molecular biology of angiogenesis may prove to be critical to progression of advanced human lesions, this topic is beyond the scope of this chapter.

The new observation that abrupt crystallization of cholesterol probably contributes majorly to acute events is highly compelling and may prove to be the single most frequent

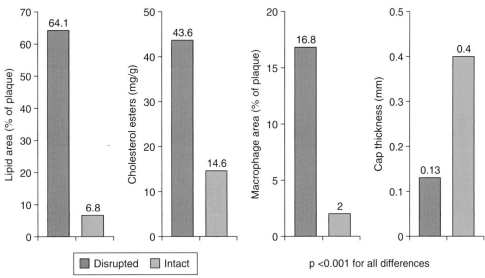

FIGURE 8-10 Composition and morphology versus stability in 668 disrupted or intact aortic plaques from 30 men with CAD. Lipid concentration correlated positively with macrophage accumulation and negatively with minimum cap thickness. *(Modified from Felton CV, Crook D, Davies MJ, Oliver MF: Relation of plaque lipid composition and morphology to the stability of human aortic plaques.* Arterioscler Thromb Vasc Biol *17:1337, 1997.)*

cause of event precipitation.[17] Prior tissue preparation techniques using ethanol dissolved the crystals and thus prevented their proper viewing. Thus, when air dried, nearly all lesions associated with acute coronary events were seen to have penetrating cholesterol crystals. There is a distinct volume expansion brought about by cholesterol crystallization, which may provide the underlying force to precipitate fissures and ruptures of the fibrous cap as well.[288,289]

With regard to vulnerable plaques, one major paradigm should be kept in mind. Among the strongest correlates of instability (if not the strongest predictor) is lipid content. This was shown strikingly in autopsy studies by Michael Davies' group (Fig. 8-10).[290] All measures of plaque vulnerability including macrophage content, degree of leukocyte activation, indices of apoptosis, MMP activity, and collagen content are improved rapidly by marked reduction of plasma lipid levels in animal models, whether by diet manipulation[7,10,291,292] or with statins.[293-295] Remarkably, rapid regression of lesions could also be achieved by infusion of cholesterol acceptors such as injected phosphatidylcholine or phospholipid micelles, which apparently mobilized cholesterol from plaques.[14]

More recently, extensive egress of foam cells was shown to occur within days of transplanting atherosclerotic vessels from genetically hyperlipidemic mice into wild-type mice.[14,296] This egress was dependent on signaling in foam cells through the CCR7 chemokine receptor and could be blocked by antibodies against the natural ligands to CCR7, namely, CCL19 and CCL21. Furthermore, expression of CCR7 was increased by LXR agonists. The hyperlipidemic environment, in some way, led to retention of foam cells in the plaque with progression through apoptosis and necrosis followed by formation of the necrotic core. If macrophages maintain their ability to egress freely from lesions, their entry and egress may enhance regression of plaque.[14] Interestingly in this regard, activation of the MAPK p38 can promote cell survival in macrophages (much as ERK1/2 does in endothelial cells through activation of Akt); activation of JNK promotes apoptosis, especially when endoplasmic reticulum stress is present. This prosurvival effect of p38 may depend on free cholesterol content and other signals (resulting in a net apoptotic signaling from p38 in some contexts).

Nevertheless, knockout of macrophage p38 nonsignificantly increased lesion area and promoted increased apoptosis, plaque necrosis, decreased collagen deposition, and thinning of the fibrous cap in apo E knockout animals.[297] These findings are reminiscent of findings, noted previously, of more advanced later complications with greater macrophage apoptosis induced by SR-A and STAT1 in already stressed macrophages.

Smooth muscle cells are important components of plaques, particularly advanced plaques. Whereas smooth muscle cells can be converted to foam cells, their presence in plaque is generally considered to promote stability, as they form the fibrous cap and are the source of most collagen and elastin in the plaque. In general, they migrate from the media into the intima like monocytes or other leukocytes in response to similar signaling from cytokines. PDGF (which exists in isoforms AA, BB, and AB) acting on the PDGF receptor is an additional important signaling pathway.

Both plasmin and MMP-9 are important in facilitating smooth muscle cell movement through the extracellular matrix. Urokinase-type plasminogen activator (u-PA) activates plasmin release by smooth muscle cells, which activates MMPs, particularly MMP-9. Interestingly, both the PDGF receptor and a u-PA receptor interact with surface lipoprotein receptors (LRP-1, LRP-1B, LR11) that regulate smooth muscle cell migration.[298] Smooth muscle cell–specific knockout of LRP-1 greatly increased atherosclerosis in LDLR knockout mice by removing a strong suppressive effect of this receptor on the PDGF receptor (which action is independent of any lipoprotein binding).[299] In contrast, LR11 appears to facilitate u-PA signaling and smooth muscle cell migration and is downregulated by statins.[298] These findings suggest that at least to some degree, smooth muscle cells can contribute to the growth of plaques.

Despite these findings, smooth muscle cells are generally considered to stabilize human lesions. They produce collagen in response to PDGF and TGF-β, which would be expected to protect against rupture. TGF-β is anti-inflammatory as well as profibrotic. Interruption of TGF-β signaling resulted in unstable plaques in apo E–deficient mice.[300,301] Suppression of smooth muscle cell production of collagen by IFN-γ from T cells is generally considered destabilizing.[12] Localized overexpression of p53 in carotid plaques of apo E–deficient mice led to an increase in smooth muscle cell apoptosis in the fibrous caps, thinning of the cap, and spontaneous rupture on hemodynamic challenge with phenylephrine.[302] In addition, activated macrophages, which are associated with unstable plaques, can produce FasL, which binds to Fas (the so-called death receptor) on smooth muscle cells, promoting smooth muscle cell apoptosis.[303] This may help explain plaque instability associated with increased macrophage numbers.

If the role of smooth muscle cells in advanced plaques seems somewhat puzzling, the potential impact of proteolytic enzymes on extracellular matrix and atherosclerosis is even less predictable. All migrating cells secrete various proteolytic enzymes to enable movement through the extracellular matrix. Such migration includes not only translocation of inflammatory cells into the intima but their egress as well. Thus, movement of many cells, even smooth muscle cells, in or out of plaque might leave it weakened.

Virtually all MMPs and cathepsins are expressed in advanced human plaques.[12] Furthermore, extracellular matrix remodeling, compensatory arterial enlargement, plaque angiogenesis, and plaque disruption will all be affected by proteolytic MMPs, tissue inhibitor of MMP (TIMP), and the highly active cathepsins. Formation of penetrating vasa vasorum seems to be stimulated by MMP-9.[304] Some effects of these various enzymes on atherosclerosis are briefly reviewed in Table 8-5. However, the interpretation of findings in animal models of advanced atherosclerosis remains controversial.[279,305]

An additional feature of smooth muscle cell behavior in advanced plaques is surprising. Intravascular ultrasound investigation of culprit plaques causing acute coronary syndromes in humans shows that plaque rupture typically occurs just proximal to (upstream of) the point of maximum stenosis. This is the area of most rapid flow.[306] This is true even though the area of slow flow just *downstream* of the stenosis is where the endothelium is activated, where monocytes penetrate, and where foam cells accumulate with resultant growth of the plaque. It appears that whereas high shear stress promotes endothelial integrity and higher NO production in this upstream area, the higher shear may promote plasmin production as well. Furthermore, underlying smooth muscle cell proliferation and collagen synthesis may be suppressed by the increased NO release. In addition, exposure of activated macrophages to NO may actually stimulate MMP release and promote smooth muscle cell apoptosis. Such changes may be involved in normal compensatory vessel enlargement in areas of rapid flow, particularly during embryogenesis; but in the context of an advanced atherosclerotic plaque, they lead to paradoxical weakening of the fibrous plaque just under the area of endothelium exposed to highest flow rates.[307,308]

Clotting and Atherosclerosis

Whereas thrombosis clearly plays a role in progression of advanced, complex plaques, resulting in demonstrable saltatory progression of obstructive lesions,[309,310] genetic predisposition to venous thrombosis does not necessarily coincide with a predilection to atherosclerosis. Furthermore, only a few animal models develop sufficiently advanced disease for hypotheses about genes related to thrombosis to be properly tested, and there are many technical difficulties in the interpretation of these models.[279] In arterial thrombosis, clots are rich in platelets and poor in fibrin; in venous thrombi, platelets are sparse, fibrin predominates, and the clots are friable and prone to large emboli. Well-recognized risk factors for the two conditions are also different.

In human studies, genetic factors clearly increasing risk of venous thromboembolism do not necessarily increase risk for arterial thrombosis, with only slightly increased but significant odds ratios for myocardial infarction associated with factor V Leiden and prothrombin 20210A in a very large meta-analysis.[311] Mothers with sons having hemophilia (essentially all heterozygotes) had measurably increased risk for bleeding episodes but only an estimated 36% decreased risk of ischemic heart disease death.[312] Nevertheless, deficiency of von Willebrand factor (vWF) and other forms of hemophilia appear to be less protective than was once thought.[313]

A full consideration of the molecular biology of thrombosis is beyond the scope of this chapter. However, the classic models of so-called intrinsic and extrinsic pathways were based on in vitro assays that have little to do with in vivo hemostasis. Thus, complete deficiency of factor XII (Hageman factor, the initiating factor of the so-called intrinsic pathway through contact with glass) does not result in any bleeding

TABLE 8–5	Genes Related to Progression of Advanced Atherosclerosis, Thrombosis, and Precipitation of Acute Events	
Gene	Effect	Gene Function
IKK2 (BMT)	↑	IKK2 activates NF-κB activation
p38 (Cre-lox)*	NS	A MAPK; antiapoptotic in macrophages
LRP-1	↑↑	Cre-lox knockout in smooth muscle cells only
MMP-1 (TG)	↓32%	Macrophage-specific TG; mice do not have MMP-1
MMP-3	↑↑	Also known as stromelysin-1
MMP-7	NS	A matrix metalloproteinase
MMP-9	↑↑	Also known as gelatinase B
MMP-12	↓↓	MMP-12 may be critical for macrophage migration
TIMP-1	NS	Tissue inhibitor of metalloproteinases
CatK	↓	Cathepsin K, an elastase
CatS	↓	One of the most potent elastases known
Cystatin C	NS	An endogenous inhibitor of cathepsins
IP	↑	PGI$_2$ receptor; vasodilating, inhibits platelet activation
TP	↓↓	TXA$_2$ receptor; vasoconstrictor, activates platelets
vWF	↓	Facilitates both platelet and macrophage adhesion
TFPI	↑	Blocks active tissue factor
Factor V	↑	FV Leiden mutation tested
Factor VIII	↓	A coagulation factor
TM	↑	Thrombomodulin activates protein C
Fibrinogen	NS to ↓↓↓	Major effect only in human Lp(a) TG mice
Plasminogen	↑↑	Precursor to plasmin
HCII	↑	Heparin cofactor II is an endogenous thrombin inhibitor
PAI-1	NS	A tissue plasminogen activator inhibitor

*The Cre-lox protocol in this study allowed knockout in macrophages only.
BMT, bone marrow transplantation; NS, not significant; TG, transgenic with overexpression.

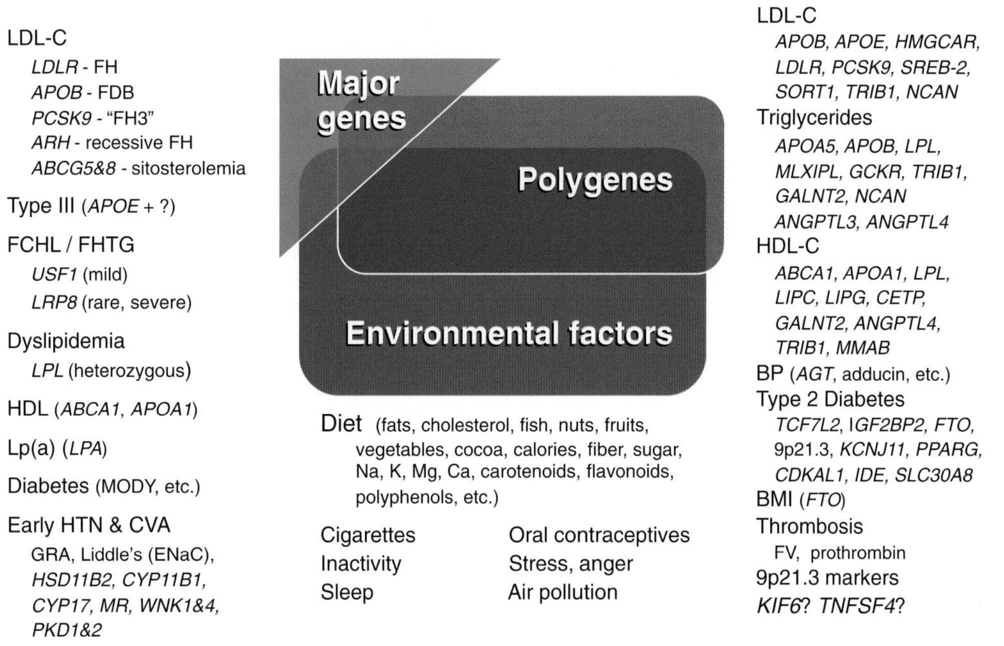

LDL-C
  LDLR - FH
  APOB - FDB
  PCSK9 - "FH3"
  ARH - recessive FH
  ABCG5&8 - sitosterolemia

Type III (*APOE* + ?)

FCHL / FHTG
  USF1 (mild)
  LRP8 (rare, severe)

Dyslipidemia
  LPL (heterozygous)

HDL (*ABCA1, APOA1*)

Lp(a) (*LPA*)

Diabetes (MODY, etc.)

Early HTN & CVA
  GRA, Liddle's (*ENaC*),
  *HSD11B2, CYP11B1,
  CYP17, MR, WNK1&4,
  PKD1&2*

Major genes

Polygenes

Environmental factors

Diet (fats, cholesterol, fish, nuts, fruits,
  vegetables, cocoa, calories, fiber, sugar,
  Na, K, Mg, Ca, carotenoids, flavonoids,
  polyphenols, etc.)

Cigarettes   Oral contraceptives
Inactivity   Stress, anger
Sleep   Air pollution

LDL-C
  *APOB, APOE, HMGCAR,
  LDLR, PCSK9, SREB-2,
  SORT1, TRIB1, NCAN*
Triglycerides
  *APOA5, APOB, LPL,
  MLXIPL, GCKR, TRIB1,
  GALNT2, NCAN
  ANGPTL3, ANGPTL4*
HDL-C
  *ABCA1, APOA1, LPL,
  LIPC, LIPG, CETP,
  GALNT2, ANGPTL4,
  TRIB1, MMAB*
BP (*AGT*, adducin, etc.)
Type 2 Diabetes
  *TCF7L2, IGF2BP2, FTO,
  9p21.3, KCNJ11, PPARG,
  CDKAL1, IDE, SLC30A8*
BMI (*FTO*)
Thrombosis
  FV, prothrombin
  9p21.3 markers
  KIF6? TNFSF4?

FIGURE 8-11 A summary of human genetic and environmental risk factors for atherosclerosis. Major genes linked to atherosclerosis are listed on the left; polygenes (genes have small, presumably cumulative effects) are listed on the right. Environmental factors are listed in the center.

tendency, nor does deficiency of high-molecular-weight kininogen or prekallikrein (cofactors with factor XII). If anything, persons deficient in factor XII have a tendency toward thrombosis, possibly through a role in activating fibrinolysis.[314] Also, these cascades fail to depict the critical participation of platelets and tissue factor–bearing cells in thrombosis. Tissue factor is expressed not just on activated macrophages but also on synthetic smooth muscle cells in atherosclerotic plaque.[315] Rather than having two possible cascades, all clotting in vivo proceeds essentially by a single, highly regulated pathway through exposure to tissue factor–bearing cells.[316,317]

Whereas activation of thrombin and subsequent thrombosis in the face of plaque rupture can obviously be expected to have adverse consequences in acute coronary syndrome, the effect of the various elements of the clotting cascade on atherogenesis at earlier or even later stages is not straightforward or predictable (see Table 8-5). Thrombin, although clearly the central player in thrombogenesis, also activates PAR1, 2, and 4 (protease-activated receptors 1, 2, and 4) and can thereby have diverse additional effects. For platelets, thrombin signaling through PAR1 and 4 is activating. In contrast, thrombin can induce PAR1-mediated forearm dilation in humans through stimulated release of NO, PGI₂, and endothelium-derived hyperpolarizing factor; yet in the context of more prolonged exposure, at least in vitro, thrombin suppresses eNOS and promotes endothelin release, stimulates fusion of Weibel-Palade bodies with the plasma membrane, promotes expression of adhesion molecules, and generally activates endothelial cells. Thrombin has multiple additional proinflammatory effects and stimulates activation of NADPH oxidase and ROS production. Finally, active thrombin may directly promote smooth muscle cell migration and proliferation directly through PAR1 on smooth muscle cells or by increasing PDGF release from endothelial cells.[318]

Interventions on thrombin have yielded contradictory findings in experimental settings. A direct thrombin inhibitor, melagatran, decreased lesion size and improved lesion stability with thicker fibrous caps, smaller necrotic cores, and decreased MMP-9 in apo E–deficient mice.[319] However,

homozygous expression of factor V Leiden or knockout of thrombomodulin, both models of impaired protein C activity and hence increased thrombin effect, led to somewhat larger but much more stable lesions in apo E knockout mice.[320] Other seemingly conflicting results regarding thrombosis have been reported. Thus, plasminogen deficiency markedly increased atherosclerosis in apo E–deficient mice[321] but decreased atherosclerosis substantially in a model of u-PA overexpression by macrophages. The plasminogen was thought to activate u-PA and thereby to promote macrophage activation.[322]

PARALLELS WITH HUMAN GENETICS

Our current understanding of the genetics of human atherosclerosis bears little resemblance to the vast and insightful literature reviewed here. Very few CAD associations with candidate gene variants have been consistently replicated.[323-325] Some candidate gene variants seem to persist with very modest associated odds ratios for CAD in large meta-analyses, but probably none can currently be considered to be clinically useful.[326-328] Other variants were found less and less predictive as better data became available.[329-337] Many of these disappointing false starts were likely due to false-positive early findings or "winner's curse." However, some of the apparent lack of measurable effects on atherosclerosis may be due, in part, to the redundancy of so many pathways affecting atherogenesis.

Effects of most of the genes that have consistently been associated with human atherosclerosis risk or risk factors are summarized in Figure 8-11. In general, recognizable major genes affect relatively few individuals but have large effects on atherosclerosis risk. Most of the recognized major genes listed in Figure 8-11 affect lipoprotein metabolism. Polygenes are probably common, but their effects have been more difficult to define or to confirm. Most of those listed on the right side of Figure 8-11 have been reported in relatively recent genome-wide association studies. Major genes, polygenes, and environmental factors all interact with each other to ultimately determine risk. On the basis of international comparisons of CAD rates, the environmental factors clearly outweigh genetic factors in determining overall population risks.

After review of the literature and the additional insights presented in Figure 8-11, it is sobering to realize that familial hypercholesterolemia provides the only example of a genetic cause of premature CAD for which a systematic, population-based approach aimed at proband identification and family screening is clearly warranted at this time. Benefits of such efforts were shown by our group, which originated the MEDPED program (Make Early Diagnoses to Prevent Early Death),[338] but the real potential for this program has been exemplified by the outstanding results of the Dutch MEDPED program.[339]

In contrast to the relatively poor showing for candidate genes, large genome-wide association studies with multiple, built-in replications have begun to provide genetic variants that are consistently associated with CAD risk. However, all these associations are very modest. The most consistently identified of these are the variants at 9p21.3 (such as rs1075724 with strong linkage disequilibrium between all the risk-associated markers at this locus). The odds ratio for CAD is approximately 1.25 for heterozygote carriers and 1.5 for homozygotes.[340] Several other less well replicated loci from genome-wide association studies include 1p13, *MIA3*, *CXCL12*, 21q22, *PHACTR1*, *WDR12*,[341] *SH2B3*,[342] and *MRAS*.[343] Still other variants are supported by associations in several populations and have not yet been clearly refuted, although lack of replication in newer genome-wide association studies is concerning. These include *KIF6* (the W719R variant)[344,345] and possibly *TNFSF4*.[325,330,332]

Whereas much has been said about the potential utility of genetic risk scores, a careful family history together with standard risk factors (together with serum lipoprotein(a) and C-reactive protein) currently remains considerably more predictive than available genetic scores.[341,346-349] The potential utility of genetic tests to guide personalized medicine in preventing or treating atherosclerosis has similarly yet to be seen. There is much hope that these limitations may be overcome in the near future. On the other hand, it may be that the strongest associations have already been found (at least for common variants). Indeed, the vast complexity of potential genetic and environmental factors and their interactions, the potential myriad contributions of rare variants, and these all working in the context of extensive redundancy of atherosclerosis-related pathways may preclude our ever being able to make greatly improved prediction of individual disease. Certainly, we must recognize currently our extremely limited ability to predict the presence of atherosclerotic disease in an individual patient before its clinical manifestation.

Ultimately, sufficiently sensitive and cost-effective noninvasive screening for atherosclerosis may obviate the need for individual risk prediction by risk factors other than for general classification into groups needing earlier or later screening. One can envision a paradigm in which vigorous medical interventions (particularly lipid-lowering medications) would be directed empirically to those with disease found by noninvasive screening and generally withheld from those with no evidence of disease. If this proves to be the most effective management model, insights gained from genetic studies would be more important as a means to clarify pathophysiology generally, to stimulate the development of innovative new therapies, and potentially even to help guide intervention. Such an outcome would arguably still justify our efforts to identify genetic associations in human populations, even if they did not ultimately prove useful for determination of individual risk.

CONCLUSION

Numerous overlapping and redundant pathways are involved in initiation, promotion, and progression of atherosclerotic plaques and precipitation of clinical events. Much recent progress has been made regarding how endothelial cells transduce changes in blood flow into intracellular signals that control the location of sites predisposed to plaque development. However, without the effect of standard risk factors, particularly at least some permissive level of dyslipidemia, atherosclerotic plaques generally do not develop, even at such predisposed sites. Recognition of multiple lipoprotein modifications, including nonoxidative, that can result in both endothelial activation and foam cell formation may illustrate the futility of using an intervention (e.g., antioxidants) that is too narrowly focused on just one aspect of atherogenesis.

The difficulty in identifying new genes associated with human atherosclerosis (particularly loci unrelated to standard risk factors) may be due, in part, to the redundancy of the pathways involved. Nevertheless, greater understanding of atherogenesis and continued progress in treatment of risk factors will undoubtedly lead to improved therapies that will further reduce clinical atherosclerotic disease.

REFERENCES

1. Gomperts BD, Kramer IM, Tatham PER: *Signal transduction*, ed 2, Burlington, Mass, 2009, Academic Press.
2. Hopkins PN, Williams RR: A survey of 246 suggested coronary risk factors. *Atherosclerosis* 40:1, 1981.
3. Subbanagounder G, Leitinger N, Schwenke DC, et al: Determinants of bioactivity of oxidized phospholipids. Specific oxidized fatty acyl groups at the sn-2 position. *Arterioscler Thromb Vasc Biol* 20:2248, 2000.
4. Suriyaphol P, Fenske D, Zahringer U, et al: Enzymatically modified nonoxidized low-density lipoprotein induces interleukin-8 in human endothelial cells: role of free fatty acids. *Circulation* 106:2581, 2002.
5. Doi H, Kugiyama K, Oka H, et al: Remnant lipoproteins induce proatherothrombogenic molecules in endothelial cells through a redox-sensitive mechanism. *Circulation* 102:670, 2000.
6. Leung WH, Lau CP, Wong CK: Beneficial effect of cholesterol-lowering therapy on coronary endothelium-dependent relaxation in hypercholesterolaemic patients. *Lancet* 341:1496, 1993.
7. Aikawa M, Sugiyama S, Hill CC, et al: Lipid lowering reduces oxidative stress and endothelial cell activation in rabbit atheroma. *Circulation* 106:1390, 2002.
8. Tabas I, Williams KJ, Boren J: Subendothelial lipoprotein retention as the initiating process in atherosclerosis: update and therapeutic implications. *Circulation* 116:1832, 2007.
9. Nofer J-R, Tepel M, Kehrel B, et al: Low-density lipoproteins inhibit the Na⁺/H⁺ antiport in human platelets. A novel mechanism enhancing platelet activity in hypercholesterolemia. *Circulation* 95:1370, 1997.
10. Kockx MM, De Meyer GR, Buyssens N, et al: Cell composition, replication, and apoptosis in atherosclerotic plaques after 6 months of cholesterol withdrawal. *Circ Res* 83:378, 1998.
11. Crisby M, Nordin-Fredriksson G, Shah PK, et al: Pravastatin treatment increases collagen content and decreases lipid content, inflammation, metalloproteinases, and cell death in human carotid plaques: implications for plaque stabilization. *Circulation* 103:926, 2001.
12. Libby P: Molecular and cellular mechanisms of the thrombotic complications of atherosclerosis. *J Lipid Res* 50:S352, 2009.
13. Wagner DD, Frenette PS: The vessel wall and its interactions. *Blood* 111:5271, 2008.
14. Williams KJ, Feig JE, Fisher EA: Rapid regression of atherosclerosis: insights from the clinical and experimental literature. *Nat Clin Pract Cardiovasc Med* 5:91, 2008.
15. Small DM: George Lyman Duff memorial lecture. Progression and regression of atherosclerotic lesions. Insights from lipid physical biochemistry. *Arteriosclerosis* 8:103, 1988.
16. Tabas I: Consequences of cellular cholesterol accumulation: basic concepts and physiological implications. *J Clin Invest* 110:905, 2002.
17. Abela GS, Aziz K, Vedre A, et al: Effect of cholesterol crystals on plaques and intima in arteries of patients with acute coronary and cerebrovascular syndromes. *Am J Cardiol* 103:959, 2009.
18. Cheng C, Tempel D, van Haperen R, et al: Atherosclerotic lesion size and vulnerability are determined by patterns of fluid shear stress. *Circulation* 113:2744, 2006.
19. Kolodgie FD, Burke AP, Nakazawa G, et al: Free cholesterol in atherosclerotic plaques: where does it come from? *Curr Opin Lipidol* 18:500, 2007.
20. Chatzizisis YS, Coskun AU, Jonas M, et al: Role of endothelial shear stress in the natural history of coronary atherosclerosis and vascular remodeling: molecular, cellular, and vascular behavior. *J Am Coll Cardiol* 49:2379, 2007.
21. Hahn C, Schwartz MA: Mechanotransduction in vascular physiology and atherogenesis. *Nat Rev Mol Cell Biol* 10:53, 2009.
22. Olgac U, Poulikakos D, Saur SC, et al: Patient-specific three-dimensional simulation of LDL accumulation in a human left coronary artery in its healthy and atherosclerotic states. *Am J Physiol Heart Circ Physiol* 296:H1969, 2009.

23. Stone PH, Coskun AU, Kinlay S, et al: Effect of endothelial shear stress on the progression of coronary artery disease, vascular remodeling, and in-stent restenosis in humans: in vivo 6-month follow-up study. *Circulation* 108:438, 2003.

24. Wentzel JJ, Corti R, Fayad ZA, et al: Does shear stress modulate both plaque progression and regression in the thoracic aorta? Human study using serial magnetic resonance imaging. *J Am Coll Cardiol* 45:846, 2005.

25. Chatzizisis YS, Jonas M, Coskun AU, et al: Prediction of the localization of high-risk coronary atherosclerotic plaques on the basis of low endothelial shear stress: an intravascular ultrasound and histopathology natural history study. *Circulation* 117:993, 2008.

26. Weinberg PD, Ross Ethier C: Twenty-fold difference in hemodynamic wall shear stress between murine and human aortas. *J Biomech* 40:1594, 2007.

27. Dancu MB, Tarbell JM: Coronary endothelium expresses a pathologic gene pattern compared to aortic endothelium: correlation of asynchronous hemodynamics and pathology in vivo. *Atherosclerosis* 192:9, 2007.

28. Berkson DM, Stamler J, Lindberg HA, et al: Heart rate: an important risk factor for coronary mortality. Ten-year experience of the Peoples Gas Co. Epidemiologic Study (1958-68). In Jones RJ, editor: *Atherosclerosis: Proceedings of the 2nd International Symposium on Atherosclerosis*, New York, 1970, Springer-Verlag, pp 382-389.

29. Chiu JJ, Usami S, Chien S: Vascular endothelial responses to altered shear stress: pathologic implications for atherosclerosis. *Ann Med* 41:19, 2009.

30. Davies PF: Hemodynamic shear stress and the endothelium in cardiovascular pathophysiology. *Nat Clin Pract Cardiovasc Med* 6:16, 2009.

31. Dai G, Kaazempur-Mofrad MR, Natarajan S, et al: Distinct endothelial phenotypes evoked by arterial waveforms derived from atherosclerosis-susceptible and -resistant regions of human vasculature. *Proc Natl Acad Sci U S A* 101:14871, 2004.

32. Mohan S, Mohan N, Sprague EA: Differential activation of NF-κB in human aortic endothelial cells conditioned to specific flow environments. *Am J Physiol Cell Physiol* 273:C572, 1997.

33. Hu YL, Chien S: Effects of shear stress on protein kinase C distribution in endothelial cells. *J Histochem Cytochem* 45:237, 1997.

34. Weinbaum S, Zhang X, Han Y, et al: Mechanotransduction and flow across the endothelial glycocalyx. *Proc Natl Acad Sci U S A* 100:7988, 2003.

35. Thi MM, Tarbell JM, Weinbaum S, Spray DC: The role of the glycocalyx in reorganization of the actin cytoskeleton under fluid shear stress: a "bumper-car" model. *Proc Natl Acad Sci U S A* 101:16483, 2004.

36. Chappell D, Jacob M, Rehm M, et al: Heparinase selectively sheds heparan sulphate from the endothelial glycocalyx. *Biol Chem* 389:79, 2008.

37. Pahakis MY, Kosky JR, Dull RO, Tarbell JM: The role of endothelial glycocalyx components in mechanotransduction of fluid shear stress. *Biochem Biophys Res Commun* 355:228, 2007.

38. White CR, Frangos JA: The shear stress of it all: the cell membrane and mechanochemical transduction. *Philos Trans R Soc Lond B Biol Sci* 362:1459, 2007.

39. Tarbell JM, Pahakis MY: Mechanotransduction and the glycocalyx. *J Intern Med* 259:339, 2006.

40. Harja E, Chang JS, Lu Y, et al: Mice deficient in PKCβ and apolipoprotein E display decreased atherosclerosis. *FASEB J* 23:1081, 2009.

41. Chang K, Weiss D, Suo J, et al: Bone morphogenic protein antagonists are coexpressed with bone morphogenic protein 4 in endothelial cells exposed to unstable flow in vitro in mouse aortas and in human coronary arteries: role of bone morphogenic protein antagonists in inflammation and atherosclerosis. *Circulation* 116:1258, 2007.

42. Liu Y, Sweet DT, Irani-Tehrani M, et al: Shc coordinates signals from intercellular junctions and integrins to regulate flow-induced inflammation. *J Cell Biol* 182:185, 2008.

43. Balligand JL, Feron O, Dessy C: eNOS activation by physical forces: from short-term regulation of contraction to chronic remodeling of cardiovascular tissues. *Physiol Rev* 89:481, 2009.

44. Tzima E: Role of small GTPases in endothelial cytoskeletal dynamics and the shear stress response. *Circ Res* 98:176, 2006.

45. Hahn C, Orr AW, Sanders JM, et al: The subendothelial extracellular matrix modulates JNK activation by flow. *Circ Res* 104:995, 2009.

46. Orr AW, Stockton R, Simmers MB, et al: Matrix-specific p21-activated kinase activation regulates vascular permeability in atherogenesis. *J Cell Biol* 176:719, 2007.

47. Gabriels JE, Paul DL: Connexin43 is highly localized to sites of disturbed flow in rat aortic endothelium but connexin37 and connexin40 are more uniformly distributed. *Circ Res* 83:636, 1998.

48. Hochleitner BW, Hochleitner EO, Obrist P, et al: Fluid shear stress induces heat shock protein 60 expression in endothelial cells in vitro and in vivo. *Arterioscler Thromb Vasc Biol* 20:617, 2000.

49. Uchiyama T, Atsuta H, Utsugi T, et al: HSF1 and constitutively active HSF1 improve vascular endothelial function (heat shock proteins improve vascular endothelial function). *Atherosclerosis* 190:321, 2007.

50. Fu Q, Wang J, Boerma M, et al: Involvement of heat shock factor 1 in statin-induced transcriptional upregulation of endothelial thrombomodulin. *Circ Res* 103:369, 2008.

51. Zhao R, Ma X, Xie X, Shen GX: Involvement of NADPH oxidase in oxidized LDL-induced upregulation of heat shock factor-1 and plasminogen activator inhibitor-1 in vascular endothelial cells. *Am J Physiol Endocrinol Metab* 297:E104, 2009.

52. Wick G, Knoflach M, Xu Q: Autoimmune and inflammatory mechanisms in atherosclerosis. *Annu Rev Immunol* 22:361, 2004.

53. Yamawaki H, Pan S, Lee RT, Berk BC: Fluid shear stress inhibits vascular inflammation by decreasing thioredoxin-interacting protein in endothelial cells. *J Clin Invest* 115:733, 2005.

54. Partridge J, Carlsen H, Enesa K, et al: Laminar shear stress acts as a switch to regulate divergent functions of NF-κB in endothelial cells. *FASEB J* 21:3553, 2007.

55. Sawada N, Salomone S, Kim HH, et al: Regulation of endothelial nitric oxide synthase and postnatal angiogenesis by Rac1. *Circ Res* 103:360, 2008.

56. Li JM, Shah AM: Endothelial cell superoxide generation: regulation and relevance for cardiovascular pathophysiology. *Am J Physiol Regul Integr Comp Physiol* 287:R1014, 2004.

57. Stocker R, Keaney JF Jr: Role of oxidative modifications in atherosclerosis. *Physiol Rev* 84:1381, 2004.

58. Zhang DX, Gutterman DD: Mitochondrial reactive oxygen species–mediated signaling in endothelial cells. *Am J Physiol Heart Circ Physiol* 292:H2023, 2007.

59. Sorop O, Spaan JA, Sweeney TE, VanBavel E: Effect of steady versus oscillating flow on porcine coronary arterioles: involvement of NO and superoxide anion. *Circ Res* 92:1344, 2003.

60. Thengchaisri N, Shipley R, Ren Y, et al: Exercise training restores coronary arteriolar dilation to NOS activation distal to coronary artery occlusion: role of hydrogen peroxide. *Arterioscler Thromb Vasc Biol* 27:791, 2007.

61. Han Z, Varadharaj S, Giedt RJ, et al: Mitochondria-derived reactive oxygen species mediate heme oxygenase-1 expression in sheared endothelial cells. *J Pharmacol Exp Ther* 329:94, 2009.

62. Veal EA, Day AM, Morgan BA: Hydrogen peroxide sensing and signaling. *Mol Cell* 26:1, 2007.

63. Berk BC: Atheroprotective signaling mechanisms activated by steady laminar flow in endothelial cells. *Circulation* 117:1082, 2008.

64. Liu Y, Min W: Thioredoxin promotes ASK1 ubiquitination and degradation to inhibit ASK1-mediated apoptosis in a redox activity–independent manner. *Circ Res* 90:1259, 2002.

65. Hosoya T, Maruyama A, Kang MI, et al: Differential responses of the Nrf2-Keap1 system to laminar and oscillatory shear stresses in endothelial cells. *J Biol Chem* 280:27244, 2005.

66. Fledderus JO, Boon RA, Volger OL, et al: KLF2 primes the antioxidant transcription factor Nrf2 for activation in endothelial cells. *Arterioscler Thromb Vasc Biol* 28:1339, 2008.

67. Davis ME, Grumbach IM, Fukai T, et al: Shear stress regulates endothelial nitric-oxide synthase promoter activity through nuclear factor κB binding. *J Biol Chem* 279:163, 2004.

68. Chen W, Bacanamwo M, Harrison DG: Activation of p300 histone acetyltransferase activity is an early endothelial response to laminar shear stress and is essential for stimulation of endothelial nitric-oxide synthase mRNA transcription. *J Biol Chem* 283:16293, 2008.

69. Reynaert NL, Ckless K, Korn SH, et al: Nitric oxide represses inhibitory κB kinase through S-nitrosylation. *Proc Natl Acad Sci U S A* 101:8945, 2004.

70. Duerrschmidt N, Stielow C, Muller G, et al: NO-mediated regulation of NAD(P)H oxidase by laminar shear stress in human endothelial cells. *J Physiol* 576:557, 2006.

71. Ramkhelawon B, Vilar J, Rivas D, et al: Shear stress regulates angiotensin type 1 receptor expression in endothelial cells. *Circ Res* 105:869, 2009.

72. Li L, Tatake RJ, Natarajan K, et al: Fluid shear stress inhibits TNF-mediated JNK activation via MEK5-BMK1 in endothelial cells. *Biochem Biophys Res Commun* 370:159, 2008.

73. Dekker RJ, van Soest S, Fontijn RD, et al: Prolonged fluid shear stress induces a distinct set of endothelial cell genes, most specifically lung Kruppel-like factor (KLF2). *Blood* 100:1689, 2002.

74. SenBanerjee S, Lin Z, Atkins GB, et al: KLF2 is a novel transcriptional regulator of endothelial proinflammatory activation. *J Exp Med* 199:1305, 2004.

75. Parmar KM, Nambudiri V, Dai G, et al: Statins exert endothelial atheroprotective effects via the KLF2 transcription factor. *J Biol Chem* 280:26714, 2005.

76. Parmar KM, Larman HB, Dai G, et al: Integration of flow-dependent endothelial phenotypes by Kruppel-like factor 2. *J Clin Invest* 116:49, 2006.

77. Hastings NE, Simmers MB, McDonald OG, et al: Atherosclerosis-prone hemodynamics differentially regulates endothelial and smooth muscle cell phenotypes and promotes pro-inflammatory priming. *Am J Physiol Cell Physiol* 293:C1824, 2007.

78. Fledderus JO, van Thienen JV, Boon RA, et al: Prolonged shear stress and KLF2 suppress constitutive proinflammatory transcription through inhibition of ATF2, *Blood* 109:4249, 2007.

79. Boon RA, Fledderus JO, Volger OL, et al: KLF2 suppresses TGF-β signaling in endothelium through induction of Smad7 and inhibition of AP-1, *Arterioscler Thromb Vasc Biol* 27:532, 2007.

80. Huddleson JP, Ahmad N, Srinivasan S, Lingrel JB: Induction of KLF2 by fluid shear stress requires a novel promoter element activated by a phosphatidylinositol 3-kinase–dependent chromatin-remodeling pathway. *J Biol Chem* 280:23371, 2005.

81. Zakkar M, Chaudhury H, Sandvik G, et al: Increased endothelial mitogen-activated protein kinase phosphatase-1 expression suppresses proinflammatory activation at sites that are resistant to atherosclerosis. *Circ Res* 103:726, 2008.

82. Garcia-Cardena G, Comander J, Anderson KR, et al: Biomechanical activation of vascular endothelium as a determinant of its functional phenotype. *Proc Natl Acad Sci U S A* 98:4478, 2001.

83. Brooks AR, Lelkes PI, Rubanyi GM: Gene expression profiling of human aortic endothelial cells exposed to disturbed flow and steady laminar flow. *Physiol Genomics* 9:27, 2002.

84. Yoshisue H, Suzuki K, Kawabata A, et al: Large scale isolation of non-uniform shear stress–responsive genes from cultured human endothelial cells through the preparation of a subtracted cDNA library. *Atherosclerosis* 162:323, 2002.

85. Passerini AG, Polacek DC, Shi C, et al: Coexisting proinflammatory and antioxidative endothelial transcription profiles in a disturbed flow region of the adult porcine aorta. *Proc Natl Acad Sci U S A* 101:2482, 2004.

86. Chu TJ, Peters DG: Serial analysis of the vascular endothelial transcriptome under static and shear stress conditions. *Physiol Genomics* 34:185, 2008.

87. Davies PF: Endothelial transcriptome profiles in vivo in complex arterial flow fields. *Ann Biomed Eng* 36:563, 2008.

88. Hajra L, Evans AI, Chen M, et al: The NF-κB signal transduction pathway in aortic endothelial cells is primed for activation in regions predisposed to atherosclerotic lesion formation. *Proc Natl Acad Sci U S A* 97:9052, 2000.
89. Schwenke DC, Carew TE: Initiation of atherosclerotic lesions in cholesterol-fed rabbits. II. Selective retention of LDL vs. selective increases in LDL permeability in susceptible sites of arteries. *Arteriosclerosis* 9:908, 1989.
90. Schwenke DC, Carew TE: Initiation of atherosclerotic lesions in cholesterol-fed rabbits. I. Focal increases in arterial LDL concentration precede development of fatty streak lesions. *Arteriosclerosis* 9:895, 1989.
91. Cushing SD, Berliner JA, Valente AJ, et al: Minimally modified low density lipoprotein induces monocyte chemotactic protein 1 in human endothelial cells and smooth muscle cells. *Proc Natl Acad Sci U S A* 87:5134, 1990.
92. Li H, Cybulsky MI, Gimbrone MA, Libby P: An atherogenic diet rapidly induces VCAM-1, a cytokine-regulatable mononuclear leukocyte adhesion molecule, in rabbit aortic endothelium. *Arterioscler Thromb* 13:197, 1993.
93. Nievelstein PF, Fogelman AM, Mottino G, Frank JS: Lipid accumulation in rabbit aortic intima 2 hours after bolus infusion of low density lipoprotein. A deep-etch and immunolocalization study of ultrarapidly frozen tissue. *Arterioscler Thromb* 11:1795, 1991.
94. van den Berg BM, Spaan JA, Rolf TM, Vink H: Atherogenic region and diet diminish glycocalyx dimension and increase intima-to-media ratios at murine carotid artery bifurcation. *Am J Physiol Heart Circ Physiol* 290:H915, 2006.
95. Florentin RA, Nam SC, Lee KT, Thomas WA: Increased H^3-thymidine incorporation into endothelial cells of swine fed cholesterol for 3 days. *Exp Mol Pathol* 10:250, 1969.
96. Navab M, Ananthramaiah GM, Reddy ST, et al: The oxidation hypothesis of atherogenesis: the role of oxidized phospholipids and HDL. *J Lipid Res* 45:993, 2004.
97. Steinberg D: The LDL modification hypothesis of atherogenesis: an update. *J Lipid Res* 50:S376, 2009.
98. Nicholls SJ, Hazen SL: Myeloperoxidase and cardiovascular disease. *Arterioscler Thromb Vasc Biol* 25:1102, 2005.
99. Napoli C, D'Armiento FP, Mancini FP, et al: Fatty streak formation occurs in human fetal aortas and is greatly enhanced by maternal hypercholesterolemia. Intimal accumulation of low density lipoprotein and its oxidation precede monocyte recruitment into early atherosclerotic lesions. *J Clin Invest* 100:2680, 1997.
100. Heinecke JW: Mechanisms of oxidative damage of low density lipoprotein in human atherosclerosis. *Curr Opin Lipidol* 8:268, 1997.
101. Nicholls SJ, Hazen SL: Myeloperoxidase, modified lipoproteins, and atherogenesis. *J Lipid Res* 50:S346, 2009.
102. Palinski W, Miller E, Witztum JL: Immunization of low density lipoprotein (LDL) receptor–deficient rabbits with homologous malondialdehyde-modified LDL reduces atherogenesis. *Proc Natl Acad Sci U S A* 92:821, 1995.
103. Freigang S, Horkko S, Miller E, et al: Immunization of LDL receptor–deficient mice with homologous malondialdehyde-modified and native LDL reduces progression of atherosclerosis by mechanisms other than induction of high titers of antibodies to oxidative neoepitopes. *Arterioscler Thromb Vasc Biol* 18:1972, 1998.
104. Binder CJ, Horkko S, Dewan A, et al: Pneumococcal vaccination decreases atherosclerotic lesion formation: molecular mimicry between *Streptococcus pneumoniae* and oxidized LDL. *Nat Med* 9:736, 2003.
105. Navab M, Imes SS, Hama SY, et al: Monocyte transmigration induced by modification of low density lipoprotein in cocultures of human aortic wall cells is due to induction of monocyte chemotactic protein 1 synthesis and is abolished by high density lipoprotein. *J Clin Invest* 88:2039, 1991.
106. Walton KA, Hsieh X, Gharavi N, et al: Receptors involved in the oxidized 1-palmitoyl-2-arachidonoyl-sn-glycero-3-phosphorylcholine–mediated synthesis of interleukin-8. A role for Toll-like receptor 4 and a glycosylphosphatidylinositol-anchored protein. *J Biol Chem* 278:29661, 2003.
107. Pasterkamp G, Van Keulen JK, De Kleijn DP: Role of Toll-like receptor 4 in the initiation and progression of atherosclerotic disease. *Eur J Clin Invest* 34:328, 2004.
108. Michelsen KS, Wong MH, Shah PK, et al: Lack of Toll-like receptor 4 or myeloid differentiation factor 88 reduces atherosclerosis and alters plaque phenotype in mice deficient in apolipoprotein E. *Proc Natl Acad Sci U S A* 101:10679, 2004.
109. Hartvigsen K, Chou M-Y, Hansen LF, et al: The role of innate immunity in atherogenesis. *J Lipid Res* 50:S388, 2009.
110. Greenberg ME, Li XM, Gugiu BG, et al: The lipid whisker model of the structure of oxidized cell membranes. *J Biol Chem* 283:2385, 2008.
111. Shi W, Wang NJ, Shih DM, et al: Determinants of atherosclerosis susceptibility in the C3H and C57BL/6 mouse model: evidence for involvement of endothelial cells but not blood cells or cholesterol metabolism. *Circ Res* 86:1078, 2000.
112. Mullick AE, Tobias PS, Curtiss LK: Modulation of atherosclerosis in mice by Toll-like receptor 2. *J Clin Invest* 115:3149, 2005.
113. Shih HH, Zhang S, Cao W, et al: CRP is a novel ligand for the oxidized LDL receptor LOX-1. *Am J Physiol Heart Circ Physiol* 296:H1643, 2009.
114. Fujita Y, Kakino A, Nishimichi N, et al: Oxidized LDL receptor LOX-1 binds to C-reactive protein and mediates its vascular effects. *Clin Chem* 55:285, 2009.
115. Mehta JL, Li D: Identification, regulation and function of a novel lectin-like oxidized low-density lipoprotein receptor. *J Am Coll Cardiol* 39:1429, 2002.
116. Mehta JL, Chen J, Hermonat PL, et al: Lectin-like, oxidized low-density lipoprotein receptor-1 (LOX-1): a critical player in the development of atherosclerosis and related disorders. *Cardiovasc Res* 69:36, 2006.
117. Li D, Mehta JL: Intracellular signaling of LOX-1 in endothelial cell apoptosis. *Circ Res* 104:566, 2009.
118. Sugimoto K, Ishibashi T, Sawamura T, et al: LOX-1–MT1–MMP axis is crucial for RhoA and Rac1 activation induced by oxidized low-density lipoprotein in endothelial cells. *Cardiovasc Res* 84:127, 2009.
119. Sangle GV, Zhao R, Shen GX: Transmembrane signaling pathway mediates oxidized low-density lipoprotein–induced expression of plasminogen activator inhibitor-1 in vascular endothelial cells. *Am J Physiol Endocrinol Metab* 295:E1243, 2008.
120. Li D, Liu L, Chen H, et al: LOX-1, an oxidized LDL endothelial receptor, induces CD40/CD40L signaling in human coronary artery endothelial cells. *Arterioscler Thromb Vasc Biol* 23:816, 2003.
121. Lu J, Yang J-H, Burns AR, et al: Mediation of electronegative low-density lipoprotein signaling by LOX-1: a possible mechanism of endothelial apoptosis. *Circ Res* 104:619, 2009.
122. Li Y, Ross-Viola JS, Shay NF, et al: Human CYP3A4 and murine Cyp3A11 are regulated by equol and genistein via the pregnane X receptor in a species-specific manner. *J Nutr* 139:898, 2009.
123. Sanchez-Quesada JL, Benitez S, Ordonez-Llanos J: Electronegative low-density lipoprotein. *Curr Opin Lipidol* 15:329, 2004.
124. Oorni K, Posio P, Ala-Korpela M, et al: Sphingomyelinase induces aggregation and fusion of small very low-density lipoprotein and intermediate-density lipoprotein particles and increases their retention to human arterial proteoglycans. *Arterioscler Thromb Vasc Biol* 25:1678, 2005.
125. Bancells C, Benitez S, Villegas S, et al: Novel phospholipolytic activities associated with electronegative low-density lipoprotein are involved in increased self-aggregation. *Biochemistry* 47:8186, 2008.
126. Shin HK, Kim YK, Kim KY, et al: Remnant lipoprotein particles induce apoptosis in endothelial cells by NAD(P)H oxidase–mediated production of superoxide and cytokines via lectin-like oxidized low-density lipoprotein receptor-1 activation: prevention by cilostazol. *Circulation* 109:1022, 2004.
127. Ishigaki Y, Katagiri H, Gao J, et al: Impact of plasma oxidized low-density lipoprotein removal on atherosclerosis. *Circulation* 118:75-83, 2008.
128. Mehta JL, Sanada N, Hu CP, et al: Deletion of LOX-1 reduces atherogenesis in LDLR knockout mice fed high cholesterol diet. *Circ Res* 100:1634, 2007.
129. Inoue K, Arai Y, Kurihara H, et al: Overexpression of lectin-like oxidized low-density lipoprotein receptor-1 induces intramyocardial vasculopathy in apolipoprotein E-null mice. *Circ Res* 97:176, 2005.
130. Kawakami A, Osaka M, Tani M, et al: Apolipoprotein CIII links hyperlipidemia with vascular endothelial cell dysfunction. *Circulation* 118:731, 2008.
131. Norata GD, Pirillo A, Callegari E, et al: Gene expression and intracellular pathways involved in endothelial dysfunction induced by VLDL and oxidised VLDL. *Cardiovasc Res* 59:169, 2003.
132. Norata GD, Grigore L, Raselli S, et al: Post-prandial endothelial dysfunction in hypertriglyceridemic subjects: molecular mechanisms and gene expression studies. *Atherosclerosis* 193:321, 2007.
133. Riehl A, Nemeth J, Angel P, Hess J: The receptor RAGE: bridging inflammation and cancer. *Cell Commun Signal* 7:12, 2009.
134. Naka Y, Bucciarelli LG, Wendt T, et al: RAGE axis: animal models and novel insights into the vascular complications of diabetes. *Arterioscler Thromb Vasc Biol* 24:1342, 2004.
135. Soro-Paavonen A, Watson AM, Li J, et al: Receptor for advanced glycation end products (RAGE) deficiency attenuates the development of atherosclerosis in diabetes. *Diabetes* 57:2461, 2008.
136. Harja E, Bu DX, Hudson BI, et al: Vascular and inflammatory stresses mediate atherosclerosis via RAGE and its ligands in $apoE^{-/-}$ mice. *J Clin Invest* 118:183, 2008.
137. van Buul JD, Hordijk PL: Signaling in leukocyte transendothelial migration. *Arterioscler Thromb Vasc Biol* 24:824, 2004.
138. Papadopoulou C, Corrigall V, Taylor PR, Poston RN: The role of the chemokines MCP-1, GRO-α, IL-8 and their receptors in the adhesion of monocytic cells to human atherosclerotic plaques. *Cytokine* 43:181, 2008.
139. Legate KR, Fassler R: Mechanisms that regulate adaptor binding to β-integrin cytoplasmic tails. *J Cell Sci* 122:187, 2009.
140. Weber C, Zernecke A, Libby P: The multifaceted contributions of leukocyte subsets to atherosclerosis: lessons from mouse models. *Nat Rev Immunol* 8:802, 2008.
141. Hansson GK, Robertson AK, Soderberg-Naucler C: Inflammation and atherosclerosis. *Annu Rev Pathol* 1:297, 2006.
142. Barlic J, Murphy PM: Chemokine regulation of atherosclerosis. *J Leukoc Biol* 82:226, 2007.
143. Galkina E, Ley K: Immune and inflammatory mechanisms of atherosclerosis. *Annu Rev Immunol* 27:165, 2009.
144. Gautier EL, Jakubzick C, Randolph GJ: Regulation of the migration and survival of monocyte subsets by chemokine receptors and its relevance to atherosclerosis. *Arterioscler Thromb Vasc Biol* 29:1412, 2009.
145. Ley K, Laudanna C, Cybulsky MI, Nourshargh S: Getting to the site of inflammation: the leukocyte adhesion cascade updated. *Nat Rev Immunol* 7:678, 2007.
146. Franscini N, Bachli EB, Blau N, et al: Gene expression profiling of inflamed human endothelial cells and influence of activated protein C. *Circulation* 110:2903, 2004.
147. Lehtonen A, Ahlfors H, Veckman V, et al: Gene expression profiling during differentiation of human monocytes to macrophages or dendritic cells. *J Leukoc Biol* 82:710, 2007.
148. Williams MR, Sakurai Y, Zughaier SM, et al: Transmigration across activated endothelium induces transcriptional changes, inhibits apoptosis, and decreases antimicrobial protein expression in human monocytes. *J Leukoc Biol* 86:1331, 2009.
149. Bobryshev YV: Dendritic cells in atherosclerosis: current status of the problem and clinical relevance. *Eur Heart J* 26:1700, 2005.
150. Bason C, Corrocher R, Lunardi C, et al: Interaction of antibodies against cytomegalovirus with heat-shock protein 60 in pathogenesis of atherosclerosis. *Lancet* 362:1971, 2003.
151. Maron R, Sukhova G, Faria AM, et al: Mucosal administration of heat shock protein-65 decreases atherosclerosis and inflammation in aortic arch of low-density lipoprotein receptor–deficient mice. *Circulation* 106:1708, 2002.
152. van Puijvelde GHM, van Es T, van Wanrooij EJA, et al: Induction of oral tolerance to HSP60 or an HSP60-peptide activates T cell regulation and reduces atherosclerosis. *Arterioscler Thromb Vasc Biol* 27:2677, 2007.
153. Boring L, Gosling J, Cleary M, Charo IF: Decreased lesion formation in $CCR2^{-/-}$ mice reveals a role for chemokines in the initiation of atherosclerosis. *Nature* 394:894, 1998.

154. Buja LM, Kovanen PT, Bilheimer DW: Cellular pathology of homozygous familial hypercholesterolemia. *Am J Pathol* 97:327, 1979.

155. Glagov S, Ozoa AK: Significance of the relatively low incidence of atherosclerosis in the pulmonary, renal and mesenteric arteries. *Ann N Y Acad Sci* 149:940, 1968.

156. Sun N, Wood NB, Hughes AD, et al: Effects of transmural pressure and wall shear stress on LDL accumulation in the arterial wall: a numerical study using a multilayered model. *Am J Physiol Heart Circ Physiol* 292:H3148, 2007.

157. Curmi PA, Juan L, Tedgui A: Effect of transmural pressure on low density lipoprotein and albumin transport and distribution across the intact arterial wall. *Circ Res* 66:1692, 1990.

158. Meyer G, Merval R, Tedgui A: Effects of pressure-induced stretch and convection on low-density lipoprotein and albumin uptake in the rabbit aortic wall. *Circ Res* 79:532, 1996.

159. Cancel LM, Fitting A, Tarbell JM: In vitro study of LDL transport under pressurized (convective) conditions. *Am J Physiol Heart Circ Physiol* 293:H126, 2007.

160. van den Berg BM, Spaan JA, Vink H: Impaired glycocalyx barrier properties contribute to enhanced intimal low-density lipoprotein accumulation at the carotid artery bifurcation in mice. *Pflugers Arch* 457:1199, 2009.

161. Durrant JR, Seals DR, Connell ML, et al: Voluntary wheel running restores endothelial function in conduit arteries of old mice: direct evidence for reduced oxidative stress, increased superoxide dismutase activity and down-regulation of NADPH oxidase. *J Physiol* 587:3271, 2009.

162. Seals DR, Desouza CA, Donato AJ, Tanaka H: Habitual exercise and arterial aging. *J Appl Physiol* 105:1323-1332, 2008.

163. DeSouza CA, Shapiro LF, Clevenger CM, et al: Regular aerobic exercise prevents and restores age-related declines in endothelium-dependent vasodilation in healthy men. *Circulation* 102:1351, 2000.

164. Okabe TA, Shimada K, Hattori M, et al: Swimming reduces the severity of atherosclerosis in apolipoprotein E deficient mice by antioxidant effects. *Cardiovasc Res* 74:537, 2007.

165. De Keulenaer GW, Chappell DC, Ishizaka N, et al: Oscillatory and steady laminar shear stress differentially affect human endothelial redox state: role of a superoxide-producing NADH oxidase. *Circ Res* 82:1094, 1998.

166. Lauer N, Suvorava T, Ruther U, et al: Critical involvement of hydrogen peroxide in exercise-induced up-regulation of endothelial NO synthase. *Cardiovasc Res* 65:254, 2005.

167. Ristow M, Zarse K, Oberbach A, et al: Antioxidants prevent health-promoting effects of physical exercise in humans. *Proc Natl Acad Sci U S A* 106:8665, 2009.

168. Marsh SA, Coombes JS: Exercise and the endothelial cell. *Int J Cardiol* 99:165, 2005.

169. Fang Y, Mohler ER III, Hsieh E, et al: Hypercholesterolemia suppresses inwardly rectifying K$^+$ channels in aortic endothelium in vitro and in vivo. *Circ Res* 98:1064, 2006.

170. Epshtein Y, Chopra AP, Rosenhouse-Dantsker A, et al: Identification of a C-terminus domain critical for the sensitivity of Kir2.1 to cholesterol. *Proc Natl Acad Sci U S A* 106:8055, 2009.

171. Meuwese MC, Mooij HL, Nieuwdorp M, et al: Partial recovery of the endothelial glycocalyx upon rosuvastatin therapy in patients with heterozygous familial hypercholesterolemia. *J Lipid Res* 50:148, 2009.

172. Alberici LC, Oliveira HC, Paim BA, et al: Mitochondrial ATP-sensitive K$^+$ channels as redox signals to liver mitochondria in response to hypertriglyceridemia. *Free Radic Biol Med* 47:1432, 2009.

173. Pacher P, Nivorozhkin A, Szabo C: Therapeutic effects of xanthine oxidase inhibitors: renaissance half a century after the discovery of allopurinol. *Pharmacol Rev* 58:87, 2006.

174. Ohtsubo T, Matsumura K, Sakagami K, et al: Xanthine oxidoreductase depletion induces renal interstitial fibrosis through aberrant lipid and purine accumulation in renal tubules. *Hypertension* 54:868, 2009.

175. Schröder K, Vecchione C, Jung O, et al: Xanthine oxidase inhibitor tungsten prevents the development of atherosclerosis in ApoE knockout mice fed a Western-type diet. *Free Radic Biol Med* 41:1353, 2006.

176. Norata GD, Catapano AL: Molecular mechanisms responsible for the antiinflammatory and protective effect of HDL on the endothelium. *Vasc Health Risk Manag* 1:119, 2005.

177. Okajima F, Sato K, Kimura T: Anti-atherogenic actions of high-density lipoprotein through sphingosine 1-phosphate receptors and scavenger receptor class B type I. *Endocr J* 56:317, 2009.

178. von Eckardstein A, Rohrer L: Transendothelial lipoprotein transport and regulation of endothelial permeability and integrity by lipoproteins. *Curr Opin Lipidol* 20:197-205, 2009.

179. Argraves KM, Argraves WS: HDL serves as a S1P signaling platform mediating a multitude of cardiovascular effects. *J Lipid Res* 48:2325, 2007.

180. Argraves KM, Gazzolo PJ, Groh EM, et al: High density lipoprotein-associated sphingosine 1-phosphate promotes endothelial barrier function. *J Biol Chem* 283:25074, 2008.

181. Zhu W, Saddar S, Seetharam D, et al: The scavenger receptor class B type I adaptor protein PDZK1 maintains endothelial monolayer integrity. *Circ Res* 102:480, 2008.

182. Terasaka N, Yu S, Yvan-Charvet L, et al: ABCG1 and HDL protect against endothelial dysfunction in mice fed a high-cholesterol diet. *J Clin Invest* 118:3701, 2008.

183. Shih DM, Lusis AJ: The roles of PON1 and PON2 in cardiovascular disease and innate immunity. *Curr Opin Lipidol* 20:288, 2009.

184. Soran H, Younis NN, Charlton-Menys V, Durrington P: Variation in paraoxonase-1 activity and atherosclerosis. *Curr Opin Lipidol* 20:265, 2009.

185. Brownlee M: The pathobiology of diabetic complications: a unifying mechanism. *Diabetes* 54:1615, 2005.

186. Brownlee M, Aiello LP, Cooper ME, et al: Complications of diabetes mellitus. In Kronenberg HM, Melmed S, Polonsky KS, Larson PR, editors: *Williams textbook of endocrinology*, ed 11, Philadelphia, 2008, Saunders Elsevier, pp 1417-1501.

187. Mathews MT, Berk BC: PARP-1 inhibition prevents oxidative and nitrosative stress-induced endothelial cell death via transactivation of the VEGF receptor 2, *Arterioscler Thromb Vasc Biol* 28:711, 2008.

188. von Lukowicz T, Hassa PO, Lohmann C, et al: PARP1 is required for adhesion molecule expression in atherogenesis. *Cardiovasc Res* 78:158, 2008.

189. Xue M, Qian Q, Adaikalakoteswari A, et al: Activation of NF-E2–related factor-2 reverses biochemical dysfunction of endothelial cells induced by hyperglycemia linked to vascular disease. *Diabetes* 57:2809, 2008.

190. Yi X, Maeda N: α-Lipoic acid prevents the increase in atherosclerosis induced by diabetes in apolipoprotein E–deficient mice fed high-fat/low-cholesterol diet. *Diabetes* 55:2238, 2006.

191. Maeda N: *Animal Models of Diabetic Complications Consortium (U01 HL087946). Annual report 2008. Dislipidemia, lipoic acid and diabetic vascular complications in humanized mice*, Chapel Hill, NC, 2008, Department of Pathology and Laboratory Medicine, University of North Carolina at Chapel Hill.

192. Bakker W, Sipkema P, Stehouwer CD, et al: Protein kinase C theta activation induces insulin-mediated constriction of muscle resistance arteries. *Diabetes* 57:706, 2008.

193. Bakker W, Eringa E, Sipkema P, van Hinsbergh V: Endothelial dysfunction and diabetes: roles of hyperglycemia, impaired insulin signaling and obesity. *Cell Tissue Res* 335:165, 2009.

194. Li G, Barrett EJ, Ko S-H, et al: Insulin and insulin-like growth factor-I receptors differentially mediate insulin-stimulated adhesion molecule production by endothelial cells. *Endocrinology* 150:3475, 2009.

195. Symons JD, McMillin SL, Riehle C, et al: Contribution of insulin and Akt1 signaling to endothelial nitric oxide synthase in the regulation of endothelial function and blood pressure. *Circ Res* 104:1085, 2009.

196. Esdaile JM, Abrahamowicz M, Grodzicky T, et al: Traditional Framingham risk factors fail to fully account for accelerated atherosclerosis in systemic lupus erythematosus. *Arthritis Rheum* 44:2331, 2001.

197. Asanuma Y, Oeser A, Shintani AK, et al: Premature coronary-artery atherosclerosis in systemic lupus erythematosus. *N Engl J Med* 349:2407, 2003.

198. Roman MJ, Shanker BA, Davis A, et al: Prevalence and correlates of accelerated atherosclerosis in systemic lupus erythematosus. *N Engl J Med* 349:2399, 2003.

199. Roman MJ, Moeller E, Davis A, et al: Preclinical carotid atherosclerosis in patients with rheumatoid arthritis. *Ann Intern Med* 144:249, 2006.

200. Duran S, Gonzalez LA, Alarcon GS: Damage, accelerated atherosclerosis, and mortality in patients with systemic lupus erythematosus: lessons from LUMINA, a multiethnic US cohort. *J Clin Rheumatol* 13:350, 2007.

201. Ahmad Y, Shelmerdine J, Bodill H, et al: Subclinical atherosclerosis in systemic lupus erythematosus (SLE): the relative contribution of classic risk factors and the lupus phenotype. *Rheumatology (Oxford)* 46:983, 2007.

202. Giles JT, Szklo M, Post W, et al: Coronary arterial calcification in rheumatoid arthritis: comparison with the Multi-Ethnic Study of Atherosclerosis. *Arthritis Res Ther* 11:R36, 2009.

203. Edwards CJ, Syddall H, Goswami R, et al: The autoantibody rheumatoid factor may be an independent risk factor for ischaemic heart disease in men. *Heart* 93:1263, 2007.

204. Khurma V, Meyer C, Park GS, et al: A pilot study of subclinical coronary atherosclerosis in systemic sclerosis: coronary artery calcification in cases and controls. *Arthritis Rheum* 59:591, 2008.

205. Gelfand JM, Neimann AL, Shin DB, et al: Risk of myocardial infarction in patients with psoriasis. *JAMA* 296:1735, 2006.

206. Ludwig RJ, Herzog C, Rostock A, et al: Psoriasis: a possible risk factor for development of coronary artery calcification. *Br J Dermatol* 156:271, 2007.

207. Gonzalez-Juanatey C, Llorca J, Amigo-Diaz E, et al: High prevalence of subclinical atherosclerosis in psoriatic arthritis patients without clinically evident cardiovascular disease or classic atherosclerosis risk factors. *Arthritis Rheum* 57:1074, 2007.

208. Robak E, Sysa-Jedrzejowska A, Robak T, et al: Tumour necrosis factor α (TNF-α), interleukin-6 (IL-6) and their soluble receptors (sTNF-α-Rp55 and sIL-6R) serum levels in systemic lupus erythematodes. *Mediators Inflamm* 5:435, 1996.

209. McKellar GE, McCarey DW, Sattar N, McInnes IB: Role for TNF in atherosclerosis? Lessons from autoimmune disease. *Nat Rev Cardiol* 6:410, 2009.

210. Aprahamian T, Rifkin I, Bonegio R, et al: Impaired clearance of apoptotic cells promotes synergy between atherogenesis and autoimmune disease. *J Exp Med* 199:1121, 2004.

211. Feng X, Li H, Rumbin AA, et al: ApoE$^{-/-}$Fas$^{-/-}$ C57BL/6 mice: a novel murine model simultaneously exhibits lupus nephritis, atherosclerosis, and osteopenia. *J Lipid Res* 48:794, 2007.

212. Minick CR: Immunologic arterial injury in atherogenesis. *Ann N Y Acad Sci* 275:210, 1976.

213. Davies DF, Davies JR, Richards MA: Antibodies to reconstituted dried cow's milk protein in coronary heart disease. *J Atheroscler Res* 9:103, 1969.

214. Epstein SE, Zhu J, Najafi AH, Burnett MS: Insights into the role of infection in atherogenesis and in plaque rupture. *Circulation* 119:3133, 2009.

215. Moazed TC, Campbell LA, Rosenfeld ME, et al: *Chlamydia pneumoniae* infection accelerates the progression of atherosclerosis in apolipoprotein E–deficient mice. *J Infect Dis* 180:238, 1999.

216. Alber DG, Powell KL, Vallance P, et al: Herpesvirus infection accelerates atherosclerosis in the apolipoprotein E–deficient mouse. *Circulation* 102:779, 2000.

217. Ott SJ, El Mokhtari NE, Musfeldt M, et al: Detection of diverse bacterial signatures in atherosclerotic lesions of patients with coronary heart disease. *Circulation* 113:929, 2006.

218. Cannon CP, Braunwald E, McCabe CH, et al: Antibiotic treatment of *Chlamydia pneumoniae* after acute coronary syndrome. *N Engl J Med* 352:1646, 2005.

219. Jespersen CM, Als-Nielsen B, Damgaard M, et al: Randomised placebo controlled multicentre trial to assess short term clarithromycin for patients with stable coronary heart disease: CLARICOR trial. *BMJ* 332:22, 2006.

220. Henderson B, Csordas A, Backovic A, et al: Cigarette smoke is an endothelial stressor and leads to cell cycle arrest. *Atherosclerosis* 201:298, 2008.
221. Ambrose JA, Barua RS: The pathophysiology of cigarette smoking and cardiovascular disease: an update. *J Am Coll Cardiol* 43:1731, 2004.
222. Kramer A, Jansen A, van Aalst-Cohen E, et al: Relative risk for cardiovascular atherosclerotic events after smoking cessation: 6-9 years excess risk in individuals with familial hypercholesterolemia. *BMC Public Health* 6:262, 2006.
223. Wannamethee SG, Lowe GDO, Shaper AG, et al: Associations between cigarette smoking, pipe/cigar smoking, and smoking cessation, and haemostatic and inflammatory markers for cardiovascular disease. *Eur Heart J* 26:1765, 2005.
224. Law MR, Wald NJ, Rudnicka AR: Quantifying effect of statins on low density lipoprotein cholesterol, ischaemic heart disease, and stroke: systematic review and meta-analysis. *BMJ* 326:1423, 2003.
225. Veniant MM, Withycombe S, Young SG: Lipoprotein size and atherosclerosis susceptibility in $APOE^{-/-}$ and $LDLR^{-/-}$ mice. *Arterioscler Thromb Vasc Biol* 21:1567, 2001.
226. Hopkins PN, Wu LL, Schumacher MC, et al: Type III dyslipoproteinemia in patients heterozygous for familial hypercholesterolemia and apolipoprotein E2. Evidence for a gene-gene interaction. *Arterioscler Thromb* 11:1137, 1991.
227. Hopkins PN, Stephenson S, Wu LL, et al: Evaluation of coronary risk factors in patients with heterozygous familial hypercholesterolemia. *Am J Cardiol* 87:547, 2001.
228. Carmena R, Roy M, Roederer G, et al: Coexisting dysbetalipoproteinemia and familial hypercholesterolemia. Clinical and laboratory observations. *Atherosclerosis* 148:113, 2000.
229. Caligiuri G, Levy B, Pernow J, et al: Myocardial infarction mediated by endothelin receptor signaling in hypercholesterolemic mice. *Proc Natl Acad Sci U S A* 96:6920, 1999.
230. Hopkins PN, Wu LL, Hunt SC, Brinton EA: Plasma triglycerides and type III hyperlipidemia are independently associated with premature familial coronary artery disease. *J Am Coll Cardiol* 45:1003, 2005.
231. Hopkins PN, Nanjee MN, Wu LL, et al: Altered composition of triglyceride-rich lipoproteins and coronary artery disease in a large case-control study. *Atherosclerosis* 207:559, 2009.
232. Smith EB: Transport, interactions and retention of plasma proteins in the intima: the barrier function of the internal elastic lamina. *Eur Heart J* 11(Suppl E):72, 1990.
233. Nakashima Y, Fujii H, Sumiyoshi S, et al: Early human atherosclerosis: accumulation of lipid and proteoglycans in intimal thickenings followed by macrophage infiltration. *Arterioscler Thromb Vasc Biol* 27:1159, 2007.
234. Brown MS, Goldstein JL: Lipoprotein metabolism in the macrophage: implications for cholesterol deposition in atherosclerosis. *Annu Rev Biochem* 52:223, 1983.
235. Batt KV, Avella M, Moore EH, et al: Differential effects of low-density lipoprotein and chylomicron remnants on lipid accumulation in human macrophages. *Exp Biol Med (Maywood)* 229:528, 2004.
236. Tabas I: Nonoxidative modifications of lipoproteins in atherogenesis. *Annu Rev Nutr* 19:123, 1999.
237. Skalen K, Gustafsson M, Rydberg EK, et al: Subendothelial retention of atherogenic lipoproteins in early atherosclerosis. *Nature* 417:750, 2002.
238. Babaev VR, Patel MB, Semenkovich CF, et al: Macrophage lipoprotein lipase promotes foam cell formation and atherosclerosis in low density lipoprotein receptor–deficient mice. *J Biol Chem* 275:26293, 2000.
239. Shimada M, Ishibashi S, Inaba T, et al: Suppression of diet-induced atherosclerosis in low density lipoprotein receptor knockout mice overexpressing lipoprotein lipase. *Proc Natl Acad Sci U S A* 93:7242, 1996.
240. Sato H, Kato R, Isogai Y, et al: Analyses of group III secreted phospholipase A_2 transgenic mice reveal potential participation of this enzyme in plasma lipoprotein modification, macrophage foam cell formation, and atherosclerosis. *J Biol Chem* 283:33483, 2008.
241. Bostrom MA, Boyanovsky BB, Jordan CT, et al: Group V secretory phospholipase A_2 promotes atherosclerosis: evidence from genetically altered mice. *Arterioscler Thromb Vasc Biol* 27:600, 2007.
242. Wooton-Kee CR, Boyanovsky BB, Nasser MS, et al: Group V $sPLA_2$ hydrolysis of low-density lipoprotein results in spontaneous particle aggregation and promotes macrophage foam cell formation. *Arterioscler Thromb Vasc Biol* 24:762, 2004.
243. Bernatchez PN, Allen BG, Gelinas DS, et al: Regulation of VEGF-induced endothelial cell PAF synthesis: role of p42/44 MAPK, p38 MAPK and PI3K pathways. *Br J Pharmacol* 134:1253, 2001.
244. Bernatchez PN, Winstead MV, Dennis EA, Sirois MG: VEGF stimulation of endothelial cell PAF synthesis is mediated by group V 14 kDa secretory phospholipase A_2. *Br J Pharmacol* 134:197, 2001.
245. Devlin CM, Leventhal AR, Kuriakose G, et al: Acid sphingomyelinase promotes lipoprotein retention within early atheromata and accelerates lesion progression. *Arterioscler Thromb Vasc Biol* 28:1723, 2008.
246. Berliner JA, Leitinger N, Tsimikas S: The role of oxidized phospholipids in atherosclerosis. *J Lipid Res* 50:S207, 2009.
247. Harkewicz R, Hartvigsen K, Almazan F, et al: Cholesteryl ester hydroperoxides are biologically active components of minimally oxidized low density lipoprotein. *J Biol Chem* 283:10241, 2008.
248. Hazen SL: Oxidized phospholipids as endogenous pattern recognition ligands in innate immunity. *J Biol Chem* 283:15527, 2008.
249. Hazen SL, Heinecke JW: 3-Chlorotyrosine, a specific marker of myeloperoxidase-catalyzed oxidation, is markedly elevated in low density lipoprotein isolated from human atherosclerotic intima. *J Clin Invest* 99:2075, 1997.
250. Apostolov EO, Shah SV, Ray D, Basnakian AG: Scavenger receptors of endothelial cells mediate the uptake and cellular proatherogenic effects of carbamylated LDL. *Arterioscler Thromb Vasc Biol* 29:1622, 2009.
251. Wang Z, Nicholls SJ, Rodriguez ER, et al: Protein carbamylation links inflammation, smoking, uremia and atherogenesis. *Nat Med* 13:1176, 2007.
252. Boyanovsky BB, Shridas P, Simons M, et al: Syndecan-4 mediates macrophage uptake of group V secretory phospholipase A_2–modified LDL. *J Lipid Res* 50:641, 2009.
253. Greaves DR, Gordon S: The macrophage scavenger receptor at 30 years of age: current knowledge and future challenges. *J Lipid Res* 50(Suppl):S282, 2009.
254. Suzuki H, Kurihara Y, Takeya M, et al: A role for macrophage scavenger receptors in atherosclerosis and susceptibility to infection. *Nature* 386:292, 1997.
255. Moore KJ, Freeman MW: Scavenger receptors in atherosclerosis: beyond lipid uptake. *Arterioscler Thromb Vasc Biol* 26:1702, 2006.
256. Manning-Tobin JJ, Moore KJ, Seimon TA, et al: Loss of SR-A and CD36 activity reduces atherosclerotic lesion complexity without abrogating foam cell formation in hyperlipidemic mice. *Arterioscler Thromb Vasc Biol* 29:19, 2009.
257. Lim WS, Timmins JM, Seimon TA, et al: Signal transducer and activator of transcription-1 is critical for apoptosis in macrophages subjected to endoplasmic reticulum stress in vitro and in advanced atherosclerotic lesions in vivo. *Circulation* 117:940, 2008.
258. Daugherty A, Rateri DL, Lu H: As macrophages indulge, atherosclerotic lesions bulge. *Circ Res* 102:1445, 2008.
259. Paul A, Chang BH-J, Li L, et al: Deficiency of adipose differentiation-related protein impairs foam cell formation and protects against atherosclerosis. *Circ Res* 102:1492, 2008.
260. Zhang WY, Gaynor PM, Kruth HS: Apolipoprotein E produced by human monocyte-derived macrophages mediates cholesterol efflux that occurs in the absence of added cholesterol acceptors. *J Biol Chem* 271:28641, 1996.
261. Shibata N, Glass CK: Regulation of macrophage function in inflammation and atherosclerosis. *J Lipid Res* 50:S277, 2009.
262. Tangirala RK, Bischoff ED, Joseph SB, et al: Identification of macrophage liver X receptors as inhibitors of atherosclerosis. *Proc Natl Acad Sci U S A* 99:11896, 2002.
263. Chawla A, Boisvert WA, Lee CH, et al: A PPARγ-LXR-ABCA1 pathway in macrophages is involved in cholesterol efflux and atherogenesis. *Mol Cell* 7:161, 2001.
264. Makowski L, Brittingham KC, Reynolds JM, et al: The fatty acid–binding protein, aP2, coordinates macrophage cholesterol trafficking and inflammatory activity. Macrophage expression of aP2 impacts peroxisome proliferator-activated receptor γ and IκB kinase activities. *J Biol Chem* 280:12888, 2005.
265. Tabas I: Apoptosis and plaque destabilization in atherosclerosis: the role of macrophage apoptosis induced by cholesterol. *Cell Death Differ* 11(Suppl 1):S12, 2004.
266. Tabas I: Phospholipid metabolism in cholesterol-loaded macrophages. *Curr Opin Lipidol* 8:263, 1997.
267. Fazio S, Major AS, Swift LL, et al: Increased atherosclerosis in LDL receptor–null mice lacking ACAT1 in macrophages. *J Clin Invest* 107:163, 2001.
268. Zhao B, Song J, Chow WN, et al: Macrophage-specific transgenic expression of cholesteryl ester hydrolase significantly reduces atherosclerosis and lesion necrosis in Ldlr mice. *J Clin Invest* 117:2983, 2007.
269. Welch CL, Sun Y, Arey BJ, et al: Spontaneous atherothrombosis and medial degradation in $Apoe^{-/-}$, $Npc1^{-/-}$ mice. *Circulation* 116:2444, 2007.
270. Tall AR: Cholesterol efflux pathways and other potential mechanisms involved in the athero-protective effect of high density lipoproteins. *J Intern Med* 263:256, 2008.
271. Rader DJ, Alexander ET, Weibel GL, et al: The role of reverse cholesterol transport in animals and humans and relationship to atherosclerosis. *J Lipid Res* 50:S189, 2009.
272. Braun A, Trigatti BL, Post MJ, et al: Loss of SR-BI expression leads to the early onset of occlusive atherosclerotic coronary artery disease, spontaneous myocardial infarctions, severe cardiac dysfunction, and premature death in apolipoprotein E–deficient mice. *Circ Res* 90:270, 2002.
273. Zhang W, Yancey PG, Su YR, et al: Inactivation of macrophage scavenger receptor class B type I promotes atherosclerotic lesion development in apolipoprotein E–deficient mice. *Circulation* 108:2258, 2003.
274. Wang X, Collins HL, Ranalletta M, et al: Macrophage ABCA1 and ABCG1, but not SR-BI, promote macrophage reverse cholesterol transport in vivo. *J Clin Invest* 117:2216, 2007.
275. Aiello RJ, Brees D, Bourassa PA, et al: Increased atherosclerosis in hyperlipidemic mice with inactivation of ABCA1 in macrophages. *Arterioscler Thromb Vasc Biol* 22:630, 2002.
276. Yvan-Charvet L, Ranalletta M, Wang N, et al: Combined deficiency of ABCA1 and ABCG1 promotes foam cell accumulation and accelerates atherosclerosis in mice. *J Clin Invest* 117:3900, 2007.
277. deGoma EM, deGoma RL, Rader DJ: Beyond high-density lipoprotein cholesterol levels evaluating high-density lipoprotein function as influenced by novel therapeutic approaches. *J Am Coll Cardiol* 51:2199, 2008.
278. Ni M, Zhang M, Ding SF, et al: Micro-ultrasound imaging assessment of carotid plaque characteristics in apolipoprotein-E knockout mice. *Atherosclerosis* 197:64, 2008.
279. Ni M, Chen WQ, Zhang Y: Animal models and potential mechanisms of plaque destabilisation and disruption. *Heart* 95:1393, 2009.
280. Eren M, Painter CA, Atkinson JB, et al: Age-dependent spontaneous coronary arterial thrombosis in transgenic mice that express a stable form of human plasminogen activator inhibitor-1. *Circulation* 106:491, 2002.
281. Davies MJ, Thomas AC: Plaque fissuring—the cause of acute myocardial infarction, sudden ischaemic death, and crescendo angina. *Br Heart J* 53:363, 1985.
282. Constantinides P: Cause of thrombosis in human atherosclerotic arteries. *Am J Cardiol* 66:37G, 1990.
283. Virmani R, Burke AP, Farb A, Kolodgie FD: Pathology of the vulnerable plaque. *J Am Coll Cardiol* 47:C13, 2006.
284. Kolodgie FD, Gold HK, Burke AP, et al: Intraplaque hemorrhage and progression of coronary atheroma. *N Engl J Med* 349:2316, 2003.
285. Tziakas DN, Chalikias GK, Stakos D, Boudoulas H: The role of red blood cells in the progression and instability of atherosclerotic plaque. *Int J Cardiol* 142:2, 2010.
286. Mayr M, Sidibe A, Zampetaki A: The paradox of hypoxic and oxidative stress in atherosclerosis. *J Am Coll Cardiol* 51:1266, 2008.

287. Sluimer JC, Gasc JM, van Wanroij JL, et al: Hypoxia, hypoxia-inducible transcription factor, and macrophages in human atherosclerotic plaques are correlated with intra-plaque angiogenesis. *J Am Coll Cardiol* 51:1258, 2008.

288. Abela GS, Aziz K: Cholesterol crystals rupture biological membranes and human plaques during acute cardiovascular events—a novel insight into plaque rupture by scanning electron microscopy. *Scanning* 28:1, 2006.

289. Vedre A, Pathak DR, Crimp M, et al: Physical factors that trigger cholesterol crystallization leading to plaque rupture. *Atherosclerosis* 203:89, 2009.

290. Felton CV, Crook D, Davies MJ, Oliver MF: Relation of plaque lipid composition and morphology to the stability of human aortic plaques. *Arterioscler Thromb Vasc Biol* 17:1337, 1997.

291. Aikawa M, Rabkin E, Okada Y, et al: Lipid lowering by diet reduces matrix metallo-proteinase activity and increases collagen content of rabbit atheroma: a potential mechanism of lesion stabilization [see comments]. *Circulation* 97:2433, 1998.

292. Aikawa M, Voglic SJ, Sugiyama S, et al: Dietary lipid lowering reduces tissue factor expression in rabbit atheroma. *Circulation* 100:1215, 1999.

293. Sakamoto H, Aikawa M, Hill CC, et al: Biomechanical strain induces class A scavenger receptor expression in human monocyte/macrophages and THP-1 cells: a potential mechanism of increased atherosclerosis in hypertension. *Circulation* 104:109, 2001.

294. Aikawa M, Rabkin E, Sugiyama S, et al: An HMG-CoA reductase inhibitor, cerivastatin, suppresses growth of macrophages expressing matrix metalloproteinases and tissue factor in vivo and in vitro. *Circulation* 103:276, 2001.

295. Fukumoto Y, Libby P, Rabkin E, et al: Statins alter smooth muscle cell accumulation and collagen content in established atheroma of Watanabe heritable hyperlipidemic rabbits. *Circulation* 103:993, 2001.

296. Trogan E, Feig JE, Dogan S, et al: Gene expression changes in foam cells and the role of chemokine receptor CCR7 during atherosclerosis regression in ApoE-deficient mice. *Proc Natl Acad Sci U S A* 103:3781, 2006.

297. Seimon TA, Wang Y, Han S, et al: Macrophage deficiency of p38a MAPK promotes apoptosis and plaque necrosis in advanced atherosclerotic lesions in mice. *J Clin Invest* 119:886, 2009.

298. Bujo H, Saito Y: Modulation of smooth muscle cell migration by members of the low-density lipoprotein receptor family. *Arterioscler Thromb Vasc Biol* 26:1246, 2006.

299. Boucher P, Gotthardt M, Li W-P, et al: Role in vascular wall integrity and protection from atherosclerosis. *Science* 300:329, 2003.

300. Mallat Z, Gojova A, Marchiol-Fournigault C, et al: Inhibition of transforming growth factor-β signaling accelerates atherosclerosis and induces an unstable plaque pheno-type in mice. *Circ Res* 89:930, 2001.

301. Lutgens E, Gijbels M, Smook M, et al: Transforming growth factor-β mediates balance between inflammation and fibrosis during plaque progression. *Arterioscler Thromb Vasc Biol* 22:975, 2002.

302. von der Thusen JH, van Vlijmen BJ, Hoeben RC, et al: Induction of atherosclerotic plaque rupture in apolipoprotein E⁻/⁻ mice after adenovirus-mediated transfer of p53. *Circulation* 105:2064, 2002.

303. Imanishi T, Han DK, Hofstra L, et al: Apoptosis of vascular smooth muscle cells is induced by Fas ligand derived from monocytes/macrophage. *Atherosclerosis* 161:143, 2002.

304. de Nooijer R, Verkleij CJ, von der Thusen JH, et al: Lesional overexpression of matrix metalloproteinase-9 promotes intraplaque hemorrhage in advanced lesions but not at earlier stages of atherogenesis. *Arterioscler Thromb Vasc Biol* 26:340, 2006.

305. Schwartz SM, Galis ZS, Rosenfeld ME, Falk E: Plaque rupture in humans and mice. *Arterioscler Thromb Vasc Biol* 27:705, 2007.

306. Fujii K, Kobayashi Y, Mintz GS, et al: Intravascular ultrasound assessment of ulcerated ruptured plaques: a comparison of culprit and nonculprit lesions of patients with acute coronary syndromes and lesions in patients without acute coronary syndromes. *Circulation* 108:2473, 2003.

307. Slager CJ, Wentzel JJ, Gijsen FJ, et al: The role of shear stress in the destabilization of vulnerable plaques and related therapeutic implications. *Nat Clin Pract Cardiovasc Med* 2:456, 2005.

308. Slager CJ, Wentzel JJ, Gijsen FJ, et al: The role of shear stress in the generation of rupture-prone vulnerable plaques. *Nat Clin Pract Cardiovasc Med* 2:401, 2005.

309. Mann J, Davies MJ: Mechanisms of progression in native coronary artery disease: role of healed plaque disruption. *Heart* 82:265, 1999.

310. Burke AP, Kolodgie FD, Farb A, et al: Healed plaque ruptures and sudden coronary death: evidence that subclinical rupture has a role in plaque progression. *Circulation* 103:934, 2001.

311. Ye Z, Liu EH, Higgins JP, et al: Seven haemostatic gene polymorphisms in coronary disease: meta-analysis of 66,155 cases and 91,307 controls. *Lancet* 367:651, 2006.

312. Sramek A, Kriek M, Rosendaal FR: Decreased mortality of ischaemic heart disease among carriers of haemophilia. *Lancet* 362:351, 2003.

313. Tuinenburg A, Mauser-Bunschoten EP, Verhaar MC, et al: Cardiovascular disease in patients with hemophilia. *J Thromb Haemost* 7:247, 2009.

314. Kitchens CS: The contact system. *Arch Pathol Lab Med* 126:1382, 2002.

315. Taubman MB, Wang L, Miller C: The role of smooth muscle derived tissue factor in mediating thrombosis and arterial injury. *Thromb Res* 122:S78, 2008.

316. Monroe DM, Hoffman M, Roberts HR: Platelets and thrombin generation. *Arterioscler Thromb Vasc Biol* 22:1381, 2002.

317. Furie B, Furie BC: Mechanisms of thrombus formation. *N Engl J Med* 359:938, 2008.

318. Borissoff JI, Spronk HM, Heeneman S, ten Cate H: Is thrombin a key player in the "coagulation-atherogenesis" maze? *Cardiovasc Res* 82:392, 2009.

319. Bea F, Kreuzer J, Preusch M, et al: Melagatran reduces advanced atherosclerotic lesion size and may promote plaque stability in apolipoprotein E–deficient mice. *Arterioscler Thromb Vasc Biol* 26:2787, 2006.

320. Seehaus S, Shahzad K, Kashif M, et al: Hypercoagulability inhibits monocyte trans-endothelial migration through protease-activated receptor-1–, phospholipase-Cβ–, phosphoinositide 3-kinase–, and nitric oxide–dependent signaling in monocytes and promotes plaque stability. *Circulation* 120:774, 2009.

321. Xiao Q, Danton MJS, Witte DP, et al: Plasminogen deficiency accelerates vessel wall disease in mice predisposed to atherosclerosis. *Proc Natl Acad Sci U S A* 94:10335, 1997.

322. Kremen M, Krishnan R, Emery I, et al: Plasminogen mediates the atherogenic effects of macrophage-expressed urokinase and accelerates atherosclerosis in apoE-knockout mice. *Proc Natl Acad Sci U S A* 105:17109, 2008.

323. Morgan TM, Krumholz HM, Lifton RP, Spertus JA: Nonvalidation of reported genetic risk factors for acute coronary syndrome in a large-scale replication study. *JAMA* 297:1551, 2007.

324. Yamada Y, Izawa H, Ichihara S, et al: Prediction of the risk of myocardial infarction from polymorphisms in candidate genes. *N Engl J Med* 347:1916, 2002.

325. Yamada Y, Matsuo H, Segawa T, et al: Assessment of genetic risk for myocardial infarction. *Thromb Haemost* 96:220, 2006.

326. Casas JP, Cooper J, Miller GJ: Investigating the genetic determinants of cardiovascular disease using candidate genes and meta-analysis of association studies. *Ann Hum Genet* 70:145, 2006.

327. Humphries SE, Cooper JA, Talmud PJ, Miller GJ: Candidate gene genotypes, along with conventional risk factor assessment, improve estimation of coronary heart disease risk in healthy UK men. *Clin Chem* 53:8, 2007.

328. Humphries SE, Yiannakouris N, Talmud PJ: Cardiovascular disease risk prediction using genetic information (gene scores): is it really informative? *Curr Opin Lipidol* 19:128, 2008.

329. Manolio TA, Boerwinkle E, O'Donnell CJ, Wilson AF: Genetics of ultrasonographic carotid atherosclerosis. *Arterioscler Thromb Vasc Biol* 24:1567, 2004.

330. Wang X, Ria M, Kelmenson PM, et al: Positional identification of TNFSF4, encoding OX40 ligand, as a gene that influences atherosclerosis susceptibility. *Nat Genet* 37:365, 2005.

331. Malarstig A, Eriksson P, Rose L, et al: Genetic variants of tumor necrosis factor super-family, member 4 (TNFSF4), and risk of incident atherothrombosis and venous throm-boembolism. *Clin Chem* 54:833, 2008.

332. Koch W, Hoppmann P, Mueller JC, et al: Lack of support for association between common variation in TNFSF4 and myocardial infarction in a German population. *Nat Genet* 40:1386; author reply 1387, 2008.

333. Clarke R, Xu P, Bennett D, et al: Lymphotoxin-α gene and risk of myocardial infarction in 6,928 cases and 2,712 controls in the ISIS case-control study. *PLoS Genet* 2:e107, 2006.

334. Lieb W, Mayer B, Konig IR, et al: Lack of association between the MEF2A gene and myocardial infarction. *Circulation* 117:185, 2008.

335. Assimes TL, Knowles JW, Priest JR, et al: Common polymorphisms of ALOX5 and ALOX5AP and risk of coronary artery disease. *Hum Genet* 123:399, 2008.

336. Shen GQ, Li L, Girelli D, et al: An LRP8 variant is associated with familial and prema-ture coronary artery disease and myocardial infarction. *Am J Hum Genet* 81:780, 2007.

337. Lieb W, Zeller T, Mangino M, et al: Lack of association of genetic variants in the LRP8 gene with familial and sporadic myocardial infarction. *J Mol Med* 86:1163, 2008.

338. Stephenson SH, Larrinaga-Shum S, Hopkins PN: Benefits of the MEDPED treatment support program for patients with familial hypercholesterolemia. *J Clin Lipidol* 3:94, 2009.

339. Versmissen J, Oosterveer DM, Yazdanpanah M, et al: Efficacy of statins in familial hypercholesterolaemia: a long term cohort study. *BMJ* 337:a2423, 2008.

340. Schunkert H, Gotz A, Braund P, et al: Repeated replication and a prospective meta-analysis of the association between chromosome 9p21.3 and coronary artery disease. *Circulation* 117:1675, 2008.

341. Kathiresan S, Voight BF, Purcell S, et al: Genome-wide association of early-onset myocardial infarction with single nucleotide polymorphisms and copy number vari-ants. *Nat Genet* 41:334, 2009.

342. Gudbjartsson DF, Bjornsdottir US, Halapi E, et al: Sequence variants affecting eosino-phil numbers associate with asthma and myocardial infarction. *Nat Genet* 41:342, 2009.

343. Erdmann J, Grosshennig A, Braund PS, et al: New susceptibility locus for coronary artery disease on chromosome 3q22.3. *Nat Genet* 41:280, 2009.

344. Shiffman D, O'Meara ES, Bare LA, et al: Association of gene variants with incident myocardial infarction in the Cardiovascular Health Study. *Arterioscler Thromb Vasc Biol* 28:173, 2008.

345. Shiffman D, Chasman DI, Zee RY, et al: A kinesin family member 6 variant is associated with coronary heart disease in the Women's Health Study. *J Am Coll Cardiol* 51:444, 2008.

346. Hunt SC, Williams RR, Barlow GK: A comparison of positive family history definitions for defining risk of future disease. *J Chronic Dis* 39:809, 1986.

347. Williams RR, Hunt SC, Heiss G, et al: Usefulness of cardiovascular family history data for population-based preventive medicine and medical research (The Health Family Tree Study and the NHLBI Family Heart Study). *Am J Cardiol* 87:129, 2001.

348. Hopkins PN, Hunt SC, Wu LL: Family history and genetic factors. In Wong ND, Black HR, Gardin JM, editors: *Preventive cardiology, a practical approach*, ed 2, New York, 2005, McGraw-Hill, pp 92-148.

349. Hopkins PN, Ellison RC, Province MA, et al: Association of coronary artery calcified plaque with clinical coronary heart disease in the National Heart, Lung and Blood Institute's Family Heart Study. *Am J Cardiol* 97:1564, 2006.

Note: Many abbreviations are traditionally not fully capitalized (such as Akt). In general, abbreviations that begin with an initial capital letter followed by lower case letters refer to the mouse gene, whereas all capitals refer to the human gene, but the literature is not consistent in this use. The most common usage is generally given here. An *s* may be added to the abbreviations shown here to indicate the plural (as in GPCRs).

ACAT1 — acyl coenzyme A:cholesterol acyltransferase (ACAT) 1; ACAT1 is in macrophages; ACAT2 is in liver and intestine, not macrophages

ADAMTS1 — a disintegrin and metalloproteinase with thrombospondin motif 1

ADFP — adipose differentiation-related protein

ADMA — asymmetric dimethylarginine

AGE — advanced glycation end products

Akt — also known as PKB; first identified as an oncogene from the AKT-8 thymoma cell line, which was derived from the AKR/J mouse

AP-1 — activator protein 1, which contains c-fos and c-Jun

ARE — antioxidant response element

ASK1 — apoptosis signal-regulating kinase 1

ASM — acid sphingomyelinase

ATF2 — activating transcription factor 2; the protein forms a homodimer or heterodimer with c-Jun and stimulates CRE-dependent transcription

ATP — adenosine triphosphate

AT₁R — angiotensin II type 1 receptor

Bad — Bcl-2–associated death promoter; a key regulatory protein for apoptosis; when phosphorylated (through growth factor receptors), it prevents apoptosis; when unphosphorylated, it promotes apoptosis

Bax — Bcl-2–associated X protein

Bcl-2 — B-cell CLL/lymphoma 2

BMP2/4 — bone morphogenic protein 2 or 4

CalDAG-GEF1 — calcium- and DAG-regulated GEF1

CaMKII — calcium/calmodulin-dependent protein kinase II

CBP — CREB-binding protein (also called p300 homologue or p300 or p300/CBP)

CCL2 — chemokine, CC motif, ligand 2 (also known as MCP-1)

CCR2 — chemokine, CC motif, receptor 2

CD14 — cluster of differentiation 14

CD40L — CD40 ligand; CD refers to "cluster of differentiation"

Cdc42 — cell division cycle 42 (a Rho family GTPase)

CEH — neutral cholesteryl ester hydrolase

CETP — cholesteryl ester transport protein

c-fos — FBJ (Finkel-Biskis-Jinkins) osteosarcoma oncogene; also known as FOS or Fos. The "c" refers to cellular as opposed to "v" for viral

c-Jun — abbreviated from Japanese, *ju-nana,* the number 17; derived from the ASV 17 provirus; also referred to as simply Jun

COX-2 — cyclooxygenase 2

CRE — cAMP response element

CREB — cAMP response element–binding protein

CRP — C-reactive protein

CSF1R — colony-stimulating factor 1 receptor; also known as FMS; receptor for M-CSF

CT — cytidine triphosphate:phosphocholine cytidylyltransferase

Cx43 — connexin 43

DAG — diacylglycerol

DIP1 — Dia-interacting protein 1

Dock2 — dedicator of cytokinesis 2

Dock180 — dedicator of cytokinesis 180; also known as Dock1; abbreviation can also mean "downstream of Crk-binding protein"

ECM — extracellular matrix

ECSIT — evolutionarily conserved signaling intermediate in toll pathways

EDHF — endothelium-derived hyperpolarizing factor

EGFR — epidermal growth factor receptor

Egr-1 — early growth response 1; a transcription factor activated by JNK

ELMO1 — engulfment and cell motility gene 1

eNOS — endothelial nitric oxide synthase

EP2 — prostaglandin E_2 receptor

ERK — extracellular signal-regulated kinase

ET-1 — endothelin 1

FAK — focal adhesion kinase

Fas — apoptosis-stimulating fragment; Fas is actually a cell receptor

FasL — Fas ligand

FGFR2 — fibroblast growth factor receptor 2

FilGAP — filamin A–associated Rho GAP

Fms — friend murine leukemia virus integration site 2; also known as CSF1R

FRS2 — fibroblast growth factor receptor substrate 2α

Gab1 — Grb2-associated binder 1

GAG — glycosaminoglycan

GAP — GTPase-activating protein (generally inactivates Ras family GTPases by converting GTP to GDP)

GAPDH — glyceraldehyde 3-phosphate dehydrogenase

GDI — G nucleotide dissociation inhibitor (inhibits dissociation of GDP or GTP from Ras-like proteins and maintains them as soluble cytosolic proteins, thereby blocking Ras or Rho signaling)

GEF — guanosine exchange factor; GEF facilitates exchange of GTP for GDP to activate Ras family proteins

GPCR — G protein–coupled receptor

Grb2 — growth factor receptor-bound protein 2 (acts as an adaptor protein between receptors and Sos)

8

GRO	growth-regulated oncogene α; also known as CXCL1GSSG
	glutathione–glutathione disulfide (oxidized glutathione)
GST	glutathione-*S*-transferase
GTP	guanosine triphosphate
H_2O_2	hydrogen peroxide
HCII	heparin cofactor II
HDL	high-density lipoprotein(s)
HETE	hydroxyeicosatetraenoic acid
HMGB1	high-mobility group box 1
4-HNE	4-hydroxy-2-nonenal
HO-1	heme oxygenase 1
HOCl	hypochlorous acid
HSF1	heat shock transcription factor 1
HSP	heat shock protein; HSP-70 aids in folding of nascent proteins; HSP-90 promotes eNOS activity; HSP-60 may be expressed in endothelial stress or activation and promote autoimmunity
IFN	interferon-γ
I B	inhibitor of NF-κB or inhibitor-κB
IKK	IκB kinase
IL	interleukin
IP3	inositol 1,4,5-triphosphate (soluble cytosolic intracellular messenger released after action of PLC)
IRAK1	interleukin-1 receptor–associated kinase 1
IRF3	interferon regulatory factor 3
JAK	Janus kinase (part of JAK-STAT pathway)
JNK	c-Jun N-terminal kinase (a MAPK)
Keap1	Kelch-like erythroid-derived cap'n'collar homology-associated protein 1
KLF2	Kruppel-like factor 2
LARG	leukemia-associated Rho GEF; also known as ARHGEF12
LDL	low-density lipoprotein(s)
LDLR	LDL receptor
LIAS	lipoic acid synthase
LIM	lin-11 isl-1 mec-3; the terms *lin* (for cell lineage), *isl*, and *mec* are genes in *Caenorhabditis elegans* that have homologous domains
LIMK	LIM domain kinase
LOX-1	lectin-like oxidized LDL receptor 1; coded by the *OLR1* gene (oxidized LDL receptor 1)
LPL	lipoprotein lipase
LpPLA₂	lipoprotein-associated phospholipase A_2; same as PAF-AH
LRP1	LDL receptor–related protein 1
MAD	mothers against decapentaplegic
MAPK	mitogen-activated protein kinase
MAPKK	MAPK kinase, also called a MEK (MAPK/ERK kinase)
MAPKKK	MAPKK kinase or MEKK (MEK kinase)
MARCO	macrophage receptor with collagenous structure
MCP-1	monocyte chemoattractant protein 1
M-CSF	monocyte colony-stimulating factor; also known as CSF-1
MD-2	origin of abbreviation obscure; also referred to as lymphocyte antigen (LY) 96; structural homology to mite allergen Der p 2
mDia1	microtubule-organizing formin diaphanous 1
MEF2C	myocyte enhancer factor 2C
MEK	MAPK/ERK kinase = MAPKK
MEKK	MEK kinase
MIF	macrophage migration inhibitory factor
MIP-1	macrophage inflammatory protein 1α; also known as CCL3
MIP-1	macrophage inflammatory protein 1β; also known as CCL4
MKK	MAP kinase kinase
MKP-1	MAPK phosphatase 1
MLCK	myosin light-chain kinase
mmLDL	minimally modified LDL
MMP	matrix metalloproteinase
MSR	macrophage scavenger receptor (name of the gene that gives rise to both SR-AI and SR-AII through alternate splicing)
MyD88	myeloid differentiation primary response protein 88
NADPH	nicotine adenine dinucleotide phosphate (H = reduced form)
NEMO	NF-κB essential modulator (part of the IKK complex); also known as IKKY
NF- B	nuclear factor-κB
NK cells	natural killer cells
Nrf2	nuclear factor erythroid 2–like related factor 2
NO	nitric oxide
O_2^-	superoxide anion
Oct1	octomer-binding transcription factor 1
OH	hydroxyl radical
OLR1	oxidized LDL receptor 1 gene
ONOO⁻	peroxynitrite radical
oxLDL	oxidized LDL (generally considered rather severely oxidized)
PAF	platelet-activating factor
PAF-AH	platelet-activating factor acyl hydrolase, also called LpPLA₂
PAK	p21-activated kinase
PAMP	pathogen-associated molecular pattern(s)
PAR1	protease-activated receptor 1 (the receptor activated by thrombin)
Par6	partitioning defective protein 6 (involved in cell polarization with Cdc42)
PARG	poly(ADP-ribose) glycohydrolase
PARP-1	poly(ADP-ribose) polymerase 1
PCAF	p300/CBP-associated factor
PDGF	platelet-derived growth factor
PDZK1	PDZ domain–containing protein 1; PDZ domains frequently involve organization of receptors, ion channels, or signaling molecules at the inner cell membrane; PDZ stands for the original recognition of shared structure in 3 proteins, PSD-95, DlgA, and ZO-1
PECAM-1	platelet and endothelial cell adhesion molecule 1
PGI₂	prostacyclin
PH	pleckstrin homology (a domain found in many proteins)
PI3K	phosphatidylinositol 3-kinase
PIP3	phosphatidylinositol 3,4,5-phosphate (membrane bound)
-PIX	Pak-interacting exchange factor beta; also known as Cool-1 and Gef7
PKB	protein kinase B (also known as Akt)
PKC	protein kinase C; there are several different isoforms: α, β1, β2, and γ are *conventional* (sensitive to calcium and DAG); δ, ε, η, and θ are *novel* (sensitive to DAG but not to calcium); ζ, ι, and λ are *atypical* (not sensitive to calcium or DAG)
PKL	paxillin-kinase linker; also known as GIT2

PLA$_2$ phospholipase A$_2$ (soluble, sPLA$_2$, and lipoprotein-associated, LpPLA$_2$, are commonly described, but other forms are also known)

PLC phospholipase C; different isoforms include β1-4 (mainly activated by the G$_q$ class of G proteins that couple to GPCRs; γ1, 2 (activated by receptor protein tyrosine kinases or nonreceptor protein tyrosine kinases and further stimulated by PIP3); δ1-4 (possibly activated by calcium or G proteins); ε (activated by Ras and Rap); and ζ (found only in mammalian sperm and sensitive to calcium)

PLD phospholipase D

PLTP phospholipid transfer protein

PPAR peroxisome proliferator-activated receptor (there are α, γ, and δ forms)

PRDX1 peroxiredoxin 1

PSGL1 P-selectin glycoprotein ligand 1

PTEN phosphatase and tensin homologue

Rac1 Ras-related C3 botulinum toxin substrate 1

RAF1 murine leukemia viral oncogene homologue 1; the derivation of the abbreviation is not clear; a MAP kinase kinase kinase or MEK kinase; typically activated by Ras but has multiple phosphorylation sites that can upregulate or downregulate activity; inactivated when bound to the 14-3-3 regulatory protein

Rag-1 recombinase activator gene 1

RAGE receptor for advanced glycation end products (AGE)

Ral Ras-like protein; also RalA

RANTES regulated on activation normal T cell expressed and secreted; also known as CCL5

Rap1 Ras-related protein 1

Ras named for a transforming oncogene found in rat sarcoma; the Ras superfamily are monomeric GTPases that act as off-on switches (off when GDP is bound, on when GTP is bound); members of the family include Ras, Rho/Rac, Rab, Rap, Arf, Ral, Ran, Rheb, Rad, Rit, and Miro; more than a hundred members are known; Ras superfamily proteins have geranyl-geranyl lipid anchors for attachment to the inner cell membrane

Rho Ras homologous; one of the members of the Ras superfamily of GTPases; RhoA, Cdc42, Rac1 are common Rho family members

ROCK Rho-associated, coiled-coil containing protein kinase; also referred to frequently as simply Rho kinase

S1P sphingosine 1-phosphate; receptors are S1P1 through 5 (also known as S1PR1-5 and "endothelial differentiation gene" or EDG receptors)

SDF1 stromal cell–derived factor 1; also known as CXCL12

SH glutathione (the –SH refers to reduced sulfur on cysteine)

SH2 Src homology domain 2 (a conserved protein domain that recognizes phosphorylated tyrosines)

Shc Src homology collagen-like; an adaptor protein whose SH2 domain binds phosphorylated tyrosine on the cytosolic domain of RTKs (receptor tyrosine kinases) and also binds Grb2

SHP-2 SH2 domain–containing tyrosine phosphatase

SMAD SMAD proteins are homologues of both the *Drosophila* protein mothers against decapentaplegic (MAD) and the *C. elegans* protein SMA; the name is a combination of the two

SMC smooth muscle cells

SOCS suppressors of cytokine signaling

SOD superoxide dismutase (Cu/Zn SOD = copper/zinc superoxide dismutase—in cytoplasm; MnSod = manganese superoxide dismutase—in mitochondria)

Sos son of sevenless; may be referred to as mSos; a GEF for Ras family proteins; binds to the adapter Grb2

SR-A scavenger receptor A (implies both AI and AII, alternate splice isoforms of the same *MSR* gene)

SR-B1 scavenger receptor B1 (an HDL receptor)

Src pronounced "sarc" (short for sarcoma), the first identified of a family of proto-oncogenic tyrosine kinases

SREC scavenger receptor expressed by endothelial cells

SR-PSOX scavenger receptor–phosphatidyl serine and oxidized lipoprotein

STAT1 signal transducer and activator of transcription 1

Syk spleen tyrosine kinase

TAB1/2 TAK1-binding protein 1 and 2

TAK1 TGF-β–activated kinase 1 (a MEKK)

tBHQ *tert*-butylhydroquinone

TBK1 TANK-binding kinase 1

TF tissue factor

TFPI tissue factor pathway inhibitor

TGF- transforming growth factor-β

TGRL triglyceride-rich lipoproteins (includes chylomicrons, VLDL, and remnants)

Th1 T-helper type 1 lymphocytes

TIAM1 T-lymphoma invasion and metastasis 1

TLR4 toll-like receptor 4

TM thrombomodulin

TNF- tumor necrosis factor-α

TRAF6 TNF receptor–associated factor 6

TRAM TRIF-related adaptor molecule

TRAP tumor necrosis factor receptor–associated protein

TRIF toll/IL-1 receptor domain–containing adaptor inducing interferon-β

Trx thioredoxin

TXNIP thioredoxin-interacting protein

UbC13 ubiquitin-conjugating enzyme 13

UEV1A ubiquitin-conjugating enzyme E2 variant 1 isoform A

uPA urokinase-type plasminogen activator

VASP vasodilator-stimulated phosphoprotein (with functions analogous to WASp)

Vav1-3 named for *vav*, the sixth letter in the Hebrew alphabet (for the sixth oncogene discovered at the laboratory that characterized the protein); the Vav proteins are GEFs for Rac

VCAM-1	vascular cell adhesion molecule 1	**vWF**	von Willebrand factor
VE-cadherin	vascular endothelial cadherin	**WASp**	Wiskott-Aldrich syndrome protein
VEGFR2	vascular endothelial growth factor receptor 2, also called Flk-1	**WAVE**	WASp family verprolin homology domain–containing protein
VLDL	very-low-density lipoprotein(s)	**ZO-1**	zona occludens 1

Blood Pressure

CHAPTER **9**

Hypertension: JNC 7 and Beyond

William J. Elliott

people with chronic kidney disease, or those with established heart disease, but the evidence for these targets is controversial.

- Despite the widespread availability of many effective and inexpensive antihypertensive drugs, hypertension control rates are

suboptimal. A concerted effort by the health care provider, patient, and health care delivery system is required to control blood pressure in the long term and to reduce the risk of cardiovascular disease.

KEY POINTS

- Reducing high blood pressure, an important and the most common cardiovascular risk factor, prevents or delays the onset of many types of cardiovascular disease.

- Measurement of blood pressure as an independent risk factor for cardiovascular disease can be easily and inexpensively accomplished in the medical office, in the home, or by sophisticated devices.

- Dietary sodium restriction reduces the long-term risk of cardiovascular disease, but weight loss is the most effective short-term lifestyle modification to lower blood pressure.

- Drug therapy for hypertension reduces the risk of cardiovascular disease more than placebo or no treatment. Different expert panels do not agree on a universally applicable treatment algorithm, but all agree that a hypertensive drug that improves prognosis can be given to the patient with a compelling indication for that drug.

- The traditional treatment target for blood pressure is <140/90 mm Hg in uncomplicated hypertensives; <130/80 mm Hg has been recommended for diabetics,

Elevated blood pressure (BP) is responsible for more deaths than any other risk factor for cardiovascular disease (CVD), which is already the leading cause of death and disability in the developed world and is expected to become the leading cause of death and disability worldwide by the year 2025.[1] Historically, "hypertension" (BP ≥140/90 mm Hg) was thought to be the major driver of these problems, but BP levels between 120-139/80-89 mm Hg (now called prehypertension) not only are more prevalent but also elevate cardiovascular risk.[1,2] Compared with many other risk factors for stroke, acute myocardial infarction, and heart failure, hypertension is among the simplest to diagnose, has the widest variety of treatment options, and (particularly in high-risk individuals) is the most cost-effective preventive strategy.[3-5] Because of its high prevalence (e.g., ~29% of adults; Fig. 9-1) in the United States,[6] hypertension ranks first among the chronic conditions for which Americans visit a health care provider.[3,7,8] One of the major reasons for the impressive reduction in age-adjusted stroke mortality (~62%) and coronary heart disease (CHD) mortality (~45%) in the United States since 1972 is the widespread acceptance of the need to treat hypertension and our increased ability to reduce BP effectively.[8]

HYPERTENSION GUIDELINES

Because of the global public health impact of hypertension, many countries and organizations have developed guidelines for its diagnosis and treatment.[3-5,9] There are major differences in how frequently these are updated, and there is little consensus among them regarding risk stratification, initial therapy, or BP targets (Table 9-1). Nonetheless, these interesting recommendations summarize our current knowledge but come to very different conclusions.

PATHOPHYSIOLOGY OF HYPERTENSION

Although several genetic forms of hypertension have been discovered and many secondary causes of hypertension identified, most hypertensive individuals have primary (or essential) hypertension, for which no specific cause can be found. Many neurohormonal systems affect BP, and many of these have been manipulated pharmacologically to assist with its control. Perhaps chief among these are the renally regulated "BP–vascular volume" concept, the renin-angiotensin-aldosterone system (RAAS), and the sympathetic nervous system (SNS).[10] Much recent work has developed the concept of dysregulation of nitric oxide (and oxidative stress) as a potential contributor to CVD, including hypertension.[11] Although animal studies, epidemiologic evidence, small cohort trials, and a few larger randomized clinical trials have implicated nitric oxide, we have few pharmacologic agents specific to this system that are clinically useful in large populations of free-living hypertensive patients. Further research is therefore necessary before the *Science Magazine* "molecule of the year" in 1998 achieves the status of the RAAS or SNS as a major contributor to elevated BP.

DEFINITION AND CLASSIFICATION OF HYPERTENSION

9

From 1974 to 1993, hypertension in the United States was defined only by diastolic BP (≥90 mm Hg) and was classified as mild, moderate, or severe. Since then, burgeoning evidence from both epidemiologic studies[12] and clinical trials[13,14] has demonstrated that systolic BP is a better predictor of future CVD and renal events than diastolic or pulse pressure is. Therefore, the focus has shifted to systolic BP, particularly

because most hypertensives (especially those older than 55 years) have pretreatment systolic BP ≥ 140 mm Hg rather than diastolic BP ≥ 90 mm Hg. Similarly, the classification system has evolved into "stages" of hypertension (Table 9-2), of which JNC 7 recognizes only two: stage 1 (systolic BP 140-159 mm Hg or diastolic BP 90-99 mm Hg) and stage 2 (systolic BP ≥ 160 mm Hg or diastolic BP ≥ 100 mm Hg).[3] This scheme is independent of gender and age, although many authorities have suggested that higher risk individuals (e.g., African Americans, diabetics, kidney and disease patients) should have BP-lowering treatment initiated at threshold BPs lower than 140/90 mm Hg. This suggestion has been carried to its logical extreme by several sets of guidelines[5,9] that base diagnosis and treatment decisions on the absolute risk of CVD for a given individual and not on any specific cutoff for BP. Proponents of the "polypill" (which contains three antihypertensive agents at moderate doses) have recommended that not only classification of BP but also measurement of BP should be abandoned in favor of BP lowering in demographically defined populations at high risk for CVD.[15] This approach denies the benefits of therapy to those who are likely to suffer target organ damage and worsened hypertension, rather than CVD events, if left untreated.

Prehypertension was defined in JNC 7 as BPs between 120-139/80-89 mm Hg,[3] but the term has been largely ignored by other guidelines. Some believe that the term is too pessimistic and deterministic, but in the Framingham cohort, more than 90% of individuals who are not already hypertensive at the age of 55 years become so during the next 25 years of follow-up.[16] Individuals with this level of BP clearly have increased CVD risk compared with normotensives (BP < 120/80 mm Hg).[2] In the most recent population-based survey of American adults, prehypertension (43% prevalence in men, 30% in women) was more common than hypertension (only 30% and 28%, respectively).[6] Because there are many more prehypertensive than hypertensive individuals in most populations,[1] the burden of BP-related illness would soar if this "disease label" was widely accepted. Although lifestyle modifications are generally recommended for these individuals,[3] and pharmacologic therapy with a moderate-dose angiotensin receptor blocker (ARB) was "feasible" (and significantly prevented the transition to frank hypertension),[17] outcomes from large clinical trials are currently lacking to address the question of whether lowering of BP in prehypertensives is effective in preventing CVD. The intent of JNC 7 in introducing the term was to highlight the elevated CVD risk and to motivate affected individuals to pursue strategies to lower their BP, not (as some have suggested) to increase the sales of antihypertensive drugs.

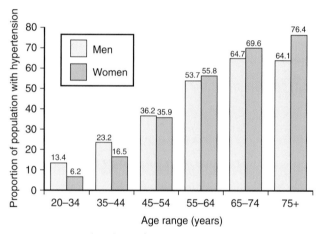

FIGURE 9-1 Age- and gender-specific prevalence of hypertension in the National Health and Nutrition Examination Survey (NHANES) 2005-2006.[8] As in all previous NHANES data sets going back to 1971, hypertension was defined as BP ≥140/90 mm Hg or taking antihypertensive medication. The overall prevalence of hypertension was about 29% (no significant change since NHANES 1999-2000), but the prevalence of the awareness, treatment, and control (to <140/90 mm Hg) of hypertension has improved to 78%, 68%, and 44%, respectively.[6]

TABLE 9–1	Recommendations of Different Sets of Hypertension Guidelines			
	JNC 7, 2003	**ASHWG, 2005**	**NICE, 2006**	**ESH/ESC, 2007**
Risk stratification	Based on BP only	Based on tests for target organ damage, not BP	Based on absolute risk	Extensive system based on absolute risk
Default initial therapy	Low-dose diuretic		Calcium channel blocker or angiotensin-converting enzyme inhibitor (age dependent)	Does not matter; most need two drugs anyway
Beta blockers	Second-line	No comment	Fourth-line	Not with diuretics in patients with metabolic syndrome
BP targets	<130/80 mm Hg for diabetics, chronic kidney disease		Lower for diabetics	<130/80 mm Hg for diabetics, even lower if renal dysfunction and proteinuria >1 g/day

JNC 7, Seventh Report of the Joint National Committee on Prevention, Detection, Evaluation, and Treatment of High Blood Pressure[3]; ASHWG, American Society of Hypertension Writing Group[9]; NICE, National Institute for Health and Clinical Excellence (British National Guidelines)[4]; ESH/ESC, European Society of Hypertension/European Society of Cardiology.[5]

JNC 7 Threshold	Setting		
	Office[3]	Home (self)[19]	24-Hour Ambulatory[23]
Prehypertension	120/80 mm Hg	115/75 mm Hg	About 114/72 mm Hg
Target for "high-risk" patients	130/80 mm Hg	130/80 mm Hg	Probably 123/77 mm Hg
Stage 1 hypertension (for diagnosis)	140/90 mm Hg	135/85 mm Hg	133/82 mm Hg
Stage 2 hypertension (for diagnosis)	160/100 mm Hg	155/95 mm Hg	About 152/93 mm Hg

TABLE 9–2 | Some Useful "Cut Points" for Blood Pressure

Modified from JNC 7,[3] the American Heart Association Scientific Statement,[19] and the European Society of Hypertension.[23]

MEASUREMENT OF BLOOD PRESSURE

Although the recommendation to eschew measurement of BP in favor of its lowering has recently been made,[15] terminology first introduced by Nicolai Korotkoff in 1905 is still used in recording of indirectly determined BPs.[18] Systolic BP is recognized when clear and repetitive tapping sounds are heard; diastolic BP is recorded when the sounds disappear. Only when audible sounds are heard down to 0 mm Hg is the "muffling" of sound (Korotkoff phase IV) recorded, between the systolic reading and zero (e.g., 178/72/0 mm Hg).

Techniques of Measuring Blood Pressure

The proper technique of accurate BP measurement is typically taught very early during medical training but seldom followed thereafter. Experience in many clinical trials has shown that retraining and at least yearly certification in BP measurement are often required to obtain meaningful BP data. One reason for including a placebo arm in registration trials of new antihypertensive drugs is to account for the many potential confounders in BP measurement, including observer expectation bias. The current push for "pay-for-performance" (which includes BP as one indicator of quality of care) is likely to lead to an overabundance of "8" as the terminal digit preference of BPs recorded by health care professionals in many office settings to ensure the greatest possible proportion of customers who are below national BP thresholds. Interestingly, current Healthcare Effectiveness Data and Information Set (HEDIS) guidelines have made achievement of BP goals more likely. Before 2007, the lowest recorded BP (systolic and diastolic) obtained simultaneously at an office visit was accepted as "the" BP for that visit. In the most recent revision, however, the lowest recorded systolic and the lowest recorded diastolic (even if obtained many minutes apart) are accepted, biasing the probability of a below-threshold BP higher.

Home Blood Pressure Measurements

Because of these and many similar challenges, more emphasis is being placed on measurements outside the medical office. Home (or self) BP monitoring is the least expensive and most widely applicable to large populations. Many convenient, inexpensive, and relatively accurate machines are now available. Some authorities think that such devices should be provided to every person with elevated BP and that

their physicians should be paid for interpreting home BP data,[19] but others are concerned about their widespread use because clinical trials have seldom based their treatment decisions solely on home readings.

Home BP readings are typically lower than measurements taken in the traditional medical environment (by about 12/7 mm Hg on average), even in normotensive subjects. Home readings are better correlated with both the extent of target organ damage and the risk of future CVD events or mortality than are readings taken in the health care provider's office. Home readings can also be helpful in evaluating symptoms suggestive of hypotension, especially if they are intermittent or infrequent. During treatment, reliable home readings can lower costs by substituting for multiple visits to health care providers.

Current recommendations advocate use of validated oscillometric devices with an appropriately sized cuff around the upper arm. The device should be calibrated against a standard sphygmomanometer (using a Y tube) and the technique of the measurer checked. At least 12 (a week of twice-daily duplicate or triplicate) readings are the minimum on which to base treatment decisions.[19] Home BP monitoring, coupled with remote monitoring and feedback by a health care professional, has improved BP control rates, perhaps by improving medication adherence.[20,21]

Ambulatory Blood Pressure Monitoring

Automatic recorders are now available that measure BP frequently in a 24-hour period, during a person's usual daily activities (including sleep). In the United States, devices that measure BP indirectly (i.e., without arterial cannulation) use either an auscultatory or an oscillometric technique. The auscultatory type uses a microphone placed over the artery to detect Korotkoff sounds in the traditional fashion. The oscillometric technique measures biophysical oscillations of the brachial artery, which are compared (by use of a proprietary algorithm) with those observed with a mercury sphygmomanometer; systolic BP is determined directly from the threshold oscillation, mean arterial pressure is estimated, and diastolic BP is calculated. Both types of monitors are lightweight (<450 g), simple to apply and to use, accurate, relatively quiet and tolerable, and powered by two to four small batteries. Data from 80 to 120 measurements of BP and pulse rate (usually every 15 to 20 minutes during waking hours and every 30 minutes during the night) typically are stored in a small microprocessor and then downloaded into a desktop computer, which then edits the readings and prints the report. Much research with the use of ambulatory blood pressure monitoring (ABPM) has suggested that this technique is the most accurate method of measuring BP, correlates most closely with target organ damage, and best predicts future cardiovascular events (even independently of office BP measurements).[22] In the research setting, ABPM readings have therefore become accepted as the "gold standard" of BP measurements. Accordingly, several expert panels have provided both correlations between ABPM results and BP measurements in other settings (see Table 9-2) and recommendations for its use (Box 9-1).[22,23] Although this method of measuring BP is becoming "standard of care" in many settings, its use is limited in the United States by restrictions on reimbursement for the procedure, which currently in the Medicare age group amounts to $60 to $90, **only** when the result is a new diagnosis of white coat hypertension.

ABPM makes it possible to measure BP routinely during sleep and has reawakened interest in the circadian variation of heart rate and BP. Most normotensives and perhaps 80% of hypertensives have at least a 10% drop in BP during sleep compared with the daytime average. Although there may be some important demographic confounders (African

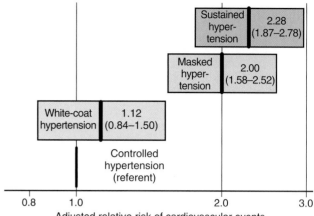

BOX 9-1 Indications for Ambulatory Blood Pressure Monitoring

Diagnosis and Prognosis
Evaluation of suspected white coat hypertension
Evaluation of refractory or resistant hypertension
Evaluation of circadian pattern of blood pressure

Symptoms
Evaluation of dizziness, presyncope, and syncope
Evaluation of relationship of blood pressure to clinical symptoms

Evaluation of Antihypertensive Agents (research based)
Evaluation of trough-to-peak ratios (and determine optimal dosing intervals)
Evaluation of antihypertensive efficacy
Evaluation of effects of timing of dosing of antihypertensive agents

Modified from Pickering et al[22] and O'Brien et al.[23]

FIGURE 9-2 Comparison of cardiovascular risk in white coat and masked hypertension with sustained and controlled hypertension. Each box corresponds to the 95% confidence limits (also given numerically within each box), and the dark vertical line within each box corresponds to the adjusted relative risk (also given numerically within each box). This meta-analysis summarizes the 912 first cardiovascular events in seven published observational studies involving 11,502 subjects with an average baseline age of 63 ± 6.5 years, during 8.0 years of mean follow-up.[24] All subjects had their blood pressures monitored in the office (where control was <140/90 mm Hg) and outside the office (where control was <135/85 mm Hg). There was no significant difference in prognosis between those whose blood pressures were controlled both at and outside the office (n = 3827, or 33.3% of the population studied) and those whose blood pressures were controlled only at home but not at the office (n = 1550, or 13.5% of the population studied). These observations support the concept that white coat hypertension has a better prognosis than sustained hypertension. The risk of individuals with masked hypertension (n = 1306, or 11.4% of the population studied: controlled blood pressure at the office but not at home) was not significantly different from that of sustained hypertensives in both locales (n = 4819, or 41.9% of the population studied), and both of these groups had a worse prognosis than that of those with controlled hypertension.

Americans and the elderly have less prominent "dips"), several prospective studies have shown an increased risk of cardiovascular events (and proteinuria in type 1 diabetics) among those with a nocturnal "nondipping" BP or pulse pattern. Several Japanese studies have raised concern that elderly persons with more than a 20% difference between nighttime and daytime average BPs ("excessive dippers") may suffer unrecognized ischemia in "watershed areas" (of the brain and other organs) during sleep if their BP declines below the autoregulatory threshold.

White Coat and Masked Hypertension

Approximately 10% to 20% of American hypertensives have substantially lower BP measurements outside the health care provider's office than in it (so-called white coat hypertension). The white coat itself is unlikely to be the only factor that increases BP. Careful studies originally done in Italy (and now corroborated elsewhere) show that BP rises in response to an approaching physician who is not previously known to the subject. The acute elevation in BP apparently is less marked if a nurse approaches the subject, even if the nurse is wearing a white coat. The pathophysiologic and psychological "reasons" for this exaggerated BP response are unclear.

The clinical consequences, prognostic significance, and amenability of white coat hypertension to drug treatment are controversial. One point of view suggests that if a person has an acute rise in BP due to "stress" from an approaching physician, similar elevations in BP are likely whenever any stressful stimulus is encountered. In several convenience samples and population-based studies, people with white coat hypertension had a greater prevalence of subclinical risk factors for CVD, including left ventricular hypertrophy, family history of hypertension and heart disease, hypertriglyceridemia, elevated fasting insulin levels, and lower HDL-cholesterol levels.

A minority view, based on more conservative definitions of the "white coat effect," proposes that some individuals consistently show a similar and marked elevation in BP in response to the health care environment. Several long-term observational studies have shown a much reduced risk of either target organ damage or major CVD sequelae among people with lower BPs measured either at home or by 24-hour BP monitoring compared with measurements taken in the same person in the physician's office. A recent meta-analysis of the seven published observational studies showed that the 1550 patients with white coat hypertension had a significantly *lower* risk of CVD than the 4819 with sustained

hypertension and a nonsignificant and only slightly higher risk than the 3827 with hypertension controlled in both the office and at home (Fig. 9-2).[24] An intermediate viewpoint is that white coat hypertension is merely regression to the mean among the subset of patients with high BP variability.

Masked hypertension is said to be present when the in-office BPs are significantly lower than those measured in other settings. Originally thought to be more common in young women with large childcare responsibilities, this condition is now found more widely, in perhaps 6% to 12% of the general population.[24] As such patients would normally not be offered drug treatment (as their in-office BPs are, by definition, below treatment thresholds), masked hypertension is associated with a higher prevalence of target organ damage and incidence of CVD events than in true normotensives. In the seven published observational studies, the 1306 patients with this form of hypertension had only a slightly (and nonsignificant) reduced risk of future CVD events compared with the 4819 patients with sustained hypertension.[24] Many have therefore recommended ABPM (or at least home readings) for **all** people at risk for hypertension as this is the only way to detect masked hypertension.

BLOOD PRESSURE AND CARDIOVASCULAR RISK

Initial estimates of how much elevated BP increases the risk of heart attack, heart failure, stroke, and other CVD events were derived from prospective epidemiologic surveys. Perhaps the most well known of these in the United States is

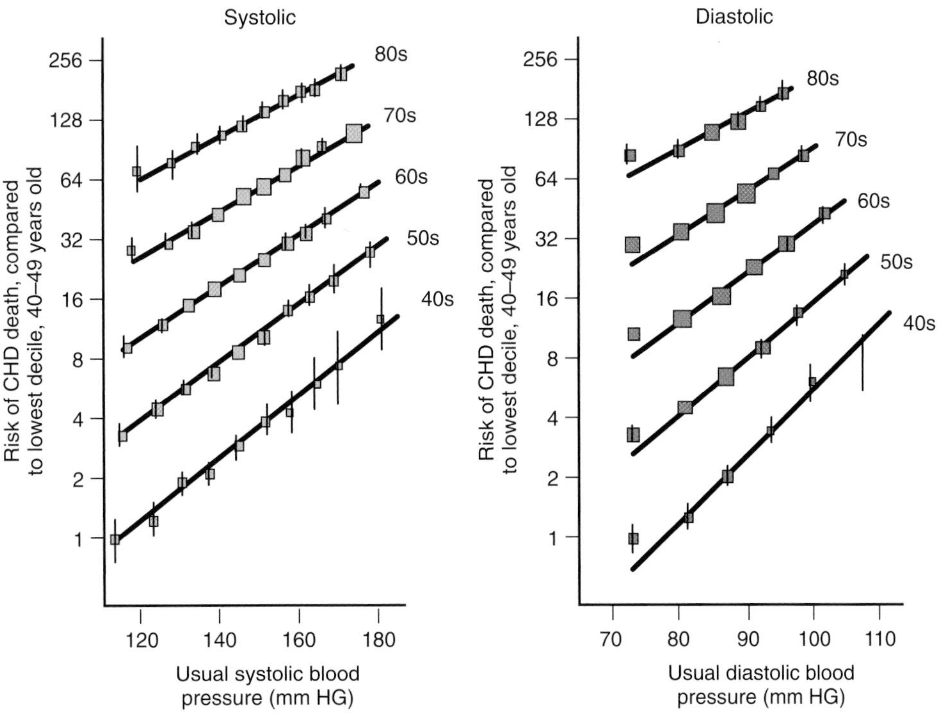

Systolic

Diastolic

FIGURE 9-3 Relationship of risk of death from CHD (on a logarithmic scale) and the initial blood pressures (systolic at left, diastolic at right) measured at the beginning of each decade of life (given at the top of each line, from 40 to 89 years) in nearly 1 million participants in 61 epidemiologic studies. Larger boxes indicate estimates with smaller 95% confidence intervals, which are indicated for smaller boxes by the vertical lines. The total number of fatal CHD deaths was 30,143. The best-fit regression line for each decade of life ignores the point corresponding to the lowest blood pressure (always <115/70 mm Hg), which includes some individuals with *very* low blood pressures. *(Modified from Prospective Studies Collaborative.* Lancet *360:1903, 2002.)*

the Framingham Heart Study, in which 5209 healthy men and women were extensively evaluated initially and then observed over time. After a sufficient number of subjects had events, a quantitative estimate could be made of the importance of hypertension in the development of these events, even after adjusting statistically for the presence of other risk factors (e.g., elevated plasma lipid levels or smoking). Data from Framingham and 60 other observational and epidemiologic data bases have been pooled (Fig. 9-3) and clearly show *a strong, positive, and continuous relationship* between the level of initial BP and the future risk of death from CHD.[12] Within each decade of life, for each BP increase of 20/10 mm Hg, beginning at 115/75 mm Hg, the risk of death from CHD, stroke, or CVD *doubles.*[12] These data also show that systolic BP is a much better predictor than diastolic BP or even pulse pressure of CVD and CHD outcomes.[12]

Perhaps more important than epidemiologic and observational studies of large numbers of people that correlate risk of death from heart disease and BP levels many years earlier are the results of prospective, randomized clinical trials that show, separately and in aggregate, that antihypertensive drug therapy reduces the risk of CHD and other CVD events during a ≤6-year time frame. Most impressive are the results of studies comparing placebo or no treatment with antihypertensive drugs (typically diuretics and beta blockers in older studies, although a few studies with angiotensin-converting enzyme [ACE] inhibitors or calcium antagonists exist). Figure 9-4 shows the results of meta-analyses of 32 clinical trials that compared placebo or no treatment with an initial diuretic, beta blocker, calcium antagonist, or ACE inhibitor in the

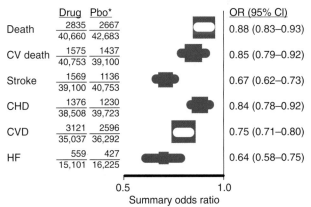

FIGURE 9-4 Results of meta-analyses of clinical trials involving placebo or no treatment compared with an *initial* low-dose diuretic, beta blocker, ACE inhibitor, or calcium antagonist in the prevention of cardiovascular events in hypertensive subjects. The results, all of which are highly significant (with no significant inhomogeneity), change only slightly if trials that gave the randomized agent as add-on therapy are included. The numbers above or below the line for each event are the numbers of subjects with that event or at risk for that event. *Pbo, placebo or no treatment; OR (95% CI), odds ratio (95% confidence interval); CV, cardiovascular; CHD, coronary heart disease; CVD, cardiovascular disease (first CHD event, stroke, or CV death); HF, heart failure. *(Updated from Elliott WJ: Cardiovascular events in clinical trials of antihypertensive drugs vs. placebo/no treatment: a meta-analysis [abstract],* J Hypertens 23[Suppl 2]:S273, 2005.)*

9

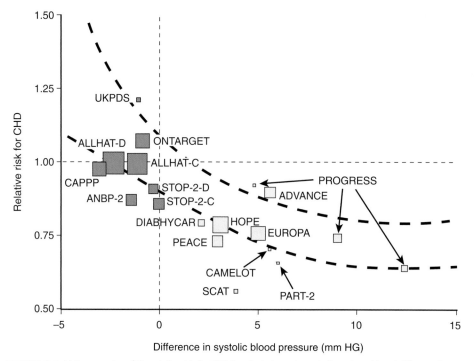

FIGURE 9-5 Meta-regression of the relative risk for CHD (*y*-axis, test agent–control) on the achieved difference in systolic blood pressure between randomized groups (control–test agent) in 27 clinical trials involving ACE inhibitors (placebo control in open squares, active control in filled squares). The regression line and its 95% confidence intervals are based on data from 27 older clinical trials.[25] ADVANCE, Action in Diabetes and Vascular disease: preterAx and diamicroN-MR Controlled Evaluation; ALLHAT-D, Antihypertensive and Lipid-Lowering treatment to prevent Heart Attack Trial–Diuretic comparison; ALLHAT-C, Antihypertensive and Lipid-Lowering treatment to prevent Heart Attack Trial–Calcium antagonist comparison; ANBP-2, Australian National Blood Pressure trial 2; CAMELOT, Comparison of AMlodipine vs. Enalapril to Limit Occurrences of Thrombosis; CAPPP, CAptopril Primary Prevention Project; DIABHYCAR, DIABetes, HYpertension, microalbuminuria or proteinuria, Cardiovascular events And Ramipril; EUROPA, EURopean Reduction Of cardiac events with Perindopril in stable coronary Artery disease; HOPE, Heart Outcomes Prevention Evaluation; ONTARGET, ONgoing Telmisartan Alone and in combination with Ramipril Global Endpoint Trial; PART-2, Prevention of Atherosclerosis with Ramipril Trial 2; PEACE, Prevention of Events with Angiotensin-Converting Enzyme inhibition; PROGRESS, Perindopril pROtection aGainst REcurrent Stroke Study; SCAT, Simvastatin/enalapril Coronary Atherosclerosis Trial; STOP-2-C, Swedish Trial in Old Patients with hypertension 2–Calcium antagonist comparison; STOP-2-D, Swedish Trial in Old Patients with hypertension 2–Diuretic or beta blocker comparison; UKPDS, United Kingdom Prospective Diabetes Study. (*Updated from Elliott WJ, Jonsson MC, Black HR: Management of hypertension: is it the pressure or the drug?* Circulation 113:2763, 2006.)

prevention of CVD in hypertensive subjects. These data indicate highly significant benefit of BP-lowering drugs in hypertensive individuals across all types of CVD *and* all-cause mortality.

Perhaps the most direct and persuasive evidence in favor of the link between BP lowering and CVD (especially CHD) events in clinical trials can be shown in one of several meta-regression analyses correlating the difference in achieved systolic BP across randomized arms in large numbers of clinical trials involving hundreds of thousands of subjects with the relative risk for the specific CVD event (Fig. 9-5).[13,14,25,26] With the exception of heart failure, these analyses generally show that a larger difference in achieved systolic BP (rather than the change in BP or initial BP) is associated with a larger difference between the randomized arms in CVD endpoints. For example, in the first such report, the differences in CHD across randomized treatment groups in trials was not at all well explained by the initial BPs of the participants in each trial ($r^2 = 0.02$; $P = 0.37$) but was instead highly significantly correlated with differences across groups in achieved systolic BP ($r^2 = 0.53$; $P = 0.0005$).[25] Such analyses also have been used to claim "benefit beyond BP control" for specific antihypertensive drug classes in preventing specific endpoints (e.g., ACE inhibitors preventing CHD),[14,27] but this is controversial.[26]

These data (both epidemiologic and those derived from clinical trials) have been interpreted in several different ways. Several groups have pointed out that elevated BP is but one (relatively minor) predictor of CVD[28]; age, for example, is a much more powerful risk factor. The sensitivity and specificity of BP are low; not everyone with elevated BP will eventually have an event, just as, regrettably, not every person with a "normal" BP will be spared. Any strategy that attempts to fix a value above which everyone should receive treatment is unlikely to be successful and cost-effective. These authorities recommend instead that treatment decisions about BP should be based on a person's *absolute* risk of CVD, which can be easily estimated by one of several country-specific risk estimators[28]; the Framingham risk equation is the most widely used of these in the United States and has been recently updated with a risk algorithm for total CVD risk.[29] For these reasons, their opinion about BP can be easily summarized: "Hypertension: Time to move on." Advocates of the polypill deem the results of BP-lowering trials so compelling that universal treatment for everyone above a gender-specific age with three moderate-dose antihypertensive drugs (and other agents) is recommended, without even measuring BP.[15] These two different approaches lead to attempts to improve the cost-effectiveness of BP treatment. The first approach would provide treatment for individuals above a certain 10-year risk level (and those below it would fund their own medical care for hypertension). The second approach uses only generically available drugs (combined in a single pill) and avoids expensive interactions with health care providers. It will be very interesting to see how JNC 8 deals with these suggestions.

PREDICTORS OF HYPERTENSION

In addition to demographic factors, many features of modern American life appear to increase the risk of becoming hypertensive. As shown in Figure 9-1, older age is probably the most powerful predictor.[8] For those younger than 55 years, men are at greater risk than women, but this reverses after the age of 55 years.[8] African Americans have a greater risk of hypertension as well as more target organ damage when it is diagnosed and a greater burden of heart disease, stroke, and end-stage renal disease, although these have been improving during the last 5 to 10 years.[6,8] Uncontrolled hypertension appears to be even more common in Mexican Americans than in other racial and ethnic groups, perhaps because of limited access to health care.[6,8] Although only a few clinical syndromes are clearly heredofamilial, a single BP measurement is about 40% predictive of inherited BP levels; longitudinal measurements increase this to about 55%.[8] Prospective longitudinal studies of the heritability of BP in male medical students show about equal inheritance from the mother or father.[30]

Although lower educational attainment, lower socioeconomic status, lower physical activity scores, smoking, dyslipidemia, inflammation, psychosocial stressors, sleep apnea, and dietary factors (including higher consumption of dietary fats, sodium, alcohol, and calories or lower potassium intake) have all been implicated in many observational studies as significant predictors of hypertension,[8] much emphasis has recently been focused on obesity, particularly in childhood and adolescence. A study of the NHANES 1988-2004 data suggests that 20% to 80% of the increase in hypertension prevalence in adults during this period could be accounted for by the alarming increase in the average body mass index.[31] Many intervention trials have also demonstrated the benefit of a low-sodium diet in preventing hypertension, particularly one that is rich in fruits and vegetables and low in saturated fat.[32] Observational studies have also shown long-term benefit in preventing hypertension (and CVD events) of dietary patterns similar to those in the Dietary Approaches to Stop Hypertension (DASH) cookbooks,[33] which are among the most popular downloads from the website of the National Institutes of Health.[3,32]

As with all diagnoses that depend on crossing a threshold of a continuous variable (e.g., BP, fasting glucose concentration), probably the most important predictor of hypertension is prehypertension (BP 120-139/80-90 mm Hg),[2,3] simply because individuals with it are closer to BP $\geq$ 140/90 mm Hg than are people with normal BPs (<120/80 mm Hg). The TRial Of Prevention of HYpertension (TROPHY) was organized to test, in humans (as had been demonstrated in rodents), whether short-term drug administration could prevent hypertension, even after the drug had been discontinued.[17] After 2 years of candesartan, the risk of hypertension was reduced by 66% compared with placebo (only three people needed treatment to prevent one from progressing); but after 2 years of receiving placebo, the benefit was much reduced (to 15.6%). Although adverse events were not significantly different, serious adverse events (including cardiovascular events: 1 versus 6) were less common in the group given candesartan. These data clearly showed that drug treatment of candesartan was feasible, but whether it is worth the cost is still debatable, particularly as a shorter Danish study showed no benefit after discontinuation of candesartan.[34]

Another important predictor of hypertension is the use of nonsteroidal anti-inflammatory drugs (NSAIDs), particularly among individuals with above-normal BPs. Hypertension incidence was originally thought to be less with the selective cyclooxygenase 2 inhibitors, but increased BP has been seen both in large observational studies and in meta-analyses of clinical trials.[35] Many attribute the increased CVD risk seen with rofecoxib in several clinical trials (against naproxen or placebo) to its higher risk of BP elevation in the long term,[35] but whether the remaining agent in this class shares these adverse effects is the topic of an ongoing, large, multicenter trial.

EVALUATION OF THE HYPERTENSIVE PATIENT

Four key issues must be addressed during the initial evaluation of a person with elevated BP readings:
- Documenting an accurate diagnosis of hypertension.[18,23,28]
- Stratifying the person's risk for CVD disease, which involves (1) defining the presence or absence of existing CVD or renal disease or target organ damage related to hypertension and (2) screening for other CVD risk factors that often accompany hypertension to obtain an estimate of global cardiac risk.[3-5,9]
- Assessing whether the person is likely to have an identifiable cause for the elevated BP (secondary hypertension) and should have further diagnostic testing for it.[3-5,9]
- Obtaining information that may be helpful in choosing appropriate therapy.[3-5,9]

Although extensive and expensive laboratory studies are rarely necessary in the evaluation of hypertensive patients, the health care provider must be able to recognize when additional studies or consultation with a specialist is appropriate and warranted. Delaying discovery of a potentially curable form of hypertension or failing to properly assess whether target organ damage or comorbidities are present puts the patient at unnecessary risk, delays implementation of specific treatment, prolongs the time to BP control, and increases CVD risk.

Documenting the Diagnosis

BP should be measured under relaxed and controlled conditions after appropriate rest (typically 5 minutes) and taken by someone whose ability to perform the measurement accurately has been certified. Because ~10% to 15% of Americans cannot properly hear and interpret Korotkoff sounds, it is unlikely that measurements reported by every observer are accurate. Excellent programs are available that can train, validate, and recertify the competency of the person performing BP measurements. Careful attention should be given to proper, standardized technique.[18]

Before the diagnosis of hypertension is made, an individual usually should have elevated BP measurements documented at least twice, at visits separated by a week or more. Each measurement should be an average of two or three readings differing by <5 mm Hg from each other, taken a few minutes apart in the seated or supine position. Patients who exhibit wide fluctuations in BP or who are hypertensive at some evaluations but normotensive at others may need additional measurements, in the office, at home, or by ABPM, to confirm that they are indeed hypertensive.[3,18-23] Treatment should generally *not* be instituted until the diagnosis is clearly proven. In some circumstances, such as when target organ damage is present, treatment may need to be started after a single set of measurements.

Stratifying Risk for Cardiovascular Disease

Before a treatment program directed at lowering of BP is begun, a thorough assessment of the person's risk for development of CVD is warranted. Little guidance is provided in JNC 7 about this,[3] but many other schemes are available to assist the physician, most of which have been developed for or adapted to European populations.[36-38] Many of these are semiquantitative, similar to those of the Framingham Heart Study's risk score,[29,36-38] and allow a reasonable estimate of the patient's 10-year risk of CVD to be calculated. The Sheffield tables, based on the Scottish national health surveys, may be the most interesting of these.[38] These reasonably well validated tables (one for men, another for women) use age and the ratio of total cholesterol to HDL-cholesterol (with 22 choices for men, 18 for women) and simply dichotomize hypertension (defined as ≥140/90 mm Hg or taking treatment), smoking, and diabetes. Perhaps surprisingly, their data indicate that hypertension (whether treated or untreated) affects overall risk of CHD only slightly; when other risk factors are incorporated into the risk equation, the absolute level of blood BP (especially at diagnosis) is nearly irrelevant.[38]

The determination of an individual's absolute risk has important implications for the selection of antihypertensive agents, the BP target, and the time to goal attainment. Individuals with the highest short-term risk of a stroke or heart attack are those who already have established CVD or renal disease (e.g., history of a recent transient ischemic attack or previous myocardial infarction). These individuals should be treated promptly, intensively, and (in general, although controversy exists[39]) to a lower BP goal than for uncomplicated hypertensive people.[3-5,9,40,41] The search for evidence of concomitant CVD or renal disease need not be extensive or expensive, however. Typically, a complete medical history, a directed physical examination, and a few routine laboratory tests (including an electrocardiogram, urinalysis, and serum chemistry panel) are sufficient.

Hypertensive people with target organ damage are also at substantial risk for cardiovascular events. Target organ damage encompasses many subclinical features of the physical examination or laboratory test results indicating that there has already been an alteration of structure or function in the eyes, heart, kidneys, or blood vessels related to hypertension. Although such individuals may not have as yet suffered an irreversible hypertension-related event (e.g., stroke), some are at substantial risk for these sequelae (e.g., those with chronic kidney disease [CKD]), and the presence of target organ damage usually indicates that hypertension has been present for some time. These people also should receive prompt and intensive efforts to lower BP, typically to a lower than usual goal. Risk calculations are useful only for reasonably low-risk individuals. People with prior CVD, diabetes, or CKD are all assumed to have a 10-year risk of CVD >20%.[3-5,9]

Other CVD risk factors (tobacco use, family history of premature CVD) are often found in hypertensive people, and central obesity, dyslipidemia, diabetes, and hypertension tend to cluster. Because other risk factors tend to be additive (if not multiplicative) in increasing the probability of CVD events, it is important to screen a newly diagnosed hypertensive person for these other risk factors to more accurately estimate cardiovascular and renal risks.

Even though age is the most important (nonmodifiable) predictor of CVD risk (see Fig. 9-3), the treatment scheme and BP goals recommended in JNC 7 are independent of the patient's age.[3] There are now good data, several meta-analyses,[41] and an important recent placebo-controlled clinical trial[42] showing that older people, even past the age of 80 years, benefit greatly from BP-lowering drug therapy.

Considering Secondary Hypertension

More than 95% of Americans with hypertension have no specific cause of their elevated BPs (i.e., idiopathic, essential, or primary hypertension). There are three reasons to consider the possibility that hypertension in a newly diagnosed patient might have a specific cause. First, BP control is often difficult to achieve in those with secondary causes of hypertension; diagnosis of it early is likely to get BP to goal more quickly. Second, and particularly important in younger people, use of specific modalities to cure the underlying disease will reduce the future burden of treatment (medical care costs, adverse effects of therapy, and quality of life). Last, routine consideration of secondary causes of hypertension when the diagnosis is originally made will ensure that these diagnostic possibilities will be entertained, and the pros and cons of further testing critically evaluated, and that the clinician will not miss a secondary cause when it is present (see later for details).

Guiding Therapy

The more than 120 antihypertensive agents and fixed-dose combinations currently available in the United States differ in BP-lowering efficacy in various situations. It is often helpful to discuss these potential confounders of treatment with the patient in an effort to "individualize" treatment according to the patient's specific dietary, medical, and personal considerations. For example, diuretics and calcium antagonists are more effective than ACE inhibitors and angiotensin II receptor antagonists when dietary sodium is excessive. JNC VI and JNC 7 both recommended treating hypertension and a concomitant illness or condition with a specific antihypertensive drug when that drug has been shown in clinical trials to improve CVD morbidity and mortality (so-called compelling indication for a specific class of antihypertensive drug).[3] Therefore, even though ACE inhibitors were not routinely recommended as initial therapy for uncomplicated hypertensives, if the patient has heart failure of the systolic type, an ACE inhibitor could be prescribed. It would be expected not only to lower the BP but also to provide the impressive benefits seen in many long-term studies in every stage of heart failure. Last, some patients are particularly fearful of specific potential adverse effects of certain antihypertensive drugs (e.g., male sexual dysfunction). If the prescriber knows this information, efforts may be taken to avoid medications with a high incidence of this particular problem.

Medical History

In addition to assessment of the risk of future CVD and renal disease, a careful medication, environmental, and nutritional history should be obtained during the initial evaluation and intermittently thereafter. It is particularly important to ascertain whether the patient is taking any agent (either by prescription or over-the-counter) or other substance that might elevate BP (Box 9-2).[43] Of particular concern are the NSAIDs, which are widely used and available over-the-counter and are sometimes not recognized as "medicines" by many patients. Sympathomimetic amines (once commonly found in weight loss, cold, and allergy preparations) have been associated with an increase in both BP and risk of intracerebral hemorrhage and stroke. Hypertensive people should avoid both NSAIDs and sympathomimetic amines and attempt to obtain relief of pain with acetaminophen and of the symptoms of nasal congestion with antihistamines, if possible. When these modalities are ineffective, short-term use of the usually prescribed drugs may be condoned, but with the recognition that BP control is

---

BOX 9-2 Substances That Can Raise Blood Pressure (Partial List)

Nonsteroidal anti-inflammatory drugs (including the newer COX-2 inhibitor celecoxib)
Corticosteroids
Sympathomimetic amines
Oral contraceptive hormones
Methylxanthines (including theophylline and caffeine*)
Cyclosporine
Erythropoietin
Cocaine
Nicotine[†]
Phencyclidine (PCP)

*Short duration (minutes to hours).
[†]Very short duration (seconds to minutes).
COX-2, cyclooxygenase 2; PCP, phenylcyclohexyl piperidine ("angel dust").
Abridged from Elliott WJ: Drug interactions and drugs affecting blood pressure control.
J Clin Hypertens (Greenwich) 8:731, 2006.

---

likely to be suboptimal during and immediately after their consumption.

Oral contraceptive pills containing estrogens and progestins may raise BP in some women, although this is much less of a problem with the lower doses in common use today. If a newly diagnosed hypertensive woman uses these pills, discontinuation for 6 months and observation of the BP may allow a decision to be made about whether the pills are the cause of hypertension. Conjugated estrogens (with or without progesterone), typically given for postmenopausal hormone replacement therapy, seldom raise BP, although they have been associated with a wide variety of other problems, including increased rates of CVD events.

Other prescription drugs can either elevate BP or interfere with certain antihypertensive agents.[43] Of the former, cyclosporine, erythropoietin, corticosteroids, cocaine, and theophylline are perhaps the most widely recognized. Of the latter, monoamine oxidase inhibitors, NSAIDs, and tricyclic antidepressants are the most common. It is important to ascertain whether a hypertensive patient has taken any of these agents as well as several other illicit drugs (e.g., phencyclidine). Some chemical elements, particularly lead and chromium, may elevate BP long after exposure; questioning about these and other environmental toxins may sometimes be helpful.

A focused dietary history is important because the most effective lifestyle modifications involve limiting either calories or sodium or both.[2-5,10,31,44,45] Dietary salt and saturated fat intake can be estimated from an informal survey of dietary habits and preferences. Many processed foods, "fast foods," "diet foods," condiments, and snack items are concentrated, often-unrecognized sources of salt. Now that most foodstuffs bear labels attesting to their high sodium content, many patients are more easily able to choose healthier foods. A sensible target (now validated in several clinical trials, notably the DASH-Sodium substudy[46] and PREMIER[47]) is 100 mEq (2.4 g or 2400 mg) of sodium per day; this can usually be achieved if the high-salt items mentioned before are avoided and the patient does not add salt either at the table or in cooking. On occasion, it is useful (and relatively inexpensive compared with formal dietary counseling) to have the patient collect a 24-hour urine sample for sodium, particularly when the patient claims to be avoiding salt but the physician is doubtful. Although not all hypertensive patients will experience a reduction in BP on a low-salt diet or an increase in BP on a high-salt diet, individuals who are "salt sensitive" (~60% of the U.S. population) will benefit from reducing dietary sodium. In general, African Americans and elderly, obese, and diabetic patients are more likely to be salt sensitive, with BPs that are more responsive to dietary salt restriction.

The nutritional history should also include questions about saturated fat consumption, dairy intake, and whether any mineral or vitamin supplements are being used. Because obesity is a major problem for many hypertensive patients, the calorie intake, eating pattern, and changes in weight should be included. Weight loss remains the most successful of all short-term lifestyle modifications for hypertension and should be a part of the therapeutic plan in all overweight hypertensives from the outset.[3,30,32,44]

Social History

Although alcohol in moderation (one drink for women and two drinks for men maximum, with each drink being 12 ounces of beer, 4 ounces of wine, or 1 ounce of spirits) appears to protect against CHD in hypertensives,[48] excessive alcohol intake (four or more drinks per day) raises both BP and all-cause mortality. In some patients, reducing or stopping alcohol ingestion can have salutary effects on BP. A clinical trial in veterans who consumed approximately six drinks per day when enrolled was unsuccessful in demonstrating a significant reduction in BP in those receiving a cognitive-behavioral alcohol reduction program, despite consuming significantly fewer drinks per day (by 1.3, on average) than the control group, who received a much less intensive educational program. Nonetheless, a meta-analysis suggests that there is a place for alcohol restriction in the nonpharmacologic therapy for hypertension.[49]

Large populations of smokers have, on average, lower BP than nonsmokers do, probably because smokers tend to be less obese than nonsmokers. Consuming tobacco has both acute and chronic adverse effects on BP and hypertensive patients. Smoking a single cigarette raises BP and heart rate acutely (within seconds to minutes) because of nicotine's stimulation of catecholamine secretion. This effect disappears in about 15 minutes, so BP should be measured at least 15 to 30 minutes after the most recent cigarette is extinguished. Chronic tobacco abuse roughly doubles the long-term risk of CVD and has an even larger effect on peripheral arterial disease (including renovascular hypertension). Inquiry about tobacco abuse and advice to discontinue it (if present) should be a part of every encounter with a health care professional. Hypertensive patients should also be questioned about a sedentary lifestyle and whether there is willingness or ability to engage in regular physical activity. Even limited aerobic exercise, including brisk walking for 30 minutes on most days, can reduce BP and the risk of all-cause and CVD mortality. Snoring, daytime sleepiness, and other clinical features of obstructive sleep apnea, especially in obese hypertensives, should lead to a Berlin Questionnaire[50] and consideration of a formal evaluation for this underappreciated and underdiagnosed form of secondary hypertension.[51]

Physical Examination

The directed physical examination of the hypertensive patient should pay special attention to weight, target organ damage, and features consistent with secondary hypertension. It should focus on items that were suggested by the medical history.

- The pattern of fat distribution should be noted. Android obesity (waist-to-hip ratio >0.95) is associated with increased CVD risk, whereas gynecoid obesity (waist-to-hip ratio <0.85) is not. Men whose waist is ≥102 cm (40 inches) and women whose waist is ≥88 cm (35 inches) are at increased risk. The International Diabetes Federation recommends lower waist circumference cut points for other populations, such as European whites and Asians, to define abdominal obesity.

- The patient's skin should be carefully examined for café au lait spots (suggesting neurofibromatosis and possible pheochromocytoma), acanthosis nigricans (suggesting insulin resistance), xanthomas at tendons, or xanthelasma (indicating dyslipidemia). Other skin signs suggesting pheochromocytoma (axillary freckles, ash-leaf patches, port-wine stains in the trigeminal distribution, and adenoma sebaceum) are uncommon, except in patients with phakomatoses.
- The many physical signs associated with other secondary causes should be sought, particularly if they are suggested by the medical history. The signs of Cushing syndrome (purple striae, moon facies, dorsocervical fat pad, atrophic skin changes) or thyroid disease (abnormal Achilles reflexes, hair quality, and eye signs) are typically difficult to ignore.
- The funduscopic examination is important in assessing the duration and severity of hypertension. The presence of hypertensive retinopathy (grade 1: arterial tortuosity, silver wiring; grade 2: arteriovenous crossing changes ["nicking"]; grade 3: hemorrhages or exudates; grade 4: papilledema) provides definitive evidence of target organ damage.
- The neck should be examined for an enlarged thyroid gland, abnormalities of the venous circulation (e.g., jugular venous distention, abnormal or cannon *a* waves), and carotid bruits.
- The chest should be auscultated for evidence of heart failure or bronchospasm; bronchospasm would likely make beta blockers contraindicated.
- The heart should be examined carefully for cardiomegaly, murmurs, and extra sounds.
- The abdominal examination is one of the most important parts of the directed physical examination because the finding of an abdominal bruit is one of the most cost-effective ways to screen for renovascular hypertension. All four abdominal quadrants and the back should be auscultated, typically with use of the pulse at the wrist as the synchronizing stimulus. Diastolic or continuous bruits are common in renovascular hypertension, but systolic bruits in young and especially thin hypertensive subjects may not be indicative of renal artery stenosis. Abdominal masses can sometimes be palpated in patients with pheochromocytoma or polycystic kidney disease.
- The groin and legs should be examined for evidence of peripheral arterial disease, which often is manifested as bruits, absent or decreased pulses, and abnormal hair growth patterns. Edema can be a sign of heart failure, renal disease, or high doses of dihydropyridine calcium antagonists.
- The neurologic examination need not be extensive in a hypertensive patient with no history of cerebrovascular disease, but it should be complete if a history of stroke or transient ischemic attack is present.

Laboratory Testing

For most hypertensives, only a few simple and inexpensive laboratory tests are needed initially. In selected patients, however, more extensive testing is not only appropriate but also necessary to diagnose secondary hypertension and to avoid delaying proper treatment. The laboratory tests that are recommended for all hypertensive persons are shown in Box 9-3 and can be divided into those that are done to assess risk, to establish etiology, to screen for important common diseases, and, finally, to guide the choice of initial therapy.

BOX 9-3 Laboratory Tests Appropriate for All Newly Diagnosed Hypertensive Patients

Assessing Risk
Lipid profile (including serum total cholesterol, HDL-cholesterol, and triglycerides)
Serum glucose concentration (preferably fasting)
Serum creatinine concentration
Urinalysis (both dipstick and microscopic)
12-Lead electrocardiogram

Establishing Cause
Serum potassium concentration
Serum creatinine concentration
Urinalysis (both dipstick and microscopic)
Thyroid-stimulating hormone (with further testing, if abnormal)

Screening for Common Asymptomatic Diseases
Complete blood count
Serum calcium concentration

Guiding Therapy
Lipid profile (including total cholesterol, HDL-cholesterol, and triglycerides)
Serum glucose concentration (preferably fasting)
Serum creatinine concentration

For uncomplicated hypertensive patients whose history and physical examination do not suggest a secondary cause, the simple battery of tests in Box 9-3 is all that is needed. A lipid profile and fasting glucose concentration are indicated in hypertensive patients because of the high prevalence of the metabolic syndrome in hypertensives. The presence of diabetes or additional risk factors not only requires institution of therapy for these conditions but also indicates substantially increased CVD risk, thus requiring more intensive therapy for hypertension, a lower goal BP, and closer follow-up.

Routine measurement of serum creatinine and a full urinalysis are recommended for three reasons. First, the urinalysis is useful to assess risk because hypertensive patients with microalbuminuria, proteinuria, or renal impairment have a distinctly worse prognosis. Second, the urinalysis may identify CKD as a secondary cause. Renal impairment (typically manifested as elevated serum creatinine) with a normal urinary sediment may be a valuable clue suggesting ischemic nephropathy, perhaps due to renal artery stenosis. Third, knowledge of the serum creatinine level frequently guides therapy[52] because loop diuretics are routinely needed and are more effective than thiazide or thiazide-like diuretics when the estimated glomerular filtration rate (eGFR) is <30 mL/min/1.73 m^2.

An electrocardiogram may provide important but limited information in most hypertensive patients. Although it may identify an occasionally important dysrhythmia or even an unsuspected old myocardial infarction, its biggest role is in screening for left ventricular hypertrophy, which is an objective measure of both the severity and duration of elevated BP. Despite a sensitivity of only 10% to 50% (depending on which criteria are used in its interpretation) in the Framingham Heart Study, electrocardiographic evidence of left ventricular hypertrophy was associated with an approximately threefold increase in incidence of CVD events. Left ventricular hypertrophy detected by echocardiography appears to be an even better predictor of future events, but this test is not recommended for routine evaluation because of its high cost and high intrinsic variability of a single procedure (~10% to 15%).

Because hypothyroidism is a cause of remediable hypertension that is subtle, especially in the elderly, a thyroid-stimulating hormone assay may be helpful. Serum calcium is useful in evaluating hyperparathyroidism and is often included in automated chemistry panels. The measurement of plasma renin activity is useful (with a plasma aldosterone concentration) in the diagnosis of mineralocorticoid excess states, such as primary hyperaldosteronism.

SECONDARY HYPERTENSION

Important clues to the presence of secondary hypertension are often provided by a carefully obtained medical history (see earlier). Many patients with primary hypertension report an isolated elevated BP reading some time in their 20s and 30s that was not reproducible or sustained until at least a decade or more later. The level of BP gradually rises until it reaches a threshold level, and then hypertension is diagnosed. In contrast, patients with an identifiable secondary cause of hypertension usually present with a very different history. Instead of the gradual onset of elevated BPs, they usually have a relatively abrupt onset of hypertension, typically presenting at a higher stage and with considerable target organ damage. The sudden onset of elevated BPs at ages before 30 years or after 50 years should alert the clinician to the possibility that the patient may have secondary hypertension. Thus, the history of the patient's presentation with hypertension should be carefully documented. At what age were the BP readings first elevated? How high were the readings? Were all prior readings within the normal range? Was it discovered during a routine office visit, or did the patient have clinical problems related to BP elevation or related target organ damage?

Because patients with secondary hypertension typically do not respond as well as patients with primary hypertension to antihypertensive drug therapy, the history of the patient's response to treatment must be ascertained. What drugs were used and at which doses? Did the patient's BP respond initially and then become resistant? A positive answer to this question is frequently found in patients with primary hypertension who later develop secondary hypertension, particularly atherosclerotic renovascular disease.

Laboratory Testing for Secondary Hypertension

All types of secondary hypertension are uncommon in the general hypertensive population, although certain factors (e.g., obesity and snoring for obstructive sleep apnea, smoking and peripheral vascular disease for renovascular hypertension) make specific diagnoses more likely. In interpreting test results in a given patient, bayesian analysis (which incorporates the pretest probability of finding disease) is therefore more important than the sensitivity of the test (i.e., the percentage of people with disease who have a positive test result). Those tests that are often recommended for the evaluation of patients for secondary hypertension are listed in Table 9-3. The proper evaluation of patients for many forms of secondary hypertension is still highly controversial despite the recent publication of guidelines for each.[53-56] Probably the most controversial are those pertaining to renovascular hypertension, for which the popular angioplasty and stenting have yet to show a significant long-term benefit in the four trials completed to date.[57-59]

TABLE 9–3	Screening and Other Tests for Common Forms of Secondary Hypertension	
Diagnosis	Preferred Screening Tests	Other Tests
Renovascular hypertension	Doppler ultrasound of renal arteries, computed tomographic angiography	Magnetic resonance angiography, renal angiography, captopril scintigraphy
Mineralocorticoid excess states	Plasma aldosterone/renin ratio, 24-hour urinary aldosterone during salt loading	Computed tomographic scan of adrenals
Pheochromocytoma	24-hour urine for vanillylmandelic acid and metanephrines	Plasma metanephrines, plasma catecholamines, T2-weighted magnetic resonance imaging
Sleep apnea	Berlin Questionnaire	Formal home nocturnal somnographic study
Cushing syndrome	8 AM plasma cortisol level	Dexamethasone suppression tests
Hypothyroidism	Thyroid-stimulating hormone	Serum thyroxine, triiodothyronine levels

Modified from recent reviews and consensus guidelines.[53-57]

BRIEF REVIEW: OUTCOMES-BASED CLINICAL TRIALS

Because so much information about hypertension and its treatment has been derived from clinical trials, many excellent, evidence-based recommendations can now be made about its diagnosis and management.[3-5,9] Although details of many of the older studies are available in an excellent monograph,[60] the results of most of these trials have been combined and summarized in other forms (e.g., meta-analyses[4,13-15,24-27,36,41,45]), which, when properly done, are said to rank higher than individual trials in the hierarchy of evidence-based medicine.

Diuretics and Beta Blockers

In the early 1990s, the most frequently cited meta-analysis compared the observed results of BP lowering in clinical trials with those expected from epidemiologic studies. Although stroke reduction in clinical trials (by about 42% ± 6%) was nearly exactly what would have been expected, prevention of CHD was substantially less (about 14% ± 5% compared with the expected 25% to 28%).[61] This led some to believe that the drugs used in the early trials (nearly exclusively diuretics and beta blockers) might be somewhat less effective in preventing CHD than stroke. A subsequent network meta-analysis of these and later trials showed that an initial diuretic or beta blocker was associated with a higher risk of incident diabetes.[62] Similarly, an initial beta blocker (particularly atenolol) has been found in meta-analyses to be significantly less effective than any other initial antihypertensive drug in preventing most types of CVD events,[63] so this class has been demoted to fourth-line therapy in the most recent British guidelines.[4]

ACE Inhibitors

Many of the placebo-controlled clinical trials of ACE inhibitors that had impressive results were performed in "high-risk patients," not all of whom had hypertension, in which the randomized agents were added to whatever other antihypertensive and other drugs were appropriate. Some therefore object to the inclusion of these studies in meta-analyses that attempt to summarize the results of BP-lowering therapies. Rather than asserting, for example, that ramipril is a better ACE inhibitor than trandolapril for prevention of CVD events, such trials can be used to illustrate the importance of concomitant therapies and residual absolute risk. In the Heart Outcomes Prevention Evaluation (HOPE),[64] only about 28%, 39%, and 76% of the patients were taking lipid-lowering agents, beta blockers, or aspirin (respectively), and the absolute risk of the primary outcome in the placebo-treated group was 39.4 events/1000 patient-years of follow-up. In the Prevention of Events with Angiotensin-Converting Enzyme inhibition (PEACE) trial, the drug use rates were 70%, 60%, and 90% (respectively), so the absolute risk with placebo was reduced to only 21.1 events/1000 patient-years of follow-up.[65] It was therefore much more likely that the HOPE investigators would see a significant benefit of ramipril compared with trandolapril in PEACE.

Several meta-analyses and meta-regressions have suggested that ACE inhibitors have a specific protective effect on CHD events, independent of BP lowering,[14,27] but this is controversial.[26] The most recent trial involving an ACE inhibitor, the ONgoing Telmisartan Alone and in combination with Ramipril Global Endpoint Trial (ONTARGET),[66] compared ramipril and telmisartan (and their combination) and showed no evidence of "benefit beyond BP control" with the ACE inhibitor (which was given along with 1.18 other antihypertensive drugs, on average). Importantly, ONTARGET also showed no significant CVD event benefit with the addition of telmisartan to ramipril, despite a slightly lower BP in subjects randomized to the combination.

Calcium Antagonists

Although fears were raised in the mid-1990s by case-control, cohort, and meta-analytic studies that calcium antagonists were associated with a significantly *higher* risk of CHD, many subsequent randomized clinical trials, especially the Antihypertensive and Lipid-Lowering treatment to prevent Heart Attack Trial (ALLHAT)[67] and the Anglo-Scandinavian Cardiac Outcomes Trial (ASCOT),[68] showed a slightly *lower* risk of CHD with amlodipine than its comparators. Furthermore, an initial calcium antagonist appears to be slightly (but not significantly) better than an initial diuretic in preventing a first stroke in hypertensive patients,[13,14,25-27,41] again allegedly independent of BP control.[27] Some attribute the benefits seen in ASCOT to the lower central aortic pressure with the amlodipine-based regimen compared with the atenolol-based regimen.[69] Conversely, both dihydropyridine and nondihydropyridine calcium antagonists are associated with a higher risk of heart failure.[13,14,25-27,41]

Angiotensin II Receptor Blockers

The evidence base for ARBs is limited, primarily because ethics prevents unconfounded comparison of this newer class of antihypertensive drugs with placebo in outcome studies. The study designs have been limited to specific indications (e.g., type 2 diabetic nephropathy or heart failure), comparisons against other BP-lowering drugs, or add-on therapy in high-risk patients (not all of whom were hypertensive).[66,70,71] Although the ARB was "noninferior" to the ACE inhibitor in ONTARGET,[66] the nonsignificant results of the two placebo-controlled trials were disappointing because these drugs are effective in lowering BP and are well tolerated.

Combination Therapy

Although nearly all clinical trials end up comparing drug regimens of multiple antihypertensive agents, two recent trials have provided data on the relative effectiveness of combination therapy. In ONTARGET, the combination of full-dose ramipril and full-dose telmisartan resulted in more BP lowering but significantly more adverse effects and renal endpoints than with ramipril alone.[66,72] The design of the Avoiding Cardiovascular events through COMBination therapy in Patients LIving with Systolic Hypertension (ACCOMPLISH) trial[73] was unique in that it set out to compare outcomes in a very high risk hypertensive population that was randomized to benazepril plus either hydrochlorothiazide (as recommended in JNC 7)[3] or amlodipine (as in the recent British guidelines).[4] The BP lowering in both groups was excellent, but the BP lowering was slightly better and CVD outcomes were less common in the group randomized to benazepril plus amlodipine. Unanswered questions about ACCOMPLISH include whether the chosen diuretic or the ACE inhibitor was optimal in dose and identity and what other explanation might be offered for the observed difference in outcomes. This trial has the potential to change the standard recommendation of JNC 7 regarding initial treatment of stage 2 hypertension, for which a diuretic and another antihypertensive drug were advised.[3]

Summary of Current Evidence from Clinical Trials

There is little doubt, on the basis of the clinical trial evidence gathered to date and summarized before[4,13-15,25-27,41,63] and updated in Figure 9-6,[74] that BP lowering is a powerful means of achieving reductions in CVD events. The initial assessment

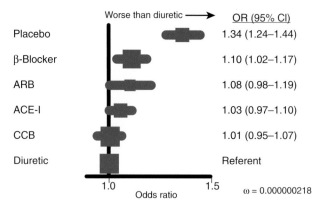

FIGURE 9-6 Results of a network meta-analysis for 23,690 first cardiovascular disease events (stroke, myocardial infarction, or cardiovascular death) comparing initial antihypertensive drug therapies and placebo or no treatment in all 55 published clinical trials that enrolled only hypertensive subjects (n = 261,051). For some trials (e.g., ALLHAT), the numbers of subjects experiencing a first event were estimated, as these data have not yet been reported. These odds ratios (OR, listed on the right, with 95% confidence intervals, 95% CI) change little (but in the expected direction) if other trials that compared add-on drug therapy (3 trials, 1889 events, 25,194 subjects) or enrolled nonhypertensive subjects (13 trials, 11,390 events, 96,332 subjects) are included in similar meta-analyses or if bayesian meta-analyses are performed. ARB, angiotensin receptor blocker; ACE-I, angiotensin-converting enzyme inhibitor; CCB, calcium channel blocker (or calcium antagonist); ω, incoherence value, reflecting how well the data "hang together" (lower values are better). *(Updated from Elliott WJ, Basu S, Meier PM: Dihydropyridine vs. non-dihydropyridine calcium antagonists as initial therapy for prevention of cardiovascular events in hypertensive patients [abstract]. J Clin Hypertens (Greenwich) 11[Suppl A]:A13, 2009.)*

of CVD risk takes on greater importance, as specific therapies are said to be more protective for different events: a diuretic to prevent heart failure, a calcium antagonist to prevent stroke,[15,27] and an ACE inhibitor to prevent CHD.[14,27] Multiple economic analyses also indicate that in addition to being effective in preventing CVD events, antihypertensive drug therapy is also relatively cost-effective compared with other commonly employed treatment strategies used in medicine today.[4]

MANAGEMENT

Successful management of hypertension requires a major commitment from the patient, the health care provider, and the health care system. The patient must continue to take what could be a costly medication with potential adverse effects and see a health care provider frequently, for an asymptomatic condition, in the belief that this will reduce the risk of a major complication or even death. The physician must help the patient achieve goal BP and maintain surveillance on this and other CVD risk factors, without being sure that such treatment will prevent an event that would have occurred without it. The health care system must fund both pharmacy and provider benefits, understanding that the 5-year number needed to treat (to prevent one expensive CVD event) is higher than its actuaries would prefer.

Lifestyle Modifications

All hypertension guidelines recommend nutritional-hygienic measures to control BP. In the short term, weight loss is the most effective,[44] but dietary sodium restriction is the only modality shown to have a long-term benefit in reducing CVD morbidity and mortality.[45] In the Trials of Hypertension Prevention, the difference in daily sodium excretion during the 18 to 48 months of follow-up between the randomized groups was only 816 to 1081 mg/day,[45] suggesting that the 2300 mg/day target recommended by guidelines and the DASH-Sodium and PREMIER trials is a good one.[46,47] Also recommended (if appropriate for the individual) are alcohol restriction to one or two drinks a day (two or three in the recent British guidelines), tobacco avoidance, major exercise (30 minutes most days of the week), reduction of caffeine (if excessive), and supplements of potassium, calcium, or magnesium (if and only if a deficiency state is present). There are few long-term controlled trials of yoga,[75] paced breathing,[76] spinal manipulation,[77] fish oil,[78] or acupuncture[79] for lowering of BP, although each can be useful for selected patients. There is limited clinical trial evidence but good public health rationale for advocating a combination of weight loss, dietary salt restriction, and other lifestyle modification methods as preventive,[80] adjunctive, and (occasionally) definitive treatment of hypertension.[32,44-49] Recidivism can be a problem for both weight loss and sodium restriction, however, and long-term adherence to such programs is uncommon in many clinics. The only study to assess outcomes using a vigorous program of lifestyle modifications with and without antihypertensive drug therapy showed significant prevention of CVD events with the combination.[81] As a result, for patients with comorbidities, target organ damage, or high 10-year risk scores, many clinicians prefer to recommend lifestyle modifications *plus* appropriate drug therapy.

Choice of Initial Drug Therapy

Initial Antihypertensive Drug Therapy for "Complicated Patients"

Since 1997, U.S. hypertension guidelines have formally recognized that many people begin treatment too late, after they have already developed CVD or other medical conditions that may be positively affected by specific antihypertensive drug therapies.[3] These have been divided into "compelling indications" and "clinical conditions." In the compelling indications (Table 9-4), a specific type of antihypertensive drug should be prescribed if clinical trials have demonstrated that class of drug to reduce morbidity or mortality for that condition.[3] Thus, for a hypertensive person with systolic heart failure, an ACE inhibitor will be likely not only to lower BP but also to reduce CVD events and hospitalizations. There are also some absolute and relative contraindications for specific antihypertensive drugs that limit their use as initial therapy in *all* hypertensives (Table 9-5). Two examples of clinical conditions for which specific antihypertensive drugs benefit certain patients are a thiazide diuretic for calcium-containing renal stones and a beta blocker for essential tremor. Although neither drug is likely to reduce CVD morbidity or mortality from these conditions, each will reduce symptoms and therefore improve adherence and BP control in the long term. JNC 7 and other hypertension treatment guidelines recognize the merits of specific antihypertensive drugs in complicated hypertensive patients, for whom an initial diuretic is sometimes not the optimal drug choice.[3-5]

Initial Antihypertensive Drug Therapy for "Uncomplicated Hypertensives"

Since the early termination of the alpha blocker (doxazosin) arm and the final results of ALLHAT, the "default choice" for initial antihypertensive drug therapy for most uncomplicated patients in the United States is a low-dose thiazide-type diuretic, which showed superiority in the secondary endpoint of combined CVD. Those who strictly adhere to evidence-based medicine will insist on chlorthalidone.[52] Perhaps because the 12.5-mg dose of chlorthalidone is not commercially available, JNC 7 did not distinguish between chlorthalidone and hydrochlorothiazide, but it did recommend a thiazide-type diuretic "for most patients." Some day, pharmacogenetic testing may be used to predict both the BP-lowering response and the preventive effect of the thiazide-like diuretic,[82] but these techniques are currently unavailable to the general population. In the United Kingdom, recommended initial antihypertensive therapy is usually an ACE inhibitor (or occasionally an ARB) for younger white patients, a calcium antagonist for older or black patients, or a diuretic for those at high risk of heart failure.[4] The European Society of Cardiology/European Society of Hypertension guidelines recognize that few patients will achieve BP control with a single agent, and therefore less importance is placed on which drug is chosen first.[5] The 2009 Canadian Hypertension Education Program guidelines stratify even further on the basis of whether the BP elevation is systolic alone or diastolic ± systolic.[83] For the former, a thiazide diuretic, long-acting calcium antagonist, or ARB is recommended, but the diuretic and calcium antagonist have the best-quality evidence. For the latter, a thiazide diuretic, beta blocker (for patients <60 years of age), ACE inhibitor, or long-acting calcium antagonist is recommended, with the thiazide having the best-quality evidence.[83]

Because the probability of achieving a reduction of more than 20/10 mm Hg in BP with a single drug is low, many hypertension guidelines recommend consideration of initiating therapy with a two-drug combination for individuals with stage 2 hypertension (or a BP ≥ 150/90 mm Hg for diabetics[3,84] or those with either CKD[3,85] or established heart disease[86]). JNC 7 suggested that a diuretic be part of such a regimen, but the ACCOMPLISH data call this strategy into question.[73] Few subjects in ACCOMPLISH were "uncomplicated stage 2 hypertensives," however.[73]

TABLE 9–4	Compelling Indications for Which Specific Antihypertensive Drug Therapy Has Reduced Morbidity or Mortality in Clinical Trials			
Compelling Indication	**Treatment Prevents or Delays**	**Recommended in 1997**	**Recommended in 2003**	**Recommended in 2010**
Heart failure (systolic type)	CV events	ACE-I (CONSENSUS, SAVE)	Beta blockers (MERIT-HF); spironolactone (RALES); ARB (Val-HeFT)	ARB (CHARM-Added)
After recent MI	Recurrent infarction or death	Beta blocker (ISIS)		
Diminished left ventricular function after recent MI	Recurrent infarction, CHF hospitalization	ACE-I (SAVE, TRACE)	Eplerenone (EPHESUS)	ARB (VALIANT)
High risk for CVD	CVD events		ACE-I (HOPE)	ARB (TRANSCEND, ONTARGET)
Type 1 diabetes mellitus	Deterioration in renal function	ACE-I (CCSG)		
Type 2 diabetes	CV events		ACE-I (MICRO-HOPE)	Diuretic + ACE-I (ADVANCE)
Type 2 diabetic nephropathy	Deterioration in renal function		ARBs (IDNT, RENAAL)	
Type 2 diabetes	Progression of microalbuminuria		ACE-I (MICRO-HOPE); ARB (IRMA-2)	Diuretic + ACE-I (ADVANCE)
Older hypertensive persons	CV events	Diuretic (SHEP); DHP-CA (Syst-Eur)	ACE-I or DHP-CA (STOP-2); DHP-CA (Syst-China); ARB (SCOPE, second-line); ARB (LIFE)	Diuretic (HYVET)
Nondiabetic renal impairment	Deterioration in renal function		ACE-I (REIN, AIPRI, AASK)	
Prior stroke, TIA	Stroke and CV events		ACE-I (PROGRESS)	ARB (ACCESS, MOSES)
Left ventricular hypertrophy (using strict criteria)	CV events (perhaps limited to stroke?)		ARB (LIFE)	

ACE-I, angiotensin-converting enzyme inhibitor; ARB, angiotensin receptor blocker; CHF, congestive heart failure; CV, cardiovascular; CVD, cardiovascular disease; DHP-CA, dihydropyridine calcium antagonist; MI, myocardial infarction; TIA, transient ischemic attack.

CONSENSUS, COoperative North Scandinavian ENalapril SUrvival Study (*N Engl J Med* 316:1429, 1987); SAVE, Survival And Ventricular Enlargement study (*N Engl J Med* 327:669, 1992); CCSG, Captopril Cooperative Study Group (*N Engl J Med* 323:1456, 1993); SHEP, Systolic Hypertension in the Elderly Program (*JAMA* 265:3255, 1991); Syst-Eur, Systolic Hypertension in Europe trial (*Lancet* 360:757, 1997); MERIT-HF, MEtoprolol Randomized Intervention Trial in congestive Heart Failure (*JAMA* 283:1295, 2000); RALES, Randomized Aldactone Evaluation Study (*N Engl J Med* 341:709, 1999); Val-HeFT, Valsartan Heart Failure Trial (*N Engl J Med* 345:1667, 2001); CHARM-Added, Candesartan in Heart failure Assessment of Reduction in Mortality and morbidity (*Lancet* 362:767, 2003); ISIS, International Study of Infarct Survival (*Lancet* 2:57, 1986); TRACE, TRAndolapril Cardiac Evaluation (*N Engl J Med* 333:1670-1676, 1995); EPHESUS = Eplerenone Post-myocardial infarction Heart Failure Efficacy and Survival Study (*N Engl J Med* 348:1309, 2003); VALIANT, VALsartan In Acute myocardial iNfarcTion (*N Engl J Med* 349:1893, 2003); HOPE, Heart Outcomes Prevention Evaluation (*N Engl J Med* 342:145, 2000); ONTARGET, ONgoing Telmisartan Alone and in combination with Ramipril Global Endpoint Trial (*Lancet* 358:1547, 2008); TRANSCEND, Telmisartan Randomised AssessmeNt Study in ACE iNtolerant subjects with cardiovascular Disease (*Lancet* 371:1174, 2008); MICRO-HOPE, MIcroalbuminuria, Cardiovascular and Renal Outcomes substudy of the Heart Outcomes Prevention Evaluation (*Lancet* 355:253, 2000); ADVANCE, Action in Diabetes and Vascular disease: preterAx and diamicroN-mr Controlled Evaluation (*Lancet* 370:829, 2007); IDNT, Irbesartan Diabetic Nephropathy Trial (*N Engl J Med* 345:841, 2001); RENAAL, Reduction of Endpoints in Non–insulin dependent diabetes mellitus with the Angiotensin II Antagonist Losartan (*N Engl J Med* 345:861, 2001); IRMA-2, IRbesartan MicroAlbuminuria study 2 (*N Engl J Med* 345:870, 2001); STOP-2, Swedish Trial in Old Patients with hypertension 2 (*Lancet* 354:1751, 1999); Syst-China, Systolic Hypertension in China trial (*J Hypertens* 16:1823, 1998); SCOPE, Study on COgnition and Prognosis in the Elderly (*J Hypertens* 21:875, 2003); LIFE, Losartan Intervention For Endpoint reduction in the Very Elderly Trial (*N Engl J Med* 358:1887, 2008); HYVET, HYpertension in the Very Elderly Trial (*N Engl J Med* 358:1887, 2008); REIN, Ramipril Evaluation In Nephropathy trial (*Lancet* 352:1252, 1998); AIPRI, Angiotensin-converting-enzyme Inhibition in Progressive Renal Insufficiency (*Kidney Int Suppl* 63:S63, 1997); AASK, African American Study of Kidney disease and hypertension (*JAMA* 288:2421, 2002); PROGRESS, Perindopril pROtection aGainst REcurrent Stroke Study (*Lancet* 358:1033, 2001); ACCESS, Acute Candesartan CilExetil therapy in Stroke Survivors (*Stroke* 34:1699, 2003); MOSES, MOrbidity and mortality after Stroke, Eprosartan compared with nitrendipine for Secondary prevention (*Stroke* 36:1218, 2005).

TABLE 9–5	Contraindications for Specific Antihypertensive Drug Classes
Antihypertensive Drug Class	**Contraindication**
Thiazide diuretic	Allergy
Beta blocker	Asthma, allergy
ACE inhibitor	Angioedema due to ACE inhibitor, pregnancy, renal artery stenosis
Calcium antagonist	Allergy
Angiotensin II receptor blocker	Pregnancy, renal artery stenosis
Alpha blocker	Orthostatic hypotension with frequent falls
Alpha$_2$-agonist (centrally acting drug)	Allergy

Add-on Drug Therapy

Perhaps because few clinical trials directly compared second-step antihypertensive drugs (after an initial diuretic), JNC 7 recommended an ACE inhibitor, ARB, beta blocker, or calcium antagonist but gave little further guidance.[3] Some would add an alpha blocker to the list, which was admittedly inferior to chlorthalidone as *initial* therapy in ALLHAT.[86] Others would routinely favor an ACE inhibitor or an ARB because of the potential synergy on serum potassium in combination with a thiazide or thiazide-like diuretic. Such a strategy has been more effective in achieving BP control during 6 months compared with traditional Canadian guidelines.[87] Beta blockers have the largest clinical trial experience as the second-line agent after a diuretic, but some object to the higher risk of incident diabetes with the combination.[4,62,68,84] Although the first published factorial-design trial of antihypertensive agents included a diuretic and calcium antagonist, and the combination was used in the Controlled ONset Verapamil INvestigation of Cardiovascular Endpoints (CONVINCE) trial,[88] the most direct evidence in its favor is a Chinese trial showing significant reduction in CVD (mostly stroke) events, comparing placebo against a calcium antagonist as second-line therapy after a diuretic.[89]

Target Blood Pressures

JNC 7 recommended only one of two BP targets. For uncomplicated hypertensives, the BP should be lowered to <140/90 mm Hg. The best clinical trial evidence in favor of this target comes from the Hypertension Optimal Treatment (HOT) study.[90] It was the largest trial to compare outcomes in subjects randomized to different target BPs. Its 18,790 hypertensive patients achieved "optimal reduction in cardiovascular risk" with an achieved BP of 138.5/82.6 mm Hg. There was no significant increase in risk by further lowering BP to a diastolic target of ≤80 mm Hg, but there was no further benefit either.[90] An open-label study of 1111 Italian nondiabetic hypertensives has recently suggested that systolic BP be lowered to <130 mm Hg because it reduced both echocardiographic left ventricular hypertrophy and cardiovascular outcomes.[91] However, because the probability of drug-related side effects often increases as the doses are increased, it is likely that the target BP of <140/90 mm Hg for uncomplicated hypertensive patients will be defensible for some time to come.

For diabetic patients or those with CKD, JNC 7 recommended a BP target of <130/80 mm Hg,[3] which is easier to justify for diabetic patients (although both are controversial).[39] The first clinical trial to demonstrate the benefit of a lower BP target for diabetics was the United Kingdom Prospective Diabetes Study (UKPDS 38).[92] During 8.4 years of follow-up, 1148 type 2 diabetics randomized to two different BP goals (<150/85 mm Hg or <180/105 mm Hg) did much better if treated to the lower goal. The achieved BP difference between groups was 10/5 mm Hg (154/87 versus 144/82 mm Hg), which if subtracted from the usual then-current BP goal for nondiabetic patients (140/90 mm Hg) gave a target for diabetics identical to that recommended in the earlier U.S. hypertension guidelines: <130/85 mm Hg! In the 1501 diabetics in the HOT study, the lowest risk of stroke, heart attack, or CVD death in the intent-to-treat analysis was seen in those randomized to a diastolic BP ≤80 mm Hg.[90] The most recent clinical trial data in favor of a lower BP target for diabetics come from the Strong Heart Study, which observed significantly lower CVD event rates among the diabetics randomized to BP <130/80 mm Hg or an LDL-cholesterol target of <100 mg/dL.[93]

There have been concerns that the lower BP goal for diabetics would be expensive, as it requires more antihypertensive pills and more visits to health care providers, but several studies show this to be untrue. A cost analysis of UKPDS showed that despite higher drug and provider costs, the strategy of the lower BP goal saved lives, strokes, limbs, *and money*. The cost-effectiveness ratio for the lower BP goal was –£720 per year of life saved and an even more impressive –£1049 per year of life without diabetic complications.

JNC 7 recommended a BP target of <130/80 mm Hg for patients with CKD, but there are few clinical trial data to support this. The most favorable long-term data came originally from the Modification of Diet in Renal Disease (MDRD) trial, which overrecruited patients with polycystic kidney disease but did show a benefit of BP <125/75 mm Hg.[94] In a patient-level meta-analysis of placebo-controlled trials of ACE inhibitors in CKD, the optimal *achieved* systolic BP to avoid doubling of serum creatinine or end-stage renal disease was 110 to 129 mm Hg.[95] In a direct comparison of BP targets for patients with hypertensive nephrosclerosis, the African

American Study of Kidney Disease and Hypertension (AASK), there was no significant benefit to reducing BP to <125/75 mm Hg (compared with <140/90 mm Hg) during the first 3 years of follow-up.[96] Unfortunately, the 10-year incidence of doubling of serum creatinine or end-stage renal disease among the cohort initially randomized to the ACE inhibitor *and* the lower BP goal was 53.5%, despite a mean BP of about 133/78 mm Hg after completion of the randomized trial.[97] The <130/80 mm Hg target for patients with CKD can be viewed as a reasonable compromise on the basis of data from MDRD, AASK, and observational studies.[3,85,95]

In 2007, an American Heart Association Scientific Statement suggested that patients with established heart disease should be treated to <130/80 mm Hg, and an "optional target" for those with heart failure is <125/75 mm Hg.[40] These recommendations are controversial because few trials randomized subjects with heart disease to different target BPs and observed subsequent outcomes.[39] Although the idea that these high-risk patients should be treated to a lower than usual BP goal is analogous to the situation for diabetics[3-5,13,25,84] and those with CKD,[3-5,85] the clearest clinical trial evidence comes from a post hoc analysis of the progression of atherosclerosis in the Comparison of AMlodipine vs. Enalapril to Limit Occurrences of Thrombosis (CAMELOT) study.[98] Although the main trial was designed to compare outcomes in 1991 CHD patients with controlled BP (baseline, 129/78 mm Hg) randomized to additional treatment with amlodipine, enalapril, or placebo,[99] a substudy of 274 patients used intravascular ultrasound to measure atherosclerosis progression or regression. Individuals with on-treatment BP ≥ 140/90 mm Hg had a significant increase in atheroma volume, patients with BP between 120-139/80-89 mm Hg had no major change, and those with BP < 120/70 mm Hg had a decrease in atheroma volume.[98] Some are still concerned, however, that lowering of BP "too far" in patients with CHD can be deleterious.[100] The most recent data to support the existence of the J-shaped curve come from a post hoc analysis of the International VErapamil/trandolapril STudy (INVEST).[101] Although there were no significant differences in outcomes among CHD patients randomized to either atenolol or verapamil, CHD events were significantly more common in those whose diastolic BP was lowered below 70 mm Hg; no such pattern was seen for stroke. The consensus is that systolic BP is more predictive for most patients, and the benefits of lowering systolic BP probably outweigh the risk of lowering diastolic BP in most hypertensives, even with CHD.[100]

Different Targets for Blood Pressure Goals?

Recent research has suggested that traditional BP measurements at the brachial artery correlate poorly with the BP experienced by the heart and brain, primarily because of disordered wave reflections, primarily in older patients with stiff arteries.[102] Many different noninvasive methods of estimating central aortic pressure have been developed, some of which are reimbursed by insurance. Several studies have shown a better prediction of CVD events with central aortic than with brachial BPs,[103] and most of the curvature in meta-regression analyses (see Fig. 9-5) disappears if estimates of central aortic systolic pressure are used on the x-axis rather than systolic BP. The largest clinical trial to prospectively measure central aortic pressure is the Conduit Artery Function Evaluation (CAFÉ),[69] a substudy of ASCOT.[68] A potential explanation for the impressive reduction in CVD events in ASCOT with the amlodipine-based regimen, despite a small difference in BP compared with the atenolol-based regimen, is that atenolol did not lower central aortic pressure nearly as well as amlodipine did. Sophisticated multivariate analyses demonstrated significant CVD benefits for every 10 mm Hg further lowering of central aortic pressure in CAFÉ.[69] Whether technically challenging serial estimations of central aortic pressure should become a target for therapy or simply a risk stratification tool (particularly in older patients) is currently controversial. Proponents tout the pathophysiologic links between the biophysics of aging arteries, collagen crosslinking, the resulting low-capacitance vessels, ventricular-vascular coupling, and the atherosclerotic process as reasons to consider central aortic pressure an appropriate target for primary prevention.[102,104]

More sophisticated technologies have also resulted in non-invasive methods of measuring pulse wave velocity, augmentation index, and aortic stiffness.[105] Whereas their utility as risk stratification tools has been demonstrated (most convincingly in the prospective Strong Heart Study), no clinical trials have yet used these measurements as targets for therapy. Because some of these parameters closely correlate with data available from 24-hour ABPM,[106] it is likely that investigators will soon reexamine their ABPM files and begin finding more data to support these measures of vascular function as prognostic tools.

Constructing a Regimen

Because most hypertensive patients will require two or more drugs to achieve the more intensive treatment goals outlined before, the health care provider probably should be concerned with choosing appropriate drug combinations more than with which specific agent is selected to begin the BP-lowering process.[5,9,15] Even in ALLHAT, which restricted enrollment to those with a high chance of being controlled on single-drug therapy (untreated BP < 180/110 mm Hg, or <160/100 on one or two drugs), an average of two medications per patient was required at the end of the study.[86]

The ideal drug regimen would have many characteristics. In addition to lowering the BP to goal, the regimen should be able to be administered once daily without regard to meals, be relatively inexpensive, cause few adverse effects (and perhaps even result in fewer side effects than single-drug therapy), and be widely available in all pharmacies and benefits plans. Several of the newer fixed-dose combination products have several of these attributes; those combining a dihydropyridine calcium antagonist and an ACE inhibitor, for instance, result in less pedal edema than the calcium channel blocker alone, even at the same doses. We now have three triple-drug combinations in the United States; one contains a diuretic, reserpine, and low-dose hydralazine; the other two combine a diuretic, amlodipine, and an ARB.

Management in Special Circumstances

Aside from patients who have a compelling indication for a particular antihypertensive drug (see Table 9-4), hypertensive patients having increased CVD risk require more attention. Those falling into this category include hypertensive patients with older age, diabetes, pregnancy, impending surgery, refractory hypertension, renal impairment, or hypertensive crisis.

Older Patients with Hypertension

There is now no question that older patients derive major benefit from antihypertensive drug therapy.[41] In fact, the number needed to treat (and similarly the cost) to prevent a single CVD event is *far* lower for older (compared with younger) patients, simply because their vintage puts them at higher absolute risk. Thus, they are also candidates for anti-platelet and lipid-lowering therapy, even if they do not have established CHD.[68,90] The decades-old controversy about whether hypertensive individuals older than 80 years benefit

from antihypertensive drug therapy has been resolved in the affirmative by the HYpertension in the Very Elderly Trial (HYVET). It was stopped after only 1.9 of the 5 years of planned follow-up because of a significant benefit on all-cause mortality, despite a final nonsignificant benefit on stroke (the primary endpoint).[42]

Diabetic Patients with Hypertension

The regimen used to treat diabetics to a BP goal of <130/80 mm Hg should include either an ACE inhibitor or an ARB (see Table 9-4).[3-5,13,14,25,36,84] An ARB can be justified if the patient is intolerant of an ACE inhibitor or if the patient has type 2 diabetes, renal impairment, and major proteinuria (e.g., patients in the Irbesartan Diabetic Nephropathy Trial [IDNT] or the Reduction of Endpoints in Non–insulin dependent diabetes mellitus with the Angiotensin II Antagonist Losartan [RENAAL] trial). The Captopril Cooperative Study Group demonstrated renoprotective effects of an ACE inhibitor in type 1 diabetics. Either an ACE inhibitor or an ARB has reduced the progression of microalbuminuria to overt proteinuria (in the MIcroalbuminuria, Cardiovascular and Renal Outcomes substudy of the Heart Outcomes Prevention Evaluation [MICRO-HOPE] and the second IRbesartan MicroAlbuminuria [IRMA-2] trial). The cardiovascular benefits of an ACE inhibitor in type 2 diabetics have been seen in MICRO-HOPE. The challenge for most diabetics is to achieve the several recommended goals (BP <130/80 mm Hg, LDL-cholesterol <100 mg/dL, A1c <7%). Unfortunately, most surveys of large groups of patients have shown worse control of BP in diabetic subjects compared with nondiabetics. However, a randomized trial carried out at the Steno Diabetes Center in Denmark showed significant reductions in both CVD events and long-term mortality among those who were given the more intensive multifactorial intervention (which included BP < 130/80 mm Hg).[107]

Pregnant Patients with Hypertension

Many of the antihypertensive drugs are either contraindicated or a potential threat to the mother or fetus.[108] Diuretics, the "preferred" first-line therapy for nonpregnant hypertensives, are generally avoided during pregnancy owing to the risk of oligohydramnios. ACE inhibitors, ARBs, and renin inhibitors are contraindicated because of the risk of renal and other fetal malformations. Nitroprusside is transformed to cyanide, which is very toxic to the fetus. As a result, time-tested and traditional antihypertensive drug therapy is usually used, including, in order, methyldopa, hydralazine, a beta blocker (typically labetalol), and then perhaps a calcium antagonist.

Hypertensive Patients with Impending Surgery

Most hypertensive patients receive closer scrutiny when elective surgery is planned. On occasion, the procedure must be postponed, especially if the BP is >160/95 mm Hg. Most anesthesiologists recommend holding the preoperative dose of an ACE inhibitor or ARB, as they increase the risk of hypotension during induction. Adding a beta blocker to reduce perioperative CVD risk is not recommended unless it was given chronically before the procedure or the patient is having major vascular surgery. Even these recommendations have been criticized on the basis of a meta-analysis of 33 trials including 12,306 patients.[109]

Patients with Refractory Hypertension

Although several definitions of refractory hypertension have been proposed, the problem is so important that an American Heart Association Scientific Statement has recently summarized our knowledge on the topic.[51] The "cause" of resistant hypertension can usually be determined for a specific patient after a proper evaluation. The causes of resistant

TABLE 9-6	Estimated Prevalence of Common Causes of Resistant Hypertension in Primary Care Versus Referral Centers	
Primary Care	Cause of Resistant Hypertension	Tertiary Center
~50%	Nonadherence to prescribed drugs	10%-20%
	Problems with blood pressure measurement	
20%-30%	White coat hypertension	10%-20%
	Medication-related causes	
~5%	Suboptimal medication regimen	30%-50%
~10%	Drug-drug interaction	<5%
<2%	Objective medication intolerance	<2%
	Interfering substances	
1%-5%	Excessive dietary sodium intake	1%-10%
1%-7%	Ethanol, NSAIDs, or illicit substances	1%-12%
	Secondary hypertension	
<5%	Sleep apnea, aldosterone excess	1%-83%
<5%	Traditional secondary causes of hypertension	5%-28%
	Psychological causes	
1%-2%	Anxiety, panic disorder, depression	1%-2%
1%-2%	Subjective medication intolerance	1%-5%

NSAIDs, nonsteroidal anti-inflammatory drugs. Medication intolerance was judged to be "objective" if the patient-reported adverse effect had been previously noted in the literature or "subjective" if it had not been previously noted (e.g., hair hurts, teeth itch).

Estimated from Calhoun[51] and other sources.

hypertension differ, depending on whether the patient is seen in a primary care setting or a referral center (Table 9-6). The most common successful pharmacologic intervention for patients with resistant hypertension in many centers is modification of the drug regimen. Adding or switching to an appropriate diuretic (a loop diuretic if the eGFR is <40 to 50 mL/min/1.73 m² or thiazide-like diuretic otherwise)[52] and adding an aldosterone antagonist or an alpha blocker are the most frequent successful changes. Research has not generated very useful solutions for the all-too-common scenarios of the older, diabetic, or autonomically challenged patient with resistant systolic hypertension who develops orthostatic hypotension on treatment. Such patients sometimes respond to individualized treatment regimens (sometimes including venous compression stockings, low-dose midodrine, or dietary salt liberalization); more commonly, the BP target has to be modified upward.

Hypertensive Patients with Chronic Kidney Disease

People with hypertension and eGFR < 60 mL/min/1.73 m² (i.e., stage 3 CKD[85]) should have their renally excreted antihypertensive drugs reduced in dose (or, less commonly, frequency of administration) and be treated to a lower target (currently <130/80 mm Hg).[3-5,85] An ACE inhibitor or ARB is highly recommended, after which a modest acute rise in serum creatinine (<25% from baseline) and usually clinically nonsignificant increase in serum potassium should be expected. An ARB delayed the progression of renal disease in type 2 diabetics in both IDNT and RENAAL[3-5,83,84]; an ACE inhibitor was more effective than the calcium antagonist or beta blocker in AASK.[96] An ACE inhibitor can be recommended for nondiabetic renal impairment.[86,95,110]

The role of albuminuria or proteinuria as a risk factor for CVD or as a target of therapy is fascinating and controversial. Many epidemiologic studies (including normotensive and nondiabetic subjects in the Framingham Heart Study[111]) and a few clinical trials have demonstrated albuminuria to be a predictor of both progression of renal disease and incident CVD.[3-5,9,85,94-97,110] The U.S. Food and Drug Administration (FDA) has never recognized albuminuria as a proper surrogate endpoint, despite the opinions of many physicians and nearly all nephrologists. As a result, no drugs are approved to reduce albuminuria, which is most commonly assessed today with an early morning urine sample sent for albumin/creatinine ratio.[85] Many clinical trials have nonetheless proved that BP lowering, ACE inhibitors, ARBs, and renin inhibitors are more likely than dihydropyridine calcium antagonists to reduce albuminuria.[112] The strongest data arguing that giving drugs to lower albuminuria reduces CVD risk may arise from the Losartan Intervention For Endpoint reduction (LIFE) trial,[113] but teasing out which attributes of a particular drug regimen have the largest effect on specific CVD events is challenging.

Patients with Hypertensive Crises

Hypertensive emergencies are best treated in the hospital (typically in the intensive care unit) with a short-acting, rapidly reversible, intravenously administered antihypertensive drug (typically nitroprusside, although the short-acting dihydropyridine calcium antagonist clevidipine, which is hydrolyzed by serum esterases, has been recently approved).[114] Hypertensive urgencies may be routinely treated in the outpatient setting with any one of a number of oral antihypertensive agents, including captopril, labetalol, and clonidine. Nifedipine capsules, which had been widely used in this setting for nearly 20 years, are now to be used "with great caution, if at all," according to an FDA advisory, because of their propensity to cause quick and excessive hypotension. Perhaps the most important aspect of the treatment of hypertensive urgency is to arrange quick follow-up for the patient where chronic, better management of BP can be ensured.

Organizing for Successful Management

The goal of hypertension management is to prevent the morbidity and mortality associated with it and to do so in the "least intrusive" manner (both physiologically and fiscally). Because hypertension is not a disease but a condition that increases CVD and renal risk, its long-term control is a continuing challenge. For many years, it was thought that most patients with hypertension have no noticeable symptoms. Recent studies using antihypertensive drugs without appreciable side effects have demonstrated a significant decrease in headache when hypertensive patients are successfully treated. The quality of life among treated hypertensives was greatest in the group that achieved the lowest BPs in both HOT[90] and the Treatment of Mild Hypertension Study,[81] suggesting that there *may* be subtle symptoms that can be attributed to an elevated BP that improve when BP is lowered. It is nonetheless often difficult to convince a person with hypertension that taking a pill or changing one's lifestyle will result in tangible benefits, especially in the short term. It is also unfortunately true that treating hypertension (even successfully) does not reduce CVD risk to the level of a normotensive person. This provides strong impetus for initiation of lifestyle modifications early, even before the levels of BP we call hypertension are present.

It is difficult to motivate patients to sustain their lifestyle modifications and to adhere long term to their prescribed medications. National survey data indicate that only 50.1% of America's hypertensives have their BPs < 140/90 mm Hg[6]; other countries have even lower control rates. Nonadherence results in wasted health care resources (~10% of costs for hypertension), unnecessary hospitalizations, preventable strokes and heart attacks, and a large portion of the admissions to nursing homes (where drug taking can be more carefully and efficiently supervised). Many suggestions have been made to increase adherence to pill taking; some have been proven successful in clinical trials. Several clinical trials in conditions besides hypertension (e.g., after myocardial infarction or in heart failure) have shown that patients who do not take the pills as directed typically suffer more CVD events than those who are adherent. Education of the patient (and family) is the cornerstone of improving adherence; patients with educational or cognitive deficits about hypertension and its treatment are unlikely to follow instructions for very long. Some clinics have improved their hypertension control rates after a health educator was added to the hypertension treatment team. Behavioral suggestions are often useful, such as integrating pill taking into the activities of daily living (e.g., taking pills when caring for teeth) or using a pill organizer (typically to organize pills according to days of the week on which they are to be consumed). Increasing social support appears to be a beneficial strategy, especially for older individuals. The family member or caretaker can remind the patient of the need to take pills and to keep office visits as well as actually measure BP with a home device.

Missing appointments for follow-up care and monitoring of hypertension treatment has been associated with poorer outcomes. Several routine procedures can help minimize this problem. Appointment reminders (either by telephone or by mail) increase return visit rates. Scheduling of a specific time and date with a known health care provider, at the end of the office visit, is more successful than "calling in for a future appointment." Decreasing waiting times, having convenient office hours, and having a solicitous, caring office staff are also helpful.

Several characteristics of physicians have an impact on patients' adherence to medications and willingness to keep appointments. Physicians who are willing to involve the patient (when appropriate) in medical decision making are more successful in controlling BP. A common example is asking whether the patient would prefer to take a less expensive pill more often or a more expensive pill just once a day. Physicians who are perceived as having effective communication skills, who encourage questions from the patient and appropriate family members, and who provide feedback about the patient's progress also achieved better results.

Much of the underachievement of BP control nationwide has been attributed to patients' unwillingness to take pills and to appear for follow-up visits, but some of the blame has been attributed to physicians and other components of the health care system. Most systems have accepted the treatment of hypertension as a worthwhile endeavor as it saves money in high-risk patients and is relatively cost-effective in others (compared with many other common medical interventions). Recent efforts to restrict pharmacy benefits, to limit the range and doses of drugs on an accepted formulary, and to reduce accessibility of health care services have led to increased costs. System-wide efforts (often called disease management programs) to encourage acceptance of generic drugs, to increase the threshold for beginning antihypertensive drug therapy in low-risk patients, to use one drug to treat both hypertension and a concomitant medical condition, and to encourage adherence to medication taking have been more successful. The workload of the health care provider involved in these efforts can be increased by some of these procedures, but it is sometimes offset by case managers and other allied health professionals who perform some of these important tasks.

CONCLUSION

Hypertension control is an important public health goal that requires a long-term commitment from the patient, the physician, and the health care system. When all work together toward a common goal, the benefits of hypertension therapy in clinical trials can be easily and effectively translated into practice. This will eventually reduce the burden of disease and adverse cardiovascular and renal outcomes that were formerly associated with untreated or undertreated hypertension.

REFERENCES

1. Lawes CM, Van der Hoorn S, Rodgers A; International Society of Hypertension: Global burden of blood-pressure-related disease, 2001. *Lancet* 371:1513, 2008.
2. Elliott WJ, Black HR: Prehypertension. *Nat Clin Pract Cardiovasc Med* 4:538, 2007.
3. Chobanian AV, Bakris GL, Black HR, et al: The Seventh Report of the Joint National Committee on Prevention, Detection, Evaluation, and Treatment of High Blood Pressure: The JNC 7 Report. *JAMA* 289:2560, 2003.
4. Littlejohns P, Ranson P, Sealey C, et al; National Collaborating Centre for Chronic Conditions: Hypertension: management of hypertension in adults in primary care (partial update of NICE Clinical Guideline 18). National Institute for Health and Clinical Excellence. Available at: www.nice.org.uk/page.aspx?o=278167. Accessed June 25, 2006.
5. Mancia G, De Backer G, Dominiczak A, et al: 2007 Guidelines for the management of arterial hypertension. Task Force for the Management of Arterial Hypertension of the European Society of Hypertension and the European Society of Cardiology. *J Hypertens* 25:1105, 2007.
6. Egan BM, Zhao Y, Axon RN: US trends in prevalence, awareness, treatment, and control of hypertension, 198-2008. *JAMA* 303:2043-2050, 2010.
7. Fang J, Alderman MH, Keenan NL, et al: Hypertension control at physicians' offices in the United States. *Am J Hypertens* 21:136, 2008.
8. Lloyd-Jones D, Adams R, Carnethon M, et al: Heart Disease and Stroke Statistics, 2009 Update. A Report from the American Heart Association Statistics Committee and Stroke Statistics Subcommittee. *Circulation* 119:e2, 2009. Available at: http://circ.ahajournals.org/cgi/reprint/CIRCULATIONAHA.108.191261. Accessed December 16, 2008.
9. Giles T, Berk B, Black HR, et al: Position Paper: Expanding the definition and classification of hypertension. *J Clin Hypertens (Greenwich)* 7:505, 2005.
10. Oparil S, Zaman A, Calhoun DA: Pathogenesis of hypertension. *Ann Intern Med* 139:761, 2003.
11. Mason RP: Nitric oxide mechanisms in the pathogenesis of global risk. *J Clin Hypertens (Greenwich)* 8(Suppl 2):31, 2006.
12. Age-specific relevance of usual blood pressure to vascular mortality: a meta-analysis of individual data for one million adults in 61 prospective studies. Prospective Studies Collaborative. *Lancet* 360:1903, 2002.
13. Turnbull F; Blood Pressure Lowering Treatment Trialists' Collaboration: Effects of different blood-pressure-lowering regimens on major cardiovascular events: Results of prospectively-designed overviews of randomised trials. *Lancet* 362:1527, 2003.
14. Turnbull F; Blood Pressure Lowering Treatment Trialists' Collaboration: Blood pressure–dependent and independent effects of agents that inhibit the renin-angiotensin system. *J Hypertens* 25:951, 2007.
15. Law MR, Morris JK, Wald NJ: Use of blood pressure lowering drugs in the prevention of cardiovascular disease: meta-analysis of 147 randomised trials in the context of expectations from prospective epidemiological studies. *BMJ* 338:b1665, 2009. doi: 101136/bmj.b1665.
16. Vasan RS, Beiser A, Seshadri S, et al: Residual lifetime risk for developing hypertension in middle-aged women and men: the Framingham Heart Study. *JAMA* 287:1003, 2002.
17. Julius S, Nesbitt SD, Egan B, et al: Feasibility of treating prehypertension with an angiotensin receptor blocker. *N Engl J Med* 354:1685, 2006.
18. Pickering TG, Hall JE, Appel LJ, et al: Recommendations for blood pressure measurement in humans and experimental animals: Part 1: Blood pressure measurement in humans: a statement for professionals from the Subcommittee of Professional and Public Education of the American Heart Association Council on High Blood Pressure Research. *Hypertension* 45:142, 2005.
19. Pickering TG, Miller NH, Ogedegbe G, et al: Call to action on use and reimbursement for home blood pressure monitoring: executive summary: a joint Scientific Statement from the American Heart Association, American Society of Hypertension, and Preventive Cardiovascular Nurses Association. *Hypertension* 52:1, 2008.
20. Parati G, Omboni S, Albini F, et al: Home blood pressure telemonitoring improves hypertension control in general practice. The TeleBPCare study. *J Hypertens* 27:198, 2009.
21. Green BB, Cook AJ, Ralston JD, et al: Effectiveness of home blood pressure monitoring, web communication, and pharmacist care on hypertension control: a randomized controlled trial. *JAMA* 299:2857, 2008.
22. Pickering TG, Shimbo D, Haas D: Current concepts: ambulatory blood-pressure monitoring. *N Engl J Med* 354:2368, 2006.
23. O'Brien E, Asmar R, Beilin L, et al: European Society of Hypertension recommendations for conventional, ambulatory and home blood pressure measurement. *J Hypertens* 21:821, 2003.
24. Fagard RH, Cornelissen VA: Incidence of cardiovascular events in white-coat, masked, and sustained hypertension compared to true normotension: a meta-analysis. *J Hypertens* 25:2193, 2007.

9

25. Staessen JA, Wang JG, Thijs L: Cardiovascular protection and blood pressure reduction: a meta-analysis. *Lancet* 358:1305, 2001.

26. Elliott WJ, Jonsson MC, Black HR: Management of hypertension: is it the pressure or the drug? *Circulation* 113:2763, 2006.

27. Verdecchia P, Reboldi G, Angeli F, et al: Angiotensin-converting enzyme inhibitors and calcium channel blockers for coronary heart disease and stroke prevention. *Hypertension* 46:386, 2005.

28. MacMahon S, Neal B, Rodgers A: Hypertension—time to move on. *Lancet* 365:1108, 2005.

29. D'Agostino RB Sr, Vasan RS, Pencina MJ, et al: General cardiovascular risk profile for use in primary care: the Framingham Heart Study. *Circulation* 117:743, 2008.

30. Wang NY, Young JH, Meoni LA, et al: Blood pressure change and risk of hypertension associated with parental hypertension: the Johns Hopkins Precursors Study. *Arch Intern Med* 168:643, 2008.

31. Cutler JA, Sorlie PD, Wolz M, et al: Trends in hypertension prevalence, awareness, treatment, and control rates in United States adults between 1988-1994 and 1999-2004. *Hypertension* 52:818, 2008.

32. Appel LJ, Brands MW, Daniels SR, et al: Dietary approaches to prevent and treat hypertension: a Scientific Statement from the American Heart Association. *Hypertension* 47:296, 2006.

33. Fung TT, Chiuve SE, McCullough ML, et al: Adherence to a DASH-style diet and risk of coronary heart disease and stroke in women. *Arch Intern Med* 168:713, 2008.

34. Skov K, Eiskjaer H, Hansen HE, et al: Treatment of young subjects at high familial risk of future hypertension with an angiotensin-receptor blocker. *Hypertension* 50:89, 2007.

35. Chan CC, Reid CM, Aw TJ, et al: Do COX-2 inhibitors raise blood pressure more than nonselective NSAIDs and placebo? An updated meta-analysis. *J Hypertens* 27:2332, 2009.

36. De Backer G, Ambrosioni E, Borch-Johnsen K, et al: Executive summary: European guidelines on cardiovascular disease prevention in clinical practice. *Eur Heart J* 24:1601, 2003.

37. Simmons RK, Sharp S, Boekholdt SM, et al: Evaluation of the Framingham Risk Score in the European Prospective Investigation of Cancer–Norfolk cohort. *Arch Intern Med* 168:1209, 2008.

38. Wallis EJ, Ramsay LE, Haq IU, et al: Coronary and cardiovascular risk estimation for primary prevention: validation of a new Sheffield table in the 1995 Scottish health survey population. *BMJ* 320:671, 2000.

39. Arguedas JA, Perez MI, Wright JM: Treatment blood pressure targets for hypertension. *Cochrane Database Syst Rev* (3):CD004349, 2009. DOI: 10.1002/14651858.CD004349. pub2. Accessed December 10, 2009.

40. Rosendorff C, Black HR, Cannon CP, et al: Treatment of hypertension in the prevention and management of ischemic heart disease. A Scientific Statement from the American Heart Association Council for High Blood Pressure Research and the Councils on Clinical Cardiology and Epidemiology and Prevention. *Circulation* 115:2761, 2007.

41. Turnbull F, Neal B, Ninomiya T, et al; Blood Pressure Lowering Treatment Trialists' Collaboration: Effects of different regimens to lower blood pressure on major cardiovascular events in older and younger adults: meta-analysis of randomised trial. *BMJ* 336:1121, 2008.

42. Beckett NS, Peters R, Fletcher AE, et al: Treatment of hypertension in patients 80 years of age or older. *N Engl J Med* 358:1887, 2008.

43. Elliott WJ: Drug interactions and drugs affecting blood pressure control. *J Clin Hypertens (Greenwich)* 8:731, 2006.

44. Dickinson HO, Mason JM, Nicolson DJ, et al: Lifestyle interventions to reduce raised blood pressure: a systematic review of randomized controlled trials. *J Hypertens* 24:215, 2006.

45. Cook NR, Cutler JA, Obarzanek E, et al: Long term effects of dietary sodium reduction on cardiovascular disease outcomes: observational follow-up of the trials of hypertension prevention (TOHP). *BMJ* 334:885, 2007.

46. Sacks FM, Svetkey LP, Vollmer WM, et al: Effects on blood pressure of reduced dietary sodium and the Dietary Approaches to Stop Hypertension (DASH) diet. *N Engl J Med* 344:3, 2001.

47. Writing Group of the PREMIER Collaborative Research Group: Effects of comprehensive lifestyle modification on blood pressure control: main results of the PREMIER clinical trial. *JAMA* 289:2083, 2003.

48. Beulens JWJ, Rimm EB, Ascherio A, et al: Alcohol consumption and risk for coronary heart disease among men with hypertension. *Ann Intern Med* 146:10, 2007.

49. Xin X, He J, Frontini MG, et al: Effects of alcohol reduction on blood pressure: a meta-analysis of randomized controlled trials. *Hypertension* 38:1112, 2001.

50. Netzer NC, Stoohs RA, Netzer CM, et al: Using the Berlin questionnaire to identify patients at high risk for the sleep apnea syndrome. *Ann Intern Med* 131:485, 1999.

51. Calhoun DA, Jones D, Textor S, et al: Resistant hypertension: diagnosis, evaluation, and treatment. A Scientific Statement from the American Heart Association Professional Education Committee of the Council for High Blood Pressure Research. *Hypertension* 51:1403, 2008.

52. Elliott WJ, Grimm RH Jr: How to use diuretics in clinical practice: one opinion [commentary]. *J Clin Hypertens (Greenwich)* 10:856, 2008.

53. Hirsch AT, Haskal ZJ, Hertzer NR, et al: ACC/AHA 2005 Practice Guidelines for the management of patients with peripheral arterial disease (lower extremity, renal, mesenteric, and abdominal aortic): a collaborative report from the American Association for Vascular Surgery/Society for Vascular Surgery, Society for Cardiovascular Angiography and Interventions, Society for Vascular Medicine and Biology, Society of Interventional Radiology, and the ACC/AHA Task Force on Practice Guidelines (Writing Committee to Develop Guidelines for the Management of Patients With Peripheral Arterial Disease): endorsed by the American Association of Cardiovascular and Pulmonary Rehabilitation; National Heart, Lung, and Blood Institute; Society for Vascular Nursing; TransAtlantic Inter-Society Consensus; and Vascular Disease Foundation. *Circulation* 113:e463, 2006.

54. Funder JW, Carey RM, Fardella C, et al: Case detection, diagnosis, and treatment of patients with primary aldosteronism: an Endocrine Society clinical practice guideline. *J Clin Endocrinol Metab* 93:3266, 2008.

55. Lenders JW, Eisenhofer G, Mannelli M, Pacak K: Phaeochromocytoma. *Lancet* 366:665, 2005.

56. Arnaldi G, Angeli A, Atkinson AB, et al: Diagnosis and complications of Cushing's syndrome: a consensus statement. *J Clin Endocrinol Metab* 88:5593, 2003.

57. Elliott WJ: Secondary hypertension: renovascular hypertension. *J Clin Hypertens (Greenwich)* 10:522, 2008.

58. Bax L, Woittiez A-JJ, Kouwenberg HJ, et al: Stent placement in patients with atherosclerotic renal artery stenosis and impaired renal function: a randomized trial. *Ann Intern Med* 150:840, 2009.

59. Wheatley K, Ives N, Kalra PA, et al; Angioplasty and Stenting for Renal Artery Lesions (ASTRAL) Investigators: Revascularization versus medical therapy for renal-artery stenosis. *N Engl J Med* 361:1953, 2009.

60. Black HR: *Clinical trials in hypertension*, New York, 2001, Marcel Dekker.

61. Collins R, Peto R, MacMahon S, et al: Blood pressure, stroke, and coronary heart disease. Part 2, Short-term reductions in blood pressure: overview of randomised drug trials in their epidemiological context. *Lancet* 335:827, 1990.

62. Elliott WJ, Meier PM: Incident diabetes in clinical trials of antihypertensive drugs: a network meta-analysis [erratum in *Lancet* 369:1518, 2007]. *Lancet* 369:201, 2007.

63. Bangalore S, Messerli FH, Kostis JB, Pepine CJ: Cardiovascular protection using beta-blockers: a critical review of the evidence. *J Am Coll Cardiol* 50:563, 2007.

64. Effects of an angiotensin-converting-enzyme inhibitor, ramipril, on death from cardiovascular causes, myocardial infarction, and stroke in high-risk patients. The Heart Outcomes Prevention Evaluation (HOPE) Study Investigators. *N Engl J Med* 342:145, 2000.

65. Braunwald E, Domanski MJ, Fowler SE, et al: Angiotensin-converting-enzyme inhibition in stable coronary artery disease. The PEACE Trial Investigators. *N Engl J Med* 351:2058, 2004.

66. Telmisartan, ramipril or both in patients at high risk for vascular events. ONTARGET Investigators. *N Engl J Med* 358:1547, 2008.

67. Major outcomes in high-risk hypertensive patients randomized to angiotensin-converting enzyme inhibitor or calcium channel blocker vs. diuretic: the Antihypertensive and Lipid Lowering Treatment to Prevent Heart Attack Trial (ALLHAT). The ALLHAT Officers and Coordinators for the ALLHAT Collaborative Research Group. *JAMA* 288:2981, 2002.

68. Dahlöf B, Sever PS, Poulter NR, et al: Prevention of cardiovascular events with an antihypertensive regimen of amlodipine adding perindopril as required versus atenolol adding bendroflumethiazide as required, in the Anglo-Scandinavian Cardiac Outcomes Trial–Blood Pressure Lowering Arm (ASCOT-BPLA): a multicentre randomised controlled trial. *Lancet* 366:895, 2005.

69. Williams B, Lacy PS, Thom SM, et al: Differential impact of blood pressure–lowering drugs on central aortic pressure and clinical outcomes: principal results of the Conduit Artery Function Evaluation (CAFE) Study. *Circulation* 113:1213, 2006.

70. Yusuf S; Telmisartan Randomised AssessmeNt Study in ACE iNtolerant subjects with cardiovascular Disease (TRANSCEND) Investigators: Effects of the angiotensin-receptor blocker telmisartan on cardiovascular events in high-risk patients intolerant to angiotensin-converting enzyme inhibitors: a randomised controlled trial. *Lancet* 371:1174, 2008.

71. Yusuf S, Diener H-C, Sacco R, et al; PRoFESS Study Group: Telmisartan to prevent recurrent stroke and cardiovascular events. *N Engl J Med* 359:1225, 2008.

72. Mann JFE, Schmieder RE, McQueen M; ONTARGET Investigators: Renal outcomes with telmisartan, ramipril, or both, in people at high vascular risk (the ONTARGET study): a multicentre, randomised, double-blind, controlled trial. *Lancet* 372:547, 2008.

73. Jamerson K, Weber MA, Bakris GL, et al; ACCOMPLISH Trial Investigators: Benazepril plus amlodipine or hydrochlorothiazide for hypertension in high-risk patients. *N Engl J Med* 359:2417, 2008.

74. Elliott WJ, Basu S, Meier PM: Dihydropyridine vs. non-dihydropyridine calcium antagonists as initial therapy for prevention of cardiovascular events in hypertensive patients [abstract]. *J Clin Hypertens (Greenwich)* 11(Suppl A):A13, 2009.

75. Patel C: Twelve-month follow-up of yoga and biofeedback in the management of hypertension. *Lancet* 1:62, 1975.

76. Elliott WJ, Izzo JL Jr, White WB, et al: Graded blood pressure reduction in hypertensive outpatients associated with use of a device to assist with slow breathing. *J Clin Hypertens (Greenwich)* 6:553, 2004.

77. Morgan JP, Dickey JL, Hunt HH, Hudgins PM: A controlled trial of spinal manipulation in the management of hypertension. *J Am Osteopath Assoc* 85:308, 1985.

78. Knapp HR, FitzGerald GA: The antihypertensive effects of fish oils: a controlled study of polyunsaturated fatty acid supplements in essential hypertension. *N Engl J Med* 320:1037, 1989.

79. Flachskampf FA, Gallasch J, Gefeller O, et al: Randomized trial of acupuncture to lower blood pressure. *Circulation* 115:3121, 2007.

80. Whelton PK, He J, Appel LJ, et al: Primary prevention of hypertension: clinical public health advisory from the National High Blood Pressure Education Program. *JAMA* 288:1882, 2002.

81. Neaton JD, Grimm RH, Prineas RJ, et al: Treatment of mild hypertension study: final results. *JAMA* 270:713, 1993.

82. Lynch AI, Boerwinkle E, Davis BR, et al: Pharmacogenetic association of the *NPPA T2238C* genetic variant with cardiovascular disease outcomes in patients with hypertension. *JAMA* 299:296, 2008.

83. Canadian Hypertension Education Program: Recommendations—2009. Available at: http://hypertension.ca/chep/recommendations-2009/. Accessed June 18, 2009.

84. American Diabetes Association: Standards of medical care in diabetes—2009. *Diabetes Care* 32(Suppl 1):S13, 2009, especially pages S28-S29.

85. Levey AS, Rocco MV, Anderson S, et al: K/DOQI clinical practice guidelines on hypertension and antihypertensive agents in chronic kidney disease. *Am J Kidney Dis* 43(Suppl 1):S1, 2004.

9

86. ALLHAT Officers and Coordinators for the ALLHAT Collaborative Research Group: Diuretic versus alpha-blocker as first-step antihypertensive therapy: final results from the Antihypertensive and Lipid-Lowering Treatment to Prevent Heart Attack Trial (ALLHAT). *Hypertension* 42:239, 2003.

87. Feldman RD, Zou GY, Vandervoort MK, et al: A simplified approach to the treatment of uncomplicated hypertension: a cluster-randomized controlled trial. *Hypertension* 53:646, 2009.

88. Black HR, Elliott WJ, Grandits G, et al; CONVINCE Research Group: Principal results of the Controlled ONset Verapamil INvestigation of Cardiovascular Endpoints (CONVINCE) Trial. *JAMA* 289:2073, 2003.

89. Liu L, Zhang Y, Liu G, et al; FEVER Study Group: The Felodipine Event Reduction (FEVER) study: a randomized long-term placebo-controlled trial in Chinese hypertensive patients. *J Hypertens* 23:2157, 2005.

90. Hansson L, Zanchetti A, Carruthers SG, et al: Effects of intensive blood pressure lowering and low-dose aspirin in patients with hypertension: principal results of the Hypertension Optimal Treatment (HOT) randomised trial: the HOT Study Group. *Lancet* 351:1755, 1998.

91. Verdecchia P, Staessen JA, Angeli F, et al; Cardio-Sis Investigators: Usual versus tight control of systolic blood pressure in non-diabetic patients with hypertension (Cardio-Sis): an open-label randomised trial. *Lancet* 374:525, 2009.

92. Tight blood pressure control and risk of macrovascular and microvascular complications in type 2 diabetes: UKPDS 38: UK Prospective Diabetes Study Group. *BMJ* 317:703, 1998.

93. Howard BV, Roman MJ, Devereux RB, et al: Effect of lower targets for blood pressure and LDL cholesterol on atherosclerosis in diabetes. *JAMA* 299:1678, 2008.

94. Sarnak MJ, Greene T, Wang X, et al: The effect of a lower target blood pressure on the progression of kidney disease: long-term follow-up of the Modification of Diet in Renal Disease study. *Ann Intern Med* 142:342, 2005.

95. Jafar TH, Stark PC, Schmid CH, et al: Progression of chronic kidney disease: the role of blood pressure control, proteinuria, and angiotensin-converting enzyme inhibition: a patient-level meta-analysis. *Ann Intern Med* 139:244, 2003.

96. Wright JT Jr, Bakris GL, Greene T, et al: Effect of blood pressure lowering and antihypertensive drug class on progression of hypertensive kidney disease: results from the AASK Trial. *JAMA* 288:2421, 2002.

97. Appel LJ, Wright JT Jr, Greene T, et al: Long-term effects of renin-angiotensin system–blocking therapy and a low blood pressure goal on progression of hypertensive chronic kidney disease in African Americans. *Arch Intern Med* 168:832, 2008.

98. Sipahi I, Tuzcu EM, Schoenhagen P, et al: Effects of normal, pre-hypertensive, and hypertensive blood pressure levels on progression of coronary atherosclerosis. *J Am Coll Cardiol* 48:833, 2006.

99. Nissen SE, Turzcu EM, Libby P, et al: Effect of antihypertensive agents on cardiovascular events in patients with coronary disease and normal blood pressure. The CAMELOT Study: a randomized controlled trial. *JAMA* 292:2217, 2004.

100. Messerli FH, Panjrath GS: The J-curve between blood pressure and coronary artery disease or essential hypertension: exactly how essential? *J Am Coll Cardiol* 54:1827, 2009.

101. Messerli FH, Mancia G, Conti CR, et al: Dogma disputed: can aggressively lowering blood pressure in hypertensive patients with coronary artery disease be dangerous? *Ann Intern Med* 144:884, 2006.

102. Agabiti-Rosei E, Mancia G, O'Rourke M, et al: Central blood pressure measurements and antihypertensive therapy: a consensus document. *Hypertension* 50:154, 2007.

103. Roman MJ, Devereux RB, Kizer JR, et al: Central pressure more strongly relates to vascular disease and outcome than does brachial pressure: the Strong Heart Study. *Hypertension* 50:197, 2007.

104. Baksi AJ, Treibel TA, Davies JE, et al: A meta-analysis of the mechanism of blood pressure change with aging. *J Am Coll Cardiol* 54:2087, 2009.

105. Smith RD, Levy PJ: New techniques for assessment of vascular function [review]. *Ther Adv Cardiovasc Dis* 2:373, 2008.

106. Schillaci G, Parati G: Ambulatory arterial stiffness index: merits and limitations of a simple surrogate measure of arterial compliance. *J Hypertens* 26:182, 2008.

107. Gaede P, Anderson HL, Parving HH, Pedersen O: Effect of a multifactorial intervention on mortality in type 2 diabetes. *N Engl J Med* 358:580, 2008.

108. Report of the National High Blood Pressure Education Program Working Group on High Blood Pressure in Pregnancy. *Am J Obstet Gynecol* 183:S1, 2000.

109. Bangalore S, Wetterslev J, Pranesh S, et al: Perioperative beta-blockers in patients having non-cardiac surgery: a meta-analysis [erratum in *Lancet* 373:1764, 2009]. *Lancet* 372:1962, 2008.

110. Kent DM, Jafar TH, Hayward RA, et al: Progression risk, urinary protein excretion, and treatment effects of angiotensin-converting enzyme inhibitors in nondiabetic kidney disease. *J Am Soc Nephrol* 18:1956, 2007.

111. Arnlöv J, Evans JC, Meigs JB, et al: Low-grade albuminuria and incidence of cardiovascular disease events in nonhypertensive and nondiabetic individuals: the Framingham Heart Study. *Circulation* 112:969, 2005.

112. Ibsen H, Wachtell K, Olsen MH, et al: Does albuminuria predict cardiovascular outcome on treatment with losartan versus atenolol in hypertension with left ventricular hypertrophy? A LIFE substudy. *J Hypertens* 22:1805, 2004.

113. Matchar DB, McCrory DC, Orlando LA, et al: Systematic review: comparative effectiveness of angiotensin-converting enzyme inhibitors and angiotensin II receptor blockers for treating essential hypertension. *Ann Intern Med* 148:16, 2008.

114. Agabiti-Rosei E, Salvetti M, Farsang C: European Society of Hypertension Scientific Newsletter: treatment of hypertensive urgencies and emergencies. *J Hypertens* 24:2482, 2006.

CHAPTER **10**

Heart Failure Prevention

Vasiliki V. Georgiopoulou, Andreas P. Kalogeropoulos,
Laurence S. Sperling, and Javed Butler

KEY POINTS

- Heart failure prevalence continues to rise in the United States and is projected to become worse with aging of the population.

- Recent therapeutic advances in heart failure have translated into only modest improvement in outcomes at the community level.

- Prevention efforts for heart failure have significantly lagged behind research for new treatment options.

- Optimal risk stratification strategies for incident heart failure continue to evolve.

- Hypertension and coronary heart disease remain the most prominent risk factors for heart failure, although cardiometabolic risk factors (e.g., obesity and diabetes) are rapidly increasing in importance.

- Several individual risk factor treatments have been shown to reduce the risk for development of heart failure.

- Further research is needed to assess optimal multiple risk factor interventions, behavior modification strategies, and novel therapeutic approaches to reduce heart failure risk in individuals with risk factors.

- Population-based promotion of healthy lifestyle at the primordial prevention level is likely to have an impact on the largest at-risk population.

The concept of "prevention" encompasses a vast spectrum ranging from primordial to primary, secondary, and tertiary prevention. For heart failure, an example of primordial prevention is avoidance of behaviors that enhance (e.g., weight gain) and embracing of behaviors that mitigate (e.g., active lifestyle) the risk for development of heart failure. Primary prevention includes control of heart failure risk factors (e.g., hypertension). Secondary prevention efforts institute interventions to reduce the risk of worsening of existing heart failure (e.g., treatment with beta blockers). Finally, tertiary prevention interventions in advanced heart failure are implemented to reduce the chances of imminent mortality (e.g., implantation of mechanical circulatory assist devices).

Most heart failure quality improvement efforts (e.g., the Get With The Guidelines program by the American Heart Association) are currently targeted at secondary prevention.[1] Similarly, most of the research efforts in heart failure are also targeted to treatment. During the last two decades, an intensified focus on the prevention of coronary artery disease has included the development of risk prediction models,[2-4] assessment of novel biomarkers,[5,6] identification of subclinical markers of coronary risk,[7,8] design of therapeutic trials for coronary disease prevention, and establishment of specific guidelines.[9,10] Despite the worsening epidemic of heart failure, however, prevention efforts in this area remain rudimentary.

Given the current and projected societal toll of heart failure, both clinically and economically, a more concentrated effort on heart failure prevention is needed. In this chapter, we focus on the primordial and primary prevention of heart failure. In recognition of the emphasis of this text, we will not discuss interventions to improve outcomes in individuals with manifest heart failure.

HEART FAILURE EPIDEMIOLOGY

Incidence, Prevalence, Outcomes, and Costs

It is estimated that more than 5.5 million subjects in the United States have heart failure, and more than 650,000 are diagnosed for the first time each year.[11] Current evidence suggests that the two major clinical subsets of heart failure (i.e., patients with impaired versus preserved left ventricular systolic function) each composes about half of the overall burden of heart failure in the community.[12] However, various studies have suggested that the proportion of heart failure with preserved ejection fraction ranges from 13% to 74% of all heart failure.[13] These studies are heterogeneous and differ considerably in patient selection criteria, diagnostic criteria for heart failure, and quantitative methods for assessment of ventricular systolic function.[14] A common finding among these studies, however, is that the proportion of heart failure with preserved ejection fraction increases with age.[12,15] Not surprisingly, there is a secular trend toward increased prevalence of heart failure with preserved ejection fraction among patients hospitalized for heart failure.[16]

Heart failure is the primary reason for 12 to 15 million office visits and 6.5 million hospital days annually. Recurrent hospitalization is a major quality of life and cost issue; the annual number of hospitalizations now exceeds more than 1 million for heart failure as a primary diagnosis and 2.4 to 3.6 million as a primary or secondary diagnosis. Heart failure patients are particularly prone to rehospitalizations, and readmission rates are near 50% within 6 months of discharge. The number of heart failure cases and deaths attributable to heart failure has increased steadily despite advances in treatment and a decline in other major cardiovascular disease during the same interval. Heart failure remains the most common Medicare diagnosis–related group, and more Medicare dollars are spent on heart failure than for any other diagnosis. It has been estimated that the total direct and indirect cost of heart failure in the United States exceeds $30 billion.[11]

Despite this, the outcomes of these patients continue to remain suboptimal at the population level, with only approximately 50% of the individuals surviving past 5 years after diagnosis.[17] Quality of life remains poor. Some temporal improvement trends in outcomes have been restricted primarily to individuals with systolic dysfunction, with no major advances in therapy for either patients with heart failure and preserved ejection fraction or those who are hospitalized for decompensated heart failure.

Future Projections

Heart failure prevalence is rising, and this trend is expected to continue. This is attributed to the increasing elderly population, improved care of acute heart diseases, and increasing prevalence of several cardiovascular risk factors like diabetes and obesity. According to the White House Conference on Aging, aging of the 78 million baby boomers will result in 1 in 5 Americans older than 65 years by 2050.[18] This trend will have a significant effect on health, health care, and health care economics because the use of formal and informal services is strongly correlated with age.

Heart failure incidence and prevalence are highest among the elderly. The incidence rate approaches 10 per 1000 population annually after the age of 65 years; 80% of patients hospitalized with heart failure are older than 65 years. Thus, the increasing age of the population is expected to significantly worsen the current heart failure epidemic. Much of heart failure research to date has focused on treatment. Considering the current epidemiologic trends and the future projections, it is imperative to further heart failure prevention efforts aggressively.

RISK FACTORS FOR HEART FAILURE

Many studies have described various risk factors for development of heart failure ranging from lifestyle factors to comorbidities, medications, laboratory and imaging characteristics, and novel biomarkers and genomic markers (Table 10-1).[19] Heart failure risk increases proportionally with advancing age. Male gender is associated with a higher risk and may in part be explained by the higher prevalence of coronary disease in men.[20] Behavioral risk factors for heart failure include lower levels of physical activity, coffee consumption, and increased dietary salt intake. Low socioeconomic status has been associated with increased risk.[20] Older age, hypertension, diabetes, obesity, and coronary artery disease are risk factors for heart failure with either reduced or preserved ejection fraction. In general, patients with preserved ejection fraction are older, are more likely to be female, and are more likely to be obese. In heart failure with preserved ejection fraction, hypertension is a more common risk factor[16]; however, a substantial proportion of patients with reduced ejection fraction have a history of hypertension also.[16] In heart failure with reduced ejection fraction, ischemic heart disease is the most common etiology, but it is also a comorbid condition among many patients with preserved ejection fraction.[16] Among patients admitted for decompensated heart failure, 63% of patients with reduced ejection fraction and 54% of patients with preserved ejection fraction have coronary artery disease.[21] Thus, from a prevention perspective,

TABLE 10–1	Risk Factors for Development of Heart Failure
Demographics	**Lifestyle factors**
Older age	Cocaine
Male gender	Tobacco use
	Excess alcohol consumption
Socioeconomic status	Excess caffeine
	Excess sodium consumption
Education	
	Echocardiographic parameters
Comorbidities	Ventricular dimension
Hypertension	Ventricular mass
Left ventricular hypertrophy	Ventricular dysfunction
Prior myocardial infarction	Diastolic filling impairment
Obesity	
Diabetes mellitus	**Biochemical markers**
Valvular heart disease	Albuminuria
Renal insufficiency	Homocysteine
Dyslipidemia	Tumor necrosis factor-α
Sleep apnea	Interleukin-6
Tachycardia	C-reactive protein
Impaired lung function	Insulin-like growth factor 1
Depression, excess stress	Natriuretic peptides
Pharmacologic exposures	**Genetic risk factors**
Chemotherapeutic agents	Adrenergic receptors α_{2C}Del322-325 deletion
Nonsteroidal anti-inflammatory drugs	Adrenergic receptors β_1Arg389 change
Thiazolidinediones	Overexpression of protein kinase C-α
Doxazosin	ACE and Ang II type 1 receptor gene polymorphisms

ACE, angiotensin-converting enzyme; Ang II, angiotensin II.

the major target risk factors for possible modification are common in both subsets of heart failure.

Hypertension and coronary artery disease are the most common and strongest risk factors, conferring a twofold to threefold increased risk for heart failure. Both elevated systolic blood pressure and elevated diastolic blood pressure have been associated with increased risk for heart failure.[22] Diabetes mellitus is associated with a higher risk, both with and without the presence of simultaneous coronary heart disease. Valvular heart disease increases risk through hemodynamic alterations on the ventricles, with either volume or pressure overload leading to myocardial dysfunction.

Obesity, through multiple mechanisms, predisposes individuals to heart failure.[23] Excessive alcohol intake increases blood pressure and is a direct myocardial toxin[24]; however, light to moderate alcohol consumption has been inversely associated with heart failure risk, especially in men.[25,26] Smoking promotes several cardiovascular risk factors and is associated with heart failure development.[17,20] Dyslipidemia predisposes to heart failure; however, it is unclear if this is primarily related to atherosclerosis or if there are alternative effects. High total cholesterol, low high-density lipoprotein cholesterol, and high triglyceride levels have all been correlated with greater left ventricular mass and impaired diastolic function.[27,28] However, observational studies investigating the association of total cholesterol with incident heart failure in individuals without prior coronary heart disease have yielded inconsistent results.[29,30]

Complications of renal dysfunction, including anemia, hypertension, arterial stiffening, sodium and water retention, endothelial dysfunction, and alteration in biomarkers profiles, are associated with elevation of the risk for development of heart failure. Anemia and sleep-disordered breathing are associated with heart failure. An increased heart rate increases heart failure odds; whether this represents a compensatory response to lower stroke volume and underlying asymptomatic systolic dysfunction or neurohumoral activation, or both, is not clearly known. Finally, several abnormalities of pulmonary function, including reduced forced vital capacity and forced expiratory volume in the first second of expiration, are associated with heart failure risk.

Microalbuminuria is associated with a threefold increased heart failure hospitalization risk. Levels of homocysteine, insulin-like growth factor, proinflammatory cytokines (e.g., tumor necrosis factor-α, interleukin-6, and C-reactive protein), and B-type natriuretic peptide are associated with an increased risk. Recently, serum resistin,[31] lipoprotein-associated phospholipase A₂,[32] and myeloperoxidase levels[33] have been associated with increased risk also.

Several chemotherapeutic agents (e.g., doxorubicin, cyclophosphamide, and 5-fluorouracil) are associated with heart failure. Doxorubicin-induced cardiotoxicity is dose related, especially when the cumulative dose exceeds 550 mg/m². Recent data show a higher risk with the use of trastuzumab. Cyclooxygenase 2 inhibitors may increase risk of myocardial infarction, raising heart failure risk concerns. Thiazolidinediones have been associated with edema and precipitation of heart failure. Recently, the Rosiglitazone Evaluated for Cardiac Outcomes and Regulation of Glycaemia in Diabetes (RECORD) study showed that thiazolidinedione use is associated with a small but clinically relevant increased risk of heart failure.[34] However, the debate continues as to whether these drugs truly predispose individuals to development of heart failure or only promote fluid retention in individuals with prevalent left ventricular dysfunction. Recreational drugs (e.g., cocaine abuse) may precipitate heart failure.

Several cardiac anatomic and physiologic measures are associated with a higher risk, including ventricular chamber dilation with an increase in end-diastolic or end-systolic dimensions, increased left ventricular mass, left ventricular diastolic filling impairment, left atrial enlargement, and asymptomatic systolic dysfunction.

Finally, there is growing interest in discovering the genomic predictors of heart failure.[19] Genetic alterations in functional pathways, such as energy production and regulation (e.g., mitochondrial mutations), calcium cycling abnormalities (e.g., *RYR2* mutations), and mutations in transcriptional regulators (e.g., Nkx2.5 leading to ventricular hypertrophy), may lead to heart failure risk. Genetic polymorphisms in sympathetic receptors, such as the genes coding for alpha$_{2C}$-adrenergic receptors (α_{2C}Del322-325) or beta$_1$-adrenergic receptors (ß$_1$Arg389), are associated with heart failure risk. Interestingly, homozygous blacks for α_{2C}Del322-325 have a fivefold higher risk. If this polymorphism is associated with homozygosity for β_1Arg389, the risk increases by 10-fold. Other polymorphisms associated with heart failure risk factors (e.g., hypertension and vascular stiffness) are angiotensin-converting enzyme and AT$_1$ receptor gene polymorphisms, which in turn may affect heart failure risk.

PREDICTING INCIDENT HEART FAILURE

Identification of High-Risk Individuals

For implementation of cost-effective preventive interventions, identification of high-risk individuals is essential. Although many heart failure risk factors have been described, determination of their role in predicting a future event is nevertheless challenging. A variable associated with a disease may be a risk marker or a risk factor. A risk factor's relative importance may change over time as the population

characteristics change (e.g., secular trends in age, treatment modalities of other risk factors, and prevalence of competing risk factors). The "independent" prognostic power of any risk factor depends largely on what it is compared against. Importantly, despite strong etiologic association with a disease, a risk factor may be limited in its prognostic role.[35]

A risk factor must have a much stronger association with disease than the usual etiologic research if it is to provide a basis for detection and prediction in an individual patient. If the distributions of the risk factor differ between two groups of patients with differing outcomes, the risk factor may be statistically associated with the outcome. However, for the risk factor to perform well as a prognostic test, the distributions in the two groups must be sufficiently separated to permit selection of a cutoff value that will discriminate between the two groups with high sensitivity and specificity.[35]

The American College of Cardiology and the American Heart Association (ACC/AHA) recently proposed a new heart failure classification scheme that includes stage A patients, those who do not have any structural heart disease but are at risk for heart failure.[36] This new classification is presented in Figure 10-1. Although individual risk factors for heart failure (e.g., hypertension) are well described, how to quantify individual risk in patients with various combinations of risk factors is not clearly described.

Multiple risk factor prediction schemes, such as the Framingham risk score, have been developed and validated for coronary events.[2] However, the heart failure syndrome represents a spectrum ranging from ischemic to nonischemic causes and normal to depressed ejection fraction. Heart failure may develop in elderly subjects as a result of age-related cardiovascular changes in the absence of traditional risk factors. High-risk subjects therefore may not be detected by coronary risk schemes. For example, in the Cardiovascular Health Study, 66% incident heart failure cases developed in subjects without baseline history of coronary heart disease, and more than half of them never had a preceding coronary event before development of heart failure.[37]

Heart Failure Risk Prediction Models

Most studies of heart failure risk factors have targeted individual risk factors. Table 10-2 summarizes the nine studies that have assessed independent risk factors for incident heart failure comparing multiple risk factors[20,37-44]; only two of them developed a prediction model for incident heart failure.[40,44] The Framingham heart failure risk score assessed the probability of development of heart failure during a 38-year period in which there were 6354 person-examinations in men and 8913 in women.[40] Although regression coefficients differed among men and women somewhat, overall predictors were similar (see Table 10-2). Interestingly, systolic blood pressure was predictive only in men and diabetes mellitus in women.

The investigators subsequently developed a 4-year event score with an event rate averaging 3.97 per 100 person-year examinations in men and 2.63 in women with a 37% increment per decade of age. There are several limitations to the use of this score. The chest radiograph and pulmonary function test requirement makes it more difficult to implement it in large population settings for screening. The model was drawn primarily on white populations, and its performance in other racial groups is not known. The model was derived on a restricted group of subjects with a known history of hypertension, coronary heart disease, or valvular heart disease; such characteristics represented less than 50% of the population in other cohorts, such as the Health, Aging, and

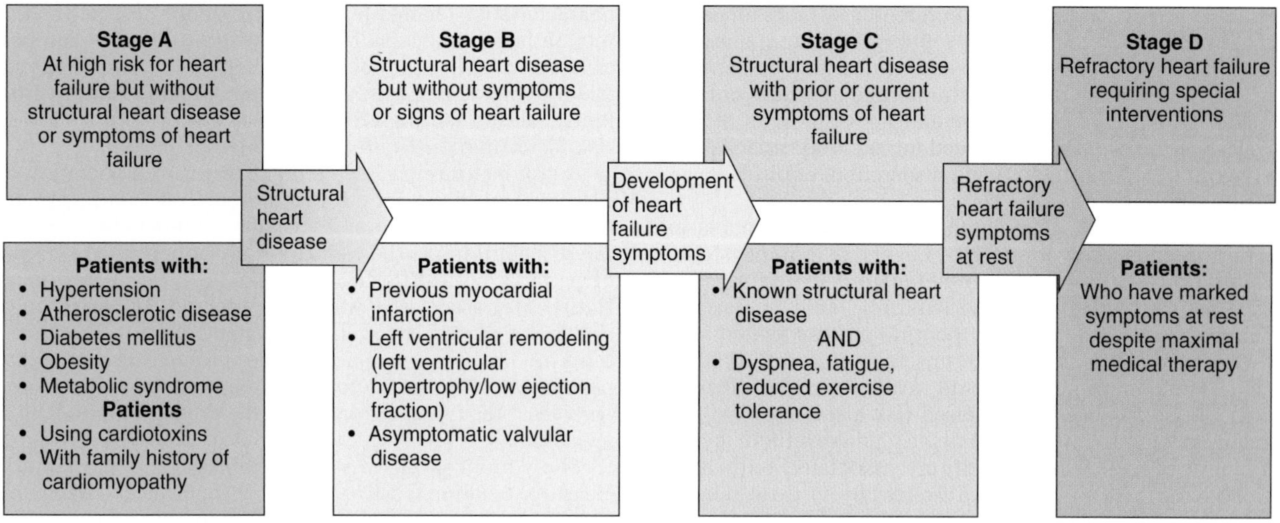

FIGURE 10-1 American Heart Association and American College of Cardiology new heart failure classification.

TABLE 10–2	Independent Risk Factors for Incident Heart Failure	
Reference	**Cohort**	**Risk Factors**
Eriksson, et al[38]	Göteborg, Sweden	Hypertension, smoking, weight, heart size, T wave abnormality, heart rate variability, peak expiratory flow rate, and psychological stress
Chen, et al[39]	EPESE	Gender, age, diabetes, pulse pressure, and body mass index
Kannel, et al[40]	Framingham Heart Study	Age, blood pressure, LVH, vital capacity, heart rate, CHD, murmurs, diabetes, cardiomegaly, and body mass index
Gottdiener, et al[37]	Cardiovascular Health Study	Age, gender, cerebrovascular disease, diabetes, blood pressure, FEV$_1$, creatinine, C-reactive protein, ankle-arm index, atrial fibrillation, LVH, abnormal ejection fraction, electrocardiographic ST-T abnormality
He, et al[20]	NHANES I	Gender, education, physical activity, smoking, weight, hypertension, diabetes, valvular disease, and CHD
Wilhelmsen, et al[41]	Göteborg, Sweden	Age, family history of infarction, diabetes, history of chest pain, smoking, coffee consumption, alcohol abuse, blood pressure, and body mass index
Bibbins-Domingo, et al[42]	Heart and Estrogen/ Progestin Replacement Study	Diabetes, atrial fibrillation, myocardial infarction, creatinine clearance, blood pressure, smoking, body mass index, left bundle branch block, and LVH
Carr, et al[43]	RENAAL and LIFE studies	Age, history of myocardial infarction, vascular disease, atrial fibrillation, urinary albumin/creatinine ratio, alcohol abuse, Cornell product, and body mass index
Butler, et al[44]	Health ABC	Age, CHD, smoking, blood pressure, heart rate, serum creatinine, fasting glucose, albumin level, and LVH on electrocardiogram

CHD, coronary heart disease; EPESE, Established Populations for Epidemiologic Studies of the Elderly; FEV$_1$, forced expiratory volume in the first second; LIFE, Losartan Intervention For Endpoint reduction in hypertension; LVH, left ventricular hypertrophy; NHANES, National Health and Nutrition Examination Survey; RENAAL, Reduction of Endpoints in Non–insulin dependent diabetes mellitus with the Angiotensin II Antagonist Losartan.

Body Composition (Health ABC) Study,[44] limiting the model's generalizability. Finally, this model was not externally validated in independent cohorts.

Recently, the Health ABC heart failure risk model was developed with the data from 2935 individuals participating in the Health ABC Study. The mean age of the population was 73.6 years, with 52% females and 41% blacks. Independent predictors of heart failure included age, history of coronary heart disease and smoking, systolic blood pressure and heart rate, serum glucose concentration, creatinine and albumin levels, and electrocardiographic left ventricular hypertrophy; the model has good discrimination (C-statistic 0.73 in the derivation data set and 0.72 by internal validation

with optimism-correction) and good calibration. A simple point score was created to predict incident heart failure risk in four risk groups corresponding to <5%, 5% to 10%, 10% to 20%, and >20% 5-year risk (Fig. 10-2).

The investigators subsequently externally validated the model in the Cardiovascular Health Study; the model retained adequate predictive capabilities.[45] The model predicted risk equally well in both men and women and in white and black races (Fig. 10-3). The utility of the Framingham heart failure risk score in predicting incident heart failure in the overall Health ABC cohort and the subcohorts in which the original score were developed (i.e., subjects with known baseline history of hypertension, coronary heart disease, or valvular

Age	
Years	**Points**
≤ 71	-1
72-75	0
76-78	1
≥ 79	2

Coronary Artery Disease	
Status	**Points**
No	0
Possible	2
Definite	5

LV Hypertrophy	
Status	**Points**
No	0
Yes	2

Systolic Blood Pressure	
mm Hg	**Points**
≤ 90	-4
95-100	-3
105-115	-2
120-125	-1
130-140	0
145-150	1
155-165	2
170-175	3
180-190	4
195-200	5
> 200	6

Heart Rate	
Bpm	**Points**
≤ 50	-2
55-60	-1
65-70	0
75-80	1
85-90	2
≥ 95	3

Smoking	
Status	**Points**
Never	0
Past	1
Current	4

Albumin	
g/dL	**Points**
≥ 4.8	-3
4.5-4.7	-2
4.2-4.4	-1
3.9-4.1	0
3.6-3.8	1
3.3-3.5	2
≤ 3.2	3

Fasting Glucose	
Mg/dL	**Points**
≤ 80	-1
85-125	0
130-170	1
175-220	2
225-265	3
≥ 270	5

Creatinine	
mg/dL	**Points**
≤ 0.7	-2
0.8-0.9	-1
1.0-1.1	0
1.2-1.4	1
1.5-1.8	2
1.9-2.3	3
> 2.3	6

Key:
Systolic BP to nearest 5 mm Hg
Heart Rate to nearest 5 bpm
Albumin to nearest 0.1 g/dL
Glucose to nearest 5 mg/dL
Creatinine to nearest 0.1 mg/dL

Health ABC HF Risk Score	HF Risk Group	5-yr HF Risk
≤ 2 Points	Low	< 5%
3-5 Points	Average	5-10%
6-9 Points	High	10-20%
≥ 10 Points	Very high	> 20%

FIGURE 10-2 The Health ABC Heart Failure (HF) Risk Score. *(From Butler J, Kalogeropoulos A, Georgiopoulou V, et al: Incident heart failure prediction in the elderly: the Health ABC Heart Failure Score.* Circ Heart Fail *1:125, 2008. Reprinted with permission of Wolters Kluwer Health.)*

heart disease) was also assessed. The Framingham heart failure risk score performance was inferior compared with the Health ABC heart failure risk model.

Challenges in Predicting Incident Heart Failure

Several unique issues make heart failure risk assessment challenging. Heart failure is a clinical diagnosis and cannot be easily diagnosed with a "test." This leads to diversity in opinions and diagnostic uncertainty in a certain proportion of cases. The most common clinical criteria used to diagnose heart failure are the Framingham criteria, which require the presence of at least two major criteria or one major criterion and two minor criteria.[46] Major criteria include paroxysmal nocturnal dyspnea, neck vein distention, rales, radiographic cardiomegaly, acute pulmonary edema, S_3 gallop, increased central venous pressure >16 cm H_2O, circulation time ≥25 seconds, hepatojugular reflux, or pulmonary edema or visceral congestion or cardiomegaly at autopsy. Minor criteria include bilateral ankle edema, nocturnal cough, dyspnea on ordinary exertion, hepatomegaly, pleural effusion, reduced vital capacity by one third from maximum, and heart rate ≥120 beats/min. Investigators from the Cardiovascular Health Study developed alternative criteria that included medication use and imaging modalities.[47] When both sets of criteria were compared, only half the patients were adjudicated to have heart failure by both criteria, whereas the other half were labeled with either one or the other but not both

criteria.[48] Similar discordance has also been shown between administrative discharge diagnoses and designation based on detailed chart review.[49]

Part of this discordance is related to diagnosis of heart failure with preserved ejection fraction. Many of the heart failure symptoms (e.g., shortness of breath) and signs (e.g., edema) are nonspecific and can be seen in other conditions (e.g., obesity and chronic lung disease). The European Society of Cardiology developed a consensus statement for diagnosis of this condition by use of biomarker- and imaging-based detailed protocols.[50] Similarly, another set of detailed clinical criteria to diagnose incident heart failure in clinical trials was recently published.[51] These criteria may be of limited usefulness from a population health perspective because of cost and logistics. Thus, these guidelines are likely to be used primarily in the clinical and research setting and not in the screening and population prevention arena.

Any clinical prediction rule is unlikely to diagnose "niche" heart failure, such as amyloidosis and hypertrophic cardiomyopathy, disorders with a distinct natural history. Similarly, whether risk prediction for heart failure differs for low versus preserved ejection fraction or stage A versus stage B heart failure is not known.

Risk Factors and Population Attributable Risk

Assessment of the population attributable risk for the common risk factors for any disease is key to prioritize prevention

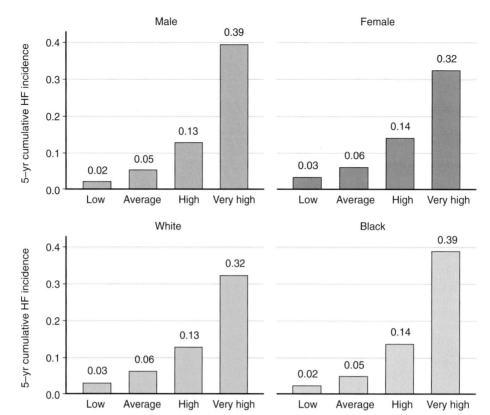

FIGURE 10-3 Health ABC Heart Failure Risk Score performance in gender- and race-stratified subgroups. Numbers represent fraction of participants with incident heart failure (HF). *(From Butler J, Kalogeropoulos A, Georgiopoulou V, et al: Incident heart failure prediction in the elderly: the Health ABC Heart Failure Score.* Circ Heart Fail *1:125, 2008. Reprinted with permission of Wolters Kluwer Health.)*

efforts cost-effectively. Population attributable risk represents the proportional reduction in disease risk that would be achieved by eliminating the risk factor from the population, assuming a causal relationship. The relative importance of risk factors in the population can help plan public health interventions; however, the absolute estimates for the population attributable risk of the various risk factors are highly dependent on the definition of risk factors and inclusion of other risk factors in the model used to derive the population attributable risks.

In a recent report from the Health ABC Study,[2] a cohort of well-functioning, community-dwelling older adults, coronary heart disease and uncontrolled blood pressure were the leading causes of heart failure in whites and blacks and in men and women. A substantial proportion of heart failure, however, was also attributed to metabolic and cardiorenal factors, including glucose and renal abnormalities. Several previous investigations have reported substantial sex- and race-related differences in population attributable risks, disease development and progression, and prognosis for heart failure.[17,52] Understanding and quantifying of these differences are important for planning appropriate preventive interventions.

The higher incidence of heart failure in black compared with white participants in the Health ABC Study was simultaneously accompanied by a higher prevalence of risk factors in black participants (Table 10-3). Interestingly, the black participants had a higher proportion not only of overall risk factors but also specifically of those risk factors that are potentially amenable to intervention, which translated the population attributable risk in general to a higher modifiable fraction in black individuals (68% versus 49% in whites). These data provide valuable information into race-based

differences and help prioritize interventions, set targets, and assess the feasibility of novel therapies.

INCIDENT HEART FAILURE RISK MODULATION

Incident heart failure risk modulation is currently targeted primarily toward risk factor management individually. For coronary artery disease, the patient's treatment plan is targeted on the basis of the individualized risk profile related to the various combinations of risk factors (e.g., blood pressure goals or low-density lipoprotein level). On the contrary, no such paradigm for heart failure risk modulation currently exists. Many heart failure risk factors (e.g., age and gender) cannot be intervened on. Other risk factors like proinflammatory states may be targets for intervention in the future. This section describes currently known interventions that directly or indirectly reduce the risk for incident heart failure. Most of these also affect other cardiovascular adverse outcomes; however, this section is focused primarily on heart failure–related data.

Lifestyle

Several studies have reported reduced risk for incident heart failure with healthy lifestyle. Maintaining healthy weight, avoiding smoking, engaging in regular exercise, and maintaining a healthy diet have been shown to favorably influence heart failure risk factors, including coronary heart disease,[53,54] diabetes mellitus,[55] and hypertension.[56] Recently, the Physicians' Health Study investigators reported that healthy lifestyle habits (i.e., normal body weight, not smoking, regular

	White (n = 1686)		Black (n = 1167)	
Risk Factors	RR (95% CI)	PAR (%)	RR (95% CI)	PAR (%)
Modifiable				
Systolic blood pressure ≥140 mm Hg	1.80 (1.27-2.55)	21.3	1.95 (1.33-2.84)	30.1
Coronary heart disease	2.72 (1.89-3.90)	23.9	3.31 (2.26-4.85)	29.5
Glucose ≥126 mg/dL	2.08 (1.35-3.22)	11.3	1.37 (0.88-2.14)	7.3
Left ventricular hypertrophy	0.90 (0.44-1.84)	–	2.20 (1.47-3.30)	19.5
Current smoking	2.04 (1.15-3.64)	5.5	2.08 (1.37-3.16)	15.0
Modifiable Fraction		48.9		67.8
Potentially Modifiable				
eGFR <60 mL/min/1.73m²	1.29 (0.88-1.87)	6.8	2.14 (1.42-3.24)	16.2
Albumin <3.8 g/dL	1.46 (0.98-2.16)	8.5	1.63 (1.09-2.44)	12.7
Heart rate >75 beats/min	1.45 (0.94-2.23)	6.7	1.97 (1.30-2.99)	15.7
Potentially Modifiable Fraction		20.5		38.6

TABLE 10–3 | **Multivariable Rate Ratios and Population Attributable Risks for Clinical Risk Factors of Incident Heart Failure in the Health ABC Study**

eGFR, estimated glomerular filtration rate; PAR, population attributable risk.

Note: Population attributable risks are *not* additive and *do not* add up to 100%.

From Kalogeropoulos A, Georgiopoulou V, Kritchevsky SB, et al: Epidemiology of incident heart failure in a contemporary elderly cohort: the health, aging, and body composition study. *Arch Intern Med* 169:708, 2009. Reproduced with permission of the American Medical Association.

exercise, moderate alcohol intake, consumption of breakfast cereals, and consumption of fruits and vegetables) were associated with a lower lifetime risk of heart failure, with the highest risk of 21.3% in men adhering to none of these lifestyle habits and the lowest risk of 10.1% in men adhering to four or more of these habits.[57]

Overweight and Obesity

Body mass index is associated with heart failure in a positive[23,58] and linear[23] fashion in both sexes. Although body mass index in the obese range (≥30 kg/m²) is clearly associated with an increased risk for heart failure,[23,58] there is controversy about body mass index in the overweight range (25 to 29.9 kg/m²).[58] Recent data, however, support that overweight is also associated with heart failure.[57,59] Abdominal obesity may be a stronger predictor for heart failure than total obesity,[60,61] even in the absence of coronary heart disease.[62] In population studies, a strong association has been found between abdominal adiposity and features of metabolic syndrome, insulin resistance, and inflammation,[63-65] all of which have been related to heart failure. Individuals with abdominal obesity have more elevated sympathetic neural activation,[66] and visceral adipose tissue has higher expression of angiotensinogen than subcutaneous adipose tissue does.[67]

The anatomic location of excess fat in the abdominal cavity may also be important as there is emerging evidence that increased intra-abdominal pressure leads to cardiac abnormalities that predispose to heart failure.[68] On the contrary, however, there are also data supporting no predictive differences between total and abdominal obesity (as evaluated by waist circumference),[69] and the association between obesity (total or abdominal) and incident heart failure may be mediated partly by insulin resistance.[69] In addition, the relation of obesity and risk of heart failure appears to become less important with age.[70] This age-related attenuation of the obesity and heart failure association needs further investigation.

Several mechanisms by which elevated body mass index increases the risk of heart failure have been proposed.[71-74] Figure 10-4 summarizes these mechanisms.

- *Alterations in cardiac loading.* Obesity is associated with hemodynamic overload with increased blood volume and cardiac output. In addition, left ventricular afterload is elevated because of both increased peripheral resistance and greater arterial stiffness.

- *Changes in cardiac structure and function.* Both overweight and obesity are associated with increased left ventricular mass, wall thickness, and dimensions, whereas longer duration and severity of increased weight accelerate remodeling. Obese individuals may fail to increase their ejection fraction with exercise secondary to abnormal diastolic function. Right ventricular afterload may be increased because of sleep-disordered breathing and left ventricular changes. Obesity is also associated with left atrial enlargement[75] and atrial fibrillation.[76] Hypertension is common in obesity and further worsens heart failure risk. In experimental studies, obesity causes lipotoxicity with myocardial steatosis and lipoapoptosis, which have been linked to cardiac dilation, reduced contractility, and diastolic dysfunction. Cardiac metabolic changes include reduced glucose and increased fatty acid oxidation; these changes increase myocardial oxygen consumption and decrease cardiac efficiency.[74]

- *Activation of neurohumoral and inflammatory pathways.* Obesity is associated with neurohumoral activation, renal sodium retention, and increased systemic and myocardial oxidative stress.[71,74,77] Sympathetic and renin-angiotensin activation directly through adipose tissue signals is common in obesity. Adipose tissue is a source of proinflammatory cytokines, such as tumor necrosis factor-α, interleukin-6, and C-reactive protein; these cytokines, which suppress cardiac function, have been associated with incident heart failure.[78,79]

- *Promotion of atherogenic conditions.* Obesity is associated with hypertension, insulin resistance, diabetes mellitus, and dyslipidemia, all of which enhance the risk of myocardial infarction[80] and also mediate or directly cause heart failure.[20,44]

- *Predisposition to sleep-disordered breathing.* Along with right ventricular changes, obstructive sleep apnea could

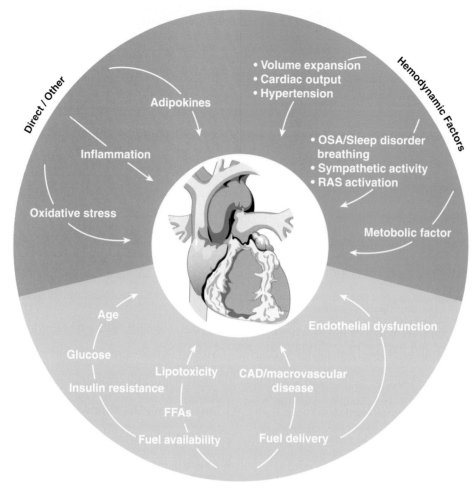

FIGURE 10-4 Multifactorial relationship between obesity and heart failure risk. CAD, coronary artery disease; FFAs, free fatty acids; OSA, obstructive sleep apnea; RAS, renin-angiotensin system. *(From Abel ED, Litwin SE, Sweeney G: Cardiac remodeling in obesity. Physiol Rev 88:389, 2008. Reprinted with permission of the American Physiological Society.)*

also lead to left ventricular hypertrophy related to exacerbation of hypertension, increased sympathetic tone, chronic hypoxemia, and exaggerated intrathoracic pressure during obstructive episodes.[81]

- *Chronic kidney disease.* Obesity is associated with an increased risk of proteinuria and renal insufficiency, presumably caused by glomerular hyperfiltration, glomerular hyperperfusion, glomerular hypertrophy, hyperlipidemia, and increased expression of vasoactive and fibrogenic substances (such as angiotensin II, insulin, leptin, and transforming growth factor-β1), all factors associated with heart failure risk.[71]

Interventions. The principal approach to cardiovascular risk reduction in obese patients should include weight control, physical activity, and control of the associated risk factors, such as hypertension, diabetes mellitus, sleep disorders, and components of the metabolic syndrome.[73] Myocardial changes with nonsurgical or surgical weight loss are feasible, and minor weight loss is efficacious; a 10% weight reduction ameliorates systolic dysfunction, and weight loss of 8 to 10 kg produces a significant decrease in left ventricular dimensions and mass index and improves diastolic function.

Substantial weight loss reduces left ventricular wall thickness and volume and filling pressures, and improves diastolic measures and left ventricular systolic function. The hemodynamic benefits of weight reduction are important and further improve ventricular structure and function related to improved ventricular loading conditions.[73] The role of metabolic and neurohumoral modification may take precedence over the hemodynamic effects as left ventricular mass or functional improvement occurs independently of loading alterations.[82] Although many metabolic and neurohumoral interventions have been implicated in animal models, the roles of the renin-angiotensin-aldosterone system antagonists, lipid-lowering therapy, and insulin-sensitizing drugs in obese humans need further study.

Sedentary Exercise Habits

Physical inactivity is an important risk factor for cardiovascular diseases including heart failure.[59] Evidence suggests that regular physical activity has important and wide-ranging health benefits like reduction in risk of cardiovascular diseases,[83] hypertension,[84] and diabetes.[85] Sitting more and performing less nonexercise activity push the risk curve upward to the left as shown in Figure 10-5, where there is the most

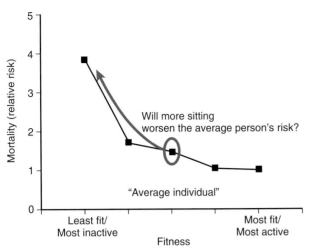

FIGURE 10-5 Sedentary lifestyle and risk for mortality. *(From Hamilton MT, Hamilton DG, Zderic TW: Role of low energy expenditure and sitting in obesity, metabolic syndrome, type 2 diabetes, and cardiovascular disease. Diabetes 56:2655, 2007.)*

risk for disease. Interestingly, emerging evidence indicates that maintaining a high level of daily low-intensity activity may be important independently of moderate to vigorous physical activity for several risk factors for coronary heart disease, such as elevated glucose, type 2 diabetes mellitus, and lipids such as triglyceride and high-density lipoprotein cholesterol levels,[86] all of which predispose to new-onset heart failure. Studies have linked prolonged sitting with cardiovascular risk independently of age or recreational energy expenditure.[83,87]

Physical activity is a key determinant of good health and an important component of weight reduction and weight maintenance,[88,89] improved lipoprotein profile,[88,90,91] and reduced risk of hypertension,[88,91,92] diabetes mellitus,[55] and coronary artery disease.[88,93] These favorable influences on cardiovascular risk profile in turn reduce the likelihood of heart failure.

Physical activity could also reduce left ventricular hypertrophy independent of body weight or blood pressure because of reduction in vascular resistance and blood volume, improved endothelial function, suppression of the renin-angiotensin and sympathetic nervous system activity, and reduction of insulin resistance.[91] Chronic physical activity reduces cytokine production by adipose tissue, skeletal muscles, endothelial cells, and blood mononuclear cells and upregulates antioxidant enzymes.[94] These modifying effects on heart failure risk factors or intermediate pathways leading to heart failure can reduce incident heart failure.

Interventions. The integration of physical activity into the daily lives of the population has proved challenging. In the United States, from 2001 to 2005, the prevalence of regular physical activity increased by 8.6% (from 43.0% to 46.7%) among women and by 3.5% (from 48.0% to 49.7%) among men.[95] The recommendations of the American College of Sports Medicine and the American Heart Association for regular physical activity in healthy adults from 18 to 65 years currently include the following.[89]

- *Aerobic activity.* Moderate-intensity aerobic physical activity for a minimum of 30 minutes on 5 days each week or vigorous-intensity aerobic activity for a minimum of 20 minutes on 3 days each week. A combination of moderate- and vigorous-intensity activity can be performed to meet this recommendation.
- *Muscle strengthening activity.* It is recommended that 8 to 10 exercises be performed on two or more nonconsecutive

days each week using the major muscle groups. To maximize strength development, a resistance (weight) should be used that allows 8 to 12 repetitions of each exercise resulting in volitional fatigue. Muscle strengthening activities include a progressive weight-training program, weight-bearing calisthenics, stair climbing, and similar resistance exercises that use the major muscle groups.
- *Activity dose.* Vigorous-intensity activities may have greater benefit than moderate-intensity physical activity.

Because walking is the preferred activity among sedentary individuals embracing physical activity and the effects of walking have been reported as beneficial in primary prevention,[96] this should be adopted by individuals who do not adhere to the current recommendations.

Alcohol Consumption

Excessive alcohol consumption regardless of beverage type is associated with alcoholic cardiomyopathy.[24,97] This entity is characterized by left ventricular dilation, increased mass, and reduced or normal wall thickness among patients with a lasting history of heavy alcohol consumption.[97] Limited data are available on the amount and duration of consumption; most studies report that patients with symptomatic heart failure had 10 years or more of exposure to heavy drinking.[97]

In animal models, excessive alcohol consumption is associated with left ventricular myocyte loss, negative inotropic effects and dysfunction of myocytes through abnormalities in calcium homeostasis, and hypertrophy through activation of cardiac beta-adrenoceptors from the elevated levels of norepinephrine. In humans, acute ethanol ingestion may also lead to depressed contractility. However, besides the direct myocardial toxicity, excessive alcohol consumption increases the risk of heart failure by promoting hypertension, myocardial infarction,[54] and diabetes.[98]

Interestingly, other data are consistent with possible benefits of moderate alcohol consumption on the risk of heart failure. The New Haven Epidemiologic Study of the Elderly program and the Cardiovascular Health Study reported a 47%[25] and a 34%[99] lower heart failure risk, respectively. The Framingham Heart Study reported a 59% lower risk among men who consumed 8 to 14 drinks per week compared with abstainers and only a modest and nonsignificant association in women.[100] Moreover, it has been reported that light to moderate alcohol consumption is associated with 40% to 50% lower risk of heart failure with previous myocardial infarction, whereas the risk of heart failure without antecedent myocardial infarction among heavy drinkers was 1.7-fold higher than in abstainers in the same study.[101]

Similar findings were reported in the Physicians' Health Study.[26] Beneficial effects of alcohol have also been reported on risk for hypertension,[102] myocardial infarction, and diabetes mellitus,[103] whereas alcohol seems to raise high-density lipoprotein cholesterol,[104] to improve insulin sensitivity,[103] to lower plasma levels of inflammatory markers and coagulation factors, and to raise plasma levels of adiponectin.[24] Furthermore, alcohol consumption has diuretic effects, which could prevent volume overload and delay onset of signs and symptoms of heart failure. Beneficial effects of light to moderate alcohol consumption on incidence of heart failure seem to be independent of the reduced incidence of myocardial infarction and could be linked to lower pulmonary artery wedge pressure, reduced afterload, systemic arterial vasodilation, and improved endothelial function.

Current evidence does not support a major role for nonethanol components of beverages on the risk of heart failure, whereas drinking patterns play an important role. Binge drinking (defined as consumption of three or more alcoholic drinks within 1 to 2 hours) has deleterious health effects, whereas light to moderate alcohol consumption (one or two drinks per day for men and one drink per day for women spread on several days of the week) appears to yield most of the beneficial health effects. Thus, for a given volume of alcohol within the moderate drinking range, it is better to be distributed evenly throughout the week than to be consumed more rapidly.

Dietary Habits

In the Dietary Approaches to Stop Hypertension (DASH) diet, individuals are encouraged to consume more (1) fruits and vegetables, (2) grains and grain products, (3) lean meats, fish, and poultry, (4) low-fat or nonfat dairy foods, and (5) nuts, seeds, and legumes and to reduce the consumption of red meat, fat, and sugar while maintaining a low-sodium intake. Initially, this diet was promoted for hypertension; however, recent evidence supports its beneficial effects on reduction of heart failure risk, with an observed 37% lower heart failure rate in women who adhere to the DASH diet.[105]

The DASH diet may contribute to heart failure prevention in some cases because of reduction in blood pressure[56,106] and incident coronary heart disease.[56,107,108] Particularly women with the highest values of a score designed to measure consistency with DASH had a 24% lower risk of coronary heart disease and an 18% lower risk of stroke[107]; using a different DASH score, Folsom and colleagues[108] did not find statistically significant associations with cardiovascular events. However, women with diets most consistent with DASH had an 18% lower rate of death from coronary heart disease and a 14% lower rate of death from stroke that is similar to the projected effect from the DASH trial.[56,108] Significantly, the DASH diet reduces low-density lipoprotein cholesterol levels and oxidative stress and exerts additional beneficial physiologic effects like estrogenic effects of phytochemicals.[105]

The relationship between several components of the DASH diet and heart failure has been investigated in human and animal studies. In prospective studies of free-living individuals, daily consumption of whole-grain breakfast cereals was associated with a 30% lower rate of heart failure compared with no consumption,[109] consumption of eggs more than twice per day was associated with a 64% higher rate,[110] consumption of fish was associated with a 20% to 31% lower heart failure rate depending on the frequency of consumption,[111] and consumption of 100 mmol or more of sodium was associated with a 26% higher rate[112]; only nut consumption[113] was not associated with an increase or decrease in heart failure. In rat models of heart failure, macronutrient intake modified the course of cardiac dysfunction. High-fat diets reduced cardiac remodeling and contractile dysfunction; however, animals fed diets high in linoleic acid survived longer than those fed diets high in carbohydrates or lard.[114,115] When high-starch, high-fructose, and high-fat diets were compared, animals fed the high-fructose diet demonstrated more cardiac remodeling and worse survival.[116]

There are several mechanisms by which whole-grain cereals can protect against heart failure risk, partially through effects on weight, hypertension, myocardial infarction, and diabetes mellitus. Nutrients contained in whole-grain cereals (e.g., potassium) may lower blood pressure, phytoestrogens may improve lipid levels and insulin sensitivity, and other constituents exert beneficial effects on lipid and homocysteine levels or possess antioxidant properties. Slowing of starch digestion or absorption and promotion of satiety are possible mechanisms by which whole-grain cereals may help control body weight.[109]

Fish consumption exerts beneficial effects on heart failure risk, with about a 20% lower risk associated with an intake of one or two times per week and about a 30% lower risk with intake of three or more times per week, compared with intake less than one time per month. Estimated intake of marine n-3 fatty acids was associated with 37% lower heart

failure risk in the highest quintile of intake compared with the lowest.[111] Fish oil favorably affects hemodynamics and reduces blood pressure, inflammation, vascular responses, and myocardial oxygen consumption at given workloads; it increases contractile recovery after ischemia-reperfusion, augments left ventricular response to exercise, prevents left ventricular remodeling, and improves left ventricular indices and diastolic filling.

Short-term trials of fish oil supplementation of 3 to 5 g/day may also reduce risk, whereas dietary doses of about 0.5 g/day may result in more modest effects that during the long term may reduce heart failure risk. The beneficial associations were most pronounced among persons consuming broiled or baked fish at least three times per week, the equivalent of about 500 mg/day of eicosapentaenoic acid and docosahexaenoic acid; fried fish intake does seem not to exert this benefit on heart failure risk. It has been reported that broiled or baked fish consumption is inversely associated with systolic blood pressure, C-reactive protein levels, and carotid intimal medial thickness, whereas fried fish intake is positively associated with them, indicating that the type of cooking could have an impact on the effects.[111]

Historically, human ancestors consumed less than 0.25 g of salt per day; humans may therefore be genetically programmed to this amount of salt.[117] The recent change to the high-salt intake of 10 to 12 g/day presents a major challenge to the physiologic systems to excrete these large amounts of salt, resulting in a rise in blood pressure, increase in the risk for cardiovascular and renal disease, bone demineralization, and stomach cancer.[118] The Department of Health and Human Services and the Department of Agriculture currently recommend that adults consume no more than 2300 mg/day of sodium (equal to approximately 1 tablespoon of salt), but specific groups (i.e., all persons with hypertension, all middle-aged and older adults, and all blacks) should consume no more than 1500 mg/day of sodium.[119] Overall, 69.2% of U.S. adults, approximately 145.5 million persons, met the criteria for the risk groups.[120]

There is overwhelming evidence for a causal relationship between salt intake and blood pressure from epidemiology, intervention, treatment, animal, and genetic studies.[106,117,118] Salt intake is also associated with increased risk for overall cardiovascular diseases. A reduction in salt intake may have other beneficial effects on the cardiovascular system, independent of and additive to its effect on blood pressure, including regression of left ventricular hypertrophy, delay in deterioration of renal function, and reduction in proteinuria.[121,122] Salt intake is also associated with incident heart failure in overweight individuals. A high dietary intake of sodium could lead to heart failure because of increased blood pressure (pressure overload) or extracellular fluid (volume overload) and left ventricular hypertrophy.

Specific strategies should be implemented to target an intake of 1500 mg/day of sodium. The food industry should be encouraged to reduce sodium used for food preparation. A public health campaign to educate consumers about the dangers of high salt intake and the need to make wise and healthy choices in the sodium content of their foods is of paramount importance. If consumers become more attuned to the sodium content of their foods and the detrimental health effects of a high-salt intake, they could demand low-sodium products, encouraging manufacturers to reduce the sodium content of their products, and they could also prepare their food with less salt. Finally, the responsibility to use fresh products and to avoid canned and other high-salt food eventually falls on individuals.

Smoking

Tobacco use is the single most prevalent preventable cause of disease and premature death in the United States. Smoking

10

is a strong and independent predictor of incident heart failure in both men and women, with 45% and 88% increased risk, respectively, after adjustment for coronary heart disease, implying a more direct effect of smoking on development of heart failure.[20] In the Coronary Artery Surgery Study, current smokers had 47% higher risk for heart failure.[123] Similarly, a cohort study in Sweden showed that smokers have a 60% higher risk for heart failure,[38] and in the Health ABC Study, current smokers had a twofold higher risk for heart failure.[17]

Smoking is carrying a considerable population attributable risk for heart failure: 17% as reported in the First National Health and Nutrition Examination Survey Epidemiologic Follow-up Study[20] and 5.5% in whites and 15% in blacks as reported in the Health ABC Study.[17] The deleterious effect of tobacco seems to be independent of the form of use (smoked or not); increased risk for cardiovascular diseases is reported in nonsmoking use of tobacco.[124] There is no "safe" level of smoking; a single cigarette may stiffen the left ventricle,[125] and as few as one to four cigarettes a day double the risk of having a myocardial infarction.[126] Moreover, cigarettes with lower yields of tar and nicotine have not been shown to lower risk of heart disease and should not be considered lower risk alternatives to regular cigarettes.

Mechanisms leading to heart failure in smokers include indirect effects (i.e., by causing or aggravating comorbidities that are strongly related with heart failure) and direct effects on the myocardium. Smoking is associated with coronary vasoconstriction, abnormal coronary endothelial function, increased ischemic burden, oxidative stress, increased peripheral vascular resistance, insulin resistance, and type 2 diabetes.[127-130] Cigarette smoke contains superoxide and other reactive oxygen species,[131] which could cause oxidative damage in endothelial cells[132] and cell death.[133] Acute inhalation of nicotine decreases nitrate, nitrite, and serum antioxidant concentrations in the plasma[134] and increases arterial stiffness.[135] Cigarettes with high- or low-nicotine content or nicotine-free cigarettes composed of synthetic material increase blood carboxyhemoglobin levels, which in turn decreases the amount of oxygen available to the myocardium. In animal models, nicotine exposure induces interstitial fibrosis in the ventricles.[136] Besides nicotine, carbon monoxide is also a significant component of tobacco smoke and causes overexpression of growth-related proteins (such as calmodulin, calcineurin, and vascular endothelial growth factor), impaired cardiac contraction-relaxation cycle, impairment in calcium handling associated with the dysfunction of the SERCA-2a calcium pump, increased cardiomyocyte cGMP, and reduction of T-tubule density, which in turn decreases the synchrony of activation and reduces the rate of calcium release during systole.[137] In healthy humans, smoking is associated with higher left ventricular mass, lower stroke volume, and lower ejection fraction[138] and impaired ventricular diastolic function.[139] All these affected pathways underscore the impact of smoking on myocardial status.

Interventions. All individuals should be asked about tobacco use, and smokers should be counseled to quit. Patients should be referred to formal cessation programs, and pharmacologic therapy should be offered to increase the success rate. Current recommended strategies include the following.

- *Medications.* Several effective medications are available for tobacco dependence, and clinicians should encourage their use by all patients attempting to quit smoking. Seven first-line medications reliably increase long-term smoking abstinence rates, including bupropion SR, nicotine gum or inhaler or lozenge or nasal spray or patch, and varenicline. Notably, none of these medications is contraindicated if cardiovascular disease exists; however, nicotine replacement therapy should be used with caution among particular cardiovascular patient groups.

- *Counseling and psychosocial support.* Individual, group, and telephone practical counseling (problem solving, skills training) and social support are effective, and their effectiveness increases with treatment intensity.
- *Combination.* The combination of counseling and medication, however, is more effective than either alone. Therefore, clinicians should encourage all individuals making a quit attempt to use both counseling and medication.

Quitting tobacco is associated with reduced morbidity and mortality. In the Studies of Left Ventricular Dysfunction trials, ex-smokers had a 30% lower mortality than that of current smokers, a benefit that accrued within 2 years after smoking cessation. This survival rate was similar to that of nonsmokers; the risk for heart failure hospitalizations and myocardial infarctions also reduced after quitting.[140] Women's risk of heart disease is reduced by one third within 2 years of quitting and by about two thirds within 5 years.[141]

Obstructive Sleep Apnea

Obstructive sleep apnea is characterized by abnormal collapse of the pharyngeal airway during sleep, causing repetitive arousals. Obesity is a major risk factor for this condition, partly because layering of fat adjacent to the pharynx narrows its lumen.[142] The Wisconsin Sleep Cohort Study,[143] a large population-based study, reported that obstructive sleep apnea affects approximately 15% of men and 5% of women between the ages of 30 and 60 years when sleep apnea is defined as an apnea-hypopnea index of ≥10 events per hour. Other studies reported similar findings[144,145] or an even higher prevalence, especially in women.[146] Several well-conducted studies provided compelling evidence that obstructive sleep apnea is related to hypertension[147] and worsening blood pressure control,[148] coronary artery disease,[149] and diabetes.[150] In addition, obstructive sleep apnea seems to induce left ventricular dysfunction independently of hypertension[151,152] and in established heart failure results in worse outcomes.[153] In the Sleep Heart Health Study, obstructive sleep apnea was found to be an independent risk factor for heart failure and was associated with a 2.38 relative risk of heart failure when the apnea-hypopnea index was ≥11 events per hour.

Obstructive sleep apnea may lead to heart failure through (1) development and worsening of comorbidities that predispose to heart failure and (2) neurohormonal abnormalities and mechanical modifications. Sleep is normally a period of cardiac rest. Apart from brief bursts of sympathetic activity in rapid eye movement (REM) sleep, sleep is characterized by decreased sympathetic and increased vagal activity, which lowers heart rate and blood pressure. In patients with obstructive sleep apnea, however, negative intrathoracic pressure generated by the inspiratory effort during obstructed breathing increases left ventricular afterload, changes venous return affecting preload and stroke volume, and increases cardiac muscle work index. In addition, sympathetic activation secondary to hypoxia increases blood pressure and heart rate, thus increasing cardiac afterload, and reduces myocardial perfusion, leading to myocardial ischemia. On the other hand, the increased venous return accompanied by acute hypoxic pulmonary vasoconstriction increases right ventricular volume and pressure and also may compromise left ventricular filling.[154] Sleep apnea treatment with devices that provide continuous positive airway pressure has been shown to improve left ventricular structure and function in patients with established left ventricular dysfunction[155] or to reverse functional ventricular abnormalities.[151]

Hypertension

Hypertension is an antecedent condition in the majority of individuals developing heart failure.[38] Systolic blood

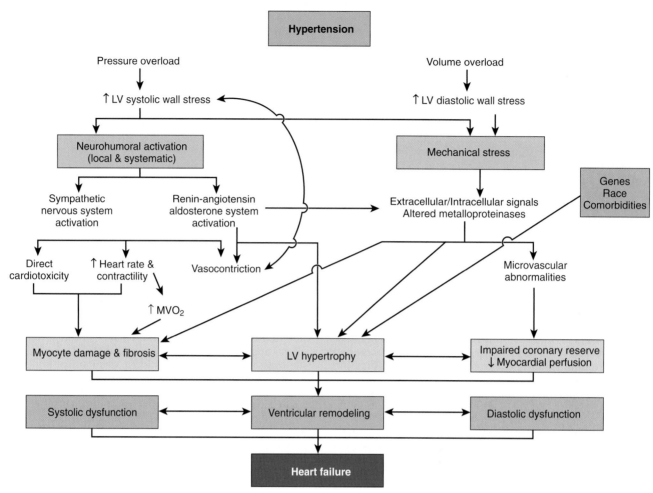

FIGURE 10-6 Hypertension and heart failure risk. LV, left ventricle; MVO₂, myocardial oxygen consumption.

pressure increases almost linearly with age, as does the overall prevalence of hypertension and the proportion of patients with isolated systolic hypertension. By the age of 75 years, almost all hypertensive individuals have isolated systolic hypertension.[156] Diastolic hypertension is more prevalent before the age of 50 years, whereas prevalent systolic hypertension increases with age and after the age of 50 years represents the most common form of hypertension.[156] Diastolic blood pressure is a more potent cardiovascular risk factor than systolic blood pressure until the age of 50 years, and thereafter systolic blood pressure becomes more important.[157] Clinical trials have demonstrated that controlling systolic hypertension reduces heart failure rates.[158] The population attributable risk of hypertension for heart failure in the general population is reported to be 39% in men and 59% in women by the Framingham investigators,[159] whereas the population attributable risk of uncontrolled blood pressure in the elderly was reported to be 21.3% in whites to 30.1% in blacks in the Health ABC Study.[17] This risk increases in a continuous fashion with increase in blood pressure.[44,159]

The lifetime risk for heart failure doubles in subjects with blood pressure >160/100 mm Hg versus those with <140/90 mm Hg, and this gradient of risk is seen in both sexes in every decade from 40 to 70 years.[160] Considering that the prevalence of hypertension is estimated to range from 25% to 60%[161] and that this proportion will likely increase with aging of the population and a sedentary lifestyle,[162] the importance of hypertension in development of heart failure cannot be overemphasized.

The progression from hypertension to structural ventricular changes and systolic and diastolic ventricular dysfunction is well established; Figure 10-6 summarizes this process. Increases in cardiac afterload, left ventricular mass, and wall stress accompanied by impairment of diastolic filling properties occur in the chronic setting. Increased peripheral vascular resistance places a greater myocardial burden leading to an increase in myocardial muscle mass.[163] The development of hypertrophy is associated with progressive degenerative changes in the myocytes and an abnormal accumulation of collagen in the interstitial spaces.[164] Initially, this leads to diastolic dysfunction with increased myocardial stiffness.[165] Also, the disproportionately increased left ventricular mass leads to inadequate microvasculature to perfuse the hypertrophied myocardium, resulting in subendocardial hypoperfusion and ischemia.[166] Hypertension also contributes to ischemia by increasing myocardial oxygen demand due to increased workload[167] and is associated with endothelial dysfunction, oxidative stress, and development of atherosclerosis. These changes increase the risk for coronary thrombosis and myocardial infarction characterized by loss of contractile function, neurohormonal activation, and ventricular remodeling, leading to the development of systolic dysfunction.[168]

Abnormalities in the neurohormonal activation and water and electrolyte balance also play a central role in the cascade that leads from hypertension to heart failure.[169] The renin-angiotensin-aldosterone system activity increases during hypertrophy[169] and heart failure. Angiotensin II is an important initiator of extracellular matrix remodeling,[169,170] which contributes to the pathogenesis of atherosclerosis and cardiac hypertrophy.[169] The heightened sympathetic nervous system predisposes to vasoconstriction, sodium retention, and ventricular hypertrophy. The ventricular hypertrophy occurs as increased norepinephrine release results in myocyte hypertrophy, increased apoptosis of cardiomyocytes, and deficits in cardiomyocyte contractility.[169] These changes are facilitated by beta-adrenergic receptor hyperactivation.

Intervention. The placebo-controlled trials and the meta-analysis arising from them demonstrate the benefit of antihypertensive therapy in reducing the incidence of cardiovascular diseases.[171] Fewer studies have specifically focused on prevention of left ventricular hypertrophy and development of heart failure. Systolic Hypertension in the Elderly Program (SHEP) demonstrated that antihypertensive treatment compared with placebo exerted a strong protective effect,[158] whereas a meta-analysis of 12 hypertension trials that included the development of heart failure and 4 that included the incidence of left ventricular hypertrophy as endpoints demonstrated significant treatment benefits.[172] The incidence of left ventricular hypertrophy was decreased by 35% (95% CI, 21% to 48%) and the incidence of heart failure was reduced by 52% (95% CI, 41% to 62%) compared with placebo subjects (Fig. 10-7).

Antihypertensive Medications

- *Diuretics.* Thiazide diuretics have been effective in preventing cardiovascular complications of hypertension. Secondary outcomes of the Antihypertensive and Lipid-Lowering Treatment to Prevent Heart Attack Trial reported a higher rate of incident heart failure with amlodipine (relative risk of 1.35) and a nonsignificant increase with lisinopril (relative risk of 1.09) compared with chlorthalidone.[173] On the contrary, the Second Australian National Blood Pressure trial[174] reported better outcomes with a regimen that was initiated with an angiotensin-converting enzyme inhibitor compared with a diuretic. Diuretics are at least as good as other classes of drugs and also enhance the antihypertensive efficacy of multidrug regimens; the Joint National Commission 7 recommend that in the absence of any other compelling indications, thiazide diuretics should be used as initial therapy for hypertension.

- *Renin-angiotensin system modulators.* Meta-analysis of double-blind trials that measured the effects of antihypertensive drugs on left ventricular mass[175] showed that the greatest reduction was achieved with angiotensin receptor blockers (Fig. 10-8). Also, these agents along with calcium channel blockers and angiotensin-converting enzyme inhibitors were more effective than beta blockers in reducing left ventricular mass. Both irbesartan- and losartan-based regimens have been shown to reduce left ventricular mass more than atenolol-based treatments.[176,177] Candesartan had efficacy similar to that of enalapril.[178] These data suggest that antihypertensive agents targeting the renin-angiotensin system are particularly effective in producing regression of left ventricular hypertrophy and that angiotensin receptor blockers are at least as effective as angiotensin-converting enzyme inhibitors. A recent meta-analysis of renin-angiotensin system inhibition showed that these agents reduce the risk for heart failure by 19% compared with calcium channel blockers.[179]

- *Beta blockers.* Although beta blockers are effective in lowering blood pressure, these medications are less effective in preventing hypertension complications, including coronary artery disease and cardiovascular and all-cause mortality,[180,181] or in reducing left ventricular mass.[176,177] However, a recent meta-analysis suggested that beta blockers are efficacious for primary prevention of heart failure in hypertension and had a similar benefit in the elderly and younger individuals compared with other agents.[182] On the other hand, the 19% increased risk for stroke in the elderly associated with beta blocker use in the same analysis tempers the enthusiasm to use them as first-line agents for heart failure prevention in hypertension.[182]

- *Calcium channel blockers.* There are limited experimental data on the effects of calcium antagonists on left ventricular mass or incident heart failure. A recent meta-analysis suggested that treatment of hypertension with calcium channel blockers is less effective for reducing heart failure for the same reduction of blood pressure[179]; the effect of this class of medications on reducing left ventricular mass was similar to that of renin-angiotensin system inhibition.[175]

Target Goals of Therapy. In patients with hypertension, systolic and diastolic blood pressure targets are

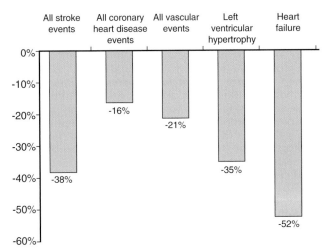

FIGURE 10-7 Hypertension treatment and its impact on cardiovascular events. Results of meta-analyses of randomized trials of antihypertensive medications therapy, indicating the impact of blood pressure reduction on reduction of cardiovascular, vascular, heart failure, and left ventricular hypertrophy events.[171,172]

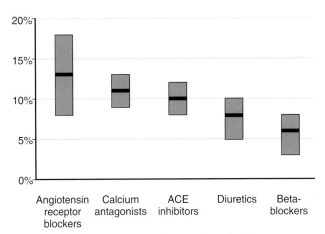

FIGURE 10-8 Alteration in left ventricular mass index with various antihypertensive medications. Angiotensin II receptor antagonists, calcium antagonists, and angiotensin-converting enzyme (ACE) inhibitors reduced left ventricular mass index more than beta blockers did. *(Reproduced from Klingbeil AU, Schneider M, Martus P, et al: A meta-analysis of the effects of treatment on left ventricular mass in essential hypertension. Am J Med 115:41, 2003.)*

<140/90 mm Hg except for patients with diabetes or renal disease, for whom the goal is <130/80 mm Hg. Because most patients with hypertension, especially those older than 50 years, will reach the diastolic blood pressure goal once systolic blood pressure is at goal, the primary focus should therefore be on systolic blood pressure. Current control rates at the population level remain far below the Healthy People 2010 goal of 50%, with 30% of patients still being unaware of their hypertension status. Recent trials have demonstrated that effective blood pressure control can be achieved in most patients, but the majority will require two or more medications in combination.[183] Data from a recent randomized trial evaluating the effect of usual versus tight control of systolic blood pressure (<130 mm Hg) in nondiabetic hypertensive individuals with left ventricular hypertrophy demonstrated additional benefit with tighter control. In particular, left ventricular hypertrophy was less frequent, but also the composite outcome of all-cause mortality, cardiovascular events, and heart failure was lower in the tight control group.[184]

Diabetes Mellitus

Diabetes mellitus is an independent risk factor for the development of heart failure in all age groups.[20,37] The relative risk for new-onset heart failure among patients with diabetes mellitus ranges from 1.3 to 2.7, increasing to 4 in patients younger than 65 years and 11 in those younger than 45 years specifically.

Several mechanisms have been proposed to explain the increased risk for heart failure among patients with diabetes mellitus. Comorbidities associated with heart failure, including obesity, hypertension, and coronary artery disease, are highly prevalent among individuals with diabetes mellitus. Insulin resistance itself may produce abnormalities in cardiac structure and function.[185] Patients with insulin resistance exhibit endothelial dysfunction and a proinflammatory state, which contribute to ventricular dysfunction, even before the development of overt diabetes mellitus. Left ventricular hypertrophy and left ventricular dysfunction are also strongly correlated with insulin resistance, and hyperinsulinemia has been associated with sympathetic nervous system activation.[185]

Several mechanisms have been proposed for the development of "diabetic cardiomyopathy"[186,187]:

- Microangiopathy and endothelial dysfunction.
- Autonomic neuropathy, which causes impaired coronary vasodilatory response to sympathetic stimulation and modulates the contractility of cardiac myocytes.
- Metabolic derangements caused by insulin resistance, such as reduced glucose and lactate metabolism and enhanced fatty acid metabolism, result in lipid accumulation in the myocardium, promoting lipotoxicity. This increased fatty acid metabolism causes increased myocardial oxygen consumption, promoting ischemia and arrhythmias, whereas lipid intermediates (e.g., ceramide) might promote apoptosis. Elevated fatty acids also activate coagulation and inflammatory pathways, enhance smooth muscle cell proliferation, and contribute to endothelial dysfunction.[188]
- Abnormalities in ion homeostasis through alteration of ion channels such as calcium and potassium channels and alteration of the function or cardiac expression of sodium-calcium exchangers, sarcoplasmic reticulum/sarcolemmal calcium-ATPases (SERCA-2a), calcium-binding proteins, and the mitochondrial calcium uniporter.
- Upregulation of the renin-angiotensin system.
- Increased oxidative stress.
- Increased glycation of interstitial proteins such as collagen, creating advanced glycosylation end products, which result in myocardial stiffness and impaired contractility.

- Activation of protein kinase C leads to alterations in cell growth and function, affecting muscle contractility and gene expression.

Interventions

Medications

- *Insulin.* Whether insulin use specifically reduces the risk for heart failure is not known. Randomized controlled trials indicate that insulin use in ACC/AHA stage A heart failure does not appear to significantly increase the risk of new-onset heart failure,[189] and insulin use in stage B heart failure does not appear to negatively affect mortality.[188]
- *Sulfonylureas.* The available data suggest that sulfonylurea therapy does not significantly increase the risk of heart failure compared with other oral antidiabetic agents, although the ADOPT (A Diabetes Outcome Progression Trial) was not powered to detect significant differences.[190]
- *Metformin.* The risk of new-onset heart failure among patients treated with metformin compared with patients treated with other oral antidiabetic medications was reported in ADOPT, and the findings were similar to those for sulfonylureas.[190]
- *Thiazolidinediones.* The hypothesis that therapies that will correct abnormal myocardial substrate metabolism in diabetes will translate to lower incidence of heart failure appears promising; however, the available data on this class of medications argue against this hypothesis. Although treatment with thiazolidinediones increased myocardial glucose uptake in patients with underlying coronary disease, and myocardial glucose uptake seems to be positively correlated with left ventricular function,[188] the Rosiglitazone Evaluated for Cardiac Outcomes and Regulation of Glycaemia in Diabetes study has indicated that thiazolidinedione use is associated with a small but clinically relevant increased risk of heart failure in patients with ACC/AHA stage A or stage B status.[34]
- *Other agents.* There are limited data regarding the risks or benefits of other antidiabetic therapies for incident heart failure, except for the α-glucosidase inhibitor acarbose, the impact of which on cardiovascular disease outcomes was evaluated in the STOP–Noninsulin-Dependent Diabetes Mellitus (STOP-NIDDM) trial.[191] Although the study was not powered to evaluate the impact of acarbose treatment on the development of heart failure, the available evidence suggests that this agent may decrease the risk of myocardial infarction and subsequent risk of heart failure.[191]

Glucose Control. The best available evidence suggests that management of hyperglycemia in patients with type 2 diabetes mellitus reduces neither cardiovascular morbidity and mortality nor the progression of heart failure. In the United Kingdom Prospective Diabetes Study (UKPDS) 33, no significant reduction in the development of macrovascular disease or heart failure was demonstrated with intensive blood glucose control.[189]

Blood Pressure Control in Diabetes Mellitus. Because hypertension further increases the risk of cardiovascular disease and heart failure in patients with diabetes, aggressive blood pressure management is essential to prevent long-term complications in this population. In UKPDS 38, tight blood pressure control with either the angiotensin-converting enzyme inhibitor or beta blocker significantly reduced the risk of cardiovascular events and diabetes-related mortality, including a 56% reduction in the risk for heart failure.[192] Notably, target blood pressure level was <150/85 mm Hg in that study, whereas the Seventh Report of the Joint National Commission on Prevention, Detection, Evaluation, and Treatment of High Blood Pressure (JNC 7) recommended more aggressive blood pressure control (target blood pressure <130/80 mm Hg) in patients with diabetes.[193]

Targeting Mechanisms Causing Diabetic Cardiomyopathy. The mechanisms leading to diabetic cardiomyopathy are complex. Medications like angiotensin-converting enzyme inhibitors, angiotensin receptor blockers, and beta blockers benefit patients with diabetes and prevent complications of diabetes including heart failure. The Heart Outcomes Prevention Evaluation (HOPE) trial[194] and the Microalbuminuria, Cardiovascular, and Renal Outcomes (MICRO-HOPE), a substudy of HOPE,[195] have shown that treatment with angiotensin-converting enzyme inhibitors reduces the relative risk for new-onset heart failure by 23% and 20%, respectively, in a population of ACC/AHA stage A or B patients, whereas the extension of HOPE study (extended follow-up period) revealed that the benefit of angiotensin-converting enzyme inhibitors for heart failure prevention is sustained over time.[196] Likewise, the Reduction of Endpoints in Non–Insulin Dependent Diabetes Mellitus with the Angiotensin II Antagonist Losartan (RENAAL) study[197] and the Losartan Intervention for Endpoint Reductions in Hypertension (LIFE) study[198] have shown a 32% and 41% reduction in the frequency of hospitalization for heart failure, respectively.

A recent meta-analysis evaluating the beneficial effects of the agents that inhibit the renin-angiotensin system on reducing the risk for new-onset heart failure showed that their favorable effect was beyond blood pressure control, and the risk was 19% lower than for calcium channel blockers.[179] Although these data are promising, there are concerns about the heterogeneity of the criteria used for assessment of heart failure in the various trials and the side effect of peripheral edema, which is common among patients receiving calcium channel blockers and may complicate diagnosis of heart failure. Recently, a randomized trial evaluating the effects of the Cu(II)-selective chelator trientine on left ventricular hypertrophy in diabetes mellitus showed a 10% decrease in left ventricular mass index after 12 months.[199] This decrease represented a ~50% restoration of left ventricular mass toward normal. In recent studies, breakers of advanced glycation end products–related protein cross-links ameliorated the adverse cardiovascular and renal changes associated with aging, diabetes, and hypertension.[200] These effects support the hypothesis that modulation of specific pathways could lead to attenuation of diabetes complications including heart failure.

Coronary Heart Disease

Coronary heart disease is a major antecedent condition predisposing to an increased risk for development of heart failure in both men and women,[44] with reported population attributable risks ranging from 56% in women to 62% in men by the First National Health and Nutrition Examination Survey Epidemiologic Follow-up Study[20] and from 23.9% in whites to 29.5% in blacks as reported in the Health ABC Study.[17] Heart failure incidence in the Framingham Heart Study changed only modestly from the 1950s through the 1990s in men but declined by about one third among women during this period. This trend was also supported by other cohort studies.[201,202] These trends in men and women may be partially attributed to sex-based differences in heart failure etiology because hypertension predominates as an etiologic risk factor for heart failure in women more so than in men, and coronary heart disease is responsible for a higher proportion of cases in men.[20,159] Increased awareness and treatment of hypertension have led to improved trends in control[203] and probably decreased heart failure incidence more so in women, especially because blood pressure control appears to be better in women.[204] On the contrary, advances in the treatment of myocardial infarction[205] have led to increasing numbers of patients surviving with residual myocardial damage, which may be partially responsible for the increase in heart failure incidence among men.[20]

Acute Myocardial Infarction

Acute myocardial infarction leads to a cascade of adaptive mechanisms that promote left ventricular remodeling. Acute loss of myocardial cells results in an increase in loading conditions on the remaining myocardium and induces a unique pattern of remodeling involving the infarcted border zone and the noninfarcted myocardium. Intracellular signaling processes initiate and modulate the reparative changes, including dilation, hypertrophy, formation of a collagen scar, neurohormonal and cytokine activation, and oxidative stress.[206]

Ventricular remodeling may continue for weeks or months until the distending forces are counterbalanced by the tensile strength of the collagen scar; this balance then determines the size, location, and transmurality of the infarct and the extent of myocardial stunning, ventricular loading conditions, and local trophic factors.[207] Although contemporary treatment attenuates remodeling,[208,209] there is a large heterogeneity in the remodeling response after an infarction. Whereas remodeling in the short term is adaptive, over time it becomes deleterious, leading to adverse structural and hemodynamic changes leading to heart failure.[209]

Initially, myocardial infarction results in the migration of circulating inflammatory cells into the infarct zone, triggering intracellular signaling and neurohormonal activation, leading to a local inflammatory response that in turn leads to cell death and degradation of the intermyocyte collagen struts, expanding infarct size.[210] Infarct expansion results in wall thinning and ventricular dilation and causes the elevation of diastolic and systolic wall stress that stimulates hypertrophy mediated by mechanoreceptors and transduces intracellular signaling, which initiates the increased synthesis of contractile assembly units.[210] Infarct expansion causes deformation of the border zone and remote myocardium, which alters the Frank-Starling response and augments shortening.[210] These changes result in alterations in circulatory hemodynamics, triggering sympathetic adrenergic and renin-angiotensin-aldosterone systems,[206] leading to myocyte hypertrophy and alterations in the ventricular architecture to distribute the increased wall stress more evenly as the extracellular matrix forms a collagen scar to stabilize the distending forces and to prevent further deformation.

Reperfusion therapy helps prevent infarct progression. However, it is associated with generation of reactive oxygen species, osmotic gradient and cell swelling, activation of the sodium-hydrogen exchanger, calcium overload–induced myocardial contracture, local inflammatory and oxidant response to reperfusion, and opening of the mitochondrial permeability transition pore that extends infarct size beyond that observed during equivalent periods of ischemia alone.[211] Thus, reperfusion injury is a possible target for interventions to reduce myocardial damage.

Chronic Coronary Artery Disease

Ischemia caused by abnormalities in coronary arteries can produce increases in the concentration of neurohormones (e.g., norepinephrine, epinephrine, endothelin, and dopamine) that results in myocardial apoptosis, fibrosis, and susceptibility to ventricular arrhythmias.[212] Thus, ischemia contributes to the progression of left ventricular systolic dysfunction even in the absence of a manifest infarct event. Chronic ischemia can result in hibernation or stunning with further progressive decline in ventricular function. These adaptive-protective mechanisms may result in myocardium rendered hypocontractile and contribute to overall left ventricular systolic dysfunction. Hibernation represents a precarious balance between perfusion and tissue viability that cannot be maintained indefinitely, and myocardial necrosis will eventually occur if blood flow is not increased.[207,212] Most patients with heart failure of ischemic origin have a substantial volume of myocardium that fails to contract because it is stunned or hibernating rather than because it is scarred. In addition, endothelial dysfunction, an inherent component of the pathophysiologic process of atherosclerosis, could directly affect ventricular function.[213] Ischemic mitral regurgitation, caused by changes in ventricular structure and function, increases left ventricular preload, leading finally to alteration of left ventricle geometry and deterioration of its function.[214]

Moreover, myocardial ischemia induces diastolic dysfunction related to impaired calcium ion sequestration into the sarcoplasmic reticulum during the energy-dependent process of relaxation[215] and through alteration of the myocardial passive compliance resulting from scarring, fibrosis, and compensatory hypertrophy of noninfarcted myocardium.[216] Diastolic dysfunction during myocardial ischemia precedes systolic dysfunction and takes longer to recover from.[212] Left ventricular diastolic dysfunction is present in the very early phases of myocardial infarction, and it is associated with the development of in-hospital heart failure and cardiac death; several studies have documented recovery of diastolic function after reperfusion therapy.[212]

Interventions. Prevention of coronary heart disease and ischemic events is a key point to maintenance of functional myocyte reserve; however, in patients with established coronary heart disease, aggressive management can reduce development of heart failure. A number of cardioprotective medications and procedures can prevent development of symptomatic heart failure in coronary heart disease. The combination of medications along with therapeutic lifestyle changes as recommended in the American Heart Association/American College of Cardiology secondary prevention guidelines[217] should be applied aggressively in all patients to reduce the risk of heart failure.

Revascularization. Mechanical (percutaneous or surgical) or pharmacologic revascularization of the infarct-related artery reduces the size of the acute infarct and prevents subsequent heart failure[208,210] if it is performed early enough for myocardial salvage. In addition, the "open artery hypothesis" proposes that late reperfusion, beyond the window for myocardial salvage, also reduces left ventricular remodeling.[218] Even after successful early revascularization, older patients are at higher risk for heart failure compared with their younger counterparts.[219]

Angiotensin-Converting Enzyme Inhibitors. Angiotensin-converting enzyme inhibitors have favorable properties in reducing left ventricular stress and progression of left ventricle enlargement, and several studies have shown them to reduce the incidence of heart failure and mortality after an acute myocardial infarction. In the third Gruppo Italiano per lo Studio della Sopravvivenza nell'Infarto Miocardico (GISSI) trial, early lisinopril therapy in acute infarction reduced mortality and left ventricular dysfunction despite therapy with aspirin, thrombolytics, and beta-adrenergic blocking agents.[220] Similar findings were demonstrated in the Survival of Myocardial Infarction Long-term Evaluation trial with zofenopril.[221] The HOPE study demonstrated a 23% reduction in risk for heart failure by ramipril in individuals with established vascular disease,[194] expanding the indication for angiotensin-converting enzyme inhibitor therapy to all patients with documented coronary heart disease, presumed coronary heart disease based on presence of other atherosclerotic vascular disease, or diabetes. The EUropean trial on Reduction Of cardiac events with Perindopril in stable coronary Artery disease (EUROPA) showed similar data with perindopril.[222] In the Survival and Ventricular Enlargement (SAVE) trial that enrolled patients with asymptomatic left ventricular dysfunction, captopril led to a 22% reduction in the risk of heart failure hospitalization.[223]

Angiotensin Receptor Blockers. Available data suggest that angiotensin receptor blockers are at least as effective as angiotensin-converting enzyme inhibitors in reducing mortality in patients with myocardial infarction complicated by left ventricular dysfunction or heart failure.[207,212] However, data on populations with atherosclerotic diseases but without heart failure are not uniform.[224,225] Because the overall evidence for the effectiveness of angiotensin receptor blockers on prevention and attenuation of post–myocardial infarction left ventricular remodeling is weaker compared with angiotensin-converting enzyme inhibitors, they may not be used as first-line therapy but limited to those individuals who do not tolerate angiotensin-converting enzyme inhibitors.

Beta Blockers. Beta blockers have been proven to be beneficial after acute myocardial infarction for more than 20 years. Notably, long-term beta blocker use is recommended for secondary prevention in patients at highest risk (e.g., those with low ejection fraction or heart failure).[226] The echocardiographic substudy of Carvedilol Post-Infarct Survival Control in Left Ventricular Dysfunction (CAPRICORN) demonstrated a beneficial effect of carvedilol on left ventricular remodeling in patients with left ventricular dysfunction after myocardial infarction over that of angiotensin-converting enzyme inhibitors.[227] The Reversal of Ventricular Remodeling with Toprol-XL (REVERT) trial gives further evidence that beta blocker use for the treatment of asymptomatic left ventricular dysfunction to prevent development of heart failure is effective and that left ventricular remodeling can be reversed.[228]

Aldosterone Antagonists. High aldosterone levels seen in patients with myocardial infarction induce ventricular remodeling.[207] Spironolactone combined with angiotensin-converting enzyme inhibitors ameliorated left ventricle remodeling after acute myocardial infarction better than angiotensin-converting enzyme inhibitors alone did in a randomized study.[207] This study also showed that spironolactone significantly suppressed transcardiac extraction of aldosterone and plasma levels of procollagen type III amino-terminal peptide, a marker of cardiac fibrosis. Aldosterone antagonists are recommended in myocardial infarction complicated by left ventricular dysfunction on the basis of the beneficial effect on mortality and cardiovascular hospitalizations seen in the Eplerenone Post–Acute Myocardial Infarction Heart Failure Efficacy and Survival Study (EPHESUS).[229]

Antiplatelet Agents. Aspirin in patients with established vascular disease has been demonstrated to reduce risk for cardiovascular events and heart failure.[212] It is recommended after acute myocardial infarction and should be continued indefinitely if no contraindications exist.[230]

Statins. Statins are of proven benefit in patients with coronary heart disease[212,231]; however, their usefulness in the setting of left ventricular dysfunction remains under investigation. Preprocedural treatment with a statin before percutaneous coronary intervention is associated with lower levels of periprocedural creatine kinase elevation.[207] Ishii and coworkers[232] reported that chronic statin therapy before the onset of the acute event is associated with improved perfusion and reduced myocardial necrosis after the intervention. Prospective studies in humans reported an effect of statins on the risk for development of heart failure in high-risk patients, most of whom were free of heart failure at enrollment. Kjekshus and associates[233] showed an 11% lower risk of new-onset heart failure in patients with stable coronary heart disease treated with statins. Similar trends were also demonstrated in other studies,[234] supporting a role for statins in the prevention of heart failure. Notably, statins appears to prevent further progression of heart failure and to decrease mortality in this population.

Novel Therapeutic Approaches. Several novel mechanistic insights into cardiac myocyte function, repair

10

mechanisms, and remodeling may lead to development of newer therapies for heart failure in the future. These include therapies targeted at nitric oxide–cGMP signaling and nitric oxide modulation, oxidative stress and antioxidant therapy, anti-inflammatory therapies, modulation of innate immunity toll-like receptors, interleukin-1 receptor antagonists, and selective matrix metalloproteinase inhibition.[231]

Stem Cell Therapy. There is also a growing interest in treatment strategies targeting angiogenesis or stem cell transfer. Coronary angiogenesis is enhanced during the acute phase of adaptive cardiac growth but is reduced as maladaptive remodeling progresses. Inhibition of angiogenesis leads to a decreased capillary density, contractile dysfunction, and impaired cardiac growth.[231] Thus, both cardiac size and function are angiogenesis dependent, and disruption of coordinated tissue growth and angiogenesis in the heart may contribute to the progression from adaptive cardiac hypertrophy to heart failure. Recent observations indicate that stem and progenitor cells can release proangiogenic factors, which in turn stimulate angiogenesis after infarction. Increased angiogenesis after stem and progenitor cell transfer has been postulated to improve infarct healing and energy metabolism in the infarct border zone.[231] Early clinical trials suggest that intracoronary delivery of bone marrow cells may improve left ventricular ejection fraction after infarction.[231] More work is needed, however, to identify the most suitable cell types and application methods and to define the impact of cell therapy on clinical endpoints and other indices of ventricular remodeling. Furthermore, other delivery strategies for proangiogenic factors after infarction need to be explored.

CONCLUSION

Considering the worsening epidemiologic trends and increase in heart failure prevalence in the society, escalating costs, and continued poor quality of life and outcomes for these patients, the importance of heart failure prevention cannot be overemphasized. This will require efforts at all levels of the prevention spectrum ranging from advocacy efforts (e.g., to reduce salt in the food chain, population screening of risk factors and their optimal control) to research in understanding novel pathophysiologic mechanisms and newer therapies to prevent heart failure in individuals with prevalent high-risk factors.

Population-level efforts at risk factor prevention and adoption of healthy lifestyle habits are essential to promote overall cardiovascular health and to reduce heart failure risk specifically. Toward this direction, the American Heart Association has taken a bold step in defining their 2020 goals, not only to achieve further reductions in mortality due to cardiovascular disease and stroke but to improve the health of the population based on a comprehensive, specifically designed metric that includes multiple healthy lifestyle parameters. Last, whether treatment goals of heart failure risk factors should be individualized on the basis of any given individual's cumulative risk profile needs further study.

REFERENCES

1. American Heart Association: Get With The Guidelines–Heart Failure. Available at: http://www.amhrt.org/downloadable/heart/1163802072170HFFactSheet.pdf. Accessed October 1, 2009.
2. Wilson PW, D'Agostino RB, Levy D, et al: Prediction of coronary heart disease using risk factor categories. *Circulation* 97:1837, 1998.
3. Hippisley-Cox J, Coupland C, Vinogradova Y, et al: Derivation and validation of QRISK, a new cardiovascular disease risk score for the United Kingdom: prospective open cohort study. *BMJ* 335:136, 2007.
4. Hippisley-Cox J, Coupland C, Vinogradova Y, et al: Predicting cardiovascular risk in England and Wales: prospective derivation and validation of QRISK2. *BMJ* 336:1475, 2008.
5. Morrow DA, Braunwald E: Future of biomarkers in acute coronary syndromes: moving toward a multimarker strategy. *Circulation* 108:250, 2003.
6. Oemrawsingh RM, Akkerhuis KM, Boersma E: Tailor-made therapy for the prevention of acute coronary syndromes: future role of biomarkers in risk stratification and disease management. *Expert Rev Cardiovasc Ther* 6:435, 2008.
7. Ikonomidis I, Stamatelopoulos K, Lekakis J, et al: Inflammatory and non-invasive vascular markers: the multimarker approach for risk stratification in coronary artery disease. *Atherosclerosis* 199:3, 2008.
8. Mancini GB, Dahlof B, Diez J: Surrogate markers for cardiovascular disease: structural markers. *Circulation* 109:IV22, 2004.
9. Smith SC Jr, Allen J, Blair SN, et al: AHA/ACC guidelines for secondary prevention for patients with coronary and other atherosclerotic vascular disease: 2006 update: endorsed by the National Heart, Lung, and Blood Institute. *Circulation* 113:2363, 2006.
10. Pearson TA, Blair SN, Daniels SR, et al: AHA Guidelines for Primary Prevention of Cardiovascular Disease and Stroke: 2002 Update: Consensus Panel Guide to Comprehensive Risk Reduction for Adult Patients Without Coronary or Other Atherosclerotic Vascular Diseases. American Heart Association Science Advisory and Coordinating Committee. *Circulation* 106:388, 2002.
11. Lloyd-Jones D, Adams R, Carnethon M, et al: Heart disease and stroke statistics—2009 update: a report from the American Heart Association Statistics Committee and Stroke Statistics Subcommittee. *Circulation* 119:e21, 2009.
12. Owan TE, Redfield MM: Epidemiology of diastolic heart failure. *Prog Cardiovasc Dis* 47:320, 2005.
13. Vasan RS, Benjamin EJ, Levy D: Prevalence, clinical features and prognosis of diastolic heart failure: an epidemiologic perspective. *J Am Coll Cardiol* 26:1565, 1995.
14. Hogg K, Swedberg K, McMurray J: Heart failure with preserved left ventricular systolic function; epidemiology, clinical characteristics, and prognosis. *J Am Coll Cardiol* 43:317, 2004.
15. Fonarow GC, Stough WG, Abraham WT, et al: Characteristics, treatments, and outcomes of patients with preserved systolic function hospitalized for heart failure: a report from the OPTIMIZE-HF Registry. *J Am Coll Cardiol* 50:768, 2007.
16. Owan TE, Hodge DO, Herges RM, et al: Trends in prevalence and outcome of heart failure with preserved ejection fraction. *N Engl J Med* 355:251, 2006.
17. Kalogeropoulos A, Georgiopoulou V, Kritchevsky SB, et al: Epidemiology of incident heart failure in a contemporary elderly cohort: the health, aging, and body composition study. *Arch Intern Med* 169:708, 2009.
18. The Booming Dynamics of Aging: The White House Conference on Aging. Available at: http://www.whcoa.gov/. Accessed August 8, 2009.
19. Butler J: Risk factors for heart failure. In Hosenpud JD, Greenberg BH, editors: *Congestive heart failure*, ed 3, Philadelphia, 2007, Lippincott Williams & Wilkins, p 263.
20. He J, Ogden LG, Bazzano LA, et al: Risk factors for congestive heart failure in US men and women: NHANES I epidemiologic follow-up study. *Arch Intern Med* 161:996, 2001.
21. Fonarow GC: The Acute Decompensated Heart Failure National Registry (ADHERE): opportunities to improve care of patients hospitalized with acute decompensated heart failure. *Rev Cardiovasc Med* 4(Suppl 7):S21, 2003.
22. Haider AW, Larson MG, Franklin SS, et al: Systolic blood pressure, diastolic blood pressure, and pulse pressure as predictors of risk for congestive heart failure in the Framingham Heart Study. *Ann Intern Med* 138:10, 2003.
23. Kenchaiah S, Evans JC, Levy D, et al: Obesity and the risk of heart failure. *N Engl J Med* 347:305, 2002.
24. Djousse L, Gaziano JM: Alcohol consumption and heart failure: a systematic review. *Curr Atheroscler Rep* 10:117, 2008.
25. Abramson JL, Williams SA, Krumholz HM, et al: Moderate alcohol consumption and risk of heart failure among older persons. *JAMA* 285:1971, 2001.
26. Djousse L, Gaziano JM: Alcohol consumption and risk of heart failure in the Physicians' Health Study I. *Circulation* 115:34, 2007.
27. Horio T, Miyazato J, Kamide K, et al: Influence of low high-density lipoprotein cholesterol on left ventricular hypertrophy and diastolic function in essential hypertension. *Am J Hypertens* 16:938, 2003.
28. Sundstrom J, Lind L, Vessby B, et al: Dyslipidemia and an unfavorable fatty acid profile predict left ventricular hypertrophy 20 years later. *Circulation* 103:836, 2001.
29. Ho KK, Pinsky JL, Kannel WB, et al: The epidemiology of heart failure: the Framingham Study. *J Am Coll Cardiol* 22:6A, 1993.
30. Dhingra R, Sesso HD, Kenchaiah S, et al: Differential effects of lipids on the risk of heart failure and coronary heart disease: the Physicians' Health Study. *Am Heart J* 155:869, 2008.
31. Butler J, Kalogeropoulos A, Georgiopoulou V, et al: Serum resistin concentrations and risk of new onset heart failure in older persons: the health, aging, and body composition (Health ABC) study. *Arterioscler Thromb Vasc Biol* 29:1144, 2009.
32. van Vark LC, Kardys I, Bleumink GS, et al: Lipoprotein-associated phospholipase A_2 activity and risk of heart failure: The Rotterdam study. *Eur Heart J* 27:2346, 2006.
33. Tang WH, Katz R, Brennan ML, et al: Usefulness of myeloperoxidase levels in healthy elderly subjects to predict risk of developing heart failure. *Am J Cardiol* 103:1269, 2009.
34. Home PD, Pocock SJ, Beck-Nielsen H, et al: Rosiglitazone evaluated for cardiovascular outcomes—an interim analysis. *N Engl J Med* 357:28, 2007.
35. Ware JH: The limitations of risk factors as prognostic tools. *N Engl J Med* 355:2615, 2006.
36. Hunt SA, Abraham WT, Chin MH, et al: ACC/AHA 2005 Guideline Update for the Diagnosis and Management of Chronic Heart Failure in the Adult: a report of the American College of Cardiology/American Heart Association Task Force on Practice Guidelines (Writing Committee to Update the 2001 Guidelines for the Evaluation and Management of Heart Failure): developed in collaboration with the American College of Chest Physicians and the International Society for Heart and Lung Transplantation: endorsed by the Heart Rhythm Society. *Circulation* 112:e154, 2005.
37. Gottdiener JS, Arnold AM, Aurigemma GP, et al: Predictors of congestive heart failure in the elderly: the Cardiovascular Health Study. *J Am Coll Cardiol* 35:1628, 2000.
38. Eriksson H, Svardsudd K, Larsson B, et al: Risk factors for heart failure in the general population: the study of men born in 1913. *Eur Heart J* 10:647, 1989.

39. Chen YT, Vaccarino V, Williams CS, et al: Risk factors for heart failure in the elderly: a prospective community-based study. *Am J Med* 106:605, 1999.
40. Kannel WB, D'Agostino RB, Silbershatz H, et al: Profile for estimating risk of heart failure. *Arch Intern Med* 159:1197, 1999.
41. Wilhelmsen L, Rosengren A, Eriksson H, et al: Heart failure in the general population of men—morbidity, risk factors and prognosis. *J Intern Med* 249:253, 2001.
42. Bibbins-Domingo K, Lin F, Vittinghoff E, et al: Predictors of heart failure among women with coronary disease. *Circulation* 110:1424, 2004.
43. Carr AA, Kowey PR, Devereux RB, et al: Hospitalizations for new heart failure among subjects with diabetes mellitus in the RENAAL and LIFE studies. *Am J Cardiol* 96:1530, 2005.
44. Butler J, Kalogeropoulos A, Georgiopoulou V, et al: Incident heart failure prediction in the elderly: the Health ABC Heart Failure Score. *Circ Heart Fail* 1:125, 2008.
45. Kalogeropoulos A, Psaty BM, Vasan RS, et al: Validation of the health ABC heart failure model for incident heart failure risk prediction: the Cardiovascular Health Study. *Circ Heart Fail* 3:495-502, 2010.
46. McKee PA, Castelli WP, McNamara PM, et al: The natural history of congestive heart failure: the Framingham study. *N Engl J Med* 285:1441, 1971.

47. Psaty BM, Kuller LH, Bild D, et al: Methods of assessing prevalent cardiovascular disease in the Cardiovascular Health Study. *Ann Epidemiol* 5:270, 1995.
48. Schellenbaum GD, Rea TD, Heckbert SR, et al: Survival associated with two sets of diagnostic criteria for congestive heart failure. *Am J Epidemiol* 160:628, 2004.
49. Schellenbaum GD, Heckbert SR, Smith NL, et al: Congestive heart failure incidence and prognosis: case identification using central adjudication versus hospital discharge diagnoses. *Ann Epidemiol* 16:115, 2006.
50. Paulus WJ, Tschope C, Sanderson JE, et al: How to diagnose diastolic heart failure: a consensus statement on the diagnosis of heart failure with normal left ventricular ejection fraction by the Heart Failure and Echocardiography Associations of the European Society of Cardiology. *Eur Heart J* 28:2539, 2007.
51. Zannad F, Stough WG, Pitt B, et al: Heart failure as an endpoint in heart failure and non–heart failure cardiovascular clinical trials: the need for a consensus definition. *Eur Heart J* 29:413, 2008.
52. O'Meara E, Clayton T, McEntegart MB, et al: Sex differences in clinical characteristics and prognosis in a broad spectrum of patients with heart failure: results of the Candesartan in Heart failure: Assessment of Reduction in Mortality and morbidity (CHARM) program. *Circulation* 115:3111, 2007.
53. Stampfer MJ, Hu FB, Manson JE, et al: Primary prevention of coronary heart disease in women through diet and lifestyle. *N Engl J Med* 343:16, 2000.
54. Yusuf S, Hawken S, Ounpuu S, et al: Effect of potentially modifiable risk factors associated with myocardial infarction in 52 countries (the INTERHEART study): case-control study. *Lancet* 364:937, 2004.
55. Knowler WC, Barrett-Connor E, Fowler SE, et al: Reduction in the incidence of type 2 diabetes with lifestyle intervention or metformin. *N Engl J Med* 346:393, 2002.
56. Appel LJ, Moore TJ, Obarzanek E, et al: A clinical trial of the effects of dietary patterns on blood pressure. DASH Collaborative Research Group. *N Engl J Med* 336:1117, 1997.
57. Djousse L, Driver JA, Gaziano JM: Relation between modifiable lifestyle factors and lifetime risk of heart failure, *JAMA* 302:394, 2009.
58. Johansson S, Wallander MA, Ruigomez A, et al: Incidence of newly diagnosed heart failure in UK general practice. *Eur J Heart Fail* 3:225, 2001.
59. Kenchaiah S, Sesso HD, Gaziano JM: Body mass index and vigorous physical activity and the risk of heart failure among men. *Circulation* 119:44, 2009.
60. Spies C, Farzaneh-Far R, Na B, et al: Relation of obesity to heart failure hospitalization and cardiovascular events in persons with stable coronary heart disease (from the Heart and Soul Study). *Am J Cardiol* 104:883, 2009.
61. Dagenais GR, Yi Q, Mann JF, et al: Prognostic impact of body weight and abdominal obesity in women and men with cardiovascular disease. *Am Heart J* 149:54, 2005.
62. Nicklas BJ, Cesari M, Penninx BW, et al: Abdominal obesity is an independent risk factor for chronic heart failure in older people. *J Am Geriatr Soc* 54:413, 2006.
63. Fox CS, Massaro JM, Hoffmann U, et al: Abdominal visceral and subcutaneous adipose tissue compartments: association with metabolic risk factors in the Framingham Heart Study. *Circulation* 116:39, 2007.
64. Piche ME, Lemieux S, Weisnagel SJ, et al: Relation of high-sensitivity C-reactive protein, interleukin-6, tumor necrosis factor-alpha, and fibrinogen to abdominal adipose tissue, blood pressure, and cholesterol and triglyceride levels in healthy postmenopausal women. *Am J Cardiol* 96:92, 2005.
65. Pou KM, Massaro JM, Hoffmann U, et al: Visceral and subcutaneous adipose tissue volumes are cross-sectionally related to markers of inflammation and oxidative stress: the Framingham Heart Study. *Circulation* 116:1234, 2007.
66. Alvarez GE, Beske SD, Ballard TP, et al: Sympathetic neural activation in visceral obesity. *Circulation* 106:2533, 2002.
67. Dusserre E, Moulin P, Vidal H: Differences in mRNA expression of the proteins secreted by the adipocytes in human subcutaneous and visceral adipose tissues. *Biochim Biophys Acta* 1500:88, 2000.
68. Sugerman HJ: Effects of increased intra-abdominal pressure in severe obesity. *Surg Clin North Am* 81:1063, vi, 2001.
69. Ingelsson E, Sundstrom J, Arnlov J, et al: Insulin resistance and risk of congestive heart failure. *JAMA* 294:334, 2005.
70. Levitan EB, Yang AZ, Wolk A, et al: Adiposity and incidence of heart failure hospitalization and mortality: a population-based prospective study. *Circ Heart Fail* 2:202, 2009.
71. Kenchaiah S, Gaziano JM, Vasan RS: Impact of obesity on the risk of heart failure and survival after the onset of heart failure. *Med Clin North Am* 88:1273, 2004.
72. Vasan RS: Cardiac function and obesity. *Heart* 89:1127, 2003.
73. Wong C, Marwick TH: Alterations in myocardial characteristics associated with obesity: detection, mechanisms, and implications. *Trends Cardiovasc Med* 17:1, 2007.
74. Abel ED, Litwin SE, Sweeney G: Cardiac remodeling in obesity. *Physiol Rev* 88:389, 2008.
75. Gottdiener JS, Reda DJ, Williams DW, et al: Left atrial size in hypertensive men: influence of obesity, race and age. Department of Veterans Affairs Cooperative Study Group on Antihypertensive Agents. *J Am Coll Cardiol* 29:651, 1997.
76. Wang TJ, Parise H, Levy D, et al: Obesity and the risk of new-onset atrial fibrillation. *JAMA* 292:2471, 2004.
77. Hall JE: The kidney, hypertension, and obesity. *Hypertension* 41:625, 2003.
78. Vasan RS, Sullivan LM, Roubenoff R, et al: Inflammatory markers and risk of heart failure in elderly subjects without prior myocardial infarction: the Framingham Heart Study. *Circulation* 107:1486, 2003.
79. Cesari M, Penninx BW, Newman AB, et al: Inflammatory markers and onset of cardiovascular events: results from the Health ABC study. *Circulation* 108:2317, 2003.
80. Anand SS, Islam S, Rosengren A, et al: Risk factors for myocardial infarction in women and men: insights from the INTERHEART study. *Eur Heart J* 29:932, 2008.
81. Quan SF, Gersh BJ: Cardiovascular consequences of sleep-disordered breathing: past, present and future: report of a workshop from the National Center on Sleep Disorders Research and the National Heart, Lung, and Blood Institute. *Circulation* 109:951, 2004.
82. MacMahon SW, Wilcken DE, Macdonald GJ: The effect of weight reduction on left ventricular mass. A randomized controlled trial in young, overweight hypertensive patients. *N Engl J Med* 314:334, 1986.
83. Manson JE, Greenland P, LaCroix AZ, et al: Walking compared with vigorous exercise for the prevention of cardiovascular events in women. *N Engl J Med* 347:716, 2002.
84. Chase NL, Sui X, Lee DC, Blair SN: The association of cardiorespiratory fitness and physical activity with incidence of hypertension in men. *Am J Hypertens* 22:417, 2009.
85. Hu FB, Li TY, Colditz GA, et al: Television watching and other sedentary behaviors in relation to risk of obesity and type 2 diabetes mellitus in women. *JAMA* 289:1785, 2003.
86. Hamilton MT, Hamilton DG, Zderic TW: Exercise physiology versus inactivity physiology: an essential concept for understanding lipoprotein lipase regulation. *Exerc Sport Sci Rev* 32:161, 2004.
87. Manini TM, Everhart JE, Patel KV, et al: Daily activity energy expenditure and mortality among older adults. *JAMA* 296:171, 2006.
88. Murphy MH, Blair SN, Murtagh EM: Accumulated versus continuous exercise for health benefit: a review of empirical studies. *Sports Med* 39:29, 2009.
89. Haskell WL, Lee IM, Pate RR, et al: Physical activity and public health: updated recommendation for adults from the American College of Sports Medicine and the American Heart Association. *Circulation* 116:108193, 2007.
90. Kraus WE, Houmard JA, Duscha BD, et al: Effects of the amount and intensity of exercise on plasma lipoproteins. *N Engl J Med* 347:1483, 2002.
91. Cornelissen VA, Fagard RH: Effects of endurance training on blood pressure, blood pressure–regulating mechanisms, and cardiovascular risk factors. *Hypertension* 46:667, 2005.
92. Kokkinos PF, Narayan P, Colleran JA, et al: Effects of regular exercise on blood pressure and left ventricular hypertrophy in African-American men with severe hypertension. *N Engl J Med* 333:1462, 1995.
93. Manson JE, Hu FB, Rich-Edwards JW, et al: A prospective study of walking as compared with vigorous exercise in the prevention of coronary heart disease in women. *N Engl J Med* 341:650, 1999.
94. Kasapis C, Thompson PD: The effects of physical activity on serum C-reactive protein and inflammatory markers: a systematic review. *J Am Coll Cardiol* 45:1563, 2005.
95. Prevalence of regular physical activity among adults—United States, 2001 and 2005. *MMWR Morb Mortal Wkly Rep* 56:1209, 2007.
96. Hamer M, Chida Y: Walking and primary prevention: a meta-analysis of prospective cohort studies. *Br J Sports Med* 42:238, 2008.
97. Lazarevic AM, Nakatani S, Neskovic AN, et al: Early changes in left ventricular function in chronic asymptomatic alcoholics: relation to the duration of heavy drinking. *J Am Coll Cardiol* 35:1599, 2000.
98. Hu FB, Manson JE, Stampfer MJ, et al: Diet, lifestyle, and the risk of type 2 diabetes mellitus in women. *N Engl J Med* 345:790, 2001.
99. Bryson CL, Mukamal KJ, Mittleman MA, et al: The association of alcohol consumption and incident heart failure: the Cardiovascular Health Study. *J Am Coll Cardiol* 48:305, 2006.
100. Walsh CR, Larson MG, Evans JC, et al: Alcohol consumption and risk for congestive heart failure in the Framingham Heart Study. *Ann Intern Med* 136:181, 2002.
101. Klatsky AL, Chartier D, Udaltsova N, et al: Alcohol drinking and risk of hospitalization for heart failure with and without associated coronary artery disease. *Am J Cardiol* 96:346, 2005.
102. Djousse L, Gaziano JM: Alcohol consumption and heart failure in hypertensive US male physicians. *Am J Cardiol* 102:593, 2008.
103. Conigrave KM, Hu BF, Camargo CA Jr, et al: A prospective study of drinking patterns in relation to risk of type 2 diabetes among men. *Diabetes* 50:2390, 2001.
104. Gaziano JM, Buring JE, Breslow JL, et al: Moderate alcohol intake, increased levels of high-density lipoprotein and its subfractions, and decreased risk of myocardial infarction. *N Engl J Med* 329:1829, 1993.
105. Levitan EB, Wolk A, Mittleman MA: Consistency with the DASH diet and incidence of heart failure. *Arch Intern Med* 169:851, 2009.
106. Sacks FM, Svetkey LP, Vollmer WM, et al: Effects on blood pressure of reduced dietary sodium and the Dietary Approaches to Stop Hypertension (DASH) diet. DASH-Sodium Collaborative Research Group. *N Engl J Med* 344:3, 2001.
107. Fung TT, Chiuve SE, McCullough ML, et al: Adherence to a DASH-style diet and risk of coronary heart disease and stroke in women. *Arch Intern Med* 168:713, 2008.
108. Folsom AR, Parker ED, Harnack LJ: Degree of concordance with DASH diet guidelines and incidence of hypertension and fatal cardiovascular disease. *Am J Hypertens* 20:225, 2007.
109. Djousse L, Gaziano JM: Breakfast cereals and risk of heart failure in the Physicians' Health Study I. *Arch Intern Med* 167:2080, 2007.

110. Djousse L, Gaziano JM: Egg consumption and risk of heart failure in the Physicians' Health Study. *Circulation* 117:512, 2008.
111. Mozaffarian D, Bryson CL, Lemaitre RN, et al: Fish intake and risk of incident heart failure. *J Am Coll Cardiol* 45:2015, 2005.
112. He J, Ogden LG, Bazzano LA, et al: Dietary sodium intake and incidence of congestive heart failure in overweight US men and women: first National Health and Nutrition Examination Survey Epidemiologic Follow-up Study. *Arch Intern Med* 162:1619, 2002.
113. Djousse L, Rudich T, Gaziano JM: Nut consumption and risk of heart failure in the Physicians' Health Study I. *Am J Clin Nutr* 88:930, 2008.
114. Chicco AJ, Sparagna GC, McCune SA, et al: Linoleate-rich high-fat diet decreases mortality in hypertensive heart failure rats compared with lard and low-fat diets. *Hypertension* 52:549, 2008.
115. Okere IC, Chess DJ, McElfresh TA, et al: High-fat diet prevents cardiac hypertrophy and improves contractile function in the hypertensive Dahl salt-sensitive rat. *Clin Exp Pharmacol Physiol* 32:825, 2005.
116. Sharma N, Okere IC, Duda MK, et al: High fructose diet increases mortality in hypertensive rats compared to a complex carbohydrate or high fat diet. *Am J Hypertens* 20:403, 2007.
117. He FJ, MacGregor GA: Salt, blood pressure and cardiovascular disease. *Curr Opin Cardiol* 22:298, 2007.
118. Intersalt: an international study of electrolyte excretion and blood pressure. Results for 24 hour urinary sodium and potassium excretion. Intersalt Cooperative Research Group. *BMJ* 297:319, 1988.
119. US Department of Health and Human Services, US Department of Agriculture: *Dietary guidelines for Americans 2005*, ed 6, Washington, DC, 2005, US Department of Health and Human Services, US Department of Agriculture. Available at: http://www.health.gov/dietaryguidelines/dga2005/document/pdf/dga2005.pdf.
120. American Heart Association: IOM Committee on Strategies to Reduce Sodium Intake, March 30, 2009. Available at: http://americanheart.org/downloadable/heart/1240425252727AHAStatementtoIOMonStrategiestoReduceSodiumIntake033009.pdf.
121. Antonios TF, MacGregor GA: Salt—more adverse effects. *Lancet* 348:250, 1996.
122. Swift PA, Markandu ND, Sagnella GA, et al: Modest salt reduction reduces blood pressure and urine protein excretion in black hypertensives: a randomized control trial. *Hypertension* 46:308, 2005.
123. Hoffman RM, Psaty BM, Kronmal RA: Modifiable risk factors for incident heart failure in the coronary artery surgery study. *Arch Intern Med* 154:417, 1994.
124. Teo KK, Ounpuu S, Hawken S, et al: Tobacco use and risk of myocardial infarction in 52 countries in the INTERHEART study: a case-control study. *Lancet* 368:647, 2006.
125. Gembala MI, Ghanem F, Mann CA, et al: Acute changes in left ventricular diastolic function: cigarette smoking versus nicotine gum. *Clin Cardiol* 29:61, 2006.
126. Willett WC, Green A, Stampfer MJ, et al: Relative and absolute excess risks of coronary heart disease among women who smoke cigarettes. *N Engl J Med* 317:1303, 1987.
127. Moliterno DJ, Willard JE, Lange RA, et al: Coronary-artery vasoconstriction induced by cocaine, cigarette smoking, or both. *N Engl J Med* 330:454, 1994.
128. Barry J, Mead K, Nabel EG, et al: Effect of smoking on the activity of ischemic heart disease. *JAMA* 261:398, 1989.
129. Burke A, Fitzgerald GA: Oxidative stress and smoking-induced vascular injury. *Prog Cardiovasc Dis* 46:79, 2003.
130. Willi C, Bodenmann P, Ghali WA, et al: Active smoking and the risk of type 2 diabetes: a systematic review and meta-analysis. *JAMA* 298:2654, 2007.
131. Tsuchiya M, Thompson DF, Suzuki YJ, et al: Superoxide formed from cigarette smoke impairs polymorphonuclear leukocyte active oxygen generation activity. *Arch Biochem Biophys* 299:30, 1992.
132. Morrow JD, Frei B, Longmire AW, et al: Increase in circulating products of lipid peroxidation (F_2-isoprostanes) in smokers. Smoking as a cause of oxidative damage. *N Engl J Med* 332:1198, 1995.
133. Ramachandran S, Xie LH, John SA, et al: A novel role for connexin hemichannel in oxidative stress and smoking-induced cell injury. *PLoS One* 2:e712, 2007.
134. Tsuchiya M, Asada A, Kasahara E, et al: Smoking a single cigarette rapidly reduces combined concentrations of nitrate and nitrite and concentrations of antioxidants in plasma. *Circulation* 105:1155, 2002.
135. Kim JW, Park CG, Hong SJ, et al: Acute and chronic effects of cigarette smoking on arterial stiffness. *Blood Press* 14:80, 2005.
136. Ahmed SS, Moschos CB, Lyons MM, et al: Cardiovascular effects of long-term cigarette smoking and nicotine administration. *Am J Cardiol* 37:33, 1976.
137. Bye A, Sorhaug S, Ceci M, et al: Carbon monoxide levels experienced by heavy smokers impair aerobic capacity and cardiac contractility and induce pathological hypertrophy. *Inhal Toxicol* 20:635, 2008.
138. Heckbert SR, Post W, Pearson GD, et al: Traditional cardiovascular risk factors in relation to left ventricular mass, volume, and systolic function by cardiac magnetic resonance imaging: the Multiethnic Study of Atherosclerosis. *J Am Coll Cardiol* 48:2285, 2006.
139. Lichodziejewska B, Kurnicka K, Grudzka K, et al: Chronic and acute effects of smoking on left and right ventricular relaxation in young healthy smokers. *Chest* 131:1142, 2007.
140. Suskin N, Sheth T, Negassa A, et al: Relationship of current and past smoking to mortality and morbidity in patients with left ventricular dysfunction. *J Am Coll Cardiol* 37:1677, 2001.
141. Kenfield SA, Stampfer MJ, Rosner BA, et al: Smoking and smoking cessation in relation to mortality in women. *JAMA* 299:2037, 2008.
142. Horner RL, Mohiaddin RH, Lowell DG, et al: Sites and sizes of fat deposits around the pharynx in obese patients with obstructive sleep apnoea and weight matched controls. *Eur Respir J* 2:613, 1989.
143. Young T, Palta M, Dempsey J, et al: The occurrence of sleep-disordered breathing among middle-aged adults. *N Engl J Med* 328:1230, 1993.
144. Bixler EO, Vgontzas AN, Lin HM, et al: Prevalence of sleep-disordered breathing in women: effects of gender. *Am J Respir Crit Care Med* 163:608, 2001.
145. Bixler EO, Vgontzas AN, Ten Have T, et al: Effects of age on sleep apnea in men: I. Prevalence and severity. *Am J Respir Crit Care Med* 157:144-148, 1998.
146. Duran J, Esnaola S, Rubio R, et al: Obstructive sleep apnea–hypopnea and related clinical features in a population-based sample of subjects aged 30 to 70 yr. *Am J Respir Crit Care Med* 163:685, 2001.
147. Peppard PE, Young T, Palta M, et al: Prospective study of the association between sleep-disordered breathing and hypertension. *N Engl J Med* 342:1378, 2000.
148. Becker HF, Jerrentrup A, Ploch T, et al: Effect of nasal continuous positive airway pressure treatment on blood pressure in patients with obstructive sleep apnea. *Circulation* 107:68, 2003.
149. Peker Y, Carlson J, Hedner J: Increased incidence of coronary artery disease in sleep apnoea: a long-term follow-up. *Eur Respir J* 28:596, 2006.
150. Reichmuth KJ, Austin D, Skatrud JB, et al: Association of sleep apnea and type II diabetes: a population-based study. *Am J Respir Crit Care Med* 172:1590, 2005.
151. Alchanatis M, Tourkohoriti G, Kosmas EN, et al: Evidence for left ventricular dysfunction in patients with obstructive sleep apnoea syndrome. *Eur Respir J* 20:1239, 2002.
152. Amin RS, Kimball TR, Bean JA, et al: Left ventricular hypertrophy and abnormal ventricular geometry in children and adolescents with obstructive sleep apnea. *Am J Respir Crit Care Med* 165:1395, 2002.
153. Wang H, Parker JD, Newton GE, et al: Influence of obstructive sleep apnea on mortality in patients with heart failure. *J Am Coll Cardiol* 49:1625, 2007.
154. Bradley TD, Floras JS: Sleep apnea and heart failure: Part I: obstructive sleep apnea. *Circulation* 107:1671, 2003.
155. Malone S, Liu PP, Holloway R, et al: Obstructive sleep apnoea in patients with dilated cardiomyopathy: effects of continuous positive airway pressure. *Lancet* 338:1480, 1991.
156. Franklin SS, Jacobs MJ, Wong ND, et al: Predominance of isolated systolic hypertension among middle-aged and elderly US hypertensives: analysis based on National Health and Nutrition Examination Survey (NHANES) III. *Hypertension* 37:869, 2001.
157. Franklin SS, Larson MG, Khan SA, et al: Does the relation of blood pressure to coronary heart disease risk change with aging? The Framingham Heart Study. *Circulation* 103:1245, 2001.
158. Kostis JB, Davis BR, Cutler J, et al: Prevention of heart failure by antihypertensive drug treatment in older persons with isolated systolic hypertension. SHEP Cooperative Research Group. *JAMA* 278:212, 1997.
159. Levy D, Larson MG, Vasan RS, et al: The progression from hypertension to congestive heart failure. *JAMA* 275:1557, 1996.
160. Lloyd-Jones DM, Larson MG, Leip EP, et al: Lifetime risk for developing congestive heart failure: the Framingham Heart Study. *Circulation* 106:3068, 2002.
161. Wolf-Maier K, Cooper RS, Banegas JR, et al: Hypertension prevalence and blood pressure levels in 6 European countries, Canada, and the United States. *JAMA* 289:2363, 2003.
162. Kearney PM, Whelton M, Reynolds K, et al: Global burden of hypertension: analysis of worldwide data. *Lancet* 365:217, 2005.
163. Drukteinis JS, Roman MJ, Fabsitz RR, et al: Cardiac and systemic hemodynamic characteristics of hypertension and prehypertension in adolescents and young adults: the Strong Heart Study. *Circulation* 115:221, 2007.
164. Weber KT, Brilla CG, Campbell SE, et al: Pathologic hypertrophy with fibrosis: the structural basis for myocardial failure. *Blood Press* 1:75, 1992.
165. Vasan RS, Levy D: The role of hypertension in the pathogenesis of heart failure. A clinical mechanistic overview. *Arch Intern Med* 156:1789, 1996.
166. Marcus ML, Harrison DG, Chilian WM, et al: Alterations in the coronary circulation in hypertrophied ventricles. *Circulation* 75:I19, 1987.
167. Brush JE Jr, Cannon RO 3rd, Schenke WH, et al: Angina due to coronary microvascular disease in hypertensive patients without left ventricular hypertrophy. *N Engl J Med* 319:1302, 1988.
168. Nolan SE, Mannisi JA, Bush DE, et al: Increased afterload aggravates infarct expansion after acute myocardial infarction. *J Am Coll Cardiol* 12:1318, 1988.
169. Wright JW, Mizutani S, Harding JW: Pathways involved in the transition from hypertension to hypertrophy to heart failure. Treatment strategies. *Heart Fail Rev* 13:367, 2008.
170. Wright JW, Harding JW: The brain angiotensin system and extracellular matrix molecules in neural plasticity, learning, and memory. *Prog Neurobiol* 72:263, 2004.
171. Hebert PR, Moser M, Mayer J, et al: Recent evidence on drug therapy of mild to moderate hypertension and decreased risk of coronary heart disease. *Arch Intern Med* 153:578, 1993.
172. Moser M, Hebert PR: Prevention of disease progression, left ventricular hypertrophy and congestive heart failure in hypertension treatment trials. *J Am Coll Cardiol* 27:1214, 1996.
173. Davis BR, Piller LB, Cutler JA, et al: Role of diuretics in the prevention of heart failure: the Antihypertensive and Lipid-Lowering Treatment to Prevent Heart Attack Trial. *Circulation* 113:2201, 2006.
174. Wing LM, Reid CM, Ryan P, et al: A comparison of outcomes with angiotensin-converting-enzyme inhibitors and diuretics for hypertension in the elderly. *N Engl J Med* 348:583, 2003.
175. Klingbeil AU, Schneider M, Martus P, et al: A meta-analysis of the effects of treatment on left ventricular mass in essential hypertension. *Am J Med* 115:41, 2003.
176. Malmqvist K, Kahan T, Edner M, et al: Regression of left ventricular hypertrophy in human hypertension with irbesartan. *J Hypertens* 19:1167, 2001.
177. Dahlof B, Devereux RB, Kjeldsen SE, et al: Cardiovascular morbidity and mortality in the Losartan Intervention for Endpoint reduction in hypertension study (LIFE): a randomised trial against atenolol. *Lancet* 359:995, 2002.
178. Cuspidi C, Muiesan ML, Valagussa L, et al: Comparative effects of candesartan and enalapril on left ventricular hypertrophy in patients with essential hypertension: the candesartan assessment in the treatment of cardiac hypertrophy (CATCH) study. *J Hypertens* 20:2293, 2002.

10

179. Verdecchia P, Angeli F, Cavallini C, et al: Blood pressure reduction and renin-angiotensin system inhibition for prevention of congestive heart failure: a meta-analysis. *Eur Heart J* 30:679, 2009.

180. Lindholm LH, Carlberg B, Samuelsson O: Should beta blockers remain first choice in the treatment of primary hypertension? A meta-analysis. *Lancet* 366:1545, 2005.

181. Bangalore S, Messerli FH, Kostis JB, et al: Cardiovascular protection using beta-blockers: a critical review of the evidence. *J Am Coll Cardiol* 50:563, 2007.

182. Bangalore S, Wild D, Parkar S, et al: Beta-blockers for primary prevention of heart failure in patients with hypertension insights from a meta-analysis. *J Am Coll Cardiol* 52:1062, 2008.

183. Cushman WC, Ford CE, Cutler JA, et al: Success and predictors of blood pressure control in diverse North American settings: the antihypertensive and lipid-lowering treatment to prevent heart attack trial (ALLHAT). *J Clin Hypertens (Greenwich)* 4:393, 2002.

184. Verdecchia P, Staessen JA, Angeli F, et al: Usual versus tight control of systolic blood pressure in non-diabetic patients with hypertension (Cardio-Sis): an open-label randomised trial. *Lancet* 374:525, 2009.

185. Masoudi FA, Inzucchi SE: Diabetes mellitus and heart failure: epidemiology, mechanisms, and pharmacotherapy. *Am J Cardiol* 99:113B, 2007.

186. Boudina S, Abel ED: Diabetic cardiomyopathy revisited. *Circulation* 115:3213, 2007.

187. Srikanthan P, Hsueh W: Preventing heart failure in patients with diabetes. *Med Clin North Am* 88:1237, 2004.

188. Choy CK, Rodgers JE, Nappi JM, et al: Type 2 diabetes mellitus and heart failure. *Pharmacotherapy* 28:170, 2008.

189. Intensive blood-glucose control with sulphonylureas or insulin compared with conventional treatment and risk of complications in patients with type 2 diabetes (UKPDS 33). UK Prospective Diabetes Study (UKPDS) Group. *Lancet* 352:837, 1998.

190. Kahn SE, Haffner SM, Heise MA, et al: Glycemic durability of rosiglitazone, metformin, or glyburide monotherapy. *N Engl J Med* 355:2427, 2006.

191. Chiasson JL, Josse RG, Gomis R, et al: Acarbose treatment and the risk of cardiovascular disease and hypertension in patients with impaired glucose tolerance: the STOP-NIDDM trial. *JAMA* 290:486, 2003.

192. Tight blood pressure control and risk of macrovascular and microvascular complications in type 2 diabetes: UKPDS 38. UK Prospective Diabetes Study Group. *BMJ* 317:703, 1998.

193. Chobanian AV, Bakris GL, Black HR, et al: The Seventh Report of the Joint National Committee on Prevention, Detection, Evaluation, and Treatment of High Blood Pressure: the JNC 7 report. *JAMA* 289:2560, 2003.

194. Yusuf S, Sleight P, Pogue J, et al: Effects of an angiotensin-converting-enzyme inhibitor, ramipril, on cardiovascular events in high-risk patients. The Heart Outcomes Prevention Evaluation Study Investigators. *N Engl J Med* 342:145, 2000.

195. Effects of ramipril on cardiovascular and microvascular outcomes in people with diabetes mellitus: results of the HOPE study and MICRO-HOPE substudy. Heart Outcomes Prevention Evaluation Study Investigators. *Lancet* 355:253, 2000.

196. Bosch J, Lonn E, Pogue J, et al: Long-term effects of ramipril on cardiovascular events and on diabetes: results of the HOPE study extension. *Circulation* 112:1339, 2005.

197. Brenner BM, Cooper ME, de Zeeuw D, et al: Effects of losartan on renal and cardiovascular outcomes in patients with type 2 diabetes and nephropathy. *N Engl J Med* 345:861, 2001.

198. Lindholm LH, Ibsen H, Dahlof B, et al: Cardiovascular morbidity and mortality in patients with diabetes in the Losartan Intervention For Endpoint reduction in hypertension study (LIFE): a randomised trial against atenolol. *Lancet* 359:1004, 2002.

199. Cooper GJ, Young AA, Gamble GD, et al: A copper(II)-selective chelator ameliorates left-ventricular hypertrophy in type 2 diabetic patients: a randomised placebo-controlled study. *Diabetologia* 52:715, 2009.

200. Cooper GJ, Phillips AR, Choong SY, et al: Regeneration of the heart in diabetes by selective copper chelation. *Diabetes* 53:2501, 2004.

201. Roger VL, Weston SA, Redfield MM, et al: Trends in heart failure incidence and survival in a community-based population. *JAMA* 292:344, 2004.

202. Djousse L, Kochar J, Gaziano JM: Secular trends of heart failure among US male physicians. *Am Heart J* 154:855, 2007.

203. Burt VL, Cutler JA, Higgins M, et al: Trends in the prevalence, awareness, treatment, and control of hypertension in the adult US population. Data from the health examination surveys, 1960 to 1991. *Hypertension* 26:60, 1995.

204. Racial/ethnic disparities in prevalence, treatment, and control of hypertension—United States, 1999-2002. *MMWR Morb Mortal Wkly Rep* 54:7, 2005.

205. Setoguchi S, Glynn RJ, Avorn J, et al: Improvements in long-term mortality after myocardial infarction and increased use of cardiovascular drugs after discharge: a 10-year trend analysis. *J Am Coll Cardiol* 51:1247, 2008.

206. Tiyyagura SR, Pinney SP: Left ventricular remodeling after myocardial infarction: past, present, and future. *Mt Sinai J Med* 73:840, 2006.

207. Ishii H, Amano T, Matsubara T, et al: Pharmacological intervention for prevention of left ventricular remodeling and improving prognosis in myocardial infarction. *Circulation* 118:2710, 2008.

208. Baks T, van Geuns RJ, Biagini E, et al: Effects of primary angioplasty for acute myocardial infarction on early and late infarct size and left ventricular wall characteristics. *J Am Coll Cardiol* 47:40, 2006.

209. Giannuzzi P, Temporelli PL, Bosimini E, et al: Heterogeneity of left ventricular remodeling after acute myocardial infarction: results of the Gruppo Italiano per lo Studio della Sopravvivenza nell'Infarto Miocardico–3 Echo Substudy. *Am Heart J* 141:131, 2001.

210. Sutton MG, Sharpe N: Left ventricular remodeling after myocardial infarction: pathophysiology and therapy. *Circulation* 101:2981, 2000.

211. Vinten-Johansen J, Zhao ZQ, Zatta AJ, et al: Postconditioning—a new link in nature's armor against myocardial ischemia-reperfusion injury. *Basic Res Cardiol* 100:295, 2005.

212. Klein L, Gheorghiade M: Coronary artery disease and prevention of heart failure. *Med Clin North Am* 88:1209, 2004.

213. Lerman A, Zeiher AM: Endothelial function: cardiac events. *Circulation* 111:363, 2005.

214. Grigioni F, Detaint D, Avierinos JF, et al: Contribution of ischemic mitral regurgitation to congestive heart failure after myocardial infarction. *J Am Coll Cardiol* 45:260, 2005.

215. Henry PD, Schuchleib R, Davis J, et al: Myocardial contracture and accumulation of mitochondrial calcium in ischemic rabbit heart. *Am J Physiol* 233:H677, 1977.

216. Ito Y, Suko J, Chidsey CA: Intracellular calcium and myocardial contractility. V. Calcium uptake of sarcoplasmic reticulum fractions in hypertrophied and failing rabbit hearts. *J Mol Cell Cardiol* 6:237, 1974.

217. Smith SC Jr, Allen J, Blair SN, et al: AHA/ACC guidelines for secondary prevention for patients with coronary and other atherosclerotic vascular disease: 2006 update endorsed by the National Heart, Lung, and Blood Institute. *J Am Coll Cardiol* 47:2130, 2006.

218. Takemura G, Nakagawa M, Kanamori H, et al: Benefits of reperfusion beyond infarct size limitation. *Cardiovasc Res* 83:269, 2009.

219. Carrabba N, Parodi G, Valenti R, et al: Comparison of effects of primary coronary angioplasty on left ventricular remodeling and heart failure in patients <70 versus > or =70 years with acute myocardial infarction. *Am J Cardiol* 104:926, 2009.

220. GISSI-3: Effects of lisinopril and transdermal glyceryl trinitrate singly and together on 6-week mortality and ventricular function after acute myocardial infarction. Gruppo Italiano per lo Studio della Sopravvivenza nell'Infarto Miocardico. *Lancet* 343:1115, 1994.

221. Ambrosioni E, Borghi C, Magnani B: The effect of the angiotensin-converting-enzyme inhibitor zofenopril on mortality and morbidity after anterior myocardial infarction. The Survival of Myocardial Infarction Long-Term Evaluation (SMILE) Study Investigators. *N Engl J Med* 332:80, 1995.

222. Fox KM: Efficacy of perindopril in reduction of cardiovascular events among patients with stable coronary artery disease: randomised, double-blind, placebo-controlled, multicentre trial (the EUROPA study). *Lancet* 362:782, 2003.

223. Pfeffer MA, Braunwald E, Moye LA, et al: Effect of captopril on mortality and morbidity in patients with left ventricular dysfunction after myocardial infarction. Results of the survival and ventricular enlargement trial. The SAVE Investigators. *N Engl J Med* 327:669, 1992.

224. Yusuf S, Teo K, Anderson C, et al: Effects of the angiotensin-receptor blocker telmisartan on cardiovascular events in high-risk patients intolerant to angiotensin-converting enzyme inhibitors: a randomised controlled trial. *Lancet* 372:1174, 2008.

225. Yusuf S, Teo KK, Pogue J, et al: Telmisartan, ramipril, or both in patients at high risk for vascular events. *N Engl J Med* 358:1547, 2008.

226. Antman EM, Hand M, Armstrong PW, et al: 2007 Focused Update of the ACC/AHA 2004 Guidelines for the Management of Patients With ST-Elevation Myocardial Infarction: a report of the American College of Cardiology/American Heart Association Task Force on Practice Guidelines: developed in collaboration With the Canadian Cardiovascular Society endorsed by the American Academy of Family Physicians: 2007 Writing Group to Review New Evidence and Update the ACC/AHA 2004 Guidelines for the Management of Patients With ST-Elevation Myocardial Infarction, Writing on Behalf of the 2004 Writing Committee. *Circulation* 117:296, 2008.

227. Doughty RN, Whalley GA, Walsh HA, et al: Effects of carvedilol on left ventricular remodeling after acute myocardial infarction: the CAPRICORN Echo Substudy. *Circulation* 109:201, 2004.

228. Colucci WS, Kolias TJ, Adams KF, et al: Metoprolol reverses left ventricular remodeling in patients with asymptomatic systolic dysfunction: the REversal of VEntricular Remodeling with Toprol-XL (REVERT) trial. *Circulation* 116:49, 2007.

229. Pitt B, Remme W, Zannad F, et al: Eplerenone, a selective aldosterone blocker, in patients with left ventricular dysfunction after myocardial infarction. *N Engl J Med* 348:1309, 2003.

230. Antman EM, Anbe DT, Armstrong PW, et al: ACC/AHA guidelines for the management of patients with ST-elevation myocardial infarction: a report of the American College of Cardiology/American Heart Association Task Force on Practice Guidelines (Committee to Revise the 1999 Guidelines for the Management of Patients with Acute Myocardial Infarction). *Circulation* 110:e82, 2004.

231. Landmesser U, Wollert KC, Drexler H: Potential novel pharmacological therapies for myocardial remodelling. *Cardiovasc Res* 81:519, 2009.

232. Ishii H, Ichimiya S, Kanashiro M, et al: Effects of receipt of chronic statin therapy before the onset of acute myocardial infarction: a retrospective study in patients undergoing primary percutaneous coronary intervention. *Clin Ther* 28:1812, 2006.

233. Kjekshus J, Pedersen TR, Olsson AG, et al: The effects of simvastatin on the incidence of heart failure in patients with coronary heart disease. *J Card Fail* 3:249, 1997.

234. Udell JA, Ray JG: Primary and secondary prevention of heart failure with statins. *Expert Rev Cardiovasc Ther* 4:917, 2006.

CHAPTER 11

Antihypertensive Drugs and Their Cardioprotective and Renoprotective Roles in the Prevention and Management of Cardiovascular Disease

Chad Kliger, Arthur Schwartzbard, Edward Fisher, and Howard Weintraub

KEY POINTS

- The complete axis of the RAAS along with intracellular RAAS components, alternative pathways, the kallikrein-kinin system, plasma renin and prorenin, and prorenin receptors play a significant role in cardiovascular and renovascular pathophysiology.

- The relationship between cardiac and renal disease is significant, with a strong but incomplete link between renoprotection and cardiovascular risk reduction.

- Proteinuria may be a potential cardiovascular risk factor and a target or indicator of therapeutic response.

- RAAS inhibitors are the primary classes of antihypertensive medications with both cardioprotective and renoprotective effects and are the cornerstone for prevention, particularly in high-risk patients.

- Combinations of different classes of RAAS inhibitors or RAAS inhibitors with calcium channel blockers provide novel ways for more complete RAAS suppression and improved end-organ protection.

Understanding of the role of the renin-angiotensin-aldosterone system (RAAS) in the genesis of cardiac and vascular disease and the close relationship between renal dysfunction and cardiovascular outcomes is increasingly important. Many classes of antihypertensive medications and their combinations have been shown to have beneficial effects, including cardioprotection and renoprotection, and are the cornerstone for primary and secondary prevention. This chapter details each class of antihypertensive medications and elaborates their roles in prevention (Table 11-1).

DIURETICS

Diuretics can be distinguished as loop or thiazide type. Loop-type diuretics have a greater ability to affect volume-overloaded states, and thiazide-type diuretics have a greater ability to reduce blood pressure. Their mechanisms of action differ. Loop diuretics inhibit the sodium-potassium-chloride (Na-K-Cl) transporter on the ascending limb of the loop of Henle. Thiazide diuretics primarily inhibit sodium reabsorption at the renal distal convoluted tubule, thereby reducing plasma volume and lowering blood pressure. Thiazide use also reduces peripheral vascular resistance and acutely stimulates the RAAS.[1,2]

Because of the thiazide diuretic role in antihypertensive treatment and its associated outcomes data, thiazides are the main class of diuretics used for primary prevention. The most commonly used thiazide in clinical practice, hydrochlorothiazide, has a short half-life of 8 to 15 hours with long-term dosing.[3] Another thiazide, chlorthalidone, has a longer half-life, 45 to 60 hours, and has been used in most clinical trials, establishing the utility of thiazides.[3] Thiazides are particularly beneficial in controlling hypertension in certain populations of

salt-sensitive patients, including African Americans, women, and the elderly.[4]

Role of Diuretics

Early literature on diuretics did not show as great a reduction in cardiovascular events as had been predicted by epidemiologic data. Many believed that such a discrepancy was explained by the shorter duration of clinical trials compared with epidemiologic studies. Others postulated that the increased risk of cardiovascular effects was attributed to the many potential adverse, metabolic effects of diuretics, which include electrolyte abnormalities, hyperlipidemia, hyperglycemia, and impaired insulin sensitivity.[5-8]

Diuretics can alter the lipid profile by increasing both serum low-density lipoprotein (LDL) and very-low-density lipoprotein (VLDL) cholesterol, without having a significant effect on high-density lipoprotein (HDL) cholesterol or the apoproteins.[8,9] The mechanism of diuretic-induced dyslipidemia is unclear, and whether this occurs for all patients taking diuretics requires further investigation. Diuretics may also impair insulin sensitivity in both diabetic and non-diabetic patients, which alone or together with resulting compensatory hyperinsulinemia can promote dyslipidemia and atherogenesis.[6-8] There may be an increased risk of new-onset diabetes or metabolic syndrome with the use of thiazides, especially at higher doses.[10]

More recent clinical trials question the role that diuretics have in reducing insulin sensitivity. Systolic Hypertension in the Elderly Program (SHEP) and Hypertension in the Very Elderly Trial (HYVET), in which diuretics were used as initial therapy or in combination with other agents, showed a significant reduction in cardiovascular events with no significant change in lipid profiles and a minimal increase in blood glucose levels.[11-13] A mean follow-up of 14.3

TABLE 11–1	Antihypertensive Classes with Examples, Mechanisms of Action, and Physiologic Effects

Antihypertensive Drug Class	Examples	Mechanisms of Action	Physiologic Effects
Diuretic (thiazide type)	Chlorthalidone Hydrochlorothiazide	Inhibits sodium reabsorption via Na^+/Cl^- channels in the distal convoluted tubule of the kidney	↓ Plasma volume ↓ Peripheral vascular resistance ↑ RAAS
Nitrate	Nitroglycerin Isosorbide mononitrate Isosorbide dinitrate	Produces active metabolite nitric oxide	↑ Vasodilation of coronary arteries, collateral vessels, veins ↓ Systemic arterial pressure ↓ Preload, myocardial wall stress, and MVO_2 ↑ Endothelial function
Calcium channel blocker	Dihydropyridines: nifedipine, amlodipine, felodipine Nondihydropyridines: diltiazem, verapamil	Reduce excess Ca^{2+} entry through voltage- and receptor-operated calcium channels in vascular smooth muscle and cardiac myocytes Improved nitric oxide production and release Increases t-PA activity Reduction in A II–mediated vasoconstriction and aldosterone production	↑ Arteriolar vasodilation including coronary arteries ↓ Inotropy (nondihydropyridine) ↑ Endothelial function ↑ RAAS
Beta blocker	Nonselective beta$_1$ and beta$_2$ antagonists: propranolol Selective beta$_1$ antagonists: atenolol, bisoprolol, metoprolol, nebivolol Alpha$_1$, beta$_1$, beta$_2$ antagonists: carvedilol, labetalol	Decrease in sympathetic activity through blockade of beta$_1$, beta$_2$, and alpha$_1$ receptors Lower plasma renin levels Reduction in endothelin and oxidative stress	↓ In catecholamine levels ↓ Myocardial workload and oxygen demand ↓ Fatty acid metabolism ↓ Inotropy, transiently Altered sympathomimetic activity
Angiotensin-converting enzyme (ACE) inhibitor	Benazepril, captopril, enalapril, fosinopril, lisinopril, perindopril, quinapril, ramipril, trandolapril	Inhibits ACE, reducing levels of A II and aldosterone Inhibits ACE-dependent metabolism of bradykinin and kallidin	Alters cardiac remodeling and vascular protective effects Modulation of adrenergic tone ↑ Bradykinin
Angiotensin receptor blocker	Candesartan, irbesartan, losartan, olmesartan, telmisartan	Block the AT$_1$ receptor Compensatory rise in A II may activate AT$_2$ receptor	↓ Vascular and cardiac hypertrophy ↓ Aldosterone secretion ↓ Vasoconstriction
Direct renin inhibitor	Aliskiren	Blocks renin, rate-limiting step of A II production Reduction in the formation of A I and A II Reduction in plasma renin activity	↓ Atherosclerosis progression* ↓ aldosterone secretion ↓ Media degeneration* ↑ Nitric oxide availability*
Mineralocorticoid receptor blocker	Eplerenone, spironolactone	Blocks aldosterone receptor	↓ Plasma volume ↓ Cardiac hypertrophy

*In animal models.

years of patients from the SHEP trial showed that diabetes that developed during the trial among subjects receiving placebo was associated with worsened cardiovascular outcomes.[14] However, diabetes that developed among subjects during diuretic therapy did not significantly affect cardiovascular mortality.

The Antihypertensive and Lipid-Lowering Treatment to Prevent Heart Attack Trial (ALLHAT) randomized more than 33,000 high-risk hypertensive patients to a regimen of chlorthalidone, amlodipine, or lisinopril as first-line therapy.[15] More than half of the patients enrolled had evidence of atherosclerotic heart disease, with one quarter having a history of myocardial infarction or stroke. No difference in cardiovascular outcomes or mortality was noted among the different agents. Although cholesterol levels and the prevalence of new-onset diabetes (11.6% versus 9.8% and 8.1%) were higher in the diuretic group up to a mean 4.9-year follow-up, these metabolic differences did not translate into increased cardiovascular events or mortality. Whether the follow-up period for ALLHAT was adequate to reveal the impact of

dyslipidemia and new-onset diabetes on outcomes remains unclear.

The SHEP, HYVET, and ALLHAT trials were performed in older populations with an average age of 67 to 84 years. Data from these trials may not be applicable to younger patients with hypertension, particularly in association with comorbid conditions such as obesity, dyslipidemia, and abnormal glucose tolerance. In contrast to ALLHAT, the Second Australian National Blood Pressure (ANBP2) trial showed a significant improvement in cardiovascular outcomes in elderly hypertensive patients who were started with an angiotensin-converting enzyme (ACE) inhibitor compared with a thiazide diuretic.[16] There were several differences between these trials, including differences in the antihypertensive agents used (enalapril instead of lisinopril and hydrochlorothiazide instead of chlorthalidone) and the population of patients studied (lower baseline risk factors). Nonetheless, thiazide diuretics appear highly effective in lowering blood pressure and reducing cardiovascular events (Table 11-2).

TABLE 11–2	**Antihypertensive Classes and Their Renoprotective Effects**	
Antihypertensive Drug Class	**Renal Trials**	**Renal Effects**
Diuretics (thiazide type)	ALLHAT (n = 33,357): chlorthalidone, amlodipine, or lisinopril versus doxazosin; diuretic with significantly increased GFR slope during 4 years compared with CCB (−0.018 versus −0.012 dL/mg per year) INSIGHT (n = 6321): nifedipine GITS versus hydrochlorothiazide + amiloride; significant decrease in GFR 2.3 mL/min SHEP (n = 4736): chlorthalidone ± atenolol; significant increase in creatinine 2.8 µmol/L	Unclear effect on proteinuria Potential worsening of renal function
Nitrates	None	None
Calcium channel blocker (CCB)	AASK (n = 1094): metoprolol, ramipril, or amlodipine; no significant difference in GFR slope; ACE inhibitor showed 38% improvement in composite GFR, ESRD, or death versus CCB ALLHAT (n = 33,357): chlorthalidone, amlodipine, or lisinopril versus doxazosin; CCB with significantly decreased GFR slope during 4 years compared with diuretic (−0.012 versus −0.018 dL/mg per year) IDNT (n = 1715): irbesartan or amlodipine versus placebo; no significant difference in renal outcomes between amlodipine and placebo	Unclear effect on proteinuria Potential preservation of renal function
Beta blocker	AASK (n = 1094): metoprolol, ramipril, or amlodipine; no significant difference in GFR slope; ACE inhibitor showed 22% improvement in composite GFR, ESRD, or death versus beta blocker GEMINI (n = 1235): carvedilol versus metoprolol; 16.2% reduction in microalbuminuria and 41% reduction in progression to microalbuminuria	Reduction in proteinuria No evidence of preservation of renal function
Angiotensin-converting enzyme (ACE) inhibitor	AASK (n = 1094): metoprolol, ramipril, or amlodipine; no significant difference in GFR slope; ACE inhibitor showed 38% improvement in composite GFR, ESRD, or death versus CCB ALLHAT (n = 33,357): chlorthalidone, amlodipine, or lisinopril versus doxazosin; ACE inhibitor showed no significant difference in the GFR slope during 4 years compared with diuretic (−0.019 versus −0.018 dL/mg per year) MICRO-HOPE (n = 3577): ramipril versus placebo; 24% reduction in overt nephropathy (>300 mg proteinuria), with and without baseline microalbuminuria REIN (n = 352): ramipril versus placebo; decline in GFR per month significantly lower with ACE inhibitor versus placebo (0.53 versus 0.88 mL/min), 55% reduction in risk of doubling of baseline creatinine or ESRD	Reduction in proteinuria Preservation of renal function
Angiotensin receptor blocker (ARB)	IDNT (n = 1715): irbesartan or amlodipine versus placebo; 20% reduction in doubling of creatinine, ESRD, creatinine >6 mg/dL, mortality compared with placebo and 23% compared with CCB MARVAL (n = 332): valsartan versus amlodipine; urine albumin excretion was 56% of baseline with valsartan and 92% of baseline with amlodipine; 29.9% valsartan versus 14.5% amlodipine reverted to normoalbuminuria RENAAL (n = 1513): losartan versus placebo; reduction in time to doubling of creatinine, ESRD, death by 16%, incidence of doubling of serum creatinine by 25%, ESRD by 28%; no impact on mortality TRANSCEND (n = 5927): telmisartan versus placebo; no significant difference in composite dialysis or creatinine doubling or change in GFR	Reduction in proteinuria Preservation of renal function
Combination		
ACE inhibitor/ARB	CALM (n = 199): candesartan, lisinopril, or combination; 50% reduction in urinary ACR with combination compared with candesartan 24% and lisinopril 39% ONTARGET (n = 8576): ramipril or telmisartan versus combination; increased ESRD, creatinine doubling, death in combination 14.5% compared with ACE inhibitor or ARB 13.5%; increase in urinary albumin excretion was 7% less in combination compared with ACE inhibitor VALERIA (n = 133): valsartan/lisinopril versus valsartan or lisinopril; 34% reduction in urine ACR in combination compared with lisinopril; 38% of combination group had normalization of microalbuminuria compared with 17% lisinopril	Reduction in proteinuria Unclear effect on renal function
Direct renin inhibitor (DRI) + ARB	AVOID (n = 599): aliskiren/losartan versus losartan; 20% reduction in urinary ACR without significant reduction in blood pressure	Reduction in proteinuria Unclear effect on renal function
ACE inhibitor or ARB/ mineralocorticoid receptor blocker (MRB)	Epstein et al (n = 268): eplerenone/enalapril versus enalapril; reduction in urine albumin excretion by 48.4% versus 7.4% Mehdi et al (n = 81): spironolactone/lisinopril versus lisinopril/losartan; reduction in urine albumin excretion with ACE inhibitor/MRB of 34% compared with ACE inhibitor/ARB 16.8%	Reduction in proteinuria Unclear effect on renal function
ACE inhibitor or ARB/ CCB	ASCOT (n = 19,257): perindopril/amlodipine versus atenolol/bendroflumethiazide; 15% reduction in development of renal impairment Fogari et al (n = 453): fosinopril, amlodipine, or combination; 67% reduction of urine albumin excretion with combination versus fosinopril 46% or amlodipine 33% at 48 months	Reduction in proteinuria Possible effect on renal function

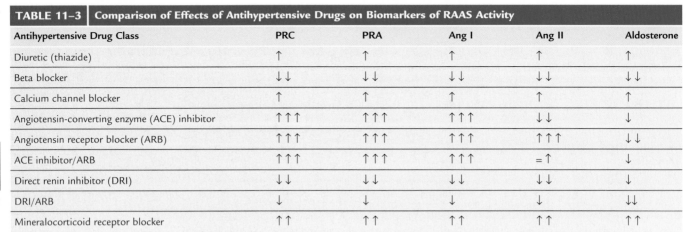

TABLE 11–3 | **Comparison of Effects of Antihypertensive Drugs on Biomarkers of RAAS Activity**

Antihypertensive Drug Class	PRC	PRA	Ang I	Ang II	Aldosterone
Diuretic (thiazide)	↑	↑	↑	↑	↑
Beta blocker	↓↓	↓↓	↓↓	↓↓	↓↓
Calcium channel blocker	↑	↑	↑	↑	↑
Angiotensin-converting enzyme (ACE) inhibitor	↑↑↑	↑↑↑	↑↑↑	↓↓	↓
Angiotensin receptor blocker (ARB)	↑↑↑	↑↑↑	↑↑↑	↑↑↑	↓↓
ACE inhibitor/ARB	↑↑↑	↑↑↑	↑↑↑	=↑	↓
Direct renin inhibitor (DRI)	↓↓	↓↓	↓↓	↓↓	↓
DRI/ARB	↓	↓	↓	↓	↓↓
Mineralocorticoid receptor blocker	↑↑	↑↑	↑↑	↑↑	↑↑

Ang, angiotensin; PRA, plasma renin activity; PRC, plasma renin concentration.

Renal Effects

Aside from altered lipid profiles and glycemic control, the SHEP and International Nifedipine GITS (INSIGHT) studies showed a greater decline in renal function with diuretic therapy, assessed by a rise in serum creatinine.[13,17] The proposed mechanisms of renal injury by diuretics are varied and include volume depletion leading to renal ischemia and stimulation of the RAAS, arteriolar vasoconstriction from endothelial dysfunction and increased oxidative stress, metabolic abnormalities leading to renal hypertrophy and fibrosis, and direct toxic effects on the distal tubular cells[18] (Table 11-3).

Summary

Diuretics are an acceptable therapy for uncomplicated hypertension. The substitution of hydrochlorothiazide with chlorthalidone in clinical practice may be indicated because of its better tolerability (longer half-life). In younger hypertensive patients and in patients with comorbid conditions, especially diabetes or when the pathophysiology of hypertension may be driven by activation of the RAAS or sympathetic activation, agents other than diuretics or diuretic combinations may be preferred (see Table 11-1).

NITRATES

Nitrates are prodrugs; their active metabolite is nitric oxide, also known as endothelium-derived relaxing factor. Nitrates relax vascular smooth muscle and have vasodilatory effects in both the systemic arteries, including the coronary arteries and collateral vessels, and the veins.[19,20] The predominant venodilatory effect of nitrates reduces ventricular preload, which in turn reduces myocardial wall stress and oxygen requirements.[21] Higher doses of nitrates may also decrease systemic arterial pressure. Other beneficial effects include improved endothelial function and a reduction in platelet adhesion and aggregation.[22,23]

Role of Nitrates

Rapid anginal improvement and the resolution of electrocardiographic signs of ischemia have promoted the use of nitrates for the treatment of angina. Trials comparing long-acting nitrates with both calcium channel blockers and beta blockers have shown no significant difference in antianginal efficacy.[24] In the treatment of heart failure, the use of nitrates reduces secondary pulmonary hypertension and improves heart failure symptoms. There are few prognostic data on nitrate therapy in heart failure. The effect of vasodilator therapy on mortality in a chronic congestive heart failure (CHF) trial (V-HeFT I) showed that when oral nitrates are used with an arterial vasodilator, hydralazine, there is a 34% reduction in overall mortality compared with alpha blockade or placebo.[25] The V-HeFT II trial compared the same combination of nitrate and hydralazine with enalapril in patients with symptomatic CHF.[26] Enalapril showed a further 28% reduction in mortality over combination therapy.

For post–myocardial infarction patients in the fibrinolytic era, trials have failed to show a significant benefit of short-term, early nitrate therapy. In the Gruppo Italiano per lo Studio della Sopravvivenza nell'Infarto Miocardico trial (GISSI-3), administration of transdermal nitroglycerin for 6 weeks after acute myocardial infarction demonstrated a non-statistically significant 6% risk reduction in overall mortality.[27] In the Fourth International Study of Infarct Survival (ISIS-4) trial, administration of oral mononitrate for 1 month after acute myocardial infarction also did not demonstrate an impact on postinfarction mortality or combined endpoint of death and heart failure or extensive ventricular dysfunction.[28] The duration of nitrate therapy and follow-up of these trials were relatively short, and the open-label use of nitrates was high in the placebo arms.

With contemporary percutaneous revascularization, one early trial evaluated the long-term nitrate treatment of post–myocardial infarction patients and suggested an increase in cardiac events.[29] Nitrate rebound during nitrate-free intervals and tolerance have been suggested as mechanisms to blunt hemodynamic effects and to increase cardiovascular events. There is also the suggestion of reflex neurohormonal activation with an increase in plasma renin activity and circulating angiotensin II (A II) levels during nitrate therapy, which attenuates the vasodilator effect of nitroglycerin during prolonged treatment.[30] Both the rebound phenomenon and tolerance may be suppressed by the use of ACE inhibitor or angiotensin receptor blocker (ARB) therapy.[31-33] More recent retrospective studies using optimal medical therapy have not identified an increase in adverse events, but a more neutral effect, further questioning the utility of nitrates in secondary prevention[34,35] (see Table 11-2).

Summary

Nitrates are effective antianginal agents used for the symptomatic therapy of all entities of myocardial ischemia. Nitrate therapy can be effective in patients with coronary vasospasm or heart failure caused by myocardial infarction. Their role in the treatment of hypertension is limited. In post–myocardial infarction patients without evidence of myocardial ischemia or heart failure, the role of nitrate therapy in secondary prevention is not well established (see Table 11-2).

CALCIUM CHANNEL BLOCKERS

Calcium channel blockers (CCBs) are classified into the dihydropyridines and the nondihydropyridines, which include phenylalkylamines and benzothiazepines. Examples of the dihydropyridines are nifedipine, felodipine, and amlodipine; examples of the nondihydropyridines are diltiazem and verapamil. Advanced generations of CCBs have modified release formulations, and specifically the newer generation dihydropyridines have higher vascular selectivity and less direct cardiac effects in comparison to short-acting nifedipine.

The CCBs act by counteracting excess calcium entry through the voltage- and receptor-operated calcium channels. CCBs cause potent arteriolar vasodilation by the reduction of calcium entry into the vascular smooth muscle. Within the cardiac myocytes, maintaining the cytosolic calcium balance and preserving ATP stores help maintain myocyte viability and delay ischemic damage.[36] Other effects of CCBs include the protection of endothelial integrity and reduction of endothelial apoptosis,[37] improved nitric oxide production and release,[38] improved fibrinolytic function through an increase in tissue-type plasminogen activator (t-PA) activity,[39] and importantly, reductions in A II–mediated vasoconstriction and decreased A II stimulatory effect on aldosterone production.[40] Many of these effects have also been attributed to inhibitors of the RAAS.

Role of Calcium Channel Blockers

Chronic Stable Angina

CCBs dilate the coronary arteries and increase coronary blood flow. Coronary blood flow is one determinant among others, including heart rate, contractility, and arterial pressure, that affects myocardial oxygen consumption, and all can be variably affected by CCBs. For chronic stable angina, three trials have evaluated the long-term effects of CCBs. Angina Prognosis Study in Stockholm (APSIS) and Total Ischaemic Burden European Trial (TIBET) compared verapamil with metoprolol and nifedipine SR with atenolol, respectively, in patients with stable angina pectoris.[41,42] Neither study found a difference in morbidity and mortality rates between CCBs and beta blockers. When long-acting nifedipine was added to optimal medical therapy including beta blockade, no difference was noted in mortality, with small reductions in the secondary endpoints of need for coronary revascularization and heart failure.[43]

Post–Myocardial Infarction

The Secondary Prevention Reinfarction Israeli Nifedipine trials (SPRINT and SPRINT II) evaluated the effect of the dihydropyridine nifedipine on cardiovascular morbidity and mortality during weeks 2 to 3 for SPRINT and within the first week for SPRINT II after an acute myocardial infarction. No significant difference was noted in morbidity or mortality for late therapy; however, early institution of calcium channel blockade was associated with an increased early mortality (within the first 6 days).

The secondary Danish Verapamil Infarction Trial (DAVIT II) showed for the first time that a nondihydropyridine reduces the incidence of death and reinfarction by approximately 20% when it is started 1 week after acute myocardial infarction.[44] A significant reduction in mortality (11.8% versus 7.7%) was noted only in patients without CHF. Interestingly, the order of magnitude of this benefit was similar to that achieved in numerous beta blocker trials. In the Multicenter Diltiazem Post-Infarction Trial (MDPIT), diltiazem nonsignificantly decreased cardiac mortality or nonfatal reinfarction by 11%.[45] However, there was a significant increase in late CHF (21% versus 11%) and an increase in cardiac events (hazard ratio, 1.41) in patients with ejection fractions less than 40%. The diltiazem-associated rise in the frequency of CHF was progressively greater with worsening decrements of ejection fraction.

Congestive Heart Failure

As potent vasodilators, CCBs have been shown to improve hemodynamic responses in CHF patients with notable decreases in pulmonary capillary wedge pressure, systemic vascular resistance, and end-diastolic ventricular pressure.[46] CCBs are also negative inotropic agents and have varying degrees of impairment in cardiac function. The differences in negative inotropy are due to differences in the binding affinity ratios of smooth to cardiac muscle, with dihydropyridines being more vascular selective. An early generation CCB, nifedipine, showed clinical effects not consistent with their hemodynamic benefit, with a significant increase in heart failure deterioration.[47] This has also been noted with the use of diltiazem after myocardial infarction in patients with ventricular dysfunction (ejection fraction <40%).[48] CHF patients who deteriorate after a CCB have been shown to have a worse prognosis, with a significant decrease in mortality at 1 year.[49]

Later generations of CCBs, felodipine and amlodipine, were developed with predominant peripheral vasodilating effects, having minimal effect on the myocardium and with longer half-lives thought to decrease reflex neurohormonal activation in patients with heart failure. The Prospective Randomized Amlodipine Survival Evaluation trials (PRAISE-1 and PRAISE-2) evaluated the long-term use of amlodipine in advanced heart failure patients.[50,51] Patients had New York Heart Association (NYHA) Class III or Class IV heart failure and ejection fractions less than 30% despite treatment with ACE inhibitor, diuretic, and digoxin. PRAISE-1 evaluated 1153 patients regardless of the cause of heart failure, and PRAISE-2 evaluated 1652 nonischemic cardiomyopathy patients. In both trials, amlodipine showed a neutral effect on mortality in patients with severe chronic heart failure.

A trial similar to PRAISE was performed with felodipine, Vasodilator–Heart Failure Trial (V-HeFT III trial).[52] This study evaluated 450 patients with NYHA Class II or Class III heart failure and ejection fractions less than 45%. Exercise capacity was not statistically significant, and no differences were noted in mortality or rates of hospitalization (see Table 11-1).

Renal Effects

CCBs have pleiotropic effects that might contribute to renal protection against hypertension-induced damage. These effects include a reduction in mesangial inflammation and proliferation and the promotion of nephrotoxic free radical removal.[53-55] At the renovascular level, CCBs preferentially dilate the glomerular afferent arteriole, with only modest action on the efferent arteriole.[56] This preferential effect, potentially noted more predominantly with dihydropyridine CCBs, may cause glomerular hypertension, increasing capillary intraglomerular pressure that could be associated with progression of renal disease.[57-59]

Given their diversity of renal effects and the potential class differences between CCBs on intraglomerular pressures, trials evaluating the effects of CCBs on nephropathy are equally divergent. The African American Study of Kidney Disease and Hypertension (AASK) showed a lesser degree of renal function preservation in African Americans with hypertensive nephrosclerosis treated with amlodipine than with the ACE inhibitor ramipril.[60] Furthermore, in this population of patients, amlodipine showed a significant increase in proteinuria compared with both metoprolol and ramipril. The ALLHAT study, on the other hand, showed that amlodipine maintained glomerular filtration rate (GFR) better than therapy with a diuretic or ACE inhibitor.[15] Overall, the use of CCBs in renal disease is safe without any evidence of further deterioration of renal function. CCBs may be better than diuretics and beta blockers, but they are not as effective as RAAS inhibitors in reducing proteinuria and preventing the progression of renal disease (see Table 11-2).

11

Summary

In patients with chronic stable angina, CCBs may be considered for adjunctive treatment but not as monotherapy unless beta blockers and RAAS inhibitors are not tolerated. Early administration of nifedipine in acute myocardial infarction, unless it is specifically indicated in vasospastic angina, is contraindicated. The nondihydropyridines, possibly because of their heart rate–lowering properties, are the only CCBs to show benefit in the post–myocardial infarction population. They also increase the risk for subsequent CHF in post–myocardial infarction patients with reduced ejection fractions and should probably be reserved for patients without heart failure who cannot tolerate a beta blocker or in whom a beta blocker is contraindicated. Amlodipine and felodipine, given their neutral effect on cardiac morbidity and mortality and ease of tolerance, may be considered in the management of hypertension or coronary artery disease (CAD) in patients with heart failure (see Table 11-1).

BETA BLOCKERS

Beta blockade reduces myocardial workload and oxygen demand through a reduction in heart rate, blood pressure, and cardiac index.[61] A decrease in sympathetic activity reduces fatty acid metabolism and reduces catecholamine levels, helping to redistribute flow to ischemic territories. In addition, beta blockers moderately lower plasma renin activity, even in patients receiving treatment with an ACE inhibitor, in whom the biologic effects of renin are already attenuated.[62]

Beta blockers differ in the degree to which they antagonize the effects of the sympathetic nervous system. The predominant effect of this class of medications is through interaction with the beta$_1$ receptor, primarily located within cardiac muscle. However, each drug has varying effects on beta$_2$ receptor antagonism regulating norepinephrine release, intrinsic sympathomimetic activity (which provides a measurable beta agonist response), and other adrenergic receptors such as the alpha$_1$ receptor. Nonselective beta antagonists block beta$_1$ and beta$_2$ receptors; an example is propranolol. Selective beta antagonists block beta$_1$ receptors; examples include atenolol metoprolol, bisoprolol, and nebivolol. Carvedilol and nebivolol block three adrenergic receptors (alpha$_1$, beta$_1$, and beta$_2$) and reduce endothelin and oxidative stress.[63]

Role of Beta Blockers

For decades, beta blockers have been widely used in the treatment of uncomplicated hypertension. However, no trial has shown that lowering of blood pressure with a beta blocker reduces the risk of cardiovascular events in patients with hypertension compared with placebo. More recently, beta blocker treatment has been associated with a substantially higher (16%) risk of stroke than treatment with other antihypertensive agents.[64] A proposed mechanism may be differences in the hemodynamic effects of beta blockade.

Treatment with a beta blocker results in reduced brachial blood pressure but does not lower central aortic blood pressure as much as treatment with an ACE inhibitor, diuretic, or CCB does.[65] Central aortic blood pressure may be more predictive of cardiovascular events than traditional brachial blood pressure measurements.[66] The outcome of both the Anglo-Scandinavian Cardiac Outcomes Trial–Blood Pressure Lowering Arm (ASCOT-BPLA) and the Losartan Intervention For Endpoint reduction in hypertension study (LIFE) showed a stroke reduction of approximately 25% when treatment with either a CCB or an ARB, respectively, was given instead of a beta blocker.[67,68]

Post–Myocardial Infarction and Chronic Stable Angina

Early beta blockade relieves chest pain and reduces infarct size and fatal arrhythmias; long-term beta blockade reduces late mortality and reinfarction.[69] Early trials and meta-analyses performed before reperfusion therapy suggested that beta blockade after myocardial infarction can reduce mortality, with the most marked reduction of about 25% occurring in the first 2 days after infarction.[70] In the Cooperative Cardiovascular Project, beta blockade showed a mortality reduction of 40% across all patient subgroups, including high-risk groups such as the elderly and patients with a severely reduced ejection fraction.[71]

The two largest pre–thrombolytic era trials examining beta blockade in acute myocardial infarction were the Metoprolol in Acute Myocardial Infarction (MIAMI) and the First International Study of Infarct Survival (ISIS-1) trials.[72,73] In the MIAMI trial, more than 5000 post–myocardial infarction patients received metoprolol within 24 hours of presentation. Mortality was 4.9% in the placebo group and 4.3% in the metoprolol group. Despite the overall nonsignificant reduction in mortality, subgroup analysis revealed a survival advantage of nearly 30% in patients considered at higher risk. ISIS-1 trial evaluated the efficacy of early atenolol in nearly 16,000 patients presenting with myocardial infarction within 12 hours of symptoms. This trial showed a 15% reduction in vascular deaths as well as a 15% reduction in early cardiac arrests and reinfarctions, predominantly noted within the first day after infarction.

This benefit of beta blockade was evident in early administration and short-term continuation, before the standard use of fibrinolytic and antiplatelet therapy. It can be attributed to the prevention of life-threatening arrhythmias and cardiac rupture. The ClOpidogrel and Metoprolol in Myocardial Infarction Trial (COMMIT) is the largest trial to date, including nearly 46,000 patients to evaluate the effects of intravenous and then oral metoprolol in acute myocardial infarction added to current antiplatelet and fibrinolytic therapy.[74] There was no significant difference noted in the rate of composite endpoint of death, reinfarction, or cardiac arrest, with overall mortality balanced by a 22% reduction in late arrhythmic death and a 29% proportional increase in early shock-related death. The overall net effect of metoprolol therapy changed from being significantly adverse during the first 2 days after admission due to shock-related death to being significantly beneficial thereafter due to a reduction in ventricular fibrillation.

In combining a retrospectively defined low-risk subgroup of COMMIT similar to the populations studied in MIAMI and ISIS-1, the overall effects were consistent, showing a significant reduction of 13% in mortality, 22% in reinfarction, or 15% in ventricular fibrillation. Beta blocker therapy for these trials among others, including the Beta Heart Attack Trial

(BHAT) and the TIMI IIB trial, was continued up to 2 years.[75,76] Furthermore, randomized trials of beta blocker therapy in patients undergoing percutaneous coronary intervention without fibrinolytic therapy have not been performed. It does seem reasonable, however, to extrapolate the results from those receiving another form of revascularization to the percutaneous coronary intervention population.

The use of beta blockade for the treatment of chronic stable angina has also been predominantly extrapolated from the evidence of improved mortality of beta blockers in the post–myocardial infarction patient. Given the lack of mortality benefit and increased risk of stroke in patients with uncomplicated hypertension, treatment of patients with chronic stable angina but no prior myocardial infarction with beta blockers is not well supported but commonly used. Other antihypertensive medications, such as CCBs and ACE inhibitors, may be equally beneficial without the potential adverse effects of beta blockade therapy.

Congestive Heart Failure

Because of transient negative inotropic effects of beta blockade, beta blockers used to be contraindicated in CHF. Many trials have since shown that patients with heart failure derive greater benefit from beta blocker therapy after myocardial infarction than do patients without heart failure. In the BHAT trial, propranolol reduced mortality equally in patients with and without systolic dysfunction by approximately 25%. However, there was a 47% reduction in sudden death in patients with heart failure, compared with 13% reduction in patients without heart failure.

The Metoprolol CR/XL Randomized Intervention Trial in Congestive Heart Failure (MERIT-HF), Cardiac Insufficiency Bisoprolol Study II (CIBIS II), and Carvedilol on Survival in Severe Chronic Heart Failure (COPERNICUS) trials evaluated the effects of beta blockade in patients with heart failure, with severely reduced ejection fractions, and receiving stable ACE inhibitor and diuretic therapy.[77-79] Metoprolol, bisoprolol, and carvedilol, respectively, showed an overall reduction in total mortality of approximately 35%. In addition to improved mortality, beta blockers, when given with ACE inhibitors, improve the patient symptoms and NYHA functional class and reduce heart failure hospitalizations (see Table 11-4).

Renal Effects

Beta$_1$ receptors alter the release of renin, and beta$_2$ and alpha$_1$ receptors alter sympathetic activity responsible for renovascular tone, important in the genesis of hypertension and progression of kidney disease. Although beta blockers improve cardiac mortality, they have not shown the same benefit on renal outcomes compared with other agents that lower blood pressure and albuminuria. Studies in both diabetic and non-diabetic nephropathy do not show a significant reduction in microalbuminuria with beta blockade compared with ACE inhibition.[80,81]

In the Glycemic Effects in Diabetes Mellitus: Carvedilol-Metoprolol Comparison in Hypertensives (GEMINI) trial, 1235 hypertensive, diabetic patients were enrolled to evaluate the effects of metoprolol versus carvedilol on glycemic control, with a secondary endpoint of change in microalbuminuria.[82] There was a 16.2% reduction in microalbuminuria for patients randomized to carvedilol compared with metoprolol despite similar blood pressure control during 3 years. Among patients with normal albuminuria at baseline, fewer in the carvedilol group (6.6%) than in the metoprolol group (11.1%) progressed to microalbuminuria. GEMINI suggests that beta blockers with alpha$_1$ receptor activity may reduce the compensatory stimulation of the sympathetic system and RAAS caused by beta blockade and may further reduce the

TABLE 11–4	Compelling Indications for Antihypertensive Drug Classes
Compelling Indication	**Therapeutic Options**
High CAD risk	Thiazide*, beta blocker, CCB*, ACE inhibitor*, ACE inhibitor/CCB, ARB/CCB
Chronic stable angina	Nitrates, CCB, ACE inhibitor, ACE inhibitor/CCB, ARB/CCB
Post–myocardial infarction	Beta blocker*, ACE inhibitor*, ARB, MRB*, nondihydropyridine CCB
Heart failure	Beta blocker*, ACE inhibitor*, ARB*, MRB*, diuretics, nitrates
Chronic kidney disease	
Reduction in proteinuria	Beta blocker, ACE inhibitor*, ARB*, DRI, ACE inhibitor/ARB, ACE inhibitor/MRB, ARB/MRB, ACE inhibitor/CCB, ARB/CCB
Preservation of renal function	CCB, ACE inhibitor*, ARB*, ACE inhibitor/CCB, ARB/CCB

*Classes recommended by the Seventh Report of the Joint National Committee (JNC7).

ACE, angiotensin-converting enzyme; ARB, angiotensin receptor blocker; CAD, coronary artery disease; CCB, calcium channel blocker; DRI, direct renin inhibitor; MRB, mineralocorticoid receptor blocker.

progression of albuminuria, providing cardiorenal protection (see Table 11-2).

Summary

Beta blockers have an established benefit for the treatment of patients after myocardial infarction or with heart failure and play an important role in secondary prevention. The role of beta blockade in the treatment of uncomplicated hypertension remains unclear, given the paucity of data and the possible mild increased risk of stroke. Delay of the initiation of beta blocker therapy until after stabilization of the patient from an acute myocardial infarction may avoid the excess risk of shock and early mortality while preserving much of its described benefits. Controversy remains as to the duration of beta blocker therapy in post–myocardial infarction patients, but if the medication remains well tolerated, discontinuation should be discouraged (see Table 11-4).

RENIN-ANGIOTENSIN-ALDOSTERONE SYSTEM

Renin is a protease produced by the juxtaglomerular cells of the kidney that line the afferent arteriole of the glomerulus. Renin is secreted principally as a result of four mechanisms: renal baroreceptors in the afferent arteriole that sense alterations in renal perfusion pressure, a change in NaCl delivery to the macula densa cells of the distal tubule, sympathetic stimulation through beta$_1$-adrenergic receptors, and negative feedback by A II on juxtaglomerular cells.[83] Outside of the kidney, renin is secreted by other tissues including the brain, adrenal gland, ovary, and adipose tissue in addition to the heart and vascular tissue. Renin is the rate-limiting step of the RAAS (Fig. 11-1).

Renin cleaves angiotensinogen to angiotensin I (A I), commonly referred to as Ang-(1-10) for its decapeptide structure. Angiotensinogen is primarily produced by the liver, but expression has been noted in tissue similar to that expressing renin, including the kidney and heart. A I is biologically inactive and is converted by ACE by the removal of a dipeptide to

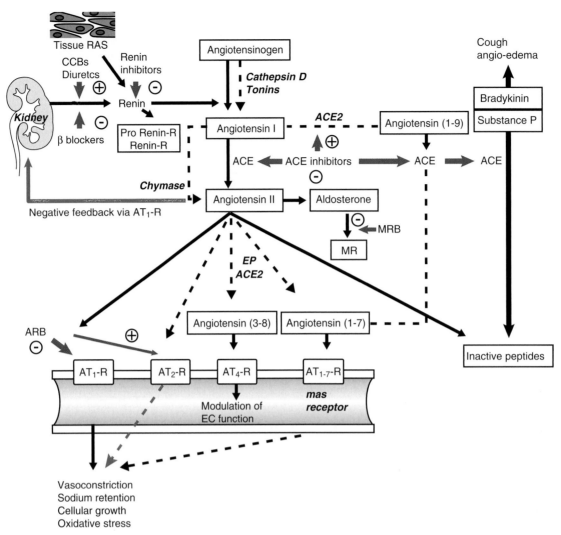

FIGURE 11-1 The renin-angiotensin-aldosterone system. ACE, angiotensin-converting enzyme; ARB, angiotensin receptor blocker; AT-R, angiotensin receptor; CCBs, calcium channel blockers; EC, endothelial cells; EP, endopeptidases; MR, mineralocorticoid receptor; MRB, mineralocorticoid receptor blocker. Black arrows show stimulation, red arrows show inhibition, and blue arrows show antihypertensive drug involvement with stimulation (+) or inhibition (−) of the pathway. Full lines represent major functional pathways, and dotted lines show alternative pathways. *(Modified from Staessen J, Li Y, Richart T: Oral renin inhibitors.* Lancet *368:1449, 2006.)*

form A II or Ang-(1-8). ACE is a membrane-bound exopeptidase predominantly localized on the membranes of the vascular endothelial and renal proximal tubular cells. ACE also metabolizes other vasodilator peptides, including bradykinin and kallidin, which may have important physiologic effects that will be described later in the chapter.

Although A II is the primary active product in the RAAS, other metabolites of A I and A II may have physiologic activity. These include angiotensin III, (Ang-[2-8]); angiotensin IV, (Ang-[3-8]); and Ang-(1-7). All metabolites are formed by removal of varying amounts of amino acids from either the N or C terminus of A II and have varying effects, some of which are unknown to date.

It is the interaction of A II with the angiotensin receptors that drives many of the RAAS effects.[83] At least four angiotensin receptors have been described; the AT$_1$ receptor mediates many of the pathophysiologic effects and therefore is a major therapeutic target for secondary prevention. AT$_1$ receptors are expressed in the kidney, adrenals, liver, brain, vasculature, and heart, and their activity includes vasoconstriction, vascular and cardiac hypertrophy, renal tubular sodium resorption, inhibition of renin release, sympathetic

activation, cell growth and proliferation, and increased inflammatory response. AT$_2$ receptors are not highly expressed in the adult and may oppose some of the AT$_1$ receptor–mediated pathways. Some physiologic effects of AT$_2$ receptors may include vasodilation, smooth muscle antiproliferation, and inhibition of cardiac remodeling. AT$_3$ receptor function is unknown, and AT$_4$ receptor function has been shown to modulate endothelial function through plasminogen activator inhibitor 1 (PAI-1).[83]

A II also stimulates, through the AT$_1$ receptor, the release of aldosterone, predominantly from the adrenal cortex, but extra-adrenal sites of aldosterone synthesis have been identified in the brain, vasculature, and heart. Aldosterone is regulated by both A II and dietary potassium.[84] It is an important hormone in sodium and fluid retention as a result of direct stimulation of the mineralocorticoid receptors in the distal renal tubules. Mineralocorticoid receptors are also as widespread as their extra-adrenal sites. Their varied proposed physiologic mechanisms include renal, vascular, and cardiac inflammation; fibrosis and hypertrophy; increases in sympathetic activation; attenuation of platelet aggregation; and impairment of endothelial dysfunction[85,86] (Fig. 11-2).

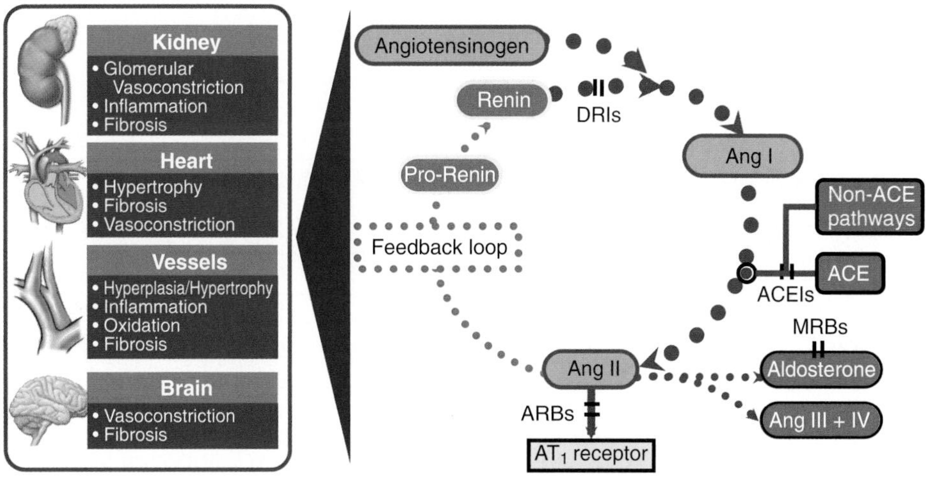

FIGURE 11-2 Classic understanding of the renin-angiotensin-aldosterone system with feedback loop activation. ACE, angiotensin-converting enzyme; ACEIs, angiotensin-converting enzyme inhibitors; Ang, angiotensin; ARBs, angiotensin receptor blockers; AT$_1$, type 1 angiotensin II receptor; DRIs, direct renin inhibitors; MRBs, mineralocorticoid receptor blockers.

Intracellular Renin-Angiotensin-Aldosterone System

Despite the multiorgan involvement, specifically in the kidney, vasculature, and heart, for the full physiologic axis of the RAAS, local tissue or intracellular RAAS has been identified and is believed to play a significant role in cardiovascular pathophysiology.[87] The intracellular RAAS is defined by a functionally active complete RAAS within a cell, including components that participate in A II production and its receptors and effector proteins. In the heart, angiotensinogen is internalized and basal expression of RAAS components is very low. Intracellular RAAS is activated in response to pathologic conditions such as pressure or volume overload, myocardial infarction, and diabetes.[88]

Potential mechanisms of action include direct intracellular A II effects on the heart, which are non–AT$_1$ receptor mediated, and intracellular A II regulation of the AT$_1$ receptor, providing an improved response to extracellular A II. These mechanisms have been suggested to have a role in left ventricular hypertrophy, activation of metalloproteinases with facilitation of plaque rupture, and pathogenesis of vascular disease.[88] Intracellular A II actions are not blocked by ACE inhibitors or ARBs because of their inability to enter the cell and to block these pathways. More complete RAAS inhibition may be provided by direct renin inhibitors that can block both extracellular and intracellular pathways.

Alternative Pathways of Angiotensin II Production

In addition to intracellular RAAS, alternative pathways of A II production independent of ACE, termed ACE escape, have been established. These include chymase and ACE-2–dependent pathways. Chymase is a protease stored within the secretory granules of mast cells; it is present within the blood vessels, the heart, and other tissues but does not circulate within the blood. In blood vessels, chymase is localized to mast cells in the adventitia, whereas ACE is localized in the vascular endothelium.[89] In normal vasculature, circulating A I does not readily penetrate into the interstitial space, and hence A I is converted to A II in an ACE-dependent fashion. In the setting of vascular injury or inflammation, mast cells are activated, allowing a chymase-dependent conversion of A I to A II.

Although chymase may have only a limited physiologic role in the generation of A II, residual A II formation may be observed in the presence of ACE inhibitor due to this chymase-dependent pathway. Other effects of chymase, outside of the A II–mediated effects, include promotion of atherosclerosis through the prevention of cholesterol removal by HDL, intimal hyperplasia of injured arteries, potential erosion and rupture of coronary atheroma leading to an acute coronary syndrome, and stimulation of transforming growth factor-β (TGF-β) leading to cardiac fibrosis.[90]

Angiotensin-converting enzyme 2 (ACE-2) is a peptidase present throughout the cardiovascular system, including in macrophages, vascular endothelium, smooth muscle cells, and potentially cardiac myocytes. It has been shown to convert A I and A II to Ang-(1-9) and Ang-(1-7), respectively.[91] The full physiologic importance of this pathway has yet to be determined. However, ACE-2 may have a counter-regulatory role with ACE in fine-tuning the RAAS system through increased production of Ang-(1-7), balancing A II vasopressor effects.[92]

Kallikrein-Kinin System

The main effector protein of the kallikrein-kinin system is bradykinin, produced by the proteolytic cleavage of a high-molecular-weight kininogen by kallikrein. Bradykinin has a variety of biologic effects, some cardioprotective. These effects are mediated through BK$_1$ and BK$_2$ receptors located on endothelial cells.[93] The BK$_1$ receptor is rarely expressed in normal tissue but is upregulated in pathologic states associated with inflammation and tissue injury.[94] It causes stimulation of smooth muscle cells, cell proliferation, and collagen synthesis. The BK$_2$ receptor, on the other hand, leads to increased stimulation of nitric oxide and prostacyclin, exerting vasodilator, anti-ischemic, and antiproliferative effects.[95] Kinins are released in the setting of ischemia, myocardial infarction, and heart failure, and the ability of ACE inhibitor to prevent the breakdown of kinins represents a potential mechanism contributing to the drug's cardioprotective effects.[96,97]

Prorenin and Prorenin Receptor

Renin is synthesized as a prohormone, prorenin, and stored in granules within the renal juxtaglomerular cells.[98] Prorenin is activated by removal of its N terminus that covers the active

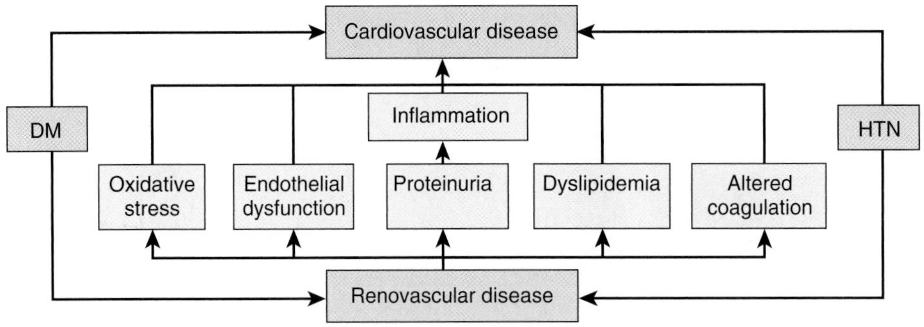

Cardiovascular disease

DM   Inflammation   HTN

Oxidative stress | Endothelial dysfunction | Proteinuria | Dyslipidemia | Altered coagulation

Renovascular disease

FIGURE 11-3 Interaction of cardiovascular and renovascular disease. DM, diabetes mellitus; HTN, hypertension.

site and blocks access to angiotensinogen.[99] The recent discovery of the prorenin receptor has expanded the physiologic role of this once believed inactive prohormone.[100] The prorenin receptor binds to both renin and prorenin and has been localized to the vascular smooth muscle, the heart, and the distal and collecting tubules of the kidney.

When renin binds to the receptor, its activity is amplified fivefold, accelerating the production of A I and in turn A II. Prorenin, when it is bound to the receptor, can undergo nonproteolytic activation by unfolding of the peptide, exposing its active site. This allows prorenin to assume full activity and to contribute to the production of A I. Independent of A II, both renin and prorenin exert physiologic effects through the prorenin receptor.[101] The activated receptor stimulates the production of TGF-β and heat shock proteins, increasing levels of PAI-1 and collagen involved in organ fibrosis and actin filament dynamics involved in contractility, hypertrophy, and apoptosis.[102]

Plasma Renin Activity

Renin is the primary effector hormone of the RAAS, the first and rate-limiting step in A II synthesis. Plasma renin concentration is a measure of the amount of renin in the circulation, and plasma renin activity is a measure of its catalytic activity.[98] Plasma renin activity correlates with the rate at which A I is generated and is a marker of the activation of the RAAS.

Early data have identified that elevated plasma renin activity has a direct relationship with adverse cardiovascular outcomes, including CHF and death, particularly in patients with CAD.[103,104] More recently, several studies by the Intermountain Heart Collaborative Study Investigators have demonstrated a correlation of plasma renin activity to both worsened ischemia and heart failure outcomes at 3 years in patients with mild and moderate coronary atherosclerosis.[105,106] The use of ACE inhibitors or ARBs can increase plasma renin activity by inhibiting the feedback loop that governs activity of the RAAS. The role and importance of prorenin, plasma renin concentration, and plasma renin activity have raised interest in the use of direct renin inhibitors (see Table 11-3).

Association Between Renal Insufficiency and Cardiovascular Disease

Many studies have demonstrated that the relationship between renal dysfunction and increased cardiovascular morbidity and mortality extends across the spectrum of renal dysfunction to include even the mildest degree of renal impairment.[107] This relationship is also maintained across varying degrees of baseline cardiovascular health. In the general population[107-109] and in patients with hypertension,[110] stable CAD,[111,112] post–myocardial infarction,[113] or heart failure,[114] there is an independent and strong correlation between worsening renal function and an increase in cardiovascular events. Baseline GFR has even been suggested to be a stronger predictor of mortality than either left ventricular ejection fraction or New York Heart Association class.[114]

The increased cardiovascular risk for individuals with renal insufficiency is explained in part by the increased prevalence and severity of diabetes and hypertension (Fig. 11-3). However, other mechanisms have been proposed to contribute to the increased risk of cardiovascular events in renal insufficiency. These mechanisms include an increase in endothelial dysfunction, an increase in oxidant stress and inflammation, progressive dyslipidemia, and stimulation of the RAAS that accompanies this disorder.[115]

In renal disease, the initial insult to the kidney results in a decline in the GFR, noted by an increase in serum creatinine concentration.[116] When nephrons are damaged, the remaining nephrons undergo hypertrophy with alterations in arteriolar tone. This in turn increases hydraulic pressure within the glomerular capillaries. The filtration capacity of the remaining nephrons increases, minimizing the functional consequences of nephron loss. The high glomerular capillary pressure enlarges the glomerular membrane pores through a process partially attributed to angiotensin (A II), which subsequently increases the number of proteins, both albumin and nonselective proteins, filtered. It is these proteins that become reabsorbed by the proximal tubular cells and may stimulate a vasoactive and inflammatory framework leading to a systemic vascular disease that can affect the kidneys as well as other arterial systems in the body, including the heart. Endothelial dysfunction, which is associated with alterations in vasomotor tone, inflammation, and oxidative stress, plays a key role in remodeling of the vasculature and increases the risk for atherosclerosis.

Described mediators of inflammation and coagulation known to be increased during renal insufficiency include C-reactive protein, fibrinogen, homocysteine, interleukin-6, factor VII/VIII, von Willebrand factor, D-dimer, and plasmin-antiplasmin complex.[117,118] These mediators, derived in part from increased A II and the modifications of lipids, directly affect endothelial function and vascular remodeling through enhanced oxidative stress. Increased oxidative stress produces reactive oxygen species mainly through the activation of nicotinamide adenine dinucleotide (NADPH) oxidase and the uncoupling of endothelial synthase. The production of reactive oxygen species directly reduces nitric oxide activity, promoting endothelial dysfunction and atherosclerosis.

Dyslipidemia associated with renal insufficiency further contributes to the production of reactive oxygen species and inflammation. Notable alterations in lipid synthesis include elevated levels of lipoprotein(a) and triglycerides, decreased levels of apo A and HDL, and the decreased ability to reduce oxidized, small dense LDL.[117] These defects are the result of a combination of overproduction and clearance defects in apo B–containing lipoproteins. The dyslipidemia of renal disease is complex, with an atherogenic profile similar to that of metabolic syndrome.[119] In general, the severity of dyslipidemia correlates with the severity of proteinuria.[120]

It has been demonstrated that the severity of atherosclerosis is highly correlated with severity of glomerulosclerosis and of renal arteriolosclerosis.[121] Renal insufficiency may be a marker for generalized atherosclerotic burden.[122] However, the presence of these altered pathways has been noted in people with renal insufficiency but with no evidence of clinical or subclinical cardiovascular disease. The prevalence of endothelial dysfunction, low-grade inflammation, dyslipidemia, and RAAS stimulation associated with renal disease may explain the acceleration of atherosclerosis.[117] In combination with hypertension and associated left ventricular hypertrophy, this may lead to a reduction in coronary reserve, explaining the prevalence of coronary ischemia and cardiovascular events in people with renal insufficiency.[118]

Association Between Proteinuria and Cardiovascular Disease

Whereas an elevated serum creatinine concentration reflects a decline in the GFR, an increased rate of albumin or protein excretion reflects a derangement in the glomerular filtration barrier.[123] The presence of abnormal quantities of albumin in the urine often precedes renal functional deterioration. Microalbuminuria, an albumin-to-creatinine ratio (ACR) of 30 to 300 mg/g, correlates with nephrosclerosis; macroalbuminuria (ACR > 300 mg/g) generally indicates established renal parenchymal damage.

Proteinuria (or albuminuria) has been shown to be an independent marker of cardiovascular risk.[124-126] The link between albuminuria and adverse cardiovascular events was first recognized with macroalbuminuria, later with microalbuminuria, and currently with any evidence of albuminuria.[127-129] It has been suggested that proteinuria is a continuous cardiovascular risk factor, whereas microalbuminuria is a designated threshold for renal functional deterioration in individuals with and without diabetes.[117,130]

Proteinuria, despite its association with renal injury, may also reflect a systemic increase in endothelial permeability or dysfunction.[131] The vascular endothelium has an important role in regulating the transport of proteins across vessel walls. Endothelial dysfunction, as a result of shear stress, may allow the deposition of lipoproteins in the subendothelial space, promoting atherogenesis. Further injury to the endothelium results in increased cell and platelet adhesiveness, greater permeability to inflammatory cells, and altered production of vasoactive mediators, specifically nitric oxide.[131] This suggests that proteinuria may be a marker of generalized damage to the peripheral vasculature, paralleling the degree of cardiac organ damage.

The Irbesartan Diabetic Nephropathy Trial (IDNT) and Reduction of Endpoints in NIDDM with the Angiotensin II Antagonist Losartan (RENAAL) trial were the first trials to help establish proteinuria as a cardiovascular risk factor.[132,133] IDNT enrolled subjects with type 2 diabetes, hypertension, and macroalbuminuria. A total of 1715 subjects were randomized to irbesartan, amlodipine, or placebo and were observed for a mean period of 2.6 years. The primary outcome was a composite of serum creatinine doubling, end-stage renal disease (ESRD), or death. Although irbesartan proved to have a significant benefit compared with other therapies, no difference was detected on a secondary outcome of cardiovascular events. Further analysis of baseline albuminuria and cardiovascular composite endpoint showed that the proportion of patients who experienced cardiovascular events progressively increased with increasing quartiles of albuminuria, a 1.3-fold increased risk for each natural log unit increase in ACR.

RENAAL enrolled the same population of subjects as IDNT did, with a total of 1513 subjects randomized to either losartan or placebo. Baseline albuminuria was again shown to be a predictor of composite cardiovascular endpoint as well as heart failure alone. In addition, the change in urinary albumin from baseline to 6 months was the only correlate of adverse cardiovascular outcomes; a 50% reduction in baseline albuminuria translated into an 18% reduction in cardiovascular events and a 27% reduction in the risk of heart failure.

Other trials, such as the Heart Outcomes Prevention Evaluation (HOPE) and the Losartan Intervention For Endpoint reduction in hypertension (LIFE), reconfirmed the association between varying degrees of proteinuria and cardiovascular risk, independent of blood pressure.[130,134] Reductions in proteinuria over time translate into improved outcomes, and it appears that proteinuria may even be more predictive than the other traditional cardiovascular risk factors. Proteinuria can be used as a potential target or indicator of therapeutic response with antihypertensive therapy.

ANGIOTENSIN-CONVERTING ENZYME INHIBITORS

After an acute myocardial infarction, a complex of changes involving neurohormonal activation and cardiac remodeling can lead to progressive heart failure and death. Left ventricular dilation is an integral part of this remodeling process, compensating for the loss of systolic function.[135] Attenuation of left ventricular dilation in combination with a reduction in preload and afterload is beneficial in CAD patients, especially in the post–myocardial infarction state. ACE inhibitor therapy alters cardiac remodeling and has a multitude of vascular protective effects through decreased levels of A II and aldosterone and upregulation of bradykinin. In addition, modulation of adrenergic tone through the effects on A II, improved endothelial function, and improved fibrinolytic balance with reduced PAI-1 and increased t-PA activity have been shown.[136-138] It is the balance of cardiac and vascular protective effects that provides the benefit of ACE inhibitor therapy.

Role of Angiotensin-Converting Enzyme Inhibitors

Post–Myocardial Infarction and Congestive Heart Failure

Early long-term trials, such as Survival and Ventricular Enlargement (SAVE), Acute Infarction Ramipril Efficacy (AIRE) study, and Trandolapril Cardiac Evaluation (TRACE), enrolled high-risk patients after myocardial infarction with heart failure, with or without symptoms, or the presence of an anterior myocardial infarction.[139-141] The results of these trials were consistent and demonstrated that the use of an ACE inhibitor significantly reduced overall heart failure and mortality by about 5% for each endpoint, with a relative reduction of approximately 20%.

In the Survival of Myocardial Infarction Long-term Evaluation (SMILE) trial, a shorter term treatment of ACE inhibitor for 6 weeks was instituted within 24 hours after an acute anterior myocardial infarction.[142] It showed a significant reduction in a combined endpoint of death and severe heart failure by 34%, attributable mainly to a decrease in the incidence of CHF. However, one of the unexpected benefits from therapy with captopril in the TRACE study was a significantly reduced likelihood of a subsequent myocardial infarction.

The Cooperative New Scandinavian Enalapril Survival Study (CONSENSUS II), GISSI-3, and ISIS-4 trials further evaluated this short-term use of early ACE inhibitor therapy but expanded the population to include all acute myocardial infarction patients.[143-145] When therapy was instituted within 24 hours, there was a less than 1% improvement in heart failure and mortality, with only GISSI-3 and ISIS-4 showing a statistically significant short-term survival benefit. Subgroup analysis showed, as in the early trials, a more pronounced benefit in patients with left ventricular dysfunction and anterior infarctions.

Coronary Artery Disease

11

ACE inhibitors have been shown to reduce cardiovascular events in patients with acute myocardial infarction and heart failure. Unexpected findings from the SAVE and Studies of Left Ventricular Dysfunction (SOLVD) trials showed a significant and consistent reduction in reinfarction rates during long-term follow-up.[139,146] Three large clinical trials have further investigated the impact of ACE inhibition in patients with stable CAD without any evidence of heart failure or left ventricular dysfunction: HOPE, EUROPA, and PEACE. In the HOPE study, high-risk patients with vascular disease including CAD or diabetes plus at least one other cardiovascular risk factor without heart failure were included.[147] The primary endpoint of cardiovascular death, myocardial infarction, or stroke occurred less frequently, approximately 4%, with a 22% risk reduction. This trial suggested that ACE inhibitor therapy is effective in the prevention of cardiovascular events in high-risk patients without left ventricular dysfunction. Not all of the benefit could be attributed to a reduction in blood pressure because a majority of the patients did not have hypertension at baseline and the mean reduction in blood pressure with treatment was relatively small.

In the European Trial on Reduction of Cardiac Events with Perindopril in Stable CAD (EUROPA) study, patients with lower risk asymptomatic stable CAD (i.e., prior myocardial infarction >3 months, percutaneous coronary intervention or coronary artery bypass grafting, >70% narrowing of at least one coronary artery, or an abnormal stress test, without heart failure or substantial hypertension) underwent treatment with an ACE inhibitor, perindopril, which was shown to reduce cardiovascular events by 20%.[148] This endpoint was predominantly driven by a significant reduction in nonfatal myocardial infarction with a lower rate of heart failure. EUROPA extended the observations of the HOPE study to a population with an improved prognosis, showing an overall similar reduction in cardiovascular events. Last, the Prevention of Events with ACE Inhibition trial (PEACE) evaluated the efficacy of the ACE inhibitor trandolapril for a reduction in atherosclerotic complications among patients with low-risk stable CAD with normal or slightly reduced left ventricular function.[149] There was no significant difference in the primary endpoint of cardiovascular death, myocardial infarction, or coronary revascularization with a median follow-up of almost 5 years.

Interpretation of the negative findings of PEACE in the context of HOPE and EUROPA is important. It has been argued that the population of patients from PEACE underwent more intensive management of baseline risk factors, with a larger proportion of patients treated with lipid-lowering agents, beta blockade, and antiplatelet therapy. In addition, a larger proportion of patients underwent coronary revascularization before enrollment. This can be noted in a much lower overall event rate in the PEACE trial compared with both EUROPA and HOPE. However, further subgroup analyses of HOPE and EUROPA reevaluating the endpoints on lipid-lowering agents, beta blockade, and antiplatelet therapy or without prior revascularization showed similar benefits. This analysis suggested that the neutral results of PEACE were probably due not to the lower risk of patients or background therapies but rather to inadequate power of the study and perhaps the relatively low dose of trandolapril that was used.

Timing and Choice of ACE Inhibition

The optimal timing of ACE inhibition after acute myocardial infarction remains controversial. ACE inhibition started relatively late (>3 days) in high-risk patients showed an important long-term benefit on heart failure and mortality. On the other hand, early institution (<24 to 36 hours) showed a relatively small short-term benefit, mainly during the first 7 days when mortality was higher.[150] The cause of death was mainly due to a higher rate of cardiac rupture, electromechanical dissociation, and pump failure after myocardial infarction in the nontreated patient. There was no overall effect on reinfarction rates in the timing of therapy, but rates of hypotension were 10% higher with early ACE inhibitor institution.

The choice of ACE inhibitor varies between many of the clinical trials. A comparison of enalapril and captopril showed that there was a significant and equivalent benefit between the ACE inhibitors. This trial, among others that had similar populations of patients but different choice of ACE inhibitors, suggested an overall class effect of ACE inhibition in excess of the benefits of optimal medical therapy. In addition, higher doses of ACE inhibition provide greater hemodynamic and symptomatic benefit than low doses do.[151] The Assessment of Treatment with Lisinopril and Survival (ATLAS) trial evaluated the effects of low-dose compared with high-dose ACE inhibitor and showed a nonsignificant 8% reduction in mortality and a significant 12% reduction in mortality or hospitalization. Overall, high doses of ACE inhibitor reduce the risk of major clinical events in patients with chronic heart failure[152] (see Table 11-4).

Renal Effects

Much of the antiproteinuric effects of RAAS blockade can be attributed to changes in glomerular hemodynamics. Both ACE inhibitors and ARBs, discussed later, induce preferential vasodilation of the efferent arteriole, decreasing glomerular capillary pressure. Blockade of A II with these agents also significantly reduces the inflammatory, proliferative, and fibrotic changes that occur in renal disease, further reducing glomerular pressure and the level of proteinuria.[153]

In the Microalbuminuria, Cardiovascular, and Renal Outcomes–Heart Outcomes Prevention Evaluation (MICRO-HOPE) trial, nearly 3600 patients with diabetes at high risk for cardiovascular events were treated with ramipril or placebo.[154] In patients without baseline microalbuminuria, the risk of new microalbuminuria was nonsignificantly reduced. There was a 24% reduction in overt nephropathy with ACE inhibitor versus control.

In nondiabetic patients with chronic nephropathy, the Ramipril Efficacy In Nephropathy (REIN) trial also noted a similar benefit.[155,156] Patients were randomized to ramipril or conventional therapy with the aim of achieving comparable blood pressure control. Results showed that in patients who had rapid progression of renal disease and macroalbuminuria at baseline, ACE inhibitor safely lowered the rate of decline in GFR and reduced by half the combined risk of creatinine doubling or progression to ESRD. The AASK trial showed a greater preservation of renal function in African Americans with hypertensive nephrosclerosis treated with ramipril than with CCB but no significant improvement in proteinuria.[60]

Not all studies with ACE inhibitors demonstrate an improvement in renal function over time. In the ALLHAT study, there was no difference in GFR with an ACE inhibitor or diuretic therapy.[15] Overall, ACE inhibitors slow renal function decline with minimal adverse events in both diabetic and nondiabetic nephropathy with various degrees of albuminuria (see Table 11-2).

Summary

The greatest benefit of ACE inhibition is noted in the selective treatment of high-risk patients, in particular patients with acute myocardial infarctions (specifically a large anterior wall), failed reperfusion therapy, and left ventricular dysfunction. ACE inhibition should be considered for all patients with left ventricular dysfunction and CAD and for patients with multiple risk factors including diabetes, metabolic syndrome, and hypertension. The magnitude of benefit from an ACE inhibitor is comparable to that observed with other proven secondary prevention measures, such as aspirin, beta blockers, and lipid-lowering agents. The institution of therapy should occur early with blood pressure parameters and close monitoring of hemodynamics. The choice of agent seems unimportant, but the dose should be maximized as tolerated by the patient (see Table 11-1).

ANGIOTENSIN RECEPTOR BLOCKERS

Despite the therapeutic success of ACE inhibitors, ARBs emerged to block the end pathway of the RAAS, the AT_1 receptor. All of the potentially damaging cardiovascular actions of A II are mediated through this receptor, including vascular and cardiac hypertrophy, aldosterone secretion, and vasoconstriction.[157] As described in an earlier section, A II can also be generated by non–ACE-mediated pathways, such that inhibition of this enzyme will not lead to complete cessation of A II synthesis. The pharmacologic rationale for interruption of the RAAS with an ARB includes a decrease in AT_1 receptor activation that mediates many of the negative cardiovascular effects and an increase in circulating A II, which undergoes a compensatory rise during ARB therapy that activates the AT_2 receptor, providing additional benefit.

Role of Angiotensin Receptor Blockers

Post–Myocardial Infarction

ACE inhibitors have been shown to reduce the risk of death and cardiovascular events after acute myocardial infarction. Two studies have assessed whether ARBs offer benefits equivalent or superior to ACE inhibitors after myocardial infarction, OPTIMAAL and VALIANT. The Optimal Trial in Myocardial Infarction with the Angiotensin II Antagonist Losartan (OPTIMAAL) evaluated the benefit of losartan compared with captopril in 5477 patients with acute myocardial infarction complicated by heart failure.[158] No significant difference was noted in all-cause mortality, cardiac mortality, or reinfarction, with losartan unable to achieve noninferiority. There was, however, a trend in event rates in favor of captopril and significantly fewer cardiovascular deaths with captopril (13.3% versus 15.3%). A lower dose of ARB in OPTIMAAL than that suggested in other ARB trials such as LIFE and RENAAL probably contributed to these results. Higher doses of losartan result in an increase in plasma renin activity and A II concentration, indicating a more potent negative feedback at the highest doses.[159] The Heart Failure Endpoint Evaluation of A II Antagonist Losartan (HEAAL) study confirmed the dose effect of losartan, with 150 mg compared with 50 mg showing a significant 10% reduction in mortality and morbidity in heart failure patients intolerant to ACE inhibitors.

The Valsartan In Acute Myocardial Infarction (VALIANT) trial evaluated the effect of the ARB valsartan versus captopril alone or in combination in 14,703 patients with acute

myocardial infarction complicated by left ventricular systolic dysfunction or heart failure.[160] The population of patients studied was identical to that enrolled in the ACE inhibitor trials after myocardial infarction, SAVE, AIRE, and TRACE, and the dose of valsartan used showed more blood pressure–lowering effects than were seen with low-dose losartan in the OPTIMAAL trial. VALIANT showed that death, reinfarction, or recurrent heart failure hospitalization was similar between the groups, around 20%. ARBs were noninferior to ACE inhibitor therapy and achieved the same benefit as ACE inhibitors noted in their respective trials.

Congestive Heart Failure

The first trial to directly compare an ARB with an ACE inhibitor in heart failure patients was the Evaluation of Losartan In The Elderly (ELITE) trial.[161] This trial compared the potential renal benefits of losartan with captopril in 722 elderly patients with heart failure. Whereas no benefit in renal function was observed in either arm, there was a significant mortality benefit in the ARB group of 46%. ELITE II trial further evaluated this benefit in more than 3000 patients with heart failure and an ejection fraction <40%.[162] This trial failed to show a benefit of losartan in reducing mortality or morbidity, with a slight nonsignificant benefit for the ACE inhibitor group.

In contrast to ELITE II, the Val-HeFT trial compared the ARB valsartan with standard heart failure therapy.[163] The majority of patients enrolled (93%) in Val-HeFT were already receiving an ACE inhibitor. There was no mortality benefit, but a significant reduction was shown in the combined endpoint of morbidity and mortality driven primarily by heart failure hospitalizations. In the subset of patients not receiving an ACE inhibitor (7%), there was a substantial 33% mortality benefit associated with valsartan. A similar reduction of cardiovascular mortality or heart failure was once again noted in CHARM-Alternative with the use of candesartan[164] (see Table 11-4).

Kinin-Mediated Side Effects

The kinin-related side effects of cough and angioedema are common with ACE inhibitors, affecting approximately 5% to 10% of patients, particularly women, African Americans, and Asians.[165,166] The use of ARBs in patients who are ACE inhibitor intolerant has been effective with minimal ACE-related adverse effects.[167] However, blocking of the AT_1 receptor with selective antagonists is known to increase plasma levels of A II. A II can then interact with other angiotensin receptors including AT_2, stimulating bradykinin release through increased kininogen activation. Cough and angioedema, mediated by bradykinin production, are less common with ARBs but not totally eliminated.[168]

Renal Effects

AT_1 receptor antagonism has been shown to improve albuminuria and to reduce progression of renal disease. The RENAAL and IDNT trials, as described, evaluated the long-term benefits of ARB therapy in patients with proteinuria and type 2 diabetes.[132,133] In RENAAL, treatment with losartan for an average of 3.4 years was associated with a 25% reduction of risk for doubling of serum creatinine and a 28% reduction in the risk for development of ESRD, independent of its blood pressure–lowering effect. IDNT showed a 20% reduction in the composite endpoint of doubling of creatinine, development of ESRD, or death with irbesartan compared with placebo and 23% reduction compared with amlodipine, for an average of 2.6 years.

Another similar trial, Microalbuminuria Reduction with Valsartan (MARVAL) in patients with type 2 diabetes mellitus, showed an improvement in proteinuria in patients (n = 332) with type 2 diabetes and microalbuminuria treated with valsartan instead of amlodipine.[169] The primary endpoint of percentage change in urine albumin excretion rate was significantly lower after 24 weeks of treatment for ARB (56%) than for CCB (92%). Valsartan lowered proteinuria in both hypertensive and normotensive subgroups, with more patients reverting to normoalbuminuria with the short-term ARB (30% versus 14.5%).

In the Telmisartan Randomised Assessment Study in ACE Intolerant Subjects with Cardiovascular Disease (TRANSCEND) trial, 5927 patients with known cardiovascular disease or diabetes without evidence of macroalbuminuria and intolerant to ACE inhibitor were treated with either telmisartan or placebo for a mean of 56 months.[170] At baseline, only 10% of patients had evidence of microalbuminuria. There was no difference in the composite renal outcome of dialysis or doubling of creatinine, changes in GFR, and changes in albuminuria. Albuminuria, however, was less likely to progress with ARB therapy.

In treatment of the hypertensive and diabetic patient, blockade of the AT_1 receptor prevents the progression of proteinuria and renal decline. The benefit in high-risk patients without significant albuminuria is less well evidenced. ARBs, like ACE inhibitors, are renoprotective, particularly in patients with type 2 diabetes and diabetic nephropathy (see Table 11-2).

Summary

ARBs are an effective alternative to ACE inhibitors in patients after myocardial infarction or with heart failure. Increased doses are needed to achieve their maximum benefit for clinical outcomes and improved heart failure symptoms. ARBs may be used for patients who are ACE inhibitor intolerant, but the risk of kinin-mediated side effects is not totally eliminated (see Table 11-1).

DIRECT RENIN INHIBITORS

The RAAS can be inhibited at different levels of the pathway. Despite treatment with ACE inhibitors and ARBs, high rates of cardiovascular events in individuals with CAD and heart failure and high rates of progression to renal failure in individuals with diabetic nephropathy persist. There is growing evidence that these drugs may not be able to optimally inhibit the RAAS because of their inability to block alternative pathways of A II production, the activation of feedback mechanisms that result in increased plasma renin concentration and plasma renin activity, and the stimulation of the prorenin receptor pathway.

In addition, intracellular A II may not be blocked by ACE inhibitors or ARBs as these drugs are unable to enter into the intracellular space. Blocking of RAAS directly at the renin level, the rate-limiting step of A II production, neutralizes any compensatory increase in plasma renin activity and prevents the formation of both A I and A II, allowing more complete RAAS suppression.[98] Decreasing plasma renin activity, perhaps the most accurate reflection of the level of RAAS activation, may further reduce the potential harmful effects of the RAAS, providing improved end-organ protection. Certainly, there appears to be cardiovascular benefit associated with lower plasma renin activity.

Role of Direct Renin Inhibitors

Aliskiren is a potent nonpeptide renin inhibitor that because of its high specificity has a low drug interaction profile.[171] It functions by binding to the enzymatic site of renin and rendering it inactive. Aliskiren binds to plasma renin before the uptake by the tissue prorenin receptor, but it is unclear whether renin inhibitors could inhibit receptor-bound, nonproteolytically activated prorenin or modify the structure of renin, altering its ability to interact with the prorenin receptor.[172] No observed changes have been shown in either renin- or prorenin-mediated prorenin receptor activation with direct renin inhibitors (DRIs), indicating that aliskiren does not affect its binding site for the prorenin receptor.[173]

The effects of DRIs are well established in animal studies. Aliskiren has been shown to prevent atherosclerosis progression compared with other antihypertensive agents with similar blood pressure–lowering effect.[174] It reduces fibrous cap thinning, creates less vulnerable plaque with decreased inflammation and lipid content, and prevents media degeneration. In untreated animals, evidence of advanced plaque with a large necrotic lipid core was found in more than 80% of cases compared with only 25% for treatment with aliskiren. Renin inhibition has also been shown to attenuate infarction-related changes, the indices of A II intracellular signaling, and cardiomyocyte apoptosis while improving left ventricular systolic and diastolic dysfunction, chamber dilation, and pulmonary congestion.[175] Furthermore, aliskiren improves nitric oxide availability and has minimal effect on platelet activity or coagulation, except for a moderate increase in antithrombin III.[176,177]

In clinical trials, aliskiren provides an effective dose-dependent and sustained reduction in blood pressure when it is used as monotherapy or in combination with other antihypertensive agents.[178-181] Left ventricular hypertrophy represents a manifestation of the effects of hypertension over time and is a predictive marker of cardiovascular events in patients with CAD risk factors. The Aliskiren in Left Ventricular Hypertrophy (ALLAY) trial assessed whether aliskiren monotherapy or combination therapy with an ARB reduced left ventricular mass in overweight, hypertensive patients with left ventricular hypertrophy.[182] The combination of a DRI with ARB did not show a statistically significant difference in the reduction of blood pressure or left ventricular mass during a 9-month follow-up period. Whether the lack of combination effect can be attributed to a lower baseline blood pressure or left ventricular mass compared with other trials, short duration of therapy, or altered renin states between these patients remains unclear. However, the reductions in left ventricular mass with DRIs were similar to those achieved with an ARB with equivalent tolerability.

Other surrogate marker trials looking at the effects of DRI in heart failure and albuminuria as well as in myocardial infarction and left ventricular remodeling have been performed. The Aliskiren Observations of Heart Failure Treatment (ALOFT) trial showed that aliskiren, added to optimal medical therapy with an ACE inhibitor or ARB and beta blocker in all patients and an aldosterone receptor antagonist in approximately one third, was associated with improvements in the heart failure markers brain natriuretic peptide (BNP), N-terminal pro-BNP (NT-proBNP), and urinary aldosterone levels.[183] There was a fivefold greater decrease in BNP levels compared with placebo. Reductions in BNP and NT-proBNP have been noted with other RAAS inhibitors and are associated with improved cardiovascular outcomes.

The Aliskiren Study in Post-MI Patients to Reduce Remodeling (ASPIRE) trial assessed the effects of DRI on left ventricular remodeling in 820 patients with ejection fractions less than 45% compared with placebo when added to standard therapy including an ACE inhibitor or ARB.[184] After 36 weeks of therapy, the addition of aliskiren within the 7 to 42 days after a myocardial infarction showed no significant improvement in left ventricular end-systolic volume or composite endpoint of cardiovascular death, CHF hospitalization, or ejection fraction reduction of greater than 6%. There was, however, a higher rate of hyperkalemia, hypotension, and renal dysfunction. Additional trials like Aliskiren and Valsartan to Reduce NT-proBNP via Renin-Angiotensin-Aldosterone System Blockade (AVANTE GARDE) will further evaluate the potential role of aliskiren after an acute myocardial infarction.

Ongoing outcomes trials include Aliskiren Trial in Type 2 Diabetes Using Cardiovascular and Renal Disease Endpoints (ALTITUDE) and Aliskiren Trial to Mediate Outcomes Prevention in Heart Failure (ATMOSPHERE).[185] The ALTITUDE trial is designed to evaluate the benefit of adding aliskiren to conventional medical therapy that includes either an ACE inhibitor or ARB long term in high-risk diabetic patients. It is an event-driven study looking at both cardiovascular and renal outcomes. The ATMOSPHERE trial will evaluate whether aliskiren can delay the time to cardiovascular death or CHF hospitalization in patients with heart failure (see Table 11-1).

Summary

Aliskiren is an effective and well-tolerated DRI for patients with hypertension. It can be added to multiple therapies with proper monitoring of electrolytes and renal function. Surrogate marker trials have suggested significant potential in the management of patients with heart failure and nephropathy. The results of future large-scale outcomes trials will help elucidate the clinically relevant protective end-organ effects of this class of medication. For now, in patients who are able to tolerate the older RAAS blockers, ACE inhibitors, or ARBs, there is no reason to prefer aliskiren. Aliskiren can be used in patients who cannot tolerate either an ACE inhibitor or an ARB. Although morbidity and mortality data are lacking, there is good evidence that combination therapy can improve blood pressure control, and ongoing randomized trials are looking at potential further event reduction with this type of combination therapy (see Table 11-1).

ALDOSTERONE RECEPTOR ANTAGONISTS/MINERALOCORTICOID RECEPTOR BLOCKERS

Early results from the CONSENSUS trial showed that in addition to sympathetic activation and increases in A II, plasma aldosterone levels predicted subsequent cardiovascular morbidity and mortality.[186] This suggested a possible role of aldosterone in the progression of systolic dysfunction. ACE inhibitor or ARB therapy has been shown to incompletely suppress aldosterone production, and an increase can be noted in up to 40% of patients with CHF.[187] Aldosterone is controlled not only by A II but also by potassium levels.[84] With a fall in A II, an increase in potassium will stimulate aldosterone production.

Role of Mineralocorticoid Receptor Blockers

The two agents used for aldosterone receptor blockade are spironolactone, the older of the two, and eplerenone. Eplerenone is 100 times more selective for the aldosterone receptor and has limited affinity for androgen and progesterone receptors.[188] There is a lower incidence of gynecomastia and breast pain in men and menstrual irregularities in women with eplerenone compared with spironolactone (<1% versus 10%). The incidence of hyperkalemia is approximately 3% to 6% for spironolactone and 1% to 3% for eplerenone. The short half-life of eplerenone and lack of active metabolites may lessen the risk of hyperkalemia.[189]

The Randomized Aldactone Evaluation Study (RALES) further evaluated the benefit of adding an aldosterone receptor antagonist to optimal medical therapy.[86] RALES enrolled 1663 subjects with NYHA Class III or Class IV heart failure with an ejection fraction of 35% or less while receiving treatment with an ACE inhibitor and a diuretic. Patients received either spironolactone or placebo, and results showed a decrease in mortality by 30% and a decrease in CHF hospitalizations by 35% with the use of spironolactone after 2 years. From RALES, the benefit of mineralocorticoid receptor blockade in subjects with CHF can be noted beyond RAAS inhibition and the diuretic effects of aldosterone blockade. However, one of the limitations of this important study was the virtual absence of beta blocker therapy, which is now considered a standard of care.

In the Eplerenone Post–Acute Myocardial Infarction Heart Failure Efficacy and Survival Study (EPHESUS), the benefit of adding eplerenone to optimal medical therapy for the treatment of heart failure after acute myocardial infarction was evaluated.[190] EPHESUS enrolled 6600 subjects with an ejection fraction of 40% or less, and treated with coronary reperfusion therapy if needed, 3 to 14 days after an acute myocardial infarction. Subjects were randomized to either eplerenone or placebo; results showed a reduced all-cause mortality by 15% and cardiovascular death or hospitalization for cardiovascular events by 13%.

The difference in risk reduction compared with RALES can potentially be attributed to subjects with a slightly improved baseline ejection fraction, successful reperfusion therapy after myocardial infarction, recovery of ventricular stunning, and improved use of beta blockade, which was 75% compared with only 12% in RALES. Nonetheless, this study expanded the use of aldosterone blockade to include post–myocardial infarction patients with impaired systolic function. Aldosterone blockade should be initiated in this population between days 3 and 14, when patients are hemodynamically stable after starting an ACE inhibitor or ARB and beta blocker therapy.

A meta-analysis evaluating 19 trials of aldosterone antagonists in CHF and post–myocardial infarction showed that aldosterone blockade reduced all-cause mortality by 20% (25% in 14 CHF trials and 15% in 4 myocardial infarction trials).[191] The trials with longer duration of follow-up were associated with the greatest reduction in all-cause mortality. From RALES and EPHESUS, aldosterone blockade has a clear mortality benefit with and without acute myocardial infarction in heart failure above standard therapy with an ACE inhibitor. Proposed mechanisms include improved endothelial function with a subsequent reduction in acute coronary events, decrease in myocardial fibrosis with a reduction in arrhythmogenic events, maintenance of potassium and magnesium levels, and improvements in fibrinolytic balance due to the direct effect of aldosterone on PAI-1[192] (see Table 11-1).

Summary

Mineralocorticoid receptor blockers (MRBs) have an important role in the treatment of heart failure, especially after an acute myocardial infarction, above standard therapy with ACE inhibition. It would seem logical that these same mechanisms and effects of aldosterone receptor antagonism, when applied to patients with CAD but no heart failure, would be evident. In addition, CAD patients without CHF would be more likely to tolerate aldosterone blockade, given their decreased likelihood of renal insufficiency and increased use of diuretics, which may further stimulate aldosterone production. No evidence is currently available that shows a benefit of aldosterone blockade in CAD patients without CHF (see Table 11-4).

11

Despite the many therapies described, a significant number of patients with cardiac and renal disease continue to progress. Incomplete blockade of the RAAS is a potential explanation for these results. Given the multiple feedback loops and alternative pathways described within the RAAS, inhibition of the RAAS at one level leads to compensatory activation at another level, which can diminish the intended therapeutic effect (see Fig. 11-2 and Table 11-3). Strategies to improve the efficacy of RAAS blockade include the combination of ACE inhibitors and ARBs. In addition, increased understanding of the role of aldosterone in vascular progression and the availability of DRIs allow varied regimens that may offer novel ways to suppress the RAAS.

Understanding of the differential effects of each therapy on the components of the RAAS is important to understand a potential means for enhanced suppression.[193] ACE inhibition reduces the levels of A II and increases A I. Increased A I may be converted to A II through non–ACE-dependent pathways, also known as the ACE escape. ARBs block the angiotensin I AT_1 receptor, causing an increase in both A I and A II. Elevated levels of A II may potentially compete with the ARB for the AT_1 receptor, maintaining AT_1 receptor signaling, and stimulate non-AT_1 receptors with unclear effects.

Both ACE inhibitors and ARBs suppress the negative feedback inhibition of renin release and cause a compensatory rise in the plasma renin concentration and plasma renin activity.[194] In addition, there is a notable secondary rise in aldosterone, irrespective of the sodium intake. Because the augmentation of bradykinin levels may also contribute to the net therapeutic benefits of ACE inhibition, combination of an ARB that stimulates bradykinin production with an ACE inhibitor that inhibits bradykinin degradation may provide a theoretical basis for augmentation of the bradykinin–nitric oxide pathway.

MRBs increase all components of RAAS: plasma renin activity, plasma renin concentration, and A I, A II, and aldosterone levels.[195,196] DRIs, on the other hand, lead to a decrease in plasma renin activity despite a compensatory increase in plasma renin concentration.[194] Renin inhibitors can antagonize the increase in plasma renin concentration induced by the ACE inhibitor, ARB, or MRB; however, nonrenin pathways of angiotensinogen–A I may limit their effectiveness.

Incomplete RAAS blockade or compensatory RAAS activation limits the potential efficacy of any one of these classes of medications on cardioprotection and renoprotection. Combinations of these medications or the addition of other antihypertensive medications, specifically CCBs, may provide more complete RAAS suppression and better end-organ protection compared with either medication alone.

Dual RAAS Blockade

ACE Inhibitor/ARB

The Val-HeFT and the Candesartan in Heart Failure (CHARM-Added) trials evaluated 5010 and 2548 patients, respectively, with NYHA Class II-IV heart failure and a left ventricular ejection fraction of less than 40% who were being treated with an ACE inhibitor.[163,197] Patients were assigned to an ARB, either valsartan or candesartan, or placebo and were observed between 23 and 41 months. In Val-HeFT, overall mortality was similar in the two groups, with a 24% reduction in heart failure hospitalization. In CHARM-Added, there was a 15% significant reduction in cardiovascular mortality or heart failure admissions. The apparent differences between the Val-HeFT and CHARM-Added trials can be potentially explained by the choice of ARB. Nonetheless, in patients with symptomatic heart failure, there is some added clinical benefit in terms of reducing the morbidity of cardiovascular disease by adding an ARB to ACE inhibitors, with a potential improvement in cardiovascular mortality.

In the VALIANT trial, the combination of valsartan and captopril showed no incremental benefit of ARB added to an ACE inhibitor in acute myocardial infarction complicated by heart failure.[160] This lack of benefit was noted in all-cause mortality and in the secondary endpoint of cardiovascular death, recurrent myocardial infarction, or heart failure hospitalization, despite additional lowering of blood pressure of 2.2 mm Hg. In the Ongoing Telmisartan Alone and in Combination with Ramipril Global Endpoint Trial (ONTARGET), 25,620 patients who had vascular disease or high-risk diabetes without heart failure, with nearly three quarters having CAD, were randomized to ramipril, telmisartan, or a combination of both.[198] No significant difference in overall mortality or rates of secondary outcomes including a composite of cardiovascular death, myocardial infarction, or stroke was noted except for a slight increased risk of renal impairment in the combination ACE inhibitor/ARB group. This lack of benefit, as in VALIANT, was also noted with a reduction in systolic blood pressure of 2 to 3 mm Hg.

The results of VALIANT and ONTARGET are discordant with those of trials like Val-HeFT and CHARM-Added. The differences in cardiovascular risk between patients with stable heart failure and patients with acute myocardial infarction, higher risk of early death and myocardial infarction, may account for the differences seen between these trials. In the latter trials, the ARB is started on a background of ACE inhibitor, not concurrently, and their doses are not titrated to proven efficacy levels. Less than half of patients were receiving full-dose ACE inhibitor therapy, and decisions about the dose and choice of an ACE inhibitor were left to individual physicians. Furthermore, all of these patients had symptomatic heart failure despite ACE inhibitor therapy (see Table 11-4).

Renal Effects. Whereas ACE inhibitors and ARBs have been shown to be renoprotective when used alone, the effect of their combined use on the progression of renal disease is less certain. Secondary endpoints from the ONTARGET trial showed that there was an increase in the composite endpoint of dialysis, doubling of serum creatinine, or death of 14.5% with ramipril/telmisartan compared with ACE inhibitor or ARB alone (13.5%).[199] This difference in renal endpoint was driven primarily by dialysis treatment for episodes of acute renal failure, not by the development of ESRD, and there was no significant difference in the incidence of creatinine doubling. Subgroup analysis showed that dual blockade was harmful only in individuals with low renal risk, without diabetes and albuminuria. This increased event rate was matched by a 7% reduction in urinary albumin excretion compared with ACE inhibitor therapy.

The Candesartan and Lisinopril Microalbuminuria (CALM) trial evaluated 199 patients with microalbuminuria, hypertension, and type 2 diabetes with 12 weeks of candesartan, lisinopril, or combination therapy.[200] There was a significant reduction in urinary ACR with ACE inhibitor/ARB compared with ACE inhibitor or ARB alone (50% versus 39% versus 24%). However, the mean reduction in blood pressure (systolic blood pressure, 25 mm Hg versus 17 mm Hg and 14 mm Hg) was significantly greater with dual versus monotherapies. Dual ACE inhibitor/ARB blockade in CALM was shown to reduce proteinuria, but it may have been explained by improved blood pressure control.

In the Valsartan in Combination with Lisinopril in Hypertensive Patients with Microalbuminuria (VALERIA) trial, 133 patients with hypertension and microalbuminuria were evaluated by ACE inhibitor/ARB combination therapy compared against high-dose ACE inhibitor or ARB monotherapy.[201] After 30 weeks of treatment, there was a 34% reduction in urine ACR with combination therapy compared with monotherapy. In the ACE inhibitor/ARB group, 38% had normalization of microalbuminuria compared with 17% in the ACE inhibitor group, with no significant difference compared with the ARB group. Hypotension was the most frequent adverse event, occurring at 9.3% for ARB and 11.6% for ACE inhibitor/ARB.

Combined therapy with ACE inhibitor and ARB results in more complete blockade of RAAS and reduction or normalization of microalbuminuria than with high-dose monotherapy. ACE inhibitor/ARB therapy in both diabetic and nondiabetic nephropathies significantly reduces proteinuria. This benefit occurs with a slightly higher incidence of adverse events. Patients at low renal risk, nondiabetics, and patients without evidence of proteinuria are at higher risk for worsened renal outcomes with combination therapy (see Table 11-2).

Summary. The benefit of combination ACE inhibitor/ARB therapy can be noted in patients with uncontrolled, symptomatic heart failure. However, there is no role for ACE inhibitor/ARB combination therapy in patients with stable CAD or in secondary prevention without heart failure. The utility of combination therapy must be weighed against the increased risk of hypotension, hyperkalemia, and renal function decline (see Table 11-1).

ACE Inhibitor/MRB or ARB/MRB

Favorable outcomes were noted by dual blockade with MRB/ACE inhibitor or MRB/ARB in patients with left ventricular dysfunction after myocardial infarction or heart failure. Evidence of this benefit was noted in their respective trials, EPHESUS and RALES, and in a meta-analysis predominantly powered by these trials. An overall all-cause mortality benefit of 20% with MRB/ACE inhibitor or MRB/ARB (25% improvement in patients with CHF and 15% improvement in patients with acute myocardial infarction) can be noted in the appropriate patients, NYHA Class III-IV heart failure with an ejection fraction <35% or acute myocardial infarction with an ejection fraction <40% (see Table 11-4).

Renal Effects. Aldosterone may promote renal fibrosis and renal dysfunction by multiple mechanisms, including an increased inflammatory state,[202] alterations in fibrinolysis,[203] stimulation of TGF-β,[204] increase in reactive oxygen species,[205] and upregulation of A II receptors.[206] By blocking aldosterone at its receptor, MRBs may attenuate the effects of aldosterone on the kidney, reducing proteinuria and renal outcomes. Several small studies have addressed the additive benefit of MRB with an ACE inhibitor or ARB. Epstein and colleagues[202] evaluated the effect of low doses (50 to 100 mg/day) of eplerenone added to enalapril on urinary ACR in patients with type 2 diabetes. A nearly 50% reduction in albumin excretion was noted from baseline as early as 4 weeks and continued for up to 12 weeks. Low-dose MRB demonstrated a similar reduction in proteinuria compared with high-dose MRB (200 mg/day) without significant hyperkalemia.[207]

Mehdi and coworkers[208] assigned 81 patients with hypertension, diabetes, and macroalbuminuria who were taking maximal doses of ACE inhibitor to either ARB (losartan, 100 mg/day) or spironolactone (25 mg/day). After 48 weeks of therapy, the urine ACR was significantly lower in patients taking ACE inhibitor/MRB (34%) versus ACE inhibitor/ARB (17%). Blood pressure did not differ between the groups, suggesting that the addition of MRB rather than ARB to maximal ACE inhibitor therapy affords greater renal protection in patients with diabetic nephropathy. Nonetheless, the long-term effect of ACE inhibitor/MRB on renal outcomes has yet to be determined. In patients with persistent proteinuria despite maximal doses of ACE inhibitor or ARB, low-dose MRB could be added to reduce proteinuria with monitoring for hyperkalemia (see Table 11-2).

ACE Inhibitor/DRI or ARB/DRI

Evidence for dual blockade with a renin inhibitor and ACE inhibitor or ARB is still minimal. In the ALOFT trial, the DRI aliskiren, when added to an ACE inhibitor or ARB and an aldosterone receptor antagonist in approximately one third, was associated with a significant improvement in intermediate endpoints of heart failure and BNP and urinary aldosterone levels. This was noted despite an absence of effect on blood pressure. Clinical outcomes for combination DRI/ACE inhibitor or DRI/ARB in patients with cardiovascular disease remain to be evaluated (see Tables 11-1 and 11-3).

Renal Effects. In the Aliskiren in the Evaluation of Proteinuria in Diabetes (AVOID) trial, the renoprotective effects of combining aliskiren with the high-dose ARB losartan, which was shown to have renoprotective effects in the RENAAL study, was evaluated in patients with hypertension, diabetes, and nephropathy.[209] Aliskiren, when added to an ARB and optimal antihypertensive treatment, provided a significant 20% further reduction in urinary ACR. Nearly twice as many patients in the aliskiren group also achieved a reduction in urinary ACR of at least 50% from baseline. These renoprotective effects were independent of the effect of DRI on blood pressure. Reductions in albuminuria in patients with diabetes and nephropathy are associated with improvements in renal outcomes and in turn potentially cardiac outcomes (see Table 11-2).

ACE Inhibitor/CCB Combination Therapy

CCBs counteract excess calcium entry through the voltage- and receptor-operated calcium channels of vascular smooth muscle. ACE inhibitors reduce the vasoconstrictive properties of A II, indirectly through sodium and water balance and directly by reducing internal calcium release. Smooth muscle vasodilation by calcium maintenance and other anti-ischemic properties including improved ATP-sparing abilities and t-PA/PAI-1 balance can potentially work synergistically for enhanced cardioprotection. The vasodilation caused by CCBs also stimulates both the RAAS and the sympathetic nervous system, which can lead to reflex vasoconstriction and tachycardia. ACE inhibition can counteract this effect.[36]

The rationale for fixed-combination ACE inhibitor and CCB therapy comes directly from the results of ASCOT, the first trial to demonstrate a difference in total mortality and cardiovascular morbidity between two antihypertensive regimens.[67] ASCOT included 19,257 hypertensive patients with at least three cardiovascular risk factors but no cardiac disease. Patients were randomized to either ACE inhibitor/CCB therapy (perindopril/amlodipine) or beta blocker/diuretic therapy (atenolol/bendroflumethiazide). The trial was stopped early because of an ~35% reduction in CHD events at a mean follow-up of about 3.3 years; there was also an 11% difference in all-cause mortality noted between the two groups at 5.5 years. Secondary endpoints included a 24% decrease in cardiovascular mortality, a 13% decrease in all coronary events, and a 23% difference in stroke.

In ASCOT, stable angina was an exclusion criterion for this study, making assessment of combination therapy on stable CAD difficult. However, there was a noted decrease in coronary events and a 32% reduction in unstable angina. The reduction of coronary and stroke events cannot entirely be explained by a reduction in blood pressure.[210] Another trial, EUROPA, conducted in stable CAD patients, showed that the ACE inhibitor perindopril significantly reduced the composite endpoint of cardiovascular death, myocardial infarction, and cardiac arrest. Post hoc analysis of this trial evaluated the effect of ACE inhibition in 2122 patients receiving CCB, 18% of the patients enrolled. The event rate for major cardiac events and mortality was reduced by 35.5% with combination ACE inhibitor/CCB therapy, with a 46% reduction in all-cause mortality.

The International Verapamil-Trandolapril Study Trial (INVEST) compared ACE inhibitor/CCB therapy (verapamil/trandolapril) with beta blocker/diuretic therapy (atenolol/hydrochlorothiazide) in 22,576 hypertensive patients with CAD.[211] The trial showed that ACE inhibitor/CCB was a well-tolerated strategy for treatment. It failed, however, to show a benefit of ACE inhibitor/CCB over beta blocker/diuretic combination therapy. In light of ASCOT, this may suggest that the effect of CCB in combination with an ACE inhibitor may not be due to a pure class effect.

In the Avoiding Cardiovascular Events through Combination Therapy in Patients Living with Systolic Hypertension (ACCOMPLISH) trial, 11,506 hypertensive patients at high risk for cardiovascular events were randomized to either ACE inhibitor/CCB (benazepril/amlodipine) or ACE inhibitor diuretic (benazepril/hydrochlorothiazide). There was a 20% risk reduction in composite endpoint of cardiovascular death, nonfatal myocardial infarction or stroke, hospitalization for angina, resuscitation after sudden cardiac arrest, and coronary revascularization. This trial showed that the combination of ACE inhibitor/CCB is superior to ACE inhibitor/diuretic in reducing cardiovascular events and death in high-risk patients. The difference in systolic blood pressure was less than 1 mm Hg between the two groups, suggesting that the difference in benefit was not related to blood pressure–lowering effects. Overall, the ACE inhibitor/CCB combination is an effective therapeutic option to optimize the management of high-risk patients with hypertension and patients with CAD (see Table 11-1).

Renal Effects. Individually, ACE inhibitors show uniform efficacy in reducing proteinuria and limiting the progression of renal disease. CCBs, as described, have more varied results. Whether this is related to the class of CCB, the underlying renal disease, or the duration of treatment has yet to be determined. Limited information is available for the effect of ACE inhibitor/CCB therapy on proteinuria and renal function, but it appears to confer an advantage.[212] Fogari and associates[213] compared the long-term effect of amlodipine and fosinopril on urine albumin excretion in 453 hypertensive, diabetic patients. In a 4-year follow-up, ACE inhibitor/CCB provided a 67% reduction in urine albumin excretion compared with monotherapy with ACE inhibitor (46%) or with CCB (33%). Furthermore, ASCOT showed a significant 15% reduction in renal impairment in the amlodipine/perindopril group versus beta blocker/diuretic.[67] These studies strengthen the recommendation for ACE inhibitor/CCB combination therapy for renoprotection in high-risk patients (see Table 11-2).

CONCLUSION

In summary, each class of antihypertensive medications has an established role in the management of hypertensive and high-risk cardiovascular patients. Understanding of the complexity of the RAAS has improved our understanding of the close interplay between cardiovascular and renovascular disease and ways to improve both cardiovascular and renal outcomes. RAAS inhibitors are the cornerstone for secondary prevention. Newer RAAS inhibitors along with combinations of different RAAS inhibitors and RAAS inhibitors with CCBs may provide more complete RAAS suppression and improve cardioprotection and renoprotection.

REFERENCES

1. Freis ED: How diuretics lower blood pressure. *Am Heart J* 106(pt 2):185, 1983.
2. Bourgoignie JJ, Catanzaro FJ, Perry HMJ, et al: Renin-angiotensin-aldosterone system during chronic thiazide therapy of benign hypertension. *Circulation* 37:27, 1968.
3. Carter BL, Ernst ME, Cohen JD: Hydrochlorothiazide versus chlorthalidone: evidence supporting their interchangeability. *Hypertension* 43:4, 2004.
4. Chapman AB, Schwartz GL, Boerwinkle E, et al: Predictors of antihypertensive response to a standard dose of hydrochlorothiazide for essential hypertension. *Kidney Int* 61:1047, 2002.
5. Siegel D, Hulley SB, Black DM, et al: Diuretics, serum and intracellular electrolyte levels, and ventricular arrhythmias in hypertensive men. *JAMA* 267:1083, 1992.
6. Perez-Stable E, Caralis PV: Thiazide-induced disturbances in carbohydrate, lipid, and potassium metabolism. *Am Heart J* 106(pt 2):245, 1983.
7. Holland OB, Pool PE: Metabolic changes with antihypertensive therapy of the salt-sensitive patient. *Am J Cardiol* 61:53H, 1988.
8. Ferrari P, Rosman J, Weidmann P: Antihypertensive agents, serum lipoproteins and glucose metabolism. *Am J Cardiol* 67:26B, 1991.
9. Weidmann P, Uehlinger DE, Gerber A: Antihypertensive treatment and serum lipoproteins [editorial review]. *J Hypertens* 3:297, 1985.
10. Lindholm LH, Persson M, Alaupovic P, et al: Metabolic outcome during 1 year in newly detected hypertensives: results of the Antihypertensive Treatment and Lipid Profile in a North of Sweden Efficacy Evaluation (ALPINE study). *J Hypertens* 21:1563, 2003.
11. SHEP Cooperative Research Group: Prevention of stroke by antihypertensive drug treatment in older persons with isolated systolic hypertension: final results of the Systolic Hypertension in the Elderly Program (SHEP). *JAMA* 265:3255, 1991.
12. Beckett NS, Peters R, Fletcher AE, et al: Treatment of hypertension in patients 80 years of age or older. *N Engl J Med* 358:1887, 2008.
13. Savage PJ, Pressel SL, Curb JD, et al: Influence of long-term, low-dose, diuretic-based antihypertensive therapy on glucose, lipid, uric acid, and potassium levels in older men and women with isolated systolic hypertension: the Systolic Hypertension in the Elderly Program. *Arch Intern Med* 158:741, 1998.
14. Kostis JB, Wilson AC, Freudenberger RS, et al: Long-term effect of diuretic-based therapy on fatal outcomes in subjects with isolated systolic hypertension with and without diabetes. *Am J Cardiol* 95:29, 2005.
15. Major outcomes in high-risk hypertensive patients randomized to angiotensin-converting enzyme inhibitor or calcium channel blocker vs diuretic: the Antihypertensive and Lipid-Lowering Treatment to Prevent Heart Attack Trial (ALLHAT). *JAMA* 288:2981, 2002.
16. Wing LM, Reid CM, Ryan P, et al: A comparison of outcomes with angiotensin-converting-enzyme inhibitors and diuretics for hypertension in the elderly. *N Engl J Med* 348:583, 2003.
17. Brown MJ, Palmer CR, Castaigne A, et al: Morbidity and mortality in patients randomised to double-blind treatment with a long-acting calcium-channel blocker or diuretic in the International Nifedipine GITS study: Intervention as a Goal in Hypertension Treatment (INSIGHT). *Lancet* 356:366, 2000.
18. Reungjui S, Pratipanawatr T, Johnson R, Nakagawa T: Do thiazides worsen metabolic syndrome and renal disease? The pivotal roles for hyperuricemia and hypokalemia. *Curr Opin Nephrol Hypertens* 17:470, 2008.
19. Goldstein RE, Stinson EB, Scherer JL, et al: Intraoperative coronary collateral function in patients with coronary occlusive disease: nitroglycerin responsiveness and angiographic correlations. *Circulation* 49:298, 1974.
20. Brown BG, Bolson E, Petersen RB, et al: The mechanisms of nitroglycerin action: stenosis vasodilatation as a major component of the drug response. *Circulation* 64:1089, 1981.
21. Parker JD, Parker JO: Nitrate therapy for stable angina pectoris. *N Engl J Med* 338:520, 1998.
22. Loscalzo J: Antiplatelet and antithrombotic effects of organic nitrates. *Am J Cardiol* 70:18B, 1992.
23. Moncada S, Higgs A: The L-arginine–nitric oxide pathway. *N Engl J Med* 329:2002, 1993.
24. Heidenreich PA, McDonald KM, Hastie T, et al: Meta-analysis of trials comparing beta-blockers, calcium antagonists, and nitrates for stable angina. *JAMA* 281:1927, 1999.
25. Cohn JN, Archibald DG, Ziesche S, et al: Effect of vasodilator therapy on mortality in chronic congestive heart failure. Results of a Veterans Administration Cooperative Study. *N Engl J Med* 314:1547, 1986.
26. Cohn JN, Johnson G, Ziesche S, et al: A comparison of enalapril with hydralazine–isosorbide dinitrate in the treatment of chronic congestive heart failure. *N Engl J Med* 325:303, 1991.
27. GISSI-3: Effects of lisinopril and transdermal glyceryl trinitrate singly and together on 6-week mortality and ventricular function after acute myocardial infarction. Gruppo Italiano per lo Studio della Sopravvivenza nell'Infarto Miocardico. *Lancet* 343:1115, 1994.
28. ISIS-4: A randomised factorial trial assessing early oral captopril, oral mononitrate, and intravenous magnesium sulphate in 58,050 patients with suspected acute myocardial infarction. ISIS-4 (Fourth International Study of Infarct Survival) Collaborative Group. *Lancet* 345:669, 1995.
29. Ishikawa K, Kanamasa K, Ogawa I, et al: Long-term nitrate treatment increases cardiac events in patients with healed myocardial infarction. Secondary Prevention Group. *Jpn Circ J* 60:779, 1996.
30. Dupuis J, Lalonde G, Lemieux R, Rouleau JL: Tolerance to intravenous nitroglycerin in patients with congestive heart failure: role of increased intravascular volume, neurohumoral activation and lack of prevention with N-acetylcysteine. *J Am Coll Cardiol* 16:923, 1990.
31. Heitzer T, Just H, Brockhoff C, et al: Long-term nitroglycerin treatment is associated with supersensitivity to vasoconstrictors in men with stable coronary artery disease: prevention by concomitant treatment with captopril. *J Am Coll Cardiol* 31:83, 1998.
32. Hirai N, Kawano H, Yasue H, et al. Attenuation of nitrate tolerance and oxidative stress by an angiotensin II receptor blocker in patients with coronary spastic angina. *Circulation* 108:1446, 2003.
33. Katz RJ, Levy WS, Buff L, Wasserman AG: Prevention of nitrate tolerance with angiotension converting enzyme inhibitors. *Circulation* 83:1271, 1991.

34. Yamauchi T, Hagiwara N, Kasanuki H, et al: Long-term nitrate use in acute myocardial infarction (the Heart Institute of Japan, Department of Cardiology nitrate evaluation program). *Cardiovasc Drugs Ther* 22:177, 2008.
35. Kojima S, Matsui K, Sakamoto T, et al: Long-term nitrate therapy after acute myocardial infarction does not improve or aggravate prognosis. *Circ J* 71:301, 2007.
36. Ferrari R: Angiotensin converting enzyme inhibitor–calcium antagonist combination: an alliance for cardioprotection? *J Hypertens Suppl* 15:S109, 1997.
37. McDonagh PF, Roberts DJ: Prevention of transcoronary macromolecular leakage after ischemia- reperfusion by the calcium entry blocker nisoldipine. Direct observations in isolated rat hearts. *Circ Res* 58:127, 1986.
38. Tanguay M, Jasmin G, Blaise G, Dumont L: Coronary and cardiac sensitivity to the vasoselective benzothiazepine-like calcium antagonist, clentiazem, in experimental heart failure. *Cardiovasc Drugs Ther* 11:71, 1997.
39. Fogari R, Zoppi A: Antihypertensive drugs and fibrinolytic function. *Am J Hypertens* 19:1293, 2006.
40. Millar JA, McLean KA, Sumner DJ, Reid JL: The effect of the calcium antagonist nifedipine on pressor and aldosterone responses to angiotensin II in normal man. *Eur J Clin Pharmacol* 24:315, 1983.
41. Rehnqvist N, Hjemdahl P, Billing E, et al: Effects of metoprolol vs verapamil in patients with stable angina pectoris: the Angina Prognosis Study in Stockholm (APSIS). *Eur Heart J* 17:76, 1996.
42. Dargie HJ, Ford I, Fox KM: Total Ischaemic Burden European Trial (TIBET): effects of ischaemia and treatment with atenolol, nifedipine SR and their combination on outcome in patients with chronic stable angina. *Eur Heart J* 17:104, 1996.
43. Poole-Wilson PA, Lubsen J, Kirwan BA, et al: Effect of long-acting nifedipine on mortality and cardiovascular morbidity in patients with stable angina requiring treatment (ACTION trial): randomised controlled trial. *Lancet* 364:849, 2004.
44. Effect of verapamil on mortality and major events after acute myocardial infarction (The Danish Verapamil Infarction Trial II—DAVIT II). *Am J Cardiol* 66:779, 1990.
45. The Multicenter Diltiazem Postinfarction Trial Research Group: The effect of diltiazem on mortality and reinfarction after myocardial infarction. *N Engl J Med* 319:385, 1988.
46. Miller AB, Conetta DA, Bass TA: Sublingual nifedipine: acute effects in severe chronic congestive heart failure secondary to idiopathic dilated cardiomyopathy. *Am J Cardiol* 55:1359, 1985.
47. Elkayam U, Amin J, Mehra A, et al: A prospective, randomized, double-blind, crossover study to compare the efficacy and safety of chronic nifedipine therapy with that of isosorbide dinitrate and their combination in the treatment of chronic congestive heart failure. *Circulation* 82:1954, 1990.
48. Goldstein RE, Boccuzzi SJ, Cruess D, Nattel S: Diltiazem increases late-onset congestive heart failure in postinfarction patients with early reduction in ejection fraction. The Adverse Experience Committee; and the Multicenter Diltiazem Postinfarction Research Group. *Circulation* 1:52, 1991.
49. Packer M, Lee WH, Medina N, et al: Prognostic importance of the immediate hemodynamic response to nifedipine in patients with severe left ventricular dysfunction. *J Am Coll Cardiol* 10:1303, 1987.
50. Packer M, O'Connor CM, Ghali JK, et al: Effect of amlodipine on morbidity and mortality in severe chronic heart failure. *N Engl J Med* 335:1107, 1996.
51. Packer M: *Prospective randomized amlodipine survival evaluation 2*, Anaheim, Calif, March 2000, American College of Cardiology.
52. Cohn JN, Ziesche S, Smith R, et al: Effect of the calcium antagonist felodipine as supplementary vasodilator therapy in patients with chronic heart failure treated with enalapril: V-HeFT III. *Circulation* 96:856, 1997.
53. Sweeney C, Shultz P, Raij L: Interactions of the endothelium and mesangium in glomerular injury. *J Am Soc Nephrol* 1(Suppl 1):S13, 1990.
54. Fukuo K, Yang J, Yasuda O, et al: Nifedipine indirectly upregulates superoxide dismutase expression in endothelial cells via vascular smooth muscle cell–dependent pathways. *Circulation* 106:356, 2002.
55. Chen L, Haught WH, Yang B, et al: Preservation of endogenous antioxidant activity and inhibition of lipid peroxidation as common mechanisms of antiatherosclerotic effects of vitamin E, lovastatin and amlodipine. *J Am Coll Cardiol* 30:569, 1997.
56. Epstein M, Loutzenhiser RD: Effects of calcium antagonists on renal hemodynamics. *Am J Kidney Dis* 16(Suppl 1):10, 1990.
57. Griffin KA, Picken MM, Bidani AK: Deleterious effects of calcium channel blockade on pressure transmission and glomerular injury in rat remnant kidneys. *J Clin Invest* 96:793, 1995.
58. Griffin KA, Picken MM, Bakris GL, Bidani AK: Class differences in the effects of calcium channel blockers in the rat remnant kidney model. *Kidney Int* 55:1849, 1999.
59. Demarie BK, Bakris GL: Effects of different calcium antagonists on proteinuria associated with diabetes mellitus. *Ann Intern Med* 113:987, 1990.
60. Wright JT Jr, Bakris G, Greene T, et al: Effect of blood pressure lowering and antihypertensive drug class on progression of hypertensive kidney disease: results from the AASK Trial. *JAMA* 288:2421, 2002.
61. Packer M: Beta-blockade in heart failure. Basic concepts and clinical results. *Am J Hypertens* 11:23S, 1998.
62. Eichhorn EJ, McGhie AL, Bedotto JB, et al: Effects of bucindolol on neurohormonal activation in congestive heart failure. *Am J Cardiol* 67:67, 1991.
63. Dandona P, Ghanim H, Brooks D: Antioxidant activity of carvedilol in cardiovascular disease. *J Hypertens* 25:731, 2007.
64. Lindholm LH, Carlberg B, Samuelsson O: Should beta blockers remain first choice in the treatment of primary hypertension? A meta-analysis. *Lancet* 366:1545, 2005.
65. Morgan T, Lauri J, Bertram D, Anderson A: Effect of different antihypertensive drug classes on central aortic pressure. *Am J Hypertens* 17:118, 2004.
66. Williams B, Lacy PS, Thom SM, et al: CAFE Investigators; Anglo-Scandinavian Cardiac Outcomes Trial Investigators; CAFE Steering Committee and Writing Committee: Differential impact of blood pressure–lowering drugs on central aortic pressure and clinical outcomes: principal results of the Conduit Artery Function Evaluation (CAFE) Study. *Circulation* 113:1213, 2006.
67. Dahlf B, Sever P, Poulter N, et al: Prevention of cardiovascular events with an antihypertensive regimen of amlodipine adding perindopril as required versus atenolol adding bendroflumethiazide as required, in the Anglo-Scandinavian Cardiac Outcomes Trial–Blood Pressure Lowering Arm (ASCOT-BPLA): a multicentre randomised controlled trial. *Lancet* 366:895, 2005.
68. Dahlf B, Devereux R, Kjeldsen S, et al: Cardiovascular morbidity and mortality in the Losartan Intervention For Endpoint reduction in hypertension study (LIFE): a randomised trial against atenolol. *Lancet* 359:995, 2002.
69. Mechanisms for the early mortality reduction produced by beta-blockade started early in acute myocardial infarction: ISIS-1. ISIS-1 (First International Study of Infarct Survival) Collaborative Group. *Lancet* 1:921, 1988.
70. Yusuf S, Peto R, Lewis J, et al: Beta blockade during and after myocardial infarction: an overview of the randomized trials. *Prog Cardiovascr Dis* 27:335, 1985.
71. Krumholz HM, Radford MJ, Wang Y, et al: National use and effectiveness of beta-blockers for the treatment of elderly patients after acute myocardial infarction: National Cooperative Cardiovascular Project. *JAMA* 280:623, 1998.
72. Metoprolol in acute myocardial infarction (MIAMI). A randomised placebo-controlled international trial. *Eur Heart J* 6:199, 1985.
73. Randomised trial of intravenous atenolol among 16,027 cases of suspected acute myocardial infarction: ISIS-1. First International Study of Infarct Survival Collaborative Group. *Lancet* 2:57, 1986.
74. Chen ZM, Pan HC, Chen YP, et al: Early intravenous then oral metoprolol in 45,852 patients with acute myocardial infarction: randomised placebo-controlled trial. *Lancet* 366:1622, 2005.
75. A randomized trial of propranolol in patients with acute myocardial infarction. I. Mortality results. *JAMA* 247:1707, 1982.
76. Roberts R, Rogers WJ, Mueller HS, et al: Immediate versus deferred beta-blockade following thrombolytic therapy in patients with acute myocardial infarction. Results of the Thrombolysis in Myocardial Infarction (TIMI) II-B Study. *Circulation* 83:422, 1991.
77. Hjalmarson A, Goldstein S, Fagerberg B, et al: Effects of controlled-release metoprolol on total mortality, hospitalizations, and well-being in patients with heart failure: the Metoprolol CR/XL Randomized Intervention Trial in congestive heart failure (MERIT-HF). MERIT-HF Study Group. *JAMA* 283:1295, 2000.
78. Packer M, Coats AJS, Fowler MB, et al: Effect of carvedilol on survival in severe chronic heart failure. *N Engl J Med* 344:1651, 2001.
79. The Cardiac Insufficiency Bisoprolol Study II (CIBIS-II): a randomised trial. *Lancet* 353:9, 1999.
80. Bjorck S, Mulec H, Johnsen SA, et al: Contrasting effects of enalapril and metoprolol on proteinuria in diabetic nephropathy. *BMJ* 300:904, 1990.
81. Wright J, Bakris G, Greene T, et al: Effect of blood pressure lowering and antihypertensive drug class on progression of hypertensive kidney disease: results from the AASK trial. *JAMA* 288:2421, 2002.
82. Bakris GL, Fonseca V, Katholi RE, et al: Differential effects of beta-blockers on albuminuria in patients with type 2 diabetes. *Hypertension* 46:1309, 2005.
83. Atlas S: The renin-angiotensin aldosterone system: pathophysiological role and pharmacologic inhibition. *J Manag Care Pharm* 13(Suppl B):9, 2007.
84. Gaddam K, Pimenta E, Husain S, Calhoun D: Aldosterone and cardiovascular disease. *Curr Probl Cardiol* 34:51, 2009.
85. Stowasser M: New perspectives on the role of aldosterone excess in cardiovascular disease. *Clin Exp Pharmacol Physiol* 28:783, 2001.
86. Pitt B, Zannad F, Remme WJ, et al: The effect of spironolactone on morbidity and mortality in patients with severe heart failure. Randomized Aldactone Evaluation Study Investigators. *N Engl J Med* 341:709, 1999.
87. Kumar R, Singh V, Baker K: The intracellular renin-angiotensin system: implications in cardiovascular remodeling. *Curr Opin Nephrol Hypertens* 17:168, 2008.
88. Re RN: Mechanisms of disease: local renin-angiotensin-aldosterone systems and the pathogenesis and treatment of cardiovascular disease. *Nat Clin Pract Cardiovasc Med* 1:42, 2004.
89. Richard V, Hurel-Merle S, Scalbert E, et al: Functional evidence for a role of vascular chymase in the production of angiotensin II in isolated human arteries. *Circulation* 104:750, 2001.
90. Bacani C, Frishman W: Chymase: a new pharmacologic target in cardiovascular disease. *Cardiol Rev* 14:187, 2006.
91. Donoghue M, Hsieh F, Baronas E, et al: A novel angiotensin-converting enzyme–related carboxypeptidase (ACE2) converts angiotensin I to angiotensin 1-9. *Circ Res* 87:e1, 2000.
92. Ishiyama Y, Gallagher PE, Averill DB, et al: Upregulation of angiotensin-converting enzyme 2 after myocardial infarction by blockade of angiotensin II receptors. *Hypertension* 43:970, 2004.
93. Marceau F, Hess JF, Bachvarov DR: The B_1 receptors for kinins. *Pharmacol Rev* 50:357, 1998.
94. Marceau F: Kinin B1 receptors: a review, *Immunopharmacology* 30:1, 1995.
95. Schachter M: ACE inhibitors, angiotensin receptor antagonists and bradykinin. *J Renin Angiotensin Aldosterone Syst* 1:27, 2000.
96. Schölkens BA: Kinins in the cardiovascular system. *Immunopharmacology* 33:209, 1996.
97. Linz W, Wiemer G, Gohlke P, et al: Contribution of kinins to the cardiovascular actions of angiotensin-converting enzyme inhibitors. *Pharmacol Rev* 47:25, 1995.
98. Gradman A, Kad R: Renin inhibition in hypertension. *J Am Coll Cardiol* 51:519, 2008.
99. Reudelhuber TL, Ramla D, Chiu L, et al: Proteolytic processing of human prorenin in renal and non-renal tissues. *Kidney Int* 46:1522, 1994.
100. Nguyen G, Burckle C, Sraer JD: The renin receptor: the facts, the promise and the hope. *Curr Opin Nephrol Hypertens* 12:51, 2003.
101. Nguyen G: Renin/prorenin receptors. *Kidney Int* 69:1503, 2006.
102. Nguyen G: The (pro)renin receptor: pathophysiological roles in cardiovascular and renal pathology. *Curr Opin Nephrol Hypertens* 16:129, 2007.

103. Alderman MH, Ooi WL, Cohen H, et al: Plasma renin activity: a risk factor for myocardial infarction in hypertensive patients. *Am J Hypertens* 10:1, 1997.
104. Latini R, Masson S, Anand I, et al: The comparative prognostic value of plasma neurohormones at baseline in patients with heart failure enrolled in Val-HeFT. *Eur Heart J* 25:292, 2004.
105. Muhlestein JB, Bair TL, May HT: *Association between baseline plasma renin activity and risk of clinical events in patients with diabetes and coronary artery disease*, New Orleans, La, 2009, American Diabetes Association 69th Scientific Sessions.
106. Bair TL, May HT, Prescott MF: *Association between baseline plasma renin activity and risk of cardiovascular events in coronary artery disease patients*, San Francisco, Calif, 2009, American Society of Hypertension.
107. Go AS, Chertow GM, Fan D, et al: Chronic kidney disease and the risks of death, cardiovascular events, and hospitalization. *N Engl J Med* 351:1296, 2004.
108. Culleton BF, Larson MG, Wilson PW, et al: Cardiovascular disease and mortality in a community-based cohort with mild renal insufficiency. *Kidney Int* 56:2214, 1999.
109. Manjunath G, Tighiouart H, Ibrahim H, et al: Level of kidney function as a risk factor for atherosclerotic cardiovascular outcomes in the community. *J Am Coll Cardiol* 41:47, 2003.
110. Shulman NB, Ford CE, Hall WD, et al: Prognostic value of serum creatinine and effect of treatment of hypertension on renal function. Results from the hypertension detection and follow-up program. The Hypertension Detection and Follow-up Program Cooperative Group. *Hypertension* 13(Suppl):I80, 1989.
111. Mann JF, Gerstein HC, Pogue J, et al: Renal insufficiency as a predictor of cardiovascular outcomes and the impact of ramipril: the HOPE randomized trial. *Ann Intern Med* 134:629, 2001.
112. Solomon S, Rice M, Jablonski K, et al: Renal function and effectiveness of angiotensin-converting enzyme inhibitor therapy in patients with chronic stable coronary disease in the Prevention of Events with ACE inhibition (PEACE) trial. *Circulation* 114:26, 2006.
113. Shlipak M, Heidenreich P, Noguchi H, et al: Association of renal insufficiency with treatment and outcomes after myocardial infarction in elderly patients. *Ann Intern Med* 137:555, 2002.
114. Hampton JR, van Veldhuisen DJ, Kleber FX, et al: Randomised study of effect of ibopamine on survival in patients with advanced severe heart failure. Second Prospective Randomised Study of Ibopamine on Mortality and Efficacy (PRIME II) Investigators. *Lancet* 349:971, 1997.
115. Fort J: Chronic renal failure: a cardiovascular risk factor. *Kidney Int Suppl* 99:S25, 2005.
116. Remuzzi G, Bertani T: Pathophysiology of progressive nephropathies. *N Engl J Med* 339:1448, 1998.
117. Schiffrin E, Lipman M, Mann JF: Chronic kidney disease: effects on the cardiovascular system. *Circulation* 116:85, 2007.
118. Shlipak MG, Fried LF, Crump C, et al: Elevations of inflammatory and procoagulant biomarkers in elderly persons with renal insufficiency. *Circulation* 107:87, 2003.
119. Chan D, Irish A, Dogra G, Watts G: Dyslipidaemia and cardiorenal disease: mechanisms, therapeutic opportunities and clinical trials. *Atherosclerosis* 196:823, 2008.
120. Kasiske BL: Hyperlipidemia in patients with chronic renal disease. *Am J Kidney Dis* 32(Suppl 3):S142, 1998.
121. Kasiske BL: Relationship between vascular disease and age-associated changes in the human kidney. *Kidney Int* 31:1153, 1987.
122. Ix JH, Shlipak M, Liu H, et al: Association between renal insufficiency and inducible ischemia in patients with coronary artery disease: the heart and soul study. *J Am Soc Nephrol* 14:3233, 2003.
123. Ruilope LM, van Veldhuisen DJ, Ritz E, Luscher TF: Renal function: the Cinderella of cardiovascular risk profile. *J Am Coll Cardiol* 38:1782, 2001.
124. Stamler J, Vaccaro O, Neaton JD, Wentworth D: Diabetes, other risk factors, and 12-yr cardiovascular mortality for men screened in the Multiple Risk Factor Intervention Trial. *Diabetes Care* 16:434, 1993.
125. Turner RC, Millns H, Neil HA, et al: Risk factors for coronary artery disease in non–insulin dependent diabetes mellitus: United Kingdom Prospective Diabetes Study (UKPDS: 23). *BMJ* 316:823, 1998.
126. Dinneen SF, Gerstein HC: The association of microalbuminuria and mortality in non–insulin-dependent diabetes mellitus. A systematic overview of the literature. *Arch Intern Med* 157:1413, 1997.
127. Kannel WB, Stampfer MJ, Castelli WP, Verter J: The prognostic significance of proteinuria: the Framingham study. *Am Heart J* 108:1347, 1984.
128. Grimm RH Jr, Svendsen KH, Kasiske B, et al: Proteinuria is a risk factor for mortality over 10 years of follow-up. MRFIT Research Group. Multiple Risk Factor Intervention Trial. *Kidney Int Suppl* 63:S10, 1997.
129. Keane WF, Eknoyan G: Proteinuria, albuminuria, risk, assessment, detection, elimination (PARADE): a position paper of the National Kidney Foundation. *Am J Kidney Dis* 33:1004, 1999.
130. Gerstein HC, Mann JF, Yi Q, et al: Albuminuria and risk of cardiovascular events, death, and heart failure in diabetic and nondiabetic individuals. *JAMA* 286:421, 2001.
131. Agrawal V, Marinescu V, Agarwal M, McCullough P: Cardiovascular implications of proteinuria: an indicator of chronic kidney disease. *Nature Rev Cardiol* 6:301, 2009.
132. Lewis EJ, Hunsicker LG, Clarke WR, et al: Renoprotective effect of the angiotensin-receptor antagonist irbesartan in patients with nephropathy due to type 2 diabetes. *N Engl J Med* 345:851, 2001.
133. Brenner BM, Cooper ME, de Zeeuw D, et al: Effects of losartan on renal and cardiovascular outcomes in patients with type 2 diabetes and nephropathy. *N Engl J Med* 345:861, 2001.
134. Ibsen H, Olsen M, Wachtell K, et al: Reduction in albuminuria translates to reduction in cardiovascular events in hypertensive patients: losartan intervention for endpoint reduction in hypertension study. *Hypertension* 45:198, 2005.
135. de Kam P, Voors A, Fici F, et al: The revised role of ACE-inhibition after myocardial infarction in the thrombolytic/primary PCI era. *J Renin Angiotensin Aldosterone Syst* 5:161, 2004.
136. Mancini GB, Henry GC, Macaya C, et al: Angiotensin-converting enzyme inhibition with quinapril improves endothelial vasomotor dysfunction in patients with coronary artery disease. The TREND (Trial on Reversing ENdothelial Dysfunction) Study. *Circulation* 94:258, 1996.
137. Vaughan DE, Rouleau JL, Ridker PM, et al: Effects of ramipril on plasma fibrinolytic balance in patients with acute anterior myocardial infarction. HEART Study Investigators. *Circulation* 96:442, 1997.
138. Minai K, Matsumoto T, Horie H, et al: Bradykinin stimulates the release of tissue plasminogen activator in human coronary circulation: effects of angiotensin-converting enzyme inhibitors. *J Am Coll Cardiol* 37:1565, 2001.
139. Pfeffer MA, Braunwald E, Moy LA, et al: Effect of captopril on mortality and morbidity in patients with left ventricular dysfunction after myocardial infarction. Results of the survival and ventricular enlargement trial. The SAVE Investigators. *N Engl J Med* 327:669, 1992.
140. Cleland JG, Erhardt L, Murray G, et al: Effect of ramipril on morbidity and mode of death among survivors of acute myocardial infarction with clinical evidence of heart failure. A report from the AIRE Study Investigators. *Eur Heart J* 18:41, 1997.
141. Kber L, Torp-Pedersen C, Carlsen JE, et al: A clinical trial of the angiotensin-converting-enzyme inhibitor trandolapril in patients with left ventricular dysfunction after myocardial infarction. Trandolapril Cardiac Evaluation (TRACE) Study Group. *N Engl J Med* 333:1670, 1995.
142. Ambrosioni E, Borghi C, Magnani B: The effect of the angiotensin-converting-enzyme inhibitor zofenopril on mortality and morbidity after anterior myocardial infarction. The Survival of Myocardial Infarction Long-Term Evaluation (SMILE) Study Investigators. *N Engl J Med* 332:80, 1995.
143. Swedberg K, Held P, Kjekshus J, et al: Effects of the early administration of enalapril on mortality in patients with acute myocardial infarction. Results of the Cooperative New Scandinavian Enalapril Survival Study II (CONSENSUS II). *N Engl J Med* 327:678, 1992.
144. GISSI-3: Effects of lisinopril and transdermal glyceryl trinitrate singly and together on 6-week mortality and ventricular function after acute myocardial infarction. *Lancet* 343:1115, 1994.
145. ISIS-4: A randomised factorial trial assessing early oral captopril, oral mononitrate, and intravenous magnesium sulphate in 58,050 patients with suspected acute myocardial infarction. *Lancet* 345:669, 1995.
146. The SOLVD Investigators: Effect of enalapril on survival in patients with reduced left ventricular ejection fractions and congestive heart failure. *N Engl J Med* 325:293, 1991.
147. Yusuf S, Sleight P, Pogue J, et al: Effects of an angiotensin-converting-enzyme inhibitor, ramipril, on cardiovascular events in high-risk patients. The Heart Outcomes Prevention Evaluation Study Investigators. *N Engl J Med* 342:145, 2000.
148. Fox KM: Efficacy of perindopril in reduction of cardiovascular events among patients with stable coronary artery disease: randomised, double-blind, placebo-controlled, multicentre trial (the EUROPA study). *Lancet* 362:782, 2003.
149. Braunwald E, Domanski M, Fowler S, et al: Angiotensin-converting-enzyme inhibition in stable coronary artery disease. *N Engl J Med* 351:2058, 2004.
150. Indications for ACE inhibitors in the early treatment of acute myocardial infarction: systematic overview of individual data from 100,000 patients in randomized trials. *Circulation* 97:2202, 1998.
151. Packer M, Poole-Wilson PA, Armstrong PW, et al: Comparative effects of low and high doses of the angiotensin-converting enzyme inhibitor, lisinopril, on morbidity and mortality in chronic heart failure. ATLAS Study Group. *Circulation* 100:2312, 1999.
152. Packer M, Poole-Wilson PA, Armstrong PW, et al: Comparative effects of low and high doses of the angiotensin-converting enzyme inhibitor, lisinopril, on morbidity and mortality in chronic heart failure. *Circulation* 100:2312, 1999.
153. Egido J: Vasoactive hormones and renal sclerosis. *Kidney Int* 49:578, 1996.
154. Heart Outcomes Prevention Evaluation Study Investigators: Effects of ramipril on cardiovascular and microvascular outcomes in people with diabetes mellitus: results of the HOPE study and MICRO-HOPE substudy. *Lancet* 355:253, 2000.
155. Remuzzi G, Chiurchiu C, Ruggenenti P: Proteinuria predicting outcome in renal disease: nondiabetic nephropathies (REIN). *Kidney Int Suppl* 92:S90, 2004.
156. Gruppo Italiano di Studi Epidemiologici in Nefrologia: Randomised placebo-controlled trial of effect of ramipril on decline in glomerular filtration rate and risk of terminal renal failure in proteinuric, non-diabetic nephropathy. *Lancet* 349:1857, 1997.
157. Unger T: The role of the renin-angiotensin system in the development of cardiovascular disease. *Am J Cardiol* 89:3A, 2002.
158. Dickstein K, Kjekshus J: Effects of losartan and captopril on mortality and morbidity in high-risk patients after acute myocardial infarction: the OPTIMAAL randomised trial. *Lancet* 360:752, 2002.
159. Gottlieb SS, Dickstein K, Fleck E, et al: Hemodynamic and neurohormonal effects of the angiotensin II antagonist losartan in patients with congestive heart failure. *Circulation* 88(pt 1):1602, 1993.
160. Pfeffer MA, McMurray JJ, Velazquez EJ, et al: Valsartan, captopril, or both in myocardial infarction complicated by heart failure, left ventricular dysfunction, or both. *N Engl J Med* 349:1893, 2003.
161. Pitt B, Segal R, Martinez FA, et al: Randomised trial of losartan versus captopril in patients over 65 with heart failure (Evaluation of Losartan in the Elderly Study, ELITE). *Lancet* 349:747, 1997.
162. Pitt B, Poole-Wilson PA, Segal R, et al: Effect of losartan compared with captopril on mortality in patients with symptomatic heart failure: randomised trial—the Losartan Heart Failure Survival Study ELITE II. *Lancet* 355:1582, 2000.
163. Cohn JN, Tognoni G, Valsartan Heart Failure Trial Investigators: A randomized trial of the angiotensin-receptor blocker valsartan in chronic heart failure. *N Engl J Med* 345:1667, 2001.

164. Granger C, McMurray JJ, Yusuf S, et al: Effects of candesartan in patients with chronic heart failure and reduced left-ventricular systolic function intolerant to angiotensin-converting-enzyme inhibitors: the CHARM-Alternative trial. *Lancet* 362:772, 2003.

165. Bart BA, Ertl G, Held P, et al: Contemporary management of patients with left ventricular systolic dysfunction. Results from the Study of Patients Intolerant of Converting Enzyme Inhibitors (SPICE) Registry. *Eur Heart J* 20:1182, 1999.

166. McDowell SE, Coleman JJ, Ferner RE: Systematic review and meta-analysis of ethnic differences in risks of adverse reactions to drugs used in cardiovascular medicine. *BMJ* 332:1177, 2006.

167. Granger CB, Ertl G, Kuch J, et al: Randomized trial of candesartan cilexetil in the treatment of patients with congestive heart failure and a history of intolerance to angiotensin-converting-enzyme inhibitors. *Am Heart J* 139:609, 2000.

168. Schachter M: ACE inhibitors, angiotensin receptor antagonists and bradykinin. *J Renin Angiotensin Aldosterone Syst* 1:27, 2000.

169. Viberti G, Wheeldon N: Microalbuminuria reduction with valsartan in patients with type 2 diabetes mellitus: a blood pressure–independent effect. *Circulation* 106:672, 2002.

170. Mann JF, Schmieder R, Dyal L, et al: Effect of telmisartan on renal outcomes: a randomized trial. *Ann Intern Med* 151:1, W1, 2009.

171. Brown M: Aliskiren. *Circulation* 118:773, 2008.

172. Krop M, Garrelds I, de Bruin RJA, et al: Aliskiren accumulates in renin secretory granules and binds plasma prorenin. *Hypertension* 52:1076, 2008.

173. Schefe J, Neumann C, Goebel M, et al: Prorenin engages the (pro)renin receptor like renin and both ligand activities are unopposed by aliskiren. *J Hypertens* 26:1787, 2008.

174. Nussberger J, Aubert JF, Bouzourene K, et al: Renin inhibition by aliskiren prevents atherosclerosis progression: comparison with irbesartan, atenolol, and amlodipine. *Hypertension* 51:1306, 2008.

175. Westermann D, Riad A, Lettau O, et al: Renin inhibition improves cardiac function and remodeling after myocardial infarction independent of blood pressure. *Hypertension* 52:1068, 2008.

176. Imanishi T, Tsujioka H, Ikejima H, et al: Renin inhibitor aliskiren improves impaired nitric oxide bioavailability and protects against atherosclerotic changes. *Hypertension* 52:563, 2008.

177. Serebruany VL, Malinin A, Barsness G, et al: Effects of aliskiren, a renin inhibitor, on biomarkers of platelet activity, coagulation and fibrinolysis in subjects with multiple risk factors for vascular disease. *J Hum Hypertens* 22:303, 2008.

178. Oh BH, Mitchell J, Herron J, et al: Aliskiren, an oral renin inhibitor, provides dose-dependent efficacy and sustained 24-hour blood pressure control in patients with hypertension. *J Am Coll Cardiol* 49:1157, 2007.

179. Gradman A, Schmieder R, Lins R, et al: Aliskiren, a novel orally effective renin inhibitor, provides dose-dependent antihypertensive efficacy and placebo-like tolerability in hypertensive patients. *Circulation* 111:1012, 2005.

180. Oparil S, Yarows S, Patel S, et al: Efficacy and safety of combined use of aliskiren and valsartan in patients with hypertension: a randomised, double-blind trial. *Lancet* 370:221, 2007.

181. Villamil A, Chrysant S, Calhoun D, et al: Renin inhibition with aliskiren provides additive antihypertensive efficacy when used in combination with hydrochlorothiazide. *J Hypertens* 25:217, 2007.

182. Solomon S, Appelbaum E, Manning W, et al: Effect of the direct renin inhibitor aliskiren, the angiotensin receptor blocker losartan, or both on left ventricular mass in patients with hypertension and left ventricular hypertrophy. *Circulation* 119:530, 2009.

183. McMurray JJ, Pitt B, Latini R, et al: Effects of the oral direct renin inhibitor aliskiren in patients with symptomatic heart failure. *Circulation* 1:17, 2008.

184. Solomon S: *The Aliskiren Study in Post-MI Patients to Reduce Remodeling (ASPIRE) Trial*, Atlanta, Georgia, 2010, American College of Cardiology.

185. Parving HH, Brenner B, McMurray JJ, et al: Aliskiren Trial in Type 2 Diabetes Using Cardio-Renal Endpoints (ALTITUDE): rationale and study design. *Nephrol Dial Transplant* 24:1663, 2009.

186. Swedberg K, Eneroth P, Kjekshus J, Snapinn S: Effects of enalapril and neuroendocrine activation on prognosis in severe congestive heart failure (follow-up of the CONSENSUS trial). CONSENSUS Trial Study Group. *Am J Cardiol* 66:40D, 1990.

187. Struthers A: The clinical implications of aldosterone escape in congestive heart failure. *Eur J Heart Fail* 6:539, 2004.

188. Davis K, Nappi J: The cardiovascular effects of eplerenone, a selective aldosterone-receptor antagonist. *Clin Ther* 25:2647, 2003.

189. Sica D: Pharmacokinetics and pharmacodynamics of mineralocorticoid blocking agents and their effects on potassium homeostasis. *Heart Fail Rev* 10:23, 2005.

190. Pitt B, Remme W, Zannad F, et al: Eplerenone, a selective aldosterone blocker, in patients with left ventricular dysfunction after myocardial infarction. *N Engl J Med* 348:1309, 2003.

191. Ezekowitz J, McAlister F: Aldosterone blockade and left ventricular dysfunction: a systematic review of randomized clinical trials. *Eur Heart J* 30:469, 2009.

192. Barr CS, Lang CC, Hanson J, et al: Effects of adding spironolactone to an angiotensin-converting enzyme inhibitor in chronic congestive heart failure secondary to coronary artery disease. *Am J Cardiol* 76:1259, 1995.

193. Bomback A, Toto R: Dual blockade of the renin-angiotensin-aldosterone system: beyond the ACE inhibitor and angiotensin-II receptor blocker combination. *Am J Hypertens* 22:1032, 2009.

194. Azizi M, Webb R, Nussberger J, Hollenberg N: Renin inhibition with aliskiren: where are we now, and where are we going? *J Hypertens* 24:243, 2006.

195. Rousseau M, Gurn O, Duprez D, et al: Beneficial neurohormonal profile of spironolactone in severe congestive heart failure: results from the RALES neurohormonal substudy. *J Am Coll Cardiol* 40:1596, 2002.

196. van de Wal RMA, Plokker HWM, Lok DJA, et al: Determinants of increased angiotensin II levels in severe chronic heart failure patients despite ACE inhibition. *Int J Cardiol* 106:367, 2006.

197. McMurray JJ, Ostergren J, Swedberg K, et al: Effects of candesartan in patients with chronic heart failure and reduced left-ventricular systolic function taking angiotensin-converting-enzyme inhibitors: the CHARM-Added trial. *Lancet* 362:767, 2003.

198. Yusuf S, Teo K, Pogue J, et al: Telmisartan, ramipril, or both in patients at high risk for vascular events. *N Engl J Med* 358:1547, 2008.

199. Mann JF, Schmieder R, McQueen M, et al: Renal outcomes with telmisartan, ramipril, or both, in people at high vascular risk (the ONTARGET study): a multicentre, randomised, double-blind, controlled trial. *Lancet* 372:547, 2008.

200. Mogensen CE, Neldam S, Tikkanen I, et al: Randomised controlled trial of dual blockade of renin-angiotensin system in patients with hypertension, microalbuminuria, and non-insulin dependent diabetes: the candesartan and lisinopril microalbuminuria (CALM) study. *BMJ* 321:1440, 2000.

201. Menne J, Farsang C, Dek L, et al: Valsartan in combination with lisinopril versus the respective high dose monotherapies in hypertensive patients with microalbuminuria: the VALERIA trial. *J Hypertens* 26:1860, 2008.

202. Epstein M, Williams G, Weinberger M, et al: Selective aldosterone blockade with eplerenone reduces albuminuria in patients with type 2 diabetes. *Clin J Am Soc Nephrol* 1:940, 2006.

203. Brown NJ, Nakamura S, Ma L, et al: Aldosterone modulates plasminogen activator inhibitor-1 and glomerulosclerosis in vivo. *Kidney Int* 58:1219, 2000.

204. Sun Y, Zhang J, Zhang JQ, Ramires FJ: Local angiotensin II and transforming growth factor-beta1 in renal fibrosis of rats. *Hypertension* 35:1078, 2000.

205. Steir CJ, Zuckerman A, Harashima H, Chander P: Antioxidants reduce aldosterone-induced renal vascular injury in stroke-prone SHR. *J Am Soc Nephrol* 10:400A, 1999.

206. Schiffrin EL, Franks DJ, Gutkowska J: Effect of aldosterone on vascular angiotensin II receptors in the rat. *Can J Physiol Pharmacol* 63:1522, 1985.

207. Epstein M, Buckalew V, Martinez F, et al: Antiproteinuric efficacy of eplerenone, enalapril, and eplerenone/enalapril combination in diabetic hypertensives with microalbuminuria. *Am J Hypertens* 15(24A), 2002.

208. Mehdi U, Adams-Huet B, Raskin P, et al: Addition of angiotensin receptor blockade or mineralocorticoid antagonism to maximal angiotensin-converting enzyme inhibition in diabetic nephropathy. *J Am Soc Nephrol* 20:2641, 2009.

209. Parving HH, Persson F, Lewis J, et al: Aliskiren combined with losartan in type 2 diabetes and nephropathy. *N Engl J Med* 358:2433, 2008.

210. Poulter NR, Wedel H, Dahlöf B, et al: Role of blood pressure and other variables in the differential cardiovascular event rates noted in the Anglo-Scandinavian Cardiac Outcomes Trial–Blood Pressure Lowering Arm (ASCOT-BPLA). *Lancet* 366:907, 2005.

211. Pepine CJ, Handberg EM, Cooper-DeHoff RM, et al: A calcium antagonist vs a non-calcium antagonist hypertension treatment strategy for patients with coronary artery disease. The International Verapamil-Trandolapril Study (INVEST): a randomized controlled trial. *JAMA* 290:2805, 2003.

212. Ferrari R: Optimizing the treatment of hypertension and stable coronary artery disease: clinical evidence for fixed-combination perindopril/amlodipine. *Curr Med Res Opin* 24:3543, 2008.

213. Fogari R, Preti P, Zoppi A, et al: Effects of amlodipine fosinopril combination on microalbuminuria in hypertensive type 2 diabetic patients. *Am J Hypertens* 15:1042, 2002.

Cholesterol/Dyslipidemia

CHAPTER **12**

Evaluation and Management of Dyslipidemia in Children and Adolescents

Christian D. Nagy and Peter O. Kwiterovich, Jr.

KEY POINTS

- Early lesions of atherosclerosis begin in childhood and are related to antecedent CVD risk factors. Environmental factors such as diet, obesity, and exercise and certain inherited dyslipidemias influence the progression of such lesions. Detection of youth at risk for atherosclerosis includes an integrated evaluation of these predisposing factors.

- Treatment starts with weight control, exercise, and a diet low in saturated fat, *trans*-fat, and cholesterol, supplemented with water-soluble fiber, plant stanols, or plant sterols.

- Drug therapy, especially with HMG-CoA reductase inhibitors or bile acid sequestrants, can be considered in those with a positive family history of premature CVD and LDL-C ≥160 mg/dL, after a period of dietary and hygienic measures. Candidates for drug therapy often include those with familial hypercholesterolemia, familial combined hyperlipidemia, the metabolic syndrome, polycystic ovarian syndrome, type 1 or 2 diabetes, and the nephrotic syndrome.

- Dietary and drug therapy appears to be safe and efficacious.

- Early identification and treatment of children with CVD risk factors and dyslipidemia are likely to retard the atherosclerotic process.

- Optimal identification and treatment of high-risk youth require an integrated universal screening, evaluation, treatment, and follow-up program.

Disorders of lipid and lipoprotein metabolism are characterized by abnormalities of the major lipoprotein classes, chylomicrons, very-low-density lipoproteins (VLDL), low-density lipoproteins (LDL), and high-density lipoproteins (HDL). Dyslipidemia can result from the expression of a mutation in a single gene that plays a significant role in lipoprotein metabolism, reflect the effects of multiple genes, or be caused by environmental influences such as excessive dietary intake of fat and calories and limited physical activity, particularly in association with overweight or obesity.

The major clinical complication of dyslipidemia is a predisposition to atherosclerosis starting early in life and leading to cardiovascular disease (CVD) in adulthood. Multiple trials in adults have demonstrated that reduction in the plasma levels of LDL results in the decreased prevalence of coronary artery disease (CAD) and stroke. Lowering of LDL also produces a decrease in the angiographic progression of CAD and even modest regression in some cases. In children with familial hypercholesterolemia, a decrease in LDL reduces carotid intima-media thickness (CIMT) and lipid screening recommendations have recently been updated by the American Academy of Pediatrics.[1]

This chapter presents a theoretical and practical approach to the diagnosis and management of dyslipidemia in children and adolescents, in the hope of preventing or retarding the progression of atherosclerosis early in life.

BACKGROUND

A number of studies strongly support the notion that atherosclerosis and CVD risk factors originate in childhood and adolescence and that treatment should begin early in life.[2] Several longitudinal pathologic studies found that early atherosclerotic lesions of fatty streaks and fibrous plaques in children, adolescents, and young adults who died of accidental deaths are significantly related to higher antecedent levels of total cholesterol (TC) and LDL-cholesterol (LDL-C), lower levels of HDL-cholesterol (HDL-C), and other CVD risk factors, such as higher blood pressure, cigarette smoking, and obesity.[2-4]

Major prospective population studies, including the Muscatine Study,[5,6] the

TABLE 12-1 | Classification and Properties of Major Plasma Lipoproteins

	Chylomicrons	Very-Low-Density Lipoproteins	Low-Density Lipoproteins	High-Density Lipoproteins
Hydrated density (g/mL)	<0.95	0.95-1.006	1.019-1.063	1.063-1.21
Electrophoretic migration	Origin	Pre-β	β	α
Molecular weight	$50\text{-}1000 \times 10^6$	$10\text{-}80 \times 10^6$	2.3×10^6	$1.8\text{-}3.6 \times 10^5$
Average composition (%)				
Cholesterol*	3	22	50	20
Triglyceride	90	55	5	5
Phospholipid	6	15	25	25
Protein	1	8	20	50
Major apolipoproteins	Apo B-48 Apo A-I, IV	Apo B-100 Apo C-I, II, III Apo E	Apo B-100	Apo A-I, II Apo C-I, II, III Apo E
Origin	Intestine	Liver	Product of VLDL catabolism	Liver, intestine
Function	Transport intestinal triglycerides and cholesterol	Transport hepatic triglycerides and cholesterol	Provide cholesterol to cells	Reverse cholesterol transport

*Includes the mass of cholesteryl ester and esterified cholesterol.

Reproduced with permission from Kwiterovich PO: Lipid, apolipoprotein and lipoprotein metabolism. In Kwiterovich PO, editor: *The Johns Hopkins textbook of dyslipidemia*, China, 2009, Wolters Kluwer, pp 1-21.

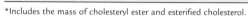

12

Bogalusa Heart Study,[7,8] the Coronary Artery Risk Development in Young Adults (CARDIA) study,[9] the Special Turku Coronary Risk Factor Intervention Project (STRIP),[10] and the Cardiovascular Risk in Young Finns Study,[11,12] demonstrated that CVD risk factors in children and adolescents, particularly LDL-C and obesity, predicted subclinical manifestations of atherosclerosis in young adults, as estimated by coronary artery calcium, CIMT, or brachial flow–mediated dilation. With respect to clinical manifestations of atherosclerosis, medical students at Johns Hopkins who had a TC level >207 mg/dL had five times the risk for development of CVD 40 years later than did those students who had a TC level <172 mg/dL.[13]

Studies in high-risk youth, selected by virtue of CVD in one parent, demonstrated the familial aggregation of dyslipidemia in such children. For example, half of the young progeny of men with premature CVD before 50 years of age had one of seven dyslipidemic profiles: elevated LDL-C alone (type IIa) or combined with high triglycerides (type IIb); elevated triglycerides alone (type IV); low HDL-C alone (hypoalphalipoproteinemia); and type IIa, type IIb, or type IV also accompanied by low HDL-C.[14] Elevated levels of apolipoprotein B, in the presence of normal LDL-C (hyperapobetalipoproteinemia), were prevalent in young offspring of adults with premature CVD and hyperapobetalipoproteinemia.[15] The levels of apolipoprotein B (apo B) and apolipoprotein A-I (apo A-I), the major apolipoproteins of LDL and HDL, respectively, and the ratio of apo B to apo A-I in young offspring from Bogalusa were stronger predictors of premature CAD in their parents than the levels of either LDL-C or HDL-C.[16]

Inherited lipoprotein disorders that often present in youth at high risk for future CVD include familial hypercholesterolemia (FH), caused by a defect in the LDL receptor (LDLR), and familial combined hyperlipidemia (FCHL) and its metabolic cousin, hyperapobetalipoproteinemia, both prototypes for overproduction of VLDL in the liver. Increased synthesis and secretion of VLDL are often driven by an increased flux of free fatty acids (FFA) from the adipose tissue to the liver, a metabolic abnormality usually accompanied by insulin resistance and the dyslipidemic triad of elevated

triglycerides, increased small, dense LDL particles (sLDL-P), and low HDL-C.

In addition, secondary accelerated atherosclerosis requiring aggressive lipid management can be encountered in certain clinical settings early in life, such as in children and adolescents with diabetes mellitus, end-stage renal disease on hemodialysis, or nephrotic syndrome; after renal or heart transplantation; in HIV-positive patients receiving protease inhibitors; in childhood cancer survivors; or in children and adolescents receiving chronic antipsychotic treatment.

LIPID AND LIPOPROTEIN CLASSIFICATION

Cholesterol, triglycerides (TG), phospholipids (PL), and cholesteryl esters (CE) are major lipid classes that are essential components found in dietary fat, plasma lipoproteins, and cells. Lipids are hydrophobic and do not circulate freely in plasma but rather as part of lipid-protein macromolecular complexes called lipoproteins. Plasma lipoproteins are generally spherical particles consisting of a core that contains nonpolar lipids, mostly TG and CE, surrounded by a surface coating consisting of proteins (apolipoproteins), and polar lipids, such as PL and unesterified (free) cholesterol (FC). Lipoproteins function as transport vehicles for water-insoluble lipids and carry them to their sites of metabolism or deposition.

Plasma lipoproteins have been classified by their density and electrophoretic mobility into chylomicrons, VLDL (density <1.006 g/mL) or pre-beta (pre-β) lipoproteins, LDL (density 1.019-1.063 g/mL) or beta (β) lipoproteins, and HDL (density 1.063-1.21 g/mL) or alpha (α) lipoproteins (Table 12-1). Intermediate-density lipoproteins (IDL; density 1.006-1.019 g/mL; also called VLDL remnants) are produced after the hydrolysis of the TG on VLDL. Electrophoresis permits the separation of the plasma lipoproteins on the basis of differences in size and electrophoretic charge. After electrophoresis, chylomicrons remain at the origin, and VLDL, LDL, and HDL migrate in the same positions as pre-β–, β-, and α-globulins, respectively. IDL migrate to a position between the pre-β– and β-globulins. The hydrated density of the

TABLE 12-2	Classification and Properties of Major Plasma Apolipoproteins		
Apolipoprotein	Molecular Weight	Chromosomal Location	Function
Apo A-I	29,016	11q23	Cofactor LCAT; facilitates both the transfer of cell cholesterol by ABCA-1 to nascent HDL and the delivery of CE and FC on HDL to liver through SR-B1
Apo A-II	17,414	1q21-23	Inhibits TG hydrolysis by HL and VLDL
Apo A-IV	44,465	11q23	Activates LCAT, promotes formation of chylomicrons
Apo A-V	39,000	11q23	Stimulates proteoglycan-bound LPL
Apo B-100	512,723	2p24-p23	Secretion of VLDL from liver; binding ligand to LDLR
Apo B-48	240,800	2p24-p23	Secretion of chylomicrons from intestine
Apo C-I	6630	19q13.2	Inhibits apo E binding to LDLR; stimulates LCAT; inhibits CETP and SR-B1
Apo C-II	8900	19q13.2	Cofactor LPL
Apo C-III	8800	11q23	Noncompetitive inhibitor of LPL; inhibits binding of apo E on TG-rich lipoproteins to LDLR
Apo D	19,000	3q26.2	Promotes reverse cholesterol transport
Apo E	34,145	19q13.2	Binding ligand for LRP on chylomicron remnants and VLDL and IDL for LDLR

CE, cholesteryl esters; CETP, cholesteryl ester transfer protein; FC, free cholesterol; HDL, high-density lipoprotein; HL, hepatic lipase; LCAT, lecithin-cholesterol acyltransferase; IDL, intermediate-density lipoprotein; LDL, low-density lipoprotein; LDLR, LDL receptor; LPL, lipoprotein lipase; LRP, LDL-like receptor protein; SR-B1, scavenger receptor B1; TG, triglycerides; VLDL, very-low-density lipoprotein.
Reproduced with permission from Kwiterovich PO: Lipid, apolipoprotein and lipoprotein metabolism. In Kwiterovich PO, editor: *The Johns Hopkins textbook of dyslipidemia*, China, 2009, Wolters Kluwer, pp 1-21.

lipoproteins is related to their chemical composition and the relative content of lipid and apolipoprotein.

Chylomicrons contain 99% lipid, mostly TG (see Table 12-1). After plasma is stored overnight in a tube, these large particles (80 to 500 nm) rise to the top, where they appear as a creamy layer. VLDL contain 90% lipid, the majority being TG, with lesser amounts of cholesterol. When they are present in plasma in increased amounts, VLDL particles are large enough (30 to 80 nm) to impart a cloudy or turbid appearance to plasma. LDL are the major carriers of cholesterol in plasma, and about 50% of their weight is CE and FC. LDL are a heterogeneous group whose size and density vary according to the core content of CE. HDL are often composed of about 50% apolipoprotein and about equal amounts of cholesterol and PL.

Apolipoproteins

Plasma lipoprotein classes are associated with a number of apolipoproteins (Table 12-2). The apolipoproteins have a number of functions; they solubilize lipids in aqueous plasma, permit secretion of chylomicrons and VLDL from intestine and liver, and serve as cofactors for important enzymes in lipoprotein metabolism, and they are responsible for the binding of lipoproteins to specific receptors. The characteristics of the 11 major apolipoproteins and their functions are summarized in Table 12-2. The nucleotide sequences of cDNA for these apolipoproteins have been determined.

LIPID AND LIPOPROTEIN METABOLISM

The transport of plasma lipids by lipoproteins may be divided into an exogenous (dietary) pathway, an endogenous (hepatic) pathway, and reverse cholesterol transport (Fig. 12-1).

Exogenous Lipid Transport

Most of the lipid in the diet is present as neutral fat or TG (75 to 150 g/day). Dietary cholesterol intake is usually about 300 to 400 mg/day but varies from 100 to 600 mg/day. In addition to dietary cholesterol, about 1100 mg of biliary cholesterol is secreted each day from the liver into the intestine (see Fig. 12-1). In the small intestine, lipids are emulsified by bile salts and hydrolyzed by pancreatic lipases. TG are broken down into FFA and 2-monoglycerides; CE are hydrolyzed into FC and FFA. These lipid components are then absorbed by the intestinal cells. Bile acids are reabsorbed by the intestinal bile acid transporter (IBAT) for return to the liver through the enterohepatic circulation (see Fig. 12-1).

The absorption of cholesterol occurs in the jejunum, through the high-affinity uptake of dietary and biliary cholesterol by the Niemann-Pick C1-like 1 (NPC1L1) protein (see Fig. 12-1). Normally, about half the dietary and biliary cholesterol is absorbed daily. Excessive cholesterol absorption is prevented by the ATP-binding cassette, subfamily G (ABCG5/ABCG8) transporters, which act together to pump excess cholesterol and plant sterols from the intestine back into the lumen for fecal excretion (see Fig. 12-1).

Inside intestinal cells, monoglyceride is re-esterified into TG and cholesterol is esterified by acyl:cholesterol acyltransferase (ACAT). Both TG and CE are packaged into chylomicrons, along with apo A-I, apo A-IV, and apo B-48. Chylomicrons are secreted into the thoracic duct, from which they enter the peripheral circulation, where they acquire apo C-II and apo E from HDL. Chylomicrons are too large to cross the endothelial barrier, and apo C-II, a cofactor for lipoprotein lipase (LPL), facilitates the hydrolysis of TG near the endothelial lining of blood vessels.

FFA that are released from the hydrolysis of TG are taken up by muscle cells for energy use or by adipose cells for re-esterification into TG and storage. As a result, a chylomicron remnant is produced that is relatively enriched in CE and apo E. This remnant is rapidly taken up by the liver by a process that involves an initial sequestration of remnant particles on hepatic cell surface proteoglycans. Receptor-mediated endocytosis of remnants follows through the interaction of apo E either with the low-density receptor–like protein (LRP, also called the chylomicron remnant receptor)

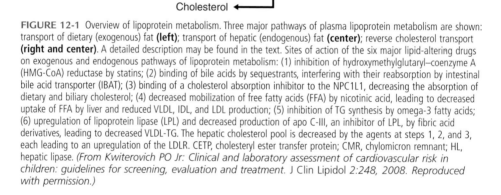

FIGURE 12-1 Overview of lipoprotein metabolism. Three major pathways of plasma lipoprotein metabolism are shown: transport of dietary (exogenous) fat **(left)**; transport of hepatic (endogenous) fat **(center)**; reverse cholesterol transport **(right and center)**. A detailed description may be found in the text. Sites of action of the six major lipid-altering drugs on exogenous and endogenous pathways of lipoprotein metabolism: (1) inhibition of hydroxymethylglutaryl–coenzyme A (HMG-CoA) reductase by statins; (2) binding of bile acids by sequestrants, interfering with their reabsorption by intestinal bile acid transporter (IBAT); (3) binding of a cholesterol absorption inhibitor to the NPC1L1, decreasing the absorption of dietary and biliary cholesterol; (4) decreased mobilization of free fatty acids (FFA) by nicotinic acid, leading to decreased uptake of FFA by liver and reduced VLDL, IDL, and LDL production; (5) inhibition of TG synthesis by omega-3 fatty acids; (6) upregulation of lipoprotein lipase (LPL) and decreased production of apo C-III, an inhibitor of LPL, by fibric acid derivatives, leading to decreased VLDL-TG. The hepatic cholesterol pool is decreased by the agents at steps 1, 2, and 3, each leading to an upregulation of the LDLR. CETP, cholesteryl ester transfer protein; CMR, chylomicron remnant; HL, hepatic lipase. *(From Kwiterovich PO Jr: Clinical and laboratory assessment of cardiovascular risk in children: guidelines for screening, evaluation and treatment. J Clin Lipidol 2:248, 2008. Reproduced with permission.)*

or with the LDLR, both on the surface of hepatic parenchymal cells (see Fig. 12-1).

The uptake of dietary and biliary cholesterol is part of a process that regulates the pool of hepatic cholesterol by downregulation of the LDLR and by inhibition of the rate-limiting enzyme of cholesterol biosynthesis, hydroxymethylglutaryl–coenzyme A (HMG-CoA) reductase (see also later). Hepatic cholesterol can be secreted into bile unchanged, converted into bile acids by 7α-hydroxylase (CYP7A1), or used for lipoprotein synthesis (see Fig. 12-1).

Endogenous Lipid Transport

In the fasting state, most TG in plasma are carried by VLDL. TG are synthesized in the liver and packaged into VLDL with other lipids and apolipoproteins (see Table 12-1), primarily apo B-100, apo E, apo C-I, apo C-II, and apo C-III, and secreted into plasma. The TG in VLDL are subsequently hydrolyzed by LPL, and its cofactor apo C-II, to produce VLDL remnants or IDL. TG can be transferred from VLDL and IDL to HDL and LDL in exchange for CE by the cholesteryl ester transfer protein (CETP; see Fig. 12-1). Compared with VLDL, IDL are

relatively enriched in CE and depleted of TG. Some IDL are taken up directly by the liver, but others are hydrolyzed by hepatic lipase to produce LDL, the final end product of VLDL metabolism (see Fig. 12-1).

The apo B-100 component of the CE-rich LDL binds with high affinity to the LDLR, in either liver or extrahepatic cells (see Fig. 12-1). Bound LDL is internalized by absorptive endocytosis. In lysosomes, apo B-100 is broken down into amino acids, CE hydrolyzed, and FC released. Cholesterol mediates the proteolytic release of a transcription factor, the sterol regulatory element–binding protein (SREBP), from the endoplasmic reticulum.[17] This effect occurs through the SREBP cleavage-activating protein (SCAP) that is both a sensor of sterols and an escort of SREBP from the endoplasmic reticulum to the Golgi.

The family of transcription factors SREBP regulates the synthesis of cholesterol and fatty acids. SREBP-2 mainly regulates cholesterol synthesis. When hepatocytes are depleted of cholesterol, SCAP transports SREBP from the endoplasmic reticulum to the Golgi, where two proteases, Site-1 protease and Site-2 protease, act in sequence to release the NH₂-terminal domain of SREBP from the membrane.[17]

The NH₂-terminal bHLH-Zip domain of SREBP enters the nucleus and binds to a sterol response element in the promoter area of the LDLR and HMG-CoA reductase genes, increasing their transcription. As the cholesterol content of the hepatocyte increases, the SREBP/SCAP complex is not incorporated into the endoplasmic reticulum, SREBP cannot reach the Golgi, and the NH₂-terminal domain of SREBP cannot be released from the membrane for transport into the nucleus, and the transcription of the LDLR and HMG-CoA reductase genes decreases.[17]

This pathway has important clinical implications. For example, excess dietary and biliary cholesterol leads to downregulation of the LDLR and HMG-CoA reductase and an increase in LDL-C. Dietary saturated fat content has a greater effect on LDL-C than dietary cholesterol does. When cholesterol is re-esterified by ACAT, SCAP senses a decrease in hepatic cholesterol, leading to upregulation of the LDLR and HMG-CoA reductase genes by SREBP. However, the preferred substrate for ACAT is oleic acid. Thus, excess saturated fatty acids decrease ACAT activity and thereby increase FC, which inhibits the proteolysis and release of SREBP; this downregulates the LDLR and HMG-CoA reductase genes, followed by an increase in LDL-C.

Decrease of dietary cholesterol and saturated fatty acids or of the hepatic cholesterol content with pharmacologic agents, such as a cholesterol absorption inhibitor or a bile acid sequestrant (see Fig. 12-1), leads to upregulation of LDLR and HMG-CoA reductase genes and lowers LDL-C. HMG-CoA reductase inhibitors (statins) also reduce hepatic cholesterol content, leading to upregulation of LDLR but without the concomitant increase in HMG-CoA reductase activity (see Fig. 12-1). The concomitant use of a statin with either a cholesterol absorption inhibitor or bile acid sequestrant provides a complementary reduction in hepatic cholesterol and consequently LDL-C.

When plasma LDL-C exceeds 100 mg/dL, the capacity to process LDL through the LDLR pathway is exceeded. Increased numbers of LDL particles cross the endothelial barrier. LDL is trapped in the vascular wall by proteoglycans and then modified by either oxidation or glycation. Such modified LDL binds to the scavenger receptors CD36 (macrophage scavenger receptor B) and SR-A (scavenger receptor A) and enters macrophages by a low-affinity, LDLR-independent mechanism (see Fig. 12-1).

This pathway is not subject to feedback inhibition of LDLR synthesis by LDL-derived cholesterol. Thus, LDL continues to be taken up in an unregulated fashion, leading to excess deposition of FC and CE in macrophages (see Fig. 12-1). Dyslipidemias that favor an increased uptake of LDL through the scavenger pathway promote the production of foam cells and their associated atherosclerosis and xanthomas.

Pathways of HDL Metabolism and Reverse Cholesterol Transport

Synthesis of HDL

Nascent HDL. Apo A-1 is released as a lipid-free protein from the intestine and liver. Apo A-1 interacts with the ATP-binding cassette transporter 1 (ABCA1) on the basolateral membranes of hepatocytes, enterocytes, and macrophages, acquiring PL and FC to form a more stable nascent HDL particle.[18]

Formation of Larger, Mature HDL Particle. The transition of HDL particles from the disc-shaped nascent HDL to the spherical "mature" HDL requires the esterification of cholesterol to create a hydrophobic core. Lecithin-cholesterol acyltransferase (LCAT) associates with HDL and catalyzes the transfer of FFA from lecithin to FC, forming CE. Apo A-I is a cofactor for this reaction (see Fig. 12-1). CE formed by this reaction constitute the neutral lipid core of mature spherical HDL₃; further activity of LCAT provides additional CE for the core of HDL₃, forming the larger HDL₂ particles (see Fig. 12-1).

Subsequent addition of cellular cholesterol to the HDL particle occurs in a number of tissues through the action of another ATP-binding cassette transporter 1 (ABCG1) and the scavenger receptor class B1 (SR-B1), molecules that prefer larger HDL as acceptors. In addition to acquiring lipids from liver and intestine, HDL also acquires lipids from chylomicrons and VLDL in the course of hydrolysis of TG by LPL. During this process, apo A-I is transferred from chylomicrons to HDL, and apo C-II and apo E on HDL are transferred to the TG-rich lipoproteins. The TG-rich lipoproteins shed excess PL and cholesterol that are transported to HDL by the phospholipid transfer protein (PLTP).[18]

Transfer of Lipid Between HDL and the Apo B–Containing Lipoproteins. CE are transferred by CETP from the core of spherical HDL to the apo B–containing lipoproteins in exchange for TG[19] (see Fig. 12-1). This process depletes CE but enriches TG in HDL particles and has important implications for HDL metabolism.[18] For example, if the TG in HDL are hydrolyzed by hepatic lipase, a smaller HDL particle is produced that is more avidly removed from plasma by cubilin in the kidney. PLTP is structurally similar to CETP and mediates the transfer of unsaturated fatty acids on PL from the apo B–containing lipoproteins to HDL, contributing to the acquisition of PL by HDL.

Reverse Cholesterol Transport

The CE on the spherical HDL can be transported back to liver by two mechanisms. CE are transferred from HDL to the apo B–containing lipoproteins by CETP, from which they are taken up by the LDLR (see Fig. 12-1). CE may also be delivered directly to the liver through SR-B1 (also called the HDL receptor). These reactions are part of a process called reverse cholesterol transport.

Once the CE is delivered to the liver and hydrolyzed into FC and FFA, the FC can be excreted directly into bile or converted into bile acids by 7α-hydroxylase. Both these pathways result in delivery of sterol from peripheral tissues and plasma into intestinal cells, promoting the excretion of sterols into the stool. Reverse cholesterol transport has been postulated to explain, at least in part, the protective effect that HDL and apo A-I have against the development of atherosclerosis. Conversely, factors that impede this process, such as a dysfunctional HDL, appear to promote atherosclerosis.

LIPID CHANGES THROUGHOUT CHILDHOOD AND ADOLESCENCE

Clearly, the plasma levels of lipids and lipoproteins result from the influence of a variety of metabolic, genetic, and environmental factors. In the general population, these levels usually follow a gaussian distribution, often skewed toward higher levels. Percentiles are therefore used to describe such data, with the 50th percentile being the median or average, the 75th to 95th percentiles borderline elevated, and >95th percentile high or elevated. To define borderline low levels, the 25th to 5th percentiles are used, and <5th percentile is a low level.[20]

Data from the Lipid Research Clinics have often been used to define such percentiles in youth, including the National Cholesterol Education Program (NCEP) Expert Panel on Blood Cholesterol Levels in Childhood in 1992.[20] Similar data are available from such studies as Bogalusa.[21] There are also data from the National Health and Nutrition Examination Survey

TABLE 12-3	Acceptable, Borderline, and High Plasma Lipid, Lipoprotein, and Apolipoprotein Concentrations for Children and Adolescents*		
Category	Acceptable	Borderline	High[†]
Total cholesterol	<170	170-199	≥200
LDL-cholesterol	<110	110-129	≥130
Non–HDL-cholesterol	<123	123-143	≥144
Apolipoprotein B	<90	90-109	≥110
Triglycerides			
0-9 years	<75	75-99	≥100
10-19 years	<90	90-129	≥130
Category	Acceptable	Borderline	Low[†]
HDL-cholesterol	>45	35-45	<35
Apolipoprotein A-I	>120	110-120	<110

* Values for plasma lipid and lipoprotein levels are from the National Cholesterol Education Program (NCEP) Expert Panel on Cholesterol Levels in Children.[20] Non–HDL-cholesterol values from Bogalusa are equivalent to NCEP Pediatric Panel cut points for LDL-cholesterol.[49] Values for plasma apolipoprotein B and A-I are from the National Health and Nutrition Examination Survey III (NHANES III).[22]

[†]The cut points for a high or low value represent approximately the 95th and 5th percentiles, respectively.[20,22,49]

12

(NHANES) on apo B and apo A-I levels[22] and more recent data on TC and LDL-C levels.[23]

Human plasma cholesterol levels are lowest during intra-uterine life.[24] At birth, the mean (1 SD) plasma levels in normal infants have been reported as follows: TC, 74 mg/dL[11]; LDL-C, 31 mg/dL[6]; HDL-C, 37 mg/dL[8]; and TG, 37 mg/dL.[15] The plasma TC and LDL-C levels increase rapidly in the first weeks of life. The kind and source of milk in the infant's diet can markedly influence cholesterol levels. After 2 years of age, the levels of the lipids and lipoproteins become constant up to adolescence.[20] During adolescence, there is a 10% to 20% fall in TC and LDL-C,[25] boys and girls being similarly affected. As well, in the second decade, the TG are higher than they are in the first decade. HDL-C decreases about 10 mg/dL in boys and stays relatively constant in girls. This information has important implications for the timing of lipid and lipoprotein screening and the cut points used because lipid concentrations are age and maturation dependent[26] and appear influenced by gender and race as well, albeit to a small degree.[27]

With use of data combined from three major population-based prospective cohort studies, TC, LDL-C, HDL-C, and TG variables in childhood and adolescence were classified on the basis of NCEP cut points[20] (Table 12-3), age and gender (not race specific), and NHANES cut points[27] and compared for their ability to predict abnormal levels in adulthood.[28] NCEP cut points (compared with NHANES cut points) were more strongly predictive of high TC, LDL-C, and TG levels in adults but less predictive of low HDL-C.

The continued use of the current NCEP cut points for TC, LDL-C, and TG levels in adolescents appears indicated. Thus, multiple cut points by single age and gender do not appear warranted. NHANES cut points (compared with NCEP cut points) were more strongly predictive of HDL-C in adults. The cut point for HDL-C might be revised upward, perhaps to 40 mg/dL, to improve the sensitivity of this measurement to predict low HDL-C in adults and to make the cut point congruent with that used in the grown-ups.

Definition of Dyslipidemia

Cut points to define elevated TC, LDL-C, apo B, non–HDL-C, and TG and low HDL-C and apo A-I in children and adolescents are found in Table 12-3. Dyslipidemia is present if one or more of these lipid, lipoprotein, or apolipoprotein factors are abnormal.

Significant percentages of children and adolescents have elevated concentrations of lipids and lipoproteins. In the Child and Adolescent Trial for Cardiovascular Health (CATCH), 13% of children in the fourth grade had TC ≥200 mg/dL, with 16% of girls and 11% of boys being affected.[29] In the 1988-1994 NHANES, approximately 10% of adolescents had TC ≥200 mg/dL.[30] Using data combined from the 1988-2002 NHANES surveys, Jolliffe and Janssen[27] found that the 95th percentile cut points for LDL-C had increased, indicating a shift in the distribution toward higher LDL-C values.

An important epidemiologic aspect of cardiovascular risk in childhood is the tracking of lipid and lipoprotein concentrations over time. Tracking indicates the likelihood that children will maintain their percentile ranking over time and has been demonstrated in a number of studies.[21,31,32] In the Muscatine Study, 75% of school-aged children who had TC >90th percentile at baseline had TC >200 mg/dL in their early 20s. In the Bogalusa Heart Study, 70% of children with elevated cholesterol continued to have increased cholesterol levels in young adulthood. The Muscatine investigators also found that onset of obesity in adolescence and young adulthood, cigarette smoking, and use of oral contraceptives may have deleterious effects on adult concentrations of lipids and lipoproteins.[31]

SCREENING FOR DYSLIPIDEMIA IN YOUTH

Two major approaches have been used to detect dyslipidemia in youth, namely, screening in the *general* population and in a *selected* population. The extensive literature related to these two screening approaches has been reviewed in detail.[33] Lipid screening recommendations have recently been updated by the American Academy of Pediatrics.[1] Traditionally, screening for dyslipidemias in high-risk children has been recommended because of multiple CVD risk factors and a family history of premature CVD or the presence of hyper-cholesterolemia. LDL-C has been the main focus of diagnosis and treatment.

Less attention has been paid to HDL-C and TG levels. With obesity, type 2 diabetes, and the metabolic syndrome increasing in the younger population,[2,30,34-39] the focus of screening is likely to be expanded to include other factors, such as obesity, low HDL-C, non–HDL-C (TC minus HDL-C), elevated TG, elevated apo B (reflecting increased numbers of LDL particles), glucose intolerance and insulin resistance, and higher blood pressure levels. Both the current and evolving concepts in screening for dyslipidemia in youth are discussed.

Selective Screening

The individualized approach identifies and treats children and adolescents at risk of having high cholesterol levels. Expanded recommendations of the NCEP Expert Panel on Blood Cholesterol Levels in Children and Adolescents[20] from 1992 include performance of selective screening if one of the following conditions is present:

1. A lipoprotein profile in youth whose parents, grand-parents, or siblings required coronary artery bypass graft

surgery or percutaneous coronary intervention before the age of 55 years because of premature CAD.

2. A lipoprotein profile in those with a family history of myocardial infarction, angina pectoris, peripheral or cerebral vascular disease, or sudden death before the age of 55 years.

3. A TC measurement in those whose parents have high TC levels (>240 mg/dL). *This recommendation might be usefully expanded to a lipoprotein profile in offspring of parents who have any genetically transmissible disorder of lipid metabolism associated with increased atherosclerosis risk, involving elevated LDL-C, non–HDL-C, apo B, TG, low HDL-C, and perhaps Lp(a).*

4. A lipoprotein profile if the parental or grandparental family history is not known and the patient has two or more other risk factors for CAD including obesity (body mass index ≥30), hypertension, cigarette smoking, low HDL-C, physical inactivity, and diabetes mellitus. *This recommendation might be usefully expanded to a lipoprotein profile if either obesity (body mass index ≥95th percentile) or overweight (body mass index 85th to 94th percentile) is present, regardless of the presence of other non-lipid CVD risk factors, to identify children and adolescents with abdominal obesity who do not meet the body mass index criterion.*

The NCEP Expert Panel on Blood Cholesterol Levels in Children and Adolescents recommendations[20] from 1992 have been modified in the most recent American Academy of Pediatrics statement,[1] which recommends screening of children with a family history of premature CVD or high cholesterol or those for whom a family history is unknown or those with other risk factors for CVD (e.g., obesity, hypertension, smoking). An optimal program would identify individuals at greatest risk for CVD in adulthood; however, there is currently no clinically applicable noninvasive screening tool available to assess this in children without familial hypercholesterolemia. Whereas the current targeted approach based on family history assumes that this information is known, with adult family members information is often not available.

Universal Screening

Universal lipid screening of all children is controversial.[1,20,33,40] There are a number of advantages and disadvantages of universal screening. What are some of the arguments in favor of universal screening? First, current screening recommendations based on family history of CVD or hypercholesterolemia will fail to detect a substantial number (17% to 90%) of children who have elevated lipid levels.[33]

Universal screening will undoubtedly detect those with undiagnosed heterozygous FH or more marked FCHL, who will require more intensive treatment, usually drug therapy. In a recent meta-analysis of screening for FH in a primary care setting, use of TC detected 88%, 94%, and 96% of cases, with false-positive rates of 0.1%, 0.5%, and 1%, respectively.[41] This approach might usefully be *combined* with a case-finding strategy in relatives of patients with FH.[41]

Identification of children and adolescents affected with hypercholesterolemia through universal screening may bring to attention their adult relatives who will have greater coronary mortality than relatives of children with normal cholesterol levels.[2,42] If universal lipid screening is combined with an assessment of obesity and high blood pressure, this can also lead to the detection of additional relatives from families at high risk for CVD.[43]

CVD risk factors cluster in childhood and persist into adulthood. Whereas offspring of parents with CVD generally have higher LDL-C and TG and lower HDL-C in both childhood and young adulthood,[44] the majority of children with

dyslipidemia and multiple risk factors will be missed by selective screening.[33]

There are some practical problems with universal screening (see later). As well, no longitudinal studies to date are available (and are unlikely ever to be available) to document that starting lipid treatment in childhood decreases adult CVD.[33] One might argue therefore that universal screening seems all the more urgent, given the epidemic of obesity and the metabolic syndrome in our youth.

What are potential concerns about universal lipid screening in childhood? The use of TC in childhood to predict TC or LDL-C in young adults, sufficiently high to warrant treatment, is often associated with suboptimal sensitivity, specificity, and predictive power of a positive test result. For example, if one uses the 75th percentile (about 170 mg/dL) as a lower TC cut point (see Table 12-3), the sensitivity (proportion of affected subjects identified) is higher and the specificity (proportion of normal subjects identified as normal) is lower, as is the predictive value of a positive test result. If one increases the cut point for TC to the 95th percentile (about 200 mg/dL), the sensitivity decreases (more children are missed who are destined to be "affected" as adults), but the predictive power of a positive test result increases (more test results above 200 mg/dL correspond to adults who will require treatment).

When one uses quantitative traits such as LDL-C values for screening, there is no simple resolution of this problem.[2,45] The use of high LDL-C (≥130 mg/dL) rather than high TC as a cut point improves the sensitivity in those with low HDL-C and the predictive power of a positive test result in those with high HDL-C.[2,45]

A number of longitudinal studies[33] found that when the 75th percentile for TC in children is used as a screening cut point, about half the individuals who will require treatment as adults are identified by universal lipid screening. In one report, the sensitivity was much lower when screening was performed during adolescence, presumably reflecting the temporary shift of LDL-C to lower values during this period of rapid growth and development.[25,46]

Another unanswered question is whether the detection of elevated TC or LDL-C in children and young adults predict those who are destined to manifest premature CVD. In the Princeton Lipid Research Clinics Prevalence follow-up study of about 30 years, the number (n = 20) of CVD events was small; the sensitivity of childhood LDL-C for prediction of adult CVD was 10.5% and specificity was 81%.[46] Use of family history information does not substantively improve these results.[46] A combined approach using other CVD risk factors, such as obesity, as part of the screening paradigm for future CVD will probably improve the detection of those adults more likely to develop premature CVD.

Health care providers need to be aware of the negative impact of labels on a child. Problems can be created where no problems may have been. Labeling can have a negative impact on a child's self-esteem, potentially predisposing one to a life that may have been different had the labeling never occurred.

Universal screening raises additional logistic issues. How will pediatricians and family practitioners handle the detection of many children and adolescents with dyslipidemias? Who will counsel in regard to dietary changes, weight loss, and regular exercise habits? Will universal screening, treatment of affected children, and follow-up be cost-effective? Clearly, national resources will be required to change the way pediatric medicine is practiced.

What to Measure

A child does not have to be fasting for TC or HDL-C to be measured. For selective screening, a lipoprotein profile after an overnight fast of 10 to 12 hours is measured for screening youth with a positive family history of premature CVD or dyslipidemia or who have obesity, have multiple CVD risk factors, or are suspected of having secondary dyslipidemia. Such a profile includes TC, TG, LDL-C, HDL-C, and non–HDL-C.

Levels of lipoproteins are typically measured and expressed in terms of their cholesterol content. LDL-C is calculated from the Friedewald equation: LDL-C = TC − (HDL-C + TG/5). Total TG in the fasting state divided by 5 is used to estimate the levels of VLDL-C. If the TG is ≥400 mg/dL, this formula should not be used and a direct LDL-C or apo B should be measured. If the patient is nonfasting, TC, HDL-C, and non–HDL-C levels can be measured. Non-HDL and apo B are valid in the nonfasting state.

Apo B and apo A-I can also be determined by well-standardized immunochemical methods.[22,47] Such measurements might provide additional useful information, particularly in youth with premature CAD in their parents.[15,16] Age- and gender-specific cut points for apo B and apo A-I empirically derived from the NHANES sample are available,[22] providing cut points that can be used to define elevated apo B and low apo A-I (see Table 12-3). Apo B provides an assessment of the total number of apo B–containing lipoprotein particles.[47]

Non–HDL-C is determined by subtracting HDL-C from TC. Non–HDL-C reflects the amount of cholesterol carried by the "atherogenic" apo B–containing lipoproteins—VLDL, IDL, LDL, and Lp(a)—and is strongly correlated with apo B. In adults, non–HDL-C is a better independent predictor of CVD than LDL-C is.[47] In children, non–HDL-C is at least as good a predictor as LDL-C of the expression of dyslipidemia in adulthood.[2,8,48] Percentiles for non–HDL-C in children are available from Bogalusa[49] (see Table 12-3).

Advanced lipoprotein testing to determine plasma levels of VLDL, LDL, and HDL subclasses has been performed in children and adolescents by nuclear magnetic resonance spectroscopy[50-52] or by vertical-spin density-gradient ultracentrifugation[53] in research studies (see also later). However, cut points derived from these methods for the diagnosis and treatment of dyslipidemia in youth are currently not available.

For universal screening, the simplest approach appears to be the measurement of TC, HDL-C, and non–HDL-C in nonfasting specimens. However, treatment algorithms in pediatrics are usually focused on fasting LDL-C. TG is usually assessed as part of the dyslipidemic triad and is often elevated in obesity and the metabolic syndrome.[30,34-39,44,54] Thus, in an ideal screening program, follow-up TC, TG, LDL-C, HDL-C, and non–HDL-C in the fasted state would be assessed after the initial nonfasting screen.

When to Sample for Dyslipidemia

Cholesterol levels are reasonably consistent after 2 years of age. Cholesterol levels are not routinely measured before the age of 2 years because no formal treatment is recommended for this age group. Ten years of age (range, 9 to 11 years) has been proposed as a good time to obtain a standard lipoprotein profile.[41] Children are older and are able to fast easier, the values are predictive of future adult lipoprotein profiles, and puberty has usually not yet started.

Because TC and LDL-C fall 10% to 20% or more during adolescence,[25,27,46] children at risk for familial dyslipidemias should ideally be screened before adolescence, between 2 and 10 years of age. In FH heterozygotes, there is a significant fall in the 1:1 ratio of affected to normal during adolescence.[55] If sampling occurs during adolescence and results are abnormal, levels are likely to be even higher after teenage years. If results during puberty are normal, sampling will need to be repeated toward the end of adolescence (16 years of age for girls and 18 years of age for boys).

The complete phenotypic expression of some disorders, such as FCHL, can be delayed until adulthood, and therefore continued evaluation of subjects from high-risk families with FCHL should occur well into adulthood. Elevated apo B is the first expression of FCHL in adolescents and young adults.[56]

PRIMARY VERSUS SECONDARY DYSLIPOPROTEINEMIA

Before a dyslipoproteinemia is considered to be primary, secondary causes must be excluded (Table 12-4). Each child with dyslipidemia should undergo routine blood testing to rule out secondary causes, including a fasting blood glucose concentration and kidney, liver, and thyroid function tests. In secondary dyslipidemia, the associated disorder producing the dyslipidemia should be treated first in an attempt to normalize lipoprotein levels. If an abnormal lipid level persists, for example, as it often does with diabetes mellitus type 1 and nephrotic syndrome, the patient requires dietary treatment and, if indicated, pharmacotherapy with use of the same guidelines as in primary dyslipidemias.

GUIDELINES FOR TREATMENT OF DYSLIPIDEMIA IN CHILDREN AND ADOLESCENTS

General guidelines for dietary and pharmacologic treatment of primary and secondary dyslipidemias in youth are

TABLE 12-4	Causes of Secondary Dyslipoproteinemia
Lifestyle	**Medication**
Obesity	Oral contraceptives
Physical inactivity	Glucocorticoids
Diet rich in fat and saturated fat	Anabolic steroids
Alcohol intake	13-*cis*-Retinoic acid
Endocrine and metabolic	Thiazide diuretics
Diabetes mellitus	Anticonvulsants
Metabolic syndrome	Antipsychotics
Hypopituitarism	Estrogen
Hypothyroidism	Testosterone
Pregnancy	Immunosuppressive agents
Polycystic ovarian syndrome	(cyclosporine)
Lipodystrophies	Protease inhibitors
Glycogen storage disease	**Others**
Acute intermittent porphyria	Anorexia nervosa
Renal	Cancer survivor
Chronic renal failure	Burns
Hemolytic-uremic syndrome	Idiopathic hypercalcemia
Nephrotic syndrome	Kawasaki disease
Hepatic	Klinefelter syndrome
Biliary atresia	Progeria (Hutchinson-Gilford
Alagille syndrome	syndrome)
Cirrhosis	Rheumatoid arthritis
Hepatitis	Systemic lupus erythematosus
	Werner syndrome

Reproduced with permission from Kwiterovich PO: Lipid, apolipoprotein and lipoprotein metabolism. In Kwiterovich PO, editor: *The Johns Hopkins textbook of dyslipidemia*, China, 2009, Wolters Kluwer, pp 143-156.

12

presented first. Specific therapies relevant to each inherited disorder of dyslipidemia are addressed in subsequent sections of this chapter.

Dietary Therapy

The first approach to therapy for children with dyslipidemia is a modified diet containing decreased amounts of total fat, saturated fat, *trans*-fat, and cholesterol. The intake of complex carbohydrates is increased, and that of simple sugars is decreased. No decrease in total protein is recommended. Adequate calories should be provided to maintain normal growth and development.

The NCEP Pediatric Panel recommended diet treatment after 2 years of age.[20] Recent data from randomized clinical trials in general populations, such as STRIP, indicate that a diet low in total fat, saturated fat, and cholesterol may be instituted safely and effectively at 6 months of age[10] (see also later).

When to Initiate Dietary Treatment

If the first fasting lipoprotein profile indicates that TC, LDL-C, non–HDL-C, or TG is elevated or the HDL-C is low (see Table 12-3), a repeated profile is obtained at least 3 weeks apart to confirm the first profile. If the dyslipidemia persists (i.e., one or more of the lipid or lipoprotein values remains elevated or the HDL-C is low), secondary causes of dyslipidemia (see Table 12-4) are ruled out and dietary treatment is initiated. A Step I diet is usually started, and the lipoprotein profile is rechecked in 6 to 8 weeks. If the dyslipidemia persists, a Step II diet is begun.

Both diets require the optimal input of a registered dietitian. This may not always be available, and the health care provider, such as the physician or nurse, may need to provide the basis for the diets in Table 12-5 along with printed materials that are available from the American Heart Association. As well, the daily estimated calories and recommended servings for grains, fruits, vegetables, and milk or dairy according to age and gender are available in tabular form from the most recent publication of the American Academy of Pediatrics.[1] Assessment of dietary intakes may become possible in the future by use of the web-based program developed by the National Cancer Institute.

The Step I diet calls for no more than 30% of calories from total fat, <10% of total calories from saturated fatty acids, <300 mg/day of cholesterol, and as little *trans*-fat as possible (only foods with no *trans*-fat on the label are acceptable); given the endemic of overweight and obesity in our society, many children will also require a reduction in simple sugars and an increase in complex carbohydrates. Adequate calories to support growth and development at a desirable body weight are necessary (this does not appear to be the problem in the United States, however). The Step I diet is evaluated for about 2 to 3 months before the Step II diet is prescribed. The Step II diet entails further reduction of saturated fatty acid intake to <7% of calories and cholesterol intake reduction to <200 mg/day.[20] For a comparison of the Step I and Step II diets, see Table 12-5.

Safety and Efficacy of Dietary Therapy in Infants, Children, and Adolescents

The efficacy and safety of diets low in total fat, saturated fat, and cholesterol to lower LDL-C levels in youth have been demonstrated across the age spectrum of pediatric patients,[2] from the age of 7 months to 15 years in STRIP[10,57-59] and from the ages of 8 to 10 years throughout adolescence in the Dietary Intervention Study in Children (DISC).[60-62] A few studies reported lower intakes of calcium, zinc, vitamin E, and phosphorus on low-fat diets.[2] Therefore, whereas

TABLE 12-5	Composition of Step I and Step II Diets	
Nutrient	**Step I Diet**	**Step II Diet**
Total fat (total daily calories)	<30%	<30%
Saturated fatty acids	<10%	<7%
Polyunsaturated fatty acids	≤10%	≤10%
Monounsaturated fatty acids	10%-15%	10%-15%
Cholesterol (daily intake)	<300 mg	<200 mg
Carbohydrates (total daily calories)	50%-60%	50%-60%
Protein (total daily calories)	10%-20%	10%-20%
Total calories	Adequate to achieve and to maintain desirable weight	Adequate to achieve and to maintain desirable weight

12

Evaluation and Management of Dyslipidemia in Children and Adolescents

normal growth is achieved and maintained on low-fat diets, adequate intake of these key nutritional elements must be considered.

Owen and colleagues[63] performed a meta-analysis of 37 publications on the effect of breast versus formula feeding on subsequent TC levels in adolescents and adults. Whereas mean TC was higher in breast-fed versus bottle-fed infants, this did not persist into childhood and adolescence, when there was no relationship of TC to infant feeding. In adults, TC of breast-fed infants was actually lower than TC of formula-fed infants. Human milk remains the "gold standard" for infant feeding.

The use of margarines (about three servings daily) high in either plant stanol esters[64,65] or plant sterol esters[66] can reduce LDL-C an additional 10% to 15% when it is added to a low-fat diet. Water-soluble fibers[67] such as psyllium[68,69] may also provide an additional 5% to 10% lowering of LDL-C. The consumption of a soy protein beverage does not lower LDL-C but may lower VLDL-C and TG and increase HDL-C.[70,71]

Compared with placebo, supplementation of a low-fat diet with an omega-3 fatty acid (docosahexaenoic acid, 1.2 g/day) did not lower LDL-C but changed the distribution between the LDL subclasses, with a significant 91% increase in the largest LDL subclass and a 48% decrease in the smallest LDL subclass 3.[72] Garlic extract therapy does not lower LDL-C in hyperlipidemic children.[73]

Overall, a diet low in fat in children with dyslipidemias appears to be both safe and efficacious when it is performed under supervision. Medical and nutritional support is necessary to reinforce good dietary behaviors and to ensure nutritional adequacy.

Effect of a Low-Fat Diet in Childhood on Future CVD in Adulthood

Prevention of CVD in adulthood by a low–saturated fat, low-cholesterol diet in childhood can be inferred only from epidemiologic studies, in which children from countries with a lower prevalence of CVD had lower TC levels than did children from countries with higher CVD and TC levels.[20] Obesity promotes insulin resistance in childhood. In that regard, a low–saturated fat dietary program starting at 7 months of age improved insulin sensitivity in 9-year-old healthy children in STRIP[74] and lowered blood pressure in 15-year-olds.[59] This same diet was associated with enhanced endothelial function in boys, but not in girls, mediated in part by the diet-induced reduction in TC.[10] After 10 years of follow-up in STRIP, 10% of the intervention girls were overweight compared with 19% of the control girls, but this significant difference was not seen in boys.[75]

Pharmacologic Therapy

Six main classes of lipid-altering drugs are used in children (see Fig. 12-1): HMG-CoA reductase inhibitors (the statins), bile acid sequestrants, cholesterol absorption inhibitors, niacin (nicotinic acid), omega-3 fatty acids (eicosapentaenoic acid and docosahexaenoic acid), and fibric acid derivatives.

Institution of Drug Therapy

The primary use of medication in the pediatric population is to lower significantly elevated LDL-C levels, predominantly but not exclusively in children from families with premature CVD or significant dyslipidemia. Drug treatment to lower LDL-C is initiated in children without other CVD risk factors if LDL-C is persistently ≥190 mg/dL despite a trial of dietary intervention. Drug treatment is started in children older than 10 years if the postdietary LDLC is ≥160 mg/dL and either one or more risk factors for CVD exist, if there is a family history of premature CVD, or if the metabolic syndrome is present. In children with type 1 or 2 diabetes mellitus, pharmacologic treatment should be considered when LDL-C is ≥130 mg/dL (see also later).

Statins and bile acid sequestrants are the two main classes of pharmaceutical agents currently used in children older than 10 years who have sufficiently elevated LDL-C. Ezetimibe, a cholesterol absorption inhibitor that blocks the absorption of cholesterol and plant sterols through the NPC1L1 protein (see Fig. 12-1), is also effective but is not approved by the Food and Drug Administration (FDA) for use in children, except in rare cases of sitosterolemia or homozygous FH (see later).

Each of these three drug classes reduces hepatic cholesterol, leading to the release of the sterol regulatory element–binding protein (SREBP) from the cytoplasm into the nucleus, where SREBP binds to the sterol response element in the promoter of the LDLR gene, increasing the number of LDLR and decreasing LDL-C.[17] Because SREBP also upregulates the gene for HMG-CoA reductase,[17] the bile acid sequestrant and cholesterol absorption inhibitor are both associated with a compensatory increase in cholesterol biosynthesis, limiting their efficacy (see Fig. 12-1). Therefore, both classes of agents might effectively be used in conjunction with statins, which reduce hepatic cholesterol by inhibiting HMG-CoA reductase and decreasing cholesterol biosynthesis.

Niacin is not routinely used in children or adolescents because of its side effects, although some FH homozygotes respond well to niacin (55 to 87 mg/kg/day in divided doses) as a result of a significant reduction of VLDL production, leading to a decreased synthesis of LDL (see Fig. 12-1). In adults, aspirin is used to ameliorate the side effects of niacin. Aspirin is not used in children because of an increased risk for development of Reye syndrome, so low-dose ibuprofen can be used if necessary to prevent flushing.

The fibrates (48 mg, 135 mg, or 145 mg/day) are also not routinely used in pediatrics, except in the adolescent with a persistently elevated TG level >500 mg/dL, who may be at increased risk for development of pancreatitis (see also later). Fish oils (2 to 4 g/day) may also be used to treat marked hypertriglyceridemia in children and adolescents by decreasing the biosynthesis of TG (see Fig. 12-1), but the prescription

version of omega-3 fatty acids is not yet approved by the FDA for use in children.

Bile Acid Sequestrants

Bile acid sequestrants were the only class of drugs recommended by the NCEP Pediatric Panel in 1992 for pharmacologic lipid-lowering therapy because of their record of safety during three decades.[20] In fact, bile acid sequestrants have never been approved by the FDA for use in children. Bile acid sequestrants suffer from significant tolerability issues and provide only a modest LDL-C reduction of about 15%.[76-78] A 17% decrease in LDL-C was reported when cholestyramine (8 g) was used to treat male and female children with heterozygous FH.[77] However, Liacouras and coworkers[78] found that 52 of 63 FH children discontinued cholestyramine treatment after an average of 22 months because of the gritty taste and gastrointestinal complaints.

The second-generation bile acid sequestrant colesevelam (625-mg tablets, three to six per day) has a greater affinity for bile salts and therefore can be used in a lower total dose. In comparison with the first-generation sequestrants, colesevelam is associated with less annoying side effects, such as constipation and gritty taste, and interferes less with absorption of other drugs.

In randomized clinical trials, cholestyramine did not affect height velocity.[77] Fat-soluble vitamins were maintained except that the bile acid sequestrant group had significantly lower 25-hydroxyvitamin D levels than the placebo group did. One girl had low folate and high homocysteine levels.

HMG-CoA Reductase Inhibitors (Statins)

Statins are widely used in adults to lower TC and LDL-C. A number of randomized, placebo-controlled trials demonstrated the safety and efficacy of statins in male and female FH adolescents.[79-87] A meta-analysis of six of these trials showed high efficacy of statins for LDL-C and apo B lowering and no increase in side effects compared with placebo.[87] Atorvastatin, lovastatin, pravastatin, rosuvastatin, and simvastatin are currently approved by the FDA for use in adolescents with FH. Usual starting doses are atorvastatin, 10 mg/day; lovastatin, 40 mg/day; pravastatin, 40 mg/day; rosuvastatin, 5 mg/day; and simvastatin, 20 mg/day. All except atorvastatin and rosuvastatin are available generically.

Wiegman and colleagues[85] studied the effect of pravastatin versus placebo on CIMT as a surrogate marker for atherosclerosis (Fig. 12-2). Children aged 8 to 18 years with heterozygous FH were randomized to pravastatin 20 to 40 mg/day (N = 106) or to placebo (N = 108). After 2 years of treatment, those taking pravastatin had a statistically significant mean reduction in LDL-C of 24% versus 0.3% in placebo. Those taking pravastatin had a significant trend toward regression of CIMT compared with those receiving placebo, who had a trend toward progression of CIMT (P < 0.01).

A follow-up study of this Dutch cohort showed that younger age (8 to 10 years) at statin initiation was an independent predictor of the beneficial effect of treatment on CIMT.[88] Early statin therapy also restored endothelial function in children with FH.[89] The American Academy of Pediatrics has recommended that statin treatment be considered in FH children starting at the age of 8 years.[1] Early intervention with statins appears likely to reduce future atherosclerosis and CVD in those with FH.

Statins may be useful in those adolescents with FCHL or with the metabolic syndrome, who have a LDL-C ≥160 mg/dL after diet and weight control, multiple risk factors, or a family history of premature CVD. Statins may also be useful in young women with polycystic ovarian syndrome (see also later), in which there is evidence of increased CIMT,[90] again suggesting that greater attention be paid to management of dyslipidemia and other CVD risk factors early in life.

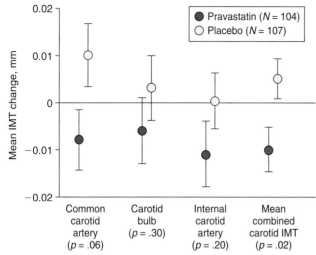

FIGURE 12-2 Mean intima-media thickness (IMT) changes from baseline to 2 years for the different carotid arterial wall segments in the pravastatin (N = 106) and placebo (N =108) groups of children (aged 8 to 18 years) with heterozygous FH. Compared with the baseline, carotid IMT showed a trend toward regression with pravastatin (mean [SD], −0.010 [0.048] mm; *P* = 0.049), whereas a trend toward progression was observed in the placebo group (mean [SD], 0.005 [0.044] mm; *P* = 0.28). The mean (SD) change in IMT between the two groups (0.014 [0.046] mm) was significant (*P* = 0.02). Pravastatin significantly reduced mean LDL-C levels compared with placebo (24.1% versus 0.3%, respectively; *P* = 0.001). *(From Wiegman A, Hutten BA, deGroot E, et al: Efficacy and safety of statin therapy in children with familial hypercholesterolemia: a randomized controlled trial. JAMA 292:331, 2004. Reproduced with permission.)*

Statin Side Effects in Children and Adolescents

Increases in liver function test results up to three times the upper limit of normal were reported in several adolescents treated with higher doses of simvastatin (40 mg/day)[82] and atorvastatin (20 mg/day).[84] In a meta-analysis,[87] the prevalence of elevated alanine aminotransferase in the statin group was 0.66% (3 per 454). Instances of asymptomatic increases (>10-fold) in creatine kinase (CK), although unusual, have been reported in adolescents receiving statin therapy.[87] No cases of rhabdomyolysis have been reported.[79-87] Adolescents are monitored for elevations in hepatic transaminases and CK concentrations. Liver function test results are checked at each clinic visit two or three times per year. CK is measured at baseline, and measurement is repeated if any myalgia develops.

Special Issues in Young Women

Adult women with FH and CAD may be more responsive than similarly affected men to LDL-C–lowering therapy, as assessed by regression of coronary plaques and tendon xanthomas.[91] The overall favorable safety profile of statin therapy in adult women with CVD is well documented; however, fewer studies have examined the effects of statins in adolescent girls.[82,85,86] Nevertheless, no adverse effects on growth and development or on adrenal and gonadal hormones have been reported.[82,85,86] One study found a small increase[81] and another study a small decrease[82] in dehydroepiandrosterone sulfate (DHEAS).

Statins are contraindicated during pregnancy because of the potential risk to a developing fetus. Hence, these drugs should be administered to adolescent girls only when they are highly unlikely to conceive. Birth control is mandatory for those who are sexually active.

Because of these concerns, the long-term commitment to therapy, and the fact that CAD often occurs after menopause, some experts believe that statins should not be used to treat adolescent girls. Although the treatment of adolescent patients with FH is indicated, especially of those with a strong family history of premature CAD, additional studies are needed to document the long-term safety of statin therapy and to determine its potential effects on the prevention of atherosclerosis and coronary events.

Metabolic Syndrome—Beyond Dyslipidemia

If LDL-C is ≥160 mg/dL despite a dietary trial, statin therapy is recommended in patients with the metabolic syndrome. In obese adolescents with metabolic syndrome and LDL-C ≤160 mg/dL, the addition of metformin to diet (low in total fat, saturated fat, *trans*-fat, cholesterol, and simple sugars), exercise, and weight reduction has been shown to be beneficial.[92,93]

Treatment of Dyslipidemia Secondary to Other Diseases

Diabetes Mellitus

Children with type 1 or type 2 diabetes mellitus are in the highest risk category for development of manifest CAD early in adult life.[40] Children with type 1 diabetes and especially type 2 often have a mixed dyslipidemia, the severity of which is related to diabetic control. The American Diabetes Association recommends dietary and other hygienic measures as the first step in the management of these children. However, if the LDL-C is ≥160 mg/dL after an adequate trial, the American Diabetes Association panel strongly recommends pharmacologic treatment, including the use of statins in adolescents.[94] This recommendation is based on the high risk of CVD in adults with diabetes mellitus type 1 and type 2 and partially on the consistent finding of abnormal CIMT in children with diabetes mellitus type 1.

Nephrotic Syndrome

The dyslipidemia in children with nephrotic syndrome is usually quite marked. The average LDL-C level is close to that found in heterozygotes with FH (Table 12-6). TG can approach 300 mg/dL. The combined elevation of LDL-C and VLDL-C can produce a hypercholesterolemia close to 400 mg/dL.[2] Twenty percent of patients with nephrotic syndrome are unresponsive to steroid administration, most cases of which can be attributed to focal segmental glomerulosclerosis. Such individuals with LDL-C ≥160 mg/dL may be at an increased risk for development of atherosclerosis and CVD[1] and may warrant treatment with a statin.

METABOLIC DISORDERS OF DYSLIPIDEMIA IN YOUTH

Disorders Affecting LDL Receptor Activity

There are five disorders expressed in children that result from either mutation in the LDLR or mutations in other genes that affect LDLR activity (Fig. 12-3). Although levels of LDL-C can vary considerably in these five conditions, each disorder manifests early atherosclerosis and premature CVD. These disorders include familial hypercholesterolemia (FH),[95,96] familial ligand defective apo B-100 (FDB),[97] autosomal recessive hypercholesterolemia (ARH),[98,99] sitosterolemia,[100-103] and mutations in proprotein convertase subtilisin/kexin type 9 (PCSK9).[104,105] Each disorder warrants diet and drug therapy in childhood in an attempt to decrease atherosclerosis and subsequent CVD.

Familial Hypercholesterolemia

FH Heterozygotes. FH is the prototype for the diagnosis and treatment of dyslipidemia in children. FH is due to

TABLE 12-6	Lipid, Lipoprotein, and Apolipoprotein B Values in Children with Common Lipoprotein Abnormalities

Lipoprotein Disorder	Age	Total Cholesterol	Triglycerides	HDL-C	LDL-C	Apo B	LDL-C/apo B
			Plasma Concentrations (mg/dL)				
FH (n = 20)	8.0 ± 4.7	323 ± 44	86 ± 36	44 ± 8	262 ± 45	219 ± 42	1.22 ± 0.22
FCHL (n = 65)	9.3 ± 4.7	220 ± 51	120 ± 91	45 ± 11	149 ± 48	153 ± 39	0.98 ± 0.19
HyperapoB (n = 11)	7.8 ± 4.6	200 ± 20	91 ± 35	52 ± 7	130 ± 16	138 ± 21	0.95 ± 0.10
Normals (n = 110)	8.7 ± 1.8	162 ± 31	70 ± 39	51 ± 10	97 ± 27	85 ± 20	1.15 ± 0.20

FH, familial hypercholesterolemia; FCHL, familial combined hyperlipidemia; hyperapoB, hyperapobetalipoproteinemia.
Modified from Cortner JA, Coates PM, Gallagher PR: Prevalence and expression of familial combined hyperlipidemia in childhood. *J Pediatr* 116:514, 1990.

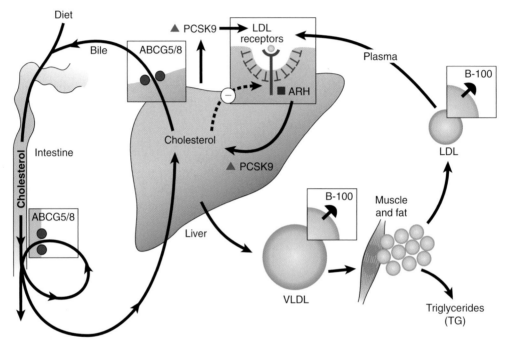

FIGURE 12-3 Schema depicting five inherited disorders of lipoprotein metabolism that are manifested early in life in childhood with marked elevations of LDL, leading to premature atherosclerosis. Apo B, the major apolipoprotein of VLDL and LDL, is necessary for the secretion of VLDL and the uptake of its catabolic product, LDL, by the LDLR. Defects in the structure of apo B-100 (familial ligand defective apo B-100) or in the LDLR (familial hypercholesterolemia) affect the normal binding, internalization, or recycling of the LDLR. Autosomal recessive hypercholesterolemia (ARH) results from a defect in the ARH protein that normally interacts with the cytoplasmic component of the LDLR, allowing the tyrosine phosphorylation and internalization of the LDLR. The PCSK9 is a serine protease that promotes the degradation of the LDLR. Gain-of-function mutations that increase PCSK9 activity decrease LDLR activity. Proposed mechanisms include targeting of the LDLR in the Golgi for degradation in the lysosome, interfering with the recycling of the LDLR after secreted PCSK9 binds to the LDLR at the cell surface, or directing the LDLR to the lysosome to be degraded. The molecular defects responsible for sitosterolemia are caused by mutations in two genes that encode the half-transporters ABCG5 and ABCG8, preventing their normal dual functions of limiting the absorption of cholesterol and plant sterols and promoting their excretion from liver into bile. ABCG5/ABCG8, ATP-binding cassette transporters G5 and G8; PCSK9, proprotein convertase subtilisin-like kexin type 9. *(Modified with permission of Goldstein JL, Brown MS: Molecular medicine. The cholesterol quartet,* Science *292:1310, 2001.)*

mutations in the LDLR gene. Heterozygotes have about a 50% reduction in LDLR, whereas homozygotes have little or no LDLR activity. Children with heterozygous FH, an autosomal dominant disorder, present at birth[24] and early in life[55] with a twofold to threefold elevation in TC and LDL-C[106,107] (see Table 12-6).

When children of an FH parent and a normal parent are screened, on average half will be affected with FH and half will be normal; in these families, the cut point for LDL-C that minimizes misclassification is about 160 mg/dL.[55] FH affects about 1 in 500 and is due to one of more than 1100 different mutations in the LDLR gene.[95,96] These mutations include

insertions, deletions, and missense and nonsense mutations, which can affect the normal synthesis, transport, LDL-binding ability, and clustering (in coated pits) of the LDLR (see Fig. 12-3).

FH heterozygous children and adolescents manifest increased CIMT,[108] decreased brachial endothelial reactivity,[109,110] but rarely overt CAD.[55] Less than 10% of FH adolescent heterozygotes develop tendon xanthomas.[55] In FH children, the null allele genotype was associated with greater CIMT, higher LDL-C, and tendency to attenuated LDL-C lowering with statin therapy compared with receptor-defective mutations.[108]

HDL-C is reduced to a certain extent in FH children compared with normals, presumably secondary to the decreased uptake of IDL by the LDLR, leading to increased IDL and enhanced transfer of TG from IDL to HDL in exchange for CE. About half of untreated adult male heterozygotes and 25% of untreated female heterozygotes will develop CAD before 50 years of age.[95,96] It is highly unusual for CAD to occur in adolescents with heterozygous FH.

Treatment of heterozygous FH includes a diet low in cholesterol, total fat, saturated fat, and *trans*-fat that can usefully be supplemented with plant stanol esters[64] or plant sterol esters[66] and water-soluble fiber.[69] Bile acid sequestrants are safe and moderately effective in FH heterozygotes,[76,77] but long-term compliance is an issue. The dose of the bile acid sequestrant required to achieve LDL-C <160 mg/dL is related to the baseline LDL-C level and *not* to body weight; an adult dose is usually required.[76]

FH heterozygous children respond well to statin therapy.[79-87] However, the addition of a bile acid sequestrant or cholesterol absorption inhibitor to a statin is often necessary to lower LDL-C to a minimum goal of <130 mg/dL. Niacin is generally not used to treat FH heterozygous children unless LDL-C is persistently elevated or unusual hypertriglyceridemia, low HDL-C, or elevated Lp(a) lipoprotein levels are present.

FH Homozygotes. About one in a million children inherit a mutant allele for FH from both parents, leading to LDL-C levels fourfold to eightfold above normal, often causing premature atherosclerosis and death from CVD in the second decade of life.[95,96,107] Atherosclerosis can also affect the aortic valve, leading to severe supravalvular aortic stenosis. Virtually all FH homozygotes have planar xanthomas by the age of 5 years, notably in the webbing of fingers and toes and over the buttocks.

Children and adolescents with the other four disorders affecting LDLR activity (see Fig. 12-3) can also present with planar, tendon, or tuberous xanthomas, as can adolescents with the dominant form of dysbetalipoproteinemia (see later). Secondary disorders of dyslipidemia associated with xanthomas usually have other clinically salient findings to distinguish them from FH homozygotes.

FH homozygotes respond somewhat to high doses of potent statins and to niacin.[111] Because FH homozygotes have markedly diminished LDLR activity, the statins and niacin both work by decreasing hepatic VLDL production, leading to decreased production of LDL-C. Cholesterol absorption inhibitors also lower LDL-C in homozygous FH, especially in combination with a more potent statin.[112] Ultimately, however, FH homozygotes will invariably require regular LDL-C apheresis every 2 weeks to effectively lower LDL-C into a less atherogenic range.[111]

Familial Ligand Defective Apo B-100

FDB results from mutations in the gene encoding apo B-100, resulting in an impaired ability of the apo B-100 ligand on LDL-C to bind to the LDLR[95-97] (see Fig. 12-3). For example, the substitution of glutamine for arginine at residue 3500 produces a defective apo B-100 molecule whose binding to LDLR is deficient, leading to decreased clearance of LDL-C from plasma and elevated LDL-C levels.

Heterozygotes for FDB are relatively common (e.g., 1 per 1000 in Europeans).[96] About 1 in 20 patients with FDB has tendon xanthomas and appears clinically similar to heterozygous FH patients. Some adult patients with FDB develop premature CAD, but FDB itself is not a common cause of premature CAD. Treatment of FDB is similar to that of heterozygous FH.

Autosomal Recessive Hypercholesterolemia

Children with ARH are clinically similar to those with homozygous FH, although LDL-C is not usually as elevated (between

350 and 550 mg/dL).[96] In contrast to homozygous FH, both parents of an ARH child usually have a normal lipoprotein profile. Results of functional assays of LDLR in cultured skin fibroblasts from children with ARH are usually normal or mildly decreased.[98]

At least six mutations have been found in the ARH gene on chromosome 1 in Sardinian and Lebanese kindred.[98] The ARH protein normally interacts with the cytoplasmic component of the LDLR and other cell surface–oriented molecules, allowing their tyrosine phosphorylation. The deficiency of the ARH protein prevents the normal internalization of the LDLR, leading to marked elevations of LDL-C (see Fig. 12-3). Those patients with ARH manifest a dramatic response to statins alone or in combination with a cholesterol absorption inhibitor.[96,98,99]

Sitosterolemia

Sitosterolemia (phytosterolemia) is a rare autosomal recessive disorder that is expressed in childhood and characterized by markedly elevated (>30-fold) plasma levels of plant sterols.[96,100,101] This is due to intestinal hyperabsorption and inefficient hepatic excretion of plant sterols and cholesterol. TC and LDL-C can be normal to markedly elevated, depending on the dietary content of cholesterol and plant sterol. Sitosterolemics absorb a higher percentage of dietary cholesterol than normals do, and they secrete less cholesterol into bile, which decreases LDLR activity and in turn increases LDL-C levels[96,100,101] (see Fig. 12-1).

The diagnosis of sitosterolemia is considered and plant sterols are measured in any child or adolescent who has xanthomas despite a disproportionately low LDL-C. Previously undiagnosed adults can mimic FH heterozygotes. Patients with sitosterolemia may develop aortic stenosis, as do those with homozygous FH.[96,100] CVD can present in the first or second decade of life; however, it is usually delayed until early to middle adulthood.

The molecular defects responsible for sitosterolemia are caused by mutations in two genes that encode the half-transporters ABCG5 and ABCG8.[96,100,101] These two genes on chromosome 2p are located in a head-to-head orientation. ABCG5 and ABCG8 are expressed exclusively in human liver and intestine, the sites of the two metabolic abnormalities in sitosterolemia (see Fig. 12-3). The dual functions of ABCG5 and ABCG8 are to limit the absorption of cholesterol and plant sterols and to promote their excretion from liver into bile.[96,100,101]

Dietary treatment of sitosterolemia is critical, and both cholesterol and plant sterols must be markedly reduced by avoidance of high-fat animal and plant products. Saturated fats are also restricted. Statins are less effective in this disorder because the high sterol content in the liver reduces cholesterol production.[96] Bile acid sequestrants are effective,[96,102,103] as is ezetimibe.[103] The combination of low-dose cholestyramine and ezetimibe in a young sitosterolemic girl led to a marked improvement in plasma sterol concentrations, complete regression of xanthomatosis, resolution of carotid bruits, and improvement in her cardiac murmur.[103]

Mutations in Proprotein Convertase Subtilisin/Kexin Type 9 (PCSK9)

PCSK9 is a serine protease that facilitates the degradation of the LDLR.[104] Gain-of-function mutations that increase PCSK9 activity decrease LDLR activity, producing a phenotype similar to FH.[104,105] Loss-of-function mutations that decrease PCSK9 activity increase LDLR activity, leading to a lifetime of low LDL-C and a markedly reduced incidence of CVD.[104]

The mechanism of action of PCSK9 on LDLR is not completely understood. One possible site of action is in the Golgi, where PCSK9 might target LDLR for degradation in the lysosome.[104] Secreted PCSK9 binds to the LDLR at the cell surface, leading to the internalization of a LDLR/PCSK9 complex in conjunction with ARH (see Fig. 12-3).

PCSK9 may interfere with the recycling of LDLR from the endosome back to the cell surface or direct LDLR to the lysosome to be degraded. It is presently unclear whether PCSK9 cleaves LDLR directly or whether catalytic activity is necessary for either of these pathways. Patients with hypercholesterolemia and the gain-of-function PCSK9 mutation respond well to treatment similar to that used for FH heterozygotes.

Disorders of VLDL and LDL Overproduction

Phenotypes of dyslipidemia that are due to VLDL overproduction include familial combined hyperlipidemia (FCHL), hyperapobetalipoproteinemia, LDL subclass pattern B, familial dyslipidemic hypertension, and syndrome X of Reaven.[113] These phenotypes are pleiotropic, but the common denominator is increased numbers of small, dense LDL. Other features can include hypercholesterolemia, hypertriglyceridemia, elevated apo B with normal or borderline LDL-C, low HDL-C, insulin resistance, diabetes mellitus type 2, glucose intolerance, and hypertension. A predilection to CVD is often present.[113]

Obesity, particularly visceral adiposity, accentuates the expression of these dyslipidemic phenotypes, indicating that the metabolic syndrome and insulin resistance are intertwined from a pathophysiologic viewpoint. No single gene defect in these syndromes has been unequivocally elucidated in humans, and oligogenic factors have been implicated. Treatment of the dyslipidemia (and other aspects) of these phenotypes can successfully start in childhood.

Familial Combined Hyperlipidemia

Goldstein and colleagues[114] described FCHL in families of survivors of myocardial infarction as an autosomal dominant disorder with delayed expression of variable lipoprotein phenotypes: elevated LDL-C level alone (type IIa); elevated LDL-C with hypertriglyceridemia (type IIb); or normal LDL-C with hypertriglyceridemia (type IV).

The prevalence of FCHL is greater than that of FH, occurring in 1 of every 200 to 300 adults. Clinically, it may be difficult to distinguish FCHL from FH if the LDL-C levels are ≥200 mg/dL and the TG levels are normal or moderately elevated. The diagnosis of FCHL is suspected when a first-degree family member has a lipoprotein phenotype different from that of the patient.

Whereas complete expression of FCHL can be delayed until adulthood,[114] it is not unusual to encounter children with FCHL who express different lipoprotein profiles in families with FCHL and premature CAD. In a pediatric lipid clinic, FCHL was three times as prevalent as FH.[106] The mean levels of TC and LDL-C are about 100 mg/dL lower in FCHL children than in children with FH (see Table 12-6). In contrast, mean TG levels are higher in FCHL than in FH children (see Table 12-6).

Total apo B can be elevated in adolescents and young adults with FCHL even before the combined dyslipidemia is fully expressed.[56] Thus, a child might have hyperapobetalipoproteinemia, as judged by an elevated apo B level, but normal LDL-C and TG levels (see Table 12-6). The ratio of LDL-C to apo B is low in FCHL and hyperapobetalipoproteinemia, indicating the presence of small, dense LDL particles, in contrast to FH, in which the LDL-C/apo B ratio is high, reflecting the underlying large LDL-C particles (see Table 12-6).

Tendon xanthomas are not present in children or adults with FCHL. Adult and even adolescent FCHL subjects can develop glucose intolerance, insulin resistance, hypertension, and visceral obesity. The dyslipidemia of FCHL is often associated with an elevated number of small, dense LDL particles out of proportion to the LDL-C level, a finding that can be evaluated beyond the standard lipid profile by measuring either apo B or the level and size of lipoprotein subclasses by nuclear magnetic resonance spectroscopy.[47]

Metabolic Basis of FCHL and Other Small, Dense LDL Syndromes. The abnormal metabolism of FFA in FCHL and other small, dense LDL syndromes may reflect the primary defect in these patients (Fig. 12-4).[113,115] Impaired insulin-mediated suppression of hormone-sensitive lipase in adipocytes leads to an elevation in FFA (see Fig. 12-4). Elevated FFA may drive hepatic overproduction of TG and apo B, leading to a twofold to threefold increased production of

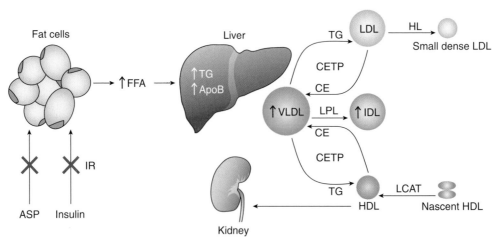

FIGURE 12-4 Mechanisms of the production of the dyslipidemic triad. An increased flux of free fatty acids (FFA) from adipose tissue can result from insulin resistance (IR) or a defect in the acylation stimulatory protein (ASP). Enhanced hepatic uptake of FFA leads to increased production of triglycerides (TG), apolipoprotein (apo B), and VLDL. The TG in VLDL is exchanged for cholesteryl esters (CE) in LDL and HDL by the cholesteryl ester transport protein (CETP), producing CE-depleted LDL and HDL. The TG in the core of LDL and HDL is then hydrolyzed by hepatic lipase (HL), producing both small, dense LDL and smaller HDL. Such HDL is more likely to be excreted by the kidney, resulting in low HDL-C levels. LCAT, lecithin-cholesterol acyltransferase; LPL, lipoprotein lipase. (From Mudd JO, Borlaug BA, Johnston PV, et al: Beyond low-density lipoprotein cholesterol: defining the role of low-density lipoprotein heterogeneity in coronary artery disease. J Am Coll Cardiol 50:1735, 2007. Reproduced with permission.)

VLDL and the dyslipidemic triad (see Fig. 12-4).[47,113,115,116] Insulin resistance also interferes with normal upregulation of LPL, leading to decreased lipolysis of TG in VLDL as well as TG in intestinally derived TG-rich lipoproteins.

This paradigm may also result from a cellular defect that prevents the normal effect of acylation stimulatory protein (see Fig. 12-4), namely, to stimulate the incorporation of FFA into TG in the adipocyte.[117] Insulin resistance may also occur in the liver, leading to an increase rather than a normal decrease in hepatic gluconeogenesis.[118] Finally, FFA and glucose compete as oxidative fuel sources in muscle, such that increased concentrations of FFA inhibit glucose uptake and result in insulin resistance.

Genetic and Molecular Defects

A number of genes (oligogenic effect)[2] may influence the expression of increased particles of small, dense LDL[119] and low HDL-C[120] in FCHL[121,122] and the other small, dense LDL syndromes.[116,121,122] Recently, an orphan G protein–coupled receptor, called C5L2, was reported to bind the acylation stimulatory protein with high affinity and promoted TG synthesis and glucose uptake[123]; however, it is not known if C5L2 is defective in hyperapobetalipoproteinemia patients.

Pajukanta and associates[124] mapped the first major gene locus of FCHL to chromosome 1q21-23 and provided strong evidence that the gene underlying the linkage is the upstream transcription factor 1 (USF-1) gene. USF-1 regulates many important genes in lipid metabolism, including the one coding for hepatic lipase, the activity of which is often increased in patients with these syndromes.

Metabolic Syndrome

There is considerable controversy about whether the metabolic syndrome is a discrete clinical entity or simply an aggregation of multiple risk factors for CVD. The characteristics of the metabolic syndrome certainly mirror the pleiotropic phenotypes found in VLDL overproduction. In the Bogalusa Heart Study, metabolic syndrome variables (i.e., body mass index, insulin resistance, ratio of TG to HDL-C, and mean arterial pressure) coexisted in terms of childhood and adulthood levels and also in long-term rates of change.[39] Thus, obesity predicted other CVD risk factors both in childhood and in adulthood and was of critical importance in the development of the metabolic syndrome.

Overweight and obesity during childhood, as determined by body mass index cutoff points, are strong predictors of obesity and CAD risk factors in young adulthood.[37] Finally, childhood obesity and LDL-C are the two strongest predictors of CIMT in young adults.[2,7] Clearly, the prevention of obesity should start in childhood.

The deleterious effects of obesity are also probably mediated through emerging (nontraditional) risk factors that include atherogenic dyslipidemia. Atherogenic dyslipidemia, also known as the lipid triad, consists of increased numbers of sLDL-P, elevated TG, and low HDL-C; insulin resistance (hyperinsulinemia); a proinflammatory state (elevation of serum high-sensitivity C-reactive protein); and a prothrombotic state (increased amount of plasminogen activator inhibitor 1).

Specific criteria to screen for multiple CVD risk factors including obesity need to be developed for children. There is no current consensus regarding the definition of the metabolic syndrome in youth. That proposed in children aged 12 to 17 years by Cook and associates[30] from the third NHANES survey is one of several. By use of NHANES data, an adolescent was considered to have the metabolic syndrome if three or more of these factors were present: TG ≥110 mg/dL; HDL-C ≤40 mg/dL; waist circumference ≥90th percentile; fasting glucose concentration ≥110 mg/dL; and blood pressure ≥90th percentile for age, sex, and height.

One alternative to waist circumference may be a body mass index >95th percentile for age and gender. Whereas waist circumference and body mass index in children are not routinely determined, recent data from the Bogalusa Heart Study[125] indicate that both body mass index and waist circumference values, when categorized by a threshold approach, independently predicted CAD risk factors.

The metabolic syndrome is of paramount interest, given its endemic nature in our children.[2,30,34-39] In the past two decades, the prevalence of adolescents with a body mass index >95th percentile increased by more than 50%.[34] The prevalence of the metabolic syndrome in adolescents increases with the severity of obesity and insulin resistance.[36] Obese adolescents with the metabolic syndrome also often have the dyslipidemic triad.[34,36] Higher blood pressure levels in such adolescents are associated with increased CIMT as a marker for occult atherosclerosis.[35]

The presence of the metabolic syndrome in childhood predicts the adult metabolic syndrome, diabetes mellitus type 2, and the development of CVD two to three decades later.[126,127] The finding of acanthosis nigricans reflects the insulin resistance that is often present. In addition, biomarkers for increased risk of atherosclerotic disease, such as high-sensitivity C-reactive protein and adiponectin, were increased and decreased, respectively, in obese children.[36]

Measurement of lipoprotein subclasses by nuclear magnetic resonance spectroscopy (despite the fact that this is not yet recommended for routine clinical practice) provides some insights into the relationship of lipoprotein heterogeneity and obesity and other components of the metabolic syndrome.[2] TG, insulin, and relative weight in children from an unselected population were positively associated with the size of VLDL and negatively associated with the size of LDL particles.[50] Large VLDL but not small VLDL was notably higher in white than in black children across quintiles of waist circumference.[51] The presence of fatty liver in obese adolescents was associated with a pronounced dyslipidemic profile characterized by large VLDL, small dense LDL, and decreased concentration of large HDL particles.[52] This proatherogenic phenotype was strongly related to the intrahepatic lipid content.

Polycystic Ovarian Syndrome

Polycystic ovarian syndrome (PCOS) often presents in adolescence as menstrual disorders, acne, and hirsutism.[2,90,128] Insulin resistance, considered one of the underlying causes of PCOS, has increased substantially in the past decade, putting more adolescent girls at risk for PCOS and its complications, including elevated LDL-C and apo B. After initial diet and weight control, a combination of estrogen and progesterone is used for treatment of PCOS.[128]

Only about one in three specialists consider metformin appropriate treatment in teenagers with PCOS; however, in obese teenagers with PCOS, almost 70% would use metformin.[128] Adults with PCOS appear to be at high risk for CVD.[90] Increased CIMT occurs in young adults with PCOS,[90] indicating that early diagnosis and treatment of PCOS in adolescence may prevent its full expression and adverse CVD complications in adulthood.

Treatment of Disorders of VLDL Overproduction

A low-fat diet reduces the burden of postprandial chylomicrons and the atherogenic chylomicron remnants (see Fig. 12-1). Reduction to ideal body weight improves insulin sensitivity and decreases overproduction of VLDL. Regular aerobic exercise is of paramount importance. Two classes of drugs, fibric acids and niacin, lower TG and increase HDL-C in adults and may also convert small, dense LDL particles into larger LDL particles.[113] However, fibrates and niacin are not ordinarily used in pediatric patients.[2,20] The statins are the most effective in lowering LDL-C and the total number of atherogenic, small, dense LDL particles.[113]

In adolescents with FCHL or with the metabolic syndrome, drug treatment with a single agent, most often a statin, is reserved for those with a more marked elevation of LDL-C >160 mg/dL (see also earlier). Cholestyramine has also been used to treat pediatric patients with FCHL who have elevated LDL-C.[78] Metformin has been used to treat obese hyperinsulinemic adolescents with the metabolic syndrome.[92,93] Metformin can enhance insulin sensitivity and reduce fasting blood glucose concentration, insulin, lipids, FFA, and leptin.[92,93]

Familial Metabolic Disorders of Triglyceride-Rich Lipoproteins

12

Metabolic disorders involving the TG-rich lipoproteins—chylomicrons, VLDL, and their remnants—are heterogeneous. Hypertriglyceridemia may result from increased synthesis or decreased catabolism of one or more of these lipoprotein classes or from a combination of enhanced synthesis and suppressed catabolism.

Most hypertriglyceridemia in children and adolescents is due to VLDL overproduction, often accompanied by obesity or overweight and other components of the metabolic syndrome (see earlier). The focus here is on inherited disorders of marked hypertriglyceridemia. The most serious complication of marked hypertriglyceridemia is pancreatitis. Some but not all families with hypertriglyceridemia will ultimately manifest CVD in middle age.

Endogenous Hypertriglyceridemia

Familial Hypertriglyceridemia. In some children, TC and LDL-C levels are normal but VLDL-C and TG are elevated (type IV lipoprotein pattern). Familial hypertriglyceridemia (FHTG) can be distinguished from FCHL by demonstrating that affected parents and siblings of the proband have normal LDL-C and apo B levels (see Table 12-3). In contrast, in relatives with FCHL, these levels are borderline high or elevated (see Table 12-5).

Whereas VLDL particles in FHTG and FCHL are both TG enriched, VLDL and apo B are not being overproduced in FHTG as they are in FCHL. HDL-C is low or normal in FHTG. Adults with FHTG often manifest glucose intolerance, obesity, hyperuricemia, and peripheral vascular disease. The disorder may be inherited as an autosomal dominant trait with reduced penetrance in childhood; for example, only one in five children younger than 20 years born to an affected parent expresses FHTG.

Exogenous Hypertriglyceridemia

Two classic inherited disorders result from absent or markedly deficient activity of LPL: a defect in LPL and a defect in apo C-II, the cofactor for LPL (see Fig. 12-1).[129] A newer unique defect of chylomicronemia has recently been described, a deficiency of glycosylphosphatidylinositol-anchored high-density lipoprotein–binding protein 1 (GPIHBP1) associated with chylomicronemia.[130] GPIHBP is an endothelial cell protein that normally binds LPL and chylomicrons. A homozygous mutation (Q115P) in *GPIHBP1* eliminates the normal binding of GPIHBP to LPL.

Defective or Missing Lipoprotein Lipase. Defective LPL produces a profound hypertriglyceridemia (as high as 10,000 mg/dL) because of the massive increases in chylomicrons and the inability to clear dietary fat.[129] Marked hypercholesterolemia (e.g., 300 to 1000 mg/dL) is also present secondary to hyperchylomicronemia, with a ratio of TG to TC of at least 5 and usually 10. VLDL-C is normal, and HDL-C and LDL-C are low. LPL activity is absent in plasma and adipose tissue of patients with this disorder (also called type I hyperlipoproteinemia).

The half-life of chylomicrons is prolonged about sixfold. The plasma levels of apo C-II, the cofactor for LPL, are normal. The diagnosis requires measurement of plasma lipolytic activity after intravenous injection of heparin (60 units/kg), which releases the membrane-bound lipases into the bloodstream (post heparin lipolytic activity [PHLA]).

This disorder usually is manifested early in the first year of life. Creamy blood is often noted after a blood draw or in a hematocrit tube after a fingerstick. Abdominal pain is a common symptom that is manifested as colic during infancy or as an acute abdominal discomfort later in childhood. Other clinical features may include eruptive xanthomas, hepatosplenomegaly, and lipemia retinalis.

Premature atherosclerosis does not occur in LPL deficiency because chylomicrons are too large to enter the vascular wall and are therefore not atherogenic. LPL deficiency is a rare recessive trait. Obligate heterozygous parents of affected children are often consanguineous and have normal lipid levels or a moderate dyslipidemia. More than 80 mutations in the LPL gene have been reported.[129]

Defect in Apolipoprotein C-II. When apo C-II, the cofactor for LPL, is deficient, hypertriglyceridemia can range from 800 to almost 10,000 mg/dL; the lipoprotein pattern may be type I, or the elevated chylomicrons may be accompanied by elevated VLDL (type V).[1,129] TC is normal or increased (151 to 980 mg/dL). LDL-C and HDL-C are low (<5th percentile). PHLA is absent or very low. Plasma apo C-II is present in only trace amounts.

If apo C-II is added to plasma in vitro or by blood or plasma transfusion in vivo, normal PHLA is restored. This disorder is a rare, autosomal recessive trait. Pancreatitis, which usually is manifested in adulthood, is the major clinical problem. Pancreatitis developed in one homozygous child by 6 years of age. Abnormalities of the apo C-II gene are caused by either small deletions or by splice-site mutations.[129]

Defect in GPIHBP1. Sixty patients with severe hypertriglyceridemia were screened for mutations in GPIHBP1, an endothelial cell protein that binds LPL and chylomicrons. Mice lacking GPIHBP1 had been found to develop TG levels above 2000 mg/dL even on a low-fat chow diet.[130] The ability of GPIHBP1-expressing CHO cells to bind LPL and chylomicrons suggested that this protein may function as a platform for lipolysis on endothelial cells in heart, skeletal muscle, and adipose tissue.

One 33-year-old man with life-long chylomicronemia was found to be homozygous for a *GPIHBP1* (Q115P) mutation. He had failure to thrive as a child but no history of pancreatitis. After a PHLA test, he had low levels of LPL at 10% of normal, the cause of which requires further study. He responded to a low-fat diet, with the TG level falling from 3366 mg/dL to 744 mg/dL.

Treatment of Profound Exogenous Hypertriglyceridemia

Stringent fat restriction to 10 to 15 g/day is required. Intake of linoleic acid as ~1% of total calories must be maintained. Medium-chain TG (MCT), which are absorbed directly through the portal vein and therefore do not require mobilization of chylomicrons from the intestine into plasma, can be added to the diet as 15% of calories to make the diet more palatable. Infants with a type I pattern may take a formula high in MCT.

A subset of LPL-deficient children with unique, possibly post-transcriptional genetic defects respond to therapy with MCT oil or omega-3 fatty acids by normalizing fasting TG levels. Thus, a therapeutic trial with MCT oil should be considered in all children presenting with the familial chylomicronemia syndrome.[2,131] A dramatic response to antioxidant therapy was reported in a small number of patients with LPL deficiency for whom dietary measures failed and in whom frequent severe episodes of pancreatitis developed.

Endogenous and Exogenous Hypertriglyceridemia

Type V Hyperlipoproteinemia

Patients with marked hypertriglyceridemia may also present with increased chylomicrons and VLDL (type V lipoprotein phenotype). Common clinical findings include pancreatitis, eruptive xanthomas, lipemia retinalis, abnormal glucose tolerance, and insulin resistance. Because LPL and apo C-II are not deficient, lipolysis of TG on both chylomicrons and VLDL occurs, albeit at a reduced rate. This leads to the production of both chylomicron remnants and VLDL remnants; thus, both peripheral and coronary atherosclerosis can develop in type V patients.

Although type V is usually expressed in young adulthood, this phenotype has been reported in several preadolescent children. Affected relatives may have either type V or type IV lipoprotein phenotypes. Autosomal dominant inheritance has been described in several large families.

Elevated VLDL may result from increased synthesis, decreased clearance, or a combination of both, but the fundamental defect in many of these patients has remained elusive. In two unrelated male and female patients with type V, Cao and colleagues[132] found two different heterozygous frameshift mutations in *CAV1* that encodes caveolin 1. Mice with a deleted *CAV1* develop adipocyte abnormalities and insulin resistance. Thus, the genomic DNA from patients with atypical lipodystrophy and hypertriglyceridemia (with no mutations in any known lipodystrophy gene) was screened for defects in the coding regions of human *CAV1*.

Dysbetalipoproteinemia (Type III Hyperlipoproteinemia)

Patients with dysbetalipoproteinemia present with elevated TC and TG levels, often above 300 mg/dL. The hyperlipidemia is caused by the accumulation of chylomicron remnants derived from intestinal lipoproteins and VLDL remnants derived from hepatic lipoproteins.

Dysbetalipoproteinemia is conventionally defined by a cholesterol-rich VLDL that has β rather than pre-β electrophoretic mobility.[2,133] Ultracentrifugation of plasma, without density adjustment (density <1.006 g/mL), is required for the diagnosis to be made. The ratio of VLDL-C to plasma total TG is usually >0.3 (normal, 0.15 to 0.25). Such "beta" VLDL reflects the accumulation of both chylomicron and VLDL remnants.

This recessive defect involves a polymorphic genetic locus that specifies the structure of apo E.[133] Apo E binds to receptors on the surface of hepatocytes, promoting uptake of both chylomicron and VLDL remnants. Human apo E exists as three major isoforms (apo E2, apo E3, and apo E4), each of which is specified by an independent allele at the locus for the apo E gene. The most common allele is apo E3. The necessary but insufficient cause of type III hyperlipoproteinemia is the presence of two copies of apo E2, which differ from the most common isoform of apo E (apo E3) by a single amino acid substitution, which is associated with the recessive form of dysbetalipoproteinemia.[133]

One in 100 people is homozygous for the apo E2 allele. Most patients with dysbetalipoproteinemia are apo E2 homozygotes; because the prevalence of the disorder is low at 1:10,000, other modifying factors, such as an overproduction of VLDL in the liver (seen in FCHL) or hormonal and environmental conditions (hypothyroidism, low-estrogen state, obesity, or diabetes mellitus), are necessary for complete clinical expression. This recessive form of dysbetalipoproteinemia has a delayed penetrance. The dominant form of dysbetalipoproteinemia can be expressed in childhood and does not require the presence of modifying factors. However, clinical features of the disease are often delayed until adulthood.

In both the recessive and dominant forms of dysbetalipoproteinemia, affected patients often develop xanthomas, particularly yellowish deposits in the palmar creases (xanthoma striatum palmare) and tuberous and tuberoeruptive xanthomas over the elbows, knees, and buttocks. Tendon xanthomas are much less frequent. Premature atherosclerosis of the coronary, carotid, abdominal, and femoral arteries is prevalent. Hyperuricemia and glucose intolerance occur in up to half the patients with this syndrome.

Treatment of the Combined Exogenous and Endogenous Triglyceride Disorders

Treatment starts with a diet low in total and saturated fat, *trans*-fat, cholesterol, and simple carbohydrates but higher in complex carbohydrates and protein (see also earlier) and weight management with reduction to ideal body mass. If TG level remains >500 mg/dL, drug therapy, including fibrates, niacin, fish oils (omega-3), and statins (see Fig. 12-1), can be considered starting in adolescence, particularly in patients who have a strong family history of premature CVD or a history of eruptive xanthomas or pancreatitis.

Familial Disorders of HDL Metabolism

In most instances, low HDL-C occurs secondary to VLDL overproduction (see Fig. 12-3) and is expressed as a component of the dyslipidemic triad. There are, however, primary HDL-C disorders that present with low HDL-C levels and CVD: familial hypoalphalipoproteinemia[134,135]; homozygous gene deletions or nonsense mutations in apo A-I[18]; missense mutations in apo A-I[136,137]; more than 100 common and rare variants in ABCA1, including the prototype, Tangier disease[138]; and LCAT deficiency.[139]

One disorder, CETP deficiency, often presents as high HDL-C, but whether this is associated with increased or reduced risk for CVD is not resolved. Inhibition of CETP with torcetrapib increased large HDL but was associated with an increased total and CVD mortality.[140]

Hypoalphalipoproteinemia

Hypoalphalipoproteinemia is defined as low HDL-C (<5th percentile or <35 mg/dL; see Table 12-3) in the presence of otherwise normal lipids and number of sLDL-P. Adults with this syndrome exhibit an increased prevalence of CVD; however, such patients do not manifest the clinical findings typical of severe forms of HDL deficiency, such as planar xanthomas, corneal clouding, and peripheral neuropathy.[18]

Primary hypoalphalipoproteinemia, although more prevalent than the rare recessive disorders, including deficiencies in HDL, is relatively uncommon.[134,135] In some families, hypoalphalipoproteinemia behaves like an autosomal dominant trait and can be associated with genetic variants.[18]

Apolipoprotein A-I Variants

A number of apo A-I variants have been described and are attributed to specific amino acid substitutions.[2,18,136,137] For example, apo A-I Milano results from a mutation in the apo A-I gene at codon 173, changing arginine to cysteine.[137] Heterozygous carriers for autosomal codominant traits often have low HDL-C but are usually asymptomatic in regard to premature CVD. Intravenous injection of recombinant apo A-I Milano weekly for 6 weeks appeared to reduce coronary atherosclerosis in adults with acute coronary syndromes.[137]

Tangier disease[138] is a rare metabolic disorder, originally described by Donald Fredrickson in two young girls from Tangier Island in the Chesapeake Bay,[141] in which HDL is both abnormal and present in severely reduced concentration. Tangier homozygotes have plasma apo A-I levels <3% of normal. Immunochemically detectable apo A-I is synthesized by intestinal cells but is rapidly degraded in plasma.

HDL in Tangier disease (termed HDL_T) is markedly abnormal; a chylomicron-like lipoprotein particle is present in the density range of HDL on a normal high-fat diet. These abnormal lipoproteins are rich in CE and are likely to be sequestered by the reticuloendothelial cells in Tangier disease. These large, flattened, lucent particles, 100 nm in diameter, disappear when a low-fat diet is consumed. These observations suggest that HDL is necessary for normal metabolism of chylomicrons.

The compositions and amounts of the other lipoproteins are also abnormal. TC is decreased, with normal or elevated TG. The lipoprotein abnormalities are accompanied by a striking deposition of CE in different tissues. The major clinical manifestations reflect the lipid storage and include enlarged orange-yellow tonsils, splenomegaly, and a relapsing peripheral neuropathy. Mild hepatomegaly, lymphadenopathy, and corneal infiltration (in adulthood) may also appear. Foam cells can be demonstrated on biopsy of the skin, bone marrow, peripheral nerves, or rectum.

The apo A-I gene is normal in Tangier disease. The basic defect resides in mutations in ABCA1.[138] Thus, ABCA1 was discovered by virtue of studies in Tangier patients from three laboratories. ABCA1 normally mediates the efflux of cellular cholesterol onto the nascent HDL particle for transport to the liver (see Fig. 12-1).

Lecithin-Cholesterol Acyltransferase Deficiency and Fish Eye Disease

LCAT is an enzyme bound to HDL-C (α-LCAT) and to a lesser extent to VLDL/LDL-C (β-LCAT) in the plasma.[139] LCAT catalyzes the formation of CE in lipoproteins. The two familial forms of LCAT deficiency are termed familial LCAT deficiency (complete LCAT deficiency) and fish eye disease (partial LCAT deficiency). Both familial LCAT deficiency and fish eye disease are autosomal recessive disorders.

In classic LCAT deficiency, both α-LCAT and β-LCAT activities are absent, resulting in a markedly reduced plasma cholesterol esterification rate, a low plasma cholesteryl ester content, and an abnormal lipoprotein profile with very low HDL-C. Clinical findings include glomerulosclerosis, normochromic anemia, corneal opacities (detectable in childhood), and premature atherosclerosis. Specific defects in the LCAT gene, including stop codons and amino acid substitutions, have been elucidated in several kindred with classic LCAT deficiency.[139]

Fish eye disease is a phenotypically distinct syndrome of LCAT deficiency in which most but not all patients appear to have a selective defect in α-LCAT activity, which is accompanied by dense corneal opacities; low HDL-C is present, but premature atherosclerosis does not develop. Several molecular defects have been described in the LCAT gene of patients with fish eye disease. An interesting mutation, LCAT(300-del), has led to the postulate that the heterogeneity in the phenotypic syndromes of LCAT deficiency may be related to the residual amounts of total plasma LCAT activity.

Treatment. In Tangier disease, a low-fat diet diminishes the abnormal lipoprotein species that are believed to be remnants of abnormal chylomicron metabolism. The large LDL-C species found in LCAT deficiency is also thought to be a remnant of abnormal chylomicron metabolism. Its disappearance on a low-fat diet may have a beneficial effect because large LDL-C may be involved in the pathogenesis of renal disease. Patients with other syndromes associated with deficiencies of HDL-C and premature atherosclerosis are also treated with a diet significantly reduced in total fat, saturated fat, *trans*-fat, and cholesterol.

Hyperalphalipoproteinemia

In distinct contrast to hypoalphalipoproteinemia, some children have very high HDL-C levels (>95th percentile), termed hyperalphalipoproteinemia. TC concentration is often elevated as a result of elevated HDL-C levels; LDL-C concentration is usually normal, and TG levels are normal or low. Hyperalphalipoproteinemia is often associated with longevity and a decreased risk of CVD. Hyperalphalipoproteinemia can be due to a defect in CETP. Lower SR-B1 levels and two SNPs in the SR-B1 gene (see Fig. 12-1) were found in subjects with hyperalphalipoproteinemia.[142]

Decreased activity of endothelial lipase due to loss-of-function mutations in *LIPG* constitutes a novel genetic basis of familial hyperalphalipoproteinemia.[143] Several kindred with hyperalphalipoproteinemia have been described in which affected members have defects in hepatic lipase (see Fig. 12-1). Mutations in hepatic lipase are associated with elevated HDL-C levels in the paradoxical presence of hypertriglyceridemia. Few data are available on the expression of hepatic lipase defects in children.

Elevated Levels of Lp(a) Lipoprotein

Lp(a) lipoprotein is a very large molecule (M_r 3×10^6) found in the density range of 1.050 to 1.080 g/mL.[144] Its lipid composition is similar to LDL, but Lp(a) contains two proteins, apo B-100 and a large glycoprotein called apo(a). Apo(a) is attached to apo B-100 through a disulfide bond. Apo(a) is homologous to plasminogen with a yet uncertain biologic function and has a variable number of repeats of the kringle 4 region, which are under genetic control. An inverse relationship exists between the size of apo(a) and the level of Lp(a).[144]

At present, most laboratories that measure Lp(a) use commercially available antibodies. Elevated Lp(a) appears to be inherited and is often strongly associated with premature CVD in some families. An Lp(a) level is usually elevated in children with strokes and should be measured as part of the workup in every child.[1] Niacin is the only lipid-altering drug that reduces Lp(a). It is currently unknown if treatment of elevated Lp(a) prevents development of future or recurrent CVD; however, current recommendations are to aggressively lower LDL-C when the Lp(a) is high.

Deficiencies in Apo B–Containing Lipoproteins

The discussion here is limited to those genetic conditions of low LDL-C levels and reduced CAD. For the rarer primary or secondary disorders of deficiencies of apo B–containing lipoproteins that present in early childhood, the reader is referred elsewhere.[145]

Hypobetalipoproteinemia

The phenotype of primary hypobetalipoproteinemia is characterized by very low levels of LDL-C, usually defined as the lower 5th percentile of a normal distribution. Plasma TC concentration is low; VLDL-C and TG levels are low or normal.

Familial Hypobetalipoproteinemia. Familial hypobetalipoproteinemia is inherited as an autosomal dominant. A relatively large number of mutations in *APOB* causing hypobetalipoproteinemia have been described.[146] Almost all of the mutations are either nonsense mutations or frameshift mutations that create a premature stop codon and a truncated apo B-100. The endogenous VLDL system (see Fig. 12-1) is defective because the apo B-100 product of the normal allele is produced at approximately 25% of normal, and the truncated apo B is cleared too rapidly from plasma.[146] This results in decreased production of apo B-100 and VLDL and low LDL-C (see Fig. 12-1).

Familial hypobetalipoproteinemia has also been linked to a susceptibility locus on the chromosome 3p21 and in some families is linked neither to *APOB* nor to chromosome 3p21.[146] Familial hypobetalipoproteinemia patients are usually asymptomatic, the prevalence of CVD is low, and often longevity is found. Those with a defect in apo B can have increased hepatic fat of about threefold.

Loss-of-Function Mutations in PCSK9. The phenotype of hypobetalipoproteinemia is also found in those with a loss-of-function mutation in the PCSK9 gene.[147] In this case, the low LDL results not from decreased production of LDL but from enhanced LDLR activity due to the decreased PCSK9 function[147,148] (see Fig. 12-3). Patients with this cause of familial hypobetalipoproteinemia also have a considerable lifelong reduction in CVD,[147,148] presumably starting at birth or early in life.

CONCLUSION

Early lesions of atherosclerosis begin in childhood and are related to antecedent CVD risk factors. Environmental factors such as diet, obesity, and exercise and certain inherited dyslipidemias influence the progression of such lesions. Detection of youth at risk for atherosclerosis includes an integrated evaluation of these predisposing factors. Treatment starts with a diet low in saturated fat, *trans*-fat, and cholesterol. Such intervention can be supplemented with water-soluble fiber, plant stanols or plant sterols, weight control, and exercise.

Drug therapy, especially with HMG-CoA reductase inhibitors or bile acid sequestrants, can be considered in those with a positive family history of premature CVD and LDL-C ≥160 mg/dL, after a period of dietary and hygienic measures. Candidates for drug therapy often include those with FH, FCHL, the metabolic syndrome, polycystic ovarian syndrome, type 1 or type 2 diabetes, and the nephrotic syndrome. Such dietary and drug therapy appears to be safe and efficacious.

The early identification and treatment of children with CVD risk factors and dyslipidemia are likely to retard the atherosclerotic process. Optimal identification and treatment of high-risk youth either from the general population or from families with premature CVD will require an integrated universal screening, evaluation, treatment, and follow-up program.

REFERENCES

1. Daniels SR, Greer FR: Lipid screening and cardiovascular health in childhood. *Pediatrics* 122:198, 2008.
2. Kwiterovich PO Jr: Clinical and laboratory assessment of cardiovascular risk in children: guidelines for screening, evaluation and treatment. *J Clin Lipidol* 2:248, 2008.
3. McGill HC Jr, McMahan CA, Zieske AW, et al: Associations of coronary heart disease risk factors with the intermediate lesion of atherosclerosis in youth. The Pathobiological Determinants of Atherosclerosis in Youth (PDAY) Research Group. *Arterioscler Thromb Vasc Biol* 20:1998, 2000.
4. Berenson GS, Srinivasan SR, Bao W, et al: Association between multiple cardiovascular risk factors and atherosclerosis in children and young adults. The Bogalusa Heart Study. *N Engl J Med* 338:1650, 1998.
5. Mahoney LT, Burns TL, Stanford W, et al: Coronary risk factors measured in childhood and young adult life are associated with coronary calcification in young adults: the Muscatine Study. *J Am Coll Cardiol* 27:277, 1996.
6. Davis PH, Dawson JD, Riley WA, et al: Carotid intimal-medial thickness is related to cardiovascular risk factors measured from childhood through middle age: The Muscatine Study. *Circulation* 104:2815, 2001.

7. Li S, Chen W, Srinivasan SR, et al: Childhood cardiovascular risk factors and carotid vascular changes in adulthood: the Bogalusa Heart Study. *JAMA* 290:17271, 2003.
8. Frontini MG, Srinivasan SR, Xu J, et al: Usefulness of childhood non–high density lipoprotein cholesterol levels versus other lipoprotein measures in predicting adult subclinical atherosclerosis: the Bogalusa Heart Study. *Pediatrics* 121:924, 2008.
9. Gidding SS, McMahan CA, McGill HC, et al: Prediction of coronary artery calcium in young adults using the Pathobiological Determinants of Atherosclerosis in Youth (PDAY) risk score: the CARDIA study. *Arch Intern Med* 166:2341, 2006.
10. Raitakari OT, Rönnemaa T, Järvisalo MJ, et al: Endothelial function in healthy 11-year-old children after dietary intervention with onset in infancy: the Special Turku Coronary Risk Factor Intervention Project for children (STRIP). *Circulation* 112:3786, 2005.
11. McMahan CA, Gidding SS, Viikari JS, et al: Association of Pathobiologic Determinants of Atherosclerosis in Youth risk score and 15-year change in risk score with carotid artery intima-media thickness in young adults (from the Cardiovascular Risk in Young Finns Study). *Am J Cardiol* 100:1124, 2007.
12. Juonala M, Viikari JSA, Rönnemaa T, et al: Associations of dyslipidemias from childhood to adulthood with carotid intima-media thickness, elasticity, and brachial flow–mediated dilatation in adulthood. The Cardiovascular Risk in Young Finns Study. *Arterioscler Thromb Vasc Biol* 28:1012, 2008. Epub 2008 Feb 28.
13. Klag MJ, Ford DE, Mead LA, et al: Serum cholesterol in young men and subsequent cardiovascular disease. *N Engl J Med* 328:313, 1993.
14. Lee J, Lauer RM, Clarke WR: Lipoproteins in the progeny of young men with coronary artery disease: children with increased risk. *Pediatrics* 78:330, 1986.
15. Sniderman AD, Teng B, Genest J, et al: Familial aggregation and early expression of hyperapobetalipoproteinemia. *Am J Cardiol* 55:291, 1985.
16. Freedman DS, Srinivasan SR, Shear CL, et al: The relation of apolipoproteins A-I and B in children to parental myocardial infarction. *N Engl J Med* 315:721, 1986.
17. Horton J, Goldstein JL, Brown MS: SREBPs: activators of the complete program of cholesterol and fatty acid synthesis in the liver. *J Clin Invest* 109:1125, 2002.
18. Rader DJ: Molecular regulation of HDL metabolism and function: implications for novel therapies. *J Clin Invest* 116:3090, 2006.
19. Tall AR, Yvan-Charvet L, Terasaka N, et al: HDL, ABC transporters, and cholesterol efflux: implications for the treatment of atherosclerosis. *Cell Metab* 7:365, 2008.
20. National Cholesterol Education Program: Report of the Expert Panel on Blood Cholesterol Levels in Children and Adolescents. *Pediatrics* 89:525, 1992.
21. Webber LS, Srinivasan SR, Wattigney WA, et al: Tracking of serum and lipids and lipoproteins from childhood to adulthood: the Bogalusa Heart Study. *Am J Epidemiol* 133:984, 1991.
22. Bachorik PS, Lovejoy KL, Carroll MD, et al: Apolipoprotein B and AI distributions in the United States. 1988-1991: Results of the National Health and Nutrition Examination Survey III (NHANES III). *Clin Chem* 43:2364, 1997.
23. Ford ES, Li C, Zhao G, et al: Concentration of low-density lipoprotein cholesterol and total cholesterol among children and adolescents in the United States. *Circulation* 119:1108, 2009.
24. Kwiterovich PO Jr, Levy RI, Fredrickson DS: Neonatal diagnosis of familial type-II hyperlipoproteinemia. *Lancet* 1:118, 1973.
25. Kwiterovich PO Jr, Barton BA, McMahon RP, et al: Effects of diet and sexual maturation of LDL-cholesterol during puberty: the Dietary Intervention Study in Children (DISC). *Circulation* 96:2526, 1997.
26. Friedman LA, Morrison JA, Daniels SR, et al: Sensitivity and specificity of pediatric lipid determinations for adult lipid status: findings from the Princeton Lipid Research Clinics Prevalence Program Follow-up Study. *Pediatrics* 118:165, 2006.
27. Jolliffe CJ, Janssen I: Distribution of lipoproteins by age and gender in adolescents. *Circulation* 114:1056, 2006.
28. Magnussen CG, Raitakari OT, Thomson R, et al: Utility of currently recommended pediatric dyslipidemia classifications in predicting dyslipidemia in adulthood: evidence from the Childhood Determinants of Adult Health (CDAH) study, Cardiovascular Risk in Young Finns Study, and Bogalusa Heart Study. *Circulation* 117:32, 2008.
29. Webber LS, Osganian V, Luepker RV, et al: Cardiovascular risk factors among third grade children in four regions of the United States. The CATCH Study: Child and Adolescent Trial for Cardiovascular Health. *Am J Epidemiol* 141:528, 1995.
30. Cook S, Weitzman M, Auinger P, et al: Prevalence of a metabolic syndrome phenotype in adolescents: findings from the third National Health and Nutrition Examination Survey, 1988-1994. *Arch Pediatr Adolesc Med* 157:821, 2003.
31. Lauer RM, Lee J, Clarke WR: Factors affecting the relationship between childhood and adult cholesterol levels: the Muscatine Study. *Pediatrics* 82:309, 1988.
32. Lauer RM, Clarke WR: Use of cholesterol measurements in childhood for the prediction of adult hypercholesterolemia: the Muscatine Study. *JAMA* 264:23034, 1990.
33. Haney EM, Huffman LH, Bougatsos C, et al: Screening and treatment for lipid disorders in children and adolescents: systematic evidence review for the US Preventive Services Task Force. *Pediatrics* 120:e189, 2007.
34. Troiano RP, Flegal KM: Overweight children and adolescents: description, epidemiology, and demographics. *Pediatrics* 101:497, 1998.
35. Vos LE, Oren A, Uiterwaal C, et al: Adolescent blood pressure and blood pressure tracking into young adulthood are related to subclinical atherosclerosis: the Atherosclerosis Risk in Young adults (ARIC) study. *Am J Hypertens* 16:549, 2003.
36. Weiss R, Dziura J, Burgert TS, et al: Obesity and the metabolic syndrome in children and adolescents. *N Engl J Med* 350:2362, 2004.
37. Janssen I, Katzmarzyk PT, Srinivasan SR, et al: Utility of childhood BMI in the prediction of adulthood disease: comparison of national and international references. *Obes Res* 13:1106, 2006.
38. Urbina EM, Kieltkya L, Tsai J, et al: Impact of multiple cardiovascular disease risk factors on brachial artery distensibility in young adults: the Bogalusa Heart Study. *Am J Hypertens* 18:767, 2005.
39. Chen W, Srinivasan SR, Li S, et al: Metabolic syndrome variables at low levels in childhood are beneficially associated with adulthood cardiovascular risk: the Bogalusa Heart Study. *Diabetes Care* 28:126, 2005.

40. Kavey RE, Allada V, Daniels SR, et al: Cardiovascular risk reduction in high-risk pediatric patients: a scientific statement from the American Heart Association Expert Panel on Population and Prevention Science; the Councils on Cardiovascular Disease in the Young, Epidemiology and Prevention, Nutrition, Physical Activity and Metabolism, High Blood Pressure Research, Cardiovascular Nursing, and the Kidney in Heart Disease; and the Interdisciplinary Working Group on Quality of Care and Outcomes Research: endorsed by the American Academy of Pediatrics. *Circulation* 114:2710, 2006.
41. Wald DS, Bestwick JP, Wald NJ: Child-parent screening for familial hypercholesterolaemia: screening strategy based on a meta-analysis. *BMJ* 335:599, 2007.
42. Schrott HG, Clarke WR, Wiebe DA: Increased coronary mortality in relatives of hypercholesterolemic school children: the Muscatine study. *Circulation* 59:320, 1979.
43. Burns TL, Moll PP, Lauer RM: Increased familial cardiovascular mortality in obese schoolchildren: the Muscatine Ponderosity Family Study. *Pediatrics* 89:262, 1992.
44. Youssef AA, Srinivasan SR, Elkasabany A: Trends of lipoprotein variables from childhood to adulthood in offspring of parents with coronary heart disease: the Bogalusa Heart Study. *Metabolism* 50:1441, 2001.
45. Kwiterovich PO Jr, Heiss G, Johnson N: Hyperlipoproteinemia in young subjects from a population-based sample, *Am J Epidemiol* 115:192, 1982.
46. Friedman LA, Morrison JA, Daniels SR: Sensitivity and specificity of pediatric lipid determinations for adult lipid status: findings from the Princeton Lipid Research Clinics Prevalence Program Follow-up Study. *Pediatrics* 118:165, 2006.
47. Mudd JO, Borlaug BA, Johnston PV, et al: Beyond low-density lipoprotein cholesterol: defining the role of low-density lipoprotein heterogeneity in coronary artery disease. *J Am Coll Cardiol* 50:1735, 2007.
48. Srinivasan SR, Frontini MG, Xu J: Utility of childhood non–high-density lipoprotein cholesterol levels in predicting adult dyslipidemia and other cardiovascular risks: the Bogalusa Heart Study. *Pediatrics* 118:201, 2006.
49. Srinivasan SR, Myers L, Berenson GS: Distribution and correlates of non–high-density lipoprotein cholesterol in children: the Bogalusa Heart Study. *Pediatrics* 110:e29, 2002.
50. Freedman DS, Bowman BA, Otvos JD: Levels and correlates of LDL and VLDL particle sizes among children: the Bogalusa heart study. *Atherosclerosis* 152:441, 2000.
51. Freedman DS, Bowman BA, Otvos JD: Differences in the relation of obesity to serum triacylglycerol and VLDL subclass concentrations between black and white children: the Bogalusa Heart Study. *Am J Clin Nutr* 75:827, 2002.
52. Cali AM, Zern TL, Taksali SE, et al: Intrahepatic fat accumulation and alterations in lipoprotein composition in obese adolescents: a perfect proatherogenic state. *Diabetes Care* 30:3093, 2007.
53. Tzou WS, Douglas PS, Srinivasan SR: Advanced lipoprotein testing does not improve identification of subclinical atherosclerosis in young adults: the Bogalusa Heart Study. *Ann Intern Med* 142:942, 2005.
54. Chen W, Srinivasan SR, Li S: Clustering of long-term trends in metabolic syndrome variables from childhood to adulthood in Blacks and Whites: the Bogalusa Heart Study. *Am J Epidemiol* 166:527, 2007.
55. Kwiterovich PO Jr, Fredrickson DS, Levy RI: Familial hypercholesterolemia (one form of familial type II hyperlipoproteinemia). A study of its biochemical, genetic and clinical presentation in childhood. *J Clin Invest* 53:1237, 1974.
56. Ter Avest E, Sniderman AD, Bredie SJH: Effect of aging and obesity on the expression of dyslipidaemia in children from families with familial combined hyperlipidemia. *Clin Sci* 112:131, 2007.
57. Kaitosaari T, Rönnemaa T, Raitakari O, et al: Effect of 7-year infancy-onset dietary intervention on serum lipoproteins and lipoprotein subclasses in healthy children in the prospective, randomized Special Turku Coronary Risk Factor Intervention Project for Children (STRIP) study. *Circulation* 108:672, 2003.
58. Rask-Nissilä L, Jokinen E, Terho P, et al: Neurological development of 5-year-old children receiving a low-saturated fat, low-cholesterol diet since infancy: a randomized controlled trial. *JAMA* 284:993, 2000.
59. Niinikoski H, Jula A, Viikari J, et al: Blood pressure is lower in children and adolescents with a low-saturated-fat diet since infancy: the special Turku coronary risk factor intervention project. *Hypertension* 53:918, 2009.
60. The DISC Collaborative Research Group: The efficacy and safety of lowering dietary intake of total fat, saturated fat, and cholesterol in children with elevated LDL-cholesterol: the Dietary Intervention Study in Children (DISC). *JAMA* 273:1429, 1995.
61. Obarzanek E, Hunsberger SA, Van Horn L, et al: Safety of a fat-reduced diet: the Dietary Intervention Study in Children (DISC). *Pediatrics* 100:51, 1997.
62. Simons-Morton DG, Hunsberger SA, Van Horn L, et al: Nutrient intake and blood pressure in children: findings from the Dietary Intervention Study in Children (DISC). *Hypertension* 29:930, 1997.
63. Owen CG, Whincup PH, Odoki K, et al: Infant feeding and blood cholesterol: a study in adolescents and a systematic review. *Pediatrics* 110:597, 2002.
64. Gylling H, Siimes MA, Miettinen TA: Sitostanol ester margarine in dietary treatment of children with familial hypercholesterolemia. *J Lipid Res* 36:1807, 1995.
65. Tammi A, Rönnemaa T, Miettinen TA, et al: Effects of gender, apolipoprotein E phenotype and cholesterol-lowering by plant stanol esters in children: the STRIP study. Special Turku Coronary Risk Factor Intervention Project. *Acta Paediatr* 91:1155, 2002.
66. Amundsen AL, Ose L, Nenseter MS, et al: Plant sterol ester–enriched spread lowers plasma total and LDL cholesterol in children with familial hypercholesterolemia. *Am J Clin Nutr* 76:338, 2002.
67. Kwiterovich PO: The role of fiber in the treatment of hypercholesterolemic children and adolescents. *Pediatrics* 96:1005, 1995.
68. Williams CL, Bollella M, Spark A, et al: Soluble fiber enhances the hypocholesterolemic effect of the step I diet in childhood. *J Am Coll Nutr* 14:251, 1995.
69. Davidson MH, Dugan LD, Burns JH, et al: A psyllium-enriched cereal for the treatment of hypercholesterolemia in children: a controlled, double-blind, crossover study. *Am J Clin Nutr* 63:96, 1996.
70. Laurin D, Jacques H, Moorjani S, et al: Effects of a soy-protein beverage on plasma lipoproteins in children with familial hypercholesterolemia. *Am J Clin Nutr* 54:98, 1991.
71. Jacques H, Laurin D, Moorjani S, et al: Influence of diets containing cow's milk or soy protein beverage on plasma lipids in children with familial hypercholesterolemia. *J Am Coll Nutr* 11:69S, 1992.
72. Engler MM, Engler MB, Malloy MJ, et al: Effect of docosahexaenoic acid on lipoprotein subclasses in hyperlipidemic children (the EARLY study). *Am J Cardiol* 95:869, 2005.
73. McCrindle BW, Helden E, Conner WT: Garlic extract therapy in children with hypercholesterolemia. *Arch Pediatr Adolesc Med* 152:1089, 1998.
74. Kaitosaari T, Rönnemaa T, Viikari J, et al: Low-saturated fat dietary counseling starting in infancy improves insulin sensitivity in 9-year-old healthy children: the Special Turku Coronary Risk Factor Intervention Project for Children (STRIP) study. *Diabetes Care* 29:781, 2006.
75. Hakanen M, Lagström H, Kaitosaari T, et al: Development of overweight in an atherosclerosis prevention trial starting in early childhood. The STRIP study. *Int J Obesity* 30:618, 2006.
76. Farah R, Kwiterovich PO, Neill CA: A study of the dose-effect of cholestyramine in children and young adults with familial hypercholesterolemia. *Lancet* 1:59, 1977.
77. Tonstad S, Knudtzon J, Sivertsen M, et al: Efficacy and safety of cholestyramine therapy in peripubertal and prepubertal children with familial hypercholesterolemia. *J Pediatr* 129:42, 1996.
78. Liacouras CA, Coates PM, Gallagher PR, et al: Use of cholestyramine in the treatment of children with familial combined hyperlipidemia. *J Pediatr* 122:477, 1993.
79. Knipscheer HC, Boelen CC, Kastelein JJ, et al: Short-term efficacy and safety of pravastatin in 72 children with familial hypercholesterolemia. *Pediatr Res* 39:867, 1996.
80. Lambert M, Lupien PJ, Gagné C, et al: Treatment of familial hypercholesterolemia in children and adolescents: effect of lovastatin. Canadian Lovastatin in Children Study Group. *Pediatrics* 97:619, 1996.
81. Stein EA, Illingworth DR, Kwiterovich PO Jr, et al: Efficacy and safety of lovastatin in adolescent males with heterozygous familial hypercholesterolemia: a randomized controlled trial. *JAMA* 281:137, 1999.
82. de Jongh S, Ose L, Szamosi T, et al: Simvastatin in Children Study Group. Efficacy and safety of statin therapy in children with familial hypercholesterolemia: a randomized, double-blind, placebo-controlled trial with simvastatin. *Circulation* 106:2231, 2002.
83. Dirisamer A, Hachemian N, Bucek RA, et al: The effect of low-dose simvastatin in children with familial hypercholesterolaemia: a 1-year observation. *Eur J Pediatr* 162:421, 2003.
84. McCrindle BW, Ose L, Marais AD: Efficacy and safety of atorvastatin in children and adolescents with familial hypercholesterolemia or severe hyperlipidemia: a multicenter, randomized, placebo-controlled trial. *J Pediatr* 143:74, 2003.
85. Wiegman A, Hutten BA, de Groot E, et al: Efficacy and safety of statin therapy in children with familial hypercholesterolemia: a randomized controlled trial. *JAMA* 292:331, 2004.
86. Clauss SB, Holmes KW, Hopkins P, et al: Efficacy and safety of lovastatin therapy in adolescent girls with heterozygous familial hypercholesterolemia. *Pediatrics* 116:682, 2005.
87. Avis HJ, Vissers MN, Stein EA, et al: A systematic review and meta-analysis of statin therapy in children with familial hypercholesterolemia. *Arterioscler Thromb Vasc Biol* 27:1803, 2007.
88. Rodenburg J, Vissers MN, Wiegman A, et al: Statin treatment in children with familial hypercholesterolemia: the younger, the better. *Circulation* 116:664, 2007.
89. de Jongh S, Lilien MR, Op't Roodt J, et al: Early statin therapy restores endothelial function in children with familial hypercholesterolemia. *J Am Coll Cardiol* 40:2117, 2002.
90. Vryonidou A, Papatheodorou A, Tavridou A, et al: Association of hyperandrogenic and metabolic phenotype with carotid intima-media thickness in young women with polycystic ovary syndrome. *J Clin Endocrinol Metab* 90:2740, 2005.
91. Kane JP, Malloy MJ, Ports TA, et al: Regression of coronary atherosclerosis during treatment of familial hypercholesterolemia with combined drug regimens. *JAMA* 264:3007, 1990.
92. Kay JP, Alemzadeh R, Langley G, et al: Beneficial effects of metformin in normoglycemic morbidly obese adolescents. *Metabolism* 50:1457, 2001.
93. Freemark M, Bursey D: The effects of metformin on body mass index and glucose tolerance in obese adolescents with fasting hyperinsulinemia and a family history of type 2 diabetes. *Pediatrics* 107:1, 2001.
94. Silverstein J, Klingensmith G, Copeland K, et al; American Diabetes Association: Care of children and adolescents with type 1 diabetes: a statement of the American Diabetes Association. *Diabetes Care* 28:186, 2005.
95. Goldstein JL, Brown MS: Molecular medicine. The cholesterol quartet. *Science* 292:1310, 2001.
96. Rader DJ, Cohen J, Hobbs HH: Monogenic hypercholesterolemia: new insights in pathogenesis and treatment. *J Clin Invest* 111:1795, 2003.
97. Innerarity TL, Mahley RW, Weisgraber KH, et al: Familial defective apolipoprotein B-100: a mutation of apolipoprotein B that causes hypercholesterolemia. *J Lipid Res* 31:1337, 1990.
98. Arca M, Zuliani G, Wilund K, et al: Autosomal recessive hypercholesterolemia in Sardinia, Italy, and mutations in ARH: a clinical and molecular genetic analysis. *Lancet* 359:841, 2002.
99. Lind S, Olsson AG, Eriksson M: Autosomal recessive hypercholesterolemia: normalization of plasma LDL cholesterol by ezetimibe in combination with statin treatment. *J Intern Med* 256:406, 2004.
100. Berge KE, Tian H, Graf GA, et al: Accumulation of dietary cholesterol in sitosterolemia caused by mutations in adjacent ABC transporters. *Science* 290:1771, 2000.
101. Lu K, Lee MH, Hazard S, et al: Two genes that map to the STSL locus cause sitosterolemia: genomic structure and spectrum of mutations involving sterolin-1 and sterolin-2, encoded by ABCG5 and ABCG8, respectively. *Am J Hum Genet* 69:278, 2001.

102. Salen G, von Bergmann K, Lütjohann D, et al; Multicenter Sitosterolemia Study Group: Ezetimibe effectively reduces plasma plant sterols in patients with sitosterolemia. *Circulation* 109:966, 2004.

103. Salen G, Starc T, Sisk CM, et al: Intestinal cholesterol absorption inhibitor ezetimibe added to cholestyramine for sitosterolemia and xanthomatosis. *Gastroenterology* 130:6853, 2006.

104. Horton JD, Cohen JC, Hobbs HH: Molecular biology of PCSK9: its role in LDL metabolism. *Trends Biochem Sci* 32:71, 2007.

105. Abifadel M, Varret M, Rabès JP, et al: Mutations in PCSK9 cause autosomal dominant hypercholesterolemia. *Nat Genet* 34:154, 2003.

106. Cortner JA, Coates PM, Gallagher PR: Prevalence and expression of familial combined hyperlipidemia in childhood. *J Pediatr* 116:514, 1990.

107. Goldstein JL, Hobbs HH, Brown MS: Familial hypercholesterolemia. In Scriver C, Beaudet A, Sly W, et al, editors: *The metabolic and molecular bases of inherited disease*, ed 8, New York, 2000, McGraw-Hill, pp 2863-2913.

108. Koeijvoets KC, Rodenburg J, Hutten BA, et al: Low-density lipoprotein receptor genotype and response to pravastatin in children with familial hypercholesterolemia: substudy of an intima-media thickness trial. *Circulation* 112:3168, 2005.

109. Mietus-Snyder M, Malloy MJ: Endothelial dysfunction occurs in children with two genetic dyslipidemias: improvement with antioxidant vitamin therapy. *J Pediatr* 133:35, 1998.

110. Slyper H: Clinical Review 168: What vascular ultrasound testing has revealed about pediatric atherogenesis, and a potential clinical role for ultrasound in pediatric risk management. *J Clin Endocrinol Metab* 89:3089, 2004.

111. Naoumova RP, Thompson GR, Soutar AK: Current management of severe homozygous FH. *Curr Opin Lipidol* 15:413, 2004.

112. Gagne C, Gaudet D, Bruckert E: Ezetimibe Study Group: Efficacy and safety of ezetimibe co-administered with atorvastatin or simvastatin in patients with homozygous familial hypercholesterolemia. *Circulation* 105:2469, 2002.

113. Kwiterovich PO: Clinical relevance of the biochemical, metabolic and genetic factors that influence low density lipoprotein heterogeneity. *Am J Cardiol* 90(Suppl 8A):30i, 2002.

114. Goldstein JL, Schrott HG, Hazzard WR: Hyperlipidemia in coronary heart disease. II. Genetic analysis of lipid levels in 176 families and delineation of a new inherited disorder, combined hyperlipidemia. *J Clin Invest* 52:1544, 1973.

115. Sniderman AD, Scantlebury T, Cianflone K: Hypertriglyceridemic hyperapoB: the unappreciated atherogenic dyslipoproteinemia in type 2 diabetes mellitus. *Ann Intern Med* 135:447, 2001.

116. Kwiterovich PO: The metabolic pathways of HDL, LDL and triglycerides. A current review. *Am J Cardiol* 86(Suppl 1):5, 2000.

117. Maslowska M, Wang HW, Cianflone K: Novel roles for acylation stimulatory protein/C3a desArg: a review of recent in vitro and in vivo evidence. *Vitam Horm* 70:309, 2005.

118. Brown MS, Goldstein JL: Selective versus total insulin resistance: a pathogenic paradox. *Cell Metab* 7:95, 2008.

119. Badzioch MD, Igo RP Jr, Gagnon F, et al: Low-density lipoprotein particle size loci in familial combined hyperlipidemia: evidence for multiple loci from a genome scan. *Arterioscler Thromb Vasc Biol* 24:1942, 2004.

120. Gagnon F, Jarvik GP, Badzioch MD, et al: Genome scan for quantitative trait loci influencing HDL levels: evidence for multilocus inheritance in familial combined hyperlipidemia. *Hum Genet* 117:594, 2005.

121. Aouizerat BE, Allayee H, Bodnar J, et al: Novel genes for familial combined hyperlipidemia. *Curr Opin Lipidol* 10:113, 1999.

122. Lusis AJ, Fogelman AM, Fonarow GC: Genetic basis of atherosclerosis: part I: new genes and pathways. *Circulation* 10:1868, 2004.

123. Kalant D, MacLaren R, Cui W, et al: C5L2 is a functional receptor for acylation stimulatory protein. *J Biol Chem* 280:23936, 2005.

124. Pajukanta P, Lilja HE, Sinsheimer JS, et al: Familial combined hyperlipidemia is associated with upstream transcription factor 1 (USF1). *Nat Genet* 36:371, 2004.

125. Janssen I, Katzmarzyk PT, Srinivasan SR, et al: Combined influence of body mass index and waist circumference on coronary artery disease risk factors among children and adolescents. *Pediatrics* 115:1623, 2005.

126. Morrison JA, Friedman LA, Wang P, et al: Metabolic syndrome in childhood predicts adult metabolic syndrome and type 2 diabetes mellitus 25 to 30 years later. *J Pediatr* 152:201, 2008.

127. Morrison JA, Friedman LA, Gray-McGuire C: Metabolic syndrome in childhood predicts adult cardiovascular disease 25 years later: the Princeton Lipid Research Clinics Follow-up Study. *Pediatrics* 120:340, 2007.

128. Guttmann-Bauman I: Approach to adolescent polycystic ovary syndrome (PCOS) in the pediatric endocrine community in the U.S.A. *J Pediatr Endocrinol Metab* 18:599, 2005.

129. Brunzell JD, Deeb SS: Familial lipoprotein lipase deficiency, apo C-II deficiency, and hepatic lipase deficiency. In Scriver C, Beaudet A, Sly W, et al, editors: *The metabolic and molecular bases of inherited disease*, ed 8, New York, 2000, McGraw-Hill, pp 2789-2816.

130. Beigneux AP, Franssen R, Bensadoun A, et al: Chylomicronemia with a mutant GPIHBP1 (Q115P) that cannot bind lipoprotein lipase. *Arterioscler Thromb Vasc Biol* 29:956, 2009.

131. Rouis M, Dugi KA, Previato L, et al: Therapeutic response to medium-chain triglycerides and omega-3 fatty acids in a patient with the familial chylomicronemia syndrome. *Arterioscler Thromb Vasc Biol* 17:1400, 1997.

132. Cao H, Alston L, Ruschman J, et al: Heterozygous CAV1 frameshift mutations (MIM 601047) in patients with atypical partial lipodystrophy and hypertriglyceridemia. *Lipids Health Dis Jan* 31:7, 2008.

133. Mahley RW, Huang Y, Rall SC Jr: Pathogenesis of type III hyperlipoproteinemia (dysbetalipoproteinemia). *J Lipid Res* 40:1933, 1999.

134. Tall AR, Breslow JL, Rubin EM: Genetic disorders affecting high-density lipoproteins. In Scriver C, Beaudet A, Sly W, et al, editors: *The metabolic and molecular bases of inherited disease*, ed 8, New York, 2000, McGraw-Hill, pp 2915-2936.

135. Cohen JC, Kiss RS, Pertsemlidis A, et al: Multiple rare alleles contribute to low plasma levels of HDL cholesterol. *Science* 305:869, 2004.

136. Assmann G, von Ekardstein A, Funcke H: High density lipoproteins, reverse cholesterol transport of cholesterol, and coronary artery disease: insights from mutations. *Circulation* 87:III28, 1993.

137. Nissen SE, Tsunoda T, Tuzcu EM, et al: Effect of recombinant Apo A-I Milano on coronary atherosclerosis in patients with acute coronary syndromes: a randomized controlled trial. *JAMA* 290:2292, 2003.

138. Brunham LR, Singaraja RR, Hayden MR: Variations on a gene: rare and common variants in ABCA1 and their impact on HDL cholesterol levels and atherosclerosis. *Annu Rev Nutr* 26:105, 2006.

139. Calabresi L, Piscotta L, Costantin A, et al: The molecular basis of lecithin:cholesterol acyltransferase deficiency syndromes. A comprehensive study of molecular and biochemical findings in 13 unrelated Italian families. *Arterioscler Thromb Vasc Biol* 25:1972, 2005.

140. Barter PJ, Caulfield M, Erikson M, et al: Effects of torcetrapib in patients at high risk for coronary events. *N Engl J Med* 357:2109, 2007.

141. Hoffman HN, Fredrickson DS: Tangier disease (familial high density lipoprotein deficiency). Clinical and genetic features in two adults. *Am J Med* 39:582, 1965.

142. West M, Greason E, Kolmakova A, et al: Scavenger receptor class B type lipoprotein as an independent predictor of high-density lipoprotein cholesterol levels in subjects with hyperalphalipoproteinemia. *J Clin Endocrinol Metab* 94:1451, 2009.

143. Edmondson AC, Brown RJ, Kathiresan S, et al: Loss-of-function variants in endothelial lipase are a cause of elevated HDL cholesterol in humans. *J Clin Invest* 119:1042, 2009.

144. Koschinsky ML: Novel insights into Lp(a) physiology and pathogenicity: more questions than answers? *Cardiovasc Hematol Disord Drug Targets* 6:267, 2006.

145. Kwiterovich PO: Disorders of lipid and lipoprotein metabolism. In Rudolph CD, Rudolph AM, Hostetter MK, et al, editors: *Rudolph's pediatrics*, ed 21, New York, 2003, McGraw-Hill, pp 693-711.

146. Schonfeld G, Lin X, Yue P: Familial hypobetalipoproteinemia: genetics and metabolism. *Cell Mol Life Sci* 62:1372, 2005.

147. Horton JD, Cohen JC, Hobbs HH: Molecular biology of PCSK9: its role in LDL metabolism. *Trends Biochem Sci* 32:71, 2007.

148. Cohen JC, Boerwinkle E, Mosley TH, et al: Sequence variations in PCSK9, low LDL, and protection against coronary heart disease. *N Engl J Med* 354:1264, 2006.

CHAPTER 13

The Role of High-Density Lipoprotein Cholesterol in the Development of Atherosclerotic Cardiovascular Disease

Puneet Gandotra and Michael Miller

KEY POINTS

- HDL-C is inversely correlated with coronary heart disease.

- In addition to its pivotal role in reverse cholesterol transport, HDL possesses anti-inflammatory, fibrinolytic, and antioxidant properties.

- Levels of HDL-C inadequately characterize HDL functionality.

- Therapies that raise HDL-C levels are associated with reduced atherosclerotic progression.

- Clinical outcome studies are evaluating whether raising of HDL-C levels independently reduces coronary heart disease risk.

EPIDEMIOLOGIC AND PATHOPHYSIOLOGIC CONSIDERATIONS

Epidemiology

During the past several decades, numerous observational studies have strongly portrayed high-density lipoprotein cholesterol (HDL-C) as an independent risk factor for coronary heart disease (CHD). In the United States, the Framingham Heart Study provided the strongest examples of this relationship.[1] As demonstrated in Figure 13-1, the risk of CHD was highest at the lowest levels of HDL-C in the Framingham Heart Study, even when low-density lipoprotein cholesterol (LDL-C) levels were not elevated (i.e., <100 mg/dL). Conversely, high levels of HDL-C conferred relative cardioprotection compared with lower HDL-C levels, even when they were accompanied by high LDL-C levels (i.e., >220 mg/dL).

Inverse relationships between HDL-C and CHD have also been demonstrated outside of the United States as exemplified in Tromsø, Norway, where a threefold greater risk of future CHD was conferred by low HDL-C independently of any other variables.[2] In western Europe, the Prospective Cardiovascular Münster (PROCAM) study observed more than 25,000 men and women without symptomatic CHD at baseline (1979-1991). Among the most prominent findings was that low HDL-C, defined as <35 mg/dL, conferred a 2.5-fold increase of incident CHD in the absence of elevated total cholesterol (<200 mg/dL) and a 5-fold increase at higher total cholesterol levels.[3]

Other prospective studies confirmed HDL-C to be inversely correlated with incident myocardial infarction even after adjustment for other risk factors, such as age, smoking, blood pressure, weight, and diabetes mellitus.[4] If low HDL-C predicted CHD events, might there be a useful metric to gauge clinical effects related to raising of HDL-C levels? In fact, before clinical outcome studies addressing the effect of raising HDL-C on CHD events (see later),

observational data from the Multiple Risk Factor Trial,[5] the Lipid Research Clinics[6] follow-up trial, the placebo arm of the Coronary Primary Prevention Trial,[7] and the Physicians' Health Study[8] suggested that an HDL-C increment of 1 mg/dL would translate into an approximate 3% reduction in CHD risk.

Taken together, observational data from prior decades (1970s-1990s), with few exceptions,[9-11] paint a vividly convincing picture in favor of HDL-C as an independent risk factor for CHD. Similarly, clinical trials assessing the effect of lipid-altering therapy on outcomes found baseline measurements of low HDL-C to be predictive of both initial and recurrent CHD events.[12] Moreover, patients with low HDL-C assigned to placebo therapy demonstrated increased atherosclerotic progression and posed the highest CHD risk in clinical trials evaluating statin therapy.[13]

Pathophysiology of High-Density Lipoprotein

In addition to reverse cholesterol transport, HDL possesses antioxidant, anti-inflammatory, and antifibrinolytic properties, all believed to contribute to its putative atheroprotective role. However, the extent to which these properties translate into clinical improvement vis-à-vis CHD outcomes awaits the results of ongoing clinical trials (see later).

The physiologic pathway underlying reverse cholesterol transport is shown in Figure 13-2.[14] Originating as an HDL precursor, lipid-depleted and hepatically or intestinally derived apolipoprotein (apo) A-I receives phospholipids and free cholesterol after hydrolysis of triglyceride-rich lipoproteins. The relatively lipid-poor pre-β (based on electrophoretic mobility) HDL interacts with the ATP transport protein ABCA1 to shuttle free cholesterol and phospholipids from peripheral cells (e.g., macrophages). Cholesterol is sequestered into the HDL core through esterification by lecithin-cholesterol acyltransferase (LCAT) to form small spherical HDL₃ (or α₂, α₃ HDL)[15] particles with approximately two molecules of apo A-I and a small percentage of particles containing hepatically derived apo A-II.[16]

Additional contributions of cholesterol mediated by ABCG1 and ABCG4 (and, to a minor extent, the scavenger receptor B1 [SR-B1]) result in HDL maturation and larger HDL₂ particles (or α₁) that contain three or four molecules of apo A-I. Whereas apo A-I plays an important role in stabilizing HDL, activating LCAT and promoting reverse cholesterol transport, the role of apo A-II in this process is less clear.[16] The fate of cholesteryl esters contained within HDL includes transfer to lower density lipoproteins (e.g., LDL, VLDL) in exchange for triglyceride, a process mediated by the cholesteryl ester transfer protein (CETP).

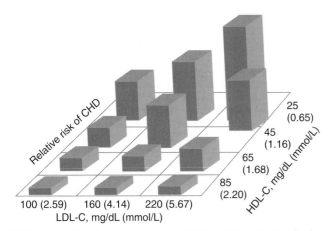

FIGURE 13-1 Risk of coronary heart disease (CHD) by HDL-C and LDL-C levels from the Framingham Heart Study. *(From Harper CR, Jacobson TA: New perspectives on the management of low levels of high-density lipoprotein cholesterol.* Arch Intern Med *159:1049, 1999.)*

The cholesteryl ester transferred to very-low-density lipoprotein (VLDL) is converted to LDL and taken up by LDL receptors for hepatobiliary delivery and excretion. Alternatively, HDL may deliver cholesteryl ester to steroidogenic tissues (liver, adrenal, testis, ovaries) by binding to a SR-B1 protein, when it may serve as a precursor for hormone and gonadal steroid production. In cases of CETP inhibition (see later), apo E–enriched HDL may also deliver hepatic cholesterol by LDL receptor–related mechanisms. Other less established contributors to reverse cholesterol transport include apo A-I uptake by high-affinity hepatic beta-chain ATP synthase receptors[17] and by the renal proximal tubule endocytic receptor cubilin.[18]

In addition to its role in reverse cholesterol transport, HDL possesses other atheroprotective properties (Fig. 13-3). Specifically, HDL downregulates expression of interstitial vascular cell adhesion molecule 1 (ICAM-1) and vascular cell adhesion molecule 1 (VCAM-1) in vascular endothelial cells. This limits transendothelial migration of monocytes and macrophage conversion, thereby reducing a proinflammatory milieu. In addition, the HDL-associated enzymes paraoxonase 1 (PON1) and platelet-activating factor acetylhydrolase (PAF-AH) inhibit LDL oxidation.[19,20] The inverse association between PON1 activity and CHD[21] validates the potential clinical relevance of non–reverse cholesterol transport characteristics of HDL.

After the discovery that apo A-I is a prostacyclin-stabilizing factor,[22] attention has been drawn to the HDL-associated phospholipid sphingosine 1-phosphate (S1P) because of an array of biologic effects on vascular endothelial and smooth muscle cells. For example, HDL-associated S1P improves arterial tone by upregulation of endothelial nitric oxide synthase. Moreover, in cellular studies and animal models, administration of HDL-associated S1P reduced infarct size and protected endothelial cells against apoptosis.[23]

HDL has also been shown to reduce platelet activation by upregulating prostacyclin and nitric oxide production and

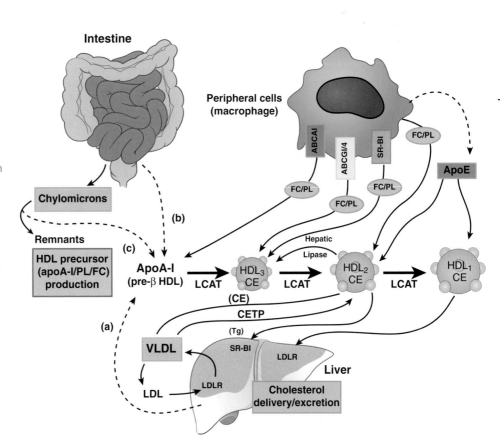

FIGURE 13-2 Role of HDL in the redistribution of lipids from cells with excess cholesterol (e.g., macrophages) to cells requiring cholesterol or to the liver for excretion. CE, cholesteryl ester; CETP, cholesteryl ester transfer protein; FC, free cholesterol; LCAT, lecithin-cholesterol acyltransferase; LDLR, LDL receptor; PL, phospholipid; SR-B1, scavenger receptor B1; Tg, triglyceride. *(From Mahley RW, Huang Y, Weisgraber KH: Putting cholesterol in its place: apo E and reverse cholesterol transport.* J Clin Invest *116:1226, 2006.)*

decreasing thromboxane A_2 synthesis as well as by down-regulating tissue factor expression.[24] Taken together, reverse cholesterol transport is likely to account for only a proportion of the cardioprotective benefit attributable to HDL.

Beyond reverse cholesterol transport and other putative atheroprotective properties is the recent identification of serine protease inhibitors and complement-modulating proteins associated with HDL (Fig. 13-4) that may protect against proteolysis and plaque rupture.[25] Although in its early developmental stages, HDL proteomics is likely to advance our understanding of the diverse roles that HDL plays in vascular biology and atherothrombosis.

GENETICS OF HIGH-DENSITY LIPOPROTEIN

13

High-Density Lipoprotein Deficiency States and Coronary Heart Disease Risk

To date, chromosomal aberrations in the APOA1/C3/A4/A5 gene complex or mutations in *ABCA1, LCAT,* and *APOAI* have been implicated in HDL deficiency states (e.g., HDL-C <10 mg/dL). Yet, in the absence of other CHD risk factors,

premature CHD, especially before the age of 40 years, has not been reported with heritable HDL deficiency. This is in marked contrast to familial hypercholesterolemia, in which, irrespective of risk factor status, homozygotes commonly develop CHD in childhood or adolescence and heterozygotes may manifest CHD before the age of 30 years.[26]

The lack of premature CHD in the absence of other risk factors (e.g., smoking, diabetes) suggests that there are other mechanisms enabling cholesterol efflux as the initial step in reverse cholesterol transport. For example, in cases of ABCA1 deficiency, cholesterol efflux occurs through SR-B1, passive diffusion, or upregulation of sterol 27-hydroxylase (CYP27A1) and caveolin 1 (Fig. 13-5).[27] Similarly, in the absence of apo A-I, other apolipoproteins such as macrophage-derived apo E may contribute to reverse cholesterol transport.[28]

A third possibility is that from a teleologic standpoint, HDL was designed to remove only excess cholesterol to maintain cellular lipid homeostasis. If this is correct, "isolated" low HDL-C as defined by physiologic levels of LDL-C and triglyceride (e.g., less than 70 mg/dL and 100 mg/dL, respectively) without traditional CHD risk factors would not be associated with increased risk of premature CHD.

In fact, as noted before, HDL-C deficiency as a consequence of monogenic abnormalities has rarely if ever been associated with premature CHD in the absence of accompanying CHD risk factors, most notably cigarette smoking.[29] Rather, the increased CHD risk associated with low levels of HDL-C may in large part be ascribed to associated metabolic perturbations (e.g., visceral adiposity, insulin resistance) that upregulate proinflammatory signaling pathways and raise overall atherothrombotic risk. This is in striking contrast to familial hypercholesterolemia, in which, in the pre–statin era, premature CHD occurred in most affected subjects, irrespective of risk factor status.

In contrast, elevated levels of HDL-C (i.e., >60 mg/dL) have been viewed as a negative CHD risk factor.[30] Yet, the association of inheritable high HDL-C (>60 mg/dL) with reduced CHD risk remains as debatable as isolated low HDL-C and premature CHD. For example, variation in the HDL regulatory gene *CETP* is associated with high HDL-C and is especially prevalent in Japan, where approximately 50% of high HDL-C is a consequence of genetic CETP deficiency.[31] Despite several case reports suggesting reduced CHD risk (Table 13-1), data are inconclusive as to whether intrinsic cardioprotection is afforded as a consequence of CETP inhibition.

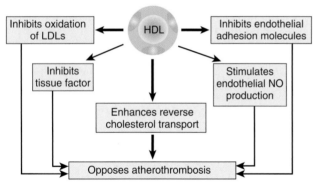

FIGURE 13-3 Other potential atheroprotective roles attributable to HDL. NO, nitric oxide. *(From Barter P: Metabolic abnormalities: high-density lipoproteins. Endocrinol Metab Clin North Am 33:393, 2004.)*

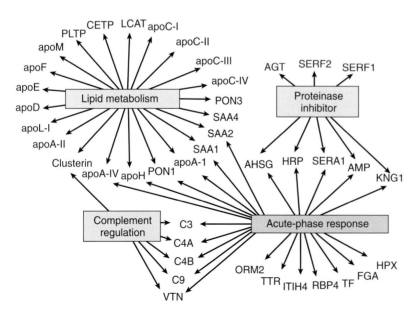

FIGURE 13-4 Global view of biologic processes and molecular functions of HDL proteins. *(From Vaisar T, Pennathur S, Green PS, et al: Shotgun proteomics implicates protease inhibition and complement activation in the antiinflammatory properties of HDL. J Clin Invest 117:746, 2007.)*

TABLE 13–1	Selected Cases of Cholesteryl Ester Transfer Protein Deficiency and Evidence of Atherogenicity*			
Mutation	Location	HDL-C (mg/dL)	Atherogenicity	Reference
Int14A	Japan	>70	↑	139
D442G	United States	≤60	↑	140
		>60	↓	
R37X	Sweden	208	↓	141
R268X	Canada	70	↓	142
IVS7+1	Netherlands	80	↑↓	143
Q87X/Q165X	Greece	194	↓	144

*Defined by history of coronary heart disease or noninvasive evaluation (carotid intima-media thickness, computed tomographic angiography).

TABLE 13–2	Novel Candidate Genes Associated with HDL-C		
Gene	Chromosome	ΔHDL	Reference
GALNT2	1	↑	145, 146
PCYT1	3	↑	147
ELOV2	6	↓	148
VNN1	6	↑	149
BMP1	8	↓	150
MMAB/MVK	12	↓	151

To address the potential benefit of CETP inhibition, a multicenter trial is currently evaluating whether the CETP inhibitor dalcetrapib reduces CHD outcomes (see later). In addition to *CETP*, variation in hepatic lipase (*LIPC*) and endothelial lipase (*LIPG*) has also been associated with high levels of HDL-C. However, *LIPC* variants have not been associated with cardioprotection,[32] and it remains unclear whether the loss-of-function *LIPG* variant Asn396Ser affects atherogenicity.[33]

In addition to loss-of-function variants that despite being rare in the general population (<1%) produce a significant phenotypic effect (e.g., very low or high HDL-C), genome-wide association studies investigate informative loci that may also contribute to HDL-C levels. In addition to known genes that regulate HDL metabolism and function, novel HDL candidates have recently been uncovered through genome-wide association studies,[34] a sample of which is represented in Table 13-2.

The potential mechanism of action of these encoded proteins on HDL metabolism is outlined in Figure 13-6. Although the impact on CHD risk has yet to be defined, the addition of genome-wide association studies to rare variant identification is likely to provide new insights related to HDL metabolism and overall atherothrombotic risk.

High-Density Lipoprotein Functionality and Classification

One of the quagmires relating HDL to CHD risk assessment is how best to assess and to represent HDL functionality. Although the level of HDL-C is most commonly used to gauge

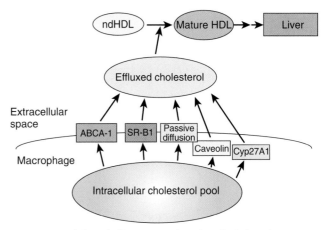

FIGURE 13-5 Cholesterol efflux may occur by at least five independent routes, including ATP-binding cassette transporter A1 (ABCA1), scavenger receptor B1 (SR-B1), caveolin, Cyp27A1, and passive diffusion. (*From Ohashi R, Mu H, Wang X, et al: Reverse cholesterol transport and cholesterol efflux in atherosclerosis. QJM 98:845, 2005.*)

CHD risk, it inadequately characterizes the HDL proteome in terms of inherent metabolic complexities and effectiveness of reverse cholesterol transport. This in part reflects the inherent difficulty in accurately quantifying the contribution of macrophage-derived fecal cholesterol, a small measure of reverse cholesterol transport. Nonetheless, the recent development of macrophage-specific reverse cholesterol transport assays in murine models[35] may hold promise as a future diagnostic tool if results are reproducible in humans.

In addition to cholesterol efflux and reverse cholesterol transport, other putative measures of HDL-mediated atheroprotection are currently under exploration. They include evaluation of reconstituted HDL, apo A-I Milano and mimetic compounds on indices of inflammation, hemostasis, thrombosis, and endothelial function.[35]

Although HDL-C levels have traditionally been used as a surrogate for reverse cholesterol transport, experimental evidence favors additional measurements that may contribute to CHD risk stratification. For example, in the setting of insulin resistance or in hypertriglyceridemic states (Fig. 13-7), free fatty acids are mobilized from adipocytes to drive hepatic VLDL production. The enhanced synthesis of triglyceride-rich lipoproteins leads to upregulation of CETP, resulting in greater exchange of triglyceride and cholesteryl ester between VLDL and HDL. Hypertriglyceridemic HDL particles exhibit reduced efficiency of cholesterol efflux[36] and are subsequently hydrolyzed by hepatic lipase to produce small, dense cholesterol-depleted HDL particles.

Apo A-I is catabolized by cubilin receptors in the proximal renal tubule,[37] and higher apo A-I fractional catabolic rates account for the reduced HDL-C levels found in postprandial states[38] as well as in obese, insulin resistance, and diabetic states. This in part reflects upregulation of CETP in triglyceride-enriched apo B–100 containing lipoproteins (most notably, VLDL), thereby permitting greater exchange of triglyceride–cholesteryl ester with HDL. The triglyceride-enriched HDL serves as an excellent substrate for hepatic lipase, resulting in small, dense, apo A-I–depleted HDL particles.[38]

Whereas greater apo A-I stability might suggest a more resounding cardioprotective effect for larger HDL particles, observational studies have been inconsistent. For example, several studies have found HDL_2 to be associated with lower CHD risk,[39] whereas others, including the Physicians' Health Study[40] and EPIC-Norfolk prospective population study,[41] failed to find significant differences between HDL particle

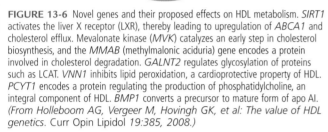

FIGURE 13-6 Novel genes and their proposed effects on HDL metabolism. *SIRT1* activates the liver X receptor (LXR), thereby leading to upregulation of *ABCA1* and cholesterol efflux. Mevalonate kinase (*MVK*) catalyzes an early step in cholesterol biosynthesis, and the *MMAB* (methylmalonic aciduria) gene encodes a protein involved in cholesterol degradation. *GALNT2* regulates glycosylation of proteins such as LCAT. *VNN1* inhibits lipid peroxidation, a cardioprotective property of HDL. *PCYT1* encodes a protein regulating the production of phosphatidylcholine, an integral component of HDL. *BMP1* converts a precursor to mature form of apo AI. *(From Holleboom AG, Vergeer M, Hovingh GK, et al: The value of HDL genetics. Curr Opin Lipidol 19:385, 2008.)*

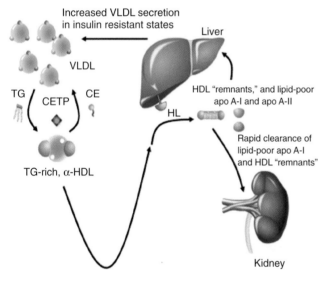

FIGURE 13-7 Mechanism of decreasing HDL-C and apo A-I in insulin-resistant and other hypertriglyceridemic states. Insulin-resistant states are associated with an increase in VLDL production and postprandial chylomicronemia. Cholesteryl ester transfer protein (CETP)–mediated exchange of HDL cholesteryl ester (CE) with triglyceride (TG) results in CE depletion and TG enrichment of HDL particles. Hepatic lipase (HL), which is also increased in insulin-resistant states, modifies TG-rich HDL, releasing lipid-poor apo A-I and forming HDL "remnant" particles. Lipid-poor apo A-I can be either recycled to form mature spherical HDL particles or filtered by the renal glomerulus and then degraded by proximal renal tubular cells. HDL remnants may also bind to putative receptors in liver or kidney that mediate HDL uptake, internalization, and degradation. *(From Rashid S, Patterson BW, Lewis GF: Thematic review series: patient-oriented research. What have we learned about HDL metabolism from kinetics studies in humans? J Lipid Res 47:1631, 2006.)*

size and risk of incident CHD after adjustment for traditional risk factors and other covariates.

A final lingering concern is the potential conversion of HDL to a proinflammatory form (Fig. 13-8).[42] For example, in the setting of an acute coronary syndrome (ACS), the enzyme myeloperoxidase released from leukocytes may bind to and oxidatively modify apo A-I. In addition to reducing the effectiveness of apo A-I in reverse cholesterol transport,[43] the associated nitration and chlorination of apo A-I convert HDL to a proinflammatory particle that may be selectively incorporated in human atheroma.[44]

Moreover, displacement of apo A-I by the acute-phase reactant serum amyloid A and associated reductions in LCAT and the HDL antioxidants PON1 and PAF-AH eliminate many of the cardioprotective properties of HDL. Statins may offset some of the adverse effects associated with proinflammatory HDL particles after ACS.[45]

THERAPIES THAT AFFECT HIGH-DENSITY LIPOPROTEIN

Lifestyle Changes Leading to Increased Levels of HDL-C (Table 13-3)

Diet and Weight Loss

The International Diabetes Federation and National Cholesterol Education Program consider abdominal adiposity and low HDL-C part of the metabolic syndrome. Weight loss, especially when it is accompanied by aerobic activity (see also later), may have a significant impact on raising HDL-C levels.[46] In the absence of weight loss, however, increasing the proportion of carbohydrates at the expense of fat reduces both HDL-C and LDL-C levels.[47] Moreover, the active process of weight loss is commonly associated with transient reductions in HDL-C, especially when a low-fat diet is prescribed,[48] because of reductions in apo A-I production.[49]

However, once weight loss has been attained and body weight stabilized, a meta-analysis of 70 diet studies found minimal increases approximating an increase of 1.6 mg/dL in HDL-C for every 10 pounds of weight lost.[50] Finally, high intake of marine-based omega-3 fatty acids has been associated with higher HDL-C in some populations,[51,52] although the overall net increase is very modest. Specifically, fish oil consumption by diet or capsule form has been associated with a 3% increase in HDL-C in subjects without hypertriglyceridemia at baseline (i.e., <177 mg/dL) compared with no increase in HDL-C among subjects with higher triglyceride levels.[52]

Exercise

Aerobic exercise has been shown to increase HDL-C levels on average by 5% to 10%, with the increase mostly related to the frequency and intensity of the exercise.[53] Increased HDL levels with exercise are associated with upregulation of lipoprotein lipase activity.[54] Overall, 10% to 20% increases in HDL-C are observed if at least 1200 kcal are expended weekly.[55]

Conditioned athletes and endurance runners often have HDL-C levels that are 30% to 50% higher than those of sedentary subjects,[56] probably reflecting the combination of enhanced lipoprotein lipase activity and increased production of pre-β HDL particles, which may facilitate reverse cholesterol transport.[57] Smaller increases (5% to 10%) are observed in subjects who have baseline low levels of HDL-C accompanied by elevated triglycerides and visceral adiposity.[58] On the other hand, isolated low HDL-C is difficult to effectively raise even after extended endurance training.[59]

Smoking Cessation

Overall, cigarette smoking impairs LCAT activity[60] and reduces levels of HDL-C. In women, 1 pack per day smokers evidenced HDL-C levels that were 10 mg/dL lower compared with those of nonsmokers, whereas an approximate differential of 3 mg/dL in HDL-C favoring nonsmokers was observed in men.[61] In contrast, a meta-analysis of 27 studies found

Myeloperoxidase

Nitrotyrosine
Chlortyrosine

Apo A-I

↓ **Apo A-I**
↓ Paraoxonase, other factors
↑ Proinflammatory factors, other factors

A   **Anti-inflammatory**   B   **Proinflammatory**

FIGURE 13-8 Model of bidirectional conversion of HDL from anti-inflammatory **(A)** to proinflammatory **(B)** and the role of myeloperoxidase in catalyzing oxidative modification of HDL, rendering it unable to effect ABCA1-mediated cholesterol transport. In association with these changes, apolipoprotein A-I (apo A-I) and paraoxonase levels decrease, whereas proinflammatory factors such as lipid oxidation products increase. *(From Ansell BJ, Fonarow GC, Fogelman AM: The paradox of dysfunctional high-density lipoprotein.* Curr Opin Lipidol *18:427, 2007.)*

TABLE 13–3	Effect of Lifestyle Modification on HDL-C Levels
Lifestyle Component	**Percentage Increase in HDL-C**
Diet and lifestyle	0-5
Weight loss	5-15
Omega-3 fatty acids	<5
Exercise	5-20
Cigarette cessation	5-10
Alcohol consumption	5-15

significant increases in HDL-C levels after smoking cessation.[62]

In a study performed by Moffatt,[63] participants who stopped smoking for 60 days saw an average increase of 12.5 mg/dL in HDL-C; reinitiation of cigarettes resulted in reversion to precessation levels.

Alcohol

Alcohol inhibits hepatic lipase, thereby raising both HDL-C and its HDL$_2$ subfraction.[64] A dose-response relationship exists; 1 ounce of alcohol consumed daily is associated with up to a 15% increase in HDL-C.[65] It has been suggested that raising of HDL levels represents approximately half of the CHD benefit attributable to alcohol use.[66]

The type of alcoholic drink does not appear to be as important as the quantity.[67] HDL-C increases due to alcohol intake may be more noteworthy in sedentary subjects compared with those who exercise on a regular basis.[68] Caution should be exercised in patients with low HDL-C who have elevated triglycerides (i.e., >200 mg/dL) as alcohol may substantially raise these levels as well.

Pharmacologic Therapy

In addition to lifestyle recommendations, medications have been employed to raise levels of HDL-C. It remains to be established whether and to what extent raising of HDL-C in and of itself reduces CHD risk. We review current and investigation agents affecting HDL metabolism as well as ongoing

clinical trials that it is hoped will provide insights into the virtue of raising HDL-C or improving its functionality.

Niacin

Nicotinic acid, or niacin (vitamin B$_3$), is currently the most potent HDL-C–raising medication in the United States, with increases ranging between 20% and 35%.[69] Of the three formulations, immediate-release (IR; three times daily), slow-release (SR; twice daily), and extended-release (ER; once daily), the IR form raises HDL-C to the greatest extent, followed by ER and SR formulations. For example, at doses of 1000 mg, the IR formulation raises HDL-C 25%, compared with 15% to 20% with ER and 10% with SR formulations.[70,71] At doses of 1500 to 2000 mg daily, observed increases range from 25% to 35% (IR) versus 20% to 30% (ER) and 10% to 20% (SR).

Niacin reduces HDL catabolism by inhibiting hepatic apo A-I removal.[72] Niacin also inhibits adipose hormone–sensitive lipase, reducing free fatty acid flux to hepatocytes, thereby decreasing VLDL production and triglyceride output.[73] Based on the inverse association between triglycerides and HDL-C, for every reduction of 50 mg/dL in triglycerides, HDL-C levels rise by approximately 1.6 mg/dL in addition to apo A-I–mediated effects.[74] Preliminary data for a combination of niacin and statin therapy found increases in HDL$_3$ levels of apo J and phospholipid transfer protein, raising the specter of improved reverse cholesterol transport, although the direct contribution by niacin (and statin) treatment remains to be determined.[75]

In the Coronary Drug Project (CDP), 3 g of IR niacin daily was associated with reduction in nonfatal myocardial infarction after 5 years and a total mortality benefit of 11% compared with placebo.[76] Coronary arteriography and studies evaluating carotid intima-media thickness have demonstrated that the addition of niacin to statin-based therapy is associated with reduced progression and in some cases regression of atherosclerotic disease.[77]

For example, in the Arterial Biology for the Investigation of the Treatment Effects of Reducing Cholesterol 3 (ARBITER 3), the addition of niacin to statin therapy resulted in decreased progression and mild regression of carotid intima-media thickness at 12 and 24 months, respectively.[78] Moreover, the HDL Atherosclerosis Treatment Study (HATS) found that the combination of niacin and statin decreased atherosclerosis by angiography as well as decreased clinical events compared with placebo.[79] In this study, despite a low sample size, those randomized to the combination (compared with placebo) had a significant 90% lower rate of recurrent cardiac events, noteworthy given that most statin studies have shown maximum event reductions on the order of 30% to 40%. HATS set the stage for the clinical outcome trial Atherothrombosis Intervention in Metabolic Syndrome with Low HDL/High Triglycerides and Impact on Global Health Outcomes (AIM-HIGH) designed to evaluate whether the combination of niacin and statin (with or without ezetimibe) is clinically superior to a predominant LDL-C–lowering regimen alone.[80]

The most common side effect of niacin therapy is the prostaglandin D_2–mediated cutaneous reaction that includes flushing and, to a lesser extent, urticaria. Pretreatment with 325 mg of chewable or nonenteric aspirin may limit or abort this reaction. Whereas the intensity of this side effect is reduced with food and ER or SR formulations and often eases with continued administration, instances of renewed flushing may occur even with long-term administration as a result of insufficient food intake, overconsumption of alcohol, overexposure to heat, and aerobic activity.

In this regard, a selective prostaglandin D_2 receptor 1 antagonist (laropiprant) that is associated with reduced flushing is currently being evaluated in a clinical outcome trial (see also later).[81] Other less frequent niacin-based side effects include dyspepsia, gout, acanthosis nigricans, toxic amblyopia, and elevation of plasma glucose concentration. However, studies suggest that diabetic subjects receiving up to 3 g IR or 2 g ER niacin had relatively modest (5% to 7%) but clinically insignificant increases in fasting glucose levels.[82-84] In fact, a CDP post hoc analysis of diabetic and metabolic syndrome patients found that niacin therapy improved CHD outcomes.[76]

The most disconcerting side effect, hepatic toxicity, has not been encountered with the ER regimen.[83,84] Nevertheless, the results of the AIM-HIGH trial and the Heart Protection Study 2–Treatment of HDL to Reduce the Incidence of Vascular Events (HPS2-THRIVE) comparing the combination of nicotinic acid/laropiprant and statin therapy versus statin-based therapy alone[85] will in large part dictate the future of this therapy in patients with vascular disease.

Fibrates

Fibrate therapy generally results in a 10% to 25% increase in HDL-C levels.[86] Fibrates are synthetic agonists of peroxisome proliferator-activated receptor α (PPARα), which stimulates expression of the hepatic apolipoprotein A-I gene[87] and modulates the transcription of other genes involved in reverse cholesterol transport, including SR-B1 and ABCA1.[88] However, the relative increase in HDL-C is largely driven by the associated reductions in triglyceride levels, the primary lipid-mediated effect of fibrates.[89] In primary prevention, the Helsinki Heart Study of 4081 asymptomatic middle-aged men with elevation of non HDL-C (>200 mg/dL) showed the fibrate gemfibrozil to be associated with a 34% overall reduction in incident CHD.[90] However, lower median HDL-C at baseline (i.e., <42 mg/dL) was associated with improved CHD outcomes despite more modest raising of HDL-C compared with higher baseline HDL-C levels.[91]

Moreover, in the secondary prevention Veterans Affairs HDL Intervention Trial (VA-HIT), recurrent CHD events were reduced by 11% with every increase of 5 mg/mL in HDL-C when patients were treated with gemfibrozil.[92] In this study, the HDL subfraction HDL_3 was correlated to a greater degree than total HDL-C levels with CHD. Moreover, gemfibrozil treatment resulted in a 10% increase in HDL particle number that correlated with a 29% reduction in CHD risk.[93]

Statins

Although statins exert a more modest effect on HDL-C levels (5% to 15% increase), they are especially effective in patients

with low HDL-C, in whom they may attenuate the elevated risk associated with reduced levels (see Fig. 13-7).[94] For example, in the Lipoprotein and Coronary Atherosclerosis Study,[13] patients with reduced HDL-C levels (on placebo) evidenced the highest rates of arteriographic progression. However, statin treatment resulted in greater decrease in progression in low versus high HDL patients that was likely a consequence of reduction in atherogenic lipoproteins and inflammation rather than raising of HDL-C.[94,95]

Statins raise HDL-C levels in part by reducing CETP activity and increasing apo A-I synthesis.[96] Among the different statins, rosuvastatin may raise HDL-C levels at the upper end of the spectrum (15%).[86] Similarly, simvastatin raises HDL-C and apo A-I levels,[97] with the most robust increases (10% to 15%) observed at the highest dose (80 mg).[98,99]

Drugs That Reduce HDL-C

Several classes of drug therapies have also been found to lower HDL-C levels. In one comprehensive review, 474 trials investigated the effects of 85 antihypertensive drugs on lipids and blood pressure. Nonselective beta blockers were shown to have a negative effect on HDL-C (10% to 20%) levels.[100,101] Subjects taking benzodiazepine derivatives have been shown to have HDL-C levels 3.3 mg/dL lower than that of nonusers.[102] However, these lipid effects may be secondary to the weight gain and accompanying increases in triglycerides.[103]

Among the most potent HDL-C–lowering agents are anabolic steroids. Testosterone increases hepatic expression of hepatic lipase and SR-B1, with resulting reductions of HDL-C up to 90%.[104,105] Fortunately, this effect can be reversed within 1 month of steroid discontinuation. Taken together, beta blockers and anabolic steroids are the two classes of drugs most associated with reductions in HDL-C.

Novel Targets of High-Density Lipoprotein Metabolism

CETP Inhibition

As described before, CETP mediates the transfer of cholesteryl esters from HDL to apo B–containing lipoproteins,[14] and inheritable CETP deficiency is associated with intrinsically high total and HDL_2 cholesterol levels. Although vaccine-based strategies are in development, early testing has yielded only modest increases in HDL-C (5% to 10%).[106] In contrast, several oral compounds have demonstrated more appreciable increases (>25%). The most well studied, torcetrapib, irreversibly bound to CETP and resulted in 50% to 100% increases in HDL-C levels.[107]

Unfortunately, the clinical trial Investigation of Lipid Level Management to Understand Its Impact in Atherosclerotic Events (ILLUMINATE) was prematurely terminated because of off-target toxicity related to aldosterone stimulation. The increase in electrolyte abnormalities (e.g., increased plasma bicarbonate and reduced potassium) was believed to contribute in part to the higher mortality rate in the torcetrapib-treated patients.[108]

Another CETP inhibitor, dalcetrapib (JTT-705), regressed aortic atherosclerosis in rabbits.[109] Dalcetrapib raises HDL-C more moderately (25% to 40%) than torcetrapib does, but it does not irreversibly bind to CETP or upregulate aldosterone secretion[110] and is currently under evaluation in a large clinical outcomes trial.[111] A third compound, anacetrapib, also exhibits potent HDL-C–raising properties without affecting aldosterone.[112] Pending the outcome of ongoing clinical studies, CETP inhibitors hold potential promise as adjuvant therapy in high-risk patients with dyslipidemia.

Apolipoprotein A-I–Targeted Therapies

On the basis of experimental evidence that intravenous HDL infusions or apo A-I overexpression reduced atherosclerosis in animals,[113,114] there has been great interest in human-based therapy targeting HDL. Several different strategies include administration of intravenous apo A-I, reconstituted phospholipid–apo A-I complexes (rHDL), oral apo A-I mimetic compounds, and phospholipid-based therapy.

The first human study to gain extensive media attention was the reduction in atheroma volume (assessed by intravenous ultrasound) after five weekly infusions of apo A-I Milano/phospholipid complex in post-ACS patients.[115] In the randomized study Effect of rHDL on Atherosclerosis Safety and Efficacy (ERASE),[116] 183 ACS patients received four weekly infusions of saline or 40 mg/kg or 80 mg/kg of HDL mimetic. Although atheroma burden was not different among the groups, there was improvement in the plaque characterization index and coronary score on quantitative coronary angiography in favor of rHDL.

Apo A-I mimetic peptides are much smaller compounds than mature apo A-I (e.g., 18 versus 243 amino acids) and possess similar apo A-I/lipid-binding domains to promote cholesterol efflux, to decrease inflammation, and to improve endothelial function.[117] For example, the mimetic D-4F improved the anti-inflammatory capacity of HDL after a single dose without altering HDL-C levels.[118]

Phospholipid administration may also be a valuable HDL-targeted therapy. For example, the synthetic compound 1,2-dimyristoyl-*sn*-glycero-3-phosphocholine (DMPC) raised HDL and apo A-I levels in association with reduced aortic lesions in a murine study.[119] Moreover, the soy-derived phospholipid phosphatidylinositol was found to raise HDL-C levels 13% to 18% during a 2-week period in normolipidemic subjects.[120]

Liver X Receptor Agonists

The liver X receptor (LXR), a nuclear hormone receptor (Fig. 13-9), forms a heterodimer with the retinoid X receptor and regulates transcription of ABCA1 and ABCG1, thereby serving an integral role in cholesterol efflux and reverse cholesterol transport.[121] Not surprisingly, therefore, synthetic activators of LXR have been pursued as a potential target to improve HDL functionality. Unfortunately, complicating the early-stage testing of LXR agonists was the induction of sterol regulatory element–binding protein 1 (SREBP-1) expression, resulting in enhanced hepatic VLDL production and hypertriglyceridemia.[122]

In contrast, selective targeting of macrophage LXR (i.e., LXRβ isoform) was associated with reduced atherosclerosis in mice.[123] Recently, a dual synthetic agonist (LXRα+β) was tested in humans and found to increase expression of ABCA1 and ABCG1 in a dose-dependent manner. However, higher doses of the compound were associated with neurologic and psychiatric side effects, including confusion, forgetfulness, decreased concentration, and paranoid ideation.[124] Although LXR-623 was withdrawn, other synthetic LXR compounds remain in clinical development.

Peroxisome Proliferator-Activated Receptor Agonists

In addition to LXR, peroxisome proliferator-activated receptors are nuclear transcription factors that also influence lipid (and glucose) homeostasis. As PPARα agonists, fibrates upregulate apo A-I transcription and promote macrophage cholesterol efflux in addition to suppressing apo C-III, resulting in increased lipoprotein lipase activity and reduced triglycerides.[87] Other more potent PPARα agonists are under investigation. They include the compound GFT505, which reduced triglycerides and cholesterol by 50% and inhibited aortic plaque formation,[125] and CP-778875, which raised HDL-C up to 14% in a diabetic cohort.[126]

The PPARγ agonists, particularly in the thiazolidinedione class, represent insulin-sensitizing agents that may raise HDL-C 5% to 15%. Of the two agents in this class, pioglitazone exerts a more favorable profile on lipids and lipoproteins, including a 15% increase in HDL-C levels compared with an 8% increase with rosiglitazone.[127] In the PROactive (PROspective Pioglitazone Clinical Trial in Macrovascular Events) study, statistically significant difference in the primary clinical endpoint was not demonstrated.[128] However, post hoc analysis found significant reduction in recurrent myocardial infarction and ACS in high-risk diabetic patients.[129] In contrast, the meta-analysis that suggested an increase in CHD events with rosiglitazone[130] was not confirmed in a recent multicenter trial.[131] The testing of dual-combination peroxisome proliferator-activated receptor agonists, specifically of the PPARα/PPARγ class, has been associated with adverse CHD events, leading to the discontinuation of several of these agents. In contrast, the PPARδ agonist GW501516 may hold promise in the treatment of low HDL-C and associated metabolic abnormalities.[132]

Other Potential High-Density Lipoprotein Therapeutic Targets and Strategies

Two additional targets to raise HDL-C include modulation of endothelial lipase and the farnesoid X receptor (FXR). Endothelial lipase is produced by vascular endothelial cells and hydrolyzes HDL phospholipids; overexpression of endothelial lipase is associated with reduced HDL-C levels.[133] Conversely, endothelial lipase inhibition is associated with increased HDL-C,[134] as are genetic loss-of-function variants,[135] raising the possibility that directed inhibition of endothelial lipase may be a potential HDL target.

The nuclear hormone receptor FXR is a transcriptional activator of several genes involved in regulation of lipid metabolism. Activation of FXR results in decreased expression of SREBP-1c, a primary regulator of triglyceride biosynthesis, thereby leading to reduced triglyceride levels. However, HDL-C levels were also reduced.[136] A natural FXR antagonist, the plant sterol guggulsterone, decreased hepatic cholesterol levels in cholesterol-fed animals,[137] although the extract gugulipid had modest LDL-C–lowering effects without affecting HDL-C or triglycerides.[138]

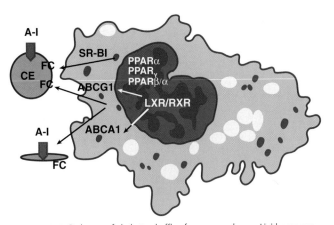

FIGURE 13-9 Pathways of cholesterol efflux from macrophages. Lipid-poor apo A-I can acquire free cholesterol (FC) from macrophages through an efflux process mediated by ABCA1. Alternatively, mature HDL can promote macrophage cholesterol efflux through the ABCG1 transporter or SR-B1. ABCA1 and ABCG1 expression is controlled by the nuclear receptor heterodimer LXR/RXR (liver X receptor/retinoid X receptor). The peroxisome proliferator-activated receptors (PPARs) may also influence the cholesterol efflux pathway. CE, cholesteryl ester. *(From Duffy D, Rader DJ: Emerging therapies targeting high-density lipoprotein metabolism and reverse cholesterol transport.* Circulation 113:1140, 2006.)

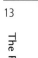

CONCLUSION

Epidemiologic studies have clearly demonstrated a strong and independent inverse relationship between HDL-C levels and risk of CHD. In addition to reverse cholesterol transport, HDL possesses other atheroprotective properties, reflecting its opposition to inflammation, oxidation, and thrombosis. However, the relationship between HDL-C levels and functionality is elusive, and it remains to be established whether and to what extent raising of HDL-C or improving its functionality reduces CHD event rates beyond non-HDL–based therapies. Ongoing clinical trials will, it is hoped, resolve these issues and justify whether targeting of HDL offers therapeutic value in secondary CHD prevention.

Acknowledgment

The work was supported by National Institutes of Health Grants HL061369 and HL094980.

REFERENCES

1. Gordon T, Castelli WP, Hjortland MC, et al: High density lipoprotein as a protective factor against coronary heart disease. The Framingham Study. *Am J Med* 62:707, 1977.
2. Miller NE, Thelle DS, Forde OH, Mjos OD: The Tromso heart-study. High-density lipoprotein and coronary heart-disease: A prospective case-control study. *Lancet* 1:965, 1977.
3. Assmann G, Cullen P, Schulte H: The Munster Heart Study (PROCAM). Results of follow-up at 8 years. *Eur Heart J* 19(Suppl A):A2, 1998.
4. Goldbourt U, Medalie JH: High density lipoprotein cholesterol and incidence of coronary heart disease—the Israeli Ischemic Heart Disease Study. *Am J Epidemiol* 109:296, 1979.
5. Watkins LO, Neaton JD, Kuller LH: Racial differences in high-density lipoprotein cholesterol and coronary heart disease incidence in the usual-care group of the Multiple Risk Factor Intervention Trial. *Am J Cardiol* 57:538, 1986.
6. Gordon DJ, Knoke J, Probstfield JL, et al: High-density lipoprotein cholesterol and coronary heart disease in hypercholesterolemic men: the Lipid Research Clinics Coronary Primary Prevention Trial. *Circulation* 74:1217, 1986.
7. Gordon DJ, Probstfield JL, Garrison RJ, et al: High-density lipoprotein cholesterol and cardiovascular disease. Four prospective American studies. *Circulation* 79:8, 1989.
8. Stampfer MJ, Sacks FM, Salvini S, et al: A prospective study of cholesterol, apolipoproteins, and the risk of myocardial infarction. *N Engl J Med* 325:373, 1991.
9. Wiklund O, Wilhelmsen L, Elmfeldt D, et al: Alpha-lipoprotein cholesterol concentration in relation to subsequent myocardial infarction in hypercholesterolemic men. *Atherosclerosis* 37:47, 1980.
10. Keys A: Alpha lipoprotein (HDL) cholesterol in the serum and the risk of coronary heart disease and death. *Lancet* 2:603, 1980.
11. Keys A, Karvonen MJ, Punsar S, et al: HDL serum cholesterol and 24-year mortality of men in Finland. *Int J Epidemiol* 13:428, 1984.
12. Berge KG, Canner PL, Hainline A, Jr: High-density lipoprotein cholesterol and prognosis after myocardial infarction. *Circulation* 66:1176, 1982.
13. Ballantyne CM, Herd JA, Ferlic LL, et al: Influence of low HDL on progression of coronary artery disease and response to fluvastatin therapy. *Circulation* 99:736, 1999.
14. Mahley RW, Huang Y, Weisgraber KH: Putting cholesterol in its place: apoE and reverse cholesterol transport. *J Clin Invest* 116:1226, 2006.
15. Asztalos BF, Schaefer EJ: HDL in atherosclerosis: actor or bystander? *Atheroscler Suppl* 4:21, 2003.
16. Gao X, Yuan S, Jayaraman S, Gursky O: Differential stability of high-density lipoprotein subclasses: effects of particle size and protein composition. *J Mol Biol* 387:628, 2009.
17. Martinez LO, Jacquet S, Esteve JP, et al: Ectopic beta-chain of ATP synthase is an apolipoprotein A-I receptor in hepatic HDL endocytosis. *Nature* 421:75, 2003.
18. Christensen EI, Birn H: Megalin and cubilin: multifunctional endocytic receptors. *Nat Rev Mol Cell Biol* 3:256, 2002.
19. Watson AD, Navab M, Hama SY, et al: Effect of platelet activating factor–acetylhydrolase on the formation and action of minimally oxidized low density lipoprotein. *J Clin Invest* 95:774, 1995.
20. Mackness B, Durrington PN, Mackness MI: Human serum paraoxonase. *Gen Pharmacol* 31:329, 1998.
21. Soran H, Younis NN, Charlton-Menys V, Durrington P: Variation in paraoxonase-1 activity and atherosclerosis. *Curr Opin Lipidol* 20:265, 2009.
22. Kawai C: Pathogenesis of acute myocardial infarction. Novel regulatory systems of bioactive substances in the vessel wall. *Circulation* 90:1033, 1994.
23. Sattler K, Levkau B: Sphingosine-1-phosphate as a mediator of high-density lipoprotein effects in cardiovascular protection. *Cardiovasc Res* 82:201, 2009.
24. Mineo C, Deguchi H, Griffin JH, Shaul PW: Endothelial and antithrombotic actions of HDL. *Circ Res* 98:1352, 2006.
25. Vaisar T, Pennathur S, Green PS, et al: Shotgun proteomics implicates protease inhibition and complement activation in the antiinflammatory properties of HDL. *J Clin Invest* 117:746, 2007.
26. Awan Z, Alrasadi K, Francis GA, et al: Vascular calcifications in homozygote familial hypercholesterolemia. *Arterioscler Thromb Vasc Biol* 28:777-785, 2008.
27. Ohashi R, Mu H, Wang X, et al: Reverse cholesterol transport and cholesterol efflux in atherosclerosis. *QJM* 98:845-856, 2005.
28. von Eckardstein A, Assmann G: High density lipoproteins and reverse cholesterol transport: lessons from mutations. *Atherosclerosis* 137(Suppl):S7-11, 1998.
29. Miller M, Aiello D, Pritchard H, et al: Apolipoprotein A-I(Zavalla) (Leu159–>Pro): HDL cholesterol deficiency in a kindred associated with premature coronary artery disease. *Arterioscler Thromb Vasc Biol* 18:1242, 1998.
30. Executive Summary of The Third Report of The National Cholesterol Education Program (NCEP) Expert Panel on Detection, Evaluation, And Treatment of High Blood Cholesterol In Adults (Adult Treatment Panel III). *JAMA* 285:2486, 2001.
31. Nagano M, Yamashita S, Hirano K, et al: Molecular mechanisms of cholesteryl ester transfer protein deficiency in Japanese. *J Atheroscler Thromb* 11:110, 2004.
32. Johannsen TH, Kamstrup PR, Andersen RV, et al: Hepatic lipase, genetically elevated high-density lipoprotein, and risk of ischemic cardiovascular disease. *J Clin Endocrinol Metab* 94:1264, 2009.
33. Edmondson AC, Brown RJ, Kathiresan S, et al: Loss-of-function variants in endothelial lipase are a cause of elevated HDL cholesterol in humans. *J Clin Invest* 119:1042, 2009.
34. Holleboom AG, Vergeer M, Hovingh GK, et al: The value of HDL genetics. *Curr Opin Lipidol* 19:385, 2008.
35. deGoma EM, deGoma RL, Rader DJ: Beyond high-density lipoprotein cholesterol levels: evaluating high-density lipoprotein function as influenced by novel therapeutic approaches. *J Am Coll Cardiol* 51:2199, 2008.
36. Greene DJ, Skeggs JW, Morton RE: Elevated triglyceride content diminishes the capacity of high density lipoprotein to deliver cholesteryl esters via the scavenger receptor class B type I (SR-BI). *J Biol Chem* 276:4804, 2001.
37. Graversen JH, Castro G, Kandoussi A, et al: A pivotal role of the human kidney in catabolism of HDL protein components apolipoprotein A-I and A-IV but not of A-II. *Lipids* 43:467, 2008.
38. Lamarche B, Uffelman KD, Carpentier A, et al: Triglyceride enrichment of HDL enhances in vivo metabolic clearance of HDL apo A-I in healthy men. *J Clin Invest* 103:1191, 1999.
39. Steenkamp HJ, Jooste PL, Benadé AJ, et al: Relationship between high density lipoprotein subfractions and coronary risk factors in a rural white population. *Arteriosclerosis* 10:1026, 1990.
40. Stampfer MJ, Sacks FM, Salvini S, et al: A prospective study of cholesterol, apolipoproteins, and the risk of myocardial infarction. *N Engl J Med* 325:373, 1991.
41. Arsenault BJ, Lemieux I, Després JP, et al: HDL particle size and the risk of coronary heart disease in apparently healthy men and women: the EPIC-Norfolk prospective population study. *Atherosclerosis* 206:276, 2009.
42. Ansell BJ, Fonarow GC, Fogelman AM: The paradox of dysfunctional high-density lipoprotein. *Curr Opin Lipidol* 18:427, 2007.
43. Nicholls SJ, Hazen SL: Myeloperoxidase, modified lipoproteins, and atherogenesis. *J Lipid Res* 50(Suppl):S346, 2009.
44. Zheng L, Nukuna B, Brennan ML, et al: Apolipoprotein A-I is a selective target for myeloperoxidase-catalyzed oxidation and functional impairment in subjects with cardiovascular disease. *J Clin Invest* 114:529, 2004.
45. Ansell BJ, Navab M, Hama S, et al: Inflammatory/antiinflammatory properties of high-density lipoprotein distinguish patients from control subjects better than high-density lipoprotein cholesterol levels and are favorably affected by simvastatin treatment. *Circulation* 108:2751, 2003.
46. Wood PD, Stefanick ML, Dreon DM, et al: Changes in plasma lipids and lipoproteins in overweight men during weight loss through dieting as compared with exercise. *N Engl J Med* 319:1173, 1988.
47. Meksawan K, Pendergast DR, Leddy JJ, et al: Effect of low and high fat diets on nutrient intakes and selected cardiovascular risk factors in sedentary men and women. *J Am Coll Nutr* 23:131, 2004.
48. Sacks FM, Katan M: Randomized clinical trials on the effects of dietary fat and carbohydrate on plasma lipoproteins and cardiovascular disease. *Am J Med* 113(Suppl 9B):13S, 2002.
49. Brinton EA, Eisenberg S, Breslow JL: A low-fat diet decreases high density lipoprotein (HDL) cholesterol levels by decreasing HDL apolipoprotein transport rates. *J Clin Invest* 85:144, 1990.
50. Dattilo AM, Kris-Etherton PM: Effects of weight reduction on blood lipids and lipoproteins: a meta-analysis. *Am J Clin Nutr* 56:320, 1992.
51. Bjerregaard P, Jørgensen ME, Borch-Johnsen K: Serum lipids of Greenland Inuit in relation to Inuit genetic heritage, westernisation and migration. Greenland Population Study. *Atherosclerosis* 174:391, 2004.
52. Harris WS: n-3 Fatty acids and lipoproteins: comparison of results from human and animal studies. *Lipids* 31:243, 1996.
53. King AC, Haskell WL, Young DR, et al: Long-term effects of varying intensities and formats of physical activity on participation rates, fitness, and lipoproteins in men and women aged 50 to 65 years. *Circulation* 91:2596, 1995.
54. Thompson PD: What do muscles have to do with lipoproteins? *Circulation* 81:1428, 1990.
55. Miller M: Raising an isolated low HDL-C level: why, how, and when? *Cleve Clin J Med* 70:553, 2003.
56. Martin DJ, Herbert PN, Thompson PD: Exercise training has little effect on HDL levels and metabolism in men with initially low HDL cholesterol. *Atherosclerosis* 137:215, 1998.
57. Gupta AK, Ross EA, Myers JN, Kashyap ML: Increased reverse cholesterol transport in athletes. *Metabolism* 42:684, 1993.
58. Couillard C, Despres JP, Lamarche B, et al: Effects of endurance exercise training on plasma HDL cholesterol levels depend on levels of triglycerides: evidence from men of the Health, Risk Factors, Exercise Training and Genetics (HERITAGE) Family Study. *Arterioscler Thromb Vasc Biol* 21:1226, 2001.
59. Zmuda JM, Yurgalevitch SM, Flynn MM, et al: Exercise training has little effect on HDL levels and metabolism in men with initially low HDL cholesterol. *Atherosclerosis* 137:215, 1998.

60. Freeman DJ, Caslake MJ, Griffin BA, et al: The effect of smoking on post-heparin lipoprotein and hepatic lipase, cholesteryl ester transfer protein and lecithin:cholesterol acyl transferase activities in human plasma. *Eur J Clin Invest* 28:584, 1998.

61. Ellison RC, Zhang Y, Qureshi MM, et al: Lifestyle determinants of high-density lipoprotein cholesterol: the National Heart, Lung, and Blood Institute Family Heart Study. *Am Heart J* 147:529, 2004.

62. Maeda K, Noguchi Y, Fukui T: The effects of cessation from cigarette smoking on the lipid and lipoprotein profiles: a meta-analysis. *Prev Med* 37:283, 2003.

63. Moffatt RJ: Effects of cessation of smoking on serum lipids and high density lipoprotein-cholesterol. *Atherosclerosis* 74:85, 1988.

64. Hartung GH, Foreyt JP, Reeves RS, et al: Effect of alcohol dose on plasma lipoprotein subfractions and lipolytic enzyme activity in active and inactive men. *Metabolism* 39:81, 1990.

65. Gaziano JM, Buring JE, Breslow JL, et al: Moderate alcohol intake, increased levels of high-density lipoprotein and its subfractions, and decreased risk of myocardial infarction. *N Engl J Med* 329:1829, 1993.

66. Klatsky AL: Alcohol, wine, and vascular diseases: an abundance of paradoxes. *Am J Physiol Heart Circ Physiol* 294:H582, 2008.

67. Gaziano JM, Hennekens CH, Godfried SL, et al: Type of alcoholic beverage and risk of myocardial infarction. *Am J Cardiol* 83:52, 1999.

68. Hartung GH, Foreyt JP, Mitchell RE, et al: Effect of alcohol intake on high-density lipoprotein cholesterol levels in runners and inactive men. *JAMA* 249:747, 1983.

69. Alderman JD, Pasternak RC, Sacks FM, et al: Effect of a modified, well-tolerated niacin regimen on serum total cholesterol, high density lipoprotein cholesterol and the cholesterol to high density lipoprotein ratio. *Am J Cardiol* 64:725, 1989.

70. Morgan JM, Capuzzi DM, Guyton JR: A new extended-release niacin (Niaspan): efficacy, tolerability, and safety in hypercholesterolemic patients. *Am J Cardiol* 82:29U, 1998.

71. McKenney J: New perspectives on the use of niacin in the treatment of lipid disorders. *Arch Intern Med* 164:697, 2004.

72. Ganji SH, Kamanna VS, Kashyap ML: Niacin and cholesterol: role in cardiovascular disease [review]. *J Nutr Biochem* 14:298, 2003.

73. Knopp RH: Drug treatment of lipid disorders. *N Engl J Med* 341:498, 1999.

74. Miller M, Langenberg P, Havas S: Impact of lowering triglycerides on raising HDL-C in hypertriglyceridemic and non-hypertriglyceridemic subjects. *Int J Cardiol* 119:192, 2007.

75. Green PS, Vaisar T, Pennathur S, et al: Combined statin and niacin therapy remodels the high-density lipoprotein proteome. *Circulation* 118:1259, 2008.

76. Canner PL, Furberg CD, McGovern ME: Benefits of niacin in patients with versus without the metabolic syndrome and healed myocardial infarction (from the Coronary Drug Project). *Am J Cardiol* 97:477, 2006.

77. Brown BG, Taylor AJ: Does ENHANCE diminish confidence in lowering LDL or in ezetimibe? *N Engl J Med* 358:1504, 2008.

78. Taylor AJ, Lee HJ, Sullenberger LE: The effect of 24 months of combination statin and extended-release niacin on carotid intima-media thickness: ARBITER 3. *Curr Med Res Opin* 22:2243, 2006.

79. Brown BG, Zhao XQ, Chait A, et al: Simvastatin and niacin, antioxidant vitamins, or the combination for the prevention of coronary disease. *N Engl J Med* 345:1583, 2001.

80. Aim-High Cholesterol Management Program. Available at: http://www.aimhigh-heart.com/background.shtml. Accessed August 14, 2009.

81. Cheng K, Wu TJ, Wu KK, et al: Antagonism of the prostaglandin D$_2$ receptor 1 suppresses nicotinic acid–induced vasodilation in mice and humans. *Proc Natl Acad Sci U S A* 103:6682, 2006.

82. Elam MB, Hunninghake DB, Davis KB, et al: Effect of niacin on lipid and lipoprotein levels and glycemic control in patients with diabetes and peripheral arterial disease: the ADMIT study: a randomized trial. Arterial Disease Multiple Intervention Trial. *JAMA* 284:1263, 2000.

83. Guyton JR, Goldberg AC, Kreisberg RA, et al: Effectiveness of once-nightly dosing of extended-release niacin alone and in combination for hypercholesterolemia. *Am J Cardiol* 82:737, 1998.

84. Guyton JR, Bays HE: Safety considerations with niacin therapy. *Am J Cardiol* 99:22C, 2007.

85. Preiss D, Sattar N: Lipids, lipid modifying agents and cardiovascular risk: a review of the evidence. *Clin Endocrinol (Oxf)* 70:815, 2009.

86. Ashen MD, Blumenthal RS: Clinical practice. Low HDL cholesterol levels. *N Engl J Med* 353:1252, 2005.

87. Staels B, Dallongeville J, Auwerx J, et al: Mechanism of action of fibrates on lipid and lipoprotein metabolism. *Circulation* 98:2088, 1998.

88. Meyers CD, Kashyap ML: Pharmacologic elevation of high-density lipoproteins: recent insights on mechanism of action and atherosclerosis protection. *Curr Opin Cardiol* 19:366, 2004.

89. Miller M, Bachorik PS, McCrindle BW, Kwiterovich PO, Jr: Effect of gemfibrozil in men with primary isolated low high-density lipoprotein cholesterol: a randomized, double-blind, placebo-controlled, crossover study. *Am J Med* 94:7, 1993.

90. Frick MH, Elo O, Haapa K, et al: Helsinki Heart Study: primary-prevention trial with gemfibrozil in middle-aged men with dyslipidemia. Safety of treatment, changes in risk factors, and incidence of coronary heart disease. *N Engl J Med* 317:1237, 1987.

91. Manninen V, Elo MO, Frick MH, et al: Lipid alterations and decline in the incidence of coronary heart disease in the Helsinki Heart Study. *JAMA* 260:641, 1988.

92. Robins SJ, Collins D, Wittes JT, et al: Relation of gemfibrozil treatment and lipid levels with major coronary events: VA-HIT: a randomized controlled trial. *JAMA* 285:1585, 2001.

93. Otvos JD, Collins D, Freedman DS, et al: Low-density lipoprotein and high-density lipoprotein particle subclasses predict coronary events and are favorably changed by gemfibrozil therapy in the Veterans Affairs High-Density Lipoprotein Intervention Trial. *Circulation* 113:1556, 2006.

94. Ballantyne CM, Rangaraj GR: The evolving role of high-density lipoprotein in reducing cardiovascular risk. *Prev Cardiol* 4:65, 2001.

95. Rezaie-Majd A, Prager GW, Bucek RA, et al: Simvastatin reduces the expression of adhesion molecules in circulating monocytes from hypercholesterolemic patients. *Arterioscler Thromb Vasc Biol* 23:397, 2003.

96. Schaefer JR, Schweer H, Ikewaki K, et al: Metabolic basis of high density lipoproteins and apolipoprotein A-I increase by HMG-CoA reductase inhibition in healthy subjects and a patient with coronary artery disease. *Atherosclerosis* 144:177, 1999.

97. Kastelein JJ, Isaacsohn JL, Ose L, et al: Comparison of effects of simvastatin versus atorvastatin on high-density lipoprotein cholesterol and apolipoprotein A-I levels. *Am J Cardiol* 86:221, 2000.

98. Crouse JR, 3rd, Frohlich J, Ose L, et al: Effects of high doses of simvastatin and atorvastatin on high-density lipoprotein cholesterol and apolipoprotein A-I. *Am J Cardiol* 83:1476, 1999.

99. Miller M, Dolinar C, Cromwell W, Otvos JD: Effectiveness of high doses of simvastatin as monotherapy in mixed hyperlipidemia. *Am J Cardiol* 87:232, 2001.

100. Kasiske BL, Ma JZ, Kalil RS, Louis TA: Effects of antihypertensive therapy on serum lipids. *Ann Intern Med* 122:133, 1995.

101. Weidmann P, Ferrier C, Saxenhofer H, Uehlinger DE, Trost BN: Serum lipoproteins during treatment with antihypertensive drugs. *Drugs* 35(Suppl 6):118, 1988.

102. Wallace RB, Hunninghake DB, Reiland S, et al: Alterations of plasma high-density lipoprotein cholesterol levels associated with consumption of selected medications. The Lipid Research Clinics Program Prevalence Study. *Circulation* 62:IV77, 1980.

103. Su KP, Wu PL, Pariante CM: A crossover study on lipid and weight changes associated with olanzapine and risperidone. *Psychopharmacology (Berl)* 183:383, 2005.

104. Wu FC, von Eckardstein A: Androgens and coronary artery disease. *Endocr Rev* 24:183, 2003.

105. Barrett-Connor EL: Testosterone and risk factors for cardiovascular disease in men. *Diabete Metab* 21:156, 1995.

106. Pal M, Pillarisetti S: HDL elevators and mimetics—emerging therapies for atherosclerosis. *Cardiovasc Hematol Agents Med Chem* 5:55, 2007.

107. Clark RW, Sutfin TA, Ruggeri RB, et al: Raising high-density lipoprotein in humans through inhibition of cholesteryl ester transfer protein: an initial multidose study of torcetrapib. *Arterioscler Thromb Vasc Biol* 24:490, 2004.

108. Barter PJ, Caulfield M, Eriksson M, et al: Effects of torcetrapib in patients at high risk for coronary events. *N Engl J Med* 357:2109, 2007.

109. Okamoto H, Yonemori F, Wakitani K, et al: A cholesteryl ester transfer protein inhibitor attenuates atherosclerosis in rabbits. *Nature* 406:203, 2000.

110. Stein EA, Stroes ES, Steiner G, et al: Safety and tolerability of dalcetrapib. *Am J Cardiol* 104:821, 2009.

111. A Study of RO4607381 in Stable Coronary Heart Disease Patients With Recent Acute Coronary Syndrome. Available at: http://clinicaltrials.gov/ct2/show/NCT00658515. Accessed September 10, 2009.

112. Bloomfield D, Carlson GL, Sapre A, et al: Efficacy and safety of the cholesteryl ester transfer protein inhibitor anacetrapib as monotherapy and coadministered with atorvastatin in dyslipidemic patients. *Am Heart J* 157:352, 2009.

113. Badimon JJ, Badimon L, Fuster V: Regression of atherosclerotic lesions by high density lipoprotein plasma fraction in the cholesterol-fed rabbit. *J Clin Invest* 85:1234, 1990.

114. Rubin EM, Krauss RM, Spangler EA, et al: Inhibition of early atherogenesis in transgenic mice by human apolipoprotein AI. *Nature* 353:265, 1991.

115. Nissen SE, Tsunoda T, Tuzcu EM, et al: Effect of recombinant ApoA-I Milano on coronary atherosclerosis in patients with acute coronary syndromes: a randomized controlled trial. *JAMA* 290:2292, 2003.

116. Tardif JC, Gregoire J, L'Allier PL, et al: Effects of reconstituted high-density lipoprotein infusions on coronary atherosclerosis: a randomized controlled trial. *JAMA* 297:1675, 2007.

117. Navab M, Shechter I, Anantharamaiah GM, et al: Structure and function of HDL mimetics. *Arterioscler Thromb Vasc Biol* 30:164, 2010.

118. Bloedon LT, Dunbar R, Duffy D, et al: Safety, pharmacokinetics, and pharmacodynamics of oral apoA-I mimetic peptide D-4F in high-risk cardiovascular patients. *J Lipid Res* 49:1344, 2008.

119. Navab M, Hama S, Hough G, Fogelman AM: Oral synthetic phospholipid (DMPC) raises high-density lipoprotein cholesterol levels, improves high-density lipoprotein function, and markedly reduces atherosclerosis in apolipoprotein E-null mice. *Circulation* 108:1735, 2003.

120. Burgess JW, Neville TA, Rouillard P, et al: Phosphatidylinositol increases HDL-C levels in humans. *J Lipid Res* 46:350, 2005.

121. Duffy D, Rader DJ: Emerging therapies targeting high-density lipoprotein metabolism and reverse cholesterol transport. *Circulation* 113:1140, 2006.

122. Schultz JR, Tu H, Luk A, et al: Role of LXRs in control of lipogenesis. *Genes Dev* 14:2831, 2000.

123. Bradley MN, Hong C, Chen M, et al: Ligand activation of LXR beta reverses atherosclerosis and cellular cholesterol overload in mice lacking LXR alpha and apoE. *J Clin Invest* 117:2337, 2007.

124. Katz A, Udata C, Ott E, et al: Safety, pharmacokinetics, and pharmacodynamics of single doses of LXR-623, a novel X-receptor agonist, in healthy participants. *J Clin Pharmacol* 49:643, 2009.

125. Fruchart JC: Peroxisome proliferator-activated receptor-α (PPARα): at the crossroads of obesity, diabetes and cardiovascular disease. *Atherosclerosis* 205:1, 2009.

126. Terra SG, Francone OL, Contant CF, et al: Efficacy and safety of a potent and selective peroxisome proliferator activated receptor alpha agonist in subjects with dyslipidemia and type 2 diabetes mellitus. *Am J Cardiol* 102:434, 2008.

127. Goldberg RB, Kendall DM, Deeg MA, et al: GLAI Study Investigators: A comparison of lipid and glycemic effects of pioglitazone and rosiglitazone in patients with type 2 diabetes and dyslipidemia. *Diabetes Care* 28:1547, 2005.

128. Dormandy JA, Charbonnel B, Eckland DJ, et al: Secondary prevention of macrovascular events in patients with type 2 diabetes in the PROactive Study (PROspective piogli-

tAzone Clinical Trial In macroVascular Events): a randomised controlled trial. *Lancet* 366:1279, 2005.

129. Erdmann E, Dormandy JA, Charbonnel B, et al: PROactive Investigators: The effect of pioglitazone on recurrent myocardial infarction in 2,445 patients with type 2 diabetes and previous myocardial infarction: results from the PROactive (PROactive 05) Study. *J Am Coll Cardiol* 49:1772, 2007.

130. Nissen SE, Wolski K: Effect of rosiglitazone on the risk of myocardial infarction and death from cardiovascular causes. *N Engl J Med* 356:2457, 2007.

131. Home PD, Pocock SJ, Beck-Nielsen H, et al: RECORD Study Team: Rosiglitazone evaluated for cardiovascular outcomes in oral agent combination therapy for type 2 diabetes (RECORD): a multicentre, randomised, open-label trial. *Lancet* 373:2125, 2009.

132. Karpe F, Ehrenborg EE: PPARδ in humans: genetic and pharmacological evidence for a significant metabolic function. *Curr Opin Lipidol* 20:333, 2009.

133. Jaye M, Lynch KJ, Krawiec J, et al: A novel endothelial-derived lipase that modulates HDL metabolism. *Nat Genet* 21:424, 1999.

134. Jin W, Millar JS, Broedl U, et al: Inhibition of endothelial lipase causes increased HDL cholesterol levels in vivo. *J Clin Invest* 111:357, 2003.

135. Edmondson AC, Brown RJ, Kathiresan S, et al: Loss-of-function variants in endothelial lipase are a cause of elevated HDL cholesterol in humans. *J Clin Invest* 119:1042, 2009.

136. Watanabe M, Houten SM, Wang L, et al: Bile acids lower triglyceride levels via a pathway involving FXR, SHP, and SREBP-1c. *J Clin Invest* 113:1408, 2004.

137. Urizar NL, Liverman AB, Dodds DT, et al: A natural product that lowers cholesterol as an antagonist ligand for FXR. *Science* 296:1703, 2002.

138. Szapary PO, Wolfe ML, Bloedon LT, et al: Guggulipid for the treatment of hypercholesterolemia: a randomized controlled trial. *JAMA* 290:765, 2003.

139. Hirano K, Yamashita S, Nakajima N, et al: Genetic cholesteryl ester transfer protein deficiency is extremely frequent in the Omagari area of Japan. Marked hyperalphalipoproteinemia caused by CETP gene mutation is not associated with longevity. *Arterioscler Thromb Vasc Biol* 17:1053, 1997.

140. Zhong S, Sharp DS, Grove JS, et al: Increased coronary heart disease in Japanese-American men with mutation in the cholesteryl ester transfer protein gene despite increased HDL levels. *J Clin Invest* 97:2917, 1996.

141. Calabresi L, Nilsson P, Pinotti E, et al: A novel homozygous mutation in CETP gene as a cause of CETP deficiency in a caucasian kindred. *Atherosclerosis* 205:506, 2009.

142. Teh EM, Dolphin PJ, Breckenridge WC, Tan MH: Human plasma CETP deficiency: identification of a novel mutation in exon 9 of the CETP gene in a Caucasian subject from North America. *J Lipid Res* 39:442, 1998.

143. van der Steeg WA, Hovingh GK, Klerkx AH, et al: Cholesteryl ester transfer protein and hyperalphalipoproteinemia in Caucasians. *J Lipid Res* 48:674, 2007.

144. Rhyne J, Ryan MJ, White C, et al: The two novel CETP mutations Gln87X and Gln165X in a compound heterozygous state are associated with marked hyperalphalipoproteinemia and absence of significant coronary artery disease. *J Mol Med* 84:647, 2006.

145. Willer CJ, Sanna S, Jackson AU, et al: Newly identified loci that influence lipid concentrations and risk of coronary artery disease. *Nat Genet* 40:161, 2008.

146. Kathiresan S, Melander O, Guiducci C, et al: Six new loci associated with blood low-density lipoprotein cholesterol, high-density lipoprotein cholesterol or triglycerides in humans. *Nat Genet* 40:189, 2008.

147. Jacobs RL, Lingrell S, Zhao Y, et al: Hepatic CTP:phosphocholine cytidylyltransferase-alpha is a critical predictor of plasma high density lipoprotein and very low density lipoprotein. *J Biol Chem* 283:2147, 2008.

148. Li X, Monda KL, Göring HH, et al: Genome-wide linkage scan for plasma high density lipoprotein cholesterol, apolipoprotein A-1 and triglyceride variation among American Indian populations: the Strong Heart Family Study. *J Med Genet* 46:472, 2009.

149. Göring HH, Curran JE, Johnson MP, et al: Discovery of expression QTLs using large-scale transcriptional profiling in human lymphocytes. *Nat Genet* 39:1208, 2007.

150. Chau P, Fielding PE, Fielding CJ: Bone morphogenetic protein-1 (BMP-1) cleaves human proapolipoprotein A1 and regulates its activation for lipid binding. *Biochemistry* 46:8445, 2007.

151. Willer CJ, Sanna S, Jackson AU, et al: Newly identified loci that influence lipid concentrations and risk of coronary artery disease. *Nat Genet* 40:161, 2008.

13

Low-Density Lipoprotein Cholesterol: Role in Atherosclerosis and Approaches to Therapeutic Management

Michael H. Davidson and Peter P. Toth

KEY POINTS

- Among patients with dyslipidemia, LDL-C is the primary target of therapy. LDL-C lowering reduces risk for CHD and its clinical sequelae, including unstable angina, ischemic stroke, myocardial infarction, and death.

- Atherogenesis is a complex disease whose etiology and progression are strongly influenced by the severity of a large number of risk factors. Low serum levels of HDL-C, hypertension, impairments in glucose metabolism, heightened systemic inflammatory tone, cigarette smoking, and others induce progressive arterial wall injury.

- The metabolic syndrome is characterized by a set of five risk factors: abdominal obesity; elevated blood pressure, triglycerides, and fasting glucose concentration; and low HDL-C. Metabolic syndrome develops secondary to the effects of insulin resistance and obesity.

- A number of preventive strategies can be used to target reductions in LDL-C to decrease the burden of CHD. The NCEP ATP III guidelines identify therapeutic lifestyle changes as the initial intervention to lower LDL-C.

- Statins, or 3-hydroxy-3-methylglutaryl-coenzyme A reductase inhibitors, are the most widely used drugs for lowering of LDL-C. The statins reduce cardiovascular morbidity and mortality.

- Bile acid sequestrants, nicotinic acid, fibrates, cholesterol absorption inhibition, and omega-3 fish oils also play important roles in LDL-C reduction and dyslipidemia management.

- Whereas LDL-C reduction has become the cornerstone of lipid management, apo B and non–HDL-C may be more accurate indicators of cardiovascular risk as well as measures by which to gauge LDL-lowering therapy.

- Clinical trials using statins and non-statin approaches to lipid lowering have demonstrated that for every 1 mg/dL reduction in serum LDL-C, there is a 1% reduction in risk for acute cardiovascular events.

Cardiovascular disease (CVD), including coronary heart disease (CHD), cerebrovascular disease, hypertension, and ischemic heart disease, is a major cause of mortality and morbidity worldwide, accounting for 17 million deaths.[1] Aggressive risk reduction therapies are indicated for patients with and without CHD to improve survival, to reduce initial or recurrent events, and to improve quality of life for these patients. Among patients with dyslipidemia, low-density lipoprotein cholesterol (LDL-C) is the primary target of therapy as research has substantiated that elevated LDL-C is a major cause of morbidity and mortality and LDL-C lowering reduces the risk for CHD and its clinical sequelae, including unstable angina, myocardial infarction, and death. This chapter reviews the role of LDL-C in the development of atherosclerosis and outlines management strategies to reduce serum levels of this lipoprotein.

HISTORICAL PERSPECTIVES ON HYPERCHOLESTEROLEMIA

The importance of hypercholesterolemia in the development of atherosclerosis can be traced historically as a medical controversy, as atherosclerosis was considered an inevitable part of aging.[2] Studies on rabbits demonstrating the impact of high-cholesterol diets on atherogenesis, published in 1913 by Anitschkow and Chalatov,[3] substantiated the role of hypercholesterolemia, yet it took a decade of research to confirm that the findings from experimental atherosclerosis in animals could be extrapolated to humans.[2]

The Framingham Heart Study and other prospective epidemiologic investigations demonstrated that risk for myocardial infarction, stroke, and death was proportional to serum cholesterol levels.[4-6] In the Seven Countries Study, a direct relationship was found between serum cholesterol and risk for CHD among 12,763 middle-aged men.[6] This relationship has been confirmed and extended in cohorts from 26 nations in the Multinational Monitoring of Trends and Determinants in Cardiovascular Disease (MONICA) study.[7] The Ni-Hon-San study evaluated the impact of migration and progressive westernization of the diet among Japanese men residing in Nippon, Japan, or in Honolulu and San Francisco.[8] As the intake of animal fat increased, serum cholesterol and risk for CHD mortality both increased. In the Multiple Risk Factor Intervention Trial (a cohort of 356,222 men), there was a clear gradient of continuously rising risk for CVD as serum cholesterol levels increased.[9] Whereas the majority of total cholesterol is composed of LDL-C in most patients, it was important to evaluate whether LDL-C is an independent predictor of CHD. The Cooperative Lipoprotein Phenotyping study,[10] the Atherosclerosis Risk in Communities study,[11] and the Framingham study[12] all demonstrated a direct and independent relationship between LDL-C and risk for cardiovascular morbidity and mortality. These relationships between total cholesterol and LDL-C and risk for CVD are remarkably consistent in populations studied throughout the world.

Acceptance of the lipid hypothesis that dyslipidemia is a causative factor in the development of atherosclerosis and CHD did not begin until the early 1960s, when research findings as well as the release of the American Heart Association's recommendation for dietary modification as a first step toward implementation of a cholesterol-lowering strategy[13] refocused attention on hypercholesterolemia. Advances in knowledge that ultimately validated the lipid hypothesis including understanding of the pathogenesis of atherosclerosis, large-scale clinical trial results including the Lipid Research Clinics Coronary Primary Prevention Trial, establishment of the National Cholesterol Education Program, and development and use of statins all led to confirmation of the role of dyslipidemia in the development of CHD.[2]

LIPOPROTEIN METABOLISM

Cholesterol derived from both biliary and dietary sources is transported into jejunal enterocytes from the intestinal lumen by a sterol translocase known as Niemann-Pick C1-like 1 protein.[14] Cholesterol, triglycerides, and phospholipids are packaged together with apoprotein B48 to form chylomicrons. Chylomicrons enter the enteric lymphatic system and are secreted into the central circulation through the lymphatic duct. The triglycerides in chylomicrons can be hydrolyzed by lipoprotein lipase in serum, yielding chylomicron remnant particles. Both chylomicrons and chylomicron remnants are taken up by hepatocytes. Intrahepatic cholesterol and lipids can be repackaged with apoprotein B100 into very-low-density lipoproteins (VLDL) and secreted into the central circulation.

The triglycerides in VLDL particles are hydrolyzed by lipoprotein lipase to yield, in sequence, intermediate-density lipoproteins (IDL) and then low-density lipoproteins (LDL). LDL particles tend to be highly enriched with cholesterol. All of the apo B100–containing lipoproteins are atherogenic. The sum of all atherogenic lipoproteins (VLDL + IDL + LDL) is defined as non–high-density lipoprotein (non-HDL). Non-HDL is a fairly sensitive measure of the total atherogenic lipoprotein burden in serum. LDL particles can be taken up into arterial walls. Alternatively, LDL particles are cleared from serum by the LDL receptor (LDLR) and LDLR-related protein expressed on the surface of hepatocytes. The cholesterol in LDL particles can then be shunted toward bile acid formation (rate-limiting step catalyzed by 7α-hydroxylase), it can be secreted into bile, or it can be repackaged into VLDL.

In patients with loss-of-function mutations in lipoprotein lipase, serum VLDL and triglyceride levels tend to be elevated. This impairs the conversion of VLDL into smaller, triglyceride-depleted lipoproteins. With this excess availability of triglyceride in VLDL, cholesteryl ester transfer protein catalyzes a 1:1 stoichiometric exchange for cholesterol between VLDL and LDL. This leads to progressive enrichment of the LDL particles with triglyceride, rendering them more vulnerable to lipolysis by the enzyme hepatic lipase. Hepatic lipase converts large buoyant LDL particles into smaller, denser and more numerous particles. Smaller LDL particles also tend to be more atherogenic: (1) biophysically, they can gain access into the subendothelial space more easily because they are smaller; (2) they are more easily oxidized than their larger counterparts; and (3) they have a lower affinity for the LDLR and hence reduced systemic clearance.

Some patients have a genetic predisposition to elevated serum levels of LDL-C. Hereditary hypercholesterolemias are frequently associated with premature multivessel coronary artery disease (CAD). Patients with familial hypercholesterolemia harbor a variety of mutations (these are indexed at *www.ucl.ac.uk/fh/*) in the gene for LDLR, resulting in reduced capacity for LDL clearance from serum.[15] Heterozygotes often present with serum LDL-C of 250 to 350 mg/dL. Homozygotes can have LDL-C levels of 500 mg/dL or more and usually require LDL apheresis to control their serum levels of this lipoprotein.

Loss-of-function mutations in cholesterol 7α-hydroxylase are also associated with elevations in LDL-C and decreased bile acid biosynthesis.[16] Patients with familial defective apo B100 have impaired capacity for LDL-C clearance secondary to polymorphisms in apo B100 (henceforth apo B), which reduce the affinity of this apoprotein for the LDLR.[17] Another fascinating group of mutations linked to hypercholesterolemia localizes to the gene coding for the enzyme proprotein convertase subtilisin/kexin type 9 (PCSK9).[18,19] This enzyme modulates the activity of the LDLR. Gain-of-function mutations lead to increased degradation of the LDLR, whereas loss-of-function mutations allow increased expression of the LDLR; these mutations are associated with increased and decreased risk for CAD, respectively.

LOW-DENSITY LIPOPROTEIN CHOLESTEROL AND ATHEROSCLEROTIC VASCULAR DISEASE

Atherogenesis is a complex disease whose etiology and progression are strongly influenced by the severity of a large number of risk factors. LDL is an apo B–containing particle (Fig. 14-1) and as such contributes to high levels of atherogenic lipoproteins (Fig. 14-2). In addition, low serum levels of high-density lipoprotein cholesterol (HDL-C), hypertension, impairments in glucose metabolism, heightened systemic inflammatory tone, cigarette smoking, and other risk factors induce progressive arterial wall injury. An early event in atherogenesis is the development of endothelial cell dysfunction. Under normal physiologic conditions, the endothelium serves as an efficient barrier between blood and the arterial wall. The endothelium produces nitric oxide (a potent vasodilator) and maintains an antithrombogenic surface by producing prostacyclin and tissue plasminogen activator. As the endothelium becomes stressed in response to risk factors, it becomes dysfunctional, resulting in a maladaptive inflammatory response (Fig. 14-3).[20,21]

Endothelial dysfunction is highly associated with atherosclerosis. Dysfunctional endothelial cells increase expression of adhesion molecules, such as vascular cell adhesion molecule 1, intercellular adhesion molecule 1, and different types of selectins.[22] These cell surface receptors interact with

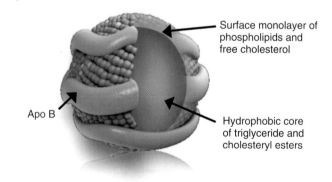

FIGURE 14-1 The structure of low-density lipoprotein. Nuclear magnetic resonance (NMR) spectroscopy of the LDL surface structure has enabled identification of a surface monolayer of phospholipids and free cholesterol and a hydrophobic core of triglyceride and cholesteryl esters. Phosphatidylcholine and sphingomyelin are tightly bound to apo B and therefore NMR invisible. *(From Murphy HC, Burns SP, White JJ, et al: Investigation of human low density lipoprotein by ¹H nuclear magnetic resonance spectroscopy: mobility of phosphatidylcholine and sphingomyelin headgroups characterizes the surface layer. Biochemistry 39:9763, 2000. Reproduced with permission.)*

Surface monolayer of phospholipids and free cholesterol

Apo B

Hydrophobic core of triglyceride and cholesteryl esters

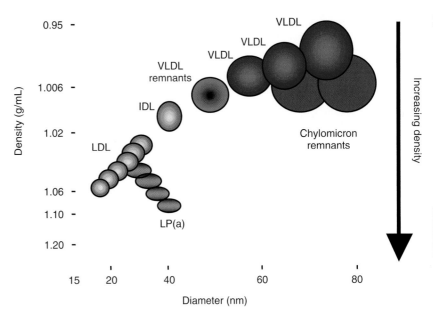

FIGURE 14-2 The atherogenicity of apo B–containing lipoproteins is related to their diameter and density. Chylomicrons are the largest lipoproteins and are produced by jejunal enterocytes. VLDL is secreted by the liver and progressively converted into IDL and then LDL by the activity of serum lipases. Atherogenic lipoproteins include chylomicron remnants, VLDL, VLDL remnants, IDL, and LDL particles. Remnants represent particles that are incompletely hydrolyzed. Lipoprotein(a) [Lp(a)] is a variant of LDL that is also atherogenic. Dyslipoproteinemia with low concentrations of HDL-C and elevated serum triglycerides with increased concentrations of small, dense LDL particles is associated with a particularly high incidence of coronary vascular disease. *(From Segrest JP, Garber DW, Brouillette CG, et al: The amphipathic alpha helix: a multifunctional structural motif in plasma apolipoproteins.* Adv Protein Chem *45:303, 1994. Reproduced with permission.)*

counterreceptors on the surface of inflammatory white blood cells, such as monocytes, T cells, and mast cells. These receptor-counterreceptor interactions facilitate the binding, rolling, and stable arrest of these cells along the endothelial surface.

Under normal conditions, endothelial cells maintain appropriate intercellular contacts through gap junctions, which allow these cells to communicate with one another and to maintain tight contacts among themselves.[23] These gap junctions also become dysfunctional and allow the transmigration of inflammatory white cells into the subendothelial space by following a gradient of monocyte chemoattractant protein 1 down into the subendothelial space. Once they are in the subendothelial space, monocytes can transform into resident macrophages in response to macrophage colony-stimulating factor. As gap junctions and endothelial cells become more dysfunctional, their barrier function becomes progressively more compromised, allowing greater influx of atherogenic lipoproteins into the arterial wall. Lipoproteins can be trapped in the vessel wall by intercellular matrix proteins such as proteoglycans, fibronectin, and vitronectin, among others.[24]

In the subendothelial space, LDL particles can be oxidized by such enzymes as myeloperoxidase, 5′-lipoxygenase, lipoprotein-associated phospholipase A_2, NADPH oxidase, and others.[25,26] T cells can present oxidized LDL to macrophages. The macrophages are activated and increase expression of families of scavenging receptors (e.g., CD36, scavenging receptor A). Scavenging receptors take up oxidized LDL, leading to foam cell formation. Foam cells can coalesce to form fatty streaks, and fatty streaks are the progenitors to the formation of atherosclerotic plaque. Macrophages can maintain a certain level of lipid homeostasis as long as there is adequate availability of HDL particles. HDL particles interact with macrophages and foam cells to promote the mobilization and externalization of intracellular lipid.[27-29]

If there is inadequate availability of HDL in the face of excess LDL in the extracellular milieu, there is continued net accumulation of lipid by the macrophage, ultimately resulting in apoptosis or programmed cell death. As cellular debris and more lipid accumulate, and as the capacity to phagocytose and clear this debris is progressively more compromised, the volume of the atherosclerotic plaque increases and develops a lipid core[30] (Fig. 14-4).

NATIONAL CHOLESTEROL EDUCATION PROGRAM GUIDELINES

A high serum level of LDL-C is an established risk factor for the development of CHD. For this reason, LDL-C reduction is the primary goal of therapy in patients with dyslipidemia. This recommendation is emphasized by the National Cholesterol Education Program Adult Treatment Panel III (NCEP ATP III),[31] the American Heart Association/American College of Cardiology guidelines for secondary prevention of CHD,[32] and the European Guidelines on Cardiovascular Disease Prevention.[33] NCEP ATP III defines an LDL-C of <100 mg/dL as optimal. Among patients in the primary prevention setting, it is recommended that 10-year projected risk for sustaining a CHD-related event be estimated with the Framingham risk score. Non–HDL-C is a surrogate measure of total atherogenic lipoprotein burden in serum and represents the sum of VLDL, IDL, LDL, and lipoprotein(a) as well as remnant particles. It is calculated by subtracting HDL-C from total cholesterol. Among patients with baseline triglycerides >200 mg/dL, non–HDL-C is the secondary target of therapy. Non–HDL-C has been shown to be a better predictor than LDL-C of risk for cardiovascular events in both men and women.[34,35] Goals for both LDL-C and non–HDL-C are risk stratified, and the goals for both of these lipoprotein fractions decrease as risk increases (Table 14-1). Among patients with CAD or a CAD risk equivalent (diabetes mellitus, abdominal aortic aneurysm, peripheral arterial disease, symptomatic carotid artery disease, or 10-year Framingham risk score >20%), it is recommended that patients achieve LDL-C <100 mg/dL and non–HDL-C <130 mg/dL. Among patients defined as very high risk (CAD complicated by a recent acute coronary syndrome, diabetes mellitus, or multiple poorly controlled risk factors), it is a therapeutic option to reduce LDL-C below 70 mg/dL and non–HDL-C below 100 mg/dL.[31] In a more recent advisory statement from the American Heart Association, it was recommended that an LDL-C target of <70 mg/dL be an option for any patient with established CAD.[36]

Evidence from clinical trials has established the merits of aggressive LDL-C risk reduction therapies for patients with CHD and other atherosclerotic vascular diseases in improving survival, reducing recurrent coronary events and need for revascularization, and improving quality of life. Data from

218

14

- Prelesional susceptible area of the arterial wall with diffuse intimal thickening (DIT)
- Lowering plasma apo B LPs and decreasing risk factors will prevent future vascular disease

- Early lipoprotein retention
- Lowering plasma apo B LPs and decreasing risk factors will readily promote removal of atherogenic components and prevent maladaptive responses and future disease

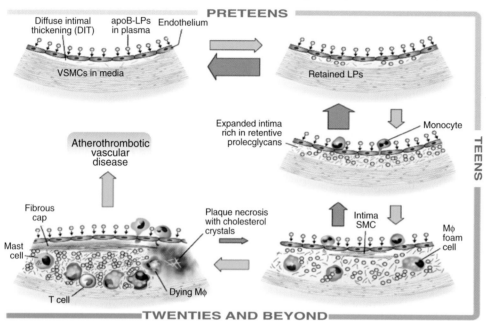

- Early responses to LP retention (e.g., monocyte entry)
- Lowering plasma apo B LPs and decreasing risk factors will readily promote removal of atherogenic components and prevent further responses and future disease
- Future strategies to prevent LP retention are likely to be most feasible up to this stage

- Advanced responses to LP retention, including maladaptive inflammation, Mϕ death, and plaque necrosis
- LP retention continues to accelerates
- Lowering plasma apo B LPs and reducing risk factors can promote removal of atherogenic components and promote regression, but reversal is more difficult and prolonged, and vascular disease may still develop

- Continued responses to LP retention, (e.g., Mϕ foam cell formation and SMC migration)
- LP retention starts to accelerate
- Lowering plasma apo B LPs and other risk factors can still promote removal of atherogenic components, promote regression, and prevent further responses and future disease

FIGURE 14-3 The continuum of developing atherosclerotic disease over a lifetime. Atherogenesis involves a complex interplay between inflammation, apo B–containing lipoproteins, and histologic components of blood vessel walls. Atherogenesis is potentiated by apo B lipoprotein retention by subendothelial extracellular matrix molecules (e.g., proteoglycans), which initiates a series of biologic reactions that develop into a maladaptive inflammatory response. As depicted in this figure, early response to lipoprotein retention begins in the preteen years and continues to accelerate in the 20s and beyond. Green arrows indicate progression; orange arrows indicate the potential for regression. The earliest stages are the most easily reversible by lowering of plasma apo B lipoproteins (large orange arrows). The complexity of advanced lesions, including accelerated lipoprotein retention, renders them less reversible (small orange arrows) as the severity of atherosclerosis advances. *(From Tabas I, Williams KJ, Borén J: Subendothelial lipoprotein retention as the initiating process in atherosclerosis: update and therapeutic implications. Circulation 116:1832, 2007. Reproduced with permission.)*

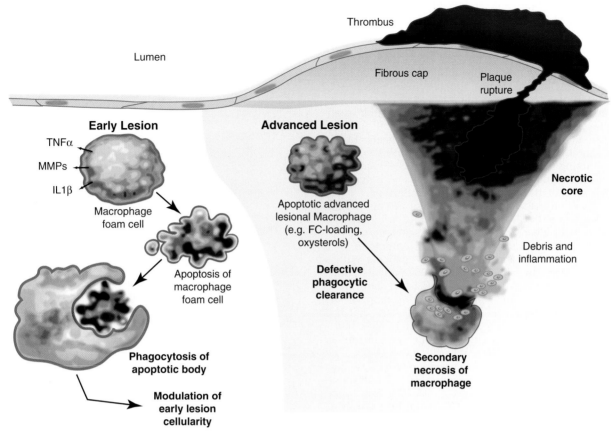

FIGURE 14-4 The role of macrophage apoptosis and atherosclerotic lesion progression. In the setting of endothelial dysfunction, atherogenic lipoproteins enter the subendothelial space, where they can aggregate and become oxidatively modified by a variety of enzymes. Oxidized LDL induces the upregulation of scavenging receptors on the surface of macrophages resident in the subendothelial space. Progressive macrophage lipid uptake results in the formation of foam cells. There is a limit to lipid uptake. Excess lipid is toxic to the cell and can result in apoptosis. Early in the course of atherogenesis, apoptotic debris is phagocytosed by other macrophages, a process that can modulate the cellularity and rate of progression of an atherosclerotic lesion. As depicted in this figure, in late lesions (right), macrophages also undergo apoptosis but are no longer cleared as efficiently. This leads to the formation of the necrotic core, which promotes inflammation, plaque instability, and acute lesional thrombosis secondary to loss of architectural integrity and rupture. *(From Tabas I: Consequences and therapeutic implications of macrophage apoptosis in atherosclerosis: the importance of lesion stage and phagocytic efficiency. Arterioscler Thromb Vasc Biol 25:2255, 2005. Reproduced with permission.)*

TABLE 14–1	LDL-C Goals and Thresholds for Initiation of Lifestyle Change and Pharmacologic Intervention		
Risk Category[1]	**LDL Goal**	**LDL Level at Which to Initiate TLC**	**LDL Level at Which to Consider Drug Therapy**
CHD or CHD risk equivalents (10-year risk >20%)	<100 mg/dL (optional goal <70)[2]	≥100 mg/dL All patients regardless of LDL	≥130 mg/dL (100-129 mg/dL: drug optional)≥100 mg/dL[3] (<100 mg/dL: drug optional)
2+ risk factors (10-year risk 10%-20%)	<130 mg/dL (optional goal <100)	≥130 mg/dL All patients regardless of LDL	≥130 mg/dL (>100 mg/dL: drug optional[4])
2+ risk factors (10-year risk ≤10%)	<130 mg/dL	≥130 mg/dL	≥160 mg/dL
0-1 risk factor	<160 mg/dL	≥160 mg/dL	≥190 mg/dL (160-189 mg/dL: LDL-lowering drug optional)

Coronary heart disease (CHD) risk equivalents include diabetes mellitus, peripheral vascular disease, carotid artery disease, and abdominal aortic aneurysm. TLC, therapeutic lifestyle changes.

[1]Risk factors included in Framingham risk evaluation are age, systolic blood pressure, total cholesterol, HDL-C, and smoking status.

[2]The optional goal of <70 mg/dL is particularly targeted at patients who are "very high" risk (e.g., patients with a recent acute coronary syndrome, poorly controlled diabetics with multiple risk factors).

[3]When statin therapy is initiated in these patients, the goal for LDL-C reduction should be 30% to 40% from baseline.

Based on Grundy SM, Cleeman JI, Merz CN, et al: Implications of recent clinical trials for the National Cholesterol Education Program Adult Treatment Panel III guidelines. *Circulation* 110:227, 2004.

studies including the Framingham Heart Study,[37] Multiple Risk Factor Intervention Trial,[9] and the Lipid Research Clinics trial[38] established the direct relationship between levels of LDL-C and the rate of development of CHD in asymptomatic patients. Other studies including the Heart Protection Study (HPS),[39] the Treating to New Targets (TNT) trial,[40] and the Incremental Decrease in Endpoints through Aggressive Lipid Lowering (IDEAL)[41] established the benefits of aggressive statin therapy in secondary prevention.

However, despite the substantial body of research establishing the benefit of LDL-C reduction, only a small percentage of patients with CHD are reaching lipid goals. In the National Cholesterol Education Program (NCEP) Evaluation Project Utilizing Novel E-Technology (NEPTUNE) survey of physicians regarding the care of 4885 patients with dyslipidemia, 75% of patients with CHD met the definition of "very high risk," yet only 18% had an LDL-C level <70 mg/dL and only 4% had an LDL-C level <70 mg/dL and a non–HDL-C level <100 mg/dL when triglycerides were >200 mg/dL.[42]

14

In a retrospective study from a national outpatient electronic medical record data base of 10,637 patients with a diagnosis of atherosclerosis, 57% of the 4067 patients with a baseline LDL-C ≥100 mg/dL were not prescribed statin treatment after diagnosis. Among patients receiving statin or any other cholesterol-lowering therapy after diagnosis who had baseline and follow-up LDL-C values (n = 682), 43% had a post-diagnosis LDL-C ≥100 mg/dL.[43] The proportion of patients with LDL-C <100 mg/dL at baseline was 46.8%, and 12% of patients had LDL-C cholesterol <70 mg/dL. Less than 5% of patients were currently receiving hypercholesterolemia therapy at the time of diagnosis, and 25% had hypercholesterolemia treatment after their condition had been diagnosed. Among patients receiving hypercholesterolemia therapy, LDL-C levels in 12 months after diagnosis of atherosclerosis were similar to levels at the time of diagnosis. These data substantiate the need for more aggressive statin therapy and implementation of combination therapy to reduce residual risk for cardiovascular events and highlight the importance of monitoring and managing lipid levels in patients with atherosclerosis.

METABOLIC SYNDROME AND CARDIOMETABOLIC RISK

In the United States, it is estimated that 35% to 40% of adults have the metabolic syndrome, a cluster of lipid and nonlipid disorders.[44,45] The metabolic syndrome is characterized by a set of five risk factors: abdominal obesity; elevated blood pressure, triglycerides, and fasting glucose concentration; and low HDL-C (Table 14-2). The presence of any three or more of the following risk factors in a single individual is diagnostic of the metabolic syndrome according to the revised ATP III/American Heart Association/National Heart, Lung, and Blood Institute definition[46]: triglycerides ≥150 mg/dL, HDL-C <40 mg/dL in men and ≤50 mg/dL in women, serum glucose concentration ≥100 mg/dL, blood pressure ≥130/85 mm Hg (can be either systolic or diastolic or on therapy with antihypertensive medication), and waist circumference ≥40 inches in men and ≥35 inches in women. Metabolic syndrome develops secondary to the effects of insulin resistance and obesity. Although the metabolic syndrome significantly increases risk for atherosclerotic disease and diabetes mellitus, it is not defined as a CAD risk equivalent.

The primary goal of clinical management of the metabolic syndrome is to reduce CHD risk and diabetes mellitus.[31] This focuses on intensified LDL-C lowering and modification of the underlying risk factors including obesity, physical inactivity, and other risk factors associated with the metabolic

TABLE 14–2	NCEP ATP III Criteria for Diagnosis of the Metabolic Syndrome*
Risk Factor	**Defining Level**
Abdominal obesity	
Men	Waist >40 inches
Women	Waist >35 inches
Triglycerides	≥150 mg/dL
HDL-C	
Men	<40 mg/dL
Women	<50 mg/dL
Blood pressure	≥130/≥85 mm Hg or taking antihypertensive medication
Fasting glucose	≥100 mg/dL or taking hypoglycemic medication

*Patients having any three of the five risk factors meet criteria for the diagnosis of the metabolic syndrome.
Modified from Toth P: Dyslipoproteinemias. *In* Rakel RE, Bope ET, editors: *Cohn's current therapy*, Philadelphia, 2006, Elsevier.

TABLE 14–3	Dietary Recommendations for Therapeutic Lifestyle Change
Dietary Component	**Recommendation Allowance**
Polyunsaturated fat	Up to 10% of total calories
Monounsaturated fat	Up to 20% of total calories
Total fat	25%-35% of total calories
Carbohydrate	50%-60% of total calories
Dietary fiber	20-30 g/day
Protein	Approximately 15% of total calories
Dietary cholesterol	<200 mg/day

syndrome, such as blood pressure control (Table 14-3).[31] The NCEP ATP III guidelines emphasize the modification of metabolic syndrome risk factors through lifestyle changes, especially because both weight loss and exercise reduce insulin resistance and favorably modify risk factors for the metabolic syndrome.[31]

THERAPEUTIC LIFESTYLE CHANGES

A number of preventive strategies can be used to target reductions in LDL-C to decrease the burden of CHD. The NCEP ATP III guidelines identify therapeutic lifestyle changes (TLC) as the initial intervention for lowering of LDL-C with a focus on smoking cessation, weight loss, total calories, physical activity to maintain desirable weight, and moderate alcohol intake (see Table 14-3). The NCEP guidelines outline TLC as a multifaceted lifestyle approach for LDL-C lowering. The recommendations for TLC include a reduction in saturated fat intake to <7% of total calories and cholesterol to <200 mg/day, weight reduction, increased physical activity, therapeutic options to enhance LDL lowering such as the use of plant stanols or sterols (2 g/day), and increased viscous (soluble) fiber (10 to 25 g/day) to reduce cholesterol absorption.[31] The aim of primary prevention is to reduce long-term risk (>10 years) as well as short-term risk (≤10 years). Whereas TLC is the basis of clinical primary prevention, pharmacologic therapy is often indicated in the management of elevated LDL-C to achieve risk-stratified target goals.

Statins, or 3-hydroxy-3-methylglutaryl-coenzyme A reductase inhibitors, have been the most widely used therapy for the treatment of dyslipidemia to reduce the risk of CHD. Statins are used to target the reduction of elevated LDL-C and to improve the lipid level profile. The statins are recognized as the first-line treatment of dyslipidemia.[31-33,47] Statins are used to target the reduction of elevated LDL-C and to improve all components of the lipid level profile.

Data from the major statin trials including the Scandinavian Simvastatin Survival Study (4S),[48] Cholesterol and Recurrent Events (CARE),[49] HPS,[39] Long-term Intervention with Pravastatin in Ischemic Disease (LIPID),[38] and TNT[40] have established that LDL-C reduction correlates with cardiovascular event reduction in a linear fashion. The HPS, the largest statin trial, demonstrated the benefits of aggressive

statin therapy with simvastatin 40 mg/day, with a 24% reduction in CVD events compared with placebo (Table 14-4). The beneficial effects of LDL-C reduction were demonstrated even in patients with baseline LDL-C levels below 100 mg/dL and in persons with diabetes.

The TNT trial additionally validated the benefit of lowering LDL-C to <100 mg/dL with treatment with atorvastatin 80 mg daily, resulting in a 22% reduction of cardiovascular events compared with atorvastatin 20 mg daily. The IDEAL[41] study established the benefit of intensive lipid lowering with statin therapy with atorvastatin 10 mg daily, resulting in a lower LDL-C level and an 11% reduction in major cardiovascular events compared with simvastatin 20 mg daily. A meta-analysis of 14 prospective randomized statin trials by the Cholesterol Treatment Trialists Collaboration showed that for every 39 mg/dL (1 mmol/L) reduction in serum LDL-C with statin therapy during a mean 5-year follow-up, there was a

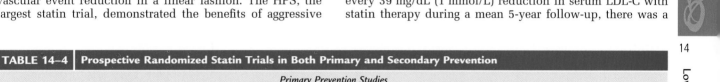

14

Low-Density Lipoprotein Cholesterol: Role in Atherosclerosis and Approaches to Therapeutic Management

TABLE 14–4	Prospective Randomized Statin Trials in Both Primary and Secondary Prevention		
Primary Prevention Studies			
Study	**Drug**	**Design**	**Outcomes**
AFCAPS/TexCAPS	Lovastatin 20 to 40 mg/day versus placebo	6605 men and women	40% reduction in fatal and nonfatal MI; 37% reduction in first ACS; 33% reduction in coronary revascularizations; and unstable angina reduced by 32%
ASCOT	Atorvastatin 10 mg/day versus placebo	10,305 hypertensive men (n = 8463) and women (n = 1942) with treated high blood pressure and no previous CAD	36% reduction in total CHD/nonfatal MI; 27% reduction in fatal and nonfatal stroke; total coronary event reduced by 29%; fatal and nonfatal stroke reduced by 27%
CARDS	Atorvastatin 10 mg/day versus placebo	2838 patients with type 2 diabetes mellitus and 1 CHD risk factor	37% reduction of major cardiovascular events; 27% reduction of total mortality; 13.4% reduction of acute cardiovascular events; 36% reduction of acute coronary events; 48% reduction of stroke
Heart Protection Study	Simvastatin 40 mg/day versus placebo	20,536 high-risk individuals (previous CHD, other vascular disease, hypertension among men aged >65 years, or diabetes)	25% reduction in all-cause and coronary death rates and in strokes; need for revascularization reduced by 24%; fatal and nonfatal stroke reduced by 25%; nonfatal MI reduced by 38%; coronary mortality reduced by 18%; all-cause mortality reduced by 13%; cardiovascular event rate reduced by 24%
PROSPER	Pravastatin 40 mg/day versus placebo	5804 men (n = 2804) and women (n = 3000) aged 70 to 82 years	15% reduction in combined endpoint (fatal/nonfatal MI or stroke); 19% reduction in total/nonfatal CHD; no effect on stroke (but 25% reduction in TIA)
WOSCOPS	Pravachol therapy 40 mg/day versus placebo	6595 men	CHD death of nonfatal MI reduced by 31%; CVD death reduced by 32%; total mortality 22% reduction
Secondary Prevention Studies			
Study	**Drug**	**Design**	**Outcomes**
4S	Simvastatin 20 mg/day versus placebo	4444 patients with angina pectoris or history of MI	Coronary mortality reduced by 42%; myocardial revascularization reduction of 37%; all-cause mortality reduced by 30%; nonfatal major coronary event reduced by 34%; fatal and nonfatal stroke reduced by 30%
AVERT	Atorvastatin 80 mg/day versus angioplasty + usual care	341 patients with stable CAD	36% reduction in ischemic event; delayed time to first ischemic event reduced by 36%
CARE	Pravastatin 40 mg/day versus placebo	3583 men and 576 women with history of MI	Death from CHD or nonfatal MI reduced by 24%; death from CHD reduced by 20%; nonfatal MI reduced by 23%; fatal MI reduced by 37%; CABG or PTCA reduced by 27%
IDEAL	Atorvastatin 80 mg/day versus simvastatin 20-40 mg/day	8888 men and women with CHD	Major cardiac events reduced by 13%; nonfatal MI reduced by 17%; revascularization reduced by 23%; peripheral arterial disease reduced by 24%

Continued

TABLE 14–4 | **Prospective Randomized Statin Trials in Both Primary and Secondary Prevention—cont'd**

		Secondary Prevention Studies	
Study	Drug	Design	Outcomes
JUPITER	Rosuvastatin 20 mg/day versus placebo	17,802 men (>50 years) and women (>60 years) with no history of CAD or diabetes mellitus, entry LDL <130 mg/dL, and CRP >2.0 mg/L	44% reduction in primary endpoint of major coronary events; 65% reduction in nonfatal MI; 48% reduction in nonfatal stroke; 46% reduction in need for revascularization; 20% reduction in all-cause mortality
LIPID	Pravachol 40 mg/day versus placebo	9014 patients	Coronary mortality reduced by 24%; stroke reduced by 19%; fatal CHD or nonfatal MI reduced by 24%; fatal or nonfatal MI reduced by 29%
LIPS	Fluvastatin 40 mg/day versus placebo	1667 men and women aged 18-80 years after angioplasty for CAD	22% lower rate of major coronary events (e.g., cardiac deaths, nonfatal MI, or reintervention procedure)
MIRACL	Atorvastatin 80 mg/day versus placebo	3086 patients with ACS	Reduction in composite endpoint by 16%; ischemia reduced by 26%; stroke reduced by 50%
PROVE IT	Atorvastatin 80 mg/day versus pravastatin 40 mg/day	4162 patient with ACS	16% reduction of composite endpoint; 14% reduction in CHD death, MI, or revascularization; revascularizations reduced by 14%; unstable angina reduced by 29%
REVERSAL	Atorvastatin 80 mg/day versus pravastatin 40 mg/day	654 patients with CAD	Atheroma: atorvastatin −0.4%, pravastatin 2.7%, difference of −3.1%, $P = 0.02$
TNT	Atorvastatin 10 mg/day versus 80 mg/day	10,003 patients with CHD and LDL cholesterol 130-250 mg/dL	22% reduction in composite endpoint; MI reduced by 22%; stroke reduced by 25%

ACS, acute coronary syndrome; CABG, coronary artery bypass grafting; CAD, coronary artery disease; CHD, coronary heart disease; CRP, C-reactive protein; LDL, low-density lipoprotein; MI, myocardial infarction; PTCA, percutaneous transluminal coronary angioplasty; TIA, transient ischemic attack.

AFCAPS/TexCAPS, Air Force/Texas Coronary Atherosclerosis Prevention Study: Implications for Preventive Cardiology in the General Adult US Population (*Curr Atheroscler Rep* 1:38, 1999); ASCOT, Anglo-Scandinavian Cardiac Outcomes Trial–Lipid Lowering Arm (*Lancet* 361:1149, 2003); CARDS, Collaborative Atorvastatin Diabetes Study (*Lancet* 364:685, 2004); Heart Protection Study (*Lancet* 360:7, 2002); PROSPER, Pravastatin in elderly individuals at risk of vascular disease (*Lancet* 360:1623, 2002); WOSCOPS, West of Scotland Coronary Prevention Study (*N Engl J Med* 333:1301, 1995); 4S, Scandinavian Simvastatin Survival Study (*Lancet* 344:1383, 1994); AVERT, Atorvastatin versus Revascularization Treatment Investigators (*N Engl J Med* 341:70, 1999); CARE, Cholesterol and Recurrent Events Trial (*N Engl J Med* 335:1001, 1996); IDEAL, Incremental Decrease in End Points Through Aggressive Lipid Lowering Study (*JAMA* 294:2437, 2005); JUPITER: The Justification for the Use of Statins in Prevention: an Intervention Trial Evaluating Rosuvastatin (*N Engl J Med* 359:2195, 2008); LIPID, Long-Term Intervention with Pravastatin in Ischemic Disease (*Am J Cardiol* 76:474, 1995); LIPS, Lescol Intervention Prevention Study (*JAMA* 287:3215, 2002); MIRACL, Myocardial Ischemia Reduction with Aggressive Cholesterol Lowering Study (*JAMA* 285:1711, 2001); PROVE IT, Pravastatin or Atorvastatin Evaluation and Infection Therapy Study (*N Engl J Med* 350:1495, 2004); REVERSAL, The REVERSing Atherosclerosis with Aggressive Lipid Lowering Study (*JAMA* 292:1, 2004); TNT, Treating to New Targets trial (*N Engl J Med* 352:1425, 2005).

From Toth PP: Management of dyslipidemia. *In* Toth PP, Cannon CP, editors: *Comprehensive cardiovascular medicine in the primary care setting*, Philadelphia, 2010, Humana-Springer. Reproduced with permission.

12% reduction in all-cause mortality, a 19% reduction in coronary mortality, a 24% reduction in myocardial infarction or coronary death, a 24% reduction in need for revascularization, and a 17% reduction in fatal or nonfatal stroke.[50]

The predominant benefits of statins on CHD risk reduction are due to their LDL-C–lowering effects, but the effects that statins have on triglycerides and HDL-C may also contribute to risk reduction. In the 4S[48] and The Air Force/Texas Coronary Atherosclerosis Prevention (AFCAPS/TexCAPS)[51] trial, apo B rather than LDL-C was a better predictor of event reduction. As apo B is contained in LDL-C, the triglyceride-containing IDL, and VLDL, the impact of statins on IDL may also affect risk reduction.

The AFCAPS/TexCAPS trial additionally demonstrated that the best overall predictor of events on treatment was the ratio apo B/apo A-I. This supports the concept that raising of HDL (the apo A-I–containing particles) also contributes to the risk-modifying benefits of statin therapy. The Justification for the Use of statins in Prevention: an Intervention Trial Evaluating Rosuvastatin (JUPITER)[52] trial demonstrated the benefit of statin therapy on dual targets of LDL-C and high-sensitivity C-reactive protein (hsCRP), with subjects receiving rosuvastatin 20 mg/day who achieved both LDL-C <70 mg/dL and hsCRP <2.0 mg/L having the lowest incidence of vascular events. The JUPITER trial also provided compelling evidence that on-treatment LDL-C level is a strong predictor of clinical benefit. Compared with placebo, participants allocated to rosuvastatin who did not achieve LDL-C <70 mg/dL had no significant reduction in vascular events (placebo event rate, 1.11%/year; participant allocated to rosuvastatin with LDL-C >70 mg/dL event rate, 0.91%/year; HR, 0.89; 95% CI, 0.65-125; $P = 0.49$). Alternatively, patients allocated to rosuvastatin who had on-treatment hsCRP >2.0 mg/L still had a significant benefit (event rate, 0.7%/year), but not as much as those who achieved an hsCRP <2.0 mg/L (event rate, 0.42%/year).

Achievement of the dual goals of LDL-C <70 mg/dL and CRP <2.0 mg/L is difficult as demonstrated in a 2-year follow-up of the Pravastatin Or atorVastatin Evaluation and Infection Therapy (PROVE-IT) study, which tested the efficacy of atorvastatin 80 mg/day and pravastatin 40 mg/day (Fig. 14-5). Whereas atorvastatin 80 mg was superior to pravastatin 40 mg/day in terms of achieving the dual goals of aggressive LDL-C and CRP reduction, neither agent brought the majority of patients below thresholds needed to maximize risk reduction.[53]

Lipid changes appear to explain the expected outcome benefits of statin therapy. The pleiotropic or added effects of statins, such as vasodilation, antithrombosis, antioxidant, antiproliferative, and anti-inflammatory effects, may also play a role in CHD risk reduction, although this is not yet firmly established. A recent meta-analysis highlighted the

FIGURE 14-5 In a 2-year follow-up study comparing the efficacy of statin regimens in achieving the dual goals of low-density lipoprotein cholesterol (LDL-C) and C-reactive protein (CRP) reduction, 44% of patients receiving atorvastatin 80 mg/day achieved the dual goals, whereas 11% of patients receiving pravastatin 40 mg/day achieved the dual goals. As shown in this figure, both groups achieved similar risk reduction, but neither agent brought the majority of patients below thresholds needed to maximize benefit, substantiating that the dual goals of LDL-C <70 mg/dL and CRP <2.0 mg/L are difficult to achieve. *(From Ridker PM, Morrow DA, Rose LM, et al: Relative efficacy of atorvastatin 80 mg and pravastatin 40 mg in achieving the dual goals of low-density lipoprotein cholesterol <70 mg/dl and C-reactive protein < 2 mg/l. J Am Coll Cardiol 45:1644, 2005. Reproduced with permission.)*

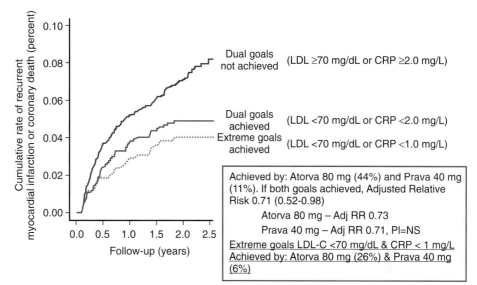

14

Low-Density Lipoprotein Cholesterol: Role in Atherosclerosis and Approaches to Therapeutic Management

association of LDL-C reduction and incidence of stroke among the major statin trials, further demonstrating the beneficial effects of statin therapy in CHD risk reduction.[54]

STATIN SAFETY

The safety of high-dose statin therapy is a clinical concern as associated adverse events include statin-associated persistent liver enzyme elevation, myotoxicity, and life-threatening rhabdomyolysis. Whereas the reported occurrence of muscle-related adverse events in clinical trials of statins is low, many of the trials were not designed or powered to detect rhabdomyolysis. Simultaneously, differing definitions of adverse events have been used in the various clinical trials. A standard definition of nonfatal rhabdomyolysis is the development of muscle symptoms plus creatine kinase >10 times the upper limit of normal. In terms of incidence rates of rhabdomyolysis, in the HPS,[39] which was the largest clinical trial of statin therapy to date, there were five cases (0.05%) of nonfatal rhabdomyolysis in patients receiving simvastatin 40 mg compared with three cases (0.03%) in patients receiving placebo. Despite the fact that the absolute event rate for rhabdomyolysis remains low at all doses for approved statins, the highest approved dose of a statin does have an increased risk for muscle adverse effects. There does not, however, appear to be a relationship between risk for myopathy and attained level of LDL-C.[40,50] It therefore becomes necessary to acknowledge the risk of statin therapy even in standard doses used to reduce cardiovascular risk. Patients should be counseled about symptoms associated with skeletal muscle and liver toxicity.

COMBINATION THERAPY

Whereas statin therapy is an established strategy of reducing death and myocardial infarction among patients with CHD, a significant number of individuals who are receiving statin therapy continue to have high residual risk. As a result, combination therapy increases the likelihood of achieving target lipid levels, especially in those patients with residual risk. Combination therapy results in a greater degree of reduction in residual risk of CVD events compared with monotherapy. Reasons for considering combination therapy include lack of achievement of LDL goals, lack of achievement of non–HDL-C goals, inadequate HDL-C elevation, and safety concerns associated with the use of high doses of statins.

Bile acid sequestrants (cholestyramine, colestipol, and colesevelam hydrochloride), niacin (extended release), and ezetimibe lower LDL-C by 15% to 20%; a 15% to 20% decrease in LDL-C is approximately equivalent to tripling the dose of a statin. For every doubling of the dose of a statin, there is a further decrease in LDL-C of approximately 6%. Therefore, the use of combination therapy is indicated to further improve the lipid profile, especially for very high risk patients who have not yet achieved the optional therapeutic target. The NCEP ATP III guidelines indicate that statin combination therapy with a bile acid sequestrant or nicotinic acid is indicated if LDL-C goals are not achieved.[31]

STATINS–BILE ACID SEQUESTRANTS

Bile acid sequestrants are a class of antihyperlipidemic drugs that augment cholesterol excretion through enhanced conversion to bile acids to lower LDL-C. By reducing intrahepatic stores of cholesterol, bile acid sequestrants stimulate increased expression of the LDLR and promote increased clearance of LDL-C. In the Lipid Research Clinics Coronary Primary Prevention Trial, lipid lowering with cholestyramine was associated with a significant 19% reduction in the composite endpoint of nonfatal myocardial infarction and death among men with no prior history of CHD.[55]

Two of the most commonly prescribed bile acid sequestrants, cholestyramine and colestipol, have established efficacy and safety as nonsystemic approaches to cholesterol reduction. Several large-scale clinical trials, including the Lipid Research Clinics Coronary Primary Prevention Trial[38] and the Familial Atherosclerosis Treatment Study,[56] have demonstrated the clinical benefit of bile acid sequestrants. Despite their known benefits, the use of bile acid sequestrants in clinical practice is hampered, in part because of issues related to poor palatability of the drugs and the occurrence of adverse gastrointestinal effects, particularly constipation, which influences therapy adherence. The incidence of constipation with colesevelam approximates that with placebo; with colestipol and cholestyramine, it is 10% and 26%, respectively.[57,58] As a result, colesevelam hydrochloride is often the preferred drug of this class.

The use of colesevelam hydrochloride in combination therapy with lovastatin,[59] simvastatin,[60] or atorvastatin[61] has demonstrated significant lowering of LDL-C levels in hypercholesterolemic patients. Low-dose combination therapy with colesevelam hydrochloride (2.3 g) and lovastatin (10 mg) was shown to reduce LDL-C by 34% (60 mg/dL; $P < 0.0001$) and 32% (53 mg/dL; $P < 0.0001$) in patients with primary hypercholesterolemia.[59] Similarly, combination therapy with simvastatin 10 mg and 20 mg and colesevelam hydrochloride 2.3 g and 3.8 g was demonstrated to reduce LDL-C. Patients treated with simvastatin–colesevelam hydrochloride combination therapy had a mean reduction in LDL-C levels of 42% (−80 mg/dL; $P < 0.0001$) compared with baseline, which surpassed reductions for simvastatin 10 mg (−26%, −48 mg/dL) or 20 mg (−34%, −61 mg/dL) alone or for colesevelam hydrochloride 2.3 g (−8%, −17 mg/dL) or 3.8 g (−16%, −31 mg/dL) alone ($P < 0.001$).[60]

Another clinical trial demonstrated that the coadministration of colesevelam hydrochloride 3.8 g and atorvastatin 10 mg or 80 mg/day resulted in LDL-C reductions of 12% to 53% in all active treatment groups ($P < 0.01$). Combination therapy resulted in significant decreases in LDL-C (48%) compared with colesevelam hydrochloride (12%) or low-dose atorvastatin (38%) alone ($P < 0.01$) but similar to those achieved with atorvastatin 80 mg/day (53%).[61]

Colesevelam hydrochloride has also been demonstrated to reduce hemoglobin A1c (HbA1c) levels in subjects with type 2 diabetes mellitus uncontrolled by existing antihyperglycemic therapy (HbA1c values of 7% to 10%). The Glucose Lowering Effect of WelChol Study (GLOWS) demonstrated that 12 weeks of colesevelam 3.75 g/day was associated with significant reductions in HbA1c in 65 subjects with type 2 diabetes.[62] In subjects with a baseline HbA1c ≥8.0%, the difference in least squares mean change in HbA1c was −1.0% (0.27; $P = 0.002$). Compared with placebo, colesevelam treatment was associated with reductions in levels of fructosamine (−29.0 [10.9] pmol/L; $P = 0.011$) and postprandial glucose (−31.5 [13.6] mg/dL; $P = 0.026$). The mean percentage change in LDL-C was −10% in the colesevelam group, compared with 2% in the placebo group (treatment difference, −12% [4.2]; $P = 0.007$). Colesevelam was also associated with significant decreases in the percentage change in apo B ($P = 0.003$) and LDL particle concentration ($P = 0.037$).[62]

In another trial, colesevelam hydrochloride 3.75 g/day in subjects with type 2 diabetes mellitus uncontrolled (HbA1c 7.5% to 9.5%) with insulin, alone or in combination with oral antihyperglycemics, those receiving treatment (n = 147) experienced a significant change in HbA1c (−0.41%) compared with controls (+0.09%, n = 140; $P < 0.0001$). Colesevelam hydrochloride also resulted in significant mean decreases in LDL-C (13%) and apo B (5%) and increases in apo A-I (2%) and median triglyceride levels (21.5%).[63] The results further supported the efficacy of colesevelam hydrochloride in enhancing glycemic control and improving lipid profiles in subjects with type 2 diabetes on an insulin-containing regimen.

NIACIN

Niacin or nicotinic acid, a potent lipid-modifying agent, is a form of vitamin B_3, one of the water-soluble B complex vitamins. Niacin was the first lipid-lowering agent to significantly reduce cardiovascular events in the Coronary Drug Project, which randomized 3908 men and demonstrated that 6 years of niacin therapy reduced the risk of nonfatal myocardial infarction and resulted in an 11% reduction in all-cause mortality (this was not significant after 5 years of follow-up; myocardial infarction [26%] and stroke [24%] reduction were significant compared with placebo).[64]

Niacin has broad-spectrum effects including LDL-C reduction, triglyceride and lipoprotein(a) reduction, and HDL elevation and is therefore used in the treatment of a variety of lipid disorders, including the metabolic syndrome, diabetes mellitus, isolated low HDL-C, and hypertriglyceridemia.[65] Niacin binds to the receptor HM74 on the surface of visceral adipocytes and helps reduce the mobilization of free fatty acid. Niacin inhibits intrahepatic triglyceride and VLDL biosynthesis, stimulates HDL secretion, reduces HDL catabolism, and increases LDL particle size and reduces LDL particle number.[66]

Despite its benefits in the management of dyslipidemia, the use of niacin has been limited by vasodilation-induced flushing. Niacin is currently available in three formulations, including immediate release, extended release, and long acting. Each differs with respect to its safety and efficacy profiles, with long-acting or extended-release niacin having less flushing. The flushing induced by niacin is mediated by prostaglandin D_1. The biosynthesis of prostaglandin D_1 can be reduced by pretreating patients with 325 mg of aspirin (generally 2 hours before nicotinic acid is taken); limiting the ingestion of hot liquids, spicy foods, and saturated fat; and avoiding alcohol. It is recommended that over-the-counter preparations of niacin be avoided, given their side effect profile and uncertain purity. Flushing is inhibited more significantly if patients use aspirin prophylaxis at 325 mg rather than 81 mg.[67]

Statin-niacin combination therapy is a recognized lipid-altering therapy used to reduce residual cardiovascular risk. Niacin is often added to a statin in patients with combined hyperlipidemia, especially if the HDL is low or lipoprotein(a) is high. Although statins have demonstrated an approximate reduction in CHD events by 30%, combination therapy with statins and niacin has resulted in relative risk reductions of ~75%.[68] This significant reduction in CHD events suggests that other effects of niacin, such as triglyceride and lipoprotein(a) lowering and HDL raising, may also contribute to the benefits.

The HDL-Atherosclerosis Treatment Study assessed the impact of simvastatin (10 to 20 mg/day) plus niacin (2 to 4 g/day) combination therapy on risk reduction for a composite of cardiovascular endpoints (death from coronary causes, confirmed myocardial infarction or stroke, or revascularization). Cardiovascular risk was decreased by 90% in the group treated with simvastatin plus niacin compared with placebo ($P = 0.03$).[69] In addition, simvastatin-niacin combination therapy resulted in a 0.4% regression in coronary stenosis, whereas progression occurred in other treatment groups receiving antioxidants alone, simvastatin plus niacin plus antioxidants, or placebo ($P < 0.001$).[68] Additional studies evaluating statin plus niacin combination therapy have also demonstrated efficacy in increasing HDL-C and reducing triglycerides and LDL-C.[70-72]

The Safety and Efficacy of A COmbination of NiAcin ER and Simvastatin in PaTients (SEACOAST) study assessed the use of two combination niacin extended-release (NER) therapies with simvastatin (1000 mg NER/20mg simvastatin and 2000 mg NER/20 mg simvastatin) in 319 dyslipidemic

14

patients. After 24 weeks of therapy, 6.5% and 9%, respectively, of patients discontinued use because of flushing. Similar results were observed in SEACOAST II, with combination NER/simvastatin in higher doses (1000 mg NER/40 mg simvastatin or 2000 mg NER/40 mg simvastatin), in which 4% and 6% (respectively) of patients withdrew because of flushing.[73] An Open-Label Evaluation of the Safety and Efficacy of a Combination of Niacin ER and Simvastatin in Patients with Dyslipidemia (OCEANS) study found comparable results with the use of NER/simvastatin (titrated to 2000/40 mg/day) during 52 weeks in 520 patients with primary type II or mixed hyperlipidemia,[74] further substantiating the benefit of statin-niacin combination therapy.

A number of trials have also demonstrated the safety of statin-niacin combination and efficacy in inhibiting the progression of atherosclerosis. Most trials have used either immediate-release niacin or extended-release niacin (Niaspan). The addition of extended-release niacin to statin therapy was evaluated in the Arterial Biology for the Investigation of the Treatment Effects of Reducing Cholesterol (ARBITER) 2 trial, which demonstrated an increase in HDL-C by 21% and slowed progression of atherosclerosis as measured by change in carotid intima-media thickness, compared with statin therapy alone in patients with known CHD and low HDL-C levels.[75]

The Arterial Biology for the Investigation of the Treatment Effects of Reducing Cholesterol 6 (ARBITER 6)–HDL and LDL Treatment Strategies in Atherosclerosis (HALTS) trial, despite some concerns about its early termination, demonstrated that in patients with CHD or CHD risk equivalent, the use of extended-release niacin 2000 mg/day in combination with long-term statin therapy caused a significant regression in carotid intima-media thickness compared with an ezetimibe-statin combination.[76]

On the basis of these surrogate outcome trials and the effect of niacin on increasing HDL-C and decreasing LDL-C and lipoprotein(a) at higher doses, niacin is a preferred treatment in combination with statin therapy to reduce cardiovascular risk. However, there is still debate as to the extent to which findings from surrogate endpoint studies can be translated into clinical benefit, and thus the completion of the clinical outcomes studies involving niacin, such as AIM-HIGH, is of great interest.

STATINS-EZETIMIBE

Combination therapy with ezetimibe, a selective cholesterol absorption inhibitor that blocks cholesterol absorption at the intestinal brush border, and statins can be used to enhance LDL-C lowering.[77,78] Ezetimibe inhibits the sterol transporter Niemann-Pick C1-like 1 protein along the luminal surface of the jejunal brush border (Fig. 14-6). Combination ezetimibe-statin therapy has been evaluated in several randomized

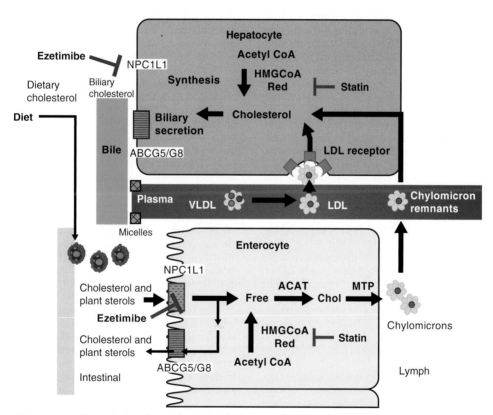

FIGURE 14-6 The mechanism of ezetimibe, a selective cholesterol absorption inhibitor. As outlined in this figure, ezetimibe reduces the small intestinal enterocyte absorption of cholesterol and plant sterols by binding to the Niemann-Pick C1-like 1 (NPC1L1) protein, which keeps cholesterol in the intestinal lumen for excretion. Excess intracellular cholesterol can also be translocated back into the intestinal lumen through the activity of the heterodimeric ATP-binding membrane cassette transport proteins G5/G8. Absorbed ezetimibe undergoes glucuronidation to a single metabolite and localizes at the intestinal wall, where it binds with higher affinity for NPC1L1 to prevent cholesterol absorption. Free cholesterol is esterified by the enzyme acyl:cholesterol acyltransferase (ACAT). Absorbed lipid, cholesteryl esters, and apo B48 are used by microsomal triglyceride transfer protein (MTP) to assemble chylomicrons. Chylomicrons are then secreted into the enteric lymphatic system and are released into the central circulation by the lymphatic duct. Chylomicrons are cleared by the liver. Ezetimibe can also reduce the hepatic reabsorption of cholesterol from bile by inhibiting NPC1L1 along the canalicular surface of the biliary tract. (From Davis HR, Veltri EP: Zetia: inhibition of Niemann-Pick C1 like 1 [NPC1L1] to reduce intestinal cholesterol absorption and treat hyperlipidemia. J Atheroscler Thromb 14:99, 2007. Reproduced with permission.)

225

14

Low-Density Lipoprotein Cholesterol: Role in Atherosclerosis and Approaches to Therapeutic Management clinical trials of patients with primary hypercholesterolemia. Ezetimibe 10 mg coadministered with simvastatin 10 mg resulted in 44% LDL-C reductions, similar to those obtained with simvastatin 80 mg alone, and coadministration of ezetimibe 10 mg with simvastatin doses of 10 to 80 mg resulted in triglyceride reductions of 26% to 31% and HDL-C increases of 8% to 11%.[79] In another study, coadministration of ezetimibe 10 mg and atorvastatin 10, 20, 40, or 80 mg compared with monotherapy resulted in significant improvements with a 12% reduction in LDL-C, 8% reduction in triglycerides, and 3% increase in HDL-C.[80]

Lovastatin monotherapy at 10, 20, or 40 mg or ezetimibe 10 mg was compared with combination therapy of ezetimibe 10 mg plus lovastatin 10, 20, or 40 mg; the coadministration of ezetimibe provided an incremental 14% decrease in LDL-C, a 5% increase in HDL-C , and a 10% decrease in triglycerides compared with pooled lovastatin alone. Ezetimibe plus lovastatin provided mean LDL-C decreases of 33% to 45%, median triglyceride decreases of 19% to 27%, and mean HDL-C increases of 8% to 9%, depending on the statin dose.[81]

In clinical practice, the prevailing recommendation is to initiate LDL-C reduction with statin therapy. If the patient cannot attain the LDL-C goal with statin monotherapy either because of an inadequate response or because of intolerance to an appropriate dose of a statin, then either niacin, a resin, or ezetimibe can be added as adjuvant therapy. Ezetimibe monotherapy can also be used in patients who are intolerant to statin therapy. For patients receiving statin therapy not at goal, the dose of the statin should generally be titrated to at least 40 mg/day before ezetimibe is added. For patients who are more than 10% above their LDL-C goal, statin titration may result in a 6% further LDL-C reduction, and ezetimibe may therefore provide enhanced ability to achieve LDL-C targets in these patients.

Ezetimibe therapy provides a level of LDL-C reduction that is equivalent to three titration steps of a statin. The efficacy of ezetimibe for reducing cardiovascular morbidity and mortality in patients with CAD is being evaluated in the IMProved Reduction of Outcomes: Vytorin Efficacy International (IMPROVE-IT) trial.[82] Unfortunately, we will probably not have clinical outcome results from this pivotal clinical trial until 2013 at the earliest.

STATIN-FIBRATE COMBINATION THERAPY

In patients with combined dyslipidemia, fibrate-statin combination therapy can be used to promote reductions in LDL-C and triglycerides and simultaneous increases in HDL-C. The fibrates activate lipoprotein lipase and promote triglyceride hydrolysis, inhibit hepatic triglyceride biosynthesis, stimulate hepatic HDL secretion, and reduce LDL particle number. Fibrate monotherapy has been shown to reduce risk for cardiovascular events[83,84] and rates of atherosclerotic disease progression.[85,86]

The Simvastatin Plus Fenofibrate for Combined Hyperlipidemia (SAFARI) trial demonstrated that combination therapy of simvastatin 20 mg/day plus fenofibrate 160 mg/day resulted in significantly decreased LDL-C levels (31%) compared with monotherapy (26%; $P < 0.001$) in patients with combined hyperlipidemia (fasting triglyceride levels ≥150 and ≤500 mg/dL and LDL cholesterol >130 mg/dL).[87] In addition, mean HDL-C levels significantly increased with combination therapy (19%) compared with monotherapy (10%; $P < 0.001$), without the occurrence of any drug-related serious adverse events.[87]

Fibrates are associated with a slightly increased risk (<1.0%) for myopathy, cholelithiasis, and venous thrombosis. When fibrate therapy is used, measurement of serum creatinine concentration is recommended before fibrate use, with dose adjustments made for renal impairment. Whereas routine monitoring of creatinine concentration is not required, a clinically important increase in creatinine without other potential causes should be reevaluated, and consideration should be given to discontinuation of fibrate therapy or reduction of the dose.[88] The efficacy of fenofibrate used in combination with simvastatin compared with simvastatin monotherapy is the Action to Control Cardiovascular Risk in Diabetes trial. Although the primary composite endpoint reduction between the two groups as a whole was not significantly different, among subjects with elevated triglycerides (>204 mg/dL) and low HDL (<34 mg/dL), there was a trend for improved benefit with combination therapy (31%).[88a]

STATIN–OMEGA-3 FATTY ACIDS

Omega-3 fatty acids, or fish oils, significantly reduce VLDL and triglyceride levels and increase LDL-C levels in patients with high triglycerides. The omega-3 fatty acids inhibit the enzyme diacylglycerol acyltransferase 2, thereby reducing intrahepatic triglyceride biosynthesis. They also stimulate mitochondrial beta-oxidation of fatty acids, decrease VLDL production and biosynthesis, and stimulate triglyceride hydrolysis by lipoprotein lipase. Dietary supplementation with the n-3 polyunsaturated fatty acids (PUFAs) eicosapentaenoic acid (EPA) and docosahexaenoic acid (DHA) has also been shown to lower the risk of death, nonfatal coronary events, and stroke after myocardial infarction.[89] In several clinical trials, PUFAs have been shown to reduce triglyceride levels by 20% to 30% and by up to 50% in patients with severe hypertriglyceridemia (triglycerides >500 mg/dL [>5.65 mmol/L]).[90,91]

Combination therapy with statins and n-3 PUFAs has demonstrated LDL-C reductions of 13% to 24% and triglyceride reductions of 27% to 30% added to pravastatin 40 mg/day[92] or simvastatin 20 mg/day.[93] Similarly, combination therapy with atorvastatin 10 mg resulted in significant reductions of the concentration of small, dense LDL particles and increases in HDL-C compared with monotherapy.[94] In a study evaluating the effects of adding prescription omega-3 acid ethyl esters 4 g/day (P-OM3; Lovaza, formerly Omacor) to simvastatin 40 mg in more than 250 patients with persistent hypertriglyceridemia, decreases in non–HDL-C were significantly greater with combination therapy than with placebo plus simvastatin (9.0% versus 2.2%, respectively; $P < 0.001$). In addition, combination therapy significantly lowered triglycerides (29.5%) and VLDL-C (27.5%), raised HDL-C (3.4%), and lowered the ratio of total cholesterol to HDL-C (9.6%; $P < 0.001$ versus placebo for all).[95]

The Japan EPA Lipid Intervention Study (JELIS) evaluated whether the addition of fish oils to patients already taking a statin would provide incremental risk reduction. Approximately 19,000 Japanese men and women with hypercholesterolemia were prospectively randomized to statin therapy with or without 1800 mg/day of EPA.[96] Combination therapy resulted in an additional 19% reduction in major coronary events at 4.6 years of follow-up compared with statin monotherapy.

BEYOND LDL-C

Whereas LDL-C has become the cornerstone of lipid diagnosis and therapy, apo B and non–HDL-C may be more accurate indicators of cardiovascular risk as well as measures by which to gauge LDL-lowering therapy.[97] The measurement of apo B provides an estimate of the number of atherosclerotic particles, and non–HDL-C represents the sum of cholesterol in VLDL and LDL, or the mass of cholesterol and cholesteryl

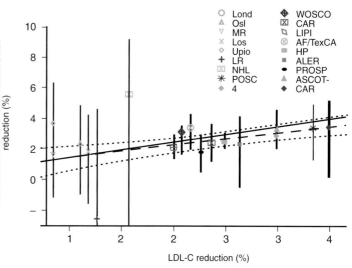

FIGURE 14-7 Estimated change in relative risk reduction for nonfatal myocardial infarction (MI) and coronary heart disease (CHD) death associated with mean LDL-C reduction. The 95% probability interval is represented by the dotted line. The crude risk estimates from individual statin trials are plotted with their 95% confidence intervals. *(From Ridker PM, Danielson E, Fonseca FA, et al: Reduction in C-reactive protein and LDL cholesterol and cardiovascular event rates after initiation of rosuvastatin: a prospective study of the JUPITER trial.* Lancet *373:1175, 2009; Robinson JG, Smith B, Maheshwari N, Schrott H: Pleiotropic effects of statins: benefit beyond cholesterol reduction?* J Am Coll Cardiol *46:1855, 2005. Reproduced with permission.)*

ester within apo B particles.[97] Defined more specifically, non–HDL-C (total cholesterol minus HDL-C) reflects the concentration of cholesterol within all lipoprotein particles currently considered atherogenic.[98] Whereas debate continues as to whether apo B or non–HDL-C directed therapy may be more effective, it is evident that both have advantages over LDL-C as predictors of cardiovascular risk.

In several epidemiologic studies and in post hoc analyses of clinical trials, apo B has been found to be a better predictor than LDL-C of CVD risk.[99,100] Additional analyses suggest that once LDL-C is lowered, apo B may be a more effective way to assess residual CVD risk and to determine the need for medication adjustments.[98] A recent consensus panel building on the guidelines of the NCEP ATP III and the American Heart Association/Centers for Disease Control for cardiovascular risk assessment recommended that for patients with diabetes mellitus and one additional risk factor, the goals of treatment should be LDL-C <70 mg/dL and non–HDL-C <100 mg/dL, with optional targets of apo B <80 mg/dL or LDL particle number (LDL-P) <1000 nmol/L.[101]

COMPLIANCE WITH MEDICATIONS

Adherence to LDL-lowering therapy is a key component in achieving target goals. A Canadian cohort of 85,020 primary prevention patients showed that after 6 and 24 months, the percentage of patients remaining on statin therapy for dyslipidemia treatment was 50% and 24%, respectively.[102] In a managed care population of high-risk patients, better compliance with statin therapy was associated with older age, being male, more frequent outpatient follow-up for lipid management, history of hospitalization for a coronary event, history of revascularization, and receiving prescriptions through the mail rather than having to pick them up monthly at a retail pharmacy.[103] The NCEP guidelines identify that adherence issues need to be addressed for the highest possible levels of CHD risk reduction to be attained. Patient education and involvement in self-monitoring, provider education and reinforcement of lipid treatment guidelines, and use of health delivery system strategies (including lipid management clinics, collaborative care with pharmacists, the use of critical care pathways, cardiac rehabilitation for patients who sustain acute cardiac events or who undergo revascularization, telehealth technologies, and nursing case management) are identified as targets for intervention to improve adherence.[31] The

need for compliance with lipid-lowering medications should be reinforced at each office visit.

CONCLUSION

The strength of LDL-C as a target for CVD risk reduction is supported by scientific evidence based on the biology of atherosclerosis, epidemiology, and clinical trial evidence with both statin- and non–statin-based approaches to serum lipid lowering. A complex set of biochemical reactions promotes the development of inflammation, LDL oxidation, and plaque progression. The absence of LDL-C elevation and other atherogenic lipoproteins is associated with less atherosclerosis in animal models. Life-long low LDL-C levels (as seen in PCSK9 loss-of-function mutations) in humans are associated with very low rates of CVD. Clinical trials using statins and non-statin approaches to lipid lowering have demonstrated that for every 1 mg/dL reduction in serum LDL-C, there is a 1% reduction in risk for acute cardiovascular events. A number of clinical trials have confirmed that LDL-C lowering predicts CVD risk reduction (Fig. 14-7).[104,105] The totality of the evidence strongly supports that LDL-C and, more recently, non–HDL-C are targets that, if achieved, result in a marked reduction in CVD. The challenge for clinicians is to identify the most appropriate patients for LDL-C or non–HDL-C treatment and maintain adherence to therapy to improve outcomes and quality of life.

On-target LDL-C predicts the benefit of treatment, and therapeutic lifestyle changes coupled with statin therapy remain the mainstay of treatment. Combination therapy has demonstrated greater benefit with lipid management, not just in terms of LDL-C but also with respect to HDL-C and triglycerides. During the next several years, ongoing clinical trials will evaluate the impact of comprehensive lipid management (modifying triglycerides, HDL-C, and other lipid parameters) compared with intensive LDL-C lowering alone and may provide further guidance on strategies to optimize cardiovascular risk reduction.

REFERENCES

1. World Health Organization: Cardiovascular disease. Available at: www.who.int/cardiovascular_diseases/en/. Accessed July 10, 2009.
2. Steinberg D: *The cholesterol wars,* New York, 2007, Elsevier.
3. Anitschkow MM, Chalatov S: Über experimentelle Cholesterinsteatose und ihre Bedeutung für die Entstehung einiger pathologischer Prozesse. *Zentralbl Allg Pathol* 24:1, 1913.

4. Kannel WB, Dawber TR, Kagan A, et al: Factors of risk in the development of coronary heart disease—six years of follow-up experience. The Framingham Study. *Ann Intern Med* 55:33, 1961.
5. Assmann G, Cullen P, Schulte H: The Munster Heart Study (PROCAM). Results of follow-up at 8 years. *Eur Heart J* 19(Suppl A):A2, 1998.
6. Verschuren WM, Jacobs DR, Bloemberg BP, et al: Serum total cholesterol and long-term coronary heart disease mortality in different cultures. Twenty-five-year follow-up of the seven countries study. *JAMA* 274:131, 1995.
7. Tunstall-Pedoe H, editor: *for the WHO MONICA Project: MONICA monograph and multimedia sourcebook*, Geneva, 2003, World Health Organization. Available at: www.ktl.fi/monica/public/monograph.html. Accessed December 29, 2009.
8. Benfante R: Studies of cardiovascular disease and cause-specific mortality trends in Japanese-American men living in Hawaii and risk factor comparisons with other Japanese populations in the Pacific region: a review. *Hum Biol* 64:791, 1992.
9. Stamler J, Wentworth D, Neaton JD: Is relationship between serum cholesterol and risk of premature death from coronary heart disease continuous and graded? Findings in 356,222 primary screenees of the Multiple Risk Factor Intervention Trial (MRFIT). *JAMA* 256:2823, 1986.
10. Castelli WP, Doyle JT, Gordon T, et al: HDL cholesterol and other lipids in coronary heart disease. The cooperative lipoprotein phenotyping study. *Circulation* 55:767, 1977.
11. Sharrett AR, Ballantyne CM, Coady SA, et al: Coronary heart disease prediction from lipoprotein cholesterol levels, triglycerides, lipoprotein(a), apolipoproteins A-I and B, and HDL density subfractions: the Atherosclerosis Risk in Communities (ARIC) Study. *Circulation* 104:1108, 2001.
12. Castelli WP: Cholesterol and lipids in the risk of coronary artery disease—the Framingham Heart Study. *Can J Cardiol* 4(Suppl A):5A, 1988.
13. American Heart Association Report of the Committee for Medical and Community Program: Dietary fat and its relation to heart attacks and strokes. *Circulation* 23:133, 1961.
14. Davis HR, Compton DS, Hoos L, et al: Ezetimibe (SCH58235) localizes to the brush border to a small intestinal enterocyte and inhibits enterocyte cholesterol uptake and absorption. *Eur Heart J Suppl* 21:636, 2000.
15. Brown MS, Goldstein JL: A receptor-mediated pathway for cholesterol homeostasis. *Science* 232:34, 1986.
16. Beigneux A, Hofmann AF, Young SG: Human CYP7A1 deficiency: progress and enigmas. *J Clin Invest* 110:29, 2002.
17. Boren J, Ekstrom U, Agren B, et al: The molecular mechanism for the genetic disorder familial defective apolipoprotein B100. *J Biol Chem* 276:9214, 2001.
18. Abifadel M, Varret M, Rabes JP, et al: Mutations in PCSK9 cause autosomal dominant hypercholesterolemia. *Nat Genet* 34:154, 2003.
19. Chen SN, Ballantyne CM, Gotto AM, Jr, et al: A common PCSK9 haplotype, encompassing the E670G coding single nucleotide polymorphism, is a novel genetic marker for plasma low-density lipoprotein cholesterol levels and severity of coronary atherosclerosis. *J Am Coll Cardiol* 45:1611, 2005.
20. Libby P: What have we learned about the biology of atherosclerosis? The role of inflammation. *Am J Cardiol* 88:3J, 2001.
21. Libby P: Inflammation in atherosclerosis. *Nature* 420:868, 2002.
22. Rao RM, Yang L, Garcia-Cardena G, Luscinskas FW: Endothelial-dependent mechanisms of leukocyte recruitment to the vascular wall. *Circ Res* 101:234, 2007.
23. Liebner S, Cavallaro U, Dejana E: The multiple languages of endothelial cell-to-cell communication. *Arterioscler Thromb Vasc Biol* 26:1431, 2006.
24. Tabas I, Williams KJ, Boren J: Subendothelial lipoprotein retention as the initiating process in atherosclerosis: update and therapeutic implications. *Circulation* 116:1832, 2007.
25. Zhang R, Brennan ML, Shen Z, et al: Myeloperoxidase functions as a major enzymatic catalyst for initiation of lipid peroxidation at sites of inflammation. *J Biol Chem* 277:46116, 2002.
26. McConnell JP, Hoefner DM: Lipoprotein-associated phospholipase A_2. *Clin Lab Med* 26:679, 2006.
27. Brewer HB, Jr, Remaley AT, Neufeld EB, et al: Regulation of plasma high-density lipoprotein levels by the ABCA1 transporter and the emerging role of high-density lipoprotein in the treatment of cardiovascular disease. *Arterioscler Thromb Vasc Biol* 24:1755, 2004.
28. Kennedy MA, Barrera GC, Nakamura K, et al: ABCG1 has a critical role in mediating cholesterol efflux to HDL and preventing cellular lipid accumulation. *Cell Metab* 1:121, 2005.
29. Toth PP: Reverse cholesterol transport: high-density lipoprotein's magnificent mile. *Curr Atheroscler Rep* 5:386, 2003.
30. Tabas I: Consequences and therapeutic implications of macrophage apoptosis in atherosclerosis: the importance of lesion stage and phagocytic efficiency. *Arterioscler Thromb Vasc Biol* 25:2255, 2005.
31. Expert Panel on Detection, Evaluation, and Treatment of High Blood Cholesterol in Adults: Executive summary of the Third Report of the National Cholesterol Education Program (NCEP) Expert Panel on Detection, Evaluation, and Treatment of High Blood Cholesterol in Adults (Adult Treatment Panel III). *JAMA* 285:2486, 2001.
32. Smith SC, Jr, Allen J, Blair SN, et al: AHA/ACC guidelines for secondary prevention for patients with coronary and other atherosclerotic vascular disease: 2006 update: endorsed by the National Heart, Lung, and Blood Institute. *Circulation* 113:2363, 2006.
33. Debacker G, Ambrosioni E, Borch-Johnsen K, et al: European guidelines on cardiovascular disease prevention in clinical practice. Third Joint Task Force of European and other Societies on Cardiovascular Disease in Clinical Practice. *Eur J Cardiovasc Prev Rehabil* 10(Suppl 1):S2, 2003.
34. Ridker PM, Rifai N, Cook NR, et al: Non-HDL cholesterol, apolipoproteins A-I and B100, standard lipid measures, lipid ratios, and CRP as risk factors for cardiovascular disease in women. *JAMA* 294:326, 2005.
35. Pischon T, Girman CJ, Sacks FM, et al: Non–high-density lipoprotein cholesterol and apolipoprotein B in the prediction of coronary heart disease in men. *Circulation* 112:3375, 2005.
36. Smith SC, Jr, Allen J, Blair SN, et al: AHA/ACC guidelines for secondary prevention for patients with coronary and other atherosclerotic vascular disease: 2006 update: endorsed by the National Heart, Lung, and Blood Institute. *Circulation* 113:2363, 2006.
37. Wilson PW, D'Agostino RB, Levy D, et al: Prediction of coronary heart disease using risk factor categories. *Circulation* 97:1837, 1998.
38. The Lipid Research Clinics Coronary Primary Prevention Trial results. I. Reduction in incidence of coronary heart disease. *JAMA* 251:351, 1984.
39. Heart Protection Study Collaborative Group: MRC/BHF Heart Protection Study of cholesterol lowering with simvastatin in 20536 high-risk individuals: a randomized placebo-controlled trial. *Lancet* 360:7, 2002.
40. LaRosa JC, Grundy SM, Waters DD, et al: Intensive lipid lowering with atorvastatin in patients with stable coronary disease. *N Engl J Med* 352:1425, 2005.
41. Pedersen TR, Faergeman O, Kastelein JJ, et al: High-dose atorvastatin vs usual-dose simvastatin for secondary prevention after myocardial infarction: the IDEAL study: a randomized controlled trial. *JAMA* 294:2437, 2005.
42. Davidson MH, Maki KC, Pearson TA, et al: Results of the National Cholesterol Education Program (NCEP) Evaluation Project Utilizing Novel E-Technology (NEPTUNE) II Survey: Implications for treatment under the recent NCEP Writing Group recommendations. *Am J Cardiol* 96:556, 2005.
43. Davidson MH, Gandhi SK, Ohsfelt RL, Fox KM: Hypercholesterolemia treatment patterns and low density lipoprotein cholesterol monitoring in patients with a diagnosis of atherosclerosis in clinical practice. *Am J Med* 122:S51, 2009.
44. Ford ES: Prevalence of the metabolic syndrome defined by the International Diabetes Federation among adults in the US. *Diabetes Care* 28:2745, 2005.
45. Toth PP: When high is low: raising low levels of high-density lipoprotein cholesterol. *Curr Cardiol Rep* 10:488, 2008.
46. Grundy SM, Cleeman JI, Daniels SR, et al: Diagnosis and management of the metabolic syndrome: an American Heart Association/National Heart, Lung, and Blood Institute scientific statement. *Curr Opin Cardiol* 21:1, 2006.
47. Grundy SM, Cleeman JI, Merz CN, et al: Implications of recent clinical trials for the National Cholesterol Education Program Adult Treatment Panel III guidelines. *Circulation* 110:227, 2004.
48. Scandinavian Simvastatin Survival Study Group: Randomised trial of cholesterol lowering in 4444 patients with coronary heart disease: the Scandinavian Simvastatin Survival Study (4S). *Lancet* 344:1383, 1994.
49. Sacks FM, Pfeffer MA, Moye LA, et al: The effect of pravastatin on coronary events after myocardial infarction in patients with average cholesterol levels. *N Engl J Med* 335:1001, 1996.
50. Baigent C, Keech A, Kearney PM, et al: Efficacy and safety of cholesterol-lowering treatment: prospective meta-analysis of data from 90,056 participants in 14 randomised trials of statins. *Lancet* 366:1267, 2005.
51. Whitney E: The Air Force/Texas Coronary Atherosclerosis Prevention Study: Implications for preventive cardiology in the general adult US population. *Curr Atheroscler Rep* 1:38, 1999.
52. Ridker PM, Danielson E, Fonseca FA, et al: Reduction in C-reactive protein and LDL cholesterol and cardiovascular event rates after initiation of rosuvastatin: a prospective study of the JUPITER trial. *Lancet* 373:1175, 2009.
53. Ridker PM, Morrow DA, Rose LM, et al: Relative efficacy of atorvastatin 80 mg and pravastatin 40 mg in achieving the dual goals of low-density lipoprotein cholesterol <70 mg/dl and C-reactive protein <2 mg/l: an analysis of the PROVE-IT TIMI-22 trial. *J Am Coll Cardiol* 45:1644, 2005.
54. Amarenco P, Labreuche J: Lipid management in the prevention of stroke: review and updated meta-analysis of statins for stroke prevention. *Lancet Neurol* 8:453, 2009.
55. The Lipid Research Clinics Coronary Primary Prevention Trial results. II. The relationship of reduction in incidence of coronary heart disease to cholesterol lowering. *JAMA* 251:365, 1984.
56. Brown G, Albers JJ, Fisher LD, et al: Regression of coronary artery disease as a result of intensive lipid lowering therapy in men with high levels of apolipoprotein B. *N Engl J Med* 323:1289, 1990.
57. Ast M, Frishman WH: Bile acid sequestrants. *J Clin Pharmacol* 30:99, 1990.
58. Armani A, Toth PP: Colesevelam hydrochloride in the management of dyslipidemia. *Expert Rev Cardiovasc Ther* 4:283, 2006.
59. Davidson MH, Toth P, Weiss S, et al: Low-dose combination therapy with colesevelam hydrochloride and lovastatin effectively decreases low-density lipoprotein cholesterol in patients with primary hypercholesterolemia. *Clin Cardiol* 24:467, 2001.
60. Knapp HH, Schrott H, Ma P, et al: Efficacy and safety of combination simvastatin and colesevelam in patients with primary hypercholesterolemia. *Am J Med* 110:352, 2001.
61. Hunninghake D, Insull W, Jr, Toth P, et al: Coadministration of colesevelam hydrochloride with atorvastatin lowers LDL cholesterol additively. *Atherosclerosis* 158:407, 2001.
62. Zieve FJ, Kalin MF, Schwartz SL, et al: Results of the glucose-lowering effect of WelChol study (GLOWS): a randomized double-blind, placebo-controlled pilot study evaluating the effect of colesevelam hydrochloride on glycemic control in subjects with type 2 diabetes. *Clin Ther* 29:74, 2007.
63. Goldberg RB, Truitt K: Colesevelam HCl improves glycemic control in type 2 diabetes mellitus subjects managed with insulin therapy. *Circulation* 114:1581, 2006.
64. Canner PL, Berge KG, Wenger NK, et al: Fifteen year mortality in coronary drug project patients: long-term benefit with niacin. *J Am Coll Cardiol* 8:1245, 1986.
65. Davidson MH: Niacin use and cutaneous flushing: mechanisms and strategies for prevention. *Am J Cardiol* 101:14B, 2008.
66. Toth PP: When high is low: raising low levels of high-density lipoprotein cholesterol. *Curr Cardiol Rep* 10:488, 2008.
67. Guyton JR, Bays HE: Safety considerations with niacin therapy. *Am J Cardiol* 99(Suppl 1):S22, 2007.

68. Davidson MH: Combination therapy for mixed dyslipidemia. Available at: MedscapeCME. http://cme.medscape.com/viewarticle/567703?src=rss. Accessed November 19, 2009.

69. Brown B, Brockenbrough A, Zhao X-Q, et al: Very intensive lipid therapy with lovastatin, niacin, and colestipol for prevention of death and myocardial infarction: a 10-year Familial Atherosclerosis Treatment Study (FATS) follow-up [abstract 3341]. *Circulation* 98:I635, 1998.

70. Yim BT, Chong PH: Niacin-ER and lovastatin treatment of hypercholesterolemia and mixed dyslipidemia. *Ann Pharmacother* 37:106, 2003.

71. Kashyap ML, McGovern ME, Berra K, et al: Long-term safety and efficacy of a once-daily niacin/lovastatin formulation for patients with dyslipidemia. *Am J Cardiol* 89:672, 2002.

72. Bays HE, Dujovne CA, McGovern ME, et al: Comparison of once-daily, niacin extended-release/lovastatin with standard doses of atorvastatin and simvastatin (the Advicor Versus Other Cholesterol-modulating Agents Trial Evaluation [ADVOCATE]). *Am J Cardiol* 91:667, 2003.

73. Ballantyne CM, Davidson MH, McKenney J, et al: Comparison of the safety and efficacy of a combination tablet of niacin extended release and simvastatin vs simvastatin monotherapy in patients with increased non-HDL cholesterol (from the SEACOAST I study). *Am J Cardiol* 101:1428, 2008.

74. Karas RH, Kashyap ML, Knopp RH, et al: Long-term safety and efficacy of a combination of niacin extended release and simvastatin in patients with dyslipidemia: the OCEANS study. *Am J Cardiovasc Drugs* 8:69, 2008.

75. Taylor AJ, Sullenberger LE, Lee HJ, et al: Arterial Biology for Investigation of the Treatment Effects of Reducing Cholesterol (ARBITER) 2: a double-blind placebo-controlled study of extended-release niacin on atherosclerosis progression in secondary prevention patients treated with statins. *Circulation* 110:3512, 2004.

76. Taylor AJ, Villines TC, Stanek EJ, et al: Extended-release niacin or ezetimibe and carotid intima-media thickness. *N Engl J Med* 361:1, 2009.

77. Dembowski E, Davidson MH: Statin and ezetimibe combination therapy in cardiovascular disease. *Curr Opin Endocrinol Diabetes Obes* 16:183, 2009.

78. Davis HR, Veltri EP: Zetia: inhibition of Niemann-Pick C1 like 1 (NPC1L1) to reduce intestinal cholesterol absorption and treat hyperlipidemia. *J Atheroscler Thromb* 14:99, 2007.

79. Davidson MH, McGarry T, Bettis R, et al: Ezetimibe coadministered with simvastatin in patients with primary hypercholesterolemia. *J Am Coll Cardiol* 40:2125, 2002.

80. Ballantyne CM, Houri J, Notarbartolo A, et al: Effect of ezetimibe coadministered with atorvastatin in 628 patients with primary hypercholesterolemia. *Circulation* 107:2409, 2003.

81. Kerzner B, Corbelli J, Sharp S, et al: Ezetimibe Study Group: Efficacy and safety of ezetimibe coadministered with lovastatin in primary hypercholesterolemia. *Am J Cardiol* 91:418, 2003.

82. Cannon CP, Giugliano RP, Blazing MA, et al: Rationale and design of IMPROVE-IT (IMProved Reduction of Outcomes: Vytorin Efficacy International Trial): comparison of ezetimibe/simvastatin versus simvastatin monotherapy on cardiovascular outcomes in patients with acute coronary syndromes. *Am Heart J* 156:826, 2008.

83. Rubins HB, Robins SJ, Collins D, et al: Gemfibrozil for the secondary prevention of coronary heart disease in men with low levels of high-density lipoprotein cholesterol. Veterans Affairs High-Density Lipoprotein Cholesterol Intervention Trial Study Group. *N Engl J Med* 341:410, 1999.

84. Huttunen JK, Heinonen OP, Manninen V, et al: The Helsinki Heart Study: an 8.5-year safety and mortality follow-up. *J Intern Med* 235:31, 1994.

85. Effect of fenofibrate on progression of coronary-artery disease in type 2 diabetes: the Diabetes Atherosclerosis Intervention Study, a randomised study. *Lancet* 357:905, 2001.

86. Frick MH, Syvanne M, Nieminen MS, et al: Prevention of the angiographic progression of coronary and vein-graft atherosclerosis by gemfibrozil after coronary bypass surgery in men with low levels of HDL cholesterol. Lopid Coronary Angiography Trial (LOCAT) Study Group. *Circulation* 96:2137, 1997.

87. Grundy SM, Vega LG, Yuan Z, et al: Effectiveness and tolerability of simvastatin plus fenofibrate for combined hyperlipidemia (the SAFARI trial). *Am J Cardiol* 95:462, 2005.

88. Davidson MH, Armani A, McKenney JM, Jacobson TA: Safety considerations with fibrate therapy. *Am J Cardiol* 99:3C, 2007.

88a. Ginsberg HN, Elam MB, Lovato LC, et al: Effects of combination lipid therapy in type 2 diabetes mellitus. *N Engl J Med* 362:1563, 2010.

89. GISSI-Prevenzione Investigators: Dietary supplementation with n-3 polyunsaturated fatty acids and vitamin E after myocardial infarction: results of the GISSI-Prevenzione trial. *Lancet* 354:447, 1999.

90. O'Keefe JH, Harris WS: From Inuit to implementation: omega-3 fatty acids come of age. *Mayo Clin Proc* 75:607, 2000.

91. Harris WS, Ginsberg HN, Arunakul N, et al: Safety and efficacy of Omacor in severe hypertriglyceridemia. *J Cardiovasc Risk* 4:385, 1997.

92. Contacos C, Barter PJ, Sullivan DR: Effect of pravastatin and omega-3 fatty acids on plasma lipids and lipoproteins in patients with combined hyperlipidemia. *Arterioscler Thromb* 13:1755, 1993.

93. Nordoy A, Bonaa KH, Niilsen H, et al: Effects of simvastatin and omega-3 fatty acids on plasma lipoproteins and lipid peroxidation in patients with combined hyperlipidaemia. *J Intern Med* 243:163, 1998.

94. Nordoy A, Hansen JB, Brox J, Svensson B: Effects of atorvastatin and omega-3 fatty acids on LDL subfractions and postprandial hyperlipemia in patients with combined hyperlipemia. *Nutr Metab Cardiovasc Dis* 11:7, 2001.

95. Davidson MH, Stein EA, Bays HE, et al: Efficacy and tolerability of adding prescription omega-3 fatty acids 4 g/d to simvastatin 40 mg/d in hypertriglyceridemic patients: an 8-week randomized, double-blind, placebo-controlled study. *Clin Ther* 29:1354, 2007.

96. Yokoyama M, Origasa H, Matsuzaki M, et al: Japan EPA lipid intervention study (JELIS) Investigators: Effects of eicosapentaenoic acid on major coronary events in hypercholesterolaemic patients (JELIS): a randomised open-label, blinded endpoint analysis. *Lancet* 369:1090, 2007.

97. Sniderman A, Williams K, Cobbaert C: ApoB versus non-HDL-C: what to do when they disagree. *Curr Atheroscler Rep* 11:358, 2009.

98. Brunzell JD, Davidson M, Furberg CD, et al: Lipoprotein management in patients with cardiometabolic risk: consensus statement from the American Diabetes Association and the American College of Cardiology Foundation. *Diabetes Care* 31:811, 2008.

99. Walldius G, Jenner I, Holmes I, et al: High apolipoprotein B, low apolipoprotein A-I, and improvement in the prediction of fatal myocardial infarction (AMORIS study): a prospective study. *Lancet* 358:2026, 2001.

100. van Lennep JE, Westerveld HT, van Lennep HW, et al: Apolipoprotein concentrations during treatment and recurrent coronary artery disease events. *Arterioscler Thromb Vasc Biol* 20:2408, 2000.

101. Davidson MH, Corson MA, Alberts MJ, et al: Consensus panel recommendation for incorporating lipoprotein-associated phospholipase A_2 testing into cardiovascular disease risk assessment guidelines. *Am J Cardiol* 101:51F, 2008.

102. Jackevicius CA, Mamdani M, Tu JV: Adherence with statin therapy in elderly patients with and without acute coronary syndromes. *JAMA* 288:462, 2002.

103. Schultz JS, O'Donnell JC, McDonough KL, et al: Determinants of compliance with statin therapy and low-density lipoprotein cholesterol goal attainment in a managed care population. *Am J Manag Care* 11:306, 2005.

104. Ridker P, Danielson E, Fonesca F, et al: Reduction in C-reactive protein and LDL cholesterol and cardiovascular event rates after initiation of rosuvastatin: a prospective study of the JUPITER trial. *Lancet* 373:1175, 2009.

105. Robinson JG, Smith B, Maheshwari N, Schrott H: Pleiotropic effects of statins: benefit beyond cholesterol reduction? A meta-regression analysis. *J Am Coll Cardiol* 46:1855, 2005.

CHAPTER 15

The Contribution of Triglycerides and Triglyceride-Rich Lipoproteins to Atherosclerotic Cardiovascular Disease

Francine K. Welty

KEY POINTS

- When TG levels are between 200 and 800 mg/dL, TG-rich particles are associated with the presence of small dense LDL, low levels of HDL-C, insulin resistance, and metabolic syndrome, all of which increase risk for atherosclerosis.

- TG-rich particles affect the size and atherogenic potential of VLDL remnants and LDL particles, both of which enter the arterial subendothelial space and contribute to atherosclerotic plaque.

- In a meta-analysis of 68 prospective studies, TG level was not a predictor of risk for nonfatal myocardial infarction and death after adjustment whereas non–HDL-C was associated with increased risk after adjustment for HDL and log TG.

- Non–HDL-C predicted risk of CHD and future cardiovascular events better than LDL-C did, probably because non–HDL-C includes all apo B–containing lipoproteins.

- Nonfasting TG levels may predict CHD better than fasting levels but are more difficult to standardize and to measure in the clinical setting; non–HDL-C can be measured in the nonfasting state.

- NCEP ATP III recommends optimal TG level <150 mg/dL. NCEP recommends calculation of non–HDL-C when TG >200 mg/dL, with the goal being 30 mg/dL higher than the LDL-C goal.

- Lifestyle changes—exercise, diet, and weight loss—are necessary to lower TG levels, especially in patients with metabolic syndrome.

- Statins, fibrates, niacin, and omega-3 fatty acids can be used to lower TG levels if lifestyle changes are insufficient to reach the goal.

The contribution of triglyceride (TG) and TG-rich lipoproteins to the development of atherosclerosis, especially as an independent predictor of cardiovascular risk, has been debated for many years. TG levels between 200 and 800 mg/dL may be associated with other lipid abnormalities that predispose to atherosclerosis, including low levels of high-density lipoprotein cholesterol (HDL-C),[1-3] small, dense low-density lipoprotein (LDL) particles, atherogenic TG-rich remnants,[4,5] and insulin resistance,[6,7] all of which increase the risk for coronary heart disease (CHD). Therefore, it is difficult to determine the independent contribution of TG and how aggressively one should treat the hypertriglyceridemia. The percentage of adults in the United States with TG levels above 150 mg/dL (1.7 mmol/L), 200 mg/dL (2.3 mmol/L), 500 mg/dL (5.7 mmol/L), and 1000 mg/dL (11.3 mmol/L) is 33%, 18%, 1.7%, and 0.4%, respectively.[8] Therefore, hypertriglyceridemia affects a significant portion of the population. Reliable assessment of the risk associated with lipid fractions is important for the development of accurate screening and treatment strategies.

This chapter reviews the epidemiologic evidence indicating that hypertriglyceridemia contributes to atherosclerosis. Lipid metabolism is then described to demonstrate the mechanisms by which the level of TG-rich lipoproteins affects the composition and size of remnant, LDL, and HDL particles and how this affects development of atherosclerosis and risk for CHD. Finally, the classification and causes of various types of hypertriglyceridemia are discussed, followed by suggestions for evaluation, treatment, and management.

EPIDEMIOLOGIC EVIDENCE LINKING TRIGLYCERIDE LEVELS WITH RISK FOR CORONARY HEART DISEASE

Several epidemiologic studies have provided important findings on the role of TGs and TG-rich lipoproteins in atherosclerosis. In 1959, Albrink and Man[9] observed that TG levels greater than 175 mg/dL were present in 70% of 100 cases of myocardial infarction (MI) compared with only 7% of 92 healthy controls. In the 8-year Prospective Cardiovascular Münster (PROCAM) study reported in 1996, elevated levels of TG were independently associated with incident CHD events after adjustment for LDL-C and HDL-C levels.[10] For this reason, elevated TG levels are in the European model for calculation of cardiovascular risk.[11] An important contribution of PROCAM was the observation that an increasing TG level is directly associated with CHD incidence up to a level of 800 mg/dL. Levels higher than 800 mg/dL are thought not to be associated with CHD because of lipoprotein particles too large to penetrate the vascular endothelium compared with smaller, atherogenic remnant particles found with mild hypertriglyceridemia. In the Framingham Heart Offspring Study, TG level was not associated with CHD after adjustment for HDL-C and other covariates in both men and women.[12] However, a later analysis showed that the cholesterol in remnant lipoproteins is an independent predictor of CHD risk in Framingham women.[13]

In 1996, the first large meta-analysis of 17 prospective, observational studies of TG and CHD events reported that an increase of 89 mg/dL (1 mmol/L) in TG level was associated with a univariate risk of 32% in men and 76% in women and was an independent risk predictor (adjusted for other covariates including HDL-C) of 14% in men and 37% in women.[14]

The Baltimore Coronary Observational Long-Term Study (COLTS), a retrospective cohort study, observed 350 individuals with CHD for up to 18 years after cardiac catheterization. After adjustment for age, gender, use of beta blockers, and other risk factors, baseline fasting TG level >100 mg/dL was associated with a 50% increased risk of subsequent events compared with those with TG <100 mg/dL (P = 0.008) and was an independent predictor of recurrent cardiovascular events in patients with CHD.[15] These results suggested that an optimal TG level is <100 mg/dL in patients with CHD.

The Copenhagen Male Study was a prospective study of 2906 white men without CHD at baseline.[16] During 8-year-follow-up, there was an increased risk for CHD with increasing TG tertiles: 4.65% for TG of 0.4 to 1.1 mmol/L; 7.7% for TG of 1.1 to 1.6 mmol/L; and 11.5% for TG of 1.6 to 2.2 mmol/L. After adjustment for age, body mass index, hypertension, smoking, alcohol, physical activity, diabetes, socioeconomic status, LDL-C, and HDL-C, the middle and highest level of TGs had a relative risk of 1.5 and 2.2, respectively, compared with the lowest tertile of TGs. Moreover, elevated TG and low HDL-C levels were predictive of CHD events in men with LDL-C both less than and greater than 170 mg/dL.[17]

In 2004, a meta-analysis pooled individual data from 96,224 subjects in 26 prospective studies in New Zealand, Australia, and several Asian countries and included 670 and 667 deaths from CHD and stroke, respectively.[18] After adjustment for age, sex, blood pressure, smoking, ratio of total cholesterol (TC) to HDL-C, and major cardiovascular risk factors, compared with those in the bottom fifth of TG levels, individuals in the top fifth of TG levels had a 70% (95% CI, 47-96) greater risk of CHD death, an 80% (95% CI, 49-119) higher risk of fatal or nonfatal CHD, and a 50% (95% CI, 29-76) increased risk of fatal or nonfatal stroke. The association between levels of TG and CHD death was similar across subgroups defined by ethnicity, age, and sex. These results suggested that serum TGs are an independent predictor of CHD and stroke risk in the Asia-Pacific region even after adjustment for HDL-C.

More recently, a meta-analysis of 29 population-based, Western prospective studies included 10,158 CHD cases from 262,525 participants. After correction of risk estimates for long-term within-individual variation in TG measurements, the risk of CHD adjusted for age, gender, and calendar period was approximately twofold higher in individuals in the top third of log TG levels compared with the bottom third.[19] The attributable risk was similar in men and women and in fasted and nonfasted participants. After adjustment for HDL-C, the odds ratio for CHD was attenuated to 1.72 but remained significant (95% CI, 1.56-1.90) in those in the top third of log TG level compared with the bottom third. An important contribution was that repeated measurements an average of 4 years apart in 1933 participants in the EPIC-Norfolk study and an average of 12 years apart in 379 participants in the Reykjavik study showed that the long-term stability of log TG values is similar to that of blood pressure and total serum cholesterol (within-person correlation coefficients of 0.64 [95% CI, 0.60-0.68] during 4 years and 0.63 [95% CI, 0.57-0.70] during 12 years).[20]

The Metabolic, Lifestyle and Nutrition Assessment in Young Adults (MELANY) study obtained two measurements of fasting TGs 5 years apart, as well as lifestyle variables, in 13,953 healthy men, aged 26 to 45 years, who were then observed for an average of 10.5 years.[21] After adjustment for eating breakfast, smoking, exercise, and changes in body mass index, those in the top quintile of TGs had a fourfold higher

risk of angiographically proven CHD compared with those in the lowest quintile. The magnitude of this risk was much greater than the average 1.7-fold increase in risk observed in the 2007 meta-analysis[19] and other large studies, a finding thought secondary to the younger age of the cohort compared with other studies. Another important finding was that change in TG level between the initial and the second measurements was positively associated with change in CHD risk.

In a recent subgroup analysis of the Treating to New Targets (TNT) study and Incremental Decrease in Endpoints through Aggressive Lipid Lowering (IDEAL) study, the utility of TGs to predict new cardiovascular events was examined.[22] IDEAL compared atorvastatin 80 mg with simvastatin 20 to 40 mg and TNT compared atorvastatin 80 mg with atorvastatin 10 mg in patients with CHD or a history of MI. After adjustment for age and gender, the risk of cardiovascular events was 63% higher in patients in the highest quintile of TG (HR, 1.63; 95% CI, 1.46-1.81) compared with the lowest quintile. The ability of TGs to predict risk was attenuated when HDL and apo B/apo A-I were in the model, and it was eliminated with inclusion of diabetes, body mass index, glucose, hypertension, and smoking (P = 0.044 and 0.621, respectively, for the trend across quintiles of TG). Similar results were observed in those in whom LDL-C had been lowered to goal.

The Pravastatin or Atorvastatin Evaluation and Infection Therapy–Thrombolysis in Myocardial Infarction (PROVE IT–TIMI 22) trial randomized patients with acute coronary syndromes to atorvastatin 80 mg or pravastatin 40 mg.[23] An on-treatment TG level <150 mg/dL was independently associated with a significant reduction in risk for the composite primary endpoint of nonfatal MI, death, and recurrent acute coronary syndrome. After adjustment for LDL-C and other covariates in a subanalysis, each 10 mg/dL decline in on-treatment TG level was associated with a 1.6% lower risk of the primary endpoint.

In summary, several studies show TGs to be an independent predictor of CHD after adjustment, whereas in others, risk of TGs is attenuated or eliminated after adjustment, especially for HDL-C levels. In the next section, potential reasons for these findings are examined on the basis of the metabolic interrelationships between levels of TG-rich lipoproteins, small dense LDL, remnant particles, and HDL particles.

LIPOPROTEIN METABOLISM

Determination of the contribution of TGs to risk for atherosclerosis is complicated by the fact that the metabolism of TG-rich lipoprotein fractions significantly affects the levels and composition of other lipoprotein fractions that also contribute to cardiovascular risk.[24] Therefore, in evaluating the role of TG and TG-rich lipoproteins in contributing to atherosclerosis, one must consider the complex interrelationships between the various lipoproteins during metabolism.

TGs (triacylglycerols) are composed of a glycerol backbone in which each of the three hydroxyl groups is esterified with a fatty acid.[25,26] TGs play an important role in lipid metabolism and are the major source of metabolic energy storage. Cholesterol and TGs are almost insoluble in plasma; therefore, they are transported in lipoprotein particles from the liver (endogenous production of very-low-density lipoprotein [VLDL]) and intestine (exogenous production of chylomicrons [CMs] from dietary fat) to various tissues—TGs for energy use in skeletal muscle or storage in adipose tissue and cholesterol for synthesis of steroid hormones, bile acid formation, and cell membrane structural integrity. Lipoprotein particles are spherical and contain a central core of varying amounts of TG and cholesteryl ester (CE) (both nonpolar lipids) covered on the surface by a monolayer of polar lipids (primarily phospholipids), one or more apolipoproteins, and unesterified cholesterol, which is also found in the core as particle size increases.[25] They are divided into five major classes on the basis of density, which is inversely related to size and lipid content: CMs, VLDL, intermediate-density lipoprotein (IDL), LDL, and HDL.[27] The main apolipoproteins include apo B (B100 and B48), apo A (A-I, A-II, A-IV, and A-V), apo C (C-I, C-II, and C-III), and apo E (E2, E3, and E4 isoforms). Apolipoproteins serve as cofactors for enzymes and ligands for receptors and therefore play key roles in the regulation of lipoprotein metabolism.

Apo B exists in two forms in plasma, apo B100 and apo B48, both of which are products of the same structural gene on chromosome 2.[27] Both apo B48 and apo B100 are constitutively synthesized; the availability of TG and CE (the core lipids) regulates their secretion. Containing mainly TG in their core, CMs and VLDL are the major TG carriers in plasma and are the two largest classes of lipoproteins. There are two pathways for the metabolism of TG-rich lipoproteins; the exogenous pathway carries dietary fats by apo B48 in CMs, whereas the endogenous pathway represents hepatic secretion of VLDL, a TG-rich apo B100–containing lipoprotein.

Endogenous Pathway: Assembly of VLDL Apo B-100 Lipoprotein Particles

The full-length apo B100 is a glycoprotein that contains 4536 amino acids. Apo B100 is synthesized by the liver and secreted in the form of VLDL, a TG-rich-lipoprotein that in plasma contains 60% TG by mass and 20% CE by mass.[27] Both fatty acids synthesized de novo from acetyl coenzyme A and fatty acids from lipolysis of stored adipose tissue TG or from core lipids of TG-rich remnant particles returning to the liver stimulate the assembly of VLDL in the liver (Fig. 15-1). Microsomal triglyceride transfer protein (MTP) transfers TGs from the cytosol to the endoplasmic reticulum containing nascent apo B during the assembly of CM and VLDL in enterocytes and hepatocytes, respectively.[28] MTP gene expression is regulated by insulin, possibly through transcriptional activity of the sterol response element–binding protein 1c (SREBP-1c). This may explain why VLDL secretion and TG levels are increased in insulin resistance syndromes.[29] In the plasma (see Fig. 15-1), VLDL particles adhere to glycosaminoglycan molecules on endothelial cells of capillaries, primarily in muscle, lung, and adipose tissue,[30,31] where interaction with lipoprotein lipase (LPL) and glycosylphosphatidylinositol-anchored high-density lipoprotein–binding protein 1 (GPIHBP1) results in hydrolysis of VLDL triglycerides to free fatty acids and glycerol.[32,33]

The removal of TG from VLDL by LPL exposes the apo E molecules on the lipoprotein surface of VLDL.[32] Apo E functions as a ligand in the receptor-mediated clearance of CM and VLDL remnants in the liver through several receptors: a remnant receptor,[34-36] the LDL receptor (an apo B/apo E receptor), the LDL receptor–related protein, the VLDL receptor, and apo E receptors.[37] With stable isotope methodology, Welty and colleagues[38] published the first study of simultaneous kinetics of apo B48 and apo B100 in human subjects and showed that about 50% of VLDL is directly removed from plasma (see Fig. 15-1) and therefore not converted to IDL or LDL. During the removal of the TG from the remaining 50% of VLDL (referred to as the delipidation cascade), the VLDL particles are hydrolyzed by LPL to smaller particles termed VLDL remnants or IDL (relatively enriched in CE but also containing TG), which then interact with hepatic lipase (HL) and are converted to CE-rich LDL, the major cholesterol-carrying lipoprotein in normal human plasma. Apo B100 is the main structural protein of LDL and contains the LDL receptor–binding domain; therefore, LDL is removed from the

circulation by binding mainly to hepatic LDL receptors (see Fig. 15-1).[27]

Exogenous Pathway: Assembly of Chylomicrons

Produced in the intestine in response to dietary fat, CMs contain apo B48, the amino-terminal 48% of apo B100, which is synthesized by the intestine and produced by a premature stop codon at the apo B100 codon 2153 by tissue-specific mRNA processing (see Fig. 15-1).[39] Genes related to sterol absorption (ABCG5)[40,41] and nuclear receptors LXR and FXR[42] in bile and sterol metabolism may affect variability in absorption of dietary fats and CM formation. Within the intestinal cell, free fatty acids combine with glycerol to form TGs, and cholesterol is esterified by acyl coenzyme A:cholesterol acyltransferase (ACAT) to form cholesterol esters.

CMs enter lacteals in the intestinal villi and travel through the lymphatics to the thoracic duct and then into the bloodstream. Similar to the metabolism of VLDL, CMs bind to LPL on the surface of endothelial cells, where most of the TGs and some surface glycerophospholipids are catabolized to form CM remnants and free fatty acid by LPL, present in capillary walls primarily of skeletal muscle, adipose tissue, and lung, with apo C-II as a cofactor and apo C-III as an inhibitor (see Fig. 15-1). Apo B48 does not contain an LDL receptor–binding domain; therefore, the CM remnants are taken up by the liver by remnant receptors[43-46] as well as by the LDL receptor that recognizes apo E.[47,48] CMs also bind to HL on the sinusoidal surface of hepatocytes, where HL further hydrolyzes remnant lipids. In the fed state, both CMs and VLDL transport TGs to peripheral organs, where, through the action of tissue-specific LPL, TG-derived free fatty acids are used as energy in muscle and in other tissues, converted to TG, or stored in adipose tissue.[49] Residual TGs (in the form of free fatty acids) and dietary cholesterol are rerouted to hepatocytes.

To transport TG and cholesterol to peripheral tissues, lipoprotein particles cross the endothelial barrier in blood vessels to reach the extracellular space (see Fig. 15-1). The subendothelial retention of apo B100–containing lipoproteins by a charge-mediated interaction with proteoglycans in the extracellular matrix is thought to be the initiating event in atherogenesis. Smaller, electronegative LDL particles penetrate the endothelial barrier 1.7-fold better than large LDL particles do; CM and VLDL remnants also can cross. All of these particles interact with positively charged intimal proteoglycans.[50,51] Oxidation, by reactive oxygen species, of fatty acids of surface phospholipids of the apo B–containing lipoprotein particles results in modification of lysine residues of apo B. Scavenger receptors on macrophages recognize modified apo B, and unregulated uptake of the modified lipoprotein particle causes macrophage accumulation of lipids, a process leading to a foamy cytoplasm and the term *foam cells* (see Fig. 15-1).[52-54] The most important scavenger receptor is CD36 (also called scavenger receptor B).[55-57] As foam cells increase in number, the fatty streak develops. VLDL particles from patients with hypertriglyceridemia are enriched in apo E, which can lead to a conformational change in the VLDL particle that facilitates binding to the macrophage scavenger receptor, resulting in unregulated uptake similar to that seen with oxidized LDL.[58] CM remnants are also small enough to enter the subendothelial space, where they are taken up by macrophages that promote atherogenesis.[59,60] Similar to LDL, IDL is taken up by macrophages and can also cause foam cell formation; endothelium-dependent vasomotor function in human coronary arteries is impaired by both IDL and LDL.[61] Several angiographic trials of cholesterol-lowering therapy

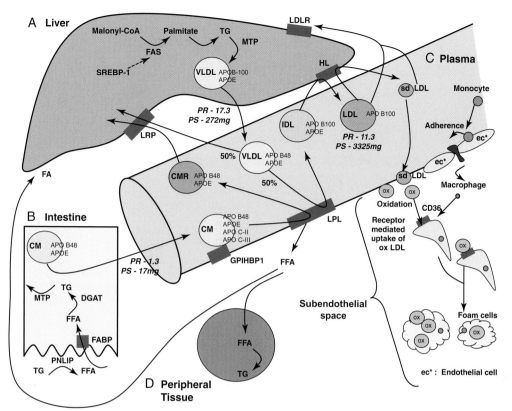

FIGURE 15-1 Schematic overview of TG-rich lipoprotein metabolism in the nonfasting (fed) state. The main sources of plasma TG are exogenous, from dietary fat, and endogenous, from the liver. In the intestine, dietary TG is hydrolyzed by pancreatic lipase (PNLIP) into monoglyceride and free fatty acids (FFA), forming micelles. Fatty acid–binding protein (FABP) transports FFA from the intestinal lumen into enterocytes, and TG is resynthesized through the sequential acyltransferase reactions, of which microsomal diacylglycerol acyltransferase (DGAT) catalyzes the terminal committed step. Microsomal triglyceride transfer protein (MTP) mediates assembly of TG with apo B48 and apo E into chylomicrons. After secretion into the blood through the lymph, chylomicrons acquire apo C-II and C-III, which modulate the plasma metabolism of TG-rich lipoproteins. Apo C-II is an obligatory cofactor for lipoprotein lipase (LPL), whereas apo C-III may interfere with LPL. Apo A-V has been shown to enhance hydrolysis of TG-rich lipoproteins, through an incompletely defined mechanism; a newly characterized protein, glycosylphosphatidylinositol-anchored high-density lipoprotein–binding protein 1 (GPIHBP1), appears to facilitate lipolysis by anchoring chylomicrons to endothelium, providing stability for LPL activity. Apo B48 is the signature protein of intestinally derived TG-rich lipoproteins. In the liver, TG is synthesized from FFA extracted from plasma, from fatty acids synthesized de novo, and from uptake of plasma lipoproteins. A central enzyme for de novo synthesis is fatty acid synthase (FAS), which catalyzes the conversion of malonyl-CoA to palmitate. FAS is induced by the membrane-bound transcription factor sterol regulatory element–binding protein 1 (SREBP-1), which is itself regulated by polyunsaturated fatty acids, glucose, and insulin. Hepatic MTP mediates TG assembly with cholesteryl esters, apo B100, and apo E to form VLDL, which is released into the space of Disse by exocytosis. Apo B48 is the signature protein of intestinally derived TG-rich lipoproteins. In adipose and muscle capillaries, TG in chylomicrons and VLDL are hydrolyzed into FFA by endothelium-bound LPL. FFA is then re-esterified and stored in adipocytes or oxidized for energy in myocytes. Chylomicrons and VLDL are remodeled, respectively, into the smaller, denser, cholesteryl ester (CE)–enriched chylomicron remnants (CMR) and VLDL remnants (also called intermediate-density lipoprotein [IDL]). CMR and some IDL are cleared by apo E–mediated endocytosis through hepatic remnant receptors (LRP). IDL can also be hydrolyzed by hepatic lipase (HL), making smaller, CE-rich LDL particles; 50% of VLDL is directly removed from plasma in normolipidemic human subjects. Production rate (PR), pool size (PS), and fractional catabolic rate for apo B48, VLDL apo B100, and LDL apo B100 are shown on a 36% fat diet. PR refers to secretion rate for VLDL apo B100 from the liver and apo B48 from the intestine. *(Modified from Hegele RA, Pollex RL: Hypertriglyceridemia: phenomics and genomics. Mol Cell Biochem 326:36, 2009.)*

have shown that serum IDL concentrations are predictive of an increased incidence of CHD[62] and an increased incidence of coronary events in those with CHD, independently of other factors.[63-65] VLDL and IDL have been identified in human atherosclerotic plaques,[66] and these particles are associated with progression of mild to moderate coronary lesions. In the Monitored Atherosclerosis Regression Study (MARS) angiographic trial, IDL, but not VLDL or LDL, was associated with progression of carotid artery intima-media thickness.[67] Moreover, the total TG level and markers for TG metabolism predicted risk of progression of low-grade but not of high-grade coronary artery lesions.[68,69]

Effect of Triglyceride-Rich Lipoproteins on Level of HDL-C in Humans

Levels of TG-rich lipoproteins also affect HDL level and particle size. HDL levels are inversely related to risk of CHD.[70-74] In contrast to LDL and VLDL, HDL has antiatherogenic properties that include reverse cholesterol transport, antioxidation (protecting apo B lipoproteins from oxidation), antithrombotic and anti-inflammatory properties, and maintenance of endothelial function. Apo A-I is secreted from the liver in a lipid-poor form. The major formation of HDL particles occurs when lipid-poor apo A-I interacts with the ABCA1

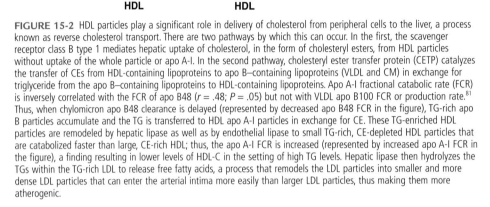

FIGURE 15-2 HDL particles play a significant role in delivery of cholesterol from peripheral cells to the liver, a process known as reverse cholesterol transport. There are two pathways by which this can occur. In the first, the scavenger receptor class B type 1 mediates hepatic uptake of cholesterol, in the form of cholesteryl esters, from HDL particles without uptake of the whole particle or apo A-I. In the second pathway, cholesteryl ester transfer protein (CETP) catalyzes the transfer of CEs from HDL-containing lipoproteins to apo B–containing lipoproteins (VLDL and CM) in exchange for triglyceride from the apo B–containing lipoproteins to HDL-containing lipoproteins. Apo A-I fractional catabolic rate (FCR) is inversely correlated with the FCR of apo B48 ($r = .48$; $P = .05$) but not with VLDL apo B100 FCR or production rate.[81] Thus, when chylomicron apo B48 clearance is delayed (represented by decreased apo B48 FCR in the figure), TG-rich apo B particles accumulate and the TG is transferred to HDL apo A-I particles in exchange for CE. These TG-enriched HDL particles are remodeled by hepatic lipase as well as by endothelial lipase to small TG-rich, CE-depleted HDL particles that are catabolized faster than large, CE-rich HDL; thus, the apo A-I FCR is increased (represented by increased apo A-I FCR in the figure), a finding resulting in lower levels of HDL-C in the setting of high TG levels. Hepatic lipase then hydrolyzes the TGs within the TG-rich LDL to release free fatty acids, a process that remodels the LDL particles into smaller and more dense LDL particles that can enter the arterial intima more easily than larger LDL particles, thus making them more atherogenic.

receptor on the surface of peripheral cells.[25] This results in transfer of free cholesterol and phospholipid to the apo A-I, forming a pre-β particle. When the free cholesterol is esterified under the action of lecithin-cholesterol acyltransferase (LCAT), this particle becomes a mature HDL particle. The majority of the proteins of HDL, apo A-I, A-II, and A-IV, are secreted as components of VLDL, which are then transferred to the apo A-I particle in the plasma. Plasma HDL is mainly assembled extracellularly during transfer of surface components of TG-rich lipoproteins, including phospholipids and cholesterol.

HDL particles play a significant role in delivery of cholesterol from peripheral cells to the liver after esterification within the particle to CE through plasma LCAT, a process known as reverse cholesterol transport. There are two pathways by which this can occur. In the first, the scavenger receptor class B type 1 (SR-B1) mediates hepatic uptake of CE from HDL particles without uptake of apo A-I or the whole HDL particle.[75] In the second pathway, cholesteryl ester transfer protein (CETP) catalyzes the transfer of CE from HDL to apo B–containing lipoproteins (VLDL and LDL) in exchange for TG from the apo B–containing lipoproteins (Fig. 15-2).[25,76,77] This exchange results in apo B–containing lipoproteins, which are enriched with CEs and depleted of TGs, and HDL particles, which are depleted of CEs and enriched with TGs. The TG-rich and CE-poor HDL particles are catabolized faster than the large, CE-rich HDL particles are[78] (apo A-I fractional catabolic rate [FCR] is increased as noted in Fig. 15-2),

resulting in lower levels of HDL-C in the setting of high TG levels. The apo B–containing lipoproteins, now enriched in CE, are taken up by the liver receptors, as previously described.[77] This exchange through CETP action is thought to be responsible for the inverse relationship between levels of TG and HDL-C.[79] The cardioprotective effect of HDL has been largely attributed to its role in reverse cholesterol transport. HL then hydrolyzes the TGs within the TG-rich LDL to release free fatty acids, a process that remodels the LDL particles into smaller and denser LDL particles that can enter the arterial intima more easily than larger LDL particles, thus making them more atherogenic (see Fig. 15-2). Small, dense LDL particles also bind less avidly to the LDL receptor, thus prolonging their half-life in the circulation, making these particles more susceptible to oxidative modification and to subsequent uptake by the macrophage scavenger receptors.[80]

Using stable isotopes in the fed (nonfasting) state in humans, Welty and colleagues[81] showed that apo A-I FCR is inversely correlated with the FCR of apo B48 (see Fig. 15-2 for details) but not with VLDL apo B100 FCR or production rate. Thus, when CM apo B48 clearance is delayed (represented by decreased apo B48 FCR in Fig. 15-2), TG-rich apo B particles accumulate and the TG is transferred to HDL apo A-I particles in exchange for CE. These results suggest that in the fed state, levels of TG-rich apo B48 of intestinal origin are more important determinants of levels of HDL-C than the amount of TG-rich lipoproteins of hepatic origin, which contain apo B100.

Mutations in Enzymes of VLDL and Chylomicron Metabolism Affecting Risk for Atherosclerosis

Alterations in the enzymes involved in lipid metabolism may affect risk for atherosclerosis. As noted earlier, LPL hydrolyzes TGs contained in the core of CMs and VLDL. In partial LPL deficiency, TG-enriched lipoproteins have a prolonged circulation time that allows more interaction with the endothelium. An Asn291Ser substitution in LPL causes impaired function of this enzyme and is associated with an increase in plasma TG. Female but not male carriers of this mutation have a twofold increase in the risk of CHD and nonfatal cerebrovascular disease.[82,83]

Apo C-II is an activator of LPL that hydrolyzes the core TGs, thereby releasing free fatty acids and making the CMs and VLDL progressively smaller and forming remnants. Apo C-II thus increases the catabolism of both CM and VLDL, thereby lowering TG levels. Apo C-III is an inhibitor of LPL, and in contrast to apo C-II, which lowers TG levels, apo C-III can raise TG levels by stimulating VLDL synthesis, inhibiting LPL, and inhibiting the binding of remnants to the LDL receptor mediated by apo E. Thus, high levels of apo C-III are associated with TG-enriched VLDL particles that are ultimately converted to TG-rich remnants. These remnants are then lipolyzed to small, dense LDL particles by HL.[59] Thus, high levels of apo C-III are associated with TG-rich VLDL particles that circulate longer and are therefore ultimately converted to TG-remnants, which are then lipolyzed by HL to small, dense LDL particles. Most patients with elevated levels of VLDL have excess amounts of both TGs and apo C-III within their lipid particles. Persons lacking apo C-III have efficient lipolysis of TGs and therefore low levels of TG.[60]

Produced in the liver, apo A-V activates proteoglycan-bound LPL and thus accelerates TG hydrolysis from VLDL and CMs independently of other apoproteins.[84] A sequence element between residues 185 and 228 functions in binding of apo A-V to heparin sulfate proteoglycans, members of the LDL receptor family and GPIHBP1.[85] Plasma levels of apo A-V are extremely low, and this factor, plus the association of apo A-V with cytosolic lipid droplets, suggests that apo A-V may modulate TG metabolism within the cell.[85] The gene for apo A-V is located at the apo A1/C3/A4/A5 gene cluster on chromosome 11q23. Several single-nucleotide polymorphisms are associated with significantly higher plasma TG levels in patients (i.e., −1131T>C, S19W, G185C).[84] The structural mutations Q139X, Q148X, and IVS3 + 3G>C predispose to familial hypertriglyceridemia and late-onset chylomicronemia.[84] Thus, apo A-V is an important regulator of plasma TG levels in humans.

Polymorphisms in HL may also affect risk for atherosclerosis. There are four common sequence polymorphisms in the HL gene promoter; the most frequent is a C to T substitution.[86] The presence of a C allele is associated with higher HL activity; smaller, denser, and more atherogenic LDL particles; and lower levels of HDL-C.[87]

CLASSIFICATION AND CAUSES OF HYPERTRIGLYCERIDEMIA

Hypertriglyceridemia can occur as an isolated hypertriglyceridemia or in combination with hypercholesterolemia (familial combined hyperlipoproteinemia and familial dysbetalipoproteinemia) (Table 15-1). Both forms can be further subdivided into primary and secondary causes. LPL, HL, and their apolipoproteins regulate levels of TG; therefore, abnormalities in any of these can affect TG levels.

Isolated Hypertriglyceridemia

Familial Hypertriglyceridemia—Severe

Familial hypertriglyceridemia is characterized by elevated TG levels with normal cholesterol and can be divided into severe and mild forms (see Table 15-1). In the severe form, TGs exceed 1000 mg/dL because of increases in both CMs and VLDL particles[25,88,89] (type V in original Fredrickson-Levy classification, also called primary mixed hypertriglyceridemia).[25] Most patients with mixed hypertriglyceridemia have familial hypertriglyceridemia due to partial deficiency of LPL or apo C-II (the ligand for LPL on CMs and VLDL) deficiency exacerbated by one or more of the secondary disorders noted in Table 15-1.

The other major primary cause of TGs >1000 mg/dL is exogenous hyperlipemia or familial chylomicronemia due to CMs (hyperlipoproteinemia type I in original Fredrickson-Levy classification).[25] The most common primary cause of type I is complete absence of either LPL activity or apo C-II.[1,90,91] When LPL is absent (prevalence is 1 in a million), TG is generally >2000 mg/dL. Patients with TGs >2000 mg/dL usually have both a genetic form of hypertriglyceridemia and a secondary cause. Similar clinical manifestations of both types I and V include hepatosplenomegaly and occasional eruptive xanthomas (see Table 15-1). Features that distinguish type I from type V include (1) presentation of type I in childhood and of type V in adulthood; (2) absence of LPL or apo C-II activity or homozygous gene mutations in type I; (3) presence of a secondary factor in type V (alcohol, obesity, type 2 diabetes mellitus, hypothyroidism, or poor diet); (4) higher prevalence of type V than of type I; and (5) increased CMs alone in type I compared with elevations in both CMs and VLDL in type V.

The primary risk associated with TG levels >1000 mg/dL is pancreatitis. Minimal atherosclerotic risk is reported for patients with hyperchylomicronemia (type I) or the severe form of familial hypertriglyceridemia (type V), probably because the lipoprotein particles are too large to enter the arterial wall.[24]

Patients with marked hypertriglyceridemia (>1000 mg/dL [11.3 mmol/L]) may develop the chylomicronemia syndrome. This can include recent memory loss, abdominal pain or pancreatitis, dyspnea, eruptive xanthoma, flushing after alcohol ingestion, and lipemia retinalis.[90]

Familial Hypertriglyceridemia—Mild

The mild form of familial hypertriglyceridemia (type IV hyperlipoproteinemia phenotype) is an autosomal dominant disorder characterized by mild to moderate elevations in TG from 200 to 500 mg/dL, often in association with insulin resistance, obesity, hyperglycemia, hypertension, hyperuricemia, and low HDL-C. Mutations in the LPL gene decrease enzyme activity and therefore delay the degradation of CMs and VLDL that carry endogenous TGs. Gly188Glu, Asp9Asn, and Asn291Ser are N-terminal mutations that reduce the activity of LPL, resulting in an increase in serum TGs by 20% to 80% and also lower levels of HDL-C.[1,91] More marked elevations require some other factor, such as one of the drugs or acquired disorders (e.g., estrogen replacement therapy in postmenopausal women).[92]

Familial hypertriglyceridemia is common in patients with premature CHD. The prevalence of familial hypertriglyceridemia with low HDL-C levels was 15% in patients undergoing coronary arteriography before the age of 55 years.[93] Among first-degree relatives of affected patients, baseline serum TG levels predicted cardiovascular mortality, independent of serum total cholesterol.[94]

15

The Contribution of Triglycerides and Triglyceride-Rich Lipoproteins to Atherosclerotic Cardiovascular Disease

TABLE 15–1 | **Classification of Hypertriglyceridemic Disorders**

Generic Designation and Elevated Lipoprotein Classes	Synonym and Prevalence	Lipid Levels	Primary Disorders	Secondary Disorders*	Clinical Manifestation
Isolated Hypertriglyceridemia					
Exogenous hyperlipemia Familial hyperchylomicronemia (↑chylomicrons with ↓LDL and ↓HDL)	Type I 1 × 10⁶	TG ≥1000 mg/dL	Familial lipoprotein lipase deficiency or familial apo C-II deficiency (95% of cases); LPL mutations[105,106]; apo C-II mutations[105] (rare)	Dysglobulinemias Systemic lupus erythematosus	Presents in childhood or adolescence; abdominal pain, pancreatitis, hepatosplenomegaly, lipemia retinalis
Endogenous hyperlipemia (↑VLDL) Familial hypertriglyceridemia	Type IV 5%-10%	TG: 200-999 mg/dL	Familial hypertriglyceridemia (mild form) Familial multiple lipoprotein type hyperlipidemia Sporadic hypertriglyceridemia Tangier disease No replicated causative or susceptibility gene	Dysglobulinemias§ Systemic lupus erythematosus§ Diabetic hyperlipemia†,§ Glycogenosis, type I§ Lipodystrophies§ Uremia§ Hypopituitarism§ Nephrotic syndrome§ (Diabetes mellitus)‡,§ (Alcoholism)§ (Estrogen use)§ (Glucocorticoid use)§ (Stress-induced)§	Asymptomatic; may be associated with increased risk of vascular disease
Primary mixed hyperlipemia (↑VLDL + ↑chylomicrons)	Type V 1 × 10³	TG ≥1000 mg/dL	Familial hypertriglyceridemia (severe form) Familial lipoprotein lipase deficiency; heterozygous LPL mutations (5%-10% of cases) or apo C-II deficiency		Presents in adulthood; hepatosplenomegaly, eruptive xanthomas, abdominal pain, pancreatitis; lipemia retinalis
Hypertriglyceridemia and Hypercholesterolemia					
Remnant hyperlipidemia (↑β-VLDL)	Type III 1 × 10²; expression is 1 × 10⁴	TG variable; can be ≥1000 mg/dL TC = 250-500 mg/dL	Familial dysbetalipoproteinemia Homozygous APOE2 mutation plus secondary genetic or medical factors	Hypothyroidism Systemic lupus erythematosus	Tuberous or tuberoeruptive xanthomas on extensor surfaces of extremities; plantar or palmar crease xanthomas; vascular disease
Familial combined hyperlipoproteinemia (↑VLDL and ↑LDL and ↓HDL)	Type IIb 5%	TG: 200-500 mg/dL TC: 200-400 mg/dL; small, dense LDL	Obligate heterozygotes for mutations of LPL or apo C-III; insulin resistance Autosomal dominant USF1[105]	Nephrotic syndrome Hypothyroidism Dysglobulinemias Cushing syndrome (Glucocorticoid use) (Stress-induced)	Premature vascular disease

*All conditions associated with VLDL or β-VLDL are aggravated by hypertrophic obesity.

†Denotes mixed hyperlipemia caused by severe, prolonged insulin deficiency.

‡Parentheses indicate conditions that frequently aggravate a primary hyperlipemia but that seldom cause hyperlipemia de novo. These conditions cause some cases of primary hypertriglyceridemia (mild form) to present as mixed hyperlipemia.

§Indicates secondary disorders that can cause type IV or type V hyperlipidemia.

Modified from Havel RJ: Approach to the patient with hyperlipidemia. *Med Clin North Am* 66:319, 1982.

15

Hypertriglyceridemia and Hypercholesterolemia

Hypertriglyceridemia can occur in two phenotypes in combination with hypercholesterolemia. The first is familial combined hyperlipoproteinemia (FCHL), and the second is familial dysbetalipoproteinemia.

Familial Combined Hyperlipoproteinemia

In FCHL (type IIb), overproduction of hepatically derived VLDL apo B100–containing lipoproteins results in plasma TG levels of 200 to 500 mg/dL and plasma cholesterol levels of 200 to 400 mg/dL and small, dense LDL.[95,96] FCHL has an autosomal dominant mode of inheritance with variable penetrance and a population prevalence of 1% to 2%.[97] It is the most common familial lipid disorder in post-MI patients[98] and accounts for one third to one half of familial causes of

CHD.[94] The molecular basis includes mutations in LPL and apo C-III and upstream stimulatory factor 1 (USF1), which encodes an upstream stimulatory factor.[99,100] FCHL is also linked with insulin resistance[101,102] due to both increased free fatty acid flux from the periphery and insulin-stimulated lipogenesis, which increases the production of VLDL.[103] Families with premature CHD often have either familial dyslipidemia (high TGs and low HDL-C [type IV]) or FCHL (high TGs, high LDL-C, and low HDL-C [type IIb]).[104]

Patients with FCHL can present with combined hypercholesterolemia and hypertriglyceridemia or either abnormality alone. Thus, subjects with FCHL who overproduce VLDL particles and also synthesize TG at an increased rate will secrete an increased number of large, TG-rich VLDL particles. If they are unable to efficiently catabolize these VLDL particles because of an LPL mutation or low LPL activity, they will have a high TG level but a normal or reduced number of LDL particles and thus a normal LDL-C level. On the other hand, with efficient catabolism of the increased numbers of large, TG-rich VLDL particles, the number of LDL particles is increased, resulting in both increased TG and LDL-C levels. Finally, subjects who synthesize a normal quantity of TG but an increased number of VLDL particles (with normal TG load) have increased numbers of LDL particles and elevated plasma LDL-C levels but a normal TG level. LPL may be responsible for part of this phenotypic variability as hypertriglyceridemia is more prominent in patients with LPL deficiency[105] or an LPL gene mutation.[106]

Familial Dysbetalipoproteinemia

As noted before, the apo E ligand is necessary for receptor-mediated catabolism of CM and VLDL remnants. There are three isoforms of the apo E allele: apo E2, apo E3, and apo E4. Apo E3/3 is the most common apo E genotype. Apo E2 differs from apo E3 by substitution of cysteine for the normal arginine at residue 158 in the receptor-binding domain. Consequently, apo E2 does not bind as well as apo E3 to the apo B/E (LDL receptor).[107] Subjects with familial dysbetalipoproteinemia have the apo E2/E2 genotype, which is an autosomal recessive disorder characterized by an accumulation of VLDL and CM remnants in the plasma due to inefficient uptake through apo E2, which binds poorly to hepatic LDL-related receptors.[108] Consequently, they have an increase in cholesterol-enriched VLDL (β-VLDL, also termed IDL) and CM remnants. The prevalence of the apo E2 isoform is 1 in 100; however, only approximately 1 in 10,000 carriers exhibits the dyslipidemia, which is thought to be triggered by a secondary cause, such as marked hyperglycemia (type 2 diabetes), hyperuricemia (gout), hypothyroidism, or obesity.[108] Classic physical findings include tuberoeruptive xanthomas and xanthomas of the palmar creases; the risk for CHD is increased.

Secondary Causes

The major secondary causes (see Table 15-1) of hypertriglyceridemia include poorly controlled type 2 diabetes, obesity, excessive alcohol intake, renal disease, pregnancy, medications (Table 15-2), excessive ingestion of saturated fats and simple sugars, nonalcoholic hepatosteatosis, and physical inactivity. Alcohol intake can cause elevated TG by inhibition of LPL[109] or increased VLDL TG production. For every gram of alcohol consumed per day, TG concentration can increase on average by 0.19 mg/dL, which is about 5.7 mg/dL for 30 g of alcohol.[110] These secondary causes must always be considered during the evaluation and treatment of hypertriglyceridemia.

Metabolic Syndrome

The association of hypertriglyceridemia with obesity and diabetes or glucose intolerance is termed the metabolic syndrome, which is defined clinically according to the National Cholesterol Education Program[111] by at least three of the following: central obesity (waist circumference >35 inches in women and >40 inches in men), fasting blood glucose concentration ≥100 mg/dL, TGs ≥150 mg/dL, low HDL-C (<40 mg/dL in men and <50 mg/dL in women), and systolic or diastolic blood pressure ≥130/≥85 mm Hg. Atherogenic dyslipidemia in metabolic syndrome and people with type 2 diabetes (termed diabetic dyslipidemia) is characterized by elevated TGs and small, dense, cholesterol-depleted LDL and HDL particles.[111] Insulin resistance increases mobilization of free fatty acids from adipose tissue to liver, where increased production of VLDL occurs; thus, hypertriglyceridemia in type 2 diabetes and metabolic syndrome is usually secondary to increased VLDL concentrations in plasma, with or without chylomicronemia.[112] Downregulation of LPL expression in

TABLE 15–2	Effects of Selected Drugs on Triglyceride and Cholesterol Levels*		
Drug	**Triglycerides**	**LDL-C**	**HDL-C**
Alcohol	Increased	No effect	Increased
Estrogens, estradiol	Increased	Decreased	Increased
Androgens, testosterone	Increased	Increased	Decreased
Progestins	Decrease	Increase	Decrease
Glucocorticoids	Increased	No effect	Increased
Cyclosporines	Increased	Increased	Increased
Tacrolimus	Increased	Increased	Increased
Thiazide diuretics	Increased	Increased	Decreased
Beta blockers	Increased	No effect	Decreased
Sertraline	Possible increase	Increased	No effect
Protease inhibitors	Increased	No effect	No effect
Valproate and related drugs	Increased	No effect	Decreased
Isotretinoin	Increased	No effect	Decreased
Clozapine, olanzapine†	Increased	No effect	Decreased

*Alcohol, estrogens, estradiol, glucocorticoids, thiazide diuretics, beta blockers, sertraline, protease inhibitors, valproate and related drugs, and isotretinoin can cause severe hypertriglyceridemia and the chylomicronemia syndrome in patients with a familial form of hypertriglyceridemia.

†Second-generation antipsychotics: clozapine and olanzapine have most effect; risperidone and quetiapine have intermediate effects; and aripiprazole and ziprasidone have least effect.

Data from Brunzell JD: Clinical practice. Hypertriglyceridemia. *N Engl J Med* 357:1009, 2007. Copyright © 2007 Massachusetts Medical Society. All rights reserved.

insulin resistance leads to decreased catabolism of TG-rich VLDL. The higher levels of TG promote CETP-mediated transfer of CE from HDL, thus producing TG-rich small, dense HDL that are catabolized more rapidly, leading to low levels of HDL-C. Small, dense HDL also have reduced antioxidant and anti-inflammatory properties. The metabolic syndrome and increased TG-rich lipoproteins are also associated with a pro-inflammatory and prothrombotic state due to the presence of atherogenic lipoproteins, clotting factors, and increased plasma viscosity.[113] In clinical practice, elevated serum TGs are most often observed in persons with the metabolic syndrome, although secondary or genetic factors can raise TG levels. Metabolic syndrome has a prevalence of 24% in U.S. adults and 43% in adults older than 60 years[114]; therefore, it is a major health problem.

LABORATORY EVALUATION OF HYPERTRIGLYCERIDEMIA

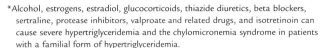

In this section, the literature on several clinical laboratory approaches to assess the risk of TGs and TG-rich lipoproteins is reviewed.

Fasting Versus Nonfasting Triglyceride Levels

The Friedewald equation is often used to estimate LDL-C levels: LDL-C = TC − (TG/5 + HDL-C); it requires measurement of fasting TG levels. TG/5 is an estimate of the cholesterol in VLDL and IDL particles (VLDL-C + IDL-C). This equation has been used for more than 40 years to calculate LDL-C; therefore, the majority of research studies have examined the association of TG with CHD on the basis of fasting TG levels. As shown earlier in the section on lipoprotein metabolism, levels of TG-rich- and apo B48–containing CMs of intestinal origin are probably more important determinants of levels of HDL-C than the amount of TG-rich lipoproteins of hepatic origin, which contain apo B100.[81] In the fasting state, very little apo B48 is being produced; therefore, it would make sense that nonfasting levels of TG might be a better predictor not only of the concentration of TG-rich lipoproteins circulating in plasma most of the time but also of the HDL-C level.

In 2007, Bansal and colleagues[115] and Nordestgaard and coworkers[116] reported that in two long-term prospective cohort studies, TG levels obtained 2 to 4 hours postprandially predicted risk of CHD better than TG levels measured after a 12- to 14-hour fast and better than LDL-C calculated by the Friedewald equation.[115-117] In both studies, elevated postprandial TG levels increased risk of CHD for both sexes; however, women had greater risk of CHD associated with hypertriglyceridemia than men did,[115,116] confirming prior studies that showed higher risk in women than in men.[14,118] Postprandial lipoproteins are TG rich, and if their catabolism is delayed (insulin resistance, LPL mutations), the products of their metabolism, CM remnants and small dense LDL, can remain in the plasma for 12 hours or more,[24] with exposure of the endothelium to TG-rich, atherogenic remnant particles, a finding accounting for the greater CHD risk with postprandial increases in TG levels.

Although postprandial TG levels may predict risk better than fasting TG levels, nonfasting TG measurements may be difficult to incorporate into clinical practice. First, a standard fat-feeding protocol would need to be developed and prepared fresh for each test. Second, a fat load may cause nausea or vomiting. Third, requirement for a 2- to 4-hour postprandial peak may not be practical in outpatient care. In the long run, fasting TG measurements may be more reliable because of controlled conditions. The strong correlation between postprandial and fasting TG levels may obviate the need for repeated postprandial measurements.[119]

Lipoprotein Particle Subclasses

Lipoprotein particle composition has been associated with differences in the relative atherogenicity of lipoproteins.[120,121] Small, dense LDL particles are more susceptible to accelerated oxidation and are incorporated more readily by vascular wall macrophages than other lipoprotein particles are.[81,122] Several prospective cohort studies have reported that the number of small, dense LDL particles is a greater predictor of CHD risk than are measured levels of serum LDL-C.[123,124] Thus, unlike the linear relationship of risk with LDL-C, the risk of CHD associated with elevated TG levels may be a function of the associated lipoprotein disorder more than a direct numerical correlation with TGs. In the Veterans Affairs High-Density Lipoprotein Intervention Trial (VA-HIT), a change in TG concentration did not predict the magnitude of reduction in risk of CHD events; rather, it was the change in LDL and HDL particles that predicted change in risk.[125]

Patients with CHD often have increases in small, dense LDL; however, LDL particle size is not an independent predictor of CHD, and in fact, the major factor regulating LDL particle size is plasma TG level.[126] Therefore, the measurement of particle size has not been proven to provide better information than standard lipid and lipoprotein measurements. Patients with TG levels >150 mg/dL generally have increased levels of small, dense LDL particles.[127] As noted

earlier, after conversion of large VLDL particles to TG-rich remnants, HL hydrolyzes the remnants to small, dense LDL particles.[128] Consequently, levels of TG and VLDL are strongly and positively correlated with levels of small, dense LDL particles.[127] In some prospective, nested case-control studies, subjects with small, dense LDL particles have an increased risk for CHD; however, other studies have concluded that increased levels of small LDL particles are not an independent predictor of CHD but rather are products of elevated levels of TG-rich lipoproteins that are associated with an atherogenic milieu—elevated TG, reduced HDL-C, and potentially other biomarkers of the metabolic syndrome.[129] Because both large and small LDL subtypes have been shown to predict CHD, apo B concentrations, which estimate particle numbers, rather than LDL particle size, may be the better predictor of CHD.[120] Moreover, apo C-III enrichment of apo B–containing lipoproteins has been linked to the atherogenicity of apo B–containing lipoproteins and therefore may also be a better predictor of CHD than particle size.[130]

Apo B

Much data supports apo B as a predictor of CHD.[131,132] Fredrickson and associates[133] recognized more than 40 years ago that atherosclerosis is more closely related to the total number of apo B–containing particles rather than to LDL-C or TG concentrations alone. One apo B molecule is present on the surface of VLDL, IDL, LDL, and lipoprotein(a), a molecule of apo B100 covalently bound to apoprotein (a)[25]; therefore, the apo B level may provide a more direct measure of circulating atherogenic lipoproteins.[134] As noted earlier, not all forms of hypertriglyceridemia are atherogenic[24]; however, the relative atherogenicity of apo B is well established by the fact that modification of lysine residues on apo B is necessary for uptake by scavenger receptors on macrophages.[52-54] However, the routine measurement of apo B is not always practical because of cost and technical limitations that preclude measurement in routine laboratory assays in hospital chemistry laboratories.

Non–HDL-C

For all of these reasons, as suggested by the National Cholesterol Education Program (NCEP) Adult Treatment Panel III (ATP III),[111] non–HDL-C is a practical and useful surrogate measure of atherogenic particle concentration[120,135] and more predictive of CHD risk than LDL-C level alone (especially when TG levels are elevated) because this measure is a sum of all atherogenic lipoproteins.[106,111] Non–HDL-C is TC − HDL-C, which is the sum of VLDL-C, IDL-C, and LDL-C. Therefore, non–HDL-C includes the cholesterol in all of the atherogenic apo B–containing lipoproteins: TG-enriched lipoproteins, CMs, CM remnants, VLDL and VLDL remnants, IDL, LDL, and lipoprotein(a). Non–HDL-C is accurate and reliable in a nonfasting state; therefore, measurement of non-HDL is practical and easy.[111] When lipid levels are normal, non–HDL-C is highly correlated with apo B levels.[136] Because high LDL-C and TG levels confer greater risk for CHD than high LDL-C alone, NCEP ATP III guidelines recommended non–HDL-C as a secondary target of therapy when the serum TG level is ≥200 mg/dL after the LDL-C target is achieved (Table 15-3).[111]

PREDICTIVE VALUE OF NON–HIGH-DENSITY LIPOPROTEIN CHOLESTEROL FOR CORONARY HEART DISEASE

Several observational and intervention studies have reported that elevated levels of non–HDL-C are predictive of

TABLE 15–3 | **LDL-C and Non–HDL-C Goals in Patients, by Risk Category***

Risk Category	LDL-C Goal	Non–HDL-C Goal†
Very high risk‡	<70 mg/dL (optional)	<100 mg/dL
High risk: CHD§ or CHD risk equivalents‖	<100 mg/dL	<130 mg/dL
Moderately high risk: ≥2 risk factors¶ (10-year risk 10%-20%)	<130 mg/dL	<160 mg/dL
Moderate risk: >2 risk factors (10-year risk <10%)	<130 mg/dL	<160 mg/dL
Lower risk: 0 or 1 risk factor	<160 mg/dL	<190 mg/dL

*NCEP ATP III guidelines for non–HDL-C state that in addition to the primary goal of LDL-C reduction, non–HDL-C is a secondary target of therapy in patients with TG levels of 200 to 499 mg/dL. Because a normal VLDL-C level is <30 mg/dL, the therapeutic goal for non–HDL-C is 30 mg/dL higher than the goal for LDL-C. Factors that place patients at very high risk favor a decision to reduce LDL-C levels to <70 mg/dL. The optional goal of <70 mg/dL does not apply to subjects who are not very high risk.

†When TGs are 200 to 499 mg/dL.

‡Presence of established cardiovascular disease plus (1) multiple major risk factors (especially diabetes mellitus), (2) severe and poorly controlled risk factors (especially continued cigarette smoking), (3) multiple risk factors for the metabolic syndrome (especially high TGs [>200 mg/dL] plus non–HDL-C >130 mg/dL with low HDL-C [<40 mg/dL]), and (4) acute coronary syndromes.

§CHD includes history of myocardial infarction, unstable angina, stable angina, coronary artery procedures, or evidence of clinically significant myocardial ischemia.

‖CHD risk equivalents include clinical manifestations of noncoronary forms of atherosclerotic disease, diabetes, and ≥2 risk factors, with 10-year risk for hard CHD >20%.

¶Risk factors include cigarette smoking, hypertension (blood pressure <140/90 mm Hg or taking antihypertensive medication), low HDL-C (<40 mg/dL), family history of premature CHD, and age (men <45 years, women <55 years).

From Miller M, Ginsberg HN, Schaefer E: Relative atherogenicity and predictive value of non-high-density lipoprotein cholesterol for coronary heart disease. *Am J Cardiol* 101:1004, 2008, with permission from Elsevier Limited.

cardiovascular disease and cardiovascular disease mortality,[131,132,137,138] similar to the predictive value of apo B and as good as or better than that of LDL-C. In the Bypass Angioplasty Revascularization Investigation (BARI), 1514 patients with multivessel CHD were observed for 5 years.[139] Non–HDL-C, but not HDL-C or LDL-C, was a significant univariate and multivariate predictor of nonfatal MI (RR, 1.049; 95% CI, 1.006-1.093; $P < 0.05$) and angina pectoris (RR,1.049; 95% CI, 1.004-1.096; $P < 0.05$) at 5 years.[139] Non–HDL-C did not predict mortality in this study. In long-term follow-up from the Lipid Research Clinics Program Follow-up Study, increases of 30 mg/dL in non–HDL-C and LDL-C levels corresponded to increases in CVD mortality of 19% and 15%, respectively, in men and 11% and 8%, respectively, in women.[131] The risk for CHD death was lowest in men and women with LDL-C levels <100 mg/dL in the Atherosclerosis Risk in Communities (ARIC) study; elevated TG levels were associated with substantially greater relative risks in women (4.7) than in men (2.1) after adjustment for LDL-C, HDL-C, and lipoprotein(a).[140] In prospective follow-up of a cohort of 15,632 healthy women older than 45 years at baseline in the Women's Health Study, non–HDL-C was as good as or better than apolipoprotein fractions for prediction of risk of a first cardiovascular event.[141] In 6-year follow-up of 18,225 men in the Health Professionals Follow-up Study free of CHD at baseline, the relative risk of CHD in the highest quintile of non–HDL-C compared with the lowest quintile was 2.76 after adjustment (95% CI, 1.66-4.58), which was better than LDL-C, 1.81 (95% CI, 1.12-2.93), but not quite as good as apo B, 3.01 (95% CI, 1.81-5.00). After mutual adjustment of non–HDL-C and LDL-C, only non–HDL-C was predictive of CHD.[137] In prospective follow-up of 1562 men and 1760 women older than 30 years and free of CHD at baseline in the Framingham Heart Study, the predictive value of non–HDL-C was better than LDL-C and comparable to apo B for prediction of risk of CHD.[132] After multivariate adjustment in a subsequent analysis of the combined original Framingham Heart Study cohort and the offspring (2693 men, 3101 women), VLDL-C was an independent predictor of risk and non–HDL-C level was a stronger predictor of CHD risk than LDL-C alone at TG levels both greater than and less than 200 mg/dL.[142] These results suggest that VLDL-C contributes to the development of CHD in addition to LDL-C and thus support the fact that both VLDL-C and LDL-C are essential in predicting CHD risk. In fact, non–HDL-C was better than LDL-C.

The Emerging Risk Factors Collaboration analyzed records of 302,430 people without initial vascular disease from 68 long-term prospective studies (Europe and North America) for a total of 12,785 cases of CHD (8857 nonfatal MIs and 3928 deaths due to CHD) during 2.79 million person-years of follow-up (median, 6.1 years to first outcome).[143] The hazard ratio for the primary outcome (nonfatal MI and CHD death) for TG was 1.37 (95% CI, 1.31-1.42) after adjustment for nonlipid risk factors. However, after further adjustment for HDL-C and non–HDL-C, the hazard ratio for TG was reduced to 0.99 (95% CI, 0.94-1.05) (Fig. 15-3). The hazard ratio for CHD with non–HDL-C was 1.56 (95% CI, 1.47-1.66) after adjustment for nonlipid risk factors. After adjustment for HDL-C and log TG, the hazard ratio for non–HDL-C remained significant at 1.50 (95% CI, 1.39-1.61) (Fig. 15-4). There was no difference between those who fasted and those who were nonfasting and no difference by gender for either TG or non–HDL-C. In a subset with available measurements, the hazard ratio for directly measured LDL-C was 1.38 (95% CI, 1.09-1.73), which was similar to the hazard ratio of 1.42 (95% CI, 1.06-1.91) for non–HDL-C in the same subset. Analysis by HDL-C showed that after adjustment for nonlipid risk factors, non–HDL-C, and log TG, the hazard ratio for CHD with HDL-C was 0.78 (95% CI, 0.74-0.82). When analyzed by quintiles of HDL-C levels, the hazard ratio was 0.35 (95% CI, 0.30-0.42) for a 15 mg/dL higher HDL-C and 80 mg/dL lower non–HDL-C; this was not changed by addition of TG level. The hazard ratios for non–HDL-C and apo B were very similar in magnitude and shape, as were those for HDL-C and apo A-I (Fig. 15-5), findings suggesting that apolipoprotein measurements are no better in predicting risk than cholesterol levels.[143] In summary, this largest meta-analysis suggests that TG level provides no additional information about risk when non–HDL-C is calculated from TC and HDL-C levels in either the fasting or nonfasting state.

NON–HIGH-DENSITY LIPOPROTEIN CHOLESTEROL TREATMENT GUIDELINES AND MANAGEMENT

ATP III presented the following classification of serum TG levels[111]:

- Normal: <150 mg/dL (1.7 mmol/L)
- Borderline-high: 150-199 mg/dL (1.7 to 2.2 mmol/L)
- High: 200-499 mg/dL (2.2 to 5.6 mmol/L)
- Very high: >500 mg/dL (>5.6 mmol/L)

The goal for non–HDL-C is 30 mg/dL higher than that for LDL-C (see Table 15-3) on the premise that a VLDL-C level <30 mg/dL is normal (a VLDL-C level of 30 mg/dL is approximately equivalent to a TG level of 150 mg/dL). Several studies

15

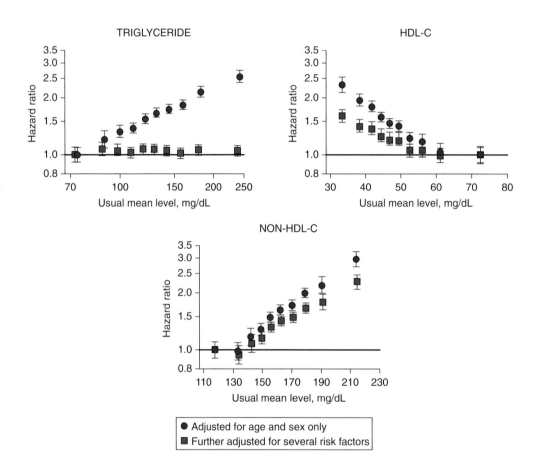

FIGURE 15-3 Hazard ratios for coronary heart disease across quantiles of usual triglyceride, HDL-C, and non–HDL-C levels. Analyses for coronary heart disease were based on 302,430 participants (involving 12,785 cases) from 68 studies. Regression analyses were stratified, where appropriate, by sex and trial group. Values with further adjustments were adjusted for age, systolic blood pressure, smoking status, history of diabetes mellitus, and body mass index; furthermore, analyses of $\log_e$ triglyceride were adjusted for HDL-C and non–HDL-C levels, analyses of HDL-C were adjusted for non–HDL-C and $\log_e$ triglyceride levels, and analyses of non–HDL-C were adjusted for HDL-C and $\log_e$ triglyceride levels. Studies with fewer than 10 cases were excluded from analysis. Sizes of data markers are proportional to the inverse of the variance of the hazard ratios. The *y*-axes are shown on a log scale. The *x*-axes for triglyceride are shown on a log scale. Referent groups are lowest quantiles for triglyceride and non–HDL-C and highest quantiles for HDL-C. Error bars indicate 95% confidence intervals. *(From Di Angelantonio E, Sarwar N, Perry P, et al; Emerging Risk Factors Collaboration: Major lipids, apolipoproteins, and risk of vascular disease.* JAMA *302:1993, 2009. Copyright © 2009 American Medical Association. All rights reserved.)*

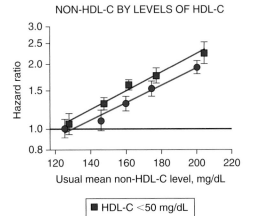

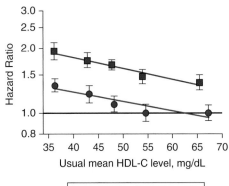

FIGURE 15-4 Hazard ratios for coronary heart disease across fifths of non–HDL-C by levels of HDL-C and fifths of HDL-C by levels of non–HDL-C. Analyses were based on 302,430 participants (involving 12,785 cases) from 68 studies. Median values in the Emerging Risk Factors Collaboration were 50 mg/dL for HDL-C and 169 mg/dL for non–HDL-C. Regression analyses were stratified, where appropriate, by sex and trial group and adjusted for age, systolic blood pressure, smoking status, history of diabetes mellitus, body mass index, and log_e triglyceride levels. Studies with fewer than 10 cases were excluded from analysis. Sizes of data markers are proportional to the inverse of the variance of the hazard ratios. The *y*-axes are shown on a log scale. Referent groups are lowest fifth of non–HDL-C in the higher level of HDL-C and highest fifth of HDL-C in the lower level of non–HDL-C. Lines are fitted by log-linear regression of log hazard ratios on mean levels. Error bars indicate 95% confidence intervals. *(From Di Angelantonio E, Sarwar N, Perry P, et al; Emerging Risk Factors Collaboration: Major lipids, apolipoproteins, and risk of vascular disease. JAMA 302:1993, 2009. Copyright ©2009 American Medical Association. All rights reserved.)*

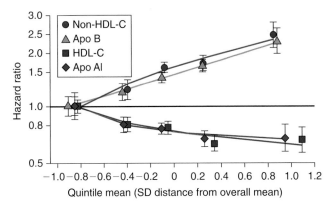

Quintile	1	2	3	4	5
Mean usual level, mg/dL					
Non–HDL-C	125	145	159	173	198
Apo B	85	99	108	118	137
HDL-C	37	44	49	55	66
Apo AL	126	139	148	158	178

FIGURE 15-5 Hazard ratios for coronary heart disease across fifths of usual lipids or apolipoproteins. Analyses were based on 91,307 participants (involving 4499 cases) from 22 studies. Regression analyses were stratified, where appropriate, by sex and trial group and adjusted for age, systolic blood pressure, smoking status, history of diabetes mellitus, and body mass index; furthermore, analyses of non–HDL-C were adjusted for HDL-C and log_e triglyceride, analyses of apo B were adjusted for apo A-I and log_e triglyceride, analyses of HDL-C were adjusted for non–HDL-C and log_e triglyceride, and analyses of apo A-I were adjusted for apo B and log_e triglyceride. Studies with fewer than 10 cases were excluded from analysis. Sizes of data markers are proportional to the inverse of the variance of the hazard ratios. Referent groups are lowest fifths. Lines are fitted by first-degree fractional polynomial regression of log hazard ratios on mean SD score. Error bars indicate 95% confidence intervals. The *y*-axis is shown on a log scale. The *x*-axis is shown on a Z-transformed scale. *(From Di Angelantonio E, Sarwar N, Perry P, et al; Emerging Risk Factors Collaboration: Major lipids, apolipoproteins, and risk of vascular disease. JAMA 302:1993, 2009. Copyright © 2009 American Medical Association. All rights reserved.)*

have shown that CHD risk begins to increase at a fasting TG concentration of 160 to 190 mg/dL (1.8 to 2.2 mmol/L), a finding that provides support for a VLDL-C level <30 mg/dL being normal (or a TG level <150 mg/dL being normal).[16,22,144] Moreover, the association of significant reduction in risk with a TG level <150 mg/dL in the PROVE-IT trial (discussed earlier) provides further support that a VLDL-C level <30 mg/dL is desirable.[23] The results of the COLTS study discussed earlier suggest that risk increases in patients with CHD at TG levels above 100 mg/dL (1.13 mmol/L),[15] a finding supporting use of the non–HDL-C goal of <100 mg/dL when the optional goal of LDL-C <70 mg/dL is used in patients with CHD.

Table 15-4 outlines a management approach to patients with hypertriglyceridemia. In evaluation of a patient with hypertriglyceridemia, thyroid-stimulating hormone, fasting glucose concentration, blood urea nitrogen, and creatinine should be measured to exclude potential secondary causes (see Table 15-1), and medications that may be raising TGs (see Table 15-2) should be stopped or switched if possible. According to the NCEP, the primary goal of therapy with borderline-high or high TG levels (150 to 499 mg/dL) is to achieve the LDL-C goal (see Table 15-3).[111] In primary prevention, lifestyle changes can be followed for at least 3 to 6 months. In secondary prevention, lifestyle changes and statins can be prescribed simultaneously. Once the LDL-C goal is achieved, the following recommendations should be observed for various levels of elevated TGs (see Table 15-4 for summary):

- When TG levels are borderline high (150 to 199 mg/dL [1.7 to 2.2 mmol/L]), emphasis is on therapeutic lifestyle changes (diet, weight reduction, and increased physical activity) as recommended by the NCEP.[111] When TG levels are high (200 to 499 mg/dL [2.2 to 5.6 mmol/L]), non–HDL-C becomes a secondary target of therapy after the LDL-C goal is achieved. If lifestyle changes do not reach the non–HDL-C goal in primary prevention, drug therapy should be considered in high-risk patients. In a consensus statement, statins remained the first-line therapy for moderate hypertriglyceridemia; the most effective TG-lowering drugs,

TABLE 15–4	Management Approach to Hypertriglyceridemia

TG 150-199 mg/dL

Counseling on lifestyle changes, diet, 30 minutes of daily aerobic exercise, and ideal body weight

TG 200-499 mg/dL; Non–HDL-C is Secondary Target After LDL-C Goal is Reached (See Table 15-3)

1. Review medications (see Table 15-2)
   Change to lipid-neutral or favorable agents when possible (e.g., alpha blockers, biguanides, thiazolidinedione).
   Lower doses of or stop drugs that increase triglycerides, such as beta blockers (particularly nonselective agents), glucocorticoids, diuretics (thiazide and loop), ticlopidine, estrogens when indicated clinically.
2. Laboratory studies: exclude secondary disorders of lipid metabolism.
   Fasting blood glucose concentration
   Serum blood urea nitrogen and creatinine levels
   Thyroid function studies (thyroid-stimulating hormone)
3. Therapeutic lifestyle changes (diet and exercise)
   Weight loss
   Avoid concentrated sugars and simple carbohydrates
   Reduce saturated fat
   Reduce or eliminate alcohol
   Increase omega-3 fatty acid intake through fish consumption
   Aerobic exercise minimum of 3 hours weekly
4. Recheck lipid profile in 3 to 6 months (give enough time for adequate weight loss).

Primary Prevention

If LDL-C goal is not reached in 3 to 6 months with steps 1 to 3, consider adding statin therapy.
Once LDL-C goal is reached, determine non–HDL-C goal.
Reinforce lifestyle changes. If still not at non–HDL-C goal, consider
   Niacin (extended release), especially if HDL-C is low; up to 2 g daily
   Fish oil (omega-3 fatty acids) up to 3.2 g EPA and DHA daily (especially if HDL-C is normal)
Repeat laboratory studies 6 to 8 weeks after dose adjustments.

Secondary Prevention

In addition to following steps 1 to 3, statin therapy should be used to reach LDL-C goal, with repeated laboratory studies 6 to 8 weeks after dose adjustments.

TG 500-999 mg/dL

Weight loss; increased exercise—follow steps 1 to 3.
Consider very-low-fat diet (<15% of calorie intake).
Remember that LDL-C cannot be estimated when TG >400 mg/dL.
Consider fibrate therapy or extended-release niacin (e.g., monitor INR on fibrate and warfarin)
   Fenofibrate
      Fenofibrate micronized 67, 134, or 200 mg/day taken with dinner
      Fenofibrate 54 or 160 mg/day; unnecessary to take with meal
      Tricor (nanocrystallized) 48 or 145 mg/day; taken without regard to meals
   Gemfibrozil (Lopid) 600-1200 mg/day (usually 600 mg bid), 30 to 60 minutes before meals
   Extended-release niacin
      Niaspan, up to 2 g daily at bedtime; take with snack; aspirin 30 minutes before limits flushing

TG ≥1000 mg/dL

Follow steps 1 to 3.
Initiate fibrate therapy—monitor serum creatinine.
With acute pancreatitis:
   Very-low-fat diet (10%-15% of energy intake)
   Cessation of alcohol
   Insulin, if indicated for glycemic control
   Admit patient to hospital if necessary.
      Nothing by mouth; IV fluid replacement
      Plasma exchange has been used.

15

fibrates and niacin, both of which also raise HDL-C (Table 15-5), were suggested for high-risk patients.[145] If patients in this category have low levels of HDL-C, nicotinic acid should be considered for its HDL-C–raising properties in addition to lowering of TG levels. When HDL-C level is normal, fish oil is another option to lower TG levels. Such patients may have a low or normal LDL-C level that increases as the serum TG concentration is reduced and may require addition of or increase in a statin drug.[146]

- When TG levels are very high (≥500 mg/dL [≥5.6 mmol/L]), the initial goal is to prevent pancreatitis by lowering TG levels with the combination of very-low-fat diets (<15% of calorie intake), weight reduction, increased physical activity, and a TG-lowering drug such as a fibrate or nicotinic acid. Once TG levels are below 500 mg/dL, the LDL-C goals should be addressed. Although pancreatitis is infrequent until the TG level is >1000 mg/dL, efforts to reduce the TG level to <500 mg/dL are important.[147]

Adult patients with a TG level ≥1000 mg/dL usually have a type V hypertriglyceridemia, although it can also result from secondary causes, such as diabetes, alcohol, and steroid hormones. Fasting glucose and thyroid-stimulating hormone concentrations must always be checked. These patients are at high risk for pancreatitis and need immediate treatment with both lifestyle changes and a fibric acid derivative.[148] Combination therapy with nicotinic acid may be necessary.

Diabetics. The American Diabetes Association has recognized the serum TG level as a surrogate for atherogenic TG-rich lipoproteins and recommends a target of <150 mg/dL in the setting of baseline statin therapy, which is recommended for all diabetics.[149] Based on NCEP, the LDL-C goal for diabetics is <100 mg/dL; therefore, the non–HDL-C goal would be <130 mg/dL (or VLDL-C <30 mg/dL, which is equivalent to a TG level of <150 mg/dL). An optional LDL-C goal for diabetics with CAD can be <70 mg/dL (see Table 15-3).

Treatment: Lifestyle Changes

Lifestyle changes—diet, exercise, and weight loss—are the cornerstone for treatment of elevated TG levels. In fact, medications can be ineffective in lowering TG levels if the patient does not make lifestyle changes, especially in patients with insulin resistance, in whom weight loss is essential to improve the insulin resistance.

Dietary changes that can improve high TG levels (and low HDL-C levels in atherogenic mixed dyslipidemia of metabolic syndrome and type 2 diabetes) include a diet low in glycemic index (eliminating white bread, white potatoes, white rice, and soda)[150] and high in omega-3 fatty acids and fiber (vegetables, fruits, and beans).[151-156] NCEP and the American Heart Association recommend total fat intake ranging from 25% to 35% with <7% saturated fat.[111,157] Polyunsaturated fat can range up to 10% in recognition of the beneficial effects of omega-3 fatty acids found in fatty fish and canola and soybean oils,[158] and monounsaturated fat can range up to 18% in recognition of the fact that replacement of saturated fat with monounsaturates leads to a smaller decrease in HDL-C than replacement with carbohydrate (especially important with low HDL-C levels). Two servings per week of fish have been shown to decrease risk of sudden death and death due to CHD in adults.[159] Additional recommendations that can lower risk for CHD and improve the lipid profile include consumption of lean meats and fat-free milk, elimination of hydrogenated or partially hydrogenated fats, elimination of *trans*-fat, and reduction of cholesterol to less than 300 mg/day.[159] Alcohol restriction is important in those with TG levels ≥500 mg/dL.

Recommended diets should be calorie restricted to promote weight loss because even moderate weight reduction can lower levels of TGs.[111] In a meta-analysis,[160] TG levels

TABLE 15–5 | **Pharmacologic Treatment of Hypertriglyceridemia**

Drug Class	Decrease in TG (%)	Decrease in LDL-C (%)	Increase in HDL-C (%)	Maintenance Regimen	Contraindications	Side Effects	Selective Decrease in Small, Dense LDL-C	Selective Increase in HDL$_2$ Cholesterol
Nicotinic acid, extended release	17-26	10-25	15-35	1500-2000 mg once a day at bedtime	Hypersensitivity, hepatic dysfunction	Flushing, pruritus, nausea, hepatitis (at higher doses), activation of migraine (rare)	Yes	Yes
Fibrate: gemfibrozil	35-50	No change to slight increase	15-25	Gemfibrozil, 600 mg twice a day	Hypersensitivity, hepatic dysfunction, end-stage renal disease	Myositis, cholelithiasis	Yes	No
Fibrate: fenofibrate	41-53	6-20	18-33	Fenofibrate, 145 mg once a day	Hypersensitivity, hepatic dysfunction, end-stage renal disease	Myositis, cholelithiasis	Yes	No
Statins	5	20-60	5-10	Multiple agents	Hypersensitivity, pregnancy, breast feeding	Myalgia, influenza-like syndrome, rhabdomyolysis (rare), weakness	No	No
Nicotinic acid and statin	20-35	30-65	20-45	Same as for individual agents	Same as for individual agents	Same as for individual agents	Yes	Yes
Statin and fibrate	35-55	20-60	15-30	Same as for individual agents	Same as for individual agents	Same as for individual agents	Yes	No
Cholesterol absorption inhibitors	No change	17	No change	Ezetimibe, 10 mg daily	Hepatic dysfunction	Hepatitis	No	No

decreased 0.015 mmol/L for each kilogram of weight lost. Small amounts of weight loss (5.3%) have been shown to result in approximately a 22% decrease in TG levels, a 9% increase in HDL-C, and a 40% decrease in small, dense LDL particles.[161,162] HL, which removes TG, can metabolize HDL to a smaller size, which has a higher FCR, thus lowering levels of HDL. In older men, reduction of intra-abdominal fat stores has resulted in lower levels of HL activity and thus higher levels of HDL-C.[161] In the Women On the Move through Activity and Nutrition (WOMAN) trial, lifestyle changes reduced the number of LDL particles as well.[163] In addition to improved lipid profiles, lifestyle interventions can lower frequency of angina[164] and need for interventions in those with CHD.[165] In the Clinical Outcomes Utilizing Revascularization and Aggressive Drug Evaluation (COURAGE) trial, two thirds of the patients with stable angina and objective evidence of myocardial ischemia in the medical treatment arm (which included a team approach with physicians, dietitians, nurses, and exercise specialists to make lifestyle changes) did well without invasive coronary intervention.[165]

Current American Heart Association guidelines for exercise recommend moderate-intensity aerobic exercise for a minimum of 30 minutes for 5 to 7 days or vigorous-intensity aerobic exercise for a minimum of 20 minutes for 3 days a week.[166] Even in the absence of weight loss, aerobic exercise has been shown to modestly reduce TG levels in a dose-dependent fashion.[167] Exercise can reduce levels of small, dense LDL particles, increase LDL particle size, raise HDL-C levels, and lower levels of TG.[168] A meta-analysis of 25 studies of walking has also shown an improvement in the lipid profile.[169] In a comparison of four types of exercise varying in intensity and frequency, the hard-intensity–high-frequency

exercise was the only one to significantly improve HDL-C (mean increase, 3.9%; $P < 0.03$).[170]

Initial weight loss and maintenance of weight loss can be difficult in clinical practice; however, Welty and coworkers[162] described a successful office-based lifestyle program for modification of lipids and blood pressure that also resulted in weight loss. The program includes a dietitian at the initial visit and at least one follow-up visit (fully reimbursable to dietitian with separate co-pay). The diet described before was recommended with additional recommendations of low sodium, fiber >25 g/day for women and 38 g/day for men, low-fat dairy products, fruits and vegetables, oils high in alpha-linolenic acid (canola and flaxseed oils), and plant sterols or stanols to 2 g/day, all geared toward lowering of TG, LDL-C, and blood pressure and raising of HDL-C. Behavioral counseling to decrease portion size included (1) eating a high-fiber breakfast daily, (2) drinking a full glass of water before each meal and with high-fiber foods to induce satiety, (3) putting the fork down between each bite and taking a sip of water or stopping a meal halfway through for 15 to 20 minutes (time for satiety signal to reach brain) geared to slowing down eating, (4) decreasing portion size by 100 calories per day (equates to 10-pound weight loss in 1 year), and (5) taking half of a restaurant portion home. Exercise prescriptions were given and included increasing 5 minutes per session weekly to a goal of 30 minutes daily. Maximum weight lost was an average of 5.6% (10.8 pounds) at a mean follow-up of 1.75 years. Sixty-four (81%) of these patients maintained significant weight loss (average weight loss, 5.3%) at a mean follow-up of 2.6 years. Those maintaining weight loss exercised significantly more.[162] Average decreases in LDL-C and TG were 9.3% and 34%, respectively, and

15

The Contribution of Triglycerides and Triglyceride-Rich Lipoproteins to Atherosclerotic Cardiovascular Disease

average increase in HDL-C was 9.6%.[161] Diastolic blood pressure decreased from a mean of 79 to 75 mm Hg ($P = 0.003$). Therefore, having a dietitian counsel patients concurrently with a physician and using the simple techniques described here may help achieve and maintain weight loss.

TREATMENT: MEDICATIONS TO TREAT HYPERTRIGLYCERIDEMIA

There are currently four major medications to treat elevated TG concentration: statins, fibrates, niacin, and fish oil. Table 15-5 summarizes average changes in lipid levels for these drugs. The following sections summarize the role of each drug in lowering TG concentration and the clinical trial evidence supporting its use.

Statins

Once the TG level is <500 mg/dL, or if the TG level is 200 to 499 mg/dL, if the LDL-C level remains above goal, statins are the drug of first choice for LDL lowering because of their reduction in cardiovascular events, stroke, coronary mortality, and total mortality without an increase in noncardiovascular mortality.[171] In an analysis of the efficacy of statins in lowering TG levels,[172] patients with baseline TG levels greater than 2.8 mmol/L had dose-dependent reductions in TGs of 22% to 45%, with atorvastatin and rosuvastatin being the most efficacious. As noted earlier, in a consensus statement, statins remained the first-line therapy for moderate hypertriglyceridemia, and other TG-lowering drugs, such as fibrates and niacin, were suggested for high-risk patients.[145]

An angiographic trial has shown that statin treatment attenuates progression of coronary atherosclerosis in those with an LPL mutation. Heterozygosity for the Asp9Asn mutation in the LPL gene (aspartic acid to an asparagine residue at position 9) causes mild defects in LPL activity leading to elevations in serum TGs and a reduction in HDL-C.[1,173] In the Regression Growth Evaluation Statin Study (REGRESS), subjects with this mutation were more likely to have a family history of cardiovascular disease ($P = 0.03$), a lower HDL-C level ($P = 0.01$), a trend toward higher TG and LDL-C levels, and progression of coronary atherosclerosis in the placebo group compared with noncarriers. Therapy with pravastatin attenuated the rate of progression of atherosclerosis in those carrying the mutation.[174]

Fibrates

By activating the nuclear transcription factor peroxisome proliferator-activated receptorα (PPARα), fibrates decrease the apo C-III concentration, which increases LPL activity, thus increasing VLDL clearance and reducing the plasma TG concentration by 30% to 50% (see Table 15-5).[175] Fibrates also increase fatty acid oxidation in liver and muscle and reduce the rate of lipogenesis in the liver, thereby reducing hepatic secretion of VLDL TGs.[175] PPARα-mediated transcription by fibrates also stabilizes apo A-I mRNA transcripts,[176-178] leading to secretion of more apo A-I–containing HDL particles, thus increasing HDL production and raising the HDL-C level by 15% to 30%, depending on baseline HDL-C level (see Table 15-5). HDL-C levels are also raised by transfer of surface apo A-I released during the enhanced catabolism of VLDL to HDL particles. The effect of fibrates on LDL-C ranges from around a 10% reduction to no change or a slight increase and an increase in LDL particle size. The accelerated clearance of TG-rich lipoproteins reduces CETP-mediated exchange, which results in less TG incorporation into LDL particles and thus limits formation of small, dense LDL and favors formation of large, cholesterol-enriched LDL particles[125,179] that

bind more efficiently to the LDL receptor than small LDL particles do. Thus, there is an overall reduction in LDL particle concentration despite a minimal change in LDL-C level.[179] Fibrates may also have anti-inflammatory and anti-atherogenic properties due to activation of PPARα.[180]

Several studies have shown that monotherapy with various fibrates reduces risk of CHD events in patients with high TGs and low HDL-C, especially in patients with diabetes mellitus or characteristics of the metabolic syndrome (summarized in Table 15-6).[181] In the Bezafibrate Infarction Prevention (BIP) trial, 3090 subjects with prior MI and HDL-C <45 mg/dL, TG <300 mg/dL, and LDL-C <180 mg/dL were randomized to bezafibrate 400 mg daily or placebo. Increasing serum TG concentrations were associated with an increase in mortality.[182] Although bezafibrate decreased levels of LDL-C by 6% and TGs by 21% and raised levels of HDL-C by 18%, there was no significant difference in the primary endpoint (fatal and nonfatal MI and sudden death) in either group. However, those patients with TG levels >200 mg/dL at baseline who had an increase in HDL of at least 5 mg/dL or a reduction in TG by >28 mg/dL had a significant 40% (13% versus 22.3% at 6.2 years; $P = 0.02$) reduction in the primary endpoint.[183]

Gemfibrozil has been studied in several trials. In the Helsinki Heart Study (HHS), a 5-year primary prevention trial, dyslipidemic men without CHD randomized to gemfibrozil had a significant 34% reduction in the incidence of fatal and nonfatal MI and cardiac death.[184] All-cause mortality did not differ significantly between the treatment group (21.9%) and the placebo group (20.7%). Those with TG levels >200 mg/dL and LDL-C/HDL-C ratio >5.0 had the greatest risk of CHD, and those in this group treated with gemfibrozil had a 71% event reduction (see Table 15-6).[185]

In VA-HIT, men with CHD and HDL-C <40 mg/dL, LDL-C <140 mg/dL, and TG <300 mg/dL were randomized to gemfibrozil or placebo. Gemfibrozil raised HDL-C by 6% (34 mg/dL versus 32 mg/dL), lowered TGs by 31% (115 mg/dL versus 166 mg/dL), and had no significant effect on LDL-C (mean 113 mg/dL in both groups). Those treated with gemfibrozil had a significant 22% reduction in the primary endpoint of nonfatal MI or death due to CHD (17.3% versus 21.7% for placebo; relative risk reduction, 22%; $P = 0.006$).[186] All-cause mortality was lower by a nonsignificant 11%. When stratified by diabetic status, diabetics had a significant 32% reduction in the combined primary endpoint ($P = 0.004$), death due to CHD ($P = 0.02$), and stroke ($P = 0.046$) compared with those without diabetes ($P = 0.07$, $P = 0.88$, and $P = 0.67$, respectively). Eight-year follow-up in VA-HIT showed a 41% reduction in CHD death ($P = 0.02$) and 26% reduction in death in those with diabetes or hyperinsulinemia at baseline. Therefore, diabetics were more likely than those without diabetes to benefit (see Table 15-6), possibly because of improvement in insulin resistance through PPARα activation.

Gemfibrozil is more likely to cause myositis in combination with a statin by raising plasma levels of statins 1.9- to 5.7-fold through inhibition of hepatic glucuronidation, which is necessary for renal excretion of lipophilic statins.[111] Fenofibrate does not inhibit glucuronidation; therefore, fenofibrate is safer to use in combination with a statin. Several trials have studied the effect of fenofibrate on cardiovascular disease outcomes. In the Diabetes Atherosclerosis Intervention Study (DAIS), 731 subjects with diabetes were randomized to micronized fenofibrate (200 mg/dL) or placebo. Those taking fenofibrate had less progression of coronary artery disease compared with those randomized to placebo.[187] Part of the benefit appeared to be related to an increase in size of LDL particles. Although the study was not powered for clinical endpoints, the rate of all-cause mortality was 2.9% in the treatment group and 4.3% in the placebo group.

The Fenofibrate Intervention and Event Lowering in Diabetes (FIELD) study was a 5-year study of 9795 patients with

TABLE 15-6 | **Cardiovascular Risk Reduction with Fibrate Monotherapy in Patients with and without Diabetes or Features of the Metabolic Syndrome**

Study	Treatment	Patients	Endpoint	Absolute Risk Reduction (%)	Relative	P Value
Primary Prevention						
HHS	Gemfibrozil 1200 mg/day	4081 men with no prior CVD	Nonfatal MI + CAD death	13.8	34	<0.02
		1146 (28% with MS)	Nonfatal MI + CAD death	27.2	71	<0.0005
		292*	Nonfatal MI + CAD death	9.1	71	0.004
FIELD	Fenofibrate 200 mg/day	9795 men and women with type 2 diabetes (some with CAD)	Nonfatal MI + CAD death	0.7	11	NS
			Total CVD events	3.2	11	0.035
		7664 without CHD	Nonfatal MI + CAD death	1.9	19	0.004
		8183 with MS	Total CVD events	1.4	11	0.052
		314 with MS and marked dyslipidemia†	Total CVD events	4.3	27	0.005
Secondary Prevention						
VA-HIT	Gemfibrozil 1200 mg/day	2531 men with CAD	Nonfatal MI, CAD death + stroke	5.6	24	<0.001
		769 (30%) with diabetes	Nonfatal MI, CAD death + stroke	10.0	32	0.004
BIP	Bezafibrate 400 mg/day	3090 men and women with previous MI	Nonfatal MI + CAD death	1.4	9.4	NS
		1470 (48%) with MS‡		4.3	25	0.03

*Patients with TG >204 mg/dL and an LDL/HDL >5 (may or may not have had diabetes mellitus or the metabolic syndrome).

†Defined as elevated triglycerides (>204 mg/dL [≥2.3 mmol/L]) and HDL <1.03 mmol/L for men and <1.29 mmol/L for women.

‡Defined as elevated triglycerides (>204 mg/dL [1 mg/dL = 0.0113 mmol/L]), low HDL-C (<42 mg/dL [1 mg/dL = 0.02586 mmol/L]), body mass index >26, and blood glucose ≥5.5 mmol/L.

BIP, Bezafibrate Infarction Prevention; CAD, coronary artery disease; CVD, cardiovascular disease; FIELD, Fenofibrate Intervention and Event Lowering in Diabetes; HHS, Helsinki Heart Study; MI, myocardial infarction; MS, metabolic syndrome; NS, not significant; VA-HIT, Veterans Affairs High-Density Lipoprotein Intervention Trial.

type 2 diabetes (78% without CVD) with TC from 116 to 251 mg/dL plus either a TC/HDL-C ratio of at least 4.0 or a TG concentration of 89 to 443 mg/dL. Those randomized to fenofibrate 200 mg/day had a nonsignificant 11% reduction (P = 0.16) in the primary endpoint of first MI or CHD death compared with those receiving placebo (see Table 15-6).[188] The initiation of statin therapy in many patients during the trial, unfortunately, confounded the results. The statin drop-in rate was higher in those with prior CVD compared with those without CVD. Analysis of patients with no prior CVD showed a significant reduction of 25% (P = 0.014) in the primary endpoint. For the overall group, significant reductions were observed in the secondary outcomes of nonfatal MI (HR, 0.76; 95% CI, 0.62-0.94), total cardiovascular disease events (HR, 0.89; 95% CI, 0.80-0.99), coronary revascularization (HR, 0.79; 95% CI, 0.68-0.93), and all revascularizations (HR, 0.80; 95% CI, 0.70-0.92). Total mortality, however, was increased by a nonsignificant 11% in those receiving fenofibrate (HR, 1.11; 95% CI, 0.95-1.29), and pancreatitis and pulmonary embolism were significantly higher in those receiving fenofibrate (P = 0.03 and 0.022, respectively) compared with those receiving placebo. In a post hoc subgroup analysis in FIELD, those with metabolic syndrome and marked dyslipidemia (TG ≥2.3 mmol/l [204 mg/dL] and low HDL-C) had the highest risk (17.8%) for development of CVD during 5 years. Fenofibrate had the greatest benefit in this group, in whom a 27% relative risk reduction in total CVD events occurred (HR, 0.73; 95% CI, 0.58-0.91; P = 0.005; number needed to treat = 23) compared with 6% in all others (HR, 0.94; 95% CI, 0.83-1.06; P = 0.321; number needed to treat =143).[189]

In a meta-analysis of 36,489 patients from 10 published randomized placebo-controlled trials including the FIELD trial, fibrates significantly reduced plasma TC and TG levels by about 8% and 30%, respectively, and raised HDL-C levels by about 9% compared with placebo.[190] The odds of all-cause mortality were higher (P = 0.08) and the odds of noncardiovascular mortality were significantly higher (P = 0.004) with

the use of fibrates. However, after exclusion of trials that used clofibrate as the study drug (because of withdrawal of clofibrate from the market more than 25 years ago due to an increase in cholangiocarcinoma and other gastrointestinal cancers), neither all-cause mortality (pooled odds ratio, 1.04; P = 0.44) nor noncardiovascular mortality (pooled odds ratio, 1.08; P = 0.20) was significantly increased with the use of fibrates. Fibrates did not significantly reduce the odds of cardiovascular mortality (P = 0.68), fatal MI (P = 0.76), or stroke (P = 0.56), and these results did not change with exclusion of clofibrate trials. However, fibrates significantly reduced the odds of nonfatal MI by about 22% (P < 0.00001), with a further slight reduction (pooled odds ratio, 0.75; P < 0.00001) with exclusion of clofibrate trials. The odds for development of cancer were not significantly higher with the use of fibrates (P = 0.98), nor were the odds of cancer-related death (P = 0.17). Another meta-analysis of 17 randomized controlled trials reported a 13% increase in risk for noncardiovascular mortality (RR, 1.13; 95% CI, 1.01-1.27); however, nine of these trials used clofibrate, and FIELD was not included.[171]

When outcome in fibrate trials is examined for patients with diabetes or metabolic syndrome, a greater benefit is seen in both primary prevention (HHS and FIELD) and secondary prevention (BIP and VA-HIT) in those with diabetes or metabolic syndrome compared with those without (see Table 15-6). Patients in the highest tertile of body mass index and TG level in follow-up in HHS had reduction of 33% in risk of death (P = 0.03) and 71% in CHD death (P = 0.0001).[191] Therefore, fibrates may have greater cardioprotective effects in patients with diabetes mellitus or features of the metabolic syndrome because of improvement in insulin resistance through PPAR agonist activation. These prior studies did not examine the role of fibrates added to statin therapy in patients with type 2 diabetes. Therefore, the Action to Control Cardiovascular Risk in Diabetes (ACCORD) study was designed to determine whether fibrate therapy provided additional benefit to statin therapy in subjects with type 2 diabetes.[192] In the trial, 10,251 patients with type 2 diabetes were randomized to either intensive or standard glycemic control, with 5518 also randomly assigned in a 2 × 2 factorial design to either simvastatin plus fenofibrate or simvastatin plus placebo. Fenofibrate plus simvastatin did not reduce the primary outcome (fatal CVD events, nonfatal MI, or nonfatal stroke) compared with simvastatin alone in the total group (2.2% versus 2.4%, respectively; HR, 0.92; 95% CI, 0.79-1.08; P = 0.32). However, those with TG levels ≥204 mg/dL (≥2.3 mmol/L) (TG level was lowered an average of 35%) and HDL level ≤34 mg/dL (HDL-C increased an average of 12.9%) randomized to fenofibrate had a 28% reduction in relative risk (12.4% event rate compared with 17.3% with placebo [P = 0.057]) compared with rates of 10.1% in both study groups for all other subjects. Therefore, although the routine use of combination therapy with fenofibrate and simvastatin did not improve outcome in subjects with type 2 diabetes, the ACCORD subgroup results suggest that the addition of fenofibrate to a statin provides additional benefit in type 2 diabetics with high TG and low HDL-C levels. In contrast to the adverse outcomes in FIELD, no increase in total mortality, pulmonary embolus, or pancreatitis was observed in the fenofibrate group compared with placebo in ACCORD; however, there was a trend toward harm in women and benefit in men in the total group.

Both gemfibrozil and fenofibrate interfere with metabolism of warfarin; therefore, warfarin dose should be decreased approximately 30%, with close monitoring of the international normalized ratio (INR).[193] Fenofibrate increases the clearance of cyclosporine, leading to an approximately 30% reduction in plasma level[188]; therefore, gemfibrozil is the preferred choice in transplant recipients. Fenofibrate lowers levels of fibrinogen and uric acid, whereas gemfibrozil has no effect.

Niacin

The extended-release form of niacin reduces TGs by 17% to 26% and raises HDL-C 15% to 35% with a dose of 2000 mg/day (see Table 15-5).[148] A 15% reduction in risk of MI occurred in 8341 men with prior MI and hypercholesterolemia who were randomized to regular-release nicotinic acid 3 g daily or placebo and observed for 6.5 years in the Coronary Drug Project.[194] Moreover, total mortality was significantly reduced 11% (P = 0.0004) and CHD mortality was reduced 12% (P < 0.05) at 15-year follow-up.[194] High doses of nicotinic acid can increase blood glucose concentration, but doses of 750 to 2000 mg/day affect glucose only modestly. In the Arterial Disease Multiple Intervention Trial (ADMIT), 2 to 3 g/day of immediate-release niacin decreased TG by 23% and raised HDL by 29% without significant worsening of glycemic control.[195] In the Assessment of Diabetes Control and Evaluation of the Efficacy of Niaspan Trial (ADVENT) in 97 patients with type 2 diabetes, 1 to 1.5 g/day of extended-release niacin resulted in no significant difference in mean fasting glucose levels during a 16-week period, although additional hypoglycemic treatment was required in some patients receiving niacin.[196] Six-year follow-up in the Coronary Drug Project showed that those with a baseline glucose concentration of ≥126 mg/dL had the greatest reduction in risk of recurrent MI (57%) compared with 30%, 24%, and 25% reductions in those with baseline fasting plasma glucose concentration <95 mg/dL, 95 to 104 mg/dL, and 105 to 125 mg/dL, respectively.

Niacin in combination with simvastatin lowered CVD events in the HDL-Atherosclerosis Treatment Study (HATS), Familial Atherosclerosis Treatment Study (FATS), and Cholesterol-Lowering Atherosclerosis Study (CLAS).[197-200] In the HATS trial, 160 patients with clinical and angiographic evidence of CHD, HDL-C <35 mg/dL, and LDL-C <145 mg/dL

were randomized to one of four regimens: simvastatin plus niacin; antioxidants; simvastatin plus niacin plus antioxidants; or placebo. Simvastatin plus niacin was associated with a 42% reduction in LDL-C and 26% increase in HDL-C and regression of proximal coronary plaque on coronary angiography (0.4% on average versus baseline) compared with a mean progression of 3.9% on placebo.[198] Those in the simvastatin plus niacin group also were significantly less likely to experience a CVD event, death, MI, stroke, or revascularization, although the numbers were small. Although niacin use is limited by flushing, taking an aspirin (325 mg) 30 minutes before extended-release niacin at bedtime, taking it with a snack, and avoiding alcohol and spicy foods limit flushing. Education of patients about the fact that flushing is also an indication that the drug is functioning and that they are properly responding to it is key to maximizing adherence. Flushing may also be transient and may decrease with time in many cases. The Atherothrombosis Intervention in Metabolic Syndrome with Low HDL-C/High Triglyceride and Impact on Global Health Outcomes (AIM-HIGH) study is examining the use of niacin plus statins and should clarify the role of niacin in the treatment of hypertriglyceridemia.[201]

Extended-release niacin can lower lipoprotein(a), an important atherogenic lipoprotein, approximately 20% at doses of 2 g daily.[202] Immediate-release niacin can lower lipoprotein(a) 38% at 4 g daily.[203] The only other medication that can lower lipoprotein(a) and is available in the United States is estrogen replacement therapy, which lowered lipoprotein(a) 17% to 23% in the Postmenopausal Estrogen/Progestin Intervention trial[204]; however, because of its potential harmful effects, estrogen replacement therapy is no longer recommended for this purpose.[205]

Omega-3 Fatty Acids

Fish oil supplements (>3 g/day of eicosapentaenoic acid [EPA] and docosahexaenoic acid [DHA], the active omega-3 fatty acids) can lower TG level by 50% or more by reducing VLDL production.[206-208] However, use can be limited by reflux and regurgitation of a "fishy taste." Placement of tablets in the refrigerator or freezer can minimize this side effect. An enteric-coated capsule is also on the market that decreases the fish odor problem. Table 15-7 outlines the number of tablets and approximate cost for each over-the-counter fish oil preparation to obtain 1 g EPA plus DHA daily. We aim for at least 2.4 g EPA plus DHA daily in our patients with hypertriglyceridemia. Over-the-counter fish oil capsules have some cholesteryl ester, whereas prescription ethyl esters of omega-3 (Lovaza) do not.

Omega-3 fatty acids can be an alternative to fibrates or niacin, although they can also be used in combination with statins, fibrates, or niacin.[111] In addition to effectively lowering TGs, omega-3 fatty acids may provide clinical benefit in patients with recent MI and may have antithrombotic and anti-inflammatory effects.[209] There are three large trials of fish oil. The largest trial with omega-3 fatty acids was the Gruppo Italiano per lo Studio della Sopravvivenza nell-Infarto Miocardico (GISSI) Prevenzione trial, which showed a 20% reduction in the combined endpoint of death, nonfatal MI, and stroke with 1 g/day of EPA plus DHA.[210] Omega-3 fatty acids also had significant antiarrhythmic effects.[210,211] In the Japan Eicosapentaenoic Acid Lipid Intervention Study (JELIS), the combination of open-label low-dose statin (pravastatin, 10 to 20 mg, or simvastatin, 5 to 10 mg, daily) with open-label eicosapentaenoic acid (1800 mg daily) reduced incident and recurrent CHD events by 19% (P = 0.011) compared with statin monotherapy.[212] There was no effect on cardiac or total mortality. LDL-C levels were reduced 25% in both groups, whereas TG levels were

TABLE 15–7 Fish Oil Supplements Providing About 1 g of EPA plus DHA

Brand or Type	No. of Capsules for ~1 g EPA + DHA	Cost for 30 Days*	Notes
GNC Triple Strength Fish Oil (647 mg EPA, 253 mg DHA per softgel)	1	$10	60 cap/$19.99[†] Size: slightly >1 inch
Vitamin World Triple Strength Omega-3 Fish Oil 1360 mg (EPA + DHA 950 mg per softgel) Same as Puritan's Pride	1	$11	60 cap/$21.99 Size: 1 inch
Lovaza 1000 mg (prescription only) (approx. 465 mg EPA and 375 mg DHA)	1	$40-$60	Insurance may not cover or may have highest co-pay
Trader Darwin's Omega 3 Fatty Acids 1100 mg (300 mg EPA, 200 mg DHA per softgel)	2	$5	Trader Joe's brand 90 cap/ $7.99 Size: 1 inch
Trader Darwin's Omega 3 Fatty Acids–Odorless 1200 mg (400 mg EPA, 200 mg DHA per softgel)	2	$6	Trader Joe's brand 90 cap/$8.99 Size: 1 inch
Kirkland Signature Fish Oil Concentrate 1200 mg enteric coated (410 mg EPA, 270 mg DHA per softgel)	2	$6	Costco's brand 180 cap/$16.99 Size: slightly >1 inch
Walgreens Finest enteric-coated One-Per-Day Omega 3 Fish Oil 1200 mg (410 mg EPA, 274 mg DHA per softgel)	2	$10	60 cap/$9.99 Size: 1 inch (enteric coated)
Nature Made Fish Oil Double Strength 1200 mg (336 mg EPA, 276 mg DHA per softgel)	2	$17	60 cap/$16.99 Size: ?
Vitamin World Premium Mini Gels Omega-3 Fish Oil (EPA + DHA 450 mg per softgel)	2	$18	60 cap/$17.99 Size: ¾ inch
Nordic Naturals Ultimate Omega, Highly Concentrated (325 mg EPA, 225 mg DHA per softgel)	2	$28	IFOS[†] Size: 1 inch (lemon flavor)
Puritan's Pride Natural Omega-3 1000 mg (300 mg EPA + DHA per softgel) Same as Vitamin World	3	$7	100 cap/$10.99 Size: 1 inch
Whole Foods molecularly distilled Omega-3 1000 mg (180 mg EPA, 120 mg DHA per softgel)	3	$10	90 cap/$9.99[†] Size: 1 inch (lemon flavor)
Gels and liquids Coromega Omega-3 Supplement (350 mg EPA, 230 mg DHA per squeeze packet)	2 packs	$20-$40	Flavors: orange, orange-chocolate, lemon-lime
Nordic Naturals Omega-3 Liquid, lemon taste (165 mg EPA, 110 mg DHA per mL)	~3/4 tsp	$12	8 oz/$24.95 Keep refrigerated, spoils easily

*Cost data were obtained from locations in the Boston, Mass, area in October 2009.

[†]ConsumerLab tested; IFOS, International Fish Oil Standards.

Most commercial brands have more than one formulation. The less expensive options are typically not as concentrated and tend to vary the EPA and DHA content with other fish oil components. Testing is not performed on all over-the-counter supplements sold; however, the majority of fish oil supplements have been shown to be free of contaminants, such as mercury. Capsules that have a strong odor may be spoiled and should not be used. To keep supplements fresh, store them in the refrigerator or freezer. Cod liver oil, which may contain excess vitamin A, is not recommended.

unchanged. In the third trial, patients with chronic heart failure had significant reductions in coronary events and cardiac and total mortality.[213]

In subjects with persistent hypertriglyceridemia, prescription omega-3 fatty acid at 4 g/day plus simvastatin 40 mg provided significant additional improvement in reducing levels of non–HDL-C (–9% versus –2.2%, respectively; $P < 0.001$), TG (29.5% versus 6.3%, respectively; $P < 0.001$), and other lipid and lipoprotein parameters to a greater extent than simvastatin alone.[214] Whether other combinations involving TG-lowering therapies are also clinically superior to statin monotherapy is a subject of intense investigation. Ongoing trials include the addition of niacin to statin, which is being investigated in AIM-HIGH[201] and HPS2-THRIVE.[215] The results of these trials are expected to help shape evidence-based guidelines to optimize management of dyslipidemia, including elevated levels of TG.

Bile Acid Sequestrants

Because of increases in VLDL synthesis and increases in TG levels, bile acid sequestrants should not be used unless TG levels are normal. Furthermore, they are normally reserved for treatment of elevated LDL-C when statins cannot be tolerated or are contraindicated or in combination with statins to achieve greater LDL-C lowering.

Hypertriglyceridemia is associated with other lipid abnormalities that predispose to atherosclerosis, including low levels of HDL-C, the presence of small, dense LDL particles and atherogenic TG-rich lipoprotein remnants, and insulin resistance. The evidence cited in this chapter suggests that non–HDL-C (TC – HDL-C) may predict risk of CHD and future cardiovascular events better than LDL-C because of the fact that non–HDL-C includes all apo B–containing lipoproteins, all of which are atherogenic. Therefore, NCEP recommends calculation of non–HDL-C when the TG level is ≥200 mg/dL, with the goal being 30 mg/dL higher than the LDL-C goal. It is also not unreasonable to consider non–HDL-C a secondary target of therapy when TG levels are in the borderline-high range (150 to 199 mg/dL) because apo B–containing lipoproteins can also be elevated in this setting. Lifestyle changes—exercise and diet with an emphasis on weight loss—are first-line therapy in lowering of TG levels, especially in patients with metabolic syndrome or type 2 diabetes. Statins, fibrates, niacin, and omega-3 fatty acids can be used to lower TG levels to reach the non–HDL-C goal if lifestyle changes are insufficient to reach goal. On the basis of the ACCORD trial results, fenofibrate can also be considered in addition to a statin in type 2 diabetics with marked dyslipidemia (TG >204 mg/dL and HDL-C <34 mg/dL) to lower risk of CVD events.[192]

REFERENCES

1. Wittrup HH, Tybjaerg-Hansen A, Nordestgaard BG: Lipoprotein lipase mutations, plasma lipids and lipoproteins, and risk of ischemic heart disease. A meta-analysis. *Circulation* 99:2901, 1999.
2. Sprecher DL, Harris BV, Stein EA, et al: Higher triglycerides, lower high-density lipoprotein cholesterol, and higher systolic blood pressure in lipoprotein lipase–deficient heterozygotes. *Circulation* 94:3239, 1996.
3. Hypertriglyceridaemia and vascular risk. Report of a meeting of physicians and scientists, University College London Medical School. *Lancet* 342:781, 1993.
4. Zilversmit DB: Atherogenesis: a postprandial phenomenon. *Circulation* 60:473, 1979.
5. Fukushima H, Kugiyama K, Sugiyama S, et al: Comparison of remnant-like lipoprotein particles in postmenopausal women with and without coronary artery disease and in men with coronary artery disease. *Am J Cardiol* 88:1370, 2001.
6. DeFronzo RA, Ferrannini E: Insulin resistance. A multifaceted syndrome responsible for NIDDM, obesity, hypertension, dyslipidemia, and atherosclerotic cardiovascular disease. *Diabetes Care* 14:173, 1991.
7. McLaughlin T, Abbasi F, Cheal K, et al: Use of metabolic markers to identify overweight individuals who are insulin resistant. *Ann Intern Med* 139:802, 2003.
8. Ford ES, Li C, Zhao G, et al: Hypertriglyceridemia and its pharmacologic treatment among US adults. *Arch Intern Med* 169:572, 2009.
9. Albrink M, Man E: Serum triglycerides in coronary artery disease. *AMA Arch Intern Med* 103:4, 1959.
10. Assmann G, Schulte H, Eckardstein AV: Hypertriglyceridemia and elevated lipoprotein(a) are risk factors for major coronary events in middle aged men. *Am J Cardiol* 77:1179, 1996.
11. Assmann G, Cullen P, Schulte H: Simple scoring scheme for calculating the risk of acute coronary events based on the 10-year follow-up of the Prospective Cardiovascular Munster (PROCAM) study. *Circulation* 105:310, 2002.
12. Wilson PW, Anderson KM, Castelli WP: Twelve-year incidence of coronary heart disease in middle-aged adults during the era of hypertensive therapy: the Framingham offspring study. *Am J Med* 90:11, 1991.
13. McNamara JR, Shah PK, Nakajima K, et al: Remnant-like particle (RLP) cholesterol is an independent cardiovascular disease risk factor in women: results from the Framingham Heart Study. *Atherosclerosis* 154:229, 2001.
14. Hokanson JE, Austin MA: Plasma triglyceride level is a risk factor for cardiovascular disease independent of high-density lipoprotein cholesterol level: a meta-analysis of population-based prospective studies. *J Cardiovasc Risk* 3:213-219, 1996.
15. Miller M, Seidler A, Moalemi A, Pearson TA: Normal triglyceride levels and coronary artery disease events. The Baltimore Coronary Observational Long-Term Study. *J Am Coll Cardiol* 31:1252, 1998.
16. Jeppesen J, Hein HO, Suadicani P, Gyntelberg F: Triglyceride concentration and ischemic heart disease: an eight year follow up in the Copenhagen Male Study. *Circulation* 97:1029, 1998.
17. Jeppesen J, Hein HO, Suadicani P, Gyntelberg F: Low triglycerides–high high-density lipoprotein cholesterol and risk of ischemic heart disease. *Arch Intern Med* 161:361, 2001.
18. Patel A, Barzi F, Jamrozik K, et al: Serum triglycerides as a risk factor for cardiovascular diseases in the Asia-Pacific region. *Circulation* 110:2678, 2004.
19. Sarwar N, Danesh J, Eiriksdottir G, et al: Triglycerides and the risk of coronary heart disease. 10,158 incident cases among 262,525 participants in 29 Western prospective studies. *Circulation* 115:450, 2006.
20. Sarwar N, Sattar N: Triglycerides and coronary heart disease: have recent insights yielded conclusive answers? *Curr Opin Lipidol* 20:275, 2009.
21. Tirosh A, Rudich A, Shochat T, et al: Changes in triglyceride levels and risk for coronary heart disease in young men. *Ann Intern Med* 147:377, 2007.
22. Faergeman O, Holme I, Fayyad R, et al: Steering Committees of IDEAL and TNT Trials: Plasma triglycerides and cardiovascular events in the Treating to New Targets and Incremental Decrease in End-Points through Aggressive Lipid Lowering trials of statins in patients with coronary artery disease. *Am J Cardiol* 104:459, 2009.
23. Miller M, Cannon CP, Murphy SA, et al: Impact of triglyceride levels beyond low-density cholesterol after acute coronary syndrome in the PROVE IT–TIMI 22 trial. *J Am Coll Cardiol* 51:724, 2008.
24. Ginsberg HN: New perspectives on atherogenesis: role of abnormal triglyceride-rich lipoprotein metabolism. *Circulation* 106:2137, 2002.
25. Havel RJ, Kane JP: Introduction: structure and metabolism of plasma lipoproteins. In Scriver CR, Beaudet AL, Sly WS, Valle D, editors: *The metabolic and molecular bases of inherited disease*, ed 7, New York, 1995, McGraw-Hill, pp 1841-1851.
26. Ducharme NA, Bickel PE: Lipid droplets in lipogenesis and lipolysis. *Endocrinology* 149:942, 2008.
27. Young SG: Recent progress in understanding apolipoprotein B. *Circulation* 82:1574, 1990.
28. Berriot-Varoqueaux N, Aggerbeck LP, Samson-Bouma M, et al: The role of the microsomal triglyceride transfer protein in abetalipoproteinemia. *Annu Rev Nutr* 20:663, 2000.
29. Sato R, Miyamoto W, Inoue J, et al: Sterol regulatory element–binding protein negatively regulates microsomal triglyceride transfer protein gene transcription. *J Biol Chem* 274:24714, 1999.
30. Hirose N, Blankenship DT, Krivanek MA, et al: Isolation and characterization of four heparin-binding cyanogen bromide peptides of human plasma apolipoprotein B. *Biochemistry* 26:5505, 1987.
31. Weisgraber KH, Rall SC, Jr: Human apolipoprotein B-100 heparin-binding sites. *J Biol Chem* 262:11097, 1987.
32. Sehayek E, Lewin-Velvert U, Chajek-Shaul T, Eisenberg S: Lipolysis exposes unreactive endogenous apolipoprotein E-3 in human and rat plasma very low density lipoprotein. *J Clin Invest* 88:553, 1991.
33. Beigneux AP, Davies BS, Gin P, et al: Glycosylphosphatidylinositol-anchored high-density lipoprotein-binding protein 1 plays a critical role in the lipolytic processing of chylomicrons. *Cell Metab* 5:279, 2007.
34. Kowal RC, Herz J, Goldstein JL, et al: Low density lipoprotein receptor–related protein mediates uptake of cholesteryl esters derived from apoprotein E–enriched lipoproteins. *Proc Natl Acad Sci U S A* 86:5810, 1989.
35. Mahley RW: Apolipoprotein E: cholesterol transport protein with expanding role in cell biology. *Science* 240:622, 1988.
36. Mahley RW, Hussain M: Chylomicron and chylomicron remnant catabolism. *Curr Opin Lipidol* 2:170-176, 1991.
37. Mahley RW, Huang Y, Rall SC: Pathogenesis of type III hyperlipoproteinemia (dysbetalipoproteinemia): questions, quandaries, and paradoxes. *J Lipid Res* 40:1933, 1999.
38. Welty FK, Lichtenstein AH, Barrett PH, et al: Human apolipoprotein (Apo) B-48 and ApoB-100 kinetics with stable isotopes. *Arterioscler Thromb Vasc Biol* 19:2966, 1999.
39. Chen SH, Habib G, Yang CY, et al: Apolipoprotein B-48 is the product of a messenger RNA with an organ-specific in-frame stop codon. *Science* 238:363, 1987.
40. Berge KE, Tian H, Graf GA, et al: Accumulation of dietary cholesterol in sitosterolemia caused by mutations in adjacent ABC transporters. *Science* 290:1771, 2000.
41. Lee MH, Lu K, Hazard S, et al: Identification of a gene, ABCG5, important in the regulation of dietary cholesterol absorption. *Nat Genet* 27:79, 2001.
42. Repa JJ, Mangelsdorf DJ: The role of orphan nuclear receptors in the regulation of cholesterol homeostasis. *Annu Rev Cell Dev Biol* 16:459, 2000.
43. Mahley RW: Apolipoprotein E: cholesterol transport protein with expanding role in cell biology. *Science* 240:622, 1988.
44. Beisiegel U, Weber W, Ihrke G, et al: The LDL-receptor–related protein, LRP, is an apolipoprotein E–binding protein. *Nature* 341:162, 1989.
45. Havel RJ, Hamilton RL: Hepatocytic lipoprotein receptors and intracellular lipoprotein catabolism. *Hepatology* 8:1689, 1988.
46. Herz J, Goldstein DK, Strickland JL, et al: 39-kDa protein modulates binding of ligands to low density lipoprotein receptor–related protein/alpha₂-macroglobulin receptor. *J Biol Chem* 266:21232, 1991.
47. Kowal RC, Herz J, Goldstein JL, et al: Low density lipoprotein receptor–related protein mediates uptake of cholesteryl esters derived from apoprotein E–enriched lipoproteins. *Proc Natl Acad Sci U S A* 86:5810, 1989.
48. Schaefer EJ, Gregg RE, Ghiselli G, et al: Familial apolipoprotein E deficiency. *J Clin Invest* 78:1206, 1986.
49. Farese RV, Jr, Yost TJ, Eckel RH: Tissue-specific regulation of lipoprotein lipase activity by insulin/glucose in normal-weight humans. *Metabolism* 40:214, 1991.
50. de Graaf J, Hak-Lemmers HL, Hectors MP, et al: Enhanced susceptibility to in vitro oxidation of the dense low density lipoprotein subfraction in healthy subjects. *Arterioscler Thromb* 11:298, 1991.
51. Hurt-Camejo E, Olsson U, Wiklund O, et al: Cellular consequences of the association of apoB lipoproteins with proteoglycans. Potential contribution to atherogenesis. *Arterioscler Thromb Vasc Biol* 17:1011, 1997.
52. Brown MS, Goldstein JL: A receptor-mediated pathway for cholesterol homeostasis. *Science* 232:34, 1986.
53. Hiltunen TP, Luoma JS, Nikkari T, et al: Expression of LDL receptor, VLDL receptor, LDL receptor–related protein, and scavenger receptor in rabbit atherosclerotic lesions. Marked induction of scavenger receptor and VLDL receptor expression during lesion development. *Circulation* 97:1079, 1998.
54. Steinberg D, Parthasarathy S, Carew TE, et al: Beyond cholesterol. Modifications of low-density lipoprotein that increase its atherogenicity. *N Engl J Med* 320:915, 1989.

55. Podrez EA, Febbraio M, Sheibani N, et al: Macrophage scavenger receptor CD36 is the major receptor for LDL modified by monocyte-generated reactive nitrogen species. *J Clin Invest* 105:1095, 2000.

56. Febbraio M, Podrez EA, Smith JD, et al: Targeted disruption of the class B scavenger receptor CD36 protects against atherosclerotic lesion development in mice. *J Clin Invest* 105:1049, 2000.

57. Febbraio M, Hajjar DP, Silverstein RL: CD36: a class B scavenger receptor involved in angiogenesis, atherosclerosis, inflammation, and lipid metabolism. *J Clin Invest* 108:785, 2001.

58. Gianturco SH, Bradley WA: A cellular basis for the potential atherogenicity of triglyceride-rich lipoproteins. In Slagov S, Newman WP, III, Schaffer SA, editors: *Pathobiology of the human atherosclerotic plaque*, New York, 1990, Springer-Verlag.

59. Rapp RJ: Hypertriglyceridemia: a review beyond low-density lipoprotein. *Cardiol Rev* 10:163, 2002.

60. Lechleitner M, Hoppichler F, Föger B, Patsch JR: Low-density lipoproteins of the post prandial state induce cellular cholesteryl ester accumulation in macrophages. *Arterioscler Thromb* 14:1799, 1994.

61. Kugiyama K, Doi H, Motoyama T, et al: Association of remnant lipoprotein levels with impairment of endothelium-dependent vasomotor function in human coronary arteries. *Circulation* 97:2519, 1998.

62. Krauss RM, Lindgren FT, Williams PT, et al: Intermediate-density lipoproteins and progression of coronary artery disease in hypercholesterolaemic men. *Lancet* 2:62, 1987.

63. Kugiyama K, Dori H, Takazoe K, et al: Remnant lipoprotein levels in fasting serum predict coronary events in patients with coronary artery disease. *Circulation* 99:2858, 1999.

64. Fukushima H, Kugiyama K, Sugiyama S, et al: Comparison of remnant-like lipoprotein particles in postmenopausal women with and without coronary artery disease and in men with coronary artery disease. *Am J Cardiol* 88:1370, 2001.

65. Masuoka H, Kamei S, Wagayama H, et al: Association of remnant-like particle cholesterol with coronary artery disease in patients with normal total cholesterol levels. *Am Heart J* 139:305, 2000.

66. Williams KJ, Petrie KA, Broacia RW, Swenson TL: Lipoprotein lipase modulates net secretory output of apolipoprotein B in vitro. *J Clin Invest* 88:1300, 1991.

67. Hodis HN, Mack WJ, Dunn M, et al: Intermediate-density lipoproteins and progression of carotid arterial wall intima-media thickness. *Circulation* 95:2022, 1997.

68. Hodis HN, Mack WJ: Triglyceride-rich lipoproteins and the progression of coronary artery disease. *Curr Opin Lipidol* 6:209, 1995.

69. Mack WJ, Krauss RM, Hodis HN: Lipoprotein subclasses in the Monitored Atherosclerosis Regression Study (MARS). Treatment effects and relation to coronary angiographic progression. *Arterioscler Thromb Vasc Biol* 16:697, 1996.

70. Castelli WP, Doyle JT, Gordon T, et al: HDL cholesterol and other lipids in coronary heart disease. The cooperative lipoprotein phenotyping study. *Circulation* 55:767, 1977.

71. Miller NE, Thelle DS, Forde OH, Mjos OD: The Tromsø Heart Study. High-density lipoprotein and coronary heart disease: a prospective case-control study. *Lancet* 1:965, 1977.

72. Gordon T, Castelli M, Hjortland MC, et al: High-density lipoprotein as a protective factor against coronary heart disease: the Framingham Study. *Am J Med* 62:707, 1977.

73. Jacobs DR, Jr, Mebane IL, Bangdiwala SI, et al: High density lipoprotein cholesterol as a predictor of cardiovascular disease mortality in men and women: the follow-up study of the Lipid Research Clinics Prevalence Study. *Am J Epidemiol* 131:32, 1990.

74. Stokes J, 3rd, Kannel WB, Wolf PA, et al: The relative importance of selected risk factors for various manifestations of cardiovascular disease among men and women from 35 to 64 years old: 30 years of follow-up in the Framingham Study. *Circulation* 75(pt 2):V65, 1987.

75. Acton S, Rigotti A, Landschulz KT, et al: Identification of scavenger receptor SR-BI as a high-density lipoprotein receptor. *Science* 271:518, 1996.

76. Tall AR: Plasma cholesteryl ester transfer protein. *J Lipid Res* 34:1255, 1993.

77. Steinberg D: A docking receptor for HDL cholesterol esters. *Science* 271:460, 1996.

78. Lamarche B, Uffelman KD, Carpentier A, et al: Triglyceride enrichment of HDL enhances in vivo metabolic clearance of HDL apo A-I in healthy men. *J Clin Invest* 103:1191, 1999.

79. Schaefer EJ, Levy RI, Anderson DW, et al: Plasma triglycerides in the regulation of HDL-cholesterol levels. *Lancet* 2:391, 1978.

80. Nigon F, Lesnik P, Rouis M, et al: Discrete subspecies of human low density lipoprotein are heterogeneous in their interaction with cellular LDL receptor. *J Lipid Res* 32:1741, 1991.

81. Welty FK, Lichtenstein AH, Barrett PHR, et al: Interrelationships between human apolipoprotein A-I and apolipoproteins B-48 and B-100 kinetics using stable isotopes. *Arterioscler Thromb Vasc Biol* 24:1703, 2004.

82. Wittrup HH, Tybjaerg-Hansen A, Abildgaard S, et al: A common substitution (Asn291Ser) in lipoprotein lipase is associated with increased risk of ischemic heart disease. *J Clin Invest* 99:1606, 1997.

83. Wittrup HH, Nordestgaard BG, Sillesen H, et al: A common mutation in lipoprotein lipase confers a 2-fold increase in risk of ischemic cerebrovascular disease in women but not in men. *Circulation* 101:2393, 2000.

84. Kluger M, Heeren J, Merkel M: Apoprotein A-V: an important regulator of triglyceride metabolism. *J Inherit Met Dis* 2008 Apr 14. [Epub ahead of print.]

85. Forte TM, Shu X, Ryan RO: The ins (cell) and outs (plasma) of apolipoprotein A-V. *J Lipid Res* 50(Suppl):S150, 2009.

86. Tahvanainen E, Syvanne M, Frick MH, et al: Association of variation in hepatic lipase activity with promoter variation in the hepatic lipase gene. The LOCAT Study Invsestigators. *J Clin Invest* 101:956, 1998.

87. Zambon A, Deeb SS, Hokanson JE, et al: Common variants in the promoter of the hepatic lipase gene are associated with lower levels of hepatic lipase activity, buoyant LDL, and higher HDL2 cholesterol. *Arterioscler Thromb Vasc Biol* 18:1723, 1998.

88. Greenberg BH, Blackwelder WC, Levy RI: Primary type V hyperlipoproteinemia. A descriptive study in 32 families. *Ann Intern Med* 87:526, 1977.

89. Ghiselli G, Schaefer EJ, Zech LA, et al: Increased prevalence of apolipoprotein E4 in type V hyperlipoproteinemia. *J Clin Invest* 70:474, 1982.

90. Santamarina-Fojo S: The familial chylomicronemia syndrome. *Endocrinol Metab Clin North Am* 27:551, 1998.

91. Nordestgaard BG, Abildgaard S, Wittrup HH, et al: Heterozygous lipoprotein lipase deficiency. Frequency in the general population, effect on plasma lipid levels, and risk of ischemic heart disease. *Circulation* 96:1737, 1997.

92. Glueck CJ, Lang J, Hamer T, Tracy T: Severe hypertriglyceridemia and pancreatitis when estrogen replacement therapy is given to hypertriglyceridemic women. *J Lab Clin Med* 123:18, 1994.

93. Genest JJ, Martin-Munley SS, McNamara JR, et al: Familial lipoprotein disorders in patients with premature coronary artery disease. *Circulation* 85:2025, 1992.

94. Austin MA, McKnight B, Edwards KL, et al: Cardiovascular disease mortality in familial forms of hypertriglyceridemia: a 20-year prospective study. *Circulation* 101:2777, 2000.

95. Kissebah AH, Alfarsi S, Adams PW: Integrated regulation of very low density lipoprotein triglyceride and apolipoprotein-B kinetics in man: normolipemic subjects, familial hypertriglyceridemia and familial combined hyperlipidemia. *Metabolism* 30:856, 1981.

96. Chait A, Albers JJ, Brunzell JD: Very low density lipoprotein overproduction in genetic forms of hypertriglyceridaemia. *Eur J Clin Invest* 10:17, 1980.

97. Cullen P, von Eckardstein A, Assmann G: Genetic and acquired abnormalities of lipoprotein metabolism. *Cardiovasc Risk Factors* 6:99, 1996.

98. Goldstein JL, Schrott HG, Hazzard WR, et al: Hyperlipidemia in coronary heart disease: II. Genetic analysis in 176 families and delineation of a new inherited disorder, combined hyperlipidemia. *J Clin Invest* 52:1544, 1973.

99. Lee JC, Lusis AJ, Pajukanta P: Familial combined hyperlipidemia: upstream transcription factor 1 and beyond. *Curr Opin Lipidol* 17:101, 2006.

100. Hegele RA: Monogenic dyslipidemias: window on determinants of plasma lipoproteins metabolism. *Am J Hum Genet* 69:1161, 2001.

101. Reaven GM: Role of insulin resistance in human disease. *Diabetes* 37:1595, 1988.

102. Reaven GM: Syndrome X: 6 years later. *J Intern Med* 736:13-22, 1994.

103. Ginsberg HN: Insulin resistance and cardiovascular disease. *J Clin Invest* 106:453, 2000.

104. Genest JJ, Jr, Martin-Munley SS, McNamara JR, et al: Familial lipoprotein disorders in patients with premature coronary artery disease. *Circulation* 85:2025, 1992.

105. Babirak SP, Brown BG, Brunzell JD: Familial combined hyperlipidemia and abnormal lipoprotein lipase. *Arterioscler Thromb* 12:1176, 1992.

106. Yang WS, Nevin DN, Peng R, et al: A mutation in the promoter of the lipoprotein lipase (LPL) gene in a patient with familial combined hyperlipidemia and low LPL activity. *Proc Natl Acad Sci U S A* 92:4462, 1995.

107. Dong LM, Parkin S, Trakhanov SD, et al: Novel mechanism for defective receptor binding of apolipoprotein E2 in type III hyperlipoproteinemia. *Nat Struct Biol* 3:718, 1996.

108. Walden CC, Hegele RA: Apolipoprotein E in hyperlipidemia. *Ann Intern Med* 120:1026, 1994.

109. Pownall HJ: Dietary ethanol is associated with reduced lipolysis of intestinally derived lipoproteins. *J Lipid Res* 35:2105, 1994.

110. Rimm EB, Williams P, Fosher K, et al: Moderate alcohol intake and lower risk of heart disease: meta analysis of effects on lipids and haemostatic factors. *BMJ* 319:1523, 1999.

111. Expert Panel on Detection, Evaluation and Treatment of High Blood Cholesterol in Adults: Third report of the National Cholesterol Education Program (NCEP) Expert Panel on Detection, Evaluation, and Treatment of High Blood Cholesterol in Adults (Adult Treatment Panel III). *Circulation* 106:3143, 2002.

112. Pollex RL, Hegele RA: Genetic determinants of the metabolic syndrome. *Nat Clin Pract Cardiovasc Med* 3:482, 2006.

113. Grundy SM: Hypertriglyceridemia, atherogenic dyslipidemia, and the metabolic syndrome. *Am J Cardiol* 81:18B, 1998.

114. Ford ES, Giles WH, Dietz WH: Prevalence of the metabolic syndrome among US adults: findings from the Third National Health and Nutrition Examination Survey. *JAMA* 287:356, 2002.

115. Bansal S, Buring JE, Rifai N, et al: Fasting compared with nonfasting triglycerides and risk of cardiovascular events in women. *JAMA* 298:309, 2007.

116. Nordestgaard BG, Benn M, Schnohr P, Tybjærg-Hansen A: Nonfasting triglycerides and risk of myocardial infarction, ischemic heart disease, and death in men and women. *JAMA* 298:299, 2007.

117. Friedewald WT, Levy RI, Fredrickson DS: Estimation of the concentration of low-density lipoprotein cholesterol in plasma, without use of the preparative ultracentrifuge. *Clin Chem* 18:499, 1972.

118. Austin MA, King MC, Vranizan KM, et al: Atherogenic lipoprotein phenotype: a proposed genetic marker for coronary heart disease risk. *Circulation* 82:495, 1990.

119. Miller M, Zhan M, Georgopoulos A: Effect of desirable fasting triglycerides on the postprandial response to dietary fat. *J Investig Med* 51:50, 2003.

120. Sacks FM: The apolipoprotein story. *Atheroscler Suppl* 7:23, 2006.

121. Carmena R, Duriez P, Fruchart JC: Atherogenic lipoprotein particles in atherosclerosis. *Circulation* 109:III2, 2004.

122. Chapman M, Guerin M, Bruckert E: Atherogenic, dense low-density lipoproteins—pathophysiology and new therapeutic approaches. *Eur Heart J* 19(Suppl):A24, 1998.

123. Otvos JD, Jeyarajah EJ, Cromwell WC: Measurement issues related to lipoprotein heterogeneity. *Am J Cardiol* 90:22i, 2002.

124. Lamarche B, Tchernof A, Moorjani S, et al: Small, dense low-density lipoprotein particles as a predictor of the risk of ischemic heart disease in men: prospective results from the Quebec Cardiovascular Study. *Circulation* 95:69, 1997.

125. Otvos JD, Collins D, Freedman DS, et al: Low-density lipoprotein and high-density lipoprotein particle subclasses predict coronary events and are favorably changed by

gemfibrozil therapy in the Veterans Affairs High-Density Lipoprotein Intervention Trial. *Circulation* 113:1556, 2006.
126. Campos H, Moye L, Glasser S, et al: Low-density lipoprotein size, pravastatin treatment, and coronary events. *JAMA* 286:1468, 2001.
127. McNamara JR, Jenner JL, Li Z, et al: Change in LDL particle size is associated with change in plasma triglyceride concentration. *Arterioscler Thromb* 12:1284, 1992.
128. Brewer H: Hypertriglyceridemia: changes in the plasma lipoproteins associated with an increased risk of cardiovascular disease. *Am J Cardiol* 83:3F, 1999.
129. Carmena R, Duriez P, Fruchart JC: Atherogenic lipoprotein particles in atherosclerosis. *Circulation* 109:III2, 2004.
130. Kawakami A, Aikawa M, Alcaide P, et al: Apolipoprotein CIII induces expression of vascular cell adhesion molecule-1 in vascular endothelial cells and increases adhesion of monocytic cells. *Circulation* 114:681, 2006.
131. Cui Y, Blumenthal R, Flaws J, et al: Non–high-density lipoprotein cholesterol level as predictor of cardiovascular disease mortality. *Arch Intern Med* 161:1413, 2001.
132. Ingelsson E, Schaefer EJ, Contois JH, et al: Clinical utility of different lipid measures for prediction of coronary heart disease in men and women. *JAMA* 298:776, 2007.
133. Fredrickson DS, Levy RI, Lees RS: Fat transport in lipoproteins—an integrated approach to mechanisms and disorders. *N Engl J Med* 276:148, 1967.
134. Barter PJ, Ballantyne CM, Carmena R, et al: Apo B versus cholesterol in estimating cardiovascular risk and in guiding therapy: report of the thirty-person/ten-country panel. *J Intern Med* 259:247, 2006.
135. Brewer H: Hypertriglyceridemia: changes in the plasma lipoproteins associated with an increased risk of cardiovascular disease. *Am J Cardiol* 83:3F, 1999.
136. Abate N, Vega GL, Grundy SM: Variability in cholesterol content and physical properties of lipoproteins containing apolipoprotein B-100. *Atherosclerosis* 104:159, 1993.
137. Pischon T, Girman CJ, Sacks FM, et al: Non–high-density lipoprotein cholesterol and apolipoprotein B in the prediction of coronary heart disease in men. *Circulation* 112:3375, 2005.
138. Shai I, Rimm EB, Hankinson SE, et al: Multivariate assessment of lipid parameters as predictors of coronary heart disease among postmenopausal women: potential implications for clinical guidelines. *Circulation* 110:2824, 2004.
139. Bittner V, Hardison R, Kelsey S, et al: Non–high-density lipoprotein cholesterol levels predict five-year outcome in the Bypass Angioplasty Revascularization Investigation (BARI). *Circulation* 106:2537, 2002.
140. Shahar E, Chambless LE, Rosamond WD, et al: Plasma lipid profile and incident ischemic stroke: the Atherosclerosis Risk in Communities (ARIC) study. *Stroke* 34:623, 2003.
141. Ridker P, Rifai N, Cook N, et al: Non–HDL cholesterol, AJC apolipoproteins A-I and B100, standard lipid measures, lipid ratios, and CRP as risk factors for cardiovascular disease in women. *JAMA* 294:326, 2005.
142. Liu J, Sempos CT, Donahue RP, et al: Non–high-density lipoprotein and very-low-density lipoprotein cholesterol and their risk predictive values in coronary heart disease. *Am J Cardiol* 98:1363, 2006.
143. Emerging Risk Factors Collaboration: Major lipids, apolipoproteins, and risk of vascular disease. *JAMA* 302:1993, 2009.
144. Stampfer MJ, Krauss RM, Ma J, et al: A prospective study of triglyceride level, low-density lipoprotein particle diameter, and risk of myocardial infarction. *JAMA* 276:882, 1996.
145. Grundy SM: Consensus statement: role of therapy with "statins" in patients with hypertriglyceridemia. *Am J Cardiol* 81:B1, 1998.
146. Ballantyne CM, Grundy SM, Oberman A, et al: Hyperlipidemia: diagnostic and therapeutic perspectives. *J Clin Endocrinol Metab* 85:2089, 2000.
147. Lloret Linares C, Pelletier AL, Czernichow S, et al: Acute pancreatitis in a cohort of 129 patients referred for severe hypertriglyceridemia. *Pancreas* 37:13, 2008.
148. Brunzell JD: Clinical practice. Hypertriglyceridemia. *N Engl J Med* 357:1009, 2007.
149. American Diabetes Association: Standards of medical care in diabetes—2008. *Diabetes Care* 31:S12, 2008.
150. Ebbeling CB, Leidig MM, Feldman HA, et al: Effects of a low-glycemic load vs low-fat diet in obese young adults: a randomized trial. *JAMA* 297:2092, 2007.
151. De Lorgeril M, Renaud S, Mamelle N, et al: Mediterranean alpha-linolenic acid rich diet in secondary prevention of coronary heart disease. *Lancet* 343:1454, 1994.
152. Leaf A: On the re-analysis of the GISSI-Prevenzione. *Circulation* 105:1874, 2002.
153. Schaefer EJ, Gleason JA, Dansinger ML: The effects of low-fat, high-carbohydrate diets on plasma lipoproteins, weight loss, and heart disease risk reduction. *Curr Atheroscler Rep* 7:421, 2005.
154. Brousseau ME, Schaefer EJ: Diet and coronary heart disease: clinical trials. *Curr Atheroscler Rep* 2:487, 2000.
155. Denke MA: Diet, lifestyle, and nonstatin trials: review of time to benefit. *Am J Cardiol* 96(Suppl):3F, 2005.
156. Parikh P, McDaniel MC, Ashen MD, et al: Diets and cardiovascular disease: an evidence-based assessment. *J Am Coll Cardiol* 45:1379, 2005.
157. Lichtenstein A, Appel LJ, Brands M, et al: Diet and lifestyle recommendations revision 2006: a scientific statement from the American Heart Association Nutrition Committee. *Circulation* 114:82, 2006.
158. Sacks FM, Katan M: Randomized clinical trials on the effects of dietary fat and carbohydrate on plasma lipoproteins and cardiovascular disease. *Am J Med* 113:13S, 2002.
159. Lichtenstein AH, Appel LJ, Brands M, et al: Summary of American Heart Association Diet and Lifestyle Recommendations revision 2006. *Arterioscler Thromb Vasc Biol* 26:2186, 2006.
160. Dattilo AM, Kris-Etherton PM: Effects of weight reduction on blood lipids and lipoproteins: a meta-analysis. *Am J Clin Nutr* 56:320, 1992.
161. Purnell JQ, Kahn SE, Albers JJ, et al: Effect of weight loss with reduction of intra-abdominal fat on lipid metabolism in older men. *J Clin Endocrinol Metab* 85:977, 2000.
162. Welty FK, Nasca MM, Lew NS, et al: Effect of onsite dietitian counseling on weight loss and lipid levels in an outpatient physician office. *Am J Cardiol* 100:73, 2007.
163. Kuller LH, Kinzel LS, Pettee KK, et al: Lifestyle intervention and coronary heart disease risk factor changes over 18 months in postmenopausal women: the Women On the Move through Activity and Nutrition (WOMAN study) clinical trial. *J Womens Health (Larchmt)* 15:962, 2006.
164. Welty FK, Stuart E, O'Meara M, Huddleston J: Effect of addition of exercise to therapeutic lifestyle changes diet in enabling women and men with coronary heart disease to reach Adult Treatment Panel III low-density lipoprotein cholesterol goal without lowering high-density lipoprotein cholesterol. *Am J Cardiol* 89:1201, 2002.
165. Boden WE, O'Rourke RA, Teo KK, et al: COURAGE Trial Research Group: Optimal medical therapy with or without PCI for stable coronary disease. *N Engl J Med* 356:1503, 2007.
166. Haskell WL, Lee IM, Pate RR, et al: Physical activity and public health: updated recommendation for adults from the American College of Sports Medicine and the American Heart Association. *Circulation* 116:1081, 2007.
167. Szapary PO, Bloedon LT, Foster GD: Physical activity and its effects on lipids. *Curr Cardiol Rep* 5:488, 2003.
168. Kraus WE, Houmard JA, Duscha BD, et al: Effects of the amount and intensity of exercise on plasma lipoproteins. *N Engl J Med* 347:1483, 2002.
169. Kelley GA, Kelley KS, Tran ZV: Walking, lipids, and lipoproteins: a meta-analysis of randomized controlled trials. *Prev Med* 38:651, 2004.
170. King AC, Haskell WL, Young DR, et al: Long-term effects of varying intensities and formats of physical activity on participation rates, fitness and lipoproteins in men and women age 50 to 65 years. *Circulation* 91:2596, 1995.
171. Studer M, Briel M, Leimenstoll B, et al: Effect of different antilipidemic agents and diets on mortality: a systematic review. *Arch Intern Med* 165:725, 2005.
172. Stein EA, Lane M, Laskarazewski P: Comparison of statins in hypertriglyceridemia. *Am J Cardiol* 81:B66, 1998.
173. Mailly F, Tugrul Y, Reymer PW, et al: A common variant in the gene for lipoprotein lipase (Asp9→Asn). Functional implications and prevalence in normal and hyperlipidemic subjects. *Arterioscler Thromb Vasc Biol* 15:468, 1995.
174. Jukema JW, van Boven AJ, Groenemeijer B, et al: REGRESS Study Group: The Asp9 Asn mutation in the lipoprotein lipase gene is associated with increased progression of coronary atherosclerosis. *Circulation* 94:1913, 1996.
175. Staels B, Dallongeville J, Auwerx J, et al: Mechanism of action of fibrates on lipid and lipoprotein metabolism. *Circulation* 98:2088, 1998.
176. Vu-Dac N, Schoonjans K, Kosykh V, et al: Fibrates increase human apolipoprotein A-II expression through activation of the peroxisome proliferator-activated receptor. *J Clin Invest* 96:741, 1995.
177. Berthou L, Duverger N, Emmanuel F, et al: Opposite regulation of human versus mouse apoprotein A-I by fibrates in human apolipoprotein A-I transgenic mice. *J Clin Invest* 97:2408, 1996.
178. Jin F-Y, Kamanna VS, Chuang M-Y, et al: Gemfibrozil stimulates apolipoprotein A-I synthesis and secretion by stabilization of mRNA transcripts in human hepatoblastoma cell line (Hep G2). *Arterioscler Thromb Vasc Biol* 16:1052, 1996.
179. Rosenson RS, Wolff DA, Huskin AL, et al: Fenofibrate therapy ameliorates fasting and postprandial lipoproteinemia, oxidative stress, and the inflammatory response in subjects with hypertriglyceridemia and the metabolic syndrome. *Diabetes Care* 30:1945, 2007.
180. Brown JD, Plutzky J: Peroxisome proliferator-activated receptors as transcriptional nodal points and therapeutic targets. *Circulation* 115:518, 2007.
181. Grundy SM, Cleeman JI, Merz CN, et al: Implications of recent clinical trials for the National Cholesterol Education Program Adult Treatment Panel III guidelines. *Circulation* 110:227, 2004.
182. Haim M, Benderly M, Brunner D, et al: BIP Study Group: Elevated serum triglyceride levels and long-term mortality in patients with coronary heart disease: the Bezafibrate Infarction Prevention (BIP) registry. *Circulation* 100:475, 1999.
183. Secondary prevention by raising HDL cholesterol and reducing triglycerides in patients with coronary heart disease: the Bezafibrate Infarction Prevention (BIP) study. *Circulation* 102:21, 2000.
184. Frick MH, Elo O, Haapa K, et al: Helsinki Heart Study: Primary-prevention trial with gemfibrozil in middle-aged men with dyslipidemia: safety of treatment, changes in risk factors, and incidence of coronary heart disease. *N Engl J Med* 317:1237, 1987.
185. Manninen V, Tenkanen L, Koskinen P, et al: Joint effects of serum triglyceride and LDL cholesterol and HDL cholesterol concentrations on coronary heart disease risk in Helsinki Heart Study. Implications for treatment. *Circulation* 85:37, 1992.
186. Rubins HB, Robins SJ, Collins D, et al: Veterans Affairs High-Density Lipoprotein Cholesterol Intervention Trial Study Group: Gemfibrozil for the secondary prevention of coronary heart disease in men with low levels of high-density lipoprotein cholesterol. *N Engl J Med* 341:410, 1999.
187. Diabetes Atherosclerosis Intervention Study Investigators: Effect of fenofibrate on progression of coronary-artery disease in type 2 diabetes: the Diabetes Atherosclerosis Intervention Study, a randomised study. *Lancet* 357:905, 2001.
188. Keech A, Simes RJ, Barter P, et al: Effects of long-term fenofibrate therapy on cardiovascular events in 9795 people with type 2 diabetes mellitus (the FIELD study): randomised controlled trial. *Lancet* 366:1849, 2005.
189. Scott R, O'Brien R, Fulcher G, et al: Fenofibrate Intervention and Event Lowering in Diabetes (FIELD) Study Investigators: Effects of fenofibrate treatment on cardiovascular disease risk in 9,795 individuals with type 2 diabetes and various components of the metabolic syndrome. *Diabetes Care* 32:493, 2009.
190. Saha SA, Kizhakepunnur LG, Bahekar A, Arora RR: The role of fibrates in the prevention of cardiovascular disease: a pooled meta-analysis of longterm randomized placebo-controlled trials. *Am Heart J* 154:943, 2007.
191. Koskinen P, Manttari M, Manninen V, et al: Coronary heart disease incidence in NIDDM patients in the Helsinki Heart Study. *Diabetes Care* 15:820, 1992.
192. The ACCORD Study Group: Effects of combination lipid therapy in type 2 diabetes mellitus. *N Engl J Med* 2010 Mar 18. [Epub ahead of print.]

193. Boissonnat P, Salen P, Guidollet J, et al: The long-term effects of the lipid-lowering agent fenofibrate in hyperlipidemic heart transplant recipients. *Transplantation* 58:245, 1994.

194. Canner PL, Berrge KG, Wenger NK, et al: Fifteen-year mortality in coronary drug project patients: long-term benefit with niacin. *J Am Coll Cardiol* 8:1245, 1986.

195. Elam MB, Hunninghake DB, Davis KB, et al: Effect of niacin on lipid and lipoprotein levels and glycemic control in patients with diabetes and peripheral arterial disease. The ADMIT study: a randomized trial. *JAMA* 284:1263, 2000.

196. Grundy SM, Vega GL, McGovern ME, et al: Diabetes Multicenter Research Group: Efficacy, safety and tolerability of once-daily niacin for the treatment of dyslipidemia associated with type 2 diabetes: results of the Assessment of Diabetes Control and Evaluation of the Efficacy of Niaspan Trial. *Arch Intern Med* 162:1568, 2002.

197. Brown G, Albers JJ, Fisher LD, et al: Regression of coronary artery disease as a result of intensive lipid-lowering therapy in men with high levels of apoB. *N Engl J Med* 323:1289, 1990.

198. Brown BG, Zhao XQ, Chait A, et al: Simvastatin and niacin, antioxidant vitamins or the combination for the prevention of coronary disease. *N Engl J Med* 345:1583, 2001.

199. Brown BG, Brockenbrough A, Zhao XQ, et al: Very intensive therapy with lovastatin, niacin, and colestipol for prevention of death and myocardial infarction: a 10-year Familial Atherosclerosis Treatment Study (FATS) follow-up. *Circulation* 98(Suppl I):I635, 1998.

200. Azen SP, Mack WJ, Cashin-Hemphill L, et al: Progression of coronary artery disease predicters clinical coronary events: long-term follow-up from the Cholesterol Lowering Atherosclerosis Study. *Circulation* 93:34-41, 1996.

201. AIM-HIGH Clinical Study: Inclusion criteria and major exclusion criteria. Available at: accelerator.axioresearch.com/aim-high/. Accessed June 12, 2008.

202. Guyton JR, Blazing MA, Hagar J, et al: Extended-release niacin vs gemfibrozil for the treatment of low levels of high-density lipoprotein cholesterol. Niaspan-Gemfibrozil Study Group. *Arch Intern Med* 160:1177, 2000.

203. Carlson LA, Hamsten A, Asplund A: Pronounced lowering of serum levels of lipoprotein Lp(a) in hyperlipidaemic subjects treated with nicotinic acid. *J Intern Med* 226:271, 1989.

204. Espeland MA, Marcovina SM, Miller V, et al: Effect of postmenopausal hormone therapy on lipoprotein(a) concentration. PEPI Investigators. Postmenopausal Estrogen/Progestin Interventions. *Circulation* 97:979, 1998.

205. Welty FK: Alternative hormone replacement regimens: is there a need for further clinical trials? *Curr Opin Lipidol* 14:585, 2003.

206. Nestel P, Connor WE, Reardon MF, et al: Suppression by diets rich in fish oil of very low density lipoprotein production in man. *J Clin Invest* 74:72, 1984.

207. Harris WS, Connor WE, Illingworth DR, et al: Effects of fish oil on VLDL triglyceride kinetics in humans. *J Lipid Res* 31:1549, 1990.

208. Durrington PN, Bhatnagar D, Mackness MI, et al: An omega-3 polyunsaturated fatty acid concentrate administered for one year decreased triglycerides in simvastatin treated patients with coronary heart disease and persisting hypertriglyceridaemia. *Heart* 85:544, 2001.

209. Nambi V, Ballantyne CM: Combination therapy with statins and omega-3 fatty acids. *Am J Cardiol* 98:34I, 2006.

210. Gruppo Italiano per lo Studio della Sopravvivenza nell'Infarto miocardico: Dietary supplementation with n-3 polyunsaturated fatty acids and vitamin E after myocardial infarction: results of the GISSI-Prevenzione trial. *Lancet* 354:447, 1999.

211. Leaf A: Omega-3 fatty acids and prevention of arrhythmias. *Curr Opin Lipidol* 18:31, 2007.

212. Yokoyama M, Origasa H, Matsuzaki M, et al: Effects of eicosapentaenoic acid on major coronary events in hypercholesterolemic patients (JELIS): a randomized open-label, blinded endpoint analysis. *Lancet* 369:1090, 2007.

213. GISSI-HF Investigators: Effect of n-3 polyunsaturated fatty acids in patients with chronic heart failure (the GISSI-HF trial): a randomized, double-blind, placebo-controlled trial. *Lancet* 372:1223, 2008.

214. Davidson M, Stein E, Bays H, et al: Combination of Prescription Omega-3 with Simvastatin (COMBOS) Investigators: An 8-week, randomized, double-blind, placebo-controlled study of the efficacy and safety of adding prescription omega-3 fatty acids 4 g/d to simvastatin 40 mg/d in hypertriglyceridemic subjects. *Clin Ther* 29:1354, 2007.

215. Clinical Trial Service Unit & Epidemiological Studies Unit: HPS2-THRIVE press release. Available at: http://www.ctsu.ox.ac.uk/pressreleases/2006-05-31/hps2-thrive-press-release. Accessed June 12, 2008.

15

The Contribution of Triglycerides and Triglyceride-Rich Lipoproteins to Atherosclerotic Cardiovascular Disease

Diet and Lifestyle Factors

CHAPTER **16**

Nutritional Approaches for Cardiovascular Disease Prevention

Alison M. Hill, Kristina A. Harris, Alison M. Coates, and
Penny M. Kris-Etherton

KEY POINTS

- A primary focus of CVD prevention is LDL-C and blood pressure lowering and improvement of other cardiometabolic risk factors.

- Current dietary guidelines for chronic disease prevention emphasize an overall healthy dietary pattern based on foods rather than on targeting specific nutrients.

- Strategies used in clinical practice for CVD prevention, specifically LDL-C and blood pressure lowering, include the Therapeutic Lifestyle Changes (TLC) and Dietary Approaches to Stop Hypertension (DASH) diets.

- Dietary patterns for weight loss are most dependent on calorie control, but modification of the macronutrient profile may target cardiovascular risk factors, including blood pressure, lipids, and lipoproteins.

- Key components of heart-healthy dietary approaches include reduced intake of saturated fatty acids, trans–fatty acids, and cholesterol and increased intake of fruits and vegetables, whole grains, reduced-fat dairy, and heart-healthy protein (from plant and low–saturated fatty acid animal sources).

- Additional dietary components (soluble fiber, sterols and stanols, soy protein, and unsaturated fats) and supplements (fish oil and niacin) improve CVD risk status.

- Food-based recommendations and their associated tools, such as MyPyramid (developed by the U.S. Department of Agriculture), assist consumers in implementing dietary guidelines and may assist clinicians in counseling patients.

NUTRITIONAL GOALS FOR PREVENTION OF CARDIOVASCULAR DISEASE

The goal of cardiovascular disease (CVD) prevention is to decrease CVD morbidity and mortality through pharmacologic and lifestyle (including dietary, behavioral, and physical) intervention. Reduction in major risk factors, which include total cholesterol and low-density lipoprotein cholesterol (LDL-C), systolic blood pressure, smoking prevalence, and physical inactivity, accounted for almost half of the decrease in coronary heart disease (CHD) mortality in the United States between 1980 and 2000.[1] Healthy lifestyle practices that improve such modifiable risk factors are therefore imperative for CVD prevention, and unlike pharmacologic treatments, lifestyle interventions are accessible to everyone and have similar efficacy in "slowing" chronic disease progression.[2] Modest dietary changes across an extended period can produce tangible results, both physically and psychologically, and may have a significant financial benefit. For example, if every adult in the United States reduced total daily calorie intake by 100 kcal, approximately 71.2 million cases of overweight and obesity could be resolved, saving an estimated $58 billion annually.[3]

The most prominent risk factors for CVD are elevated serum total cholesterol and LDL-C, hypertension, diabetes, and cigarette smoking.[4,5] Randomized controlled trials have shown that lowering of LDL-C and blood pressure, in particular, reduces risk for CVD.[6,7] Statin drug trials demonstrate that for every 25 mg/dL lowering of serum LDL-C, there is a decrease in major vascular (−14%) and coronary (−16%) events.[8] A linear relationship also exists between hypertension and CVD risk, which doubles with every increment of 20/10 mm Hg in systolic blood pressure (SBP)/diastolic blood pressure (DBP).[6] Currently, the primary aim of nonpharmacologic dietary interventions is a reduction in LDL-C, with a secondary aim of lowering non–high-density lipoprotein cholesterol and blood pressure. Other CVD risk factors, such as increased serum triglycerides (TG) and glucose, decreased high-density lipoprotein cholesterol (HDL-C), hypertension, and increased waist circumference, which cluster as part of the metabolic syndrome, also are targets for intensive lifestyle therapy in an effort to optimize CVD prevention.[9] Evidence for nontraditional risk factors, such as markers of thrombosis and inflammation, LDL-C particle size, and apolipoproteins, is emerging,[10] and additional research will establish their contribution to overall CVD risk.

Current dietary guidelines advocate a food-based approach for optimal health and chronic disease risk reduction.[11] Indeed, the American Heart Association (AHA) recommends a diet consistent with current guidelines to meet their 2020 Impact Goal to "improve the cardiovascular health of all Americans by 20% while reducing deaths from cardiovascular diseases and stroke by 20%."[12] The *Dietary Guidelines for Americans, 2005* emphasize a balanced diet that incorporates a variety of foods that are consumed in moderation. Therefore, although specific foods and nutrients have been identified as being more or less "healthful," it is the total dietary package that is most important. This chapter discusses the efficacy of a range of heart-healthy dietary patterns that have been scientifically evaluated for overall health promotion and CVD risk reduction. In particular, it reviews specific dietary patterns, such as the Therapeutic Lifestyle Changes (TLC)[9] and Dietary Approaches to Stop Hypertension (DASH)[13] diets, that are used in clinical practice for LDL-C and blood pressure lowering, respectively. Dietary strategies for weight loss also are reviewed. In evaluating dietary patterns, it is evident that a number of common foods exist between diets. The evidence supporting the benefits of specific foods and supplements on cardiovascular risk factors, with a particular focus on reducing LDL-C and blood pressure, is discussed. The information presented in this chapter will assist clinicians in implementing dietary strategies to manage CVD risk status in at-risk patients.

DIETARY PATTERNS TO REDUCE CARDIOVASCULAR DISEASE RISK

Therapeutic Lifestyle Changes Diet

LDL-C has long been identified by the National Cholesterol Education Program (NCEP) as the primary target for CHD risk reduction. Recommendations by NCEP for testing and management of high blood cholesterol have been published in reports by the Expert Panel on Detection, Evaluation, and Treatment of High Blood Cholesterol in Adults (Adult Treatment Panel III).[9] The evidence base for such recommendations is primarily from randomized clinical trials that have demonstrated that LDL-C lowering substantially reduces risk for CHD. Since the publication of the Adult Treatment Panel III (ATP III) guidelines, the results from several large-scale clinical trials have reinforced ATP III recommendations for therapeutic LDL-C lowering in high-risk and very-high-risk individuals.[14] ATP III recommends TLC for the clinical management of LDL-C in persons from all risk classifications (see Table 16-1 for summary of key components).[9] TLC may further reduce the incidence of CHD by modifying other cardiovascular risk factors beyond LDL-C. The primary focus of TLC is a reduction in saturated fatty acids (SFA) to <7% of total calories, *trans*–fatty acids to as low as possible, and cholesterol to <200 mg/day. Guidelines also are provided for monounsaturated fatty acid (MUFA) and polyunsaturated fatty acid (PUFA) intake (up to 20% and 10% of total calories, respectively), carbohydrate intake (50% to 60% of total calories), protein intake (approximately 15% of total calories), and dietary fiber intake (20 to 30 g/day). Additional therapeutic options for lowering of LDL-C include viscous fiber (10 to 25 g/day) and plant stanols or sterols (2 g/day). Achieving or maintaining a healthy body weight (by calorie manipulation) and participating in regular physical activity (enough moderate exercise to expend at least 200 kcal/day) also are essential TLC features. The combination of TLC with other LDL-C–lowering options may collectively reduce LDL-C levels by

TABLE 16–1	Key Components of Therapeutic Lifestyle Changes as Recommended by ATP III
Component	**Recommendation**
LDL-raising nutrients	
Saturated fatty acids	<7% of total calories
Cholesterol	<200 mg/day
Therapeutic options for LDL lowering	
Increased viscous (soluble) fiber	10-25 g/day
Plant stanols and sterols (2 g/day)	2 g/day
Energy intake	Adjust calorie intake to achieve a healthy body weight or to prevent weight gain
Physical activity	Participate in enough moderate exercise to expend at least 200 kcal/day
Macronutrients	
Monounsaturated fatty acids	Up to 20% of total calories
Polyunsaturated fatty acids	Up to 10% of total calories
Total fat	25%-35% of total calories
Carbohydrate	50%-60% of total calories
Protein	Approximately 15% of total calories
Dietary fiber	20-30 g/day

Modified from *Third Report of the National Cholesterol Education Program (NCEP) Expert Panel on Detection, Evaluation, and Treatment of High Blood Cholesterol in Adults (Adult Treatment Panel III). Final Report.* Bethesda, Md, 2002, National Heart, Lung and Blood Institute. NIH publication 02-5215.

TABLE 16–2	Cumulative Effect of Cholesterol-Lowering Strategies on LDL-C Levels	
Dietary Component	**Dietary Change**	**Approximate LDL Reduction**
Saturated fat	<7% of calories	8%-10%
Trans-fat	<1% of calories	1%-2%
Dietary cholesterol	<200 mg/day	3%-5%
Weight reduction	Lose 10 pounds	5%-8%
Soy protein		3%-5%
Other LDL-lowering options		
Viscous fiber	5 to 10 g/day	3%-5%
Plant sterol and stanol esters	2 g/day	6%-15%
Cumulative estimate		**24%-37%**

Modified from *Third Report of the National Cholesterol Education Program (NCEP) Expert Panel on Detection, Evaluation, and Treatment of High Blood Cholesterol in Adults (Adult Treatment Panel III). Final Report.* Bethesda, Md, 2002, National Heart, Lung, and Blood Institute. NIH publication 02-5215.

24% to 37% (Table 16-2). The magnitude of these effects has been established in well-controlled dietary intervention trials and further evaluated in free-living settings. The TLC dietary guidelines have been translated to food-based recommendations that are consistent with the AHA Diet and Lifestyle Recommendations 2006 (see Box 16-1, discussed later in this chapter). Numerous dietary patterns that meet current nutrient recommendations for CVD risk reduction have been evaluated and shown to be efficacious relative to improving major risk factors for CVD. Several of these dietary patterns are discussed on the following pages.

Portfolio Diet

The portfolio diet incorporates four key cholesterol-lowering strategies, plant sterols (1.0 g/1000 calories), viscous fiber (8.2 g/1000 calories), soy protein (22.7 g/1000 calories), and almonds (14 g/1000 calories), within a reduced total fat diet (<30% of total calories).[15] The portfolio diet is largely vegetarian, and SFA is limited to <7% of total calories and cholesterol to <200 mg/day. Sources of viscous fiber include eggplant and okra, oat bran, barley grains, and psyllium. Soy protein is obtained from soy milk and other soy products (such as soy burgers and sausages), and beans, chick peas, and lentils provide additional vegetable protein.

In a controlled 1-month dietary intervention with hyperlipidemic individuals, the portfolio diet reduced LDL-C by 29%, compared with an 8% reduction achieved by a low SFA (<7% of total calories) and cholesterol (<200 mg/day) diet alone (also known as a Step II diet).[15] A subsequent trial compared the effectiveness of the portfolio diet on LDL-C lowering with statin therapy.[16] In this study, subjects completed three 1-month intervention treatments in a randomized crossover design: a very low saturated fat diet (control or Step II diet), a control diet plus 20 mg lovastatin (statin), and the portfolio diet. LDL-C was reduced by 8%, 33%, and 29% following the control, statin, and portfolio diets, respectively. These results clearly illustrate the effectiveness of the portfolio diet over a traditional cholesterol-lowering diet and suggest that in controlled settings, the portfolio diet may be as potent as first-generation statin drugs for lowering of LDL-C. However, this dietary pattern is limited in its effects on HDL-C and TG.[15,16]

When the portfolio diet is implemented in a free-living setting, its effectiveness is reduced. In a 12-month study, subjects were instructed to follow a self-selected low-fat diet (Step II diet) that incorporated the portfolio of cholesterol-lowering foods (plant sterols, viscous fiber, soy protein, and almonds).[17] Subjects were advised to follow a vegetarian diet (without eggs, dairy products, or meat) that included 5 to 10 servings of fruits and vegetables per day, with additional plant protein and fiber from dried legumes. If meat or dairy products were consumed, subjects were counseled to choose options with reduced SFA and cholesterol. After 12 months, LDL-C was reduced by 12.8%. This reduction is appreciably less than that achieved in the metabolically controlled study, which is probably due to dietary compliance. The authors reported a significant correlation between total dietary adherence and change in LDL-C, and by 12 months, the majority of subjects had returned to an omnivorous diet (59 of 66).

When the individual components of the portfolio diet were evaluated, subjects were most compliant for almonds (79%) and plant sterol–enriched margarine (67%), whereas compliance for viscous fiber and soy protein was 55% and 51%, respectively. Despite these challenges, 32% of subjects experienced LDL-C reductions of >20%. The results of this study demonstrate the difficulty of adhering to a plant-based diet in a free-living setting. However, for subjects who do achieve this, the portfolio diet is particularly effective at lowering LDL-C. For other individuals, a focus on the incorporation of individual components (such as almonds or plant sterol–enriched margarine) may be most efficacious, particularly as plant sterols were identified as the primary LDL-C–lowering dietary component of the portfolio diet.[18]

In addition to effects on LDL-C, the portfolio diet targets other CVD risk factors, such as LDL particle size and C-reactive protein (CRP) level. The portfolio diet significantly reduces small LDL-C subfractions <25.5 nm (–0.69 mmol/L); this effect is comparable to that achieved by statins and greater than that by a Step II diet alone and translates to a 19% reduction in 13-year risk for CHD.[19] Interestingly, this study reported that baseline CRP levels predicted LDL-C particle size change in response to the portfolio diet. Individuals with plasma CRP levels <3.0 mg/L at baseline showed significant reductions in LDL-C particle <25.5 nm concentration, with no change in individuals with CRP levels >3.0 mg/L. When individuals with high CRP levels (>3.5 mg/L) were removed from the analysis, CRP level was significantly reduced by statins (16%) and portfolio diet (24%) but not by the Step II diet (15%).[20] These outcomes illustrate the importance of therapeutic interventions, such as the portfolio diet, that address multiple CVD risk factors, both traditional and emerging.

DASH and DASH-Sodium Trials

The DASH trial was a randomized controlled feeding intervention that evaluated the effects of three dietary patterns on blood pressure, lipids, and lipoproteins.[13,21] The DASH dietary pattern, which is rich in fruits and vegetables (8 to 10 servings/day) and low-fat dairy products (2 or 3 servings/day), includes whole grains, legumes, fish, and poultry and is limited in added sugars and fats. It is high in dietary fiber (~30 g/day), magnesium, potassium, and calcium and low in total fat (27% of total calories), SFA (<7% of total calories), and cholesterol (150 mg/day). In this study, 459 adults with mildly elevated blood pressure (SBP <160 mm Hg and DBP 80 to 95 mm Hg) were randomized to consume a Western diet (control diet; 48% carbohydrate, 15% protein, 37% total fat, 16% SFA), a fruits and vegetables diet (which provided more fruits and vegetables and fewer snacks and sweets than in the control diet but otherwise had a similar macronutrient distribution), or the DASH diet for 8 weeks. Sodium intake (3000 mg/day) was similar across all diets, and body weight remained constant throughout the intervention.

Compared with a Western diet, the DASH diet lowered SBP and DBP by –5.5 mm Hg and –3.0 mm Hg, respectively.[13] It also reduced total cholesterol (–9.5%), LDL-C (–9.1%), and HDL-C (–9.2%), with no change in TG.[21] Smaller reductions in blood pressure were observed in subjects consuming the fruits and vegetables diet (SBP, –2.8 mm Hg; DBP, –1.1 mm Hg); total cholesterol, LDL-C, HDL-C, and TG did not change. Stratified by hypertension status, the DASH diet reduced SBP and DBP by –11.6 mm Hg and –5.3 mm Hg, respectively, in stage 1 hypertensives (SBP >140 mm Hg, DBP >90 mm Hg, or both), with less dramatic effects in normotensive individuals (SBP/DBP, –3.5/–2.2 mm Hg).[22] The most substantial reductions were observed in hypertensive African Americans; the DASH diet reduced SBP by –13.2 mm Hg and DBP by –6.1 mm Hg.[22]

Additional hypotensive benefits can be achieved by following a DASH diet with further reductions in sodium. The DASH-Sodium trial compared the hypotensive effects of three levels of sodium restriction (high, 3200 mg/day; intermediate, 2300 mg/day; and low, 1500 mg/day) within a Western or DASH diet.[23] In both the Western and DASH diets, sodium restriction progressively lowered blood pressure; however, the effect of sodium on blood pressure was more pronounced in subjects following the Western than the DASH dietary pattern (Fig. 16-1). From highest to lowest sodium level, the reduction in SBP/DBP was 6.7/3.5 mm Hg on the Western diet and 3.0/1.6 mm Hg on the DASH diet.

For each level of sodium restriction, the DASH diet elicited lower blood pressure responses than the Western diet did, with the lowest blood pressure observed in subjects consuming the DASH diet with the lowest sodium level. The hypotensive effects of sodium restriction alone or with the DASH diet were consistent across several subgroups, including African Americans, hypertensive individuals (SBP ≥140 mm Hg or DBP ≥90 mm Hg), older adults (>45 years), and women, with mean reductions of 9.6 to 11.6 mm Hg for SBP and 4.7 to 5.7 mm Hg for DBP.[24]

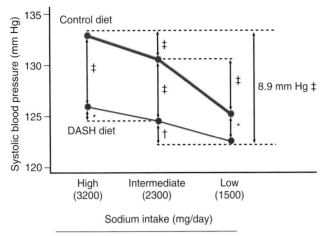

FIGURE 16-1 Change in systolic blood pressure in the DASH-Sodium trial. *(Modified from Sacks FM, Svetkey LP, Vollmer WM, et al: Effects on blood pressure of reduced dietary sodium and the Dietary Approaches to Stop Hypertension [DASH] diet. N Engl J Med 344:3, 2001. Copyright © 2001 Massachusetts Medical Society. All rights reserved.)*

Mediterranean-Style Diets

The Mediterranean diet is a whole food–based dietary pattern that has been associated with a reduced incidence of CVD and its associated risk factors.[25] This dietary pattern is representative of the traditions of Crete, Greece, and southern Italy in the 1960s, when the incidence of chronic disease was substantially lower than that of other countries. Key components of this dietary pattern include olive oil as the principal dietary fat source, abundant plant foods (fruits, vegetables, grains, cereals, nuts, and seeds), fish and shellfish, dairy in low to moderate amounts, poultry, eggs, and limited amounts of red meat and sweets. Moderate wine consumption (one or two 5-ounce glasses/day for men and one 5-ounce glass/day for women) also was allowed.

The cardioprotective benefits of the Mediterranean diet may in part be attributed to its nutrient profile, low SFA and high MUFA (from olive oil), and high fiber and phytosterol intake (>400 mg/day) from plants. Several clinical intervention trials have been undertaken to evaluate the benefits of the Mediterranean diet on CVD risk; however, comparisons among studies are challenging as each trial has differed with respect to nutrient profile and the specific foods used to implement the diet.

Lyon Diet Heart Study

The Lyon Diet Heart Study demonstrated that a Mediterranean-type diet, rich in α-linolenic acid, was more effective than a modified-fat diet in secondary prevention of coronary events.[26] This study randomized 605 post–myocardial infarction patients to consume either a Mediterranean-type diet (30% of total calories from fat, 8% from SFA, 13% from MUFA, and 5% from PUFA and 203 mg/day of cholesterol) or a modified-fat diet consistent with a Step I diet with a mean follow-up of 46 months. Patients in the Mediterranean-type diet intervention group received instructions from the study dietitian and cardiologist to increase their intake of bread, fish, and root and green vegetables; to consume fruit daily; to eat less meat (beef, lamb, and pork to be replaced with poultry); and to replace butter and cream with margarine supplied by the study. The fatty acid composition of the margarine was similar to that of olive oil, except that it was higher in linoleic acid (16.4% versus 8.6% kcal) and α-linolenic acid (4.8% versus 0.6% kcal). Control group subjects followed a diet that provided 34% of calories from fat,

12% from SFA, 11% from MUFA, and 6% from PUFA and 312 mg/day of cholesterol. After 48 months, subjects consuming the Mediterranean-type diet (n = 219) had a 50% to 70% lower risk of mortality from heart disease than did subjects consuming a low-fat diet (n = 204). These outcomes occurred despite similar plasma lipids and lipoproteins, blood pressure, body mass index, and smoking status in the two groups, indicating that other risk factors, such as thrombogenesis, are involved in coronary protection.

Medi-RIVAGE Study

The Mediterranean Diet, Cardiovascular Risks and Gene Polymorphisms (Medi-RIVAGE) study is a 12-month, parallel dietary intervention trial designed to compare the effects of a Mediterranean-type diet and a low-fat diet on CVD risk factors.[27] The low-fat diet was based on AHA guidelines and aimed for a total fat intake of <30% of total calories with equal contributions (10% each) from SFA, MUFA, and PUFA. A higher dietary fat intake (35% to 38% of total calories) was recommended for subjects in the Mediterranean-type diet arm, with an emphasis on MUFA (18% to 20% of total calories) from olive oil. SFA and PUFA each contributed 10% of total calories. The low-fat and Mediterranean-type diets were similar in their relative contributions from protein (~15%), carbohydrate (~55% to 60%), and cholesterol (<300 mg/day). However, the Mediterranean-type diet was higher in fiber (25 g/day compared with 20 g/day in the low-fat group) and allowed two glasses of wine per day for men and one glass for women. Alcohol was to be avoided in the low-fat group.

After 3 months of intervention, both groups (total n = 212) had similarly reduced their total fat, SFA, and cholesterol intake.[28] The only macronutrient that differed between the groups was MUFA, which was higher in the Mediterranean-type diet group (15.6%) than in the low-fat diet group (13.4%). Significant reductions in total cholesterol were observed in both groups (Mediterranean-type diet, −7.5%; low-fat diet, −4.5%), with a trend toward reductions in LDL-C (Mediterranean-type diet, −11.4%; low-fat diet, −5.0%). Compared with baseline, both groups showed a decrease in triglycerides, glucose, and insulin, although these did not differ between groups. This lack of distinction between the two diets is not surprising given their similar macronutrient composition at 3 months of intervention.

PREDIMED Study

The Prevención con Dieta Mediterránea (PREDIMED) study is an ongoing multicenter clinical trial designed to evaluate the effects of a Mediterranean diet on the primary prevention of CVD in 7000 asymptomatic subjects (*www.predimed.org*). Men (55 to 80 years) and women (60 to 80 years) with diabetes or three or more major cardiovascular risk factors will be randomized to consume either a low-fat diet (total fat <30%, based on AHA dietary guidelines) or a Mediterranean-type diet supplemented with either 30 g/day of mixed nuts (15 g walnuts, 7.5 g hazelnuts, and 7.5 g almonds) or 1 L/week of olive oil. Participants will be observed for a median duration of >5 years and evaluated for primary clinical outcomes (cardiovascular death, myocardial infarction, and stroke).

A pilot group of 772 participants (339 men, 433 women) was evaluated for changes in lipids and lipoproteins, blood pressure, and glucose after 3 months of intervention.[29] Compared with the low-fat group, the Mediterranean diet with nuts reduced total cholesterol by 6.2 mg/dL and TG by 13 mg/dL. HDL-C was increased by 2.9 mg/dL and 1.6 mg/dL on the Mediterranean diet with olive oil and nuts, respectively. Both diets also produced favorable changes in SBP/DBP (nuts, −7.1/−2.6 mm Hg; olive oil, −5.9/−1.6 mm Hg) and glucose concentration (nuts, −5.4 mg/dL; olive oil, −7.0 mg/dL) compared with the low-fat diet. Although it appears that a

Mediterranean diet is advantageous, the results of the PRE-DIMED study should be interpreted with caution as both Mediterranean intervention groups received intensive behavioral counseling and nutrition education intervention, whereas the low-fat group received simple dietary advice only.

Dietary Patterns That Emphasize Specific Macronutrients

OmniHeart Trial

The OmniHeart trial was a three-period, 6-week crossover, controlled feeding study involving 164 prehypertensive or stage 1 hypertensive subjects that evaluated the cardiovascular benefits of substituting SFA with carbohydrate, protein, or unsaturated fat.[30] Each diet period emphasized the intake of one specific macronutrient—high carbohydrate (58% of total calories), moderate to high protein (25% of total calories, 50% of which were from plant proteins), or high unsaturated fat (31% of total calories, predominantly MUFA)—thereby enabling direct comparison of these macronutrients. Increasing unsaturated fat intake caused a 9.2% reduction in TG and a 10.3% reduction in LDL-C but no change in HDL-C (–0.6%). Protein elicited a similar response, although this was more effective than unsaturated fat in lowering TG (–16.2%) and LDL-C (–11.0%) but also caused a modest reduction in HDL-C (–5.2%).

In comparison, the high-carbohydrate diet was effective only in reducing LDL-C (–9.0%) and was accompanied by a reduction in HDL-C (–2.8%). Compared with baseline, all diets decreased SBP (–8.2, –9.5, –9.3 mm Hg, carbohydrate, protein, and unsaturated fat, respectively) and DBP (–4.1, –5.2, –4.8 mm Hg, carbohydrate, protein, and unsaturated fat, respectively); however, on stratification by hypertension status, subgroup analysis showed that in both prehypertensive and stage 1 hypertensive subjects, the moderate- to high-protein and unsaturated-fat diets reduced blood pressure more than the carbohydrate diet did. On the basis of these results, partial replacement of SFA with protein or unsaturated fat appears to be more effective than replacement with carbohydrate in improving lipids and reducing blood pressure.

DIETARY STRATEGIES FOR WEIGHT LOSS

Dietary guidelines issued by the U.S. government and other prominent health organizations, such as the U.S. Department of Agriculture (USDA)[11] and the AHA,[31] emphasize the importance of achieving and maintaining a healthy body weight for prevention of chronic disease. However, there continues to be some debate as to the most effective way to achieve weight loss and subsequently to maintain weight loss. In the design of dietary interventions for weight loss, one important aspect that has emerged in recent years is the relative contribution of fat, protein, and carbohydrate. The macronutrient profile of a diet may facilitate dietary adherence, thereby promoting weight loss, and it could promote specific changes in blood pressure, lipids, and lipoproteins as the results from the OmniHeart trial suggest. Thus far, clinical intervention trials have yielded mixed results, and studies are often thwarted by small subject numbers and inadequate follow-up; few studies have evaluated outcomes beyond 1 year, when weight regain is most pronounced. The following section discusses CVD risk factor outcomes from select weight loss trials. In reviewing these dietary effects, it is important to acknowledge the role that additional strategies, such as physical activity and behavioral therapy, may have played in improving weight loss outcomes and preventing weight regain.[32]

Low-Fat Diets

Diabetes Prevention Program and Look AHEAD

The Diabetes Prevention Program (DPP) compared the efficacy of three treatments in preventing type 2 diabetes and metabolic syndrome in individuals at high risk on the basis of elevated fasting blood glucose concentration and impaired glucose tolerance.[33,34] Participants (n = 3234) were randomized to receive either standard lifestyle recommendations (written material advising lifestyle changes) plus placebo or metformin (850 mg twice daily) or intensive lifestyle intervention (education curriculum covering diet, exercise, and behavior modification), which aimed to achieve 7% weight loss through a healthy low-calorie, low-fat diet (<25% of total calories) and 150 min/wk of physical activity.

At 1 year, participants in the lifestyle intervention group had lost substantially more weight (~6.5 kg) than either the placebo (~0 kg) or metformin (~2.2 kg) groups. Weight loss was a strong predictor of reduced diabetes incidence; each kilogram of weight lost contributed to a 16% reduction in risk,[35] and diabetes incidence was 58% and 31% lower in the lifestyle and metformin groups compared with placebo. Intensive lifestyle therapy also was most effective in preventing the development of metabolic syndrome; at 3 years, incidence rates for metabolic syndrome were 38% for the lifestyle group, 47% for metformin, and 53% for placebo. The low-fat diet (as part of the lifestyle intervention) reduced the prevalence of the individual criteria of metabolic syndrome (i.e., HDL-C was increased; TG, blood pressure, and glucose levels were reduced).

The Look AHEAD (Action for Health in Diabetes) trial, an ongoing multicenter clinical trial modeled on the DPP, is investigating the long-term effects (11.5-year follow-up) of an intensive lifestyle intervention program in 5145 individuals with type 2 diabetes.[36] This lifestyle intervention program is similar to the DPP in that it combines dietary modification, behavior therapy (based on programs employed in DPP), and increased physical activity (175 min/wk moderate exercise) to achieve a 10% (minimum 7%) reduction in body weight. However, whereas the DPP focused on fat restriction to decrease calories, the primary method to achieve weight loss in Look AHEAD is through calorie restriction (although fat intake is considered; total fat <30% of calories, SFA <10% of calories). In addition to the "toolbox" of adherence strategies used in the DPP, Look AHEAD encourages weight loss medication (orlistat) for patients who do not meet their weight loss goals in the first 6 months. Patients randomized to the intensive lifestyle program are compared with those receiving usual care of diabetes support and education.

After 1 year of intervention, participants in the lifestyle group lost 8.6% of body weight, compared with 0.7% in the diabetes support and education group. Substantially greater improvements in glucose control (–21.5 mg/dL), SBP and DBP (–6.8/–3.0 mm Hg), TG (–30.3 mg/dL), and HDL-C (+3.4 mg/dL) were observed in the lifestyle intervention group. The primary determinants for weight loss success were greater self-reported physical activity, attendance at sessions, and consumption of meal replacements.[37]

PREMIER Trial

Recommendations for hypertension management include weight loss, sodium reduction (<100 mg/day), increased physical activity (180 min/wk), moderate alcohol consumption for those who drink alcohol (two drinks/day for men and one drink/day for women), and the DASH diet[6] (see Table 16-3 for approximate reductions in SBP). The PREMIER (Prevention of Myocardial Infarction Early Remodeling) trial evaluated the effectiveness of these management strategies in combination, with or without the DASH diet, on blood

TABLE 16–3 | **JNC 7 Report: Lifestyle Changes and Associated Reductions in Systolic Blood Pressure[6]**

Modification	Recommendation	SBP Reduction (Range)
Weight reduction	Maintain normal body weight (body mass index 18.5 to 24.9 kg/m²)	5-20 mm Hg/10 kg
Adopt DASH eating plan	Consume a diet rich in fruits, vegetables, and low-fat dairy products with a reduced saturated fatty acid and total fat content	8-4 mm Hg
Dietary sodium restriction	Reduce sodium intake to no more than 100 mmol/day (2.4 g sodium or 6 g sodium chloride)	2-8 mm Hg
Physical activity	Engage in regular aerobic physical activity such as brisk walking (at least 30 min/day, most days)	4-9 mm Hg
Moderation of alcohol consumption	Limit consumption to no more than 2 drinks/day (e.g., 24 oz beer, 10 oz wine, 3 oz 80-proof whiskey) in most men, no more than 1 drink/day in women and lighter weight men	2-14 mm Hg

16

pressure and weight loss.[38] Individuals with untreated, elevated blood pressure (SBP 120 to 159 mm Hg and DBP 80 to 95 mm Hg) were randomized to one of three intervention groups: advice only (control), established lifestyle recommendations (as described before), or DASH plus established lifestyle recommendations. At 6 months, weight loss was significantly greater in the established (−4.9 kg) and DASH plus established (−5.8 kg) groups compared with control (−1.1 kg), although both groups experienced weight regain by 18 months (+1.1-1.5 kg).[39]

Similar group treatment effects were observed at 6 months for blood pressure, which was reduced by 10.5/5.5 mm Hg in the established group and 11.1/6.4 mm Hg in the DASH plus established group. However, by 18 months, these changes were not significantly different compared with those observed in the advice-only group, although this is likely due to the unexpected improvement in several lifestyle factors in this group rather than to the limited effectiveness of the interventions.

Fasting insulin, glucose, lipid, and lipoprotein changes have been reported in a secondary analysis that stratified individuals according to presence of metabolic syndrome.[40] This analysis revealed highly variable effects that differed by treatment group and metabolic syndrome status. The established and DASH plus established interventions compared with the control group lowered total cholesterol in subjects with (−7.98 and −5.91 mg/dL, respectively) and without (−7.41 and −7.06 mg/dL, respectively) metabolic syndrome. The established intervention reduced TG in both subpopulations (log transformed: with metabolic syndrome, −0.16 mg/dL; without, −0.10 mg/dL) but lowered LDL-C only in individuals without metabolic syndrome (−6.89 mg/dL). The DASH plus established group also lowered LDL-C only in individuals without metabolic syndrome (−5.13 mg/dL). Neither intervention influenced HDL-C. Insulin resistance (as

determined by homeostasis model assessment) was improved by both the established and DASH plus established interventions, in subjects with and without metabolic syndrome. Despite such variable effects on independent cardiovascular risk factors, these combined behavioral interventions have a profound influence on CHD risk. Compared with advice alone, the established and DASH plus established interventions reduced estimated 10-year CHD risk by 12% and 14%, respectively.[41]

Very-Low-Fat Diets

Multicenter Lifestyle Demonstration Project

The Multicenter Lifestyle Demonstration Project (MLDP) was a comprehensive intervention that examined the combined effects of diet, exercise, stress management, and group support on medical and psychosocial characteristics in 440 patients with coronary artery disease (CAD).[42] The dietary component of MLDP consisted of a low-fat (<10% of total calories), high-carbohydrate (70% to 75% of total calories), moderate-protein (15% to 20% of calories), predominantly vegetarian diet that emphasized fruits, vegetables, grains, legumes, and soy products. Animal products were limited to nonfat dairy products and egg whites. Other intervention components included participation in 1 hr/day of stress management, 3 hr/wk of moderate exercise (according to American College of Sports Medicine guidelines for CAD patients), and twice-weekly group support sessions.

At 3 months, subjects had reduced their total fat intake to ~7% of total calories and increased time spent in physical activity (~3 to 4.0 hr/wk) and stress management (~5.5 hr/wk). Body weight was reduced by 4 kg in men and 4.6 kg in women. Significant improvements in other cardiovascular risk factors were achieved; blood pressure (men, −5/−5 mm Hg; women, −6/−3 mm Hg), total cholesterol (men, −18 mg/dL; women, −14 mg/dL), and LDL-C (men, −19 mg/dL; women, −17 mg/dL) were reduced. These behavioral changes and cardiovascular risk factor improvements remained at 12 months. Subjects experienced a substantial reduction in angina (from 42% at baseline to 20% at 1 year for men and 53% to 27% in women), and 20% of individuals with diabetes mellitus reduced their use of glucose-lowering medication.[43]

Popular Diets

The majority of popular diets promote extreme carbohydrate or fat restriction to achieve weight loss. Three recent trials have evaluated the efficacy of popular diets (with significantly different macronutrient compositions) for weight loss and improvements in CVD risk factors. In a 12-month randomized controlled trial involving 160 overweight or obese individuals, Dansinger and colleagues[44] compared the effects of four popular diets: Atkins (very low carbohydrate), Zone (macronutrient balance), Ornish (very low fat), and Weight Watchers (calorie control). The low-carbohydrate diets (Atkins and Zone) achieved the greatest short-term (2 month) reductions in TG, glucose concentration, and DBP, whereas reductions in LDL-C and total cholesterol were observed in the higher carbohydrate groups (Ornish and Weight Watchers). These between-group differences were not present at 12 months. Short- and long-term weight loss (2-month range, 3.5 to 3.8 kg; 12-month range, 2.1 to 3.3 kg) were similar for all diet groups; the magnitude of weight loss was strongly associated with dietary adherence rather than with diet type.

The A to Z weight loss study[45] compared the effects of three popular diets (Ornish, Zone, and Atkins) and a conventional low-fat (<10% of energy from SFA), high-carbohydrate diet (Lifestyle, Exercise, Attitudes, Relationships, and Nutrition [LEARN]) on weight loss in 311 premenopausal women.

Women following the Atkins diet achieved greater short-term weight loss (2 months, 4.4 kg; 6 months, 5.6 kg) than did women following the Ornish, Zone, and LEARN diets, although only differences between the Atkins (4.7 kg) and Zone (1.6 kg) diets were significant at 12 months. Again, for each diet, weight loss was associated with greater dietary adherence.[46] By 12 months, the Atkins diet produced substantially greater changes in TG (−29.3 mg/dL, significantly different from Zone), HDL-C (+4.9 mg/dL, significantly different from Ornish), SBP (−7.7 mm Hg, significantly different from all other diets), and DBP (−4.4 mm Hg, significantly different from Ornish).

Sacks and colleagues[47] recently published outcomes from the Preventing Overweight Using Novel Dietary Strategies (POUNDS LOST) study, a 2-year trial comparing the effects of three primary macronutrients on weight loss. The study design allowed direct comparison of two levels of fat (20% and 40%) and protein (15% and 25%) intake and a dose-response evaluation of carbohydrate (35% to 65% of total calories). All diets were reduced by 750 kcal from baseline and were standardized to include 8% of calories from SFA, at least 20 g/day of dietary fiber, and ≤150 mg of cholesterol per 1000 kcal.

Weight loss was similar for participants in each group at 6 months (~6 kg, 7% of initial weight) and 2 years (2.9 to 3.6 kg, intention-to-treat analysis). Dietary analysis showed that participants were equally compliant across the four diets; however, in general, participants failed to attain the required calorie reduction and specific macronutrient targets. At 2 years, LDL-C decreased more with the low-fat diets and the highest carbohydrate diet than with the high-fat diets or the lowest carbohydrate diet. The lowest carbohydrate diet increased HDL-C compared with the highest carbohydrate diet. TG, insulin, and blood pressure levels were reduced by all diets (except the highest carbohydrate diet did not lower insulin). These changes are not entirely consistent with the macronutrient effects reported in the OmniHeart study, which may be due to the substantial macronutrient overlap between the diet groups. The results of these three studies collectively suggest that calorie restriction is more important than macronutrient distribution for weight loss; however, modification of macronutrient intake may be instrumental for targeting of cardiovascular risk factors such as elevated blood pressure, lipids, and lipoproteins.

KEY FOODS AND NUTRIENTS

The dietary patterns showcased in the previous section have a number of similarities: a focus on weight control; reduced intake of SFA, trans-fat, and cholesterol; and increased intake of fruits, vegetables, whole grains, protein, and reduced-fat dairy. In combination with a heart-healthy dietary pattern, these components have profound effects on blood pressure, lipids, and lipoproteins; yet there is evidence for their independent benefits. The inclusion of other dietary factors, such as increased intake of unsaturated fats, sterols and stanols, soy protein, and fiber, allows greater flexibility for personal preference and additional targeting of specific risk factors. For patients who require a gradual introduction to dietary change, incorporation of one or a few of these strategies may elicit beneficial effects on CVD risk factors.

Key Dietary Components

Cholesterol, Saturated Fatty Acids, and Trans–Fatty Acids

Diets high in SFA and trans-fat contribute to elevated levels of total cholesterol in the blood.[48] Sources of SFA are high-fat and processed meats, poultry or game (with skin), high-fat dairy products, butter, gravy, and palm and coconut oils.

Trans-fats are commonly found in processed and fast foods, shortening, margarines, fried tortilla chips, commercial or store-bought baked goods, salad dressings, candy, and energy bars. Substituted for carbohydrate, SFA increase both LDL-C and HDL-C, whereas trans-fats increase LDL-C and decrease HDL-C.[49]

Dietary cholesterol is naturally present in any animal food source. Dietary cholesterol raises LDL-C; however, its effects are less than those of SFA and trans–fatty acids.[50] Whereas total fat per se does not affect LDL-C (i.e., the guidelines are built on specific fatty acid recommendations to meet LDL-C goals), it is prudent to control total fat intake within current recommended ranges (because fat is the most concentrated energy source in the diet) to achieve weight loss. Weight loss can lower LDL-C by 5% to 8%.[9] Therefore, reduction of the intake of foods that increase LDL-C or decrease HDL-C is an important part of a heart-healthy diet. Furthermore, replacement of SFA and trans-fats in the diet with healthful foods that include unsaturated fats, proteins, or complex carbohydrates will accentuate the health benefits gained by the reduction in SFA and trans-fat intake.[30]

Fruits and Vegetables

Fruits and vegetables are nutrient-dense and low-calorie foods that are an essential part of a healthy diet. The most abundant nutrients in fruits and vegetables are vitamin C, vitamin E, vitamin A, folate, fiber, and potassium. Many of these are antioxidants and reduce oxidative stress in the body by neutralizing damaging free radicals. Studies using antioxidants in supplement form have not been able to demonstrate their value for reduction of CVD risk[51]; interactions between the antioxidants and other nutrients in the whole food may be necessary to have the desired effect. For protection against chronic disease and to maintain good health, the Dietary Guidelines for Americans, 2005[11] recommends consumption of at least 4.5 cups (nine servings) of fruits and vegetables per day for the reference 2000-calorie level (higher or lower amounts can be consumed for other calorie levels).

Fruit and vegetable intake consistently has been associated with decreased risk for CVD in epidemiologic studies. In an analysis of more than 125,000 participants from the Nurses' Health Study and the Health Professionals Follow-up Study, persons who ate eight or more servings of fruits and vegetables per day had a 20% reduction in risk of CHD (RR = 0.80; 95% CI, 0.69-0.93) compared with those who ate three or fewer servings per day.[52] With each increase in serving of fruit or vegetable per day, the risk of CHD decreased by 4%; leafy greens and fruits and vegetables high in vitamin C contributed most to this effect. Consistent with these data, the Physicians' Health Study found that men who consumed two or more servings per day of vegetables had a 22% lower risk of CHD than did men who ate less than one serving per day (RR = 0.77; 95% CI, 0.60-0.98).[53] Furthermore, for each additional serving of vegetables per day, CHD risk was reduced by 17% (RR = 0.83; 95% CI, 0.71-0.98). In the Women's Health Study, fruit and vegetable consumption was inversely associated with CVD risk (RR = 0.45 for highest versus lowest quintile of intake; 95% CI, 0.22-0.91).[54] Whereas the epidemiologic studies are convincing, there is limited clinical evidence because of the paucity of controlled, nutritional prevention trials varying only in fruit and vegetable intake.[55] Nevertheless, the DASH dietary intervention studies (described earlier) clearly demonstrate the benefit of increasing fruit and vegetable intake for the management of hypertension.[13] In addition, because of their low energy density, fruits and vegetables may play a key role in weight loss and maintenance.[56]

Whole Grains

Whole grains are defined as intact, ground, cracked, or flaked fruit of the grains whose principal components—the starchy endosperm, germ, and bran—are present in the same relative proportions as they exist in the intact grain.[57] If they are processed correctly, wheat, oats, barley, brown and wild rice, corn, rye, and sorghum are whole grains. To be considered a good source of whole grains, foods must be at least 51% whole grain by weight per reference amount commonly consumed and have a whole-grain source as the first ingredient on the food label. Whereas all whole grains have many bioactive components (such as fiber, folate, phenolic compounds, lignan, and sterols), each type of grain has different levels of these components, and therefore they cannot be equated. For example, oats, barley, bulgur, rye, and whole wheat are high in fiber (>10 g fiber/100 g food), whereas brown rice, wild rice, corn, and sorghum are lower in fiber (<8 g fiber/100 g food).[57] Soluble and insoluble fibers have different effects on and mechanisms of action in improving CVD risk factors. Specifically, soluble (viscous) fiber has been shown to reduce LDL-C levels,[58] whereas insoluble fiber may increase short-chain fatty acid synthesis, which reduces endogenous cholesterol production.[59] See the section on soluble (viscous) fiber for additional information.

Similar to fruit and vegetable intake, epidemiologic studies have shown whole-grain intake to be protective against CHD. These associations may be due to the various vitamins (B and E), minerals (calcium, magnesium, potassium, phosphorus, selenium, manganese, zinc, and iron), phytochemicals (such as fiber), phenolic compounds, and phytoestrogens (lignans) found in whole grains. An analysis of the Health Professionals Follow-up Study, which included more than 40,000 men, found an inverse association between higher habitual whole-grain intake and incidence of CHD (HR = 0.82; 95% CI, 0.70-0.96); indeed, there was a 6% decrease in CHD risk with every increase of 20 g in daily whole-grain intake (95% CI, 0%-13%).[60] Higher intakes of whole grains (lowest versus highest quartiles) have been associated with a lower incidence of metabolic syndrome, fasting plasma glucose concentration, and body mass index in older adults.[61] Although it appears that whole-grain intake is associated with a reduced risk for CVD, these results may be confounded by lifestyle characteristics. Jensen and colleagues[60] reported that individuals who had higher intakes of whole grains generally had a lower body mass index, were more physically active, had less hypertension, and ate more fruits and vegetables and protein.

Randomized controlled trials designed to evaluate whether whole grains are protective against CVD generally have shown a beneficial effect, albeit with mixed results. In a recent review of both observational and intervention studies, 11 of 15 intervention studies reported that whole grains were protective against CVD events.[57] Of note is that oats and barley were more effective than whole wheat in improving CVD risk factors such as total cholesterol, LDL-C, and blood pressure. The difference in effect between the whole grains is attributed to the compositions of the grain, as oats and barley are higher in fiber, especially insoluble fiber, and have unique phytochemicals. NCEP ATP III recommends 5 to 10 g/day of soluble (viscous) fiber to lower LDL-C by 3% to 5%.[9] Currently, the *Dietary Guidelines for Americans, 2005* advise that at least half of the recommended grain servings come from whole grains and state that "consuming at least 3-ounce equivalents of whole grains per day can reduce the risk of CHD, may help with weight maintenance, and may lower risk for other chronic diseases."[11] Switching from refined to whole-grain products is becoming increasingly easier as more products are being made with whole grains; thus, three servings of whole grains per day is an attainable health goal.

Heart-Healthy Protein Sources

Reduction of meat intake, especially red meat, is often recommended to decrease intake of SFA and cholesterol. Animal products are the predominant source of SFA and cholesterol in the diet, but processed foods like fast food and snack foods contribute significantly.[62] Animal products also are excellent sources of protein, and increased protein intake, from plant or animal sources, has been linked to lower blood pressure and TG, higher HDL-C, and a healthier body weight.[30,63] Protein is low in energy density (4 kcal/g), and therefore replacement of fatty acids with protein may help with satiety and weight loss.

The Nurses' Health Study found that women with a higher protein intake (~24% of total energy) were at reduced risk for ischemic heart disease (RR = 0.75; 95% CI, 0.61-0.92) compared with women with lower intakes (~14% of total energy).[64] However, in an analysis of the nutritional profiles of 18- to 30-year old men and women from the Coronary Artery Risk Development in Young Adults (CARDIA) study, adults who ate meat or poultry less than once per week had lower serum TG, total cholesterol, and LDL-C levels than did those who ate meat more frequently, although the low-meat intake group also had a lower body mass index, increased reported physical activity, and a diet higher in fiber and certain vitamins.[63,65]

Until recently, there have been no specific recommendations for intake of protein from animal products with regard to CVD health, other than to consume reduced-fat products. Protein intake of 10% to 20% of total daily calories from either plant or animal sources is widely accepted[63]; The Dietary Guidelines For Americans, 2010, however, emphasizes the importance of plant-based dietary patterns for CVD risk reduction.[65a] For all individuals, the challenge is finding good sources of low-fat protein in the diet. Meats that are high in SFA are high-fat red meat cuts and processed meats, such as hamburger, hotdogs, and bacon, and these should be limited in the diet. Full-fat dairy products also are a rich source of SFA. Low-SFA animal protein sources are lean meats (beef, ham), poultry (trimmed and without skin), fish, cottage cheese, and reduced-fat milk and dairy products. Plant protein may provide a healthier protein alternative in the diet as it is lower in SFA. Common sources of plant protein are soy, seeds, nuts, and legumes.

Reduced-Fat Dairy

Overall, epidemiologic studies of dairy intake have shown no association with increased risk for CVD, even when full-fat dairy products high in SFA are consumed.[66] However, an analysis of the contribution of different fatty acids to CVD risk showed that an increase in the ratio of high-fat to low-fat dairy products increased risk for CVD in the Nurses' Health Study.[67] This suggests either a protective or minimal effect of low-fat dairy products on CVD risk. In a meta-analysis and systematic review of dairy consumption, high dairy consumers had a 29% reduced risk for metabolic syndrome and 14% reduced risk for type 2 diabetes compared with low dairy consumers.[68]

The main mechanism by which low-fat dairy products reduce CVD risk is by lowering of blood pressure, although increased insulin sensitivity, decreased inflammation, and weight loss are emerging benefits. Dairy products are an excellent dietary vehicle for protein, vitamin A, vitamin D, vitamin B_{12}, riboflavin, niacin, potassium, phosphorus, magnesium, and calcium. Increased intake of calcium, potassium, magnesium, and dairy protein has been shown to decrease blood pressure.[2,69] According to a meta-analysis of 12 intervention studies, short peptide chains found in milk improve CVD outcomes by decreasing SBP (–4.8 mm Hg) and DBP (–2.2 mm Hg).[70] These nutrients appear to be more effective when they are provided as foods, such as low-fat dairy products, than when they are taken in supplement form.[51] This is a key principle of dietary patterns such as the DASH diet, which incorporate low-fat or nonfat dairy products within a heart-healthy diet.[13]

By virtue of reducing the amount of fat in dairy products, it is possible to enjoy the nutritional benefits and to limit SFA intake. Replacement of high-SFA dairy foods, such as butter and ice cream, with low-fat options, like yogurt and skim milk, provides complete proteins and essential vitamins and minerals for the maintenance of health. Incorporation of low-fat dairy products into any diet increases nutritional quality without markedly increasing calories; however, consumption of fat-free dairy foods may limit the amount of fat-soluble vitamins that are absorbed. The DASH diet and TLC advise two or three servings of low-fat dairy products per day to achieve a healthy diet and to decrease risk of CVD.[31]

Other Beneficial Dietary Components

Soluble (Viscous) Fiber

Foods rich in water-soluble (viscous) fiber include oats, barley, legumes, some fruits (such as apples and pears), and psyllium seeds. Soluble fibers have been recognized since the 1960s as having lipid-lowering effects, and there is growing evidence to support an association between intake of whole grains and decreased incidence of fatal and nonfatal CHD.[60] The cholesterol-reducing effects of whole-grain foods such as oats and barley are associated with the soluble fiber component, beta-glucan.

Although not all individual studies have found positive outcomes, several meta-analyses concluded that regular consumption of oats can lower cholesterol.[58,71] Brown and colleagues[58] reported that 3 g/day of soluble fiber decreases total cholesterol and LDL-C by ~0.13 mmol/L. Health claims for cholesterol reduction have been approved for both oat fiber[72] and barley fiber.[73] The exact mechanism by which water-soluble fibers lower serum LDL-C levels is not known. Water-soluble fibers may interfere with lipid or bile acid metabolism[74] by downregulating genes involved in fatty acid synthesis and transport.[75] Oat bran with beta-glucan also has been shown to increase exclusion of bile acids.[76] Another suggested mechanism is the inhibition of hepatic cholesterol synthesis by fermentation products.[77] Short-chain fatty acids also may regulate hepatic AMP-activated protein kinase in the liver, thereby stimulating fatty acid oxidation and inhibiting lipogenesis and glucose production.[78] As well as having beneficial effects on lowering cholesterol, soluble fiber may reduce CVD risk by acting on glucose regulation and insulin sensitivity, body weight, inflammation, endothelial function, and blood pressure.[79-81]

Sterols and Stanols

Several observational studies have evaluated the relationship between plasma phytosterol levels and CVD risk, with two large cohorts reporting a reduced risk of coronary events in individuals with higher plasma sitosterol levels.[82,83] However, the Prospective Cardiovascular Münster (PROCAM) study reported a 1.8-fold increased risk of coronary events in subjects with sitosterol levels in the upper quartile compared with the lower three quartiles.[84] CVD effects may be due to the ability of stands to inhibit cholesterol absorption, thereby reducing plasma total cholesterol and LDL-C.[85] The greatest benefit is observed in individuals with unfavorable lipid profiles.[86] In a meta-analysis of supplementation studies, subjects with familial hypercholesterolemia who consumed fat spreads enriched with 2.3 g of phytosterols per day significantly reduced their total cholesterol and LDL-C by 7% to 11% and 10% to 15%, respectively, compared with control.[87]

At least 1 g/day of phytosterols is necessary to obtain a significant 5% to 8% LDL-C reduction.[88] A meta-analysis of 41 trials showed that 2 g/day of stanols or sterols reduced LDL-C by 10%, although higher intakes added little to this

effect.[89] This outcome supports the level of plant sterols or stanols (2 g/day) recommended in the NCEP ATP III guideline for lowering of LDL-C.[9] As the typical daily dietary intake of phytosterols in Western cultures ranges from 150 to 400 mg/day, it is necessary to consider dietary supplementation to reach the recommended intake.[89] Phytosterols are well tolerated, can easily be incorporated into a range of foods, and are not associated with any adverse effects.[90]

Efficacy is similar for sterols and stanols, but food form may substantially affect LDL-C reduction.[91] Sterols incorporated into fat spreads, mayonnaise and salad dressing, milk, and yogurt appear to be more advantageous at lowering LDL-cholesterol than in food products such as croissants and muffins, orange juice, nonfat beverages, cereal bars, and chocolate. The effects of sterols or stanols on LDL-C lowering are additive with diet or drug interventions; previous studies reported greater reductions in LDL-C when statin use is combined with foods enriched with plant sterols or stanols[92,93] compared with doubling of the dose of statins.[94] Despite such positive effects on cholesterol reduction, sterols have not been shown to be effective at reducing oxidative stress and endothelial dysfunction,[95] and there are mixed reports in the literature on their ability to reduce low-grade inflammation.[95,96]

Soy Protein

There has been extensive investigation about the effects of soy protein on lipids and lipoproteins during the past decade.[88] On the basis of the outcomes of a meta-analysis of 38 trials,[97] the U.S. Food and Drug Administration approved the following health claim: "25 g of soy protein a day, as part of a diet low in saturated fat and cholesterol, may reduce the risk of heart disease."[98] The average consumption of soy protein in the studies reviewed in the Anderson meta-analysis[97] was 47 g/day, which is almost double that recommended in the U.S. health claim. This amount was associated with significant reductions in total cholesterol (9.3%), LDL-C (12.9%), and TG (10.5%). The magnitude of reduction in total cholesterol and LDL-C was associated with baseline levels, such that individuals with higher serum cholesterol levels at baseline had the greatest reduction.

More recent meta-analyses have concluded that the extent of cholesterol reduction is much less than was initially reported.[99] In 2006, the AHA assessed 22 randomized controlled trials since 1999 and found that consumption of isolated soy protein with isoflavones resulted in a small reduction in LDL-C (3%) but had no effect on HDL-C, TG, lipoprotein(a), or blood pressure.[100] Taku and associates[101] found no effect of soy isoflavones (without concurrent consumption of soy protein) on total cholesterol and LDL-C in menopausal women. Randomized controlled trials conducted since these reviews have reported similar, modest reductions in LDL-C or total cholesterol.[102,103] The variable effect of soy isoflavones on cholesterol reduction may be due to the different doses of isoflavones used[104] or may be related to the ability of individuals to convert the isoflavone daidzein into equol through bacterial fermentation in the large intestine.[105] However, evidence to support the latter is not consistent.[106]

Unsaturated Fats

Both the quantity and quality of dietary fat influence the risk of CVD. Intake of unsaturated fats, namely, MUFA and PUFA, is associated with a more favorable CVD risk profile as they reduce total cholesterol and LDL-C[107] and may improve blood pressure regulation.[108] Clinical studies have since found that when it is substituted for SFA in the diet, MUFA reduces total cholesterol and LDL-C and relative to carbohydrate increases HDL-C and reduces TG.[30,107] MUFAs principally are found in vegetable oils such as olive, rapeseed (canola), and peanut oils as well as in poultry, meat, nuts, and avocado.

PUFAs are composed of two classes: omega-6 (n-6) fatty acids, found in vegetable oils and nuts, and omega-3 (n-3) fatty acids, found in fatty fish, such as salmon and anchovies, and in walnuts and flax. Three of the main dietary sources of unsaturated fat and their effects on CVD risk are discussed in greater detail.

Fish (and Fish Oil). Numerous epidemiologic and clinical studies have demonstrated associations between increased intake of marine-derived n-3 fatty acids from fish or fish oil and reduced incidence of CVD.[109] In the U.S. Health Professionals Study, regular fish consumption was associated with a significantly lower risk of total CVD in men.[110] It also is associated with reduced progression of coronary artery atherosclerosis in men and women with CAD,[111,112] reduced risk of CAD and total mortality in diabetic women,[113] reduced risk of thrombotic infarction,[114] and reduced risk of cardiac arrhythmias resulting in sudden cardiac death.[115] The n-3 fatty acids in fish are the key nutrients thought to be responsible for the benefits described, although it is plausible that the interactions between these fats and other nutrients, including trace elements, vitamins, and amino acids, also may be important to reduce CVD risk.[116] Marine-derived n-3 fatty acids elicit cardioprotective benefits through mechanisms such as antiarrhythmic effects, TG and blood pressure lowering, reduced platelet function and aggregation, improved vascular function, and decreased inflammation. Consequently, regular consumption of marine-derived n-3 fatty acids is recommended for healthy persons and those with CHD.

Recommendations to eat fish and other seafood are included in most national dietary guidelines because of their beneficial health effects. Seafood is an important dietary source of marine-derived n-3 fatty acids, protein, vitamins D and E, and iodine. Seafood is low in SFA. Because of this unique nutrient profile, regular fish consumption is recommended as part of a healthy diet. The American Dietetic Association and Dietitians of Canada recommend two servings of fish per week, preferably fatty fish.[117] The AHA also recommends two servings of oily fish per week (equivalent to 400 to 500 mg of marine-derived n-3 fatty acids per day) for optimal health.[31,118] However, fish intake in Western cultures is typically very low (about one fish meal per week) and frequently is from sources that are low in marine-derived n-3 fatty acids (e.g., shrimp, cod, and other white fish).[119]

Oily fish rich in marine-derived n-3 fatty acids include tuna, salmon, mackerel, sardines, herring, and trout. The amount of eicosapentaenoic acid (EPA) and docosahexaenoic acid (DHA) is shown for a variety of fish species (both fresh and farmed) in Table 16-4. Farmed fish provides as much EPA and DHA as wild fish do, if not more. As the fatty acid profiles of diets for farmed fish can be closely monitored, their lipid is less affected by seasonal variations and location of catch. Moreover, the EPA and DHA content of farmed salmon and trout has been reported to be ~15% higher than that of wild catch.[118] The nutritional content of farmed fish has been found to be at least as beneficial as that of wild fish in terms of prevention of CVD, with additional benefits arising from greater control over pollutants (including heavy metals and polychlorinated biphenyls).[120]

Fish oil supplementation is advised when dietary intake of fish is low, particularly for individuals with a history of CHD or hypertriglyceridemia (TG levels >500 mg/dL). The AHA recommends 1 g/day or 2 to 4 g/day of marine-derived n-3 fatty acids for individuals with CHD or hypertriglyceridemia, respectively, under supervision of a physician. On the basis of data from a meta-analysis of 72 placebo-controlled trials, this level of supplementation (3 to 4 g/day) will reduce TG levels by 25% to 35%, with more substantial reductions in hypertriglyceridemic individuals.[121] The mechanism by which marine-derived n-3 fatty acids lower TG levels is unclear. There is evidence that they increase TG clearance

TABLE 16-4	Amount of Marine-Derived n-3 Fatty Acids (EPA and DHA) in Select Species of Fish	
Fish	**EPA and DHA (g/3-ounce Serving, Edible Portion)**
Tuna	
Light, canned in water, drained	0.26
White, canned in water, drained	0.73
Fresh	0.24-1.28
Sardines	0.98-1.70
Salmon	
Chum	0.68
Sockeye	0.68
Pink	1.09
Chinook	1.48
Atlantic, farmed	1.09-1.83
Atlantic, wild	0.9-1.56
Mackerel	0.34-1.57
Herring	
Pacific	1.81
Atlantic	1.71
Trout, rainbow	
Farmed	0.98
Wild	0.84

Data from Kris-Etherton PM, Harris WS, Appel LJ: Fish consumption, fish oil, omega-3 fatty acids, and cardiovascular disease. *Circulation* 106:2747, 2002.

from circulating very-low-density lipoprotein (VLDL) particles by increasing lipoprotein lipase activity. Some studies have shown a small increase in HDL-C (11% to 14%) with high doses of marine-derived n-3 fatty acids (4 g/day).[122]

Nuts. Nuts are energy- and nutrient-dense foods that have macronutrient and micronutrient profiles that are cardioprotective.[123,124] They have a healthy fatty acid profile, containing high levels of the 18-carbon MUFA oleic acid and low amounts of SFA, and some varieties (e.g., brazil nuts, pine nuts, and walnuts) are important sources of n-6 and n-3 fatty acids.[125] Nuts are rich in plant protein, fiber, and micronutrients (such as potassium, calcium, and magnesium). Tree nuts and peanuts also contain numerous phytochemicals, including phytosterols, tocopherols, antioxidant vitamins, and flavonoids (e.g., resveratrol in peanuts).[125,126] These constituents may reduce oxidative stress and counteract any potential pro-oxidative effects of the unsaturated fatty acids and in turn elicit potential antiatherogenic effects.

Frequent consumption of nuts or peanut butter has been associated with decreased CVD risk in several large, prospective cohort studies including the Adventist Health Study,[127] the Iowa Women's Health Study,[128] the Nurses' Health Study,[129] and the Physicians' Health Study.[130] Collectively, the evidence suggests that the risk of CHD is 37% lower for people consuming nuts more than four times per week compared with those who never or seldom consume nuts, with an average reduction of 8.3% for each weekly serving of nuts.[131] However, the evidence supporting a reduced risk of heart failure with regular nut consumption is less strong.[132]

A range of cardiometabolic health benefits are likely to contribute to these epidemiologic observations.[124] Both tree nuts and peanuts have lipid-lowering properties. Clinical studies have demonstrated that when nuts are included as part of a healthy diet that is low in SFA and cholesterol, they elicit favorable effects on lipids and lipoproteins compared with a control diet (typically either a low-fat diet or an average American/Western diet). The primary outcome is a reduction in plasma LDL-C and TG, along with an increase in HDL-C.[133] Nuts also have been found to reduce oxidation and inflammation and to improve glucose regulation and endothelial function,[134-136] and they may be protective against the development of hypertension.[137] However, this area of research is less advanced than that for lipids and lipoproteins, and consequently the effects of tree nuts and peanuts on oxidative stress, inflammation, and blood pressure generally are inconsistent.

Olive Oil. Epidemiologic and clinical studies have reported that the traditional Mediterranean-style diet is associated with significantly lower mortality from CAD.[26] Although it is difficult to isolate individual dietary factors, cumulative evidence suggests that olive oil, which is the primary source of fat used by Mediterranean populations, may play a key role in the observed cardiovascular benefit.[138] Olive oil is rich in oleic acid (typically about 75% of total fatty acids), and virgin (unrefined) olive oil contains a significant amount of antioxidants (α-tocopherol) and phytochemicals.

There are multiple mechanisms by which olive oil may affect the development of atherosclerosis. The unsaturated fatty acid profile of olive oil lowers LDL-C and increases HDL-C. It also contains polyphenols that reduce oxidative stress as they are able to scavenge free radicals and to protect LDL from oxidation. Results of the EUROLIVE study[139] have provided evidence for the protective role of phenolic compounds from olive oil on in vivo LDL oxidation in humans. Regular olive oil consumption also has been shown to be protective against hypertension in some epidemiologic studies, including the Seguimiento Universidad de Navarra (SUN) study[140] and the Greek European Prospective Investigation into Cancer and Nutrition (EPIC) study.[141]

Omega-6/Omega-3 Ratio. Both n-3 and n-6 fatty acids are essential PUFAs that are necessary for proper growth and development. The n-3 fatty acids in cell membranes produce anti-inflammatory, pro-resolutary eicosanoids, whereas n-6 fatty acids are the precursors to proinflammatory prostaglandins.[142] Eicosanoids and prostaglandins affect a number of pathways associated with CVD progression, such as thrombosis, inflammation, and vasoconstriction. Thus, it is hypothesized that a balanced ratio of n-6/n-3 fatty acids will attenuate inflammatory and vasoconstrictive pathways, resulting in lowered CVD risk. However, a number of studies have reported no relationship between n-6 fatty acid intake and inflammatory markers.[143,144] Moreover, in a study conducted by Ferrucci and coworkers,[145] certain proinflammatory markers were decreased and an anti-inflammatory marker was elevated with increasing serum levels of arachidonic acid (a metabolite of linoleic acid) as well as serum levels of EPA and DHA.

As noted by Harris,[146] the concept of balancing the n-6/n-3 fatty acids ratio in the diet is conceptually flawed. It overlooks the absolute levels and chain-length differences within each fatty acid class. For example, an n-6/n-3 ratio of 5 can be achieved by vastly different amounts of linoleic acid and n-3 PUFAs, the latter of which could include widely differing amounts of α-linolenic acid, EPA, and DHA. Currently, it is estimated that the ratio of n-6/n-3 fatty acids in the Western diet is 15 to 20:1. All current recommendations advocate that n-3 intake be increased. Thus, the n-6/n-3 ratio as a measure of diet quality is flawed for a number of reasons. The best advice is to consume adequate amounts of both n-6 and n-3 fatty acids, thereby focusing on the total amounts of both n-3 and n-6 fatty acids. The AHA supports the recommendation that at least 5% to 10% of total daily calories be provided by n-6 fatty acids, and individuals who consume less may have a higher risk for CVD events.[147] Thus, a higher PUFA diet that emphasizes both n-3 and n-6 fatty acids is the current recommendation to reduce CVD risk.

Red Wine and Alcohol

Epidemiologic studies have indicated that moderate red wine consumption is associated with reduced rates of cardiovascular morbidity and mortality.[148] There has been some debate as to whether the protective effects of red wine result from the alcohol content or the antioxidant properties of the flavonoids found at high concentrations in some red wines.[149] The protective effect of alcohol may partly be attributed to alcohol-associated increases in HDL-C by stimulation of reverse cholesterol transport pathways[150] and reduced platelet aggregation.[148] Although the concentration of antioxidant polyphenols is higher in red than in white wine, some studies have found that both types of wine[151] as well as other alcoholic beverages[152,153] provide a similar extent of cardiovascular protection.

The role of resveratrol (*trans*-3,4′,5-trihydroxystilbene) also is being investigated. Resveratrol is a natural polyphenol present in red wine that has purported atheroprotective properties.[154] There is evidence that resveratrol can act through several mechanisms, including inhibition of platelet aggregation[155] and smooth muscle cell proliferation,[156] reduction of LDL oxidation, and enhanced cholesterol efflux.[157] Several studies have reported a decrease in the susceptibility of LDL particles to oxidation in healthy subjects after the daily consumption of 375 to 400 mL of red wine for 2 weeks,[158] although this was not reported in another study.[159] The inconsistency of these results may be related to variations in the polyphenol concentration of the red wine used in the different studies. It is unclear whether polyphenols from red wine can provide additional cardiovascular benefits beyond that of ethanol alone.

FOOD-BASED DIETARY RECOMMENDATIONS

Food guides translate recommendations on nutrient intake into food-based guidance. Such information is presented in a framework that promotes the selection of a variety of foods that together provide a nutritionally adequate diet. These dietary principles help people to maintain and improve their health and to reduce their risk for major chronic diseases. Graphic presentations, such as the pyramid, often are used to convey important guidelines about food intake to help consumers implement dietary recommendations.

MyPyramid

MyPyramid was developed by the USDA to incorporate recommendations from the *Dietary Guidelines for Americans, 2005*.[160] The MyPyramid symbol conveys a personalized approach to diet and physical activity for healthy individuals and promotes several key messages: variety, proportion, and moderation (Fig. 16-2). The colored bands (orange, green, red, blue, purple) represent the five food groups of the pyramid (grains, vegetables, fruits, milk, meat and beans) and oils (yellow) and suggest that a variety of foods be consumed from each of these groups. The varying width of each band serves as a guide to the proportion of food that should be consumed from each band (actual serving size can be determined by visiting *www.MyPyramid.gov*). For example, the greater width of the orange grain band indicates that people should eat more foods from this group than from the purple meat and beans group. Moderation is represented by the narrowing of each food group toward the top of the pyramid. Foods that are lower in total or solid fats and added sugars form the base of the pyramid and should be chosen more often. The narrower area represents foods that are high in solid fats and added sugar. People who are more active can consume more of these foods. Other features of MyPyramid designed to assist consumers in choosing a healthier diet include ranges in the number of servings from each group (to account for different energy and nutrient levels by age, sex, and activity level) and expression of serving sizes in household measures and amounts commonly eaten (e.g., one serving of milk is 1 cup).

DASH Pyramid

The DASH diet is low in total fat, SFA, and cholesterol and rich in fruits, vegetables, and reduced-fat dairy products. It also includes whole grains, nuts, fish, and poultry and therefore promotes foods that are rich in blood pressure–lowering nutrients, such as potassium, magnesium, calcium, and fiber. It is reduced in sodium, red meat, sweets, added sugars, and fats. The DASH diet has been modified by the Center for Science in the Public Interest's *Nutrition Action Healthletter*[161] to fit the Food Guide Pyramid model first published by the USDA in 1992. The DASH pyramid has a base of fruits and vegetables (8 to 10 servings/day) and grains (preferably whole grains, 7 to 8 servings/day) at level 2. Level 3 is shared by low-fat dairy (2 to 3 servings/day) and seafood, poultry, and lean meat (0 to 2 servings/day). Legumes, nuts, and seeds (1 serving/day) and oils (for healthy fats; 2 to 3 servings/day) make up level 4. The final level is composed of sweets (no more than 5 servings/week). Lower salt foods should be chosen from all categories. The DASH pyramid developed by the Center for Science in the Public Interest also provides examples of servings for each food group, which may be a useful resource for meal planning.

Mediterranean Pyramid

The Mediterranean dietary pattern emphasizes vegetables, fruits, grains, nuts and seeds, unsaturated fats (primarily from olive oil), fish, and shellfish. Poultry, eggs, and dairy are eaten regularly but in low to moderate amounts. Intake of red meat and sweets is limited. Use of herbs and spices is encouraged as they add flavor to foods and reduce the need to add salt or fat during cooking. These food choices are reflected in the Mediterranean Diet Pyramid (Fig. 16-3).[162] Regular, moderate wine consumption (one or two 5-ounce glasses/day for men

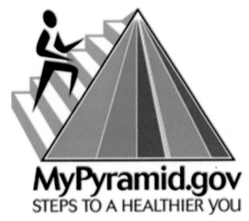

FIGURE 16-2 The USDA Food Guide Pyramid.

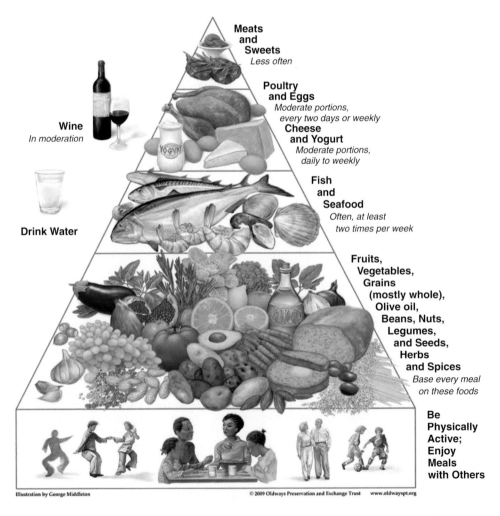

FIGURE 16-3 The Mediterranean Diet Pyramid. (© *Oldways Preservation and Exchange Trust.*[162])

and one 5-ounce glass/day for women), participation in daily physical activity, adequate water intake, and enjoying meals in the company of others are also important components. The visual display of the Mediterranean Diet Pyramid assists consumers in determining portion size and frequency of consumption of various foods; foods in the bottom section of the pyramid may be eaten in larger amounts and more often, whereas the portion size and frequency of consumption decline in the upper section of the pyramid.

SUPPLEMENTS

Dietary supplement use in the United States is increasing.[163] In the NHANES 1999-2000 survey, 52% of adults reported taking a dietary supplement in the last month, the most prominent of which were multivitamin and multimineral supplements (35% of individuals).[164] However, there are limited data supporting the use of nutritional supplements for CVD risk reduction, and some supplements may even have adverse effects.[51] Several prominent organizations have determined that the evidence for the prevention of CVD by vitamin E, selenium, and multivitamins (containing folic acid) is inconclusive,[165] and the AHA also does not recommend antioxidant supplementation for CVD risk reduction.[166] The following section briefly discusses the evidence for use of select dietary supplements to improve CVD risk factors and to reduce CVD mortality and morbidity.

Niacin

Niacin is a broad-spectrum lipid-regulating drug that has well-established effects on CVD risk. In pharmacologic doses of 2 to 4 g/day, niacin reduces total cholesterol (20%), TG (25% to 50%), VLDL (45%), LDL-C (5% to 25%), and lipoprotein(a) (40%) and increases HDL-C (25% to 50%).[167,168] Niacin, alone or in combination with other lipid-lowering agents, significantly reduces total mortality and coronary events, retards progression, and induces regression of atherosclerosis.[167-169] However, outcomes from the HDL–Atherosclerosis Treatment Study (HATS) suggest that antioxidant vitamins (800 IU vitamin E, 1000 mg vitamin C, 25 mg beta carotene, and 100 μg selenium) may blunt any beneficial effects of simvastatin and niacin treatment on lipids and stenosis regression.[169] Niacin (1 to 2 g/day) currently is recommended for the treatment of elevated TG and LDL-C levels and low HDL-C.[9] Despite such broad beneficial effects on lipids and atherosclerosis, the clinical use of niacin is limited in some patients because of adverse effects, such as flushing and hepatotoxicity. Over-the-counter formulations that promote "no flushing" vary widely in quality and do not have the same benefits as prescription niacin. For this reason and because of the risks associated with niacin supplementation beyond standard vitamin doses, it is advised that only prescription niacin be considered and administered under medical supervision.

B Vitamins (Folate, B$_6$, B$_{12}$)

Elevated levels of homocysteine are associated with an increased risk for ischemic heart disease, stroke, peripheral vascular disease, and thrombosis, possibly because of increased oxidative stress, thrombosis, and vascular dysfunction. Several factors, including an inadequate dietary intake of B vitamins (folic acid, B$_{12}$, and B$_6$), have been associated with increased homocysteine concentrations, and supplementation with B vitamins may therefore provide a means to reduce CVD risk.

A meta-analysis of 25 randomized controlled trials reported that 0.2 to 5.0 mg/day of folic acid reduced homocysteine by 13% to 25%.[170] The addition of vitamin B$_{12}$ (mean dose, 0.4 mg/day) produced a further 7% reduction, but vitamin B$_6$ had no effect. However, several long-term clinical trials demonstrate that homocysteine lowering with B vitamin supplementation does not necessarily translate to reduced risk for stroke, myocardial infarction, or cardiovascular mortality. The VISP (Vitamin Intervention for Stroke Prevention) trial randomized 3680 adults with nondisabling cerebral infarction to receive either high-dose (2.5 mg folic acid, 400 μg B$_{12}$, and 25 mg B$_6$) or low-dose (20 μg folic acid, 6 μg B$_{12}$, and 200 μg B$_6$) B vitamins.[171] Despite a reduction in homocysteine after 2 years of follow-up, there was no effect on vascular outcomes.

The NORVIT (Norwegian Vitamin) trial evaluated clinical outcomes during 3.5 years in 3749 patients with a recent myocardial infarction.[172] Patients were randomized to one of four groups and received daily folic acid (0.8 mg) and B vitamins (40 mg B$_6$ and 0.4 mg B$_{12}$), folic acid (0.8 mg/day) and B$_{12}$ (0.4 mg), B$_6$ (40 mg), or placebo. Despite a reduction in homocysteine, there was no significant effect on recurrent CVD in any of the treatment groups. A trend toward an increased risk was observed in the combined folic acid and B vitamin group (B$_6$ and B$_{12}$). The Heart Outcomes Prevention Evaluation (HOPE) 2 study reported that daily supplementation with folic acid (2.5 mg), B$_6$ (50 mg), and B$_{12}$ (1 mg) in patients with diabetes or vascular disease for 5 years had no effect on overall cardiovascular mortality or combined cardiovascular risk.[173] Other studies also have reported no effect of folic acid (0.8 mg), B$_{12}$ (0.4 mg), or B$_6$ supplementation (40 mg) on cardiovascular events or total mortality in patients with CAD.[174] Homocysteine lowering (18.5% more than placebo) with a combination supplement of folic acid (2.5 mg), B$_6$ (50 mg), and B$_{12}$ (1 mg) also failed to reduce cardiovascular events in high-risk women.[175]

Antioxidants (Vitamin E, Vitamin C, Carotenoids)

Antioxidants from dietary sources, such as vitamin E, vitamin C, and carotenoids, have been studied for their potential to protect against oxidative stress. Prospective cohort studies have shown promising inverse associations between intake of antioxidants, particularly carotenoids and vitamin E, and risk for CVD.[176] However, findings from clinical intervention studies have reported null and even adverse effects on CVD outcomes from intake of large doses of single and combination antioxidant supplements.[166,177-179] A recent meta-analysis of 68 randomized trials with 232,606 participants reported that antioxidant supplements taken daily or on alternate days (mean duration, 2.7 years) had no significant effect on mortality.[177] However, when only low-bias risk trials (those with high methodologic quality) were included in the analysis, beta carotene (mean dose, 17.8 mg), vitamin A (mean dose, 20,219 IU), and vitamin E (mean dose, 569 IU/day), singly or combined, significantly increased mortality. There was no effect of vitamin C (mean, 488 mg) or selenium (mean, 99 μg) on cardiovascular mortality. These outcomes are supported by more extensive analysis as part of a *Cochrane Review* of antioxidant supplementation and mortality prevention.[178] The AHA advocates the consumption of antioxidant-rich foods such as fruits, vegetables, whole grains, and nuts rather than antioxidant supplements for CVD risk reduction.[31]

Vitamin D

Vitamin D is a fat-soluble vitamin that is produced by skin exposed to ultraviolet B rays or is found in foods like salmon and fortified milk. The main function of vitamin D is to maintain appropriate calcium and phosphorus levels in the blood through the regulation of calcium absorption from the diet, resorption from bones, and reabsorption in the kidneys. Recent evidence suggests that vitamin D also plays a role in neuromuscular function, immune function, blood pressure, and inflammation as well. Low levels of vitamin D in the blood are associated with increased risk for cancer, multiple sclerosis, and Parkinson disease.[180]

Thus far, clinical trials have not been able to prove causation, although there is plausible biologic and robust epidemiologic evidence to support the role of vitamin D in the prevention of CVD. A large cross-sectional study of patients who were referred for coronary angiography showed that those with vitamin D deficiency (<25 nmol/L) compared with those with optimal vitamin D levels (>75 nmol/L) had a hazard ratio of 2.84 (95% CI, 1.20-6.74) and 5.05 (95% CI, 2.13-11.97) for death by heart failure and sudden cardiac death, respectively.[181] In a prospective cohort study (Framingham Offspring cohort) of 1739 adults with no history of CVD, low levels of serum vitamin D ($\leq$15 ng/dL) were associated with an increased risk for cardiovascular events (HR, 1.62; 95% CI, 1.11-2.36) compared with those with normal vitamin D levels (>15 ng/dL).[182] This relationship was present in individuals with hypertension (2.13; 95% CI, 1.30-3.48) but not in those without hypertension (95% CI, 0.55-1.96). Overall, multiple meta-analyses show a strong link between low vitamin D status and increased CVD risk[183,184]; however, the intervention studies designed to test the effect of vitamin D supplementation on CVD outcomes currently are being conducted.

The sun provides much of the vitamin D needed by the body, and 5 to 10 minutes of exposure of bare face, arms, and hands per day should be sufficient to obtain the recommended dietary allowance for vitamin D (200 IU, for those younger than 50 years).[185] However, this conversion depends on a multitude of factors including skin color, time of year, location, and genetics. Currently, a committee from the Food and Science Board of the Institute of Medicine is reviewing the recent literature with regard to vitamin D recommendations and may increase the dietary reference intake in the coming year. Some experts now recommend 800 to 1000 IU/day of vitamin D_3 from supplements or diet for adults and children to avoid vitamin D deficiency when sunlight exposure is not sufficient.[186] Because the majority of vitamin D is from the sun and dietary records cannot capture vitamin D intake well, direct measures of serum vitamin D levels (25-hydroxyvitamin D) are important for diagnosis of insufficient or inadequate vitamin D status. Unfortunately, there has been difficulty in standardizing measurement methodology. This is problematic when trying to correlate vitamin D status with health outcomes, and additional research is needed to prove causation between vitamin D status and CVD.

AMERICAN HEART ASSOCIATION DIETARY GUIDELINES REVISION 2006

It is evident that healthy diet and lifestyle behaviors markedly decrease risk of CVD. Consequently, the AHA historically has been at the forefront of issuing diet and lifestyle recommendations for heart health. The most recent diet and lifestyle recommendations were issued in 2006.[31] The 2006 goals are presented in Box 16-1 and target major risk factors for CVD including overweight and obesity, abnormal lipids and lipoproteins, high blood pressure, high blood glucose levels, sedentary behavior, and exposure to tobacco products.

The AHA 2006 Diet and Lifestyle Recommendations are presented in Box 16-2 and target the major CVD risk factors. Achievement of a healthy body weight will reduce risk of

---

BOX 16-1 American Heart Association 2006 Diet and Lifestyle Goals for Cardiovascular Disease Risk Reduction

Consume an overall healthy diet.
Aim for a healthy body weight.
Aim for recommended levels of LDL-C, HDL-C, and triglycerides.
Aim for a normal blood pressure.
Aim for a normal blood glucose level.
Be physically active.
Avoid use of and exposure to tobacco products.

Reprinted from Lichtenstein AH, Appel LJ, Brands M, et al: Diet and lifestyle recommendations revision 2006: a scientific statement from the American Heart Association Nutrition Committee. *Circulation* 114:82, 2006. ©2006, American Heart Association, Inc.

BOX 16-2 American Heart Association 2006 Diet and Lifestyle Recommendations

Balance calorie intake and physical activity to achieve or maintain a healthy body weight.
Consume a diet rich in vegetables and fruits.
Choose whole-grain, high-fiber foods.
Consume fish, especially oily fish, at least twice a week.
Limit your intake of saturated fat to <7% of energy, *trans*-fat to <1% of energy, and cholesterol to <300 mg per day by:
   choosing lean meats and vegetable alternatives;
   selecting fat-free (skim), 1%-fat, and low-fat dairy products; and
   minimizing intake of partially hydrogenated fats.
Minimize your intake of beverages and foods with added sugars.
Choose and prepare foods with little or no salt.
If you consume alcohol, do so in moderation.
When you eat food that is prepared outside of the home, follow the AHA Diet and Lifestyle Recommendations.

Reprinted from Lichtenstein AH, Appel LJ, Brands M, et al: Diet and lifestyle recommendations revision 2006: a scientific statement from the American Heart Association Nutrition Committee. *Circulation* 114:82, 2006. ©2006, American Heart Association, Inc.

CVD and facilitate achievement of a recommended lipid and lipoprotein profile, blood pressure, and glucose level. Limiting SFA, *trans*–fatty acids, and cholesterol also will help achieve a recommended lipid and lipoprotein profile. Limiting sodium (<1500 mg/day) will help achieve a normal blood pressure. Fruit and vegetable, whole-grain, and fatty fish recommendations will decrease CVD risk by providing a mineral-rich, fiber-rich diet high in long chain n-3 fatty acids, all of which have been shown to be cardioprotective. Minimizing added sugar will help with calorie control as well. Moderating alcohol consumption can be of benefit to heart health.

Food-based recommendations consistent with the 2006 Diet and Lifestyle Recommendations are presented in Table 16-5. Specific food-based recommendations have been made for the DASH dietary pattern and the TLC diet that promote the AHA Diet and Lifestyle Recommendations 2006. These diets are comparable and recommend a dietary pattern that is high in vegetables and fruits, whole grains, fat-free or low-fat dairy products, lean meats and poultry, fish (preferably oily), nuts, seeds, legumes, and liquid vegetable oils.

	Eating Pattern			
Food Group	DASH	TLC	USDA Dietary Guidelines	Serving Size
Vegetables	4-5 servings/day	5 servings/day	5 servings/day	1 c raw leafy vegetables, ½ c cut-up raw or cooked vegetables, ½ c vegetable juice
Fruits	4-5 servings/day	4 servings/day	4 servings/day	1 medium fruit; ¼ c dried fruit; ½ c fresh, frozen, or canned fruit; ½ c fruit juice
Grains	6-8 servings/day	7 servings/day	7 servings/day	1 slice bread, 1 oz dry cereal, ½ c cooked rice or pasta
Fat-free or low-fat milk products	2-3 servings/day	2-3 servings/day	3 servings/day	1 c milk, 1 c yogurt, ⅕ oz cheese
Lean meats, poultry, fish	<6 oz/day	≤5 oz/day	5.5 oz/day	1 oz cooked
Nuts, seeds, legumes	4-5 servings/day	Counted in vegetable servings	Counted in lean meats, poultry and fish, and vegetable servings*	⅓ c, 2 tbsp peanut butter or seeds, ½ c dry beans or peas
Fats and oils	2-3 servings/day	Amount depends on daily calorie level	Liquid oils: amount depends on daily calorie level; Solid fats: counted in discretionary calorie allowance (~10% total kcal)	1 tsp soft margarine, 1 tbsp mayonnaise, 1 tsp vegetable oil, 2 tbsp salad dressing
Sweets and added sugars	≤5 servings/day	No recommendation	Counted in discretionary calorie allowance (~10% total kcal)	1 tbsp sugar, jelly, or jam; ½ c sorbet; 1 c lemonade

TABLE 16–5 | Examples of Dietary Patterns That Are Consistent with American Heart Association Dietary Guidelines*

*For daily calorie intake of 2000 kcal.

Modified from Lichtenstein AH, Appel LJ, Brands M, et al: Diet and lifestyle recommendations revision 2006: a scientific statement from the American Heart Association Nutrition Committee. *Circulation* 114:82, 2006. ©2006, American Heart Association, Inc.

AMERICAN HEART ASSOCIATION STRATEGIC IMPACT GOALS THROUGH 2020

The AHA 2020 Impact Goals are "to improve the cardiovascular health of all Americans by 20% while reducing deaths from cardiovascular diseases and stroke by 20%."[12] To meet this goal, the AHA recommends the consumption of an overall healthy dietary pattern that is consistent with a DASH-type eating plan. Key components include but are not limited to the following:

- Fruits and vegetables: ≥4.5 cups per day
- Fish: two or more 3.5-ounce servings per week (preferably oily fish)
- Fiber-rich whole grains (≥1.1 g of fiber per 10 g of carbohydrate): three or more 1-ounce equivalent servings per day
- Sodium: <1500 mg/day
- Sugar-sweetened beverages: ≤450 kcal (36 ounces) per week.

Secondary dietary goals that support cardiovascular health and are consistent with a DASH-like diet include the following:

- Nuts, legumes, and seeds: ≥4 servings per week
- Processed meats: none or ≤2 servings per week
- Saturated fat: <7% of total energy intake

SIMPLE STRATEGIES TO IMPLEMENT AND TO MAINTAIN HEALTHFUL DIETARY CHANGES

Behavior change is central to achievement of diet and lifestyle recommendations for heart health. Much research is being done to identify effective behavior change strategies, and there are some strategies that seem to work. It all starts with knowing if a patient is "ready" to make changes in a sustained way. If not, then work is needed to "get" the individual to a stage of change state. The Stages of Change model[187] is an integrative model of intentional behavior change. It is used to describe how people can achieve a desirable behavior or modify a problem behavior. In attempting to change a specific behavior, a person typically cycles through a series of five stages: pre-contemplation, contemplation, preparation, action, and maintenance. Identification of what stage an individual is in will assist in determining what techniques will be most successful in moving the individual to the next stage of change. Motivational interviewing is widely used in practice to evaluate stage of change and to enhance intrinsic motivation to change by exploring and resolving ambivalence.[188] In addition, motivational interviewing is effective at identifying reluctance to change and helps the individual "see" that needed change can be attained.

Presuming the individual is ready to change, important steps to follow include goal setting (ensuring that goals are realistic), self-monitoring strategies (such as keeping food records, body weight measurements), and ensuring that social support is available. These strategies promote self-efficacy (i.e., helping patients see that they can attain short-term goals and pursue longer term goals). Inherent to modifying behavior is that change strategies need to be individualized and monitored closely for behavior change to be sustained. We encourage readers to refer to a recent scientific statement published by the American Heart Association, which provides an excellent review of interventions to promote physical activity and dietary lifestyle changes for the reduction of CVD risk factors.[189]

NATIONAL AND COMMUNITY INITIATIVES AND RESOURCES

Many resources are available to the public to implement current diet and lifestyle recommendations for heart health. The government is actively promoting educational programs that promote heart health. Likewise, professional organizations have many programs available for different target groups. In addition, the private sector is committed to improving the health of Americans. Communities and work sites have ongoing programs that target heart health. Examples of programs available are presented here.

Federal Government

- *Dietary Guidelines for Americans, 2005.* The *Dietary Guidelines for Americans* is published jointly every 5 years by the Department of Health and Human Services and the USDA. The guidelines provide authoritative advice for people 2 years and older about how good dietary habits can promote health and reduce risk for major chronic diseases. They serve as the basis for federal food and nutrition education programs. Visit *http://www.health.gov/DietaryGuidelines/dga2005/document/default.htm.*
- *Dietary Guidelines for Americans,* 2010. Provides the most recent dietary guidelines for Americans. Visit *http://www.cnpp.usda.gov/dietaryguidelines.htm*
- *MyPyramid.gov.* MyPyramid offers personalized eating plans and interactive tools that help plan and assess healthy food choices based on the *Dietary Guidelines for Americans.* Visit *http://www.mypyramid.gov/.*
- Health and Human Services Small Step Adult and Teen program. Information is presented about steps to take to improve health and well-being. Visit *http://www.smallstep.gov/.*
- National Heart, Lung, and Blood Institute (NHLBI)
  - National Cholesterol Education Program. The goal of the NCEP is to reduce illness and death from CHD in the United States by reducing the percentage of Americans with high blood cholesterol. Through educational efforts directed at health professionals and the public, the NCEP aims to raise awareness and understanding about high blood cholesterol as a risk factor for CHD and the benefits of lowering cholesterol levels as a means of preventing CHD. Visit *http://www.nhlbi.nih.gov/about/ncep/.*
  - Hearts N' Parks program is a national, community-based program supported by the NHLBI and the National Recreation and Park Association that is designed to encourage heart-healthy lifestyles in communities. Visit *http://www.nhlbi.nih.gov/health/prof/heart/obesity/hrt_n_pk/index.htm.*
  - Seventh Report of the Joint National Committee on Prevention, Detection, Evaluation, and Treatment of High Blood Pressure. Updated guidelines for hypertension for the health care professional. The report provides new evidence for treating high blood pressure. Visit *http://www.nhlbi.nih.gov/guidelines/hypertension/jnc7full.htm.*
- Centers for Disease Control and Prevention
  - Healthy weight program is designed to help individuals achieve and maintain a healthy weight. Visit *http://www.cdc.gov/healthyweight/index.html.*
  - Nutrition program helps individuals follow a healthy diet. Visit *http://www.cdc.gov/nutrition/index.html.*
  - Physical activity program helps individuals learn about recommendations for active living. Visit *http://www.cdc.gov/physicalactivity/index.html.*
  - Cholesterol website provides information about blood cholesterol levels and risk of heart disease. Visit *http://www.cdc.gov/cholesterol/.*
- Food and Drug Administration, food labeling and nutrition programs. Information is presented about labeling requirements for foods under the Federal Food Drug and Cosmetic Act and its amendments. Included in this is information about the nutrition facts panel, health claims/qualified health claims, and nutrient content claims. Visit *http://www.fda.gov/Food/LabelingNutrition/default.htm.*

Professional Organizations

- American Heart Association
  - Heart-Healthy Grocery Shopping Made Simple program provides a tool for consumers to use that simplifies selection of heart-healthy foods at the supermarket. Visit *http://www.americanheart.org/presenter.jhtml?identifier=2115.*
  - Delicious Decisions program provides heart-healthy recipes online. Visit *http://www.americanheart.org/deliciousdecisions/jsp/home/home.jsp?_requestid=1884425.*
  - Start! program is a new daily walking program that is designed to improve fitness. Visit *http://www.startwalkingnow.org/.*
  - My Life Check assists individuals in assessing their current health status, and in establishing a customized action plan to improve heart health and quality of life. Visit *http://mylifecheck.heart.org/AboutUs.aspx?NavID=2&CultureCode=en-US.*
- American Dietetic Association website provides food and nutrition information for individuals of all ages. In addition, there is a link for consumers to find a registered dietitian. Visit *http://www.eatright.org/.*

Other Programs

Many local, regional, and state programs provide information about a healthy lifestyle. One example is the YMCA Activate America program that is designed to create and to sustain healthier communities. Ways to locate these programs include asking health professionals in the community, searching the Internet and print media, and calling the local or state public health office.

CONCLUSION

Clinical intervention trials have demonstrated the efficacy of diet intervention, notably by TLC and DASH, for treatment of elevated LDL-C and blood pressure. These dietary patterns are reduced in SFA and *trans*–fatty acids, cholesterol, and total fat and emphasize increased consumption of fruits and vegetables, whole grains, heart-healthy protein, and reduced-fat dairy. Additional LDL-C lowering is expected with the addition of plant sterols and stanols, unsaturated fatty acids, soy protein, and fiber. Such dietary approaches also improve the metabolic syndrome profile and beneficially affect nontraditional risk factors, such as markers of thrombosis and inflammation, LDL-C particle size, and apolipoproteins. The Mediterranean diet is another treatment strategy to improve CVD risk status.

Many of the dietary factors emphasized by the TLC, DASH, and Mediterranean diets are included in the *Dietary Guidelines for Americans, 2005, 2010.* These guidelines ensure that energy and nutrient requirements are met through foods, although the inclusion of fortified foods and supplements may afford greater dietary flexibility and help some individuals meet specific nutrient needs or target certain risk factors. However, it is important to carefully evaluate the efficacy of supplements promoted for CVD risk reduction. Certain dietary supplements, such as fish oil and niacin, have shown promising cardiovascular effects, but there is insufficient evidence for others (such as B vitamins and antioxidants). Clinicians should therefore encourage a food-based approach to CVD risk reduction.

Maintaining a healthy body weight is a key component of cardiovascular health. Many studies have demonstrated that dietary modification (specifically calorie restriction) is a key facilitator of weight loss, and modest changes in body weight

16

(–10%) are associated with improvements in LDL-C and blood pressure. Of recent interest has been the relative contribution of specific macronutrients to weight loss; however, data from large-scale clinical trials demonstrate that reduction in total calories is the single most important step for weight loss, although macronutrients may induce differential effects on cardiovascular risk factors. Whereas calorie restriction alone is effective for short-term weight loss, interventions that combine diet therapy and physical activity with continued professional support (including behavioral intervention, diet and physical activity counseling) are most efficacious in the long term.[32]

REFERENCES

1. Ford ES, Ajani UA, Croft JB, et al: Explaining the decrease in U.S. deaths from coronary disease, 1980-2000. N Engl J Med 356:2388, 2007.
2. Kris-Etherton PM: Adherence to dietary guidelines: benefits on atherosclerosis progression. Am J Clin Nutr 90:13, 2009.
3. Dall TM, Fulgoni VL, Zhang Y, et al: Potential health benefits and medical cost savings from calorie, sodium, and saturated fat reductions in the American diet. Am J Health Promot 23:412, 2009.
4. Mariotti S, Capocaccia R, Farchi G, et al: Age, period, cohort and geographical area effects on the relationship between risk factors and coronary heart disease mortality. 15-year follow-up of the European cohorts of the Seven Countries study. J Chronic Dis 39:229, 1986.
5. Stamler J, Wentworth D, Neaton JD: Is relationship between serum cholesterol and risk of premature death from coronary heart disease continuous and graded? Findings in 356,222 primary screenees of the Multiple Risk Factor Intervention Trial (MRFIT). JAMA 256:2823, 1986.
6. The Seventh Report of the Joint National Committee on Prevention, Detection, Evaluation, and Treatment of High Blood Pressure, Bethesda, Md, 2004, National Heart, Lung, and Blood Institute. NIH publication 04-5230.
7. Turnbull F, Neal B, Ninomiya T, et al: Effects of different regimens to lower blood pressure on major cardiovascular events in older and younger adults: meta-analysis of randomised trials. BMJ 336:1121, 2008.
8. Delahoy PJ, Magliano DJ, Webb K, et al: The relationship between reduction in low-density lipoprotein cholesterol by statins and reduction in risk of cardiovascular outcomes: an updated meta-analysis. Clin Ther 31:236, 2009.
9. Third Report of the National Cholesterol Education Program (NCEP) Expert Panel on Detection, Evaluation, and Treatment of High Blood Cholesterol in Adults (Adult Treatment Panel III). Final Report, Bethesda, Md, 2002, National Heart, Lung, and Blood Institute. NIH publication 02-5215.
10. Hackam DG, Anand SS: Emerging risk factors for atherosclerotic vascular disease: a critical review of the evidence. JAMA 290:932, 2003.
11. U.S. Department of Health and Human Services and U.S. Department of Agriculture: Dietary guidelines for Americans, ed 6, Washington, DC, 2005, U.S. Government Printing Office.
12. Lloyd-Jones DM, Hong Y, Labarthe D, et al: Defining and setting national goals for cardiovascular health promotion and disease reduction: the American Heart Association's strategic Impact Goal through 2020 and beyond. Circulation 121:586, 2010.
13. Appel LJ, Moore TJ, Obarzanek E, et al: A clinical trial of the effects of dietary patterns on blood pressure. DASH Collaborative Research Group. N Engl J Med 336:1117, 1997.
14. Grundy SM, Cleeman JI, Merz CN, et al: Implications of recent clinical trials for the National Cholesterol Education Program Adult Treatment Panel III guidelines. Arterioscler Thromb Vasc Biol 24:e149, 2004.
15. Jenkins DJ, Kendall CW, Faulkner D, et al: A dietary portfolio approach to cholesterol reduction: combined effects of plant sterols, vegetable proteins, and viscous fibers in hypercholesterolemia. Metabolism 51:1596, 2002.
16. Jenkins DJ, Kendall CW, Marchie A, et al: Direct comparison of a dietary portfolio of cholesterol-lowering foods with a statin in hypercholesterolemic participants. Am J Clin Nutr 81:380, 2005.
17. Jenkins DJ, Kendall CW, Faulkner DA, et al: Assessment of the longer-term effects of a dietary portfolio of cholesterol-lowering foods in hypercholesterolemia. Am J Clin Nutr 83:582, 2006.
18. Jenkins DJ, Kendall CW, Nguyen TH, et al: Effect of plant sterols in combination with other cholesterol-lowering foods. Metabolism 57:130, 2008.
19. Gigleux I, Jenkins DJ, Kendall CW, et al: Comparison of a dietary portfolio diet of cholesterol-lowering foods and a statin on LDL particle size phenotype in hypercholesterolaemic participants. Br J Nutr 98:1229, 2007.
20. Jenkins DJ, Kendall CW, Marchie A, et al: Direct comparison of dietary portfolio vs statin on C-reactive protein. Eur J Clin Nutr 59:851, 2005.
21. Obarzanek E, Sacks FM, Vollmer WM, et al: Effects on blood lipids of a blood pressure–lowering diet: the Dietary Approaches to Stop Hypertension (DASH) trial. Am J Clin Nutr 74:80, 2001.
22. Svetkey LP, Simons-Morton D, Vollmer WM, et al: Effects of dietary patterns on blood pressure: subgroup analysis of the Dietary Approaches to Stop Hypertension (DASH) randomized clinical trial. Arch Intern Med 159:285, 1999.
23. Sacks FM, Svetkey LP, Vollmer WM, et al: Effects on blood pressure of reduced dietary sodium and the Dietary Approaches to Stop Hypertension (DASH) diet. N Engl J Med 344:3, 2001.
24. Vollmer WM, Sacks FM, Ard J, et al: Effects of diet and sodium intake on blood pressure: subgroup analysis of the DASH-Sodium trial. Ann Intern Med 135:1019, 2001.
25. Giugliano D, Esposito K: Mediterranean diet and metabolic diseases. Curr Opin Lipidol 19:63, 2008.
26. de Lorgeril M, Salen P, Martin J-L, et al: Mediterranean diet, traditional risk factors, and the rate of cardiovascular complications after myocardial infarction: final report of the Lyon Diet Heart Study. Circulation 99:779, 1999.
27. Vincent S, Gerber M, Bernard MC, et al: The Medi-RIVAGE study (Mediterranean Diet, Cardiovascular Risks and Gene Polymorphisms): rationale, recruitment, design, dietary intervention and baseline characteristics of participants. Public Health Nutr 7:531, 2004.
28. Vincent-Baudry S, Defoort C, Gerber M, et al: The Medi-RIVAGE study: reduction of cardiovascular disease risk factors after a 3-mo intervention with a Mediterranean-type diet or a low-fat diet. Am J Clin Nutr 82:964, 2005.
29. Estruch R, Martinez-Gonzalez MA, Corella D, et al: Effects of a Mediterranean-style diet on cardiovascular risk factors: a randomized trial. Ann Intern Med 145:1, 2006.
30. Appel LJ, Sacks FM, Carey VJ, et al: Effects of protein, monounsaturated fat, and carbohydrate intake on blood pressure and serum lipids: results of the OmniHeart randomized trial. JAMA 294:2455, 2005.
31. Lichtenstein AH, Appel LJ, Brands M, et al: Diet and lifestyle recommendations revision 2006: a scientific statement from the American Heart Association Nutrition Committee. Circulation 114:82, 2006.
32. Franz MJ, VanWormer JJ, Crain AL, et al: Weight-loss outcomes: a systematic review and meta-analysis of weight-loss clinical trials with a minimum 1-year follow-up. J Am Diet Assoc 107:1755, 2007.
33. Knowler WC, Barrett-Connor E, Fowler SE, et al: Reduction in the incidence of type 2 diabetes with lifestyle intervention or metformin. N Engl J Med 346:393, 2002.
34. Orchard TJ, Temprosa M, Goldberg R, et al: The effect of metformin and intensive lifestyle intervention on the metabolic syndrome: the Diabetes Prevention Program randomized trial. Ann Intern Med 142:611, 2005.
35. Hamman RF, Wing RR, Edelstein SL, et al: Effect of weight loss with lifestyle intervention on risk of diabetes. Diabetes Care 29:2102, 2006.
36. Pi-Sunyer X, Blackburn G, Brancati FL, et al: Reduction in weight and cardiovascular disease risk factors in individuals with type 2 diabetes: one-year results of the Look AHEAD trial. Diabetes Care 30:1374, 2007.
37. Wadden TA, West DS, Neiberg RH, et al: One-year weight losses in the Look AHEAD study: factors associated with success. Obesity 17:713, 2009.
38. Appel LJ, Champagne CM, Harsha DW, et al: Effects of comprehensive lifestyle modification on blood pressure control: main results of the PREMIER clinical trial. JAMA 289:2083, 2003.
39. Elmer PJ, Obarzanek E, Vollmer WM, et al: Effects of comprehensive lifestyle modification on diet, weight, physical fitness, and blood pressure control: 18-month results of a randomized trial. Ann Intern Med 144:485, 2006.
40. Lien LF, Brown AJ, Ard JD, et al: Effects of PREMIER lifestyle modifications on participants with and without the metabolic syndrome. Hypertension 50:609, 2007.
41. Maruthur NM, Wang NY, Appel LJ: Lifestyle interventions reduce coronary heart disease risk. Results from the PREMIER trial. Circulation 119:2026, 2009.
42. Koertge J, Weidner G, Elliott-Eller M, et al: Improvement in medical risk factors and quality of life in women and men with coronary artery disease in the Multicenter Lifestyle Demonstration Project. Am J Cardiol 91:1316, 2003.
43. Pischke CR, Weidner G, Elliott-Eller M, et al: Comparison of coronary risk factors and quality of life in coronary artery disease patients with versus without diabetes mellitus. Am J Cardiol 97:1267, 2006.
44. Dansinger ML, Gleason JA, Griffith JL, et al: Comparison of the Atkins, Ornish, Weight Watchers, and Zone diets for weight loss and heart disease risk reduction: a randomized trial. JAMA 293:43, 2005.
45. Gardner CD, Kiazand A, Alhassan S, et al: Comparison of the Atkins, Zone, Ornish, and LEARN diets for change in weight and related risk factors among overweight premenopausal women: the A TO Z Weight Loss Study: a randomized trial. JAMA 297:969, 2007.
46. Alhassan S, Kim S, Bersamin A, et al: Dietary adherence and weight loss success among overweight women: results from the A TO Z weight loss study. Int J Obes (Lond) 32:985, 2008.
47. Sacks FM, Bray GA, Carey VJ, et al: Comparison of weight-loss diets with different compositions of fat, protein, and carbohydrates. N Engl J Med 360:859, 2009.
48. Grundy SM, Denke MA: Dietary influences on serum lipids and lipoproteins. J Lipid Res 31:1149, 1990.
49. Mensink RP, Zock PL, Kester AD, et al: Effects of dietary fatty acids and carbohydrates on the ratio of serum total to HDL cholesterol and on serum lipids and apolipoproteins: a meta-analysis of 60 controlled trials. Am J Clin Nutr 77:1146, 2003.
50. Hawthorne VM, Hegsted DM, Shekelle RB, et al: Plasma cholesterol, coronary heart disease, and cancer. Lancet 334:736, 1989.
51. Lichtenstein AH: Nutrient supplements and cardiovascular disease: a heartbreaking story. J Lipid Res 50(Suppl):S429, 2009.
52. Joshipura KJ, Hu FB, Manson JE, et al: The effect of fruit and vegetable intake on risk for coronary heart disease. Ann Intern Med 134:1106, 2001.
53. Liu S, Lee IM, Ajani U, et al: Intake of vegetables rich in carotenoids and risk of coronary heart disease in men: the Physicians' Health Study. Int J Epidemiol 30:130, 2001.
54. Liu S, Manson JE, Lee IM, et al: Fruit and vegetable intake and risk of cardiovascular disease: the Women's Health Study. Am J Clin Nutr 72:922, 2000.
55. Dauchet L, Amouyel P, Dallongeville J: Fruits, vegetables and coronary heart disease. Nat Rev Cardiol 6:599, 2009.
56. Ello-Martin JA, Roe LS, Ledikwe JH, et al: Dietary energy density in the treatment of obesity: a year-long trial comparing 2 weight-loss diets. Am J Clin Nutr 85:1465, 2007.
57. De Moura FF, Lewis KD, Falk MC: Applying the FDA definition of whole grains to the evidence for cardiovascular disease health claims. J Nutr 139:2220S, 2009.
58. Brown L, Rosner B, Willett WW, et al: Cholesterol-lowering effects of dietary fiber: a meta-analysis. Am J Clin Nutr 69:30, 1999.
59. Schneeman BO: Gastrointestinal physiology and functions. Br J Nutr 88:S159, 2002.

60. Jensen MK, Koh-Banerjee P, Hu FB, et al: Intakes of whole grains, bran, and germ and the risk of coronary heart disease in men. *Am J Clin Nutr* 80:1492, 2004.

61. Sahyoun NR, Jacques PF, Zhang XL, et al: Whole-grain intake is inversely associated with the metabolic syndrome and mortality in older adults. *Am J Clin Nutr* 83:124, 2006.

62. Li D, Siriamornpun S, Wahlqvist ML, et al: Lean meat and heart health. *Asia Pac J Clin Nutr* 14:113, 2005.

63. Hecker KD: Effects of dietary animal and soy protein on cardiovascular disease risk factors. *Curr Atheroscler Rep* 3:471, 2001.

64. Hu FB, Stampfer MJ, Manson JE, et al: Dietary protein and risk of ischemic heart disease in women. *Am J Clin Nutr* 70:221, 1999.

65. Slattery ML, Jacobs DR, Jr, Hilner JE, et al: Meat consumption and its associations with other diet and health factors in young adults: the CARDIA study. *Am J Clin Nutr* 54:930, 1991.

65a. U.S. Department of Health and Human Services and U.S. Department of Agriculture: Report of the Dietary Guidelines Advisory Committee on the Dietary Guidelines for Americans, 2010. Washington, DC, 2010. Available at: http://www.cnpp.usda.gov/DietaryGuidelines.htm. Accessed October 29, 2010.

66. German JB, Gibson RA, Krauss RM, et al: A reappraisal of the impact of dairy foods and milk fat on cardiovascular disease risk. *Eur J Nutr* 48:191, 2009.

67. Hu FB, Stampfer MJ, Manson JE, et al: Dietary saturated fats and their food sources in relation to the risk of coronary heart disease in women. *Am J Clin Nutr* 70:1001, 1999.

68. Pittas AG, Lau J, Hu FB, et al: The role of vitamin D and calcium in type 2 diabetes. A systematic review and meta-analysis. *J Clin Endocrinol Metab* 92:2017, 2007.

69. Beyer FR, Dickinson HO, Nicolson DJ, et al: Combined calcium, magnesium and potassium supplementation for the management of primary hypertension in adults. *Cochrane Database Syst Rev* (3):CD004805, 2006.

70. Xu JY, Qin LQ, Wang PY, et al: Effect of milk tripeptides on blood pressure: a meta-analysis of randomized controlled trials. *Nutrition* 24:933, 2008.

71. Castro IA, Barroso LP, Sinnecker P: Functional foods for coronary heart disease risk reduction: a meta-analysis using a multivariate approach. *Am J Clin Nutr* 82:32, 2005.

72. FDA allows whole oat foods to make health claim on reducing the risk of heart disease. *FDA Talk Paper*, January 21, 1997.

73. FDA allows barley products to claim reduction in risk of coronary heart disease. *FDA News*, December 23, 2005.

74. Andersson M, Ellegard L, Andersson H: Oat bran stimulates bile acid synthesis within 8 h as measured by 7α-hydroxy-4-cholesten-3-one. *Am J Clin Nutr* 76:1111, 2002.

75. Drozdowski LA, Reimer RA, Temelli F, et al: β-Glucan extracts inhibit the in vitro intestinal uptake of long-chain fatty acids and cholesterol and down-regulate genes involved in lipogenesis and lipid transport in rats. *J Nutr Biochem* 21:695, 2010.

76. Ellegard L, Andersson H: Oat bran rapidly increases bile acid excretion and bile acid synthesis: an ileostomy study. *Eur J Clin Nutr* 61:938, 2007.

77. van Bennekum AM, Nguyen DV, Schulthess G, et al: Mechanisms of cholesterol-lowering effects of dietary insoluble fibres: relationships with intestinal and hepatic cholesterol parameters. *Br J Nutr* 94:331, 2005.

78. Hu GX, Chen GR, Xu H, et al: Activation of the AMP activated protein kinase by short-chain fatty acids is the main mechanism underlying the beneficial effect of a high fiber diet on the metabolic syndrome. *Med Hypotheses* 74:123, 2010.

79. Flint AJ, Hu FB, Glynn RJ, et al: Whole grains and incident hypertension in men. *Am J Clin Nutr* 90:493, 2009.

80. Steffen LM, Jacobs DR, Jr, Murtaugh MA, et al: Whole grain intake is associated with lower body mass and greater insulin sensitivity among adolescents. *Am J Epidemiol* 158:243, 2003.

81. Whelton SP, Hyre AD, Pedersen B, et al: Effect of dietary fiber intake on blood pressure: a meta-analysis of randomized, controlled clinical trials. *J Hypertens* 23:475, 2005.

82. Fassbender K, Lutjohann D, Dik MG, et al: Moderately elevated plant sterol levels are associated with reduced cardiovascular risk—the LASA study. *Atherosclerosis* 196:283, 2008.

83. Pinedo S, Vissers MN, von Bergmann K, et al: Plasma levels of plant sterols and the risk of coronary artery disease: the prospective EPIC-Norfolk Population Study. *J Lipid Res* 48:139, 2007.

84. Assmann G, Cullen P, Erbey J, et al: Plasma sitosterol elevations are associated with an increased incidence of coronary events in men: results of a nested case-control analysis of the Prospective Cardiovascular Münster (PROCAM) study. *Nutr Metab Cardiovasc Dis* 16:13, 2006.

85. Ostlund RE, Jr: Phytosterols in human nutrition. *Annu Rev Nutr* 22:533, 2002.

86. Naumann E, Plat J, Kester AD, et al: The baseline serum lipoprotein profile is related to plant stanol induced changes in serum lipoprotein cholesterol and triacylglycerol concentrations. *J Am Coll Nutr* 27:117, 2008.

87. Moruisi KG, Oosthuizen W, Opperman AM: Phytosterols/stanols lower cholesterol concentrations in familial hypercholesterolemic subjects: a systematic review with meta-analysis. *J Am Coll Nutr* 25:41, 2006.

88. Nguyen TT: The cholesterol-lowering action of plant stanol esters. *J Nutr* 129:2109, 1999.

89. Katan MB, Grundy SM, Jones P, et al: Efficacy and safety of plant stanols and sterols in the management of blood cholesterol levels. *Mayo Clinic Proc* 78:965, 2003.

90. Van Horn L, McCoin M, Kris-Etherton PM, et al: The evidence for dietary prevention and treatment of cardiovascular disease. *J Am Diet Assoc* 108:287, 2008.

91. Abumweis SS, Barake R, Jones PJ: Plant sterols/stanols as cholesterol lowering agents: a meta-analysis of randomized controlled trials. *Food Nutr Res* 52, 2008.

92. de Jong A, Plat J, Lutjohann D, et al: Effects of long-term plant sterol or stanol ester consumption on lipid and lipoprotein metabolism in subjects on statin treatment. *Br J Nutr* 100:937, 2008.

93. Plat J, Brufau G, Dallinga-Thie GM, et al: A plant stanol yogurt drink alone or combined with a low-dose statin lowers serum triacylglycerol and non-HDL cholesterol in metabolic syndrome patients. *J Nutr* 139:1143, 2009.

94. Jones P, Kafonek S, Laurora I, et al: Comparative dose efficacy study of atorvastatin versus simvastatin, pravastatin, lovastatin, and fluvastatin in patients with hypercholesterolemia (the CURVES study). *Am J Cardiol* 81:582, 1998.

95. De Jong A, Plat J, Bast A, et al: Effects of plant sterol and stanol ester consumption on lipid metabolism, antioxidant status and markers of oxidative stress, endothelial function and low-grade inflammation in patients on current statin treatment. *Eur J Clin Nutr* 62:263, 2008.

96. Devaraj S, Autret BC, Jialal I: Reduced-calorie orange juice beverage with plant sterols lowers C-reactive protein concentrations and improves the lipid profile in human volunteers. *Am J Clin Nutr* 84:756, 2006.

97. Anderson JW, Johnstone BM, Cook-Newell ME: Meta-analysis of the effects of soy protein intake on serum lipids. *N Engl J Med* 333:276, 1995.

98. Food and Drug Administration: Food labeling health claims; soy protein and coronary heart disease. *Fed Regist* 64:57700, 1999.

99. Zhan S, Ho SC: Meta-analysis of the effects of soy protein containing isoflavones on the lipid profile. *Am J Clin Nutr* 81:397, 2005.

100. Sacks FM, Lichtenstein A, Van Horn L, et al: Soy protein, isoflavones, and cardiovascular health: an American Heart Association Science Advisory for professionals from the Nutrition Committee. *Circulation* 113:1034, 2006.

101. Taku K, Umegaki K, Ishimi Y, et al: Effects of extracted soy isoflavones alone on blood total and LDL cholesterol: meta-analysis of randomized controlled trials. *Ther Clin Risk Manag* 4:1097, 2008.

102. Matthan NR, Jalbert SM, Ausman LM, et al: Effect of soy protein from differently processed products on cardiovascular disease risk factors and vascular endothelial function in hypercholesterolemic subjects. *Am J Clin Nutr* 85:960, 2007.

103. Pipe EA, Gobert CP, Capes SE, et al: Soy protein reduces serum LDL cholesterol and the LDL cholesterol:HDL cholesterol and apolipoprotein B:apolipoprotein A-I ratios in adults with type 2 diabetes. *J Nutr* 139:1700, 2009.

104. Taku K, Umegaki K, Sato Y, et al: Soy isoflavones lower serum total and LDL cholesterol in humans: a meta-analysis of 11 randomized controlled trials. *Am J Clin Nutr* 85:1148, 2007.

105. Setchell KD: Soy isoflavones—benefits and risks from nature's selective estrogen receptor modulators (SERMs). *J Am Coll Nutr* 20:354S; discussion 81S, 2001.

106. Thorp AA, Howe PR, Mori TA, et al: Soy food consumption does not lower LDL cholesterol in either equol or nonequol producers. *Am J Clin Nutr* 88:298, 2008.

107. Kris-Etherton PM: AHA science advisory: monounsaturated fatty acids and risk of cardiovascular disease. *J Nutr* 129:2280, 1999.

108. Rasmussen BM, Vessby B, Uusitupa M, et al: Effects of dietary saturated, monounsaturated, and n-3 fatty acids on blood pressure in healthy subjects. *Am J Clin Nutr* 83:221, 2006.

109. Psota TL, Gebauer SK, Kris-Etherton P: Dietary omega-3 fatty acid intake and cardiovascular risk. *Am J Cardiol* 98:3, 2006.

110. Virtanen JK, Mozaffarian D, Chiuve SE, et al: Fish consumption and risk of major chronic disease in men. *Am J Clin Nutr* 88:1618, 2008.

111. Erkkila AT, Lehto S, Pyorala K, et al: n-3 Fatty acids and 5-y risks of death and cardiovascular disease events in patients with coronary artery disease. *Am J Clin Nutr* 78:65, 2003.

112. Erkkila AT, Lichtenstein AH, Mozaffarian D, et al: Fish intake is associated with a reduced progression of coronary artery atherosclerosis in postmenopausal women with coronary artery disease. *Am J Clin Nutr* 80:626, 2004.

113. Hu FB, Cho E, Rexrode KM, et al: Fish and long-chain omega-3 fatty acid intake and risk of coronary heart disease and total mortality in diabetic women. *Circulation* 107:1852, 2003.

114. Iso H, Rexrode KM, Stampfer MJ, et al: Intake of fish and omega-3 fatty acids and risk of stroke in women. *JAMA* 285:304, 2001.

115. Mozaffarian D, Stein PK, Prineas RJ, et al: Dietary fish and omega-3 fatty acid consumption and heart rate variability in US adults. *Circulation* 117:1130, 2008.

116. He K: Fish, long-chain omega-3 polyunsaturated fatty acids and prevention of cardiovascular disease—eat fish or take fish oil supplement? *Prog Cardiovasc Dis* 52:95, 2009.

117. Kris-Etherton PM, Innis S: American Dietetic Association, Dietitians of Canada: Position of the American Dietetic Association and Dietitians of Canada: dietary fatty acids. *J Am Diet Assoc* 107:1599, 2007.

118. Kris-Etherton PM, Harris WS, Appel LJ: Fish consumption, fish oil, omega-3 fatty acids, and cardiovascular disease. *Circulation* 106:2747, 2002.

119. York R, Gossard MH: Cross-national meat and fish consumption: exploring the effects of modernization and ecological context. *Ecological Economics* 48:293, 2004.

120. Cahu C, Salen P, de Lorgeril M: Farmed and wild fish in the prevention of cardiovascular diseases: assessing possible differences in lipid nutritional values. *Nutr Metab Cardiovasc Dis* 14:34, 2004.

121. Harris WS: n-3 Fatty acids and serum lipoproteins: human studies. *Am J Clin Nutr* 65:1645S, 1997.

122. Bays HE, Tighe AP, Sadovsky R, et al: Prescription omega-3 fatty acids and their lipid effects: physiologic mechanisms of action and clinical implications. *Expert Rev Cardiovasc Ther* 6:391, 2008.

123. Coates AM, Howe PR: Edible nuts and metabolic health. *Curr Opin Lipidol* 18:25, 2007.

124. Kris-Etherton PM, Hu FB, Ros E, et al: The role of tree nuts and peanuts in the prevention of coronary heart disease: multiple potential mechanisms. *J Nutr* 138:1746S, 2008.

125. U.S. Department of Agriculture, Agricultural Research Service: USDA national nutrient database for standard reference, release 22. Available at: http://www.nal.usda.gov/fnic/foodcomp/search/. Accessed December 20, 2009.

126. Chen CY, Blumberg JB: Phytochemical composition of nuts. *Asia Pac J Clin Nutr* 17(Suppl 1):329, 2008.

127. Fraser GE, Sabate J, Beeson WL, Strahan TM: A possible protective effect of nut consumption on risk of coronary heart disease. The Adventist Health Study. *Arch Intern Med* 152:1416, 1992.

128. Ellsworth JL, Kushi LH, Folsom AR: Frequent nut intake and risk of death from coronary heart disease and all causes in postmenopausal women: the Iowa Women's Health Study. *Nutr Metab Cardiovasc Dis* 11:372, 2001.

129. Hu F, Stampfer M, Manson J, et al: Frequent nut consumption and risk of coronary heart disease in women: prospective cohort study. *BMJ* 317:1341, 1998.

130. Albert CM, Gaziano JM, Willett WC, et al: Nut consumption and decreased risk of sudden cardiac death in the Physicians' Health Study. *Arch Intern Med* 162:1382, 2002.

131. Kelly JH, Jr, Sabate J: Nuts and coronary heart disease: an epidemiological perspective. *Br J Nutr* 96(Suppl 2):S61, 2006.

132. Djousse L, Rudich T, Gaziano JM: Nut consumption and risk of heart failure in the Physicians' Health Study I. *Am J Clin Nutr* 88:930, 2008.

133. Griel AE, Kris-Etherton P: Tree nuts and the lipid profile: a review of clinical studies. *Br J Nutr* 96:S68, 2006.

134. Jiang R, Jacobs DR, Jr, Mayer-Davis E, et al: Nut and seed consumption and inflammatory markers in the multi-ethnic study of atherosclerosis. *Am J Epidemiol* 163:222, 2006.

135. Ros E, Nunez I, Perez-Heras A, et al: A walnut diet improves endothelial function in hypercholesterolemic subjects: a randomized crossover trial. *Circulation* 109:1609, 2004.

136. Sari I, Baltaci Y, Bagci C, et al: Effect of pistachio diet on lipid parameters, endothelial function, inflammation, and oxidative status: a prospective study. *Nutrition* 26:399, 2010.

137. Djousse L, Rudich T, Gaziano JM: Nut consumption and risk of hypertension in US male physicians. *Clin Nutr* 28:10, 2009.

138. Covas MI: Olive oil and the cardiovascular system. *Pharmacol Res* 55:175, 2007.

139. Covas MI, Nyyssonen K, Poulsen HE, et al: The effect of polyphenols in olive oil on heart disease risk factors: a randomized trial. *Ann Intern Med* 145:333, 2006.

140. Alonso A, Martinez-Gonzalez MA: Olive oil consumption and reduced incidence of hypertension: the SUN study. *Lipids* 39:1233, 2004.

141. Psaltopoulou T, Naska A, Orfanos P, et al: Olive oil, the Mediterranean diet, and arterial blood pressure: the Greek European Prospective Investigation into Cancer and Nutrition (EPIC) study. *Am J Clin Nutr* 80:1012, 2004.

142. Galli C, Calder PC: Effects of fat and fatty acid intake on inflammatory and immune responses: a critical review. *Ann Nutr Metab* 55:123, 2009.

143. Lennie TA, Chung ML, Habash DL, et al: Dietary fat intake and proinflammatory cytokine levels in patients with heart failure. *J Card Fail* 11:613, 2005.

144. Pischon T, Hankinson SE, Hotamisligil GS, et al: Habitual dietary intake of n-3 and n-6 fatty acids in relation to inflammatory markers among US men and women. *Circulation* 108:155, 2003.

145. Ferrucci L, Cherubini A, Bandinelli S, et al: Relationship of plasma polyunsaturated fatty acids to circulating inflammatory markers. *J Clin Endocrinol Metab* 91:439, 2006.

146. Harris WS: The omega-6/omega-3 ratio and cardiovascular disease risk: uses and abuses. *Curr Atheroscler Rep* 8:453, 2006.

147. Harris WS, Mozaffarian D, Rimm E, et al: Omega-6 fatty acids and risk for cardiovascular disease: a science advisory from the American Heart Association Nutrition Subcommittee of the Council on Nutrition, Physical Activity, and Metabolism; Council on Cardiovascular Nursing; and Council on Epidemiology and Prevention. *Circulation* 119:902, 2009.

148. Renaud S, de Lorgeril M: Wine, alcohol, platelets, and the French paradox for coronary heart disease. *Lancet* 339:1523, 1992.

149. Hansen AS, Marckmann P, Dragsted LO, et al: Effect of red wine and red grape extract on blood lipids, haemostatic factors, and other risk factors for cardiovascular disease. *Eur J Clin Nutr* 59:449, 2005.

150. Senault C, Betoulle D, Luc G, et al: Beneficial effects of a moderate consumption of red wine on cellular cholesterol efflux in young men. *Nutr Metab Cardiovasc Dis* 10:63, 2000.

151. Whelan AP, Sutherland WH, McCormick MP, et al: Effects of white and red wine on endothelial function in subjects with coronary artery disease. *Intern Med J* 34:224, 2004.

152. de Jong HJ, de Goede J, Oude Griep LM, et al: Alcohol consumption and blood lipids in elderly coronary patients. *Metabolism* 57:1286, 2008.

153. Mukamal KJ, Conigrave KM, Mittleman MA, et al: Roles of drinking pattern and type of alcohol consumed in coronary heart disease in men. *N Engl J Med* 348:109, 2003.

154. Das DK, Maulik N: Resveratrol in cardioprotection: a therapeutic promise of alternative medicine. *Mol Interv* 6:36, 2006.

155. Olas B, Wachowicz B, Saluk-Juszczak J, et al: Effect of resveratrol, a natural polyphenolic compound, on platelet activation induced by endotoxin or thrombin. *Thromb Res* 107:141, 2002.

156. Poussier B, Cordova AC, Becquemin JP, et al: Resveratrol inhibits vascular smooth muscle cell proliferation and induces apoptosis. *J Vasc Surg* 42:1190, 2005.

157. Berrougui H, Grenier G, Loued S, et al: A new insight into resveratrol as an atheroprotective compound: inhibition of lipid peroxidation and enhancement of cholesterol efflux. *Atherosclerosis* 207:420, 2009.

158. Lapointe A, Couillard C, Lemieux S: Effects of dietary factors on oxidation of low-density lipoprotein particles. *J Nutr Biochem* 17:645, 2006.

159. de Rijke YB, Demacker PN, Assen NA, et al: Red wine consumption does not affect oxidizability of low-density lipoproteins in volunteers. *Am J Clin Nutr* 63:329, 1996.

160. U.S. Department of Agriculture: MyPyramid.gov: Steps to a healthier you. Washington, DC, 2005. Available at: http://www.mypyramid.gov/. Accessed June 20, 2009.

161. A DASHing Pyramid. *Nutrition Action Healthletter*, May 8, 2003.

162. Oldways Preservation and Exchange Trust: Mediterranean Diet Pyramid. Available at: http://www.oldwayspt.org/med_pyramid.html. Accessed November 20, 2009.

163. Rock CL: Multivitamin-multimineral supplements: who uses them? *Am J Clin Nutr* 85:277S, 2007.

164. Radimer K, Bindewald B, Hughes J, et al: Dietary supplement use by US adults: data from the National Health and Nutrition Examination Survey, 1999-2000. *Am J Epidemiol* 160:339, 2004.

165. Morris CD, Carson S: Routine vitamin supplementation to prevent cardiovascular disease: a summary of the evidence for the U.S. Preventive Services Task Force. *Ann Intern Med* 139:56, 2003.

166. Kris-Etherton PM, Lichtenstein AH, Howard BV, et al: Antioxidant vitamin supplements and cardiovascular disease. *Circulation* 110:637, 2004.

167. Carlson LA: Nicotinic acid: the broad-spectrum lipid drug. A 50th anniversary review. *J Intern Med* 258:94, 2005.

168. Meyers CD, Kamanna VS, Kashyap ML: Niacin therapy in atherosclerosis. *Curr Opin Lipidol* 15:659, 2004.

169. Brown BG, Zhao X-Q, Chait A, et al: Simvastatin and niacin, antioxidant vitamins, or the combination for the prevention of coronary disease. *N Engl J Med* 345:1583, 2001.

170. Homocysteine Lowering Trialists Collaboration: Dose-dependent effects of folic acid on blood concentrations of homocysteine: a meta-analysis of the randomized trials. *Am J Clin Nutr* 82:806, 2005.

171. Toole JF, Malinow MR, Chambless LE, et al: Lowering homocysteine in patients with ischemic stroke to prevent recurrent stroke, myocardial infarction, and death: the Vitamin Intervention for Stroke Prevention (VISP) randomized controlled trial. *JAMA* 291:565, 2004.

172. Bonaa KH, Njolstad I, Ueland PM, et al: Homocysteine lowering and cardiovascular events after acute myocardial infarction. *N Engl J Med* 354:1578, 2006.

173. Lonn E, Yusuf S, Arnold MJ, et al: Homocysteine lowering with folic acid and B vitamins in vascular disease. *N Engl J Med* 354:1567, 2006.

174. Ebbing M, Bleie O, Ueland PM, et al: Mortality and cardiovascular events in patients treated with homocysteine-lowering B vitamins after coronary angiography: a randomized controlled trial. *JAMA* 300:795, 2008.

175. Albert CM, Cook NR, Gaziano JM, et al: Effect of folic acid and B vitamins on risk of cardiovascular events and total mortality among women at high risk for cardiovascular disease: a randomized trial. *JAMA* 299:2027, 2008.

176. Willcox BJ, Curb JD, Rodriguez BL: Antioxidants in cardiovascular health and disease: key lessons from epidemiologic studies. *Am J Cardiol* 101:S75, 2008.

177. Bjelakovic G, Nikolova D, Gluud LL, et al: Mortality in randomized trials of antioxidant supplements for primary and secondary prevention: systematic review and meta-analysis. *JAMA* 297:842, 2007.

178. Bjelakovic G, Nikolova D, Gluud LL, et al: Antioxidant supplements for prevention of mortality in healthy participants and patients with various diseases. *Cochrane Database Syst Rev* (2):CD007176, 2008.

179. Miller ER, III, Pastor-Barriuso R, Dalal D, et al: Meta-analysis: high-dosage vitamin E supplementation may increase all-cause mortality. *Ann Intern Med* 142:37, 2005.

180. Moats C, Rimm EB: Vitamin intake and risk of coronary disease: observation versus intervention. *Curr Atheroscler Rep* 9:508, 2007.

181. Pilz S, Marz W, Wellnitz B, et al: Association of vitamin D deficiency with heart failure and sudden cardiac death in a large cross-sectional study of patients referred for coronary angiography. *J Clin Endocrinol Metab* 93:3927, 2008.

182. Wang TJ, Pencina MJ, Booth SL, et al: Vitamin D deficiency and risk of cardiovascular disease. *Circulation* 117:503, 2008.

183. Autier P, Gandini S: Vitamin D supplementation and total mortality: a meta-analysis of randomized controlled trials. *Arch Intern Med* 167:1730, 2007.

184. Parkera J, Hashmia O, Dutton D, et al: Levels of vitamin D and cardiometabolic disorders: systematic review and meta-analysis. *Maturitas* 65:225, 2009.

185. Moats C, Rimm EB: Vitamin intake and risk of coronary disease: observation versus intervention. *Curr Atheroscler Rep* 9:508, 2007

186. Holick MF, Chen TC: Vitamin D deficiency: a worldwide problem with health consequences. *Am J Clin Nutr* 87:1080S, 2008.

187. Prochaska JQ, DiClemente CC: Stages of change in the modification of problem behaviors. In Hersen M, Eisler RM, Miller PM, editors: *Progress in behavior modification*, Sycamore, Ill, 1992, Sycamore Press, pp 184-214.

188. Miller W, Rollnick S: Motivational interviewing: preparing people for change, ed 2, New York, 2002, Guilford Press.

189. Artinian NT, Fletcher GF, Mozaffarian D, et al: Interventions to promote physical activity and dietary lifestyle changes for cardiovascular risk factor reduction in adults: A scientific statement from the American Heart Association. *Circulation* 122:406, 2010.

CHAPTER 17

Integrative Medicine in the Prevention of Cardiovascular Disease

John C. Longhurst and Rebecca B. Costello

KEY POINTS

- Integrative medicine, which blends standard Western and nontraditional medical practices, is used by 38% of adults and 12% of children in the United States.

- Placebo responses, inherent in all conventional and integrative medical therapies, account for as much as 20% to 50% of clinical outcomes.

- Traditional Chinese medicine, incorporating acupuncture and herbals, reduces elevated systolic blood pressure and oxygen demand to improve supply-demand imbalances and myocardial ischemia. Tai Chi and Qigong, two forms of Chinese energy medicine, frequently involve a component of exercise that also may reduce blood pressure.

- Ayurvedic medicine, originating from India, includes lifestyle changes, particularly dietary and herbal prescriptions, as well as stress reduction through yoga and meditation.

- Chinese and Ayurvedic medicines, with a long history of traditional use, require further study to assess their actions on cardiovascular risk factors.

- Observational studies on single-nutrient dietary supplements suggest reduced cardiovascular risk that has not yet been validated by randomized trials.

- Blood pressure, body mass index, and cholesterol level are improved by a program of yoga incorporating vegetarian diet and stress management with meditation.

- Behavioral and cognitive training, guided imagery, meditation, biofeedback, and

progressive muscle relaxation appear to be capable of reducing blood pressure.

- Naturopathic medicine incorporates a number of natural practices, such as dietary manipulation and exercise, to prevent disease and to promote healing; other naturopathic practices,

like homeopathy, require validation before they can be recommended.

- Chelation therapy, which seeks to lower calcium and to alter atherosclerosis progression, has the potential for serious side effects and is not recommended on the basis of currently available evidence.

Complementary and alternative medicine (CAM) consists of a diverse group of practices and health care systems that generally are not considered to be part of usual Western or allopathic medical practices (Box 17-1). Most academic medical centers in the United States have adopted the term *integrative medicine*, recognizing the usefulness of combining conventional and CAM practice. There is a large diversity of disciplines that make up CAM therapies (see Box 17-1), and because scientific and clinical studies supporting their mechanisms of action and clinical utility vary tremendously, most academically based centers tend to focus on only a few that are supported by evidence.

This chapter discusses areas of integrative medicine that are supported by evidence (Box 17-2) and that can be used in preventive approaches to cardiovascular disease, particularly coronary artery disease. Some therapies have little rationale or support for efficacy in preventive cardiovascular medicine and are discussed only briefly (Box 17-3). Most guidelines (48%) that have been developed are based on recommendations that are less scientifically rigorous and expert opinion, case studies, or standards of care.[1] Despite the absence of high-quality prospective randomized clinical trials on cardiovascular prevention in integrative medicine, experimental studies have identified the mechanisms by which these therapies may reduce cardiovascular risk and, by extension, establish the potential for their clinical action.

In addition to its action on traditional cardiovascular risk factors, the influence of CAM on stress is discussed throughout this chapter because it is linked to many aspects

of coronary disease,[2] including blood pressure dysregulation, diabetes, and elevated cholesterol.[3,4] This chapter, therefore, provides a brief overview of available clinical and basic science evidence for the use of integrative approaches to reduce cardiovascular disease risk, focusing on our current Western understanding of CAM rather than on traditional CAM theory, which can be found in recent texts.[5-8] Dietary and nutritional approaches are considered in Chapter 16, although a discussion of supplements, including herbals and vitamins as they relate to cardiovascular risk reduction, is provided here.

USE OF INTEGRATIVE MEDICINE IN THE UNITED STATES

The National Center for Complementary and Alternative Medicine (NCCAM) recently released an update on the use of CAM practices in the United States, taken from data collected in the National Health Interview Survey of 2007.[9] Approximately 38% of adults and 12% of children use some form of CAM. CAM is used with higher frequency by women and children of families that use CAM. The most common uses are for pain, anxiety or stress, hypercholesterolemia, and insomnia (Fig. 17-1). A major issue is the absence of communication between patients using integrative medical therapies and their physicians, in part because access is obtained outside the standard medical environment and because of the lack of approval of many of these unconventional therapies by the medical profession. Thus, interest in CAM is driven by the lay community more than by the medical community.

Despite the absence of acceptance in the past, there is increasing use and referral by some practitioners, mainly family physicians and other primary care providers, as they are encouraged by their patients, as studies begin to appear, and as many schools begin to introduce CAM education into their curriculum.[10] It is apparent, however, that there are only a limited number of cardiologists who use or refer patients for CAM therapy and fewer yet who study it.[6-8,11] The skepticism of many physicians stems from a common belief that much if not all of the clinical effect of CAM is equivalent to that of a placebo.

ROLE OF PLACEBO IN COMPLEMENTARY AND ALTERNATIVE MEDICINE

Placebo, translated from the Latin phrase "I shall please," is part of every clinical intervention, whether standard Western therapy or CAM procedure, and clearly has been well recognized in many forms of cardiovascular medicine.[12-14] Simple interaction between a provider and a patient frequently leads to clinical improvement unrelated to the intervention in many diseases.[15] In fact, between 20% and 50% of response to any medical treatment, including standard Western therapies for cardiovascular disease, may be ascribed to a placebo effect, either because of a physiologic placebo-related response or because of regression to the mean with repetitive testing.[16,17] Furthermore, placebo responses are more likely to occur in trials comparing continuous variables like pain and blood pressure.

Chronic stable angina improves by 30% to 50%[18] and blood pressure can be reduced by as much as 20 to 40 mm Hg by reassurance or placebo interventions.[19] In integrative medicine, the concern is that most if not all of the effect is a nonspecific response to placebo, that is, there is no active intervention. This belief is reinforced by the fact that many

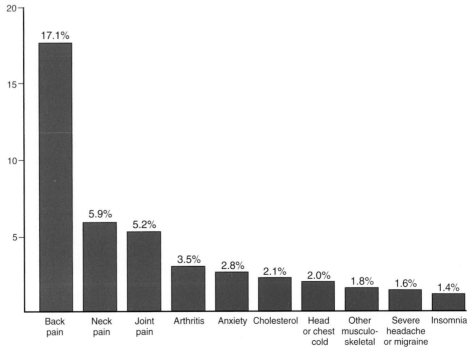

FIGURE 17-1 Diseases and conditions for which CAM is most frequently used among adults, 2007. (*From Barnes P, Bloom B, Nahin R: Complementary and alternative medicine use among adults and children: United States, 2007.* Natl Health Stat Report *12:1, 2008.*)

Diseases/conditions for which CAM is most frequently used among adults—2007 of the symptoms and diseases treated in cardiovascular medicine, such as angina and stress responses, have improved with placebo therapy.[20] Compounding the difficulty in distinguishing between active and placebo responses is the finding that both operate through the endogenous opioid system, including shared regions of the brain like the periaqueductal gray that are activated by acupuncture and placebo.[21-25] Furthermore, unwarranted or exaggerated expectation in patients using CAM interventions may heighten the placebo response.[26]

Double-blind controls, placebo interventions, and nontreatment arms have been used to detect placebo responses.[27] It is frequently difficult to truly blind the practitioner, however; for example, the acupuncturist has to know where to place the needle to achieve an optimal response. Furthermore, the use of no or inadequate controls has limited the interpretation of many clinical CAM trials. More than 50% of trials coming from Asian countries are limited by the absence of adequate controls, and once many trials use a suitable control, some studies have found little difference between the sham and the true (verum) intervention.[28]

Despite the inherent problems with control intervention in studies of integrative medicine, they are extremely important, and many suitable control interventions have been devised. One example of a suitable control is in the study of electroacupuncture regulation of elevated blood pressure, in which a needle is placed in an acupoint known to exert biologic effects but is not stimulated. Alternatively, needles can be placed in acupoints known not to exert responses.[29] In the first control, afferent nerves are not stimulated, and hence any response is related to interaction between the therapist and the subject. The latter control is associated with sensory stimulation, but neural input to the central nervous system does not involve the areas known to regulate blood pressure.[28,30]

Uninformed study subjects cannot differentiate between control and active interventions.[31] By use of this paradigm, 30 minutes of low-frequency, low-intensity acupuncture at active acupoints, but not sham acupuncture with either type of control intervention described earlier, lowers elevated blood pressure in experimental studies.[29]

TRADITIONAL CHINESE MEDICINE

Traditional Chinese medicine, originating more than 2000 years ago, incorporates several diverse treatment options, including acupuncture and acupressure, Chinese herbals, moxibustion (local heat with a Chinese herb), massage, Tai Chi, Qigong, and dietary therapy. Acupuncture, Tai Chi, and Qigong are forms of energy-based medicine, the energy referred to as *Qi*.

Acupuncture, Acupressure, and Moxibustion

Acupuncture and its derivatives, acupressure and moxibustion, are based on a system of 12 principal channels or meridians that lie along the body surface. Along these meridians are small nodes or acupuncture points (acupoints) that direct the therapist where to place the needle to exert pressure or heat. Although neither the meridians nor the acupoints have a physical basis, they are useful because they direct the therapist to where stimulation should occur.

Mechanism of Action

Many if not all meridians lie over major neural pathways that contain both motor and, more important, sensory nerves. Thus, from a physiologic perspective, acupuncture needles penetrate the skin and in most circumstances are positioned through underlying nerves or sufficiently near the mixed nerve bundles that contain both sensory and motor fibers. Although stimulation of the muscle motor fibers is not important in the acupuncture effect because paralytic agents do not alter acupuncture's action on the cardiovascular system, fine muscle contractions are helpful in alerting the practitioner that the needle is positioned in a proper location near the nerve bundle. Conversely, activation of sensory neural pathways provides input to regions of the central nervous system that regulate cardiovascular function.[28]

Transection of the afferent pathway central to needle insertion eliminates all but the placebo response to acupuncture. More specifically, acupuncture-related activation of thin-fiber somatic sensory pathways provides strong input to the spinal cord, ventral hypothalamus, midbrain periaqueductal gray, and both pressor and depressor regions that regulate sympathetic (and probably parasympathetic) outflow in the medulla, located in the lower brainstem.

Manual acupuncture or low-frequency, low-intensity electroacupuncture is capable of causing the release of a number of modulatory (inhibitory) neuropeptides in the brain, including opioids (endorphins and enkephalins), γ-aminobutyric acid, nociceptin, serotonin, and endocannabinoids as well as excitatory amino acids like glutamate and acetylcholine, that ultimately inhibit sympathetic (and probably parasympathetic) outflow to the heart and vascular system.[32,33] In the spinal cord, acupuncture appears to inhibit sensory inflow and sympathetic outflow through both opioid and nociceptin mechanisms of blockade.[34,35]

Two important concepts in acupuncture are acupoint specificity and the nature of its action. Point specificity is the differential clinical response to stimulation of specific acupoints.[32] For example, some acupoints, like those along the pericardial meridian overlying the median nerve in the wrist, exert a stronger influence on the cardiovascular system than other points do.[36] The extent of influence is determined by the amount of input to regions of the brain that control cardiovascular function. The nature of acupuncture's action is determined by the mode of sensory nerve stimulation, the duration of stimulation, and the extent of release of neurotransmitters in the central nervous system.

Low-frequency electrical (2 to 6 Hz) or manual acupuncture for 30 to 45 minutes seems to be most effective, reducing sympathetic outflow after 10 to 15 minutes of stimulation and lasting for many minutes to hours or even days after acupuncture, depending on the model of investigation and extent of repetitive stimulation. Thus, the cardiovascular influence of electroacupuncture can last for 1 to 2 hours in anesthetized experimental animal studies and for 10 to 12 hours in awake animals, whereas repetitive acupuncture in patients can exert an influence on blood pressure for several weeks.[28]

Acupuncture's Action on Cardiovascular Risk Factors

A number of cardiovascular risk factors, including hypertension, obesity, and hypercholesterolemia, potentially may be influenced by acupuncture. In addition, there is some evidence that acupuncture may be efficacious in stroke and coronary as well as peripheral arterial disease.[28]

Because acupuncture can decrease sympathetic outflow and sympathoexcitatory reflex responses associated with elevated blood pressure, there is a rationale to use it for treatment of mild to moderate hypertension.[32] However, the results of clinical trials are mixed. Experimental studies in quadriplegic rats suggest that transcutaneous electrical stimulation (TENS), which shares some features of stimulation and physiologic response with electroacupuncture, decreases the exaggerated blood pressure responses associated with colon distention.[37] Although acupuncture appears to be safe,[38] no clinical trials are available on its effect in spinal patients experiencing large fluctuations in blood pressure associated with autonomic dysreflexia. Blood pressure in spontaneously hypertensive rats is reduced by acupuncture at an acupoint located over the deep peroneal nerve for periods lasting up to 12 hours.[39] A small study of 50 patients suggested that 30 minutes of acupuncture lowered both systolic and diastolic pressure.[40] Conversely, the SHARP (Stop Hypertension with Acupuncture Research Program) trial, which treated patients with moderate hypertension during a 12-week period, demonstrated no influence on blood pressure over and above the response to an invasive sham control when blood pressure was measured intermittently with manual mercury sphygmomanometers.[41] However, large and small trials incorporating ambulatory monitoring have demonstrated more consistent decreases in blood pressure in patients with mild to moderate hypertension, especially if acupoints that have been shown to have a strong cardiovascular influence (P5, P6, St36, St37, referring to points along the pericardial and stomach meridians overlying the median and deep peroneal nerves) are used.[42,43] Acupuncture appears to influence systolic and mean blood pressure more than diastolic blood pressure. The onset of action is slow, frequently requiring several acupuncture treatments before a sustained decrease in blood pressure is observed. Blood pressure decreases by 5 to 20 mm Hg and tends to remain low for several weeks after cessation of treatment.

In addition to hypertension, experimental studies demonstrate that acupuncture can lower cholesterol. Daily acupuncture for a 2-week period reduces the increase in cholesterol in experimental animal models fed high-cholesterol diets.[44,45] There are no good randomized controlled clinical trials, but a small nonrandomized, unblinded trial of electroacupuncture that did not incorporate a control acupoint group demonstrated similar or greater weight loss, low-density lipoprotein cholesterol (LDL-C) and triglyceride reductions compared with a control group fed a low-calorie diet.[46]

Although stimulation of auricular acupoints to treat overweight patients provides input to regions of the brain that regulate food ingestion,[47] its ability to assist with weight loss in obesity is less certain. Experimental studies[48,49] in rats show that auricular (ear) acupuncture leads to a 5% loss in weight during a period of 2 to 3 weeks. However, clinical trials are mixed, with uncontrolled studies showing small decreases[49-52] and controlled trials[53-56] showing either very modest or no weight loss that could be ascribed to acupuncture. Many of the trials lacked suitable controls.

Because acupuncture leads to the release of endogenous opioids, it has been thought that it may be useful in treating addictive habits like smoking. In this regard, acupuncture reduces symptoms in subjects addicted to opiates like morphine.[57,58] However, meta-analyses of relevant clinical trials reveal that many are of low quality, are frequently short term, lack suitable controls, and do not provide sufficient information to assess their quality.[59] Thus, at present, insufficient data are available to determine the efficacy of acupuncture in smoking cessation.

Cardiovascular Responses to Transcutaneous Electrical Stimulation and Acupuncture

Through an opioid mechanism, acupuncture lowers myocardial oxygen demand and hence can reduce demand-supply imbalances and ventricular dysfunction in experimental myocardial ischemia.[60,61] Similarly, both TENS and acupuncture reduce myocardial ischemia occurring during exercise in patients with angina and electrocardiographic evidence of ischemia.[62-71] TENS shares some similarities with but is not exactly equivalent to acupuncture because much higher stimulation intensities and frequencies are used during the noninvasive TENS stimulation that is not directed at specific locations (acupoints) over neural pathways. Although there

is some debate about whether acupuncture can increase coronary blood flow, the preponderance of evidence suggests that it mainly reduces ischemia by reducing the increase in blood pressure and double product (but not the elevated heart rate) associated with exercise, hence lowering myocardial oxygen demand.[31]

Acupuncture also lowers the reflex excitatory responses to mental stress.[72] The influence of acupuncture is not universal because it occurs in only 70% of individuals.[31] This raises the question of which individuals are most likely to respond. Whereas there is no definitive answer to this question, those individuals demonstrating changes in pain threshold and skin finger temperature in response to acupuncture appear most likely to respond.[73,74] Acupuncture's action on skin temperature signals its action on the sympathetic nervous system, more specifically cutaneous vasomotor fibers.

Application of acupuncture over a course of several weeks decreases nitroglycerin consumption and the rate of anginal attacks in patients with stable angina.[71,73-75] Finally, a prospective nonrandomized study of patients in whom acupuncture was administered as part of a lifestyle program incorporating stress reduction and healthy eating and living found reduced in-patient days, medication use, and accumulated mortality rate.[70,71,76] The independent contribution of acupuncture to these beneficial effects was not determined.

TENS increases the survival of skin flaps in experimental models as well as in patients undergoing reconstructive surgery.[77,78] Spinal cord stimulation, which may involve stimulation of many of the same central neural systems as in acupuncture,[79] increases skin temperature and reduces pain, ulcer formation, and tissue salvage in patients with peripheral vascular insufficiency.[80-82] No trials of acupuncture's influence in patients with peripheral vascular disease have been published.

Tai Chi and Qigong

Energy medicine stems from the belief that all living organisms radiate energy, although there is no sound scientific evidence that demonstrates the existence of bioenergy fields.[2] Tai Chi and Qigong, belonging to energy medicine, are part of traditional Chinese medicine. Like yoga, they include slow movements of the body, diaphragmatic breathing exercises, and mental concentration that have an impact on the autonomic nervous system, catecholamines, and blood pressure. Chi or Qi is considered to be energy that helps maintain homeostasis. According to traditional Chinese medicine theory, this energy flows through channels called meridians. Although somewhat controversial, most modern scientists recognize that these meridians, rather than forming a physical entity, represent a road map overlying neural pathways that provide sensory input to the central nervous system when they are stimulated.[32] A unique traditional Chinese medicine view is that the physical and emotional hearts are included as a single concept, taking into account our understanding that the brain (and spinal cord) strongly controls autonomic and hence cardiovascular function.[83,84]

Qigong means Qi training or Qi practice. Of the different forms of Qigong, medical Qigong is most applicable to treatment of cardiovascular disease and risk factors that promote cardiovascular disease. A typical session of Qigong includes meditation (see later), deep breathing and relaxation, guided imagery, mindful focus, and exercise and is practiced in a quiet place in fresh air. Thus, practitioners seek to relax their muscles, to regulate their breathing, and to concentrate their mind. Exercise consists of small postural movements of the limbs, walking, and larger movements.

A number of studies have evaluated the influence of Qigong on blood pressure in patients with mild to moderate hypertension.[85,86] For example, two small studies show that

Qigong lowers serum catecholamines and blood pressure in patients with essential hypertension.[87,88] However, in general, the quality of these studies is low, and they need to be repeated with larger numbers of patients, better blinding, randomization, and concealment of allocation.

Tai Chi is a type of Qigong that involves meditation, breathing, and slow movements of the limbs. It has roots in dance as well as in martial arts. Although there are many styles of Tai Chi, it can be modified for physical disability. Typically, the degree of exercise stress is considered mild to moderate, increasing heart rate reserve in one study by 58% and oxygen consumption to 55% of peak capacity.[89] Tai Chi increases aerobic capacity to the greatest extent in deconditioned subjects.[90] A small study has shown that compared with sedentary age-matched controls, during a 5-year period, elderly male and female subjects who regularly use Tai Chi experience smaller decrements in peak oxygen consumption and weight gain and smaller increments in body mass index and body fat as measured by skinfold thickness, although differences between the control and intervention groups were small.[91]

During a 12-week period, Tai Chi mildly lowers systolic and diastolic arterial blood pressure (–7/2 mm Hg) much like moderate exercise in patients with mild hypertension.[92] Decreases in anxiety and in total cholesterol and LDL-C and elevations in HDL-C, in addition to the blood pressure reduction, have been noted in hypertensive patients participating in a 12-week program of Tai Chi.[93,94] However, a review of approximately 70 articles on Qigong for hypertension suggests that most reports are in low-level scientific journals, conference proceedings, book excerpts, and informal reports that were not peer reviewed. Only five studies reported a randomized design.[95]

A few studies have investigated the role of Tai Chi and Qigong in patients with coronary artery disease. Patients randomized to Tai Chi and Qigong 3 weeks after an acute myocardial infarction demonstrate a reduction in systolic blood pressure similar to that of a music exercise group and show a greater reduction in diastolic blood pressure.[96]

Reiki and therapeutic touch are two other forms of energy medicine. Reiki uses what is believed to be "healing energy" to improve health by inducing deep relaxation. However, there are no studies demonstrating that a practitioner can "transfer energy" through strategic points (chakras) to cause a demonstrable cardiovascular response.[97,98] In contrast, therapeutic touch, in which the hands are used to direct healing energy, in several studies has demonstrated reduction of anxiety in coronary care unit patients.[97] There is no evidence showing that there is any direction of energy in therapeutic touch. The responses most likely are simply a "placebo" interaction involving reassurance and stress reduction that occurs between the therapist and the patient.[99]

Chinese Herbs

Traditional Chinese medicine employs herbs as frequently as acupuncture and frequently in conjunction with acupuncture. Herbs in traditional Chinese medicines are used to correct energy flow and balance as noted earlier for acupuncture and other traditional Chinese medicine therapies. Most commonly, herbs are taken as a fixed formula or in a fixed combination of several herbs. Each individual herb is thought to address a particular imbalance. In the less formal practice of Chinese folk medicine, herbs are used more simply, somewhat in the manner of Western herbal medicine.

Herbs most commonly used include astragalus (Astragalus mongholicus); danshen, commonly referred to as Chinese salvia (Salvia miltiorrhiza); dong quai (Angelica sinensis); ginger (Zingiber officinale); kudzu (Pueraria lobata); licorice (Glycyrrhiza glabra); lycium (Lycium chinense); Asian ginseng (Panax ginseng); and schizandra (Schisandra sphenanthera)

(see Appendix). Herbal preparations may be administered in many forms, including as a tea, tablet, capsule, or decoction; as such, their standardization and use in clinical trials have been challenging. In China today, traditional Chinese medicine is used alongside conventional pharmaceutical treatment in a holistic approach to treatment.

In a recent review[100] of 167 randomized controlled trials on the use of traditional Chinese medicine involving more than 18,000 participants, the authors noted that the overall methodologic quality of the trials was rated poor because of lack of description or incorporation of adequate sample sizes, randomization, allocation and blinding procedures, and disclosure of sample size estimates. Description of the quality control of herbal products also has been lacking from randomized controlled clinical trials reported in the literature addressing such issues as quality of the herbs selected, growing conditions, methods of preparation, testing for heavy metals and microbial contaminants, and use of good manufacturing processes.[101]

Despite some severe limitations with traditional Chinese medicine herbal interventions used in clinical trials, a number of compounds have been reported to be efficacious for treatment of cardiovascular conditions (Table 17-1), such as angina pectoris (danshen, compound salvia, suxiao jiuxin wan, tongxinluo) and hyperlipidemia (preparations of red yeast rice).

Danshen

According to traditional Chinese medicine, chronic stable angina belongs within the scope of pectoral pain and stuffiness (obstruction of Qi and blood in the chest). The traditional Chinese medicine herbal danshen, obtained from the dried root of Salvia miltiorrhiza, promotes blood circulation and relieves blood stasis. It is one of the most versatile traditional Chinese medicine herbals that has been used for hundreds of years in the treatment of numerous ailments. Much of the early research on the pharmacologic actions of danshen has been documented through intravenous use in animal models and human subjects.[102] Because of its properties related to improving microcirculation, enhancing coronary vasodilation, and protecting against myocardial ischemia through its negative chronotropic effects as well as suppressing the formation of thromboxane and inhibiting platelet adhesion and aggregation, danshen is widely used either alone or in combination with other herbals.

Danshen has also been studied with respect to its actions on lipid lowering (inhibition of LDL oxidation) and hypertension (inhibition of angiotensin-converting enzyme).[102] It is indicated for use for patients with coronary artery disease and other cardiovascular diseases in China and to a lesser extent in Japan, the United States, and other European countries. In China, danshen is used to treat angina pectoris, hyperlipidemia, and acute ischemic stroke.

The primary active ingredients containing tanshinones and phenolic compounds in danshen are found in dried root and rhizome preparations. Although danshen has no major side effects, it has the potential to interact with anticoagulants[103] and antiplatelet drugs or supplements with those properties.[104] Hence, it may increase the international normalized ratio (INR) and the risk of bleeding and should be avoided in patients taking warfarin. Danshen also may interfere with serum digoxin measurements.[105] Side effects include pruritus, upset stomach, and reduced appetite.[102]

Evidence to support use of danshen preparations is too weak for any judgment to be made about its effects. Collectively, evidence from randomized controlled trials is insufficient and of low quality. The first documented systematic review on the quality of randomized trials of danshen was recently published according to the CONSORT standards (Consolidated Standards for Reporting of Trials for

| TABLE 17–1 | Composition of Popular Traditional Chinese Medicines for Cardiovascular Indications |

Common Name	Latin Name	Active Constituents	Uses	Purported Actions
Single-ingredient Preparations				
Danshen	*Salvia miltiorrhizae*	Tanshinones, phenolic compounds	Angina pectoris	Coronary vasodilation
Red rice yeast	*Monascus purpureus*	Monocolin K	Lipid lowering	HMG-CoA reductase inhibitor
Compound-ingredient Preparations				
Compound salvia preparations			Angina pectoris	
Danshen	*Salviae miltiorrhizae*	Tanshinones, phenolic compounds		Coronary vasodilation
Sanqui	*Panax notoginseng*	Ginsenosides		
Borneol	*Cinnamomum camphora*			
Suxiao jiuxin wan			Angina pectoris	
Radix chuanxiong	*Ligusticum chuanxiong Hort*			Coronary vasodilation
Borneol (synthetic formulation)	*Borneolum syntheticum*			Increase plasma levels of radix chuanxiong
Tongxinluo			Angina pectoris	
Ren shen	*Radix ginseng*, 10%-20%	Ginsenosides		Increase cardiac contractility
Scorpion	*Scorpio*, 10%-20%			Decrease blood pressure
Leech	*Hirudo*, 20%-30%			Anticoagulant
Ground beetle	*Eupolyphaga seu steleophage*, 10%-20%			Increase cardiac output
Centipede	*Scolopendra*, 6%-15%			Increase cardiac contractility, decrease blood pressure
Cicada slough	*Periostracum cicadae*, 10%-20%			Decrease heart rate
Root of common peony	*Radix paeoniae rubra*, 5%-15%			Anticoagulant, coronary vasodilation
Borneol (synthetic formulation)	*Borneolum syntheticum*, 2%-10%			Analgesic and sedative

Modified from Wu T, Harrison RA, Chen X, et al: Tongxinluo (Tong xin luo or Tong-xin-luo) capsule for unstable angina pectoris. *Cochrane Database Syst Rev* (4):CD004474, 2006.

Traditional Chinese Medicine), which used the Jadad quality scale, for studies published in China from 1998 to 2007. A total of 150 studies were identified, with only 6.7% of the randomized controlled trials being identified as high quality (Jadad score ≥4). The authors concluded that the overall quality of these trials has not improved over time, and the evidence base for danshen is still poorly developed. More evidence from high-quality trials is needed to support the clinical use of danshen preparations.[106]

Recommendation. Evidence to support the use of danshen preparations is weak. Collectively, information from randomized controlled trials is insufficient and of low quality. Danshen has the potential to potentiate the effects of warfarin, and as such, it is prudent not to combine use of danshen with any anticoagulant or antiplatelet drugs.

Salvia

Compounded salvia has been promoted to improve blood circulation and is one of the alternative therapies widely used in China when long-acting nitrates are not an option. The primary herbal ingredients in this formulation include danshen *(Salviae miltiorrhizae),* sanqi *(Panax notoginseng),* and borneol *(Cinnamomum camphora).*[107] The principal active component in the compound is danshen (see Table 17-1). A recent meta-analysis supported by the Chinese Cochrane Center of 27 randomized trials (n = 3722) to evaluate the effectiveness of compounded salvia preparations (danshen pill) compared with isosorbide dinitrate concluded that the salvia preparations demonstrated a significant improvement in angina symptoms along with electrocardiographic improvements and few adverse events. The adverse event rate was significantly less than that of nitrates (2.4% versus 29.7%), leading to greater withdrawal of patients from the nitrate intervention compared with the salvia intervention group. However, there was significant heterogeneity in study endpoints, such as anginal symptoms and electrocardiographic changes.[108] Methodologic improvements with more well defined outcomes are needed. A subsequent

systematic review of 17 randomized controlled trials in patients with unstable angina noted significant improvement with compounded salvia in combination with standard therapy. Salvia preparations compared with standard therapy alone demonstrate greater improvement in electrocardiographic parameters and reduced anginal symptoms.[109] Again, the methodologic quality of the studies was low, thus limiting the clinical application of this herbal preparation.

Recommendation. Compounded salvia may be a viable alternative to standard therapy for the control of anginal symptoms if other standard therapies fail. However, the data are not robust, and caution should be used in patients receiving warfarin or other anticoagulants.

Suxiao Jiuxin Wan

Another popular Chinese herbal that has been used for the treatment of angina pectoris is suxiao jiuxin wan. This preparation may cause remission of angina pectoris, improve anginal symptoms, and reduce the use of nitroglycerin.[110] The ingredients in suxiao jiuxin wan include radix chuanxiong *(Ligusticum chuanxiong)* and borneol *(Borneolum syntheticum)* (see Table 17-1). A recent *Cochrane Review* identified 15 randomized controlled trials ranging from 4 weeks to 2 years in 1776 patients comparing the effects of suxiao jiuxin wan with nitroglycerin, danshen, and isosorbide dinitrate by evaluating electrocardiographic and angina endpoints. Unfortunately, the treatment regimen varied tremendously. In 10 studies, suxiao jiuxin wan provided better electrocardiographic results, better improvement in anginal symptoms, and less nitroglycerin use compared with patients randomized to nitroglycerin alone. Two studies reported electrocardiographic improvements with suxiao jiuxin wan compared with danshen. Clinical symptoms of angina were also improved with suxiao jiuxin wan. The one study that compared suxiao jiuxin wan with isosorbide dinitrate noted no improvement in the electrocardiographic or anginal symptoms. As noted before, studies tended to be of poor quality and lacked clinically relevant event outcomes that varied between trials. Headaches and bradycardia were reported in some studies, but none required medical management.[111]

Recommendation. Suxiao jiuxin wan is not recommended for cardiovascular use until further well-controlled trials with clinically relevant endpoints can substantiate benefits and reduction of anginal symptoms comparable to that of current standard therapies.

Tongxinluo

A new drug studied clinically only since 1995 for its efficacy in reducing episodes of angina pectoris is tongxinluo. Studies have demonstrated that tongxinluo possesses pleiotropic effects that are cardioprotective, including the improvement of endothelial function, lipid lowering, antioxidation, vasodilation, antithrombosis, anti-inflammation, antiapoptosis, and enhancement of angiogenesis.[112-115] These effects are similar to those of statin therapies.[116]

In a study using a rabbit model of induced atherosclerosis, tongxinluo in a dose-dependent manner increased the thickness of fibrous caps and plaque contents of smooth muscle cells and collagen; reduced serum lipoprotein levels, inflammatory biomarkers, and mRNA expression of matrix metalloproteinases; and decreased the incidence of plaque rupture.[117] Tongxinluo capsules contain both herbal and insect (scorpion, leech, and centipede) ingredients (see Table 17-1).

A systematic review performed by the Cochrane Collaboration identified 18 short-term studies (15 randomized) involving 1413 subjects that evaluated the benefit of tongxinluo with or without other treatments (danshen, isosorbide mononitrate, or low-molecular-weight heparin) in patients with unstable angina. The caliber of the studies was rated low, and thus no definitive conclusions were drawn about its efficacy with respect to myocardial infarction, angioplasty, or coronary artery bypass grafting. However, the authors noted some benefit in reduction of angina and electrocardiographic improvement. Although there were no recorded severe adverse events, slight gastrointestinal discomfort and ecchymoses were noted in a few cases. The safety of tongxinluo remains to be evaluated in appropriately designed trials. Additional efficacy studies are necessary for a thorough evaluation of this herbal preparation.[118]

Recommendation. Data are preliminary and weak; the safety of tongxinluo remains to be determined. Use of this combination product is not recommended.

Red Yeast Rice

Perhaps the most well known traditional Chinese medicine herbal therapy in Western clinical practice is red yeast rice (*Monascus purpureus*), used to treat hypercholesterolemia. Single herbs touted for lipid lowering include tumeric (*Curcuma longa*), hawthorn fruit (*Crataegus monogyna*), coptis or goldthread (*Coptis deltoidea*), soybean (*Glycine max*), five-leaf gynostemma (*Gynostemma pentaphyllum*), green tea (*Camellia sinensis*), Chinese rhubarb (*Rheum palmatum*), fleece flower tuber (*Polygonum multiflorum*), cassia seed (*Cinnamomum aromaticum*), and *Panax ginseng* (see Appendix). A number of compound recipes for lipid lowering have been used in recent years and have shown therapeutic effects by improving either clinical signs and symptoms or pathologic changes.[119]

Red yeast rice is derived from a yeast that grows on rice. It has been an Asian food staple and traditional remedy for thousands of years. One of the active ingredients in the yeast, monacolin K or lovastatin, is an inhibitor of HMG-CoA reductase, the rate-limiting enzyme in the pathway of cholesterol synthesis. The concentration of lovastatin varies in red rice yeast but averages nearly 0.4% by weight.

A meta-analysis of 93 randomized controlled trials (n = 9625) using three different commercial preparations of red yeast rice (cholestin, xuezhikang, and zhibituo) demonstrated a mean reduction in total cholesterol of 0.91 mmol/L, LDL-C of 0.73 mmol/L, and triglyceride of 0.41 mmol/L and a mean rise in HDL-C of 0.15 mmol/L compared with placebo. These levels are comparable to those achieved by many of the standard pharmacologic lipid-lowering agents,[120] except for the most powerful statins.

Xuezhikang, a commercial red yeast rice product containing 0.8% lovastatin, or approximately equivalent to 10 mg of lovastatin, has shown impressive results in clinical studies. The China Coronary Secondary Prevention Study carried out in 65 hospitals in China randomized 4870 patients with a prior history of myocardial infarction to either xuezhikang 600 mg twice daily or placebo for a mean duration of 4.5 years. The primary endpoints of nonfatal myocardial infarction and fatal coronary events, cardiovascular mortality, and total mortality were significantly reduced in the treatment group. The need for coronary revascularization was similarly reduced. Total cholesterol was reduced by 13% and LDL-C by 20%, with a noted 4.2% rise in HDL-C. No treatment-related serious adverse events or deaths were reported during the study period.[13]

It is possible that other monacolins or lovastatin hydroxyl acid, plant sterols, isoflavones, and isoflavone glycosides present in xuezhikang also could have cardioprotective effects in addition to that attributed to monacolin K. Reported side effects to red rice yeast are limited but include gastrointestinal upset, headaches, and dizziness. Similar cautions typical of HMG-CoA reductase inhibitors regarding potential side effects, including myopathy, hepatitis, and rhabdomyolysis, should be considered with red rice yeast products and will depend on the levels of monacolin K present.[121] As different concentrations of monacolins exist in an array of red yeast rice products, clinicians should examine the specifications of individual products before prescribing. Purity of products also may be variable; some may possess a toxic byproduct of yeast fermentation called citrinin.[122] Future use of xuezhikang as well as of other traditional Chinese recipes for lowering of cholesterol will depend on the separation, identification, characterization, and development of carefully formulated preparations. Additional well-controlled trials are needed before clinicians can use these products confidently. Although red yeast rice remains available in the United States, it is now fermented by a different process and the active ingredient has been removed, making its ability to lower cholesterol questionable.[104]

Recommendation. Red yeast rice products lower cholesterol and may be recommended to patients who prefer alternative treatments or who cannot tolerate standard drug therapies. Choice of products should be carefully scrutinized, and standard laboratory monitoring as used for HMG-CoA reductase inhibitors should be employed.

Conclusion

Collectively, the data on the effectiveness of Chinese herbs in the treatment of angina pectoris is not compelling, except possibly for danshen, which must be used with care when it is combined with conventional medications. Herbs used to treat hyperlipidemia (red yeast rice) are supported by limited data for efficacy. Additional well-controlled clinical trials with standardized preparations in appropriately studied population groups are needed to further define the efficacy and safety of these products.

AYURVEDIC MEDICINE

Ayurvedic medicine is one of the oldest systems of natural medicine (originating 4000 to 5000 years ago), older even than traditional Chinese medicine because Chinese and other medical systems originated from it.[123,124] It originated in India, and the Sanskrit word *ayurveda* means knowledge or science of life. The principal concept in ayurveda is living in harmony with the universe (environment) across one's life span. The original Vedic text, forming the foundation for this system, provides treatment of disease that includes diet, herbals, lifestyle, and disease prevention. Disease occurs when there is an imbalance between the body and the mind. Treatment, based on mind-body constitutions called *doshas,* uses dietary, lifestyle, and herbal prescriptions to evoke natural healing. There is a strong correspondence to traditional Chinese medicine and other integrative therapies like naturopathy. Heart disease, called *hydroga,* is related to several different causes, including, among others, emotional turmoil, dietary indiscretion, and sedentary lifestyle.

Ayurvedic therapies include yoga and transcendental meditation (a variant of yoga) in addition to dietary alterations and herbals. Yoga means "to join" and includes breath control, physical exercise, and meditation. A 3-month residential yoga program, which includes a vegetarian diet and regular yoga practice, can improve a number of cardiovascular risk factors, including blood pressure, weight (body mass index), and LDL-C.[125,126] These responses are similar to those noted in small early studies of lifestyle modification that incorporated dietary modification, exercise, and stress management.[127] Patients with angiographic coronary disease, not receiving lipid-lowering therapy, who practice yoga experience less angina and improved exercise capacity in association with atherosclerosis regression or reduced progression of disease.[128] Small controlled and uncontrolled studies suggest that yoga reduces blood pressure in patients with hypertension.[129-131] Regular yoga enhances mood and emotional well-being, indicating improved quality of life.[132] Much of the yoga relaxation response is related to reduced neuroendocrine stress as measured by urinary catecholamines, dopamine, and aldosterone or by heart rate and skin conductance.[133] The long-term cardiovascular influence of yoga has not been adequately studied.

Herbs in Ayurvedic Medicine

The medical system of Ayurveda is popular worldwide, not just in India. Recent analysis of the U.S. National Health Interview Survey 2007 Complementary and Alternative Medicine Supplement estimates that 214,000 adults used an Ayurvedic product in the past 12 months, a 28% increase from the 2002 survey on CAM use.[9] Herbs, minerals, and metals are used in Ayurvedic herbal products. Ayurvedic medicines are divided into two major types: herbal only and *rasa shastra*. In the practice of *rasa shastra,* herbs are combined with metals, minerals, and gems and appear to have been used safely for centuries when they are properly prepared. A number of the more popular Westernized Ayurvedic preparations with randomized controlled trials have been evaluated for efficacy, quality, and product effectiveness. Among these preparations are garlic *(Allium sativum)* for hyperlipidemia and hypertension and guggul *(Commiphora mukul)* and arjuna *(Terminalia arjuna)* for hyperlipidemia.

Garlic (Allium sativum)

Garlic has long been touted as a natural product useful for modulation of immune system activity, treatment of hyperlipidemia and hypertension, and primary and secondary prevention of myocardial infarction. Allicin, the bioactive component responsible for the cardiovascular activity of garlic, is rapidly formed from the allyl sulfur compounds (such as alliin) in the garlic. Raw crushed garlic has the highest concentration of allicin. Multiple mechanisms of action have been proposed, including decreases in cholesterol and fatty acid synthesis and cholesterol absorption as well as potent antioxidant properties.

Epidemiologic studies have shown an inverse correlation between garlic consumption and a reduced risk of cardiovascular disease progression.[134,135] Clinical studies of garlic's efficacy in lipid lowering, however, have yielded mixed results, with significant design flaws compromising the trials of garlic's effectiveness. Short-term studies have shown some benefit in lipid lowering, whereas long-term studies of 6 months or more fail to show sustained benefit when garlic is used as a single agent.[136] A recent well-designed randomized controlled trial using highly characterized diet and supplement interventions comparing the effects of raw garlic, powdered garlic supplement, aged garlic supplement, and placebo in 192 moderately hypercholesterolemic adults demonstrated no significant difference in LDL-C between treatment groups.[137] A systematic review of 21 garlic studies to evaluate the reporting quality, safety, and efficacy of randomized controlled trials for lipid lowering demonstrated that 53% of the garlic trials reported positive efficacy with a mean safety score of 63 of 100.[138]

Studies of garlic's effectiveness in hypertension also have suffered from poor methodology, and results have revealed small, mostly insignificant decreases in blood pressure. A meta-analysis published in 1994 reported promising results in subjects with mild hypertension but found insufficient evidence to recommend garlic for clinical therapy.[134] A subsequent systematic review of 27 small, randomized controlled trials of at least 4 weeks' duration comparing garlic with placebo, no garlic, or another active agent reported mixed effects of various garlic preparations on blood pressure.[136] Two meta-analyses published in 2008[139,140] concluded that compared with placebo, garlic significantly lowered systolic blood pressure in hypertensive individuals but not in normotensive individuals. However, the sample sizes of these two meta-analyses of hypertensive patients were not large. Garlic preparations and doses of 600 to 900 mg/day, providing 3.6 to 5.4 mg of allicin, were common in both meta-analyses. The level of blood pressure lowering was comparable to reductions seen with some antihypertensive drugs, suggesting that garlic may be a nonpharmacologic alternative for individuals with borderline or mild hypertension. However, additional studies with adequate sample size and standardized garlic preparations are needed to confirm these findings. Evidence for supplementation with garlic for either primary or secondary prevention of heart disease is not sufficient for its use to be recommended for hypertension.

Garlic preparations have been used in clinical studies for up to 4 years without reports of toxicity. The concomitant use of garlic with herbs or drugs that have warfarin constituents or affect platelet aggregation could increase INR and risk of bleeding. Garlic combined with fish oils and eicosapentaenoic acid (EPA) may increase antithrombotic effects. As such, individuals taking warfarin should be monitored more closely if they are consuming garlic supplements.[104] Additive effects on cholesterol lowering have been seen when garlic is taken with prescription drugs.

Recommendation. Garlic at best may offer modest cardiovascular risk reduction for lowering of blood pressure. It is not recommended for cholesterol lowering. Consumption of dietary sources of garlic is safe and can be incorporated into a heart-healthy dietary plan. Pharmacologic treatment guidelines should be followed for individuals identified with cardiovascular risk factors. Garlic as adjuvant therapy may be an option for some patients, although the American Heart Association notes that garlic has "no major role" in lipid lowering (total cholesterol and LDL-C).[141]

Guggul is the gummy resin derived from the bark of the mukul myrrh tree in India but can also be found in countries extending from northern Africa to central Asia. In fact, the mukul myrrh tree has been placed on the Red Data List[142] for further evaluation as it is on the threatened list in two regions in India where it is found because of excessive harvesting. It has played a role in Ayurvedic medicine for several thousand years and, in addition to its cardiovascular role, is used in the treatment of arthritis and digestive, skin, and menstrual problems.

The cardiovascular therapeutic benefits for guggul appear to be due to its multiple pharmacologic activities, notably the hypolipidemic, antioxidant, and anti-inflammatory effects. Gugulipid is the ethyl acetate extract of the gum containing 4.09 *Z*- and *E*-guggulsterones per 100 g. The lipid-lowering effect of gugulipid and guggulsterone, the bioactive constituent of guggul, has been consistently demonstrated in a number of animal species.

Guggulsterone has been identified as an antagonist to the farnesoid X nuclear receptor (FXR),[143,144] a key transcriptional regulator of cholesterol and bile acid homeostasis.[145-147] More recently, guggulsterone has also been shown to be an antagonist at the mineralocorticoid, glucocorticoid, and androgen receptors and an agonist of the pregnane X receptor (PXR), progesterone, and estrogen receptors (ERα).[148,149]

Clinical studies of guggul have demonstrated significant reductions in total cholesterol and LDL-C of 15% to 23% and triglyceride reduction of 20%, but results have been variable because populations under study have had different ethnic backgrounds, dietary habits, body weight, and severity of existing hyperlipidemia. The largest clinical study to date with 205 hypercholesterolemic or hypertriglyceridemic patients was conducted in 1989. After an 8-week diet and placebo lead-in, patients were randomized to gugulipid or placebo daily for 12 weeks. Total serum cholesterol was lowered by 24% and triglycerides were decreased by 23% in 70% to 80% of patients taking gugulipid.[150] In a subsequent 12-week crossover study of 125 patients taking gugulipid compared with a comparable dose of clofibrate, gugulipid decreased serum cholesterol by 11% and triglycerides by 17% compared with clofibrate reductions of 10% and 22%, respectively. Unlike clofibrate, gugulipid increased HDL levels by 60%. A longer term study (24 weeks) administering 100 mg of gugulipid daily, as guggulsterone, in conjunction with dietary modification also has shown significant reductions in lipid levels in hypercholesterolemic patients but no improvement in HDL-C.[151] In a randomized placebo-controlled trial of gugulipid in the United States, 103 healthy adults with hypercholesterolemia were given 1000 mg (low dose) or 2000 mg (high dose) gugulipid containing 2.5% guggulsterones for 8 weeks. Patients treated with gugulipid experienced no improvement in their lipid levels. In fact, their LDL levels increased by 4%, whereas patients who received placebo experienced a 5% decrease in LDL levels. The effects of gugulipids on HDL were mixed. Also noted was a median serum high-sensitivity C-reactive protein level that was decreased by 29% in the high-dose gugulipid group, whereas it increased by 25% in the placebo group, thus suggesting that gugulipid may also possess anti-inflammatory effects. A hypersensitivity rash was reported in a small number of subjects.[152] A systematic review of seven guggul studies (133 subjects) to evaluate the reporting quality, safety, and efficacy of published randomized controlled trials for lipid lowering concluded that 86% of the guggul trials reported positive efficacy with a mean safety score of 71 of 100.[138] It appears that individuals on a Western-style diet may achieve less of a lipid-lowering effect from gugulipid compared with those consuming a more traditional Indian diet.

Currently, no clinical studies have been conducted to evaluate the safety of long-term use of guggul or guggulsterone, but gugulipids have been shown to cause gastrointestinal upset, headache, mild nausea, belching, hiccups, and rash, depending on the dose and formulation (gugulipid versus crude guggul). Currently, 2.5% guggulsterone content is the minimum standard for quality gugulipid preparations.[153] Concomitant oral administration can reduce propranolol and diltiazem bioavailability and hence may reduce the therapeutic effects of these drugs.[154] Guggul also may have antiplatelet effects.[121]

Recommendation. Data on the efficacy of guggul for treatment of cardiovascular risk factors are mixed and limited. At this time, guggul is not recommended as a substitute for standard pharmacologic therapies for lipid lowering.

Terminalia arjuna

This is a deciduous tree found throughout India. Its bark has been used in Ayurvedic medicine for more than three centuries, primarily as a cardiac tonic. Arjuna is purported to be useful in alleviating anginal pain, hypercholesterolemia, heart failure, and coronary artery disease. It has been shown in animal studies and clinical trials to have cardiotonic, antihypertensive, antihyperlipidemic, antioxidant, and anticoagulant properties.

Among the bioactive constituents in arjuna are tannins, triterpenoid saponins, flavonoids, gallic acid, ellagic acid, oligomeric proanthocyanidins, phytosterols, and several minerals (calcium, magnesium, zinc, and copper).[155] The antioxidant cardioprotective effects are attributed to flavonoids and oligomeric proanthocyanidins; the positive inotropic effects may be caused by saponin glycosides.[156]

A systematic review of six studies of *Terminalia arjuna* incorporating 390 patients to evaluate the reporting quality, safety, and efficacy of published randomized controlled trials for lipid lowering demonstrated that 100% of the trials reported benefit and had a mean safety score of 20 of 100.[138] *Terminalia arjuna* has been shown to be efficacious in a small randomized clinical trial to evaluate the effectiveness of an extract in patients with stable angina compared with placebo and isosorbide mononitrate.[157] The arjuna preparation used in these studies was a commercial herbal-mineral compound containing more than eight different herbs, making it uncertain whether the cardioprotective benefit was due solely to arjuna.

Recommendation. Data for *Terminalia arjuna* are limited to a single product formulation evaluated in a small number of subjects. Additional well-controlled comparative trials are needed, and safety profiles must be established before its use can be recommended.

Conclusion

Several studies have shown poor quality control of some Ayurvedic medications, particularly some *rasa shastra* Ayurvedic medicines containing high levels of lead, mercury, and arsenic.[158] More than 80 cases of lead poisoning associated with Ayurvedic medicine use have been reported worldwide since 1978.[159,160] A recent random sample of commercially prepared Ayurvedic medicines purchased from the Internet had high metal concentrations determined by x-ray fluorescence spectroscopy. One fifth of both the U.S.- and Indian-manufactured medicines contained detectable lead, mercury, or arsenic exceeding at least 1 regulatory standard for acceptable daily metal intake. The presence of metals in non–*rasa shastra* medicines is also of concern because 17% of these have been determined to have higher levels of metals, the consequence of environmental contamination of the herbs or incidental contamination during manufacturing.[158] *Rasa shastra* experts claim that these medicines have been used for centuries and, if properly prepared and administered, are safe and therapeutic.[161,162]

Collectively, the data on the effectiveness of Ayurvedic herbs in the treatment of hyperlipidemia or hypertension are not compelling. Additional well-controlled clinical trials with standardized preparations in appropriately studied population groups are needed to further define the efficacy and safety of these products.

MEDITATION AND STRESS REDUCTION

During meditation, there is concentration on a word or a phrase, called a mantra. Meditation reduces blood pressure, heart rate, oxygen consumption, and plasma cortisol as subjects relax.[163-166] Likewise, meditation in elderly subjects with congestive heart failure is associated with reduced catecholamine production and improvement in the quality of life.[167] Depression, which predisposes to poor outcome after myocardial infarction, due in part to low adherence to a low-fat diet, regular exercise, and stress management,[168] can be reduced by mindfulness-based stress reduction.[123] However, cognitive therapy for these patients may not improve survival after a myocardial infarction.[169] Conversely, rehabilitation programs that include emotional support can reduce anxiety and improve mortality by up to 25%.[170-173] One phase of deep relaxation that has been called the fourth state of consciousness, to distinguish it from waking, dreaming, and sleeping, is characterized by reduced plasma cortisol and lactate levels, decreased metabolism, reduced breathing, increased brain alpha wave activity, and increased cerebral blood flow.[174,175] Many publications come from international journals or American CAM journals with relatively low impact factors because studies in this area are small, frequently inadequately controlled, and often not blinded.

Substantial research has examined the effects of lifestyle modification involving stress relaxation on blood pressure. These studies have used a number of different methods, such as autogenic training, cognitive and behavioral therapy, guided imagery, meditation, biofeedback, progressive muscle relaxation, and yoga. There is substantial overlap between the various techniques of relaxation. Autogenic training, for example, includes focusing on a physiologic sensation like the heartbeat and self-suggestion, which also can be used during meditation. Cognitive therapy involves control of irrational thought processes; behavioral reinforcement rewards certain behaviors that promote relaxation. Guided imagery focuses on calming images. A review of more than 25 randomized trials suggests that relaxation lowers systolic and diastolic blood pressure a small amount, ranging from 2 to 8 mm Hg.[176] However, many trials have been poorly constructed, and the use of so many different techniques to lower stress makes comparison difficult. Furthermore, 15 of the trials that compared relaxation with sham demonstrated an insignificant decrease in blood pressure. More rigorous evaluation of this commonly included aspect of lifestyle modification is warranted.

NATUROPATHIC MEDICINE

Naturopathic medicine is both a health system and a philosophy (Box 17-4). It originated from a number of traditional medical systems from India (Ayurvedic), China (traditional Chinese medicine), Greece (Hippocratic), and Germany (homeopathy, hydrotherapy), among others. It is largely based on the belief that the body can heal itself and thus subscribes to the healing power of nature. The goal is to live as naturally as possible and to use healing practices that support normal physiologic function rather than drugs that

BOX 17-4 Healing Practices in Naturopathic Medicine

- Consuming natural unrefined and organically grown foods
- Sufficient exercise
- Living a lifestyle that is in moderation
- Thinking constructive thoughts and emotions
- Avoiding environmental toxins
- Maintaining proper elimination

would be considered an artificial enhancement. Naturopathic physicians believe that most (not all) disease is the result of violation of natural laws of living. Thus, healing results from a variety of practices that support normal function.

Naturopathy consists of health maintenance, disease prevention, education, and self-responsibility. The practice of naturopathy relies on diagnosis and the use of natural therapies that evoke the body's endogenous healing mechanisms. Naturopaths function as primary care physicians; because they realize that not all disease can be prevented or treated by the natural approach, practitioners will employ office surgery, prescription drugs, and referrals as appropriate. Clinical nutrition, botanical medicine, acupuncture, hydrotherapy, physical medicine, and counseling form the most compelling therapies. Homeopathy, although practiced by most naturopaths, has little documented value for cardiovascular disease.

Clinical nutrition uses the diet as therapy and in prevention of disease. It is the foundation of naturopathic practice. Botanicals, including herbals, can be used in place of some drugs, but they are more commonly used to support natural healing of the body. In fact, nutritional training in naturopathy generally is much greater than that received by allopathic students. Other chapters in this textbook provide information that would be recommended by naturopathic practitioners, including dietary fiber, omega fatty acids, walnuts and almonds to reduce LDL-C, soy-based foods, and the Mediterranean diet.[177-180]

Chelation Therapy

Chelation therapy with disodium ethylenediaminetetraacetic acid (EDTA), which is used by some naturopathic practitioners, has clear clinical value in treating lead intoxication. It also has been used "off label" for more than 30 years to treat atherosclerosis. Chelation therapy with EDTA, supplemented with some vitamins, heparin, and magnesium, has been promoted by the American College for Advancement in Medicine. EDTA binds divalent and trivalent cations, including calcium. Proposed mechanisms of action, including lowering of calcium from plaques, inhibition of platelet aggregation, mobilization of parathyroid hormone to remove calcium, vascular antioxidant effects including chelation of iron, and transient lowering of cholesterol, are unproven. Because calcification of plaques tends to occur late in plaque development, mobilization of serum calcium is not likely to be effective in altering atherosclerotic progression.

EDTA infusion carries a risk of congestive heart failure because EDTA is administered in large volumes as the disodium salt. Renal toxicity, hypoglycemia, and hypocalcemia and tetany also can occur if the infusion rate is too rapid.[181] There also is evidence that EDTA may be a pro-oxidant.[182] Studies show that 100,000 to 800,000 individuals in the United States have received this therapy.[183,184]

Clinical trials of chelation therapy are few, small in size, and poorly designed.[185] The majority of the studies of coronary or peripheral arterial disease are case reports and case studies, most uncontrolled and retrospective. One large study and a smaller follow-up study of patients with peripheral vascular disease found no difference between control and treatment groups in symptomatic relief[186] or in angiographic disease and transcutaneous oxygen tension.[187] Three prospective randomized trials of chelation therapy have been published. A Danish trial of 153 patients in 1992 reported no long-term therapeutic effect at 3 or 6 months; a small trial of 32 patients from New Zealand showed some improvement in patients with peripheral vascular disease at 3 months.[186-190] Both trials had significant methodologic deficiencies that preclude accurate conclusions. A final 6-month prospective study called the PATCH trial (Program to Assess Alternative Treatment Strategies to Achieve Cardiac Health) of 39 patients with well-documented coronary disease observed no significant difference in clinical outcome or quality of life score.[190] Unfortunately, this study was underpowered, and the placebo arm contained vitamin C, which may have provided an antioxidant effect. A larger randomized trial to assess chelation therapy (TACT) is ongoing. It is unclear why NCCAM funded this $30 million trial without definitive mechanistic evidence for the action of EDTA infusion or support from previous clinical trials.

Recommendation. Given the lack of firm evidence supporting a beneficial effect of chelation therapy and the potential for serious side effects, the American College of Cardiology and the American Heart Association have not endorsed its use in chronic stable angina.[191]

NUTRITIONAL SUPPLEMENTS

It is estimated that 52% of adults participating in the 1999-2000 National Health and Nutrition Examination Survey (NHANES) had consumed some form of a dietary supplement within a month before participating in the survey; 35% took a multivitamin-multimineral supplement.[192] Dietary supplement use in individuals with coronary artery disease or risk factors for coronary artery disease is common; 60% of adults with coronary artery disease, stroke, hypertension, or elevated cholesterol used at least one dietary supplement within the month preceding the survey. Individuals with a history of coronary artery disease or stroke commonly report the use of vitamin E, folic acid, and niacin; those with a history of hypertension or elevated cholesterol report higher use of herbals, commonly ginseng, as tabulated from the 1999-2002 NHANES data.[193]

A number of popular dietary supplements with a significant evidence base lack public health recommendations for primary or secondary prevention of cardiovascular disease. These include B vitamins, the antioxidant vitamins C and E, vitamin D, and magnesium. On occasion, as appropriate, these supplements may be warranted for individual use.

Other nutrient supplements purported for cardiovascular disease or prevention that have been less well studied in clinical trials, or for which there is a lack of data from the United States, remain alternative therapies and should be integrated with great care. Supplements in this category include α-lipoic acid, L-arginine, L-carnitine, nonprescription niacin products, and selenium (see Appendix). Dietary supplements continue to be popular as documented by the spending of more than $23.7 billion by Americans on products in 2007. The most popular products for heart health are shown in Table 17-2.

B Vitamins

Moderate elevations of plasma homocysteine levels have been associated with an enhanced risk for atherosclerotic

TABLE 17–2	Sales of Dietary Supplements for Heart Health		
	Supplements	**$ Million**	**% of Sales**
1	Fish/animal oils	326	25
2	CoQ10	272	21
3	Multivitamins	225	17
4	Vitamin E	125	9
5	Plant oils	109	8
6	B vitamins	104	8
7	Potassium	58	4
8	Magnesium	41	3
9	Homeopathics	39	3
10	Vitamin A/beta carotene	31	2

Source: Nutrition Business Journal's 2008 Business Report.

disease.[194-197] The metabolism of homocysteine requires several B vitamins as cofactors, specifically vitamin B_6, vitamin B_{12}, and folate. Homocysteine levels can be decreased by the administration of supplemental folate, with or without vitamin B_6 or B_{12}. Although epidemiologic studies suggest potential cardiovascular benefit with B vitamin supplementation, most intervention trials (such as HOPE-2, VISP, and NORVIT) using combined B vitamin therapy of folic acid and vitamins B_6 and B_{12} have shown no benefit.[198-200]

More recently, results from the Women's Antioxidant and Folic Acid Cardiovascular Study, a secondary prevention trial of 5442 women, revealed that combination B vitamin therapy, including 2.5 mg folic acid, 50 mg vitamin B_6, and 1 mg vitamin B_{12}, after 7 years of treatment and follow-up demonstrated no reduction in total cardiovascular events compared with placebo.[201] A meta-analysis of four randomized, controlled trials of B vitamin therapy found no evidence that B vitamin supplements slowed the progression of atherosclerosis.[202] However, it has been postulated that folic acid supplementation, through lowering of homocysteine levels, may positively influence vascular function in the early stages of cardiovascular disease by modulating endothelial dysfunction. A recent meta-analysis of 14 intervention trials in which high doses of folic acid were administered for 4 months or more and flow was measured demonstrated that folic acid improved flow-mediated dilation by only 1.08% compared with placebo.[203]

A protocol for a collaborative meta-analysis of homocysteine-lowering trials for prevention of vascular disease has been proposed by the B-Vitamin Treatment Trialists' Collaboration. By pooling of the data from 12 B vitamin supplementation trials for the prevention of coronary heart disease and stroke, it is hoped that more definitive recommendations on the use of folic acid and vitamin B_{12} for prevention of cardiovascular disease will emerge. Presently, seven studies with 33,755 subjects are being monitored for major coronary events.[204] Until such time, the American Heart Association notes that the available evidence is inadequate for the recommendation of folic acid and other B vitamin supplements as a means of primary or secondary prevention of cardiovascular disease.[205]

Recommendation. Current evidence is inadequate for the recommendation of folic acid and other B vitamin supplements for primary or secondary prevention of cardiovascular disease.[205] However, they can be used to lower plasma homocysteine levels in high-risk subjects.

Antioxidant Vitamins

Despite a large body of epidemiologic evidence suggesting a favorable association between a diet high in antioxidants and reduced risk of coronary heart disease, no clinical trial has confirmed such benefit. Higher overall intake of vitamin C was associated with lower rates of coronary disease in some cohort studies with information on supplemental vitamin C intake[206] but not in others.[207] Improved endothelial function has been observed with vitamin C supplementation in patients at risk for cardiovascular disease.[208] An inverse relationship between vitamin E intake and the risk of coronary disease demonstrated that 30 IU/day of vitamin E potentially can lower coronary disease risk by 4%. Supplementation with vitamin E alone also has shown an inverse correlation with coronary heart disease.[207]

Randomized trials have evaluated antioxidant supplements in varying doses for lowering of coronary heart disease risk. In the Heart Protection Study, 20,536 patients with coronary artery disease or diabetes were randomized to antioxidant vitamins (600 mg of vitamin E, 250 mg of vitamin C, and 20 mg of beta carotene) versus placebo. Although the vitamin regimen was found to be safe, there was no evidence for a therapeutic effect after 5 years of treatment.[209] Similarly, the Physicians' Health Study follow-up also found that neither vitamin C nor vitamin E reduced the incidence of major cardiovascular events, myocardial infarction, stroke, or cardiovascular mortality after 8 years of study. Furthermore, use of vitamin E was associated with an increased risk of hemorrhagic stroke.[210]

In contrast, the Antioxidant Supplementation in Atherosclerosis Prevention (ASAP) study in hypercholesterolemic patients randomized to twice-daily supplements of 136 IU of vitamin E, 250 mg of slow-release vitamin C, both, or placebo demonstrated that only combined supplementation of vitamin E and vitamin C slowed the progression of common carotid intima-media thickness (25% decrease).[211] However, in the Women's Angiographic Vitamin and Estrogen study, postmenopausal women with some degree of coronary stenosis who took vitamin E and vitamin C twice a day or placebo for more than 4 years experienced no cardiovascular benefit, and in fact, all-cause mortality was significantly higher in women taking the supplements.[212] Whereas this latter observation may have been a chance finding, it follows a trend toward an increase in mortality that was observed in the Heart Protection Study.[209]

Randomized clinical trials also have cast doubt on the efficacy of vitamin E as monotherapy to prevent coronary disease. Although the Cambridge Heart Antioxidant Study (CHAOS) demonstrated a reduction in events of the combined endpoint of death or nonfatal myocardial infarction by 47%,[213] HOPE and HOPE-2 provide strong evidence that moderately high doses of vitamin E supplements do not reduce the risk of serious cardiovascular events among men and women with established heart disease or diabetes. In fact, participants taking vitamin E in the HOPE-2 trial were 13% more likely to experience and 21% more likely to be hospitalized for heart failure, an unexpected and statistically significant finding.[214] Possible explanations for this harmful effect of vitamin E could relate to the potential for α-tocopherol to become a pro-oxidant in an oxidative environment, thereby depressing myocardial function,[215] or to the higher doses than those normally consumed in the diet employed in the study.

Data from randomized controlled trials in women have provided much needed information for clinicians to make appropriate therapeutic choices in the management of cardiovascular risk in women. The Women's Heath Study of 39,876 apparently healthy women aged 45 years and older found that vitamin E (600 IU on alternate days) reduced cardiovascular death, a secondary endpoint, by 24% but had no effect on total cardiovascular events, myocardial infarction, or stroke.[216] In further analysis of the same data, women randomized to vitamin E demonstrated an overall 21% reduced risk of venous thromboembolism. The observed risk reduction was 44% among those with prothrombotic mutations or a personal history of venous thromboembolism. Overall, vitamin E was associated with lower risk of bleeding than that observed for low-dose aspirin.[217]

The American Heart Association concluded in their 2007 update of the women's prevention guidelines that antioxidant vitamin supplements should not be used for the primary or secondary prevention of cardiovascular disease.[218] However, as observed in the Women's Heath Study, there may be certain populations, such as the elderly (>65 years) or those with a history of venous embolism, that could benefit from targeted therapy.

A number of meta-analyses have evaluated a range of cardiovascular disease outcomes for varying forms and doses of vitamin E in a number of populations of patients.[219-223] Most analyses concluded that vitamin E provided no benefit and no increased risk. Lacking from most antioxidant intervention trials are plasma measures of vitamins or determination of a subject's baseline oxidative stress status. Future studies should determine whether those with marginal vitamin status based on measurements will benefit from supplementation.

Recommendation. The American Heart Association does not recommend the use of antioxidant vitamin supplements for the primary or secondary prevention of cardiovascular disease. Patients should be encouraged to supplement their diet with foods rich in antioxidants and to consume a multivitamin-mineral supplement if they are concerned that their diets are inadequate.

Vitamin D

Recent literature suggests that vitamin D inadequacy is pandemic, and a growing body of evidence is emerging to show that low levels of vitamin D may adversely affect the cardiovascular system. In this regard, data are accumulating in populations with elevated cardiovascular disease risk factors, such as hypertension[224-227] and metabolic syndrome,[228-230] as well as in subjects with established disease, such as diabetes,[231,232] coronary heart disease,[233] peripheral arterial disease,[234] stroke,[235] congestive heart failure,[236,237] and cardiovascular mortality associated with low vitamin D.[238] In 1739 participants in the Framingham Offspring Heart Study, researchers found that those with vitamin D blood levels <15 ng/mL had twice the risk of a cardiovascular event in the next 5 years compared with those with higher levels of vitamin D.[227] Interestingly, the risk remained significant after adjustment for traditional cardiovascular disease risk factors. Calcium and vitamin D supplementation was found neither to increase nor to decrease coronary or cerebrovascular risk in generally healthy postmenopausal women participating in the Women's Health Initiative.[239]

Low circulating levels of 25-hydroxyvitamin D also are associated with increased evidence of inflammation, oxidative burden, and cell adhesion, suggesting that vitamin D plays a role in processes that contribute to cardiovascular risk and mortality.[240] Unfortunately, no dose-response studies with supplemental vitamin D are available yet to test the association of vitamin D with cardiovascular disease. Unlike the data and association of vitamin D with osteoporosis, the cardiovascular data are mixed and less robust and thus lack the evidence base to suggest causation. It is premature to recommend screening for at-risk individuals and supplementation with vitamin D above the recommended levels.

There is considerable discussion of the appropriate serum concentrations of 25-hydroxyvitamin D associated with deficiency versus optimal overall health (Table 17-3). The current

TABLE 17–3	Serum 25-Hydroxyvitamin D Concentrations and Health	
ng/mL*	nmol/L*	Health Status
<11	<27.5	Associated with vitamin D deficiency and rickets in infants and young children
<10-15	<25-37.5	Generally considered inadequate for bone and overall health in healthy individuals
≥30	≥75	Proposed by some as desirable for overall health and disease prevention, although a recent government-sponsored expert panel concluded that insufficient data are available to support these higher levels.
Consistently >200	Consistently >500	Considered potentially toxic, leading to hypercalcemia and hyperphosphatemia, although human data are limited. In an animal model, concentrations ≤400 ng/mL (≤1000 nmol/L) demonstrated no toxicity.

*Serum concentrations of 25-hydroxyvitamin D are reported in both nanograms per milliliter (ng/mL) and nanomoles per liter (nmol/L).

level of variability in 25-hydroxyvitamin D measurements calls into question the stability of 25-hydroxyvitamin D assays and their ability to reflect accurately the vitamin D status in individuals.[241,242]

No clinical practice guidelines have been issued regarding the use of vitamin D for conditions of cardiovascular disease. Current recommendations set by the Institute of Medicine are 400 IU/day for individuals 50 to 70 years and 600 IU/day for individuals 70 years and older. Newer clinical trials conducted in healthy adults suggest that a dose as high as 10,000 IU/day has been used without ill effects, but the upper level of intake established by the Institute of Medicine of 2000 IU/day is considered safe.[243] Although vitamin D supplementation above recommended levels given in clinical trials has not shown harm, most trials have not been designed to assess harm.[244] In the Women's Health Initiative, increased risk of hypercalcemia and hypercalciuria was not clinically significant, but it was associated with a 17% increase in the risk of kidney stones.[226]

Recommendation. Vitamin D is not recommended at this time for prevention or treatment of cardiovascular disease. However, supplementation with 400 to 600 IU/day and no more than 2000 IU of 1,25-dihydroxyvitamin D_3 for low circulating levels of vitamin D or those with poor dietary intakes and low sun exposure can safely be recommended for patients with cardiovascular disease.

Magnesium

Magnesium is cardioprotective. Aging, decreases in dietary intake, and polypharmacy coupled with decreases in intestinal magnesium absorption and increases in urinary magnesium losses place older adults at risk for magnesium deficiency. According to the U.S. Department of Agriculture, less than 60% of adult men and women have an adequate dietary intake of magnesium.[245]

Trials of magnesium therapy in acute myocardial infarction have produced mixed results, and chronic use has focused on the role of magnesium as an antihypertensive. A review of more than 28,000 women enrolled in the Women's Health Study indicated that those in the highest quintile of magnesium intake had a decreased risk for hypertension compared with those in the lowest quintile.[246] A recent review of nutritional effects on blood pressure indicated that high levels of magnesium as well as of potassium, calcium, and soy seem to have beneficial effect on hypertension.[247] A *Cochrane Review* evaluating the effect of combined calcium, potassium, and magnesium supplementation for management of primary hypertension in adults failed to find robust evidence to support a role for these supplements in the treatment of hypertension.[248]

There is insufficient evidence to recommend magnesium supplementation for treatment of cardiovascular risk factors. However, the Joint National Committee on Prevention, Detection, Evaluation, and Treatment of High Blood Pressure states that diets that provide plenty of magnesium represent positive lifestyle modifications for individuals with hypertension.[249] General multivitamin-mineral supplements often provide approximately 25% (100 mg) of the daily recommended need for magnesium, an amount considered safe but that may not be adequate to sustain magnesium stores in the body for at-risk individuals. A small well-controlled feeding study in a group of healthy postmenopausal women suggested that consumption of this amount of dietary magnesium daily for 58 days was inadequate as shown by the onset of cardiac arrhythmias.[250] Supplementation with the recommended dietary allowance (420 mg for men and 320 mg for women) of magnesium typically is safe in individuals without compromised kidney function but may cause diarrhea, depending on the formulation.

Recommendation. Dietary supplementation of magnesium is not recommended for treatment of cardiovascular risk factors but can be recommended in the form of a general multivitamin-mineral supplement for those with consistently poor dietary intakes.

Conclusion

In general, clinical trials have not provided sufficient evidence supporting routine use of antioxidants, B vitamins, or other nutrient supplements to prevent cardiovascular disease or to reduce morbidity and mortality. Some investigators have suggested that understanding of the potential utility of vitamin E and vitamin C in prevention of coronary disease might require longer studies in younger participants taking higher doses of the supplement.[251] Further research is needed to determine whether dietary supplements have any protective value for younger, healthier people without risk factors for coronary heart disease.

NONVITAMIN, NONMINERAL SUPPLEMENTS

Nearly 18% of participants in the National Health Interview Survey revealed that the most common CAM therapies used were nonvitamin, nonmineral natural products, including fish oil or omega-3 or docosahexaenoic acid (DHA), glucosamine, echinacea, flaxseed oil or pills, and ginseng.[9] Among the dietary supplements with possible cardiovascular benefit not endorsed by national public health recommendations but with a developing base of evidence on which randomized clinical trials can be planned or guidelines for use might be formulated include coenzyme Q10, French pine bark, horse chestnut seed extract, and *Ginkgo biloba*. As appropriate, these supplements can be integrated into clinical practice and are discussed here. Other supplements purported for cardiovascular disease prevention that have been less well studied in controlled clinical trials or that lack data in U.S. population groups remain alternative therapies and should be integrated into medical practice with great care. Supplements in this category include artichoke leaf, fenugreek, green tea, gugulipid (described earlier), and policosanol for lipid lowering, and hawthorn for angina pectoris and mild heart failure (see Table 17-1).

Because nonvitamin, nonmineral supplements lack public health recommendations and, except for soy, are not used extensively in the United States, clinicians should keep abreast of the changing literature on their use. If they are prescribed, frequent checks of reputable resources should be made for contraindications and adverse event reports.

Soy and Soy Isoflavones

Approximately 30% of women use acupuncture, natural estrogens, herbal supplements, or plant estrogens to treat symptoms and discomforts related to menopause.[252] This number was actually higher for women participating in the Study of Women's Health Across the Nation, in which 66% and 37% of the women, respectively, used nutritional remedies or herbal remedies for menopausal symptoms.[253] Alternative treatments include phytoestrogens (from soy and red clover), black cohosh, and progesterone creams; only soy and soy isoflavones are discussed here.

Soy protein and soy isoflavones have not been shown to improve vasomotor symptoms of menopause because they do not have sufficient estrogenic activity to have an important impact on vasomotor symptoms of estrogen deficiency in perimenopausal women.[254] With regard to cardiovascular disease prevention, diets substituted with soy protein in place of animal protein can produce significant reductions in LDL-C and triglycerides.[255] Whether this reflects a unique benefit of soy or isoflavones in particular or merely is the result of a reduction in dietary animal protein and fat is unclear. Much of the most favorable evidence on this intervention is observational. A meta-analysis of 10 studies of the effect of soy isoflavones on cholesterol concentrations in well-controlled trials substituting soy proteins for dairy or animal protein for at least 14 days found that consumption of soy isoflavones was not related to changes in LDL-C or HDL-C.[256] A review of the benefits of soy protein and isoflavones has been published by the American Heart Association Nutrition Committee.[254] A total of 22 randomized trials evaluated the effects of soy protein and, in aggregate, found a small decrease in LDL-C with no effects on other lipid fractions or blood pressure. Soy isoflavones, also believed to be efficacious in reducing cardiovascular disease risk, were evaluated in 19 studies and did not alter lipids or blood pressure. The American Heart Association concluded that no meaningful benefit of soy consumption could be demonstrated for HDL-C, triglycerides, or lipoprotein(a). However, the National Cholesterol Education Program Adult Treatment Panel III recommends replacement of products containing animal fats with soy protein to enhance cholesterol lowering.[257]

Recommendation. Supplementation with soy or its constituent isoflavones is not warranted and should not be encouraged for cardiovascular disease risk reduction. However, increasing soy food consumption in the diet is safe and is encouraged by some authorities.

Coenzyme Q10

Coenzyme Q10 (CoQ10) is involved in cellular oxidative phosphorylation and the generation of ATP. In addition, CoQ10 acts as a free radical scavenger and a membrane stabilizer. CoQ10 may improve the efficiency of energy production in heart tissue and thus assist the heart during times of physical or oxidative stress.[258-261] Several meta-analyses reviewing the data with regard to CoQ10 therapy in patients with congestive heart failure have reached mixed conclusions about efficacy. Of more interest are the reduced plasma or serum levels of CoQ10 that have been documented in observational studies and randomized clinical trials in patients receiving statin therapies.[262-266] Decreases in blood CoQ10 levels with statin treatment may be related to reduced synthesis as well as to a decrease in circulating levels of CoQ10, as it is carried in the blood by LDL-C.[267] A recent systematic review on the role of CoQ10 in statin-associated myopathy confirmed that statin treatment reduced circulating levels of CoQ10 and that supplementation can raise circulating levels of CoQ10.[268] However, overall data on CoQ10 blood levels are contradictory.

The largest trial of 1049 patients noted reductions in plasma CoQ10 levels after 52 weeks of treatment with either atorvastatin (38% reduction) or lovastatin (27% reduction).[264] Supplementation with CoQ10 (100 mg/day for 30 days) decreased muscle pain by 40% in patients with myopathic symptoms associated with statin treatment. However, 200 mg/day in another study did not improve statin-induced myalgia.[269] Additional well-designed clinical trials are required to address this issue. At this time, routine use of CoQ10 is questionable in statin-treated patients, although it may be an alternative for patients taking statins with myalgia who cannot be satisfactorily treated with other agents.

In general, CoQ10 appears to be safe. No significant side effects have been found, even in studies that lasted a year. CoQ10 chemically resembles vitamin K. However, because vitamin K counters the anticoagulant effect of warfarin, it is not surprising that case reports associate CoQ10 therapy with decreased INR in patients receiving warfarin therapy.[121] On the other hand, 100 mg of CoQ10 daily did not alter the INR in patients taking warfarin in a randomized, double-blind, placebo-controlled, crossover trial.[270] Typical doses range from 100 to 200 mg, two or three times daily. Caution is advised if patients take CoQ10 and warfarin as CoQ10 has the potential to decrease the effectiveness of warfarin.

Recommendation. Routine use of CoQ10 currently is questionable in statin-treated patients, although it may be an alternative for patients taking statins with myalgia who cannot be satisfactorily treated with other agents. CoQ10 otherwise is not recommended for the prevention of cardiovascular disease. Caution is advised in patients taking CoQ10 and warfarin.

Cocoa (Theobroma cacao)

Cocoa belongs to a class of natural compounds, called polyphenols, rich in a number of plant foods. Flavanols, a subclass of polyphenols, are abundant in raw cocoa. Epidemiologic studies in the Kuna Indians, a population with low cardiovascular event rates compared with their Panamanian neighbors, peaked interest in the antihypertensive effects of cocoa.[271] In the Zutphen Elderly Study, the median cocoa intake among users was 2.11 g/day, which was found to be inversely associated with blood pressure and 15-year cardiovascular and all-cause mortality.[272] Chocolate and cocoa products inhibit LDL oxidation and platelet activation, positively affect eicosanoid synthesis, and promote endothelium-dependent relaxation. Cocoa flavanols enhance flow-mediated dilation through a nitric oxide–dependent mechanism.[273] Large interindividual variations in absorption of flavanols have been observed, thus limiting interpretation of study results.

Consumption of flavanol-rich cocoa for 6 weeks in 101 healthy volunteers failed to improve blood pressure (as shown in earlier studies in normotensive subjects),[274-276] lipid parameters, or C-reactive protein levels.[277] However, chronic administration of 6.3 g/day of dark chocolate containing 30 mg of polyphenols or matching polyphenol-free chocolate in 44 healthy prehypertensive or stage 1 hypertensive adults for 18 weeks demonstrated small but significant reductions in systolic and diastolic blood pressures. Reductions in oxidative stress and improved formation of nitric oxide also were observed.[278] A 2-week intervention trial administering a flavanol-rich cocoa drink (150 mL twice a day, approximately 900 mg flavanols per day) did not reduce blood pressure or improve insulin resistance in 20 subjects with essential hypertension but did enhance insulin-mediated vasodilation.[279]

A recent meta-analysis of five randomized trials (173 normotensive and hypertensive subjects) evaluated cocoa intake and blood pressure in studies with a median duration of 2 weeks. Of the five studies, four reported reductions in systolic and diastolic blood pressure with cocoa consumption. The polyphenol content administered was 500 mg/day in three of the five studies and roughly half that in the other two studies. Compared with the cocoa-free control, the pooled decrease was −4.7 mm Hg in systolic blood pressure and −2.8 mm Hg in diastolic blood pressure for those randomized to cocoa.[280] Similar blood pressure reductions were confirmed in a subsequent meta-analysis.[281] Chocolate or cocoa also increased flow-mediated dilation by 4% after acute administration (six studies) and by 1.45% after chronic administration (two studies).[281]

Clinical data on consumption of cocoa for cardiac protection appear favorable for blood pressure lowering in individuals with mild hypertension, but the response is not robust. Additional studies are warranted before clinical endorsements can be issued regarding supplemental use beyond incorporation of traditional foods containing cocoa or chocolate into a daily diet plan.

Recommendation. Intake of supplements containing cocoa or its active constituents should be discouraged for disease prevention or reduction of risk factors.

Ginkgo biloba (Ginkgo Leaf Extract)

Ginkgo is one of the most popular herbal therapies in Germany and France, where physicians prescribe it for memory lapses, dizziness, anxiety, headaches, tinnitus, and other problems. It has been used for relief of intermittent claudication in patients with peripheral arterial occlusive disease.[159] Compared with placebo, Ginkgo biloba extract appears to be effective in patients with intermittent claudication (Fontaine stage II peripheral arterial disease). Doses employed in clinical trials ranged from 120 to 160 mg/day. Pain-free walking distance and maximal walking distance were often the monitored outcomes of interest. As with other phytomedicines, several constituents of ginkgo extracts may contribute to its therapeutic effect. Ginkgo leaf and its extracts contain several bioactive constituents including flavonoids, terpenoids, and organic acids.[282] Flavonoids reduce capillary permeability and fragility and serve as free radical scavengers. The terpenes, which include the active principle ginkgolides, inhibit platelet-activating factor, decrease vascular resistance, and improve circulatory flow.[283]

A small benefit for ginkgo in the treatment of peripheral arterial disease was confirmed by two meta-analyses reporting a statistically significant increase in walking distance averaging nearly 25 meters.[284,285] The most common dosage is 40 mg of standardized extract of ginkgo leaf three times daily. Ginkgo is considered relatively safe and well tolerated and has only a few documented adverse effects, including mild gastrointestinal upset, nausea, dyspepsia, and headache. Ginkgo has been reported to increase both spontaneous and trauma-related bleeding during surgery and other procedures.[286,287] Ginkgo does not appear to interact or adversely affect concomitant therapy with cardiac glycosides. The combined use of ginkgo with herbs or drugs with anticoagulant or antiplatelet potential should be avoided. Ginkgo may increase plasma levels of nifedipine.[104]

Recommendation. Ginkgo should not be used in place of standardized pharmacologic therapies for peripheral vascular disease but may be an alternative for patients who do not tolerate or are resistant to standard therapy.

Horse Chestnut (Aesculus hippocastanum)

The horse chestnut tree is found worldwide. Horse chestnut seed extract (HCSE) contains saponins, coumarins, flavonoids, and tannins.[283] Biologic activity has been shown to be related to the saponins, notably aescin, which has mild anti-inflammatory properties.[288] The mechanism of action of HCSE involves sensitization to calcium ions to increase the resistance of small-vessel permeability to water.[289]

With respect to cardiovascular therapy, research has focused on HCSE for the relief of chronic venous insufficiency. A systematic review of 17 randomized placebo-controlled trials was completed recently.[290] Most studies used a prepared extract containing a daily dose of 100 mg aescin. Leg pain in six trials (n = 543) was significantly reduced compared with placebo. Four of five trials (n = 420) reported a significant decrease in edema in patients treated with HCSE compared with placebo. Calf and ankle circumference also were reduced by HCSE. One trial found HCSE to be as efficacious as compression stockings. Symptoms of fatigue and tenderness also were reduced with HCSE. An effective dose of HCSE is standardized to 100 to 150 mg aescin daily, which is reduced to 35 to 70 mg daily after improvement.[291] Side effects are uncommon but can include gastrointestinal irritation, dizziness, nausea, headache, and pruritus. Contraindications include hypersensitivity to aescin or horse chestnut and renal or hepatic dysfunction. Aescin has antithrombotic effects and might increase the risk of bleeding or bruising.[292] The German Commission E has approved the use of HCSE in chronic venous insufficiency and has listed no precautions or known drug reactions.[283] Commercial preparations are available in the United States.

Recommendation. HCSE may be an efficacious alternative to standardized pharmacologic therapies for patients with chronic venous insufficiency who are not able to tolerate or are resistant to standard therapy. Monitor with concomitant use of anticoagulants and antiplatelet drugs.

French Pine Bark (Pinus pinaster extract)

A common extract made from the bark of the French maritime pine tree is used for chronic venous insufficiency. The strongest evidence for efficacy of this extract relates to improvement in heart health and treatment of chronic venous insufficiency, but formulations also have been evaluated for the reduction of venous complications of diabetes.[293] The extract consists of a mixture of bioflavonoids and has been shown to have potent antioxidant properties. In a small clinical study of healthy young men, 180 mg/day of French pine bark administered for 2 weeks was shown to augment endothelium-dependent vasodilation by increasing nitric oxide production.[294] In chronic venous insufficiency, it is thought that procyanidins in French tree bark reduce capillary permeability by cross-linking capillary wall proteins to reduce edema and microbleeding.[121] The extract also might lower capillary permeability because several of its constituents have antioxidant effects.[121] French tree bark generally is well tolerated, and serious adverse effects have not been recorded. Possible side effects include mild gastrointestinal complaints and decreased blood glucose levels. It may significantly decrease serum thromboxane concentrations, so caution is advised with anticoagulant or antiplatelet agents.[104] An ongoing U.S. clinical trial will provide additional data on the efficacy of this preparation.

Recommendation. French tree bark extract should not be used as a substitute for standardized pharmacologic therapies for venous insufficiency but may be an efficacious alternative for patients who cannot tolerate or are resistant to standard therapy.

Omega-3 Fatty Acids

The extensive data from experimental studies, prospective observational studies, and randomized controlled trials are remarkably consistent for a cardioprotective role for omega-3 fatty acids. The anti-inflammatory effects of omega-3 fats may partially explain their cardioprotective benefit because incorporation of these fats in cell membranes promotes vasodilation, provides antiarrhythmic effects, and promotes vascular patency.[295,296]

Numerous large diet studies support cardiovascular benefits of omega-3 fats. Several meta-analyses have shown a favorable effect of fish and omega-3 fatty acid intake on stroke and fatal coronary heart disease.[297-299] A new pooled analysis of prospective cohort studies that included only healthy individuals without established coronary disease determined that an intake of 250 mg/day of eicosapentaenoic acid (EPA) and docosahexaenoic acid (DHA) reduced risk for coronary heart disease.[300] In addition, a meta-analysis of prospective U.S. studies determined that an intake of approximately 500 mg/day afforded significant protection from coronary disease,[301] which is consistent with the American Heart Association recommendation to consume two fish meals per week for cardiovascular disease protection.[205]

The Japan EPA Lipid Intervention Study (JELIS), which was in part a primary prevention trial, randomized more than 18,000 patients with hyperlipidemia on statin therapy to receive 1.8 g/day EPA or control. After 4.6 years, the primary endpoint of "major coronary events" was reduced by 19% in the EPA group.[302] By far the largest secondary prevention trial, the GISSI-Prevenzione Study, enrolled more than 11,000 patients who had survived a recent infarction. Treatment with 850 mg EPA and DHA per day and 300 mg vitamin E per day resulted in a 20% reduction in total mortality, predominantly by reducing sudden cardiac death (45%).[303]

Short-term administration of 1 to 2 g/day of EPA and DHA in randomized trials also documented favorable effects on blood pressure, resting heart rate, heart rate variability, and triglyceride levels.[304] However, omega-3 fatty acids compared with placebo did not mitigate the effects of intermittent claudication in a review of six randomized controlled trials (n = 313). This study found some hematologic benefits but no improvement in ankle-brachial pressure index or walking distance.[305] Lacking from the evidence base are primary prevention outcome studies in U.S. population groups.

It is unclear to what extent omega-3 fatty acids affect coagulation status. Clinical evidence suggests that fish oil does not affect coagulation even when it is taken with anticoagulant therapy, but diets containing salmon oil, mackerel oil, or cod liver oil have been reported to prolong bleeding times.[104] Concomitant use of omega-3 preparations with anticoagulant or antiplatelet drugs should be monitored.

Recommendation. An intake of 1 g/day EPA and DHA for secondary prevention, treatment after myocardial infarction, and prevention of sudden cardiac death is prudent; higher intakes are recommended for lowering triglyceride levels.[306] EPA and DHA therapy should be administered under a physician's care.[307]

Bioidentical Hormones

Results from the Heart and Estrogen/Progestin Replacement Study (HERS) and the Estrogen Replacement for Atherosclerosis trial suggested that synthetic estrogens plus progestin may pose adverse cardiovascular disease risk to women.[308,309] The Women's Health Initiative trial confirmed that risks were higher in women using conventional hormone replacement therapy and outweighed the benefits for some.[310] Since the Women's Health Initiative, there has been increased interest in the use of bioidentical hormones, which are a derivative of plant extracts chemically modified to be structurally identical to human endogenous hormones.

Many bioidentical hormone products require a prescription because they are compounded by pharmacists. Compounded preparations of bioidentical hormones may include estriol, estrone, estradiol, testosterone, DHEA, thyroxine, cortisol, or progesterone. Some clinical studies and studies in postmenopausal cynomolgus monkeys suggest beneficial physiologic changes in lipid metabolism,[311-313] blood clotting,[312,314,315] and coronary vasoreactivity.[316-318] However, there is minimal scientific evidence, and rigorous controlled clinical studies are lacking. The bioidentical hormones can be expected to have the same adverse effect profile as that of conventional hormone replacement therapy.[319] There are proponents who believe that bioidentical hormones remain the preferred method of hormone replacement therapy until it is proved otherwise.[320,321]

Recommendation. Bioidentical hormones are not recommended for the reduction of risk in patients with cardiovascular disease.

Homeopathy

Homeopathy is a distinct formal system of medicine that has a long history of use in America. At the turn of the twentieth century, 8% of U.S. physicians used homeopathy. There were 20 homeopathic medical schools and more than 140 homeopathic hospitals.[322] Samuel Hahnemann introduced the practice based on the principle of similars. That is, if a substance in large amounts caused a certain condition, then the same substance in small amounts could cure the condition. Treatments are usually patient specific and individualized. Most homeopathic products contain little or no active ingredient and therefore possess little risk and require minimal oversight by the Food and Drug Administration. Homeopathy has been used worldwide as therapy for an array of chronic and acute cardiovascular conditions. However, data from randomized controlled trials and meta-analyses have major methodologic limitations, and therefore interpretation of results of therapeutic efficacy is questionable.[323] Five systematic reviews and meta-analyses evaluated clinical trials of the effectiveness of homeopathic remedies compared with placebo. "The reviews found that, overall, the quality of clinical research in homeopathy is low. But, when high-quality studies were selected for analysis, a surprising number showed positive results."[324]

Recommendation. Homeopathy should not be used in place of standardized and conventional therapy for the treatment or prevention of cardiovascular disease.

Supplements for Weight Loss

Obesity is one of the major risk factors for cardiovascular disease and predisposes to numerous cardiac conditions, such as coronary disease, heart failure, and sudden death. No prospective weight loss studies have demonstrated increased survival. However, strong evidence does suggest that weight loss in overweight and obese individuals reduces risk for development of diabetes and cardiovascular disease.[325] A higher body mass index has been associated with a higher likelihood of angiographic progression of coronary artery disease.[326]

Liquid protein diets and very-low-calorie diets have been associated with adverse cardiac events independent of the biologic and nutritional value of the products' constituents.[325] Current prescription weight loss products, such as sibutramine hydrochloride and orlistat, have shown some success but may be contraindicated in some patients with cardiovascular diseases.[327]

Survey data suggest that adults with higher body mass index are no more likely to use CAM therapies for weight loss than normal-weight individuals are.[328] Herbal antiobesity products as a class are heterogeneous in composition and often have unpredictable levels of active ingredients. Potentially harmful are toxic herbs such as *Aristolochia* species, ephedra or ma huang and bitter orange *(Citrus aurantium)* because of their sympathomimetic stimulatory activity, and herbal laxatives (anthraquinones, anthrones, and dianthrones) that may cause hepatotoxicity and nephrotoxicity or electrolyte depletion. A number of herbal weight loss blends contain caffeine in higher levels than typically would be consumed if the ingredients were taken individually, presumably to increase energy expenditure. These include ingredients such as guarana, kola nut, cacao, and yerba mate. The cardiovascular and central nervous system effects of ephedra are magnified when it is consumed with caffeine-containing products.[185] Last, there is also the potential for intentional as well as unintentional (misidentification) adulteration of ingredients, including the addition of drugs or other natural products.[329]

Recommendation. The mainstay for weight loss remains decreased calorie intake and increased physical activity or caloric expenditure. The only appropriate supplements for weight loss are those prescribed by knowledgeable clinicians, which may include a multivitamin-mineral supplement to compensate for those nutrients lost in calorie-restricted diets.

CONCLUSION

Integrative medicine consists of a large number of diverse practices used widely by adults and less so by children in the United States today. Interest in these nontraditional therapies stems from general dissatisfaction with current Western methods of healing and increased ownership that the public has assumed in their own health care. Furthermore, the American public is bombarded with advertisements and claims of efficacy, when in reality strong clinical trials showing efficacy are relatively scarce (Table 17-4).

TABLE 17-4	Summary of Alternative Therapies with Potential Use to Reduce the Risk of Cardiovascular Disease					
	Blood Pressure	Blood Lipids	Stress Reduction	Coronary Artery Disease or Angina Pectoris	Venous or Vascular Insufficiency	Obesity
Traditional Chinese medicine						
Acupuncture, acupressure, moxibustion	Yes	Yes	Possibly	Yes		Yes
Energy therapies						
Tai Chi, Qigong	Yes		Possibly	Yes		
Chinese herbs						
Danshen		Yes*		Yes*		
Compounded *Salvia*		Yes*		Yes*		
Suxiao jiuxin wan					No	
Tongxinluo					No	
Red yeast rice		Yes				
Ayurvedic medicine						
Yoga	Yes		Possibly			
Herbs						
Garlic	Possibly	No				
Guggul		No				
Terminalia arjuna		No				
Meditation and stress reduction	Yes		Yes			
Naturopathic medicine	Lacks evidence-based data to determine efficacy					
Chelation therapy				No		
Nutritional supplements						
B vitamins				No		
Antioxidants				No		
Vitamin D				No		
Magnesium	No			No		
Omega-3 fatty acids	Yes	Yes		Yes		
Nonvitamin, nonmineral supplements						
Soy		No		No		
Coenzyme Q10				Yes*		
Cocoa	No					
Ginkgo biloba					Yes*	
Horse chestnut seed extract					Yes	
French pine bark					Yes	
Bioidentical hormones		No		No		
Homeopathy	Lacks evidence-based data to determine efficacy					
Weight loss supplements						No

*Indicates beneficial use in some patients under some conditions; review contraindications and concomitant medications.

Fortunately, in some areas, such as acupuncture, yoga, and some nutritional approaches, the mechanisms of action are beginning to be elucidated. This fundamental approach to demonstrate how these therapies work along with rigorous clinical trials will be necessary before the medical community accepts these new therapies as advantageous over current Western approaches to medical practice. However, despite the lack of basic and clinical information, there may be utility in adopting an integrative approach to health care that employs both conventional and nonconventional treatments, if they have a positive impact on chronic conditions for which Western medicine often has proved to be inadequate.

There is emerging evidence that many of the therapies can reduce stress and associated cardiovascular responses, such as hypertension, that frequently accompany disease. Furthermore, the preventive approaches advocated in naturopathic, traditional Chinese, and Ayurvedic medicine seem to coincide with Western epidemiologic studies indicating that reduction of cardiovascular risk by improving nutrition, increasing exercise, and lowering body weight can reduce future morbidity. In fact, some of the most promising data in the areas of nutrition and positive health outcomes relate to dietary patterns and not dietary supplements. There are insufficient data to justify an alteration in public health policy from one that emphasizes food and diet to one that emphasizes supplements.[330] However, use of well-characterized dietary supplements in targeted individuals at risk for development of cardiovascular disease may serve to complement conventional therapies. We believe that to foster healthier lifestyles in their patients, clinicians will need to become more involved in helping patients remove barriers and adopt lifestyle measures that meet their needs and at the same time reduce their cardiovascular risk.

Acknowledgment

The authors thank Dr. Jay Udani for his careful review.

REFERENCES

1. Tricoci P, Allen J, Kramer J, Califf R, et al: Scientific evidence underlying the ACC/AHA clinical practice guidelines, *JAMA* 301:831, 2009.
2. Vogel J, Bolling SF, Costello R, et al: Integrating complementary medicine into cardiovascular medicine. A report of the American College of Cardiology Foundation Task Force on Clinical Expert Consensus Documents (Writing Committee to Develop an Expert Consensus Document on Complementary and Integrative Medicine), *J Am Coll Cardiol* 46:184-221, 2005.
3. Friedman M, Rosenman RH: Association of specific overt behavior pattern with blood and cardiovascular findings; blood cholesterol level, blood clotting time, incidence of arcus senilis, and clinical coronary artery disease, *JAMA* 169:1286, 1959.
4. van Doornen LJ, Orlebeke KE: Stress, personality and serum-cholesterol level, *J Human Stress* 8:24, 1989.
5. Jonas WB, Levin JS: *Essentials of complementary and alternative medicine*, Philadelphia, 1999, Lippincott Williams & Wilkins.
6. Stein RA, Oz M: *Complementary and alternative cardiovascular medicine: clinical handbook*, Totowa, NJ, 2004, Humana Press.
7. Frishman W, Weintraub M, Micozzi MS: *Complementary and integrative therapies for cardiovascular disease*, St Louis, 2005, Elsevier/Mosby.
8. Vogel J, Krucoff M: *Integrative cardiology: complementary and alternative medicine for the heart*, New York, 2007, McGraw Hill Medical.
9. Barnes P, Bloom B, Nahin R: Complementary and alternative medicine use among adults and children: United States, 2007, *Natl Health Stat Report* 12:1, 2008.
10. Longhurst JC: Academic integrative medical centers of excellence. In Vogel J, Krucoff M, editors: *Integrative cardiology: complementary and alternative medicine for the heart*, New York, 2007, McGraw Hill Medical, pp 49-62.
11. Soong Y: The treatment of exogenous obesity employing auricular acupuncture, *Am J Chin Med* 3:285, 1975.
12. Beecher HK: The powerful placebo, *JAMA* 159:1602, 1955.
13. Lu Z, Kou W, Du B, et al: Effect of Xuezhikang, an extract from red yeast Chinese rice, on coronary events in a Chinese population with previous myocardial infarction, *Am J Cardiol* 101:1689, 2008.
14. Olshansky B: Placebo and nocebo in cardiovascular health: implications for healthcare, research, and the doctor-patient relationship, *J Am Coll Cardiol* 49:415, 2007.
15. Walsh BT, Seidman SN, Sysko R, Gould M: Placebo response in studies of major depression: variable, substantial, and growing, *JAMA* 287:1840, 2002.
16. Archer T, Leier CV: Placebo treatment in congestive heart failure, *Cardiology* 81:125, 1992.
17. Frishman W, Wolff A, Lee W, et al: The placebo effect in cardiovascular disease. In Frishman W, Weintraub M, Micozzi MS, editors: *Complementary and integrative therapies for cardiovascular disease*, St. Louis, 2005, Elsevier/Mosby, pp 2-28.
18. Amsterdam EA, Wolfson S, Gorlin R: New aspects of the placebo response in angina pectoris, *Am J Cardiol* 24:305, 1969.
19. Chasis H, Goldring W, Schreiner GE, Smith HW: Reassurance in the management of benign hypertensive disease, *Circulation* 14:260, 1956.
20. Beecher HK: The powerful placebo, *JAMA* 159:1602, 1955.
21. Kong J, Gollub RL, Rosman IS, et al: Brain activity associated with expectancy-enhanced placebo analgesia as measured by functional magnetic resonance imaging, *J Neurosci* 26:381, 2006.
22. Zubieta JK, Bueller JA, Jackson LR, et al: Placebo effects mediated by endogenous opioid activity on mu-opioid receptors, *J Neurosci* 25:7754, 2005.
23. Wager TD, Scott DJ, Zubieta JK: Placebo effects on human mu-opioid activity during pain, *Proc Natl Acad Sci U S A* 104:11056, 2007.
24. Petrovic P, Kalso E, Petersson KM, Ingvar M: Placebo and opioid analgesia— imaging a shared neuronal network, *Science* 295:1737, 2002.
25. Pariente J, White P, Frackowiak RS, Lewith G: Expectancy and belief modulate the neuronal substrates of pain treated by acupuncture, *Neuroimage* 25:1161, 2005.
26. Kaptchuk TJ: The placebo effect in alternative medicine: can the performance of a healing ritual have clinical significance? *Ann Intern Med* 136:817, 2002.
27. Hróbjartsson A, Gøtzsche PC: Is the placebo powerless? An analysis of clinical trials comparing placebo with no treatment, *N Engl J Med* 344:1594, 2001.
28. Longhurst JC: Acupuncture. In Vogel J, Krucoff M, editors: *Integrative cardiology: complementary and alternative medicine for the heart*, New York, 2007, McGraw Hill Medical, pp 113-131.
29. Zhou W, Fu LW, Tjen-A-Looi SC, et al: Afferent mechanisms underlying stimulation modality-related modulation of acupuncture-related cardiovascular responses, *J Appl Physiol* 98:872, 2005.
30. Zhou W, Tjen-A-Looi S, Longhurst JC: Brain stem mechanisms underlying acupuncture modality-related modulation of cardiovascular responses in rats, *J Appl Physiol* 99:851, 2005.
31. Li P, Ayannusi O, Reed C, Longhurst J: Inhibitory effect of electroacupuncture (EA) on the pressor response induced by exercise stress, *Clin Auton Res* 14:182, 2004.
32. Longhurst JC: Integrative cardiology: mechanisms of cardiovascular action of acupuncture. In Vogel J, Krucoff M, editors: *Integrative cardiology: complementary and alternative medicine for the heart*, New York, 2007, McGraw Hill Medical, pp 382-398.
33. Longhurst JC: Central and peripheral neural mechanisms of acupuncture in myocardial ischemia. In Sato A, Li P, Campbell JL, editors: *Acupuncture: is there a physiological basis?* Boston, 2002, Elsevier, pp 79-87.
34. Zhou W, Hsiao I, Lin V, Longhurst J: Modulation of cardiovascular excitatory responses in rats by transcutaneous magnetic stimulation: role of the spinal cord, *J Appl Physiol* 100:926, 2006.
35. Zhou W, Mahajan A, Longhurst JC: Spinal nociceptin mediates electroacupuncture-related modulation of visceral sympathoexcitatory reflex responses in rats, *Am J Physiol Heart Circ Physiol* 297:H859, 2009.
36. Tjen-A-Looi SC, Li P, Longhurst JC: Medullary substrate and differential cardiovascular response during stimulation of specific acupoints, *Am J Physiol* 287:R852, 2004.
37. Collins H, DiCarlo S: TENS attenuates response to colon distension in paraplegic and quadriplegic rats, *Am J Physiol Heart Circ Physiol* 283:H1734, 2002.
38. Averill A, Cotter AC, Nayak S, et al: Blood pressure response to acupuncture in a population at risk for autonomic dyreflexia, *Arch Phys Med Rehabil* 81:1494, 2000.
39. Yao T, Andersson S, Thoren P: Long-lasting cardiovascular depression induced by acupuncture-like stimulation of the sciatic nerve in unanaesthetized spontaneously hypertensive rats, *Brain Res* 240:77, 1982.
40. Chiu YJ, Chi A, Reid IA: Cardiovascular and endocrine effects of acupuncture in hypertensive patients, *Clin Exp Hypertens* 19:1047, 1997.
41. Macklin EA, Wayne PM, Kalish LA, et al: Stop Hypertension with the Acupuncture Research Program (SHARP): results of a randomized, controlled clinical trial, *Hypertension* 48:838, 2006.
42. Flachskampf FA, Gallasch J, Gefeller O, et al: Randomized trial of acupuncture to lower blood pressure, *Circulation* 115:3121, 2007.
43. Li P, Tjen-A-Looi S, Longhurst J: Rostral ventrolateral medullary opioid receptor subtypes in the inhibitory effect of electroacupuncture on reflex autonomic response in cats, *Auton Neurosci* 89:38, 2001.
44. Wu C-C, Hsu CJ: Neurogenic regulation of lipid metabolism in the rabbit. A mechanism for the cholesterol-lowering effect of acupuncture, *Atherosclerosis* 33:153, 1979.
45. Li M, Zhang Y: Modulation of gene expression in cholesterol-lowering effect of electroacupuncture at Fenglong acupoint (ST40): a cDNA microarray study, *Int J Mol Med* 19:617, 2007.
46. Cabioglu MT, Ergene N: Electroacupuncture therapy for weight loss reduces serum total cholesterol, triglycerides, and LDL cholesterol levels in obese women, *Am J Chin Med* 33:525, 2005.
47. Shiraishi T, Onoe M, Kojima T, et al: Effects of auricular stimulation on feeding-related hypothalamic neuronal activity in normal and obese rats, *Brain Res Bull* 36:141, 2009.
48. Asamoto S, Takeshige C: Activation of the satiety center by auricular acupuncture point stimulation, *Brain Res Bull* 29:157, 1992.
49. Sacks LL: Drug addiction, alcoholism, smoking, obesity, treated by auricular staplepuncture, *Am J Acupuncture* 3:147, 1975.
50. Soong Y: The treatment of exogenous obesity employing auricular acupuncture, *Am J Chin Med* 3:285, 1975.
51. Dung HC: Role of the vagus nerve in weight reduction through auricular acupuncture, *Am J Acupuncture* 14:249, 1986.
52. Huang MH, Yang RC, Hu Sh: Preliminary results of triple therapy for obesity, *Int J Obes Relat Metab Disord* 20:830, 1996.
53. Sun Q, Xu Y: Simple obesity and obesity hyperlipemia treated with otoacupoint pellet pressure and body acupuncture, *J Tradit Chin Med* 13:22, 1993.
54. Shafshak TS: Electroacupuncture and exercise in body weight reduction and their application in rehabilitating patients with knee osteoarthritis, *Am J Chin Med* 23:15, 1995.

55. Mazzoni R, Mannucci E, Rizzello SM, ea: Failure of acupuncture in the treatment of obesity: a pilot study, *Eat Weight Disord* 4:198, 1999.
56. Mok MS, Parker LN, Voina S, Bray GA: Treatment of obesity by acupuncture, *Am J Clin Nutr* 29:832, 1976.
57. Wen HL, Cheung SYC: Treatment of drug addiction by acupuncture and 14 electrical stimulation, *Asian J Med* 9:138, 1973.
58. Han JS, Zhang RL: Suppression of morphine abstinence syndrome by body electroacupuncture of different frequencies in rats, *Drug Alcohol Depend* 31:169, 1993.
59. White AR, Resch KL, Ernst E: A meta-analysis of acupuncture techniques for smoking cessation, *Tob Control* 8:393, 1999.
60. Li P, Pitsillides K, Rendig S, et al: Reversal of reflex-induced myocardial ischemia by median nerve stimulation: a feline model of electroacupuncture, *Circulation* 97:1186, 1998.
61. Chao DM, Shen LL, Tjen-A-Looi S, Pitsillides KF et al: Naloxone reverses inhibitory effect of electroacupuncture on sympathetic cardiovascular reflex responses, *Am J Physiol* 276:H2127-H2134, 1999.
62. Mannheimer C, Carlsson C-A, Emanuelsson H, et al: The effects of transcutaneous electrical nerve stimulation in patients with severe angina pectoris, *Circulation* 71:308, 1985.
63. Mannheimer C, Emanuelsson H, Waagstein F, Wilhelmsson C: Influence of naloxone on the effects of high frequency transcutaneous electrical nerve stimulation in angina pectoris induced by atrial pacing, *Br Heart J* 62:36, 1989.
64. Mannheimer C, Carlsson C-A, Eriksson K, et al: Transcutaneous electrical nerve stimulation in severe angina pectoris, *Eur Heart J* 3:297, 1982.
65. Emanuelsson H, Mannheimer C, Waagstein F, Wilhelmsson C: Catecholamine metabolism during pacing-induced angina pectoris and the effect of transcutaneous electrical nerve stimulation, *Am Heart J* 114:1360, 1987.
66. Ballegaard S, Pedersen F, Pietersen A, et al: Effects of acupuncture in moderate stable angina pectoris, *J Intern Med* 227:25, 1990.

67. Ballegaard S, Meyer CN, Trojaborg W: Acupuncture in angina pectoris: does acupuncture have a specific effect? *J Intern Med* 229:357, 1991.
68. Ballegaard S, Johannessen A, Karpatschof B, Nyeboe J: Addition of acupuncture and self-care education in the treatment of patients with severe angina pectoris may be cost beneficial: an open, prospective study, *J Altern Complement Med* 5:405, 1999.
69. Ballegaard S, Karpatschof B, Holck JA, et al: Acupuncture in angina pectoris. Do psycho-social and neurophysiological factors relate to the effect? *Acupunct Electrother Res* 20:101, 1995.
70. Ballegaard S, Norrelund S, Smith DF: Cost benefit of combined use of acupuncture, Shiatsu and lifestyle adjustment for treatment of patients with severe angina pectoris, *Acupunct Electrother Res* 21:187, 1996.
71. Richter A, Herlitz J, Hjalmarson A: Effect of acupuncture in patients with angina pectoris, *Eur Heart J* 12:175, 1991.
72. Middlekauff HR, Yu JL, Hui K: Acupuncture effects on reflex responses to mental stress in humans, *Am J Physiol Regul Integr Comp Physiol* 280:R1462, 2001.
73. Ballegaard S, Pedersen F, Pietersen A, et al: Effects of acupuncture in moderate stable angina pectoris, *J Intern Med* 227:25, 1990.
74. Ballegaard S, Meyer CN, Trojaborg W: Acupuncture in angina pectoris: does acupuncture have a specific effect? *J Intern Med* 229:357, 1991.
75. Liu F, Li J, Liu G, et al: Clinical observation of effect of acupuncture on angina pectoris. In Chang HT, editor: *Research on acupuncture, moxibustion and acupuncture anesthesia*, Beijing, 1986, Science Press and Springer-Verlag, pp 861-875.
76. Ballegaard S, Borg E, Karpatschof B, et al: Long-term effects of integrated rehabilitation in patients with advanced angina pectoris: a nonrandomized comparative study, *J Altern Complement Med* 10:777, 2004.
77. Cramp FL, McCullough GR, Lowe AS, Walsh DM: Transcutaneous electric nerve stimulation: the effect of intensity on local and distal cutaneous blood flow and skin temperature in healthy subjects, *Arch Phys Med Rehabil* 83:5, 2002.
78. Lundeberg T, Kjartansson J, Samuelson UE: Effect of electrical nerve stimulation on healing of ischaemic skin flaps, *Lancet* 24:712, 1998.
79. Longhurst J: Alternative approaches to the medical management of cardiovascular disease: acupuncture, electrical nerve and spinal cord stimulation, *Heart Dis* 3:236, 2001.
80. Augustinsson LE, Carlson CA, Holm J, Jivegard L: Epidural electrical stimulation in severe limb ischemia: pain relief, increased blood flow and possible limb saving effect, *Ann Surg* 202:104, 1985.
81. Jivegard LD, Augustinsson LE, Carlsson C-A, Holm J: Long-term results by epidural spinal electrical stimulation (ESES) in patients with inoperable severe lower limb ischaemia, *Eur J Vasc Surg* 1:345, 1987.
82. Noguchi E, Ohsawa H, Kobayashi S, et al: The effect of electro-acupuncture stimulation on the muscle blood flow of the hindlimb in anesthetized rats, *J Auton Nerv Syst* 75:78, 1999.
83. Jahnke R: Qigong and Tai Chi: traditional Chinese health promotion practices in the prevention and treatment of cardiovascular disease. In Frishman W, Weintraub M, Micozzi MS, editors: *Complementary and integrative therapies for cardiovascular disease*, St. Louis, 2005, Elsevier/Mosby, pp 204-219.
84. Whitemont R, Mamtani R: Homeopathy with a special focus on treatment of cardiovascular diseases. In Frishman W, Weintraub M, Micozzi MS, editors: *Complementary and integrative therapies for cardiovascular disease*, St. Louis, 2005, Elsevier/Mosby, pp 232-256.
85. Lee MS, Pittler MH, Guo R, Ernst E: Qigong for hypertension: a systematic review of randomized clinical trials, *J Hypertens* 25:1525, 2007.
86. Guo X, Zhou B, Nishimura T, et al: Clinical effect of qigong practice on essential hypertension: a meta-analysis of randomized controlled trials, *J Altern Complement Med* 14:27, 2008.
87. Lee MS, Lee MS, Kim HJ, Moon SR: Qigong reduced blood pressure and catecholamine levels of patients with essential hypertension, *Int J Neurosci* 113:1691, 2003.
88. Lee MS, Lee MS, Choi ES, Chung HT: Effects of Qigong on blood pressure, blood pressure determinants and ventilatory function in middle-aged patients with essential hypertension, *Am J Chin Med* 31:489, 2003.
89. Lan C, Chen SY, Lai JS: The exercise intensity of Tai Chi Chuan, *Med Sports Sci* 52:9, 2008.
90. Taylor-Piliae RE, Froelicher ES: Effectiveness of Tai Chi exercise in improving aerobic capacity: a meta-analysis, *J Cardiovas Nurs* 19:48, 2004.
91. Lan C, Chen SY, Lai JS: Changes of aerobic capacity, fat ratio and flexibility in older TCC practitioners: a five-year follow-up, *Am J Chin Med* 36:1041, 2008.
92. Young DR, Appel LJ, Jee S, Miller ER 3rd: The effects of aerobic exercise and T'ai Chi on blood pressure in older people: results of a randomized trial, *J Am Geriatr Soc* 47:277, 1999.
93. Tsai JC, Wang WH, Chan P, et al: The beneficial effects of Tai Chi Chuan on blood pressure and lipid profile and anxiety status in a randomized controlled trial, *J Altern Complement Med* 9:747, 2003.
94. Lee MS, Huh HJ, Kim BG, et al: Effects of Qi-training on heart rate variability, *Am J Chin Med* 30:463, 2002.
95. Mayer M: Qigong and hypertension: a critique of research, *J Altern Complement Med* 5:371, 1999.
96. Channer KS, Barrow D, Barrow R, et al: Changes in haemodynamic parameters following Tai Chi Chuan and aerobic exercise in patients recovering from acute myocardial infarction, *Postgrad Med J* 72:349, 1996.
97. Astin JA, Harkness E, Ernst E: The efficacy of "distant healing": a systematic review of randomized trials, *Ann Intern Med* 132:903, 2000.
98. Sharma VG, Sanghvi C, Mehta Y, Trehan N: Efficacy of reiki on patients undergoing coronary artery bypass graft surgery, *Ann Card Anaesth* 3:12, 2000.
99. Ernst E: Distant healing—an "update" of a systematic review, *Wien Klin Wochenschr* 115:241, 2003.
100. Wang QC: Research direction for syndromes of traditional Chinese medicine: differentiating diseases from syndromes and differentiating syndromes from diseases, *J Chin Integr Med (Zhong Xi Yi Jie He Xue Bao)* 4:225, 2006.
101. Bian Z: Improving the quality of randomized controlled trials in Chinese herbal medicine, Part 1: clinical trial design and methodology, *J Chin Integr Med (Zhong Xi Yi Jie He Xue Bao)* 4:120, 2006.
102. Cheng TO: Cardiovascular effects of Danshen, *Int J Cardiol* 121:9, 2007.
103. Cheng TO: Warfarin danshen interaction, *Ann Thorac Surg* 67:894, 1999.
104. Ulbricht C, Chao W, Costa D, et al: Clinical evidence of herb-drug interactions: a systematic review by the natural standard research collaboration, *Curr Drug Metab* 9:1063, 2008.
105. Wahed A, Dasgupta A: Positive and negative in vitro interference of Chinese medicine dan shen in serum digoxin measurement. Elimination of interference by monitoring free digoxin concentration, *Am J Clin Pathol* 116:403, 2001.
106. Yu S, Zhong B, Zheng M, et al: The quality of randomized controlled trials on DanShen in the treatment of ischemic vascular disease, *J Altern Complement Med* 15:557, 2009.
107. Guo ZX, Jia W, Gao WY, et al: Clinical investigation of composite danshen pill for the treatment of angina pectoris, *Chin J Nat Med (Zhongguo Tianran Yaowu)* 1:124, 2003.
108. Wang G, Wang L, Xiong ZY, et al: Compound salvia pellet, a traditional Chinese medicine, for the treatment of chronic stable angina pectoris compared with nitrates: a meta-analysis, *Med Sci Monit* 12:SR1, 2006.
109. Junhua Z, Hongcai S, Xiumei G, et al: Methodology and reporting quality of systematic review/meta-analysis of traditional Chinese medicine, *J Altern Complement Med* 13:797, 2007.
110. Yuan G: Curative effect observations on Suxiao jiuxin wan compound to Xiao xin tong for angina pectoris, *Med J Heal Heart Vessel* 9:71, 2002.
111. Wu T, Duan X, Zhou L, et al: Chinese herbal medicine suxiao jiuxin wan for angina pectoris, *Cochrane Database Syst Rev* (1):CD004473, 2008.
112. Xu GC, Gao RL, Wu YL: Clinical study on tongxinluo capsule in treatment of patients with angina pectoris caused by coronary heart disease, *Zhongguo Zhong Xi Yi Jie He Za Zhi* 17:414, 1997.
113. Zhang L, Wu Y, Jia Z, et al: Protective effects of a compound herbal extract (Tong Xin Luo) on free fatty acid induced endothelial injury: implications of antioxidant system, *BMC Complement Altern Med* 8:39, 2008.
114. Wu YL, You JH, Yuan GQ, et al: The effects of Tongxinluo Supermicro Powder on nuclear factor-κB, intercellular adhesion molecule-1 and vascular cell adhesion molecule-1 expression in aorta of rabbits fed with high-lipid diet, *Zhonghua Xin Xue Guan Bing Za Zhi* 35:271, 2007.
115. Liu JX, Shang XH, Wang G: Effect of tongxinluo capsule on experimental myocardial ischemia, arrhythmia and hyperlipidemia, *Zhongguo Zhong Xi Yi Jie He Za Zhi* 17:425, 1997.
116. Li Z, Yang YJ, Qin XW, et al: Effects of Tongxinluo and simvastatin on the stabilization of vulnerable atherosclerotic plaques of aorta in aortic atherosclerosis and molecular mechanism thereof: a comparative study with rabbits, *Zhonghua Yi Xue Za Zhi* 86:3146, 2006.
117. Zhang L, Liu Y, Lu XT, et al: Traditional Chinese herbal medicine Tongxinluo dose-dependently enhances stability of vulnerable plaques: a comparison with a high-dose simvastatin therapy, *Am J Physiol Heart Circ Physiol* 297:H2004, 2009.
118. Wu T, Harrison RA, Chen X, et al: Tongxinluo (Tong xin luo or Tong-xin-luo) capsule for unstable angina pectoris, *Cochrane Database Syst Rev* (4):CD004474, 2006.
119. Dou XB, Wo XD, Fan CL: Progress of research in treatment of hyperlipidemia by monomer or compound recipe of Chinese herbal medicine, *Chin J Integr Med* 14:71, 2008.
120. Liu J, Zhang J, Shi Y, et al: Chinese red yeast rice *(Monascus purpureus)* for primary hyperlipidemia: a meta-analysis of randomized controlled trials, *Chin Med* 1:4, 2006.
121. Jellin JM, Gregory PJ, Batz F, et al: *Pharmacist's letter/prescriber's letter natural medicines comprehensive database*, ed 10, Stockton, Calif, 2008, Therapeutic Research Faculty.

122. Heber D, Lembertas A, Lu QY, et al: An analysis of nine proprietary Chinese red yeast rice dietary supplements: implications of variability in chemical profile and contents, *J Altern Complement Med* 7:133, 2001.

123. Modir S, Leopold D: An Ayurvedic approach to cardiovascular disease. In Vogel J, Krucoff M, editors: *Integrative cardiology: complementary and alternative medicine for the heart*, New York, 2007, McGraw Hill Medical, pp 257-277.

124. Mamtani R, Mamtani R: Ayurveda and yoga in cardiovascular diseases. In Frishman W, Weintraub M, Micozzi MS, editors: *Complementary and integrative therapies for cardiovascular disease*, St. Louis, 2005, Elsevier/Mosby, pp 168-181.

125. Schmidt T, Wijga A, Von Zur Mühlen A, et al: Changes in cardiovascular risk factors and hormones during a comprehensive residential three month kriya yoga training and vegetarian nutrition, *Acta Physiol Scand Suppl* 640:158, 1997.

126. Mahajan AS, Reddy KS, Sachdeva U: Lipid profile of coronary risk subjects following yogic lifestyle intervention, *Indian Heart J* 51:37, 1999.

127. Ornish D, Scherwitz LW, Doody RS, et al: Effects of stress management training and dietary changes in treating ischemic heart disease, *JAMA* 249:54, 1983.

128. Manchanda SC, Narang R, Reddy KS, e a: Retardation of coronary atherosclerosis with yoga lifestyle intervention. *J Assoc Physicians India* 48:687, 2000.

129. Raub JA: Psychophysiologic effects of Hatha Yoga on musculoskeletal and cardiopulmonary function: a literature review, *J Altern Complement Med* 8:797, 2009.

130. Patel C: 12-month follow-up of yoga and bio-feedback in the management of hypertension, *Lancet* 1:62, 2009.

131. Murugesan R, Govindarajulu N, Bera TK: Effect of selected yogic practices on the management of hypertension, *Indian J Physiol Pharmacol* 44:207, 2000.

132. Ananda S: *The complete book of yoga: harmony of body and mind*, Delhi, 2005, Orient Paperbacks.

133. Vempati RP, Telles S: Yoga-based guided relaxation reduces sympathetic activity judged from baseline levels, *Psychol Rep* 90:487, 2002.

134. Silagy CA, Neil HA: A meta-analysis of the effect of garlic on blood pressure, *J Hypertens* 12:463, 1994.

135. Banerjee SK, Maulik SK: Effect of garlic on cardiovascular disorders: a review, *Nutr J* 1:4, 2002.

136. Ackermann RT, Mulrow CD, Ramirez G, et al: Garlic shows promise for improving some cardiovascular risk factors, *Arch Intern Med* 161:813, 2001.

137. Gardner CD, Lawson LD, Block E, et al: Effect of raw garlic vs commercial garlic supplements on plasma lipid concentrations in adults with moderate hypercholesterolemia: a randomized clinical trial, *Arch Intern Med* 167:346, 2007.

138. Singh BB, Vinjamury SP, Der-Martirosian C, et al: Ayurvedic and collateral herbal treatments for hyperlipidemia: a systematic review of randomized controlled trials and quasi-experimental designs, *Altern Ther Health Med* 13:22, 2007.

139. Reinhart KM, Coleman CI, Teevan C, et al: Effects of garlic on blood pressure in patients with and without systolic hypertension: a meta-analysis, *Ann Pharmacother* 42:1766, 2008.

140. Ried K, Frank OR, Stocks NP, et al: Effect of garlic on blood pressure: a systematic review and meta-analysis, *BMC Cardiovasc Disord* 8:13, 2008.

141. Fletcher B, Berra K, Ades P, et al: Managing abnormal blood lipids: a collaborative approach, *Circulation* 112:3184, 2005.

142. CAMP Workshops on Medicinal Plants, India 1998: *Commiphora wightii*. IUCN Red List of Threatened Species. Version 2009.1. Available at: http://www.iucnredlist.org/. Accessed June 24 2009.

143. Urizar NL, Liverman AB, Dodds DT, et al: A natural product that lowers cholesterol as an antagonist ligand for FXR, *Science* 296:1703, 2002.

144. Wu J, Xia C, Meier J, Li S, et al: The hypolipidemic natural product guggulsterone acts as an antagonist of the bile acid receptor, *Mol Endocrinol* 16:1590, 2002.

145. Ory DS: Nuclear receptor signaling in the control of cholesterol homeostasis: have the orphans found a home? *Circ Res* 95:660, 2004.

146. Kalaany NY, Mangelsdorf DJ: LXRS and FXR: the yin and yang of cholesterol and fat metabolism, *Annu Rev Physiol* 68:159, 2006.

147. Cai SY, Boyer JL: FXR: a target for cholestatic syndromes? *Expert Opin Ther Targets* 10:409, 2006.

148. Brobst DE, Ding X, Creech KL, et al: Guggulsterone activates multiple nuclear receptors and induces CYP3A gene expression through the pregnane X receptor, *J Pharmacol Exp Ther* 310:528, 2004.

149. Burris TP, Montrose C, Houck KA, et al: The hypolipidemic natural product guggulsterone is a promiscuous steroid receptor ligand, *Mol Pharmacol* 67:948, 2005.

150. Nityanand S, Srivastava JS, Asthana OP: Clinical trials with gugulipid. A new hypolipidaemic agent, *J Assoc Physicians India* 37:323, 1989.

151. Singh RB, Niaz MA, Ghosh S: Hypolipidemic and antioxidant effects of *Commiphora mukul* as an adjunct to dietary therapy in patients with hypercholesterolemia, *Cardiovasc Drugs Ther* 8:659, 1994.

152. Szapary PO, Wolfe ML, Bloedon LT, et al: Guggulipid for the treatment of hypercholesterolemia: a randomized controlled trial, *JAMA* 290:765, 2003.

153. Deng R: Therapeutic effects of guggul and its constituent guggulsterone: cardiovascular benefits, *Cardiovasc Drug Rev* 25:375, 2007.

154. Dalvi SS, Nayak VK, Pohujani SM, et al: Effect of gugulipid on bioavailability of diltiazem and propranolol, *J Assoc Physicians India* 42:454, 1994.

155. Terminalia arjuna, *Altern Med Rev* 4:436, 1999.

156. Enomoto Y, Ito K, Kawagoe Y, et al: Positive inotropic action of saponins on isolated atrial and papillary muscles from the guinea-pig, *Br J Pharmacol* 88:259, 1986.

157. Bharani A, Ganguli A, Mathur LK, et al: Efficacy of *Terminalia arjuna* in chronic stable angina: a double-blind, placebo-controlled, crossover study comparing *Terminalia arjuna* with isosorbide mononitrate, *Indian Heart J* 54:170, 2002.

158. Saper RB, Phillips RS, Sehgal A, et al: Lead, mercury, and arsenic in US- and Indian-manufactured Ayurvedic medicines sold via the Internet, *JAMA* 300:915, 2008.

159. Ernst E: The risk-benefit profile of commonly used herbal therapies: ginkgo, St. John's Wort, ginseng, echinacea, saw palmetto, and kava, *Ann Intern Med* 136:42, 2002.

160. Centers for Disease Control and Prevention: Lead poisoning associated with ayurvedic medications—five states, 2000-2003, *MMWR Morb Mortal Wkly Rep* 53:582, 2004.

161. Satpute AD: *Rasa Ratna Samuchaya of Vagbhatta*, trans, Varanasi, India, 2003, Chaukhamba Sanskrit Pratishtana.

162. Shastri K: *Rasa Tarangini of Sadanand Sharma*, trans, New Delhi, India, 1979, Motilal Banarsidass Publishers.

163. Malec J, Sipprelle CN: Physiological and subjective effects of Zen meditation and demand characteristics, *J Consult Clin Psychol* 45:339, 1977.

164. Barnes VA, Treiber FA, Johnson MH: Impact of transcendental meditation on ambulatory blood pressure in African-American adolescents, *Am J Hypertens* 17:366, 2004.

165. Delmonte MM: Physiological responses during meditation and rest, *Biofeedback Self Regul* 9:181, 1984.

166. Zamarra JW, Schneider RH, Besseghini I, et al: Usefulness of the transcendental meditation program in the treatment of patients with coronary artery disease, *Am J Cardiol* 77:867, 1996.

167. Curiati JA, Bocchi E, Freire JO, et al: Meditation reduces sympathetic activation and improves the quality of life in elderly patients with optimally treated heart failure: a prospective randomized study, *J Altern Complement Med* 11:465, 2005.

168. Ziegelstein RC, Fauerbach JA, Stevens SS, et al: Patients with depression are less likely to follow recommendations to reduce cardiac risk during recovery from a myocardial infarction, *Arch Intern Med* 160:1818, 2000.

169. National Heart, Lung, and Blood Institute: Study finds no reduction in deaths or heart attacks in heart disease patients treated for depression and low social support, *NIH News Release*, November 12, 2001.

170. Hedback B, Perk J, Wodlin P: Long-term reduction of cardiac mortality after myocardial infarction: 10-year results of a comprehensive rehabilitation programme, *Eur Heart J* 14:831, 1993.

171. Burgess AW, Lerner DJ, D'Agostino RB, et al: A randomized control trial of cardiac rehabilitation, *Soc Sci Med* 24:359, 2009.

172. Mayou R: Rehabilitation after heart attack, *BMJ* 313:1498, 1996.

173. Denollet J, Brutsaert DL: Enhancing emotional well-being by comprehensive rehabilitation in patients with coronary heart disease, *Eur Heart J* 16:1070, 1995.

174. Sharma HS, Clark C: *Contemporary Ayurveda: medicine and research in Maharishi Ayur-Veda*, New York, 1997, Churchill Livingstone.

175. Jevning R, Wilson AF: Behavioral increase of blood flow, *Physiologist* 21:60, 1978.

176. Dickinson H, Campbell F, Beyer F, et al: Relaxation therapies for the management of primary hypertension in adults: a Cochrane review, *J Hum Hypertens* 12:809, 2008.

177. Albert C, Gaziano J, Willett W, Manson J: Nut consumption and decreased risk of sudden cardiac death in the Physicians' Health Study, *Arch Intern Med* 162:1382, 2002.

178. Ros E, Núñez I, Pérez-Heras A, et al: A walnut diet improves endothelial function in hypercholesterolemic subjects: a randomized crossover trial, *Circulation* 109:1609, 2004.

179. Jenkins DJ, Kendall CW, Marchie A, et al: Effects of a dietary portfolio of cholesterol-lowering foods vs lovastatin on serum lipids and C-reactive protein, *JAMA* 290:502, 2003.

180. Crawford P, Paden SL, Park MK: Clinical inquiries: what is the dietary treatment for low HDL cholesterol? *J Fam Pract* 55:1076, 2006.

181. Atwood KC, Woeckner E, Baratz RS, Sampson WI: Why the NIH Trial to Assess Chelation Therapy (TACT) should be abandoned, *Medscape J Med* 10:115, 2008.

182. Green S, Sampson W: EDTA chelation therapy for atherosclerosis and degenerative diseases: implausibility and paradoxical oxidant effects, *Sci Rev Altern Med* 6:17, 2002.

183. Grier MT, Meyers DG: So much writing, so little science: a review of 37 years of literature on edetate sodium chelation therapy, *Ann Parmacother* 27:1504, 1993.

184. Quan H, Galbraith PD, Norris CM, et al: Opinions on chelation therapy in patients undergoing coronary angiography: cross-sectional survey, *Can J Cardiol* 23:635, 2007.

185. Halbert S: Chelation therapy and CVD. In Stein RA, Oz M, editors: *Complementary and alternative cardiovascular medicine: clinical handbook*, Totowa, NJ, 2004, Humana Press, pp 189-200.

186. Guldager B, Jelnes R, Jørgensen SJ, et al: EDTA treatment of intermittent claudication——a double-blind, placebo-controlled study, *J Intern Med* 231:261, 1992.

187. Sloth-Nielsen J, Guldager B, Mouritzen C, et al: Arteriographic findings in EDTA chelation therapy on peripheral arteriosclerosis, *Am J Surg* 162:122, 1991.

188. Udvalgene vedrørende Videnskabelig Uredelighed, the Committee on Scientific Dishonesty: Conclusions concerning complaints in connection with trial of EDTA versus placebo in the treatment of atherosclerosis, 1994.

189. van Rij AM, Solomon C, Packer SG, Hopkins WG: Chelation therapy for intermittent claudication. A double-blind, randomized, controlled trial, *Circulation* 90:1194, 1994.

190. Knudtson ML, Wyse DG, Galbraith PD, et al: Chelation therapy for ischemic heart disease: a randomized controlled trial, *JAMA* 287:481, 2002.

191. Gibbons RJ, Abrams J, Chatterjee K, et al: ACC/AHA 2002 guideline update for the management of patients with chronic stable angina—summary article: a report of the American College of Cardiology/American Heart Association Task Force on practice guidelines (Committee on the Management of Patients With Chronic Stable Angina), *J Am Coll Cardiol* 41:159, 2003.

192. Radimer K, Bindewald B, Hughes J, et al: Dietary supplement use by US adults: data from the National Health and Nutrition Examination Survey, 1999-2000, *Am J Epidemiol* 160:3399, 2004.

193. Buettner C, Phillips RS, Davis RB, et al: Use of dietary supplements among United States adults with coronary artery disease and atherosclerotic risks, *Am J Cardiol* 99:661, 2007.

194. Nygard O, Nordrehaug JE, Refsum H, et al: Plasma homocysteine levels and mortality in patients with coronary artery disease, *N Engl J Med* 337:230, 1997.

195. Selhub J, Jacques PF, Bostom AG, et al: Association between plasma homocysteine concentrations and extracranial carotid-artery stenosis, *N Engl J Med* 332:286, 1995.

196. Stampfer MJ, Malinow MR, Willett WC, et al: A prospective study of plasma homocyst(e)ine and risk of myocardial infarction in US physicians, *JAMA* 268:877, 1992.

197. Wald NJ, Watt HC, Law MR, et al: Homocysteine and ischemic heart disease: results of a prospective study with implications regarding prevention, *Arch Intern Med* 158:862, 1998.
198. Lonn E, Yusuf S, Arnold MJ, et al: Homocysteine lowering with folic acid and B vitamins in vascular disease, *N Engl J Med* 354:1567, 2006.
199. Toole JF, Malinow MR, Chambless LE, et al: Lowering homocysteine in patients with ischemic stroke to prevent recurrent stroke, myocardial infarction, and death: the Vitamin Intervention for Stroke Prevention (VISP) randomized controlled trial, *JAMA* 291:565, 2004.
200. Bonaa KH, Njolstad I, Ueland PM, et al: Homocysteine lowering and cardiovascular events after acute myocardial infarction, *N Engl J Med* 354:1578, 2006.
201. Albert CM, Cook NR, Gaziano JM, et al: Effect of folic acid and B vitamins on risk of cardiovascular events and total mortality among women at high risk for cardiovascular disease: a randomized trial, *JAMA* 299:2027, 2008.
202. Bleys J, Miller ER III, Pastor-Barriuso R, et al: Vitamin-mineral supplementation and the progression of atherosclerosis: a meta-analysis of randomized controlled trials, *Am J Clin Nutr* 84:880, 2006.
203. de Bree A, van Mierlo LA, Draijer R: Folic acid improves vascular reactivity in humans: a meta-analysis of randomized controlled trials, *Am J Clin Nutr* 86:610, 2007.
204. Clarke R, Armitage J, Lewington S, Collins R: Homocysteine-lowering trials for prevention of vascular disease: protocol for a collaborative meta-analysis, *Clin Chem Lab Med* 45:1575, 2007.
205. Lichtenstein AH, Appel LJ, Brands M, et al: Diet and lifestyle recommendations revision 2006: a scientific statement from the American Heart Association Nutrition Committee, *Circulation* 114:82, 2006.
206. Knekt P, Ritz J, Pereira MA, et al: Antioxidant vitamins and coronary heart disease risk: a pooled analysis of 9 cohorts, *Am J Clin Nutr* 80:1508, 2004.
207. Ye Z, Song H: Antioxidant vitamins intake and the risk of coronary heart disease: meta-analysis of cohort studies, *Eur J Cardiovasc Prev Rehabil* 15:26, 2008.
208. Ting HH, Timimi FK, Haley EA, et al: Vitamin C improves endothelium-dependent vasodilation in forearm resistance vessels of humans with hypercholesterolemia, *Circulation* 95:2617, 1997.
209. Heart Protection Study Collaborative Group: MRC/BHF Heart Protection Study of antioxidant vitamin supplementation in 20,536 high-risk individuals: a randomised placebo-controlled trial, *Lancet* 360:23, 2002.
210. Sesso HD, Buring JE, Christen WG, et al: Vitamins E and C in the prevention of cardiovascular disease in men: the Physicians' Health Study II randomized controlled trial, *JAMA* 300:2123, 2008.
211. Salonen RM, Nyyssonen K, Kaikkonen J, et al: Six-year effect of combined vitamin C and E supplementation on atherosclerotic progression: the Antioxidant Supplementation in Atherosclerosis Prevention (ASAP) Study, *Circulation* 107:947, 2003.
212. Waters DD, Alderman EL, Hsia J, et al: Effects of hormone replacement therapy and antioxidant vitamin supplements on coronary atherosclerosis in postmenopausal women: a randomized controlled trial, *JAMA* 288:2432, 2002.
213. Stephens NG, Parsons A, Schofield PM, et al: Randomised controlled trial of vitamin E in patients with coronary disease: Cambridge Heart Antioxidant Study (CHAOS), *Lancet* 347:781, 1996.
214. Lonn E, Bosch J, Yusuf S, et al: Effects of long-term vitamin E supplementation on cardiovascular events and cancer: a randomized controlled trial, *JAMA* 293:1338, 2005.
215. Bowry VW, Ingold KU, Stocker R: Vitamin E in human low-density lipoprotein. When and how this antioxidant becomes a pro-oxidant, *Biochem J* 288:341, 1992.
216. Lee IM, Cook NR, Gaziano JM, et al: Vitamin E in the primary prevention of cardiovascular disease and cancer: the Women's Health Study: a randomized controlled trial, *JAMA* 294:56, 2005.
217. Glynn RJ, Ridker PM, Goldhaber SZ, et al: Effects of random allocation to vitamin E supplementation on the occurrence of venous thromboembolism: report from the Women's Health Study, *Circulation* 116:1497, 2007.
218. Mosca L, Banka CL, Benjamin EJ, et al: Evidence-based guidelines for cardiovascular disease prevention in women: 2007 update, *J Am Coll Cardiol* 49:1230, 2007.
219. Vivekananthan DP, Penn MS, Sapp SK, et al: Use of antioxidant vitamins for the prevention of cardiovascular disease: meta-analysis of randomised trials, *Lancet* 361:2017, 2003.
220. Bjelakovic G, Nikolova D, Gluud LL, et al: Mortality in randomized trials of antioxidant supplements for primary and secondary prevention: systematic review and meta-analysis, *JAMA* 297:842, 2007.
221. Miller ER III, Pastor-Barriuso R, Dalal D, et al: Meta-analysis: high-dosage vitamin E supplementation may increase all-cause mortality, *Ann Intern Med* 142:37, 2005.
222. Huang HY, Caballero B, Chang S, et al: The efficacy and safety of multivitamin and mineral supplement use to prevent cancer and chronic disease in adults: a systematic review for a National Institutes of Health state-of-the-science conference, *Ann Intern Med* 145:372, 2006.
223. Shekelle PG, Morton SC, Jungvig LK, et al: Effect of supplemental vitamin E for the prevention and treatment of cardiovascular disease, *J Gen Intern Med* 19:380, 2004.
224. Forman JP, Giovannucci E, Holmes MD, et al: Plasma 25-hydroxyvitamin D levels and risk of incident hypertension, *Hypertension* 49:1063, 2007.
225. Martins D, Wolf M, Pan D, et al: Prevalence of cardiovascular risk factors and the serum levels of 25-hydroxyvitamin D in the United States: data from the Third National Health and Nutrition Examination Survey, *Arch Intern Med* 167:1159, 2007.
226. Pfeifer M, Begerow B, Minne HW, et al: Effects of a short-term vitamin D_3 and calcium supplementation on blood pressure and parathyroid hormone levels in elderly women, *J Clin Endocrinol Metab* 86:1633, 2001.
227. Wang TJ, Pencina MJ, Booth SL, et al: Vitamin D deficiency and risk of cardiovascular disease, *Circulation* 117:503, 2008.
228. Ford ES, Ajani UA, McGuire LC, Liu S: Concentrations of serum vitamin D and the metabolic syndrome among U.S. adults, *Diabetes Care* 28:1228, 2005.
229. Liu S, Song Y, Ford ES, et al: Dietary calcium, vitamin D, and the prevalence of metabolic syndrome in middle-aged and older U.S. women, *Diabetes Care* 28:2926, 2005.
230. Reis JP, von Muhlen D, Kritz-Silverstein D, et al: Vitamin D, parathyroid hormone levels, and the prevalence of metabolic syndrome in community-dwelling older adults, *Diabetes Care* 30:1549, 2007.
231. Pittas AG, Dawson-Hughes B, Li T, et al: Vitamin D and calcium intake in relation to type 2 diabetes in women, *Diabetes Care* 29:650, 2006.
232. Pittas AG, Lau J, Hu FB, Dawson-Hughes B: The role of vitamin D and calcium in type 2 diabetes. A systematic review and meta-analysis, *J Clin Endocrinol Metab* 92:2017, 2007.
233. Scragg R, Jackson R, Holdaway IM, et al: Myocardial infarction is inversely associated with plasma 25-hydroxyvitamin D_3 levels: a community-based study, *Int J Epidemiol* 19:559, 1990.
234. Melamed ML, Muntner P, Michos ED, et al: Serum 25-hydroxyvitamin D levels and the prevalence of peripheral arterial disease: results from NHANES 2001 to 2004, *Arterioscler Thromb Vasc Biol* 28:1179, 2008.
235. Poole KE, Loveridge N, Barker PJ, et al: Reduced vitamin D in acute stroke, *Stroke* 37:243, 2006.
236. Zittermann A, Schleithoff SS, Tenderich G, et al: Low vitamin D status: a contributing factor in the pathogenesis of congestive heart failure? *J Am Coll Cardiol* 41:105, 2003.
237. Schleithoff SS, Zittermann A, Tenderich G, et al: Vitamin D supplementation improves cytokine profiles in patients with congestive heart failure: a double-blind, randomized, placebo-controlled trial, *Am J Clin Nutr* 83:754, 2006.
238. Dobnig H, Pilz S, Scharnagl H, et al: Independent association of low serum 25-hydroxyvitamin D and 1,25-dihydroxyvitamin D levels with all-cause and cardiovascular mortality, *Arch Intern Med* 168:1340, 2008.
239. Hsia J, Heiss G, Ren H, et al: Calcium/vitamin D supplementation and cardiovascular events, *Circulation* 115:846, 2007.
240. Giovannucci E, Liu Y, Hollis BW, Rimm EB: 25-Hydroxyvitamin D and risk of myocardial infarction in men: a prospective study, *Arch Intern Med* 168:1174, 2008.
241. Binkley N, Krueger D, Gemar D, Drezner MK: Correlation among 25-hydroxy-vitamin D assays, *J Clin Endocrinol Metab* 93:1804, 2008.
242. Centers for Disease Control and Prevention: *Analytical note for NHANES 2000-2006 and NHANES III (1988-1994)—25-hydroxyvitamin D analysis*, Atlanta, Ga, 2009, Centers for Disease Control and Prevention.
243. Institute of Medicine, Food and Nutrition Board. *Dietary Reference Intakes: Calcium, phosphorus, magnesium, vitamin d, and fluoride*, Washington, DC, 1997, National Academy Press.
244. Cranney A, Horsley T, O'Donnell S, et al: Effectiveness and safety of vitamin D in relation to bone health, *Evid Rep Technol Assess (Full Rep)* 158:1, 2007.
245. Dietary Guidelines Advisory Committee, Agricultural Research Service: *Report of the Dietary Guidelines Advisory Committee on the Dietary Guidelines for Americans, 2005*, U.S. Department of Agriculture (USDA).
246. Song Y, Sesso HD, Manson JE, et al: Dietary magnesium intake and risk of incident hypertension among middle-aged and older US women in a 10-year follow-up study, *Am J Cardiol* 98:1616, 2006.
247. Myers VH, Champagne CM: Nutritional effects on blood pressure, *Curr Opin Lipidol* 18:204, 2007.
248. Beyer FR, Dickinson HO, Nicolson D, et al: Combined calcium, magnesium and potassium supplementation for the management of primary hypertension in adults. *Cochrane Database Syst Rev* (3):CD004805, 2006.
249. Chobanian AV, Bakris GL, Black HR, et al: Seventh report of the Joint National Committee on Prevention, Detection, Evaluation, and Treatment of High Blood Pressure, *Hypertension* 42:1206, 2003.
250. Nielsen FH, Milne DB, Klevay LM, et al: Dietary magnesium deficiency induces heart rhythm changes, impairs glucose tolerance, and decreases serum cholesterol in post menopausal women, *J Am Coll Nutr* 26:121, 2007.
251. Blumberg JB, Frei B: Why clinical trials of vitamin E and cardiovascular diseases may be fatally flawed. Commentary on "The relationship between dose of vitamin E and suppression of oxidative stress in humans," *Free Radic Biol Med* 43:1374, 2007.
252. Kaufert P, Boggs PP, Ettinger B, et al: Women and menopause: beliefs, attitudes, and behaviors. The North American Menopause Society 1997 Menopause Survey, *Menopause* 5:197, 1998.
253. Bair YA, Gold EB, Zhang G, et al: Use of complementary and alternative medicine during the menopause transition: longitudinal results from the Study of Women's Health Across the Nation, *Menopause* 15:32, 2008.
254. Sacks FM, Lichtenstein A, Van Horn L, et al: Soy protein, isoflavones, and cardiovascular health: an American Heart Association Science Advisory for professionals from the Nutrition Committee, *Circulation* 113:1034, 2006.
255. Anderson JW, Johnstone BM, Cook-Newell ME: Meta-analysis of the effects of soy protein intake on serum lipids, *N Engl J Med* 333:276, 1995.
256. Weggemans RM, Trautwein EA: Relation between soy-associated isoflavones and LDL and HDL cholesterol concentrations in humans: a meta-analysis, *Eur J Clin Nutr* 57:940, 2003.
257. Introduction to the TLC diet, Bethesda, Md, 2006, National Heart, Lung, and Blood Institute.
258. Barbiroli B, Frassineti C, Martinelli P, et al: Coenzyme Q10 improves mitochondrial respiration in patients with mitochondrial cytopathies. An in vivo study on brain and skeletal muscle by phosphorous magnetic resonance spectroscopy, *Cell Mol Biol (Noisy-le-grand)* 43:741, 1997.
259. Crane FL: Biochemical functions of coenzyme Q10, *J Am Coll Nutr* 20:591, 2001.
260. Kaikkonen J, Tuomainen TP, Nyyssonen K, Salonen JT: Coenzyme Q10: absorption, antioxidative properties, determinants, and plasma levels, *Free Radic Res* 36:389, 2002.
261. Rosenfeldt F, Marasco S, Lyon W, et al: Coenzyme Q10 therapy before cardiac surgery improves mitochondrial function and in vitro contractility of myocardial tissue, *J Thorac Cardiovasc Surg* 129:25, 2005.
262. Bargossi AM, Battino M, Gaddi A, et al: Exogenous CoQ10 preserves plasma ubiquinone levels in patients treated with 3-hydroxy-3-methylglutaryl coenzyme A reductase inhibitors, *Int J Clin Lab Res* 24:171, 1994.

263. De Pinieux G, Chariot P, Ammi-Said M, et al: Lipid-lowering drugs and mitochondrial function: effects of HMG-CoA reductase inhibitors on serum ubiquinone and blood lactate/pyruvate ratio, *Br J Clin Pharmacol* 42:333, 1996.
264. Davidson M, McKenney J, Stein E, et al: Comparison of one-year efficacy and safety of atorvastatin versus lovastatin in primary hypercholesterolemia, *Am J Cardiol* 79:1475, 1997.
265. Ghirlanda G, Oradei A, Manto A, et al: Evidence of plasma CoQ10-lowering effect by HMG-CoA reductase inhibitors: a double-blind, placebo-controlled study, *J Clin Pharmacol* 33:226, 1993.
266. Mortensen SA, Leth A, Agner E, Rohde M: Dose-related decrease of serum coenzyme Q10 during treatment with HMG-CoA reductase inhibitors, *Mol Aspects Med* 18(Suppl):S137, 1997.
267. Berthold HK, Naini A, Di Mauro S, et al: Effect of ezetimibe and/or simvastatin on coenzyme Q10 levels in plasma: a randomised trial, *Drug Saf* 29:703, 2006.
268. Marcoff L, Thompson PD: The role of coenzyme Q10 in statin-associated myopathy: a systematic review, *J Am Coll Cardiol* 49:2231, 2007.
269. Young JM, Florkowski CM, Molyneux SL, et al: Effect of coenzyme Q_{10} supplementation on simvastatin-induced myalgia, *Am J Cardiol* 100:1400, 2007.
270. Engelsen J, Nielsen JD, Winther K: Effect of coenzyme Q10 and *Ginkgo biloba* on warfarin dosage in stable, long-term warfarin treated outpatients. A randomised, double blind, placebo-crossover trial, *Thromb Haemost* 87:1075, 2002.
271. Hollenberg NK, Martinez G, McCullough M, Meinking T et al: Aging, acculturation, salt intake, and hypertension in the Kuna of Panama, *Hypertension* 29:171, 1997.
272. Buijsse B, Feskens EJ, Kok FJ, Kromhout D: Cocoa intake, blood pressure, and cardiovascular mortality: the Zutphen Elderly Study, *Arch Intern Med* 166:411, 2006.
273. Corti R, Flammer AJ, Hollenberg NK, Luscher TF: Cocoa and cardiovascular health, *Circulation* 119:1433, 2009.
274. Grassi D, Lippi C, Necozione S, et al: Short-term administration of dark chocolate is followed by a significant increase in insulin sensitivity and a decrease in blood pressure in healthy persons, *Am J Clin Nutr* 81:611, 2005.
275. Murphy KJ, Chronopoulos AK, Singh I, et al: Dietary flavanols and procyanidin oligomers from cocoa *(Theobroma cacao)* inhibit platelet function, *Am J Clin Nutr* 77:1466, 2003.
276. Fisher ND, Hughes M, Gerhard-Herman M, Hollenberg NK: Flavanol-rich cocoa induces nitric-oxide-dependent vasodilation in healthy humans, *J Hypertens* 21:2281, 2003.
277. Crews WD, Jr, Harrison DW, Wright JW: A double-blind, placebo-controlled, randomized trial of the effects of dark chocolate and cocoa on variables associated with neuropsychological functioning and cardiovascular health: clinical findings from a sample of healthy, cognitively intact older adults, *Am J Clin Nutr* 87:872, 2008.
278. Taubert D, Roesen R, Lehmann C, et al: Effects of low habitual cocoa intake on blood pressure and bioactive nitric oxide: a randomized controlled trial, *JAMA* 298:49, 2007.
279. Muniyappa R, Hall G, Kolodziej TL, et al: Cocoa consumption for 2 wk enhances insulin-mediated vasodilatation without improving blood pressure or insulin resistance in essential hypertension, *Am J Clin Nutr* 88:1685, 2008.
280. Taubert D, Roesen R, Schomig E: Effect of cocoa and tea intake on blood pressure: a meta-analysis, *Arch Intern Med* 167:626, 2007.
281. Hooper L, Kroon PA, Rimm EB, et al: Flavonoids, flavonoid-rich foods, and cardiovascular risk: a meta-analysis of randomized controlled trials, *Am J Clin Nutr* 88:38, 2008.
282. Schulz V, Hansel R, Tyler VE: *Rational phytotherapy: a physician's guide to herbal medicine*, Berlin, 1996, Springer-Verlag.
283. Blumenthal M, editor: *The Complete German Commission E monographs: therapeutic guide to herbal medicines*, Austin, Texas, 1998, American Botanical Council.
284. Moher D, Pham B, Ausejo M, et al: Pharmacological management of intermittent claudication: a meta-analysis of randomised trials, *Drugs* 59:1057, 2000.
285. Pittler MH, Ernst E: *Ginkgo biloba* extract for the treatment of intermittent claudication: a meta-analysis of randomized trials, *Am J Med* 108:276, 2000.
286. Rowin J, Lewis SL: Spontaneous bilateral subdural hematomas associated with chronic *Ginkgo biloba* ingestion, *Neurology* 46:1775, 1996.
287. Fessenden JM, Wittenborn W, Clarke L: Gingko biloba: a case report of herbal medicine and bleeding postoperatively from a laparoscopic cholecystectomy, *Am Surg* 67:33, 2001.
288. Sirtori CR: Aescin: pharmacology, pharmacokinetics and therapeutic profile, *Pharmacol Res* 44:183, 2001.
289. Arnould T, Janssens D, Michiels C, Remacle J: Effect of aescine on hypoxia-induced activation of human endothelial cells, *Eur J Pharmacol* 315:227, 1996.
290. Pittler MH, Ernst E: Horse chestnut seed extract for chronic venous insufficiency, *Cochrane Database Syst Rev* (1):CD003230, 2006.
291. Tyler VE, editor: *Herbs of choice: the therapeutic use of phytomedicinals*, Binghamton, NY, 1994, Pharmaceutical Product Press.
292. Brinker FJ: *Herb contraindications and drug interactions*, ed 3, Sandy, Oregon, 1998, Eclectic Medical Publications.
293. Cesarone MR, Belcaro G, Rohdewald P, et al: Improvement of diabetic microangiopathy with pycnogenol: a prospective, controlled study, *Angiology* 57:431, 2006.
294. Nishioka K, Hidaka T, Nakamura S, et al: Pycnogenol, French maritime pine bark extract, augments endothelium-dependent vasodilation in humans, *Hypertens Res* 30:775, 2007.
295. Calder PC: Polyunsaturated fatty acids and inflammation, *Prostaglandins Leukot Essent Fatty Acids* 75:197, 2006.
296. de Lorgeril M: Essential polyunsaturated fatty acids, inflammation, atherosclerosis and cardiovascular diseases, *Subcell Biochem* 42:283, 2007.
297. He K, Song Y, Daviglus ML, et al: Accumulated evidence on fish consumption and coronary heart disease mortality: a meta-analysis of cohort studies, *Circulation* 109:2705, 2004.
298. Whelton SP, He J, Whelton PK, Muntner P: Meta-analysis of observational studies on fish intake and coronary heart disease, *Am J Cardiol* 93:1119, 2004.
299. Bucher HC, Hengstler P, Schindler C, Meier G: n-3 Polyunsaturated fatty acids in coronary heart disease: a meta-analysis of randomized controlled trials, *Am J Med* 112:298, 2002.
300. Harris WS, Mozaffarian D, Lefevre M, et al: Towards establishing dietary reference intakes for eicosapentaenoic and docosahexaenoic acids, *J Nutr* 139:804S, 2009.
301. Harris WS, Kris-Etherton PM, Harris KA: Intakes of long-chain omega-3 fatty acid associated with reduced risk for death from coronary heart disease in healthy adults, *Curr Atheroscler Rep* 10:503, 2008.
302. Yokoyama M, Origasa H, Matsuzaki M, et al: Effects of eicosapentaenoic acid on major coronary events in hypercholesterolaemic patients (JELIS): a randomised open-label, blinded endpoint analysis, *Lancet* 369:1090, 2007.
303. GISSI-Prevenzione Investigators: Dietary supplementation with n-3 polyunsaturated fatty acids and vitamin E after myocardial infarction: results of the GISSI-Prevenzione trial, *Lancet* 354:447, 1999.
304. Mozaffarian D, Geelen A, Brouwer IA, et al: Effect of fish oil on heart rate in humans: a meta-analysis of randomized controlled trials, *Circulation* 112:1945, 2005.
305. Sommerfield T, Price J, Hiatt WR: Omega-3 fatty acids for intermittent claudication, *Cochrane Database Syst Rev* (4):CD003833, 2007.
306. Smith SC, Jr, Allen J, Blair SN, et al: AHA/ACC guidelines for secondary prevention for patients with coronary and other atherosclerotic vascular disease: 2006 update: endorsed by the National Heart, Lung, and Blood Institute, *Circulation* 113:2363, 2006.
307. McKenney JM, Sica D: Role of prescription omega-3 fatty acids in the treatment of hypertriglyceridemia, *Pharmacotherapy* 5:715, 2007.
308. Hulley S, Grady D, Bush T, et al: Randomized trial of estrogen plus progestin for secondary prevention of coronary heart disease in postmenopausal women. Heart and Estrogen/progestin Replacement Study (HERS) Research Group, *JAMA* 280:605, 1998.
309. Herrington DM, Reboussin DM, Brosnihan KB, et al: Effects of estrogen replacement on the progression of coronary-artery atherosclerosis, *N Engl J Med* 343:522, 2000.
310. Rossouw JE, Anderson GL, Prentice RL, et al: Risks and benefits of estrogen plus progestin in healthy postmenopausal women: principal results from the Women's Health Initiative randomized controlled trial, *JAMA* 288:321, 2002.
311. The Writing Group for the PEPI Trial: Effects of estrogen or estrogen/progestin regimens on heart disease risk factors in postmenopausal women. The Postmenopausal Estrogen/Progestin Interventions (PEPI) Trial, *JAMA* 273:199, 1995.
312. Ottosson UB: Oral progesterone and estrogen/progestogen therapy. Effects of natural and synthetic hormones on subfractions of HDL cholesterol and liver proteins, *Acta Obstet Gynecol Scand Suppl* 127:1, 1984.
313. Ottosson UB, Johansson BG, von Schoultz B: Subfractions of high-density lipoprotein cholesterol during estrogen replacement therapy: a comparison between progestogens and natural progesterone, *Am J Obstet Gynecol* 151:746, 1985.
314. Toy JL, Davies JA, Hancock KW, McNicol GP: The comparative effects of a synthetic and a "natural" oestrogen on the haemostatic mechanism in patients with primary amenorrhoea, *Br J Obstet Gynaecol* 85:359, 1978.
315. Stephenson K, Price C, Kurdowska A, et al: Topical progesterone cream does not increase thrombotic and inflammatory factors in postmenopausal women, *Blood* 104:Abstr. 5318, 2004.
316. Minshall RD, Stanczyk FZ, Miyagawa K, et al: Ovarian steroid protection against coronary artery hyperreactivity in rhesus monkeys, *J Clin Endocrinol Metab* 83:649, 1998.
317. Miyagawa K, Rosch J, Stanczyk F, Hermsmeyer K: Medroxyprogesterone interferes with ovarian steroid protection against coronary vasospasm, *Nat Med* 3:324, 1997.
318. Mishra RG, Hermsmeyer RK, Miyagawa K, et al: Medroxyprogesterone acetate and dihydrotestosterone induce coronary hyperreactivity in intact male rhesus monkeys, *J Clin Endocrinol Metab* 90:3706, 2005.
319. Fugh-Berman A, Bythrow J: Bioidentical hormones for menopausal hormone therapy: variation on a theme, *J Gen Intern Med* 22:1030, 2007.
320. Moskowitz D: A comprehensive review of the safety and efficacy of bioidentical hormones for the management of menopause and related health risks, *Altern Med Rev* 11:208, 2006.
321. Holtorf K: The bioidentical hormone debate: are bioidentical hormones (estradiol, estriol, and progesterone) safer or more efficacious than commonly used synthetic versions in hormone replacement therapy? *Postgrad Med* 121:73, 2009.
322. Rothstein WG: *American physicians in the nineteenth century; from sects to science*, Baltimore, Md, 1972, Johns Hopkins University Press.
323. Novella S, Roy R, Marcus D, et al: A debate: homeopathy—quackery or a key to the future of medicine? *J Altern Complement Med* 14:9, 2008.
324. Whole medical systems: an overview, National Center for Complementary and Alternative Medicine, National Institutes of Health, U.S. Department of Health and Human Services, 2007.
325. Poirier P, Giles TD, Bray GA, et al: Obesity and cardiovascular disease: pathophysiology, evaluation, and effect of weight loss: an update of the 1997 American Heart Association Scientific Statement on Obesity and Heart Disease from the Obesity Committee of the Council on Nutrition, Physical. *Circulation* 113:898, 2006.
326. Wee CC, Girotra S, Weinstein AR, et al: The relationship between obesity and atherosclerotic progression and prognosis among patients with coronary artery bypass grafts the effect of aggressive statin therapy, *J Am Coll Cardiol* 52:620, 2008.
327. Costello RB, Dwyer JT: Obesity and weight loss: an overview of diet, drugs and dietary supplements. In Vogel JH, Krucoff MW, editors: *Integrative cardiology: complementary and alternative medicine for the heart*, New York, 2007, McGraw-Hill, pp 447-467.
328. Bertisch SM, Wee CC, McCarthy EP: Use of complementary and alternative therapies by overweight and obese adults, *Obesity (Silver Spring)* 16:1610, 2008.
329. Chan TY: Potential risks associated with the use of herbal anti-obesity products, *Drug Saf* 32:453, 2009.
330. Lichtenstein AH, Russell RM: Essential nutrients: food or supplements? Where should the emphasis be? *JAMA* 294:351, 2005.

Reported Uses and Potential Interactions Between Dietary Supplement Products and Conventional Medications

Supplement	Reported Uses	Active Ingredient	Potential Interactions	Comments and Suggested Guidelines of Use
Arginine	Improve peripheral and coronary blood flow and as adjuvant therapy for CAD, CHF, PVD, angina pectoris, and hypertension	L-Arginine	Has been shown to have additive hypotensive effects if combined with hypertensive drugs, but data is limited	L-Arginine is the precursor of nitric oxide and has been shown to improve coronary and brachial artery endothelial function. Short-term efficacy for intermittent claudication due to PVD was not replicated in a longer term trial. Efficacy of oral L-arginine for CHD awaits confirmation.
Artichoke leaf extract (*Cynara cardunculus*)	Lower blood cholesterol	Phenolic acids (chlorogenic acid, cynarin, and caffeic acid), sesquiterpene lactones, and flavonoids (scolymoside, cynaroside, and luteolin)	No known interactions with herbs and other dietary supplements, drugs, foods, or laboratory tests	In the United States, artichoke has GRAS use in foods. Few data from rigorous clinical trials exist. Beneficial effects are reported but not compelling. Cynaroside and its derivative, luteolin, might also indirectly inhibit HMG-CoA reductase. Potential adverse effects include flatulence and allergenic dermatitis.
Astragalus, root (*Astragalus membranaceus*)	Used as an anti-inflammatory, antioxidant, diuretic, vasodilator, and hypotensive agent	Saponins (astragaloside), flavonoids (isoflavones, pterocarpans, and isoflavans), polysaccharides, trace minerals, amino acids, and coumarins	No known interactions with herbs and other dietary supplements, drugs, foods, or laboratory tests. However, certain isoflavones affect alcohol dehydrogenase.	Astragalus is most commonly used in combination with other herbs. Small clinical studies have found astragalus to be effective for relief of angina pectoris. As astragalus may stimulate immune function, theoretically it might decrease the effects of immunosuppressive therapy.
Carnitine	Reduce symptoms of angina pectoris and PVD Adjunct therapy for heart failure	L-Carnitine, acetyl-L-carnitine, and propionyl-L-carnitine	Concomitant use with acenocoumarol may potentiate (decrease) anticoagulant effects. It is unknown if interactions occur with warfarin.	L-Carnitine is naturally found in the body. D- or DL-carnitine should not be substituted for L-carnitine. Potential side effects include GI upset, diarrhea, body odor, and seizures. The FDA approved L-carnitine for use in primary carnitine deficiency. CHF clinical trials are under way in Italy. Monitor INRs in patients receiving anticoagulant therapies. ACC/AHA Practice Guidelines note that effectiveness of propionyl-L-carnitine as a therapy to improve walking distance in patients with intermittent claudication is not well established (Level of Evidence: B).

Continued

Supplement	Reported Uses	Active Ingredient	Potential Interactions	Comments and Suggested Guidelines of Use
Danshen (*Salvia miltiorrhiza*)	Reduce symptoms of angina pectoris	Main components derived from the root include protocatechualdehyde and 3,4-dihydrophenyl-lactic acid, which may alter vasoactivity; the tanshinone derivatives, diterpenoids miltirone and salvinone, may have anticoagulant properties	Concomitant use is discouraged as anticoagulant (warfarin) or antiplatelet drugs might ↑ the risks of bleeding. May interact with digoxin and ↑ arrhythmias	Collectively, evidence from randomized controlled trials is insufficient and of low quality and use is discouraged.
Dong quai (*Angelica sinensis*)	Reduce symptoms of menopause Lower blood pressure	Root contains coumarin derivatives (angelol, angelicone, osthol, psoralen, oxypeucedanin, and bergapten) and other constituents such as ferulic acid and ligusticide	Limited data suggests interaction with warfarin and may increase risk of bleeding and ↑ INR and prothrombin time. Note that not all coumarin derivatives have anticoagulant potential.	This popular TCM preparation is generally well tolerated. Avoid use in patients taking warfarin. It has been used safely in a clinical trial lasting up to 24 weeks. Preliminary research suggests that dong quai might protect against ischemia-reperfusion injury.
Fenugreek (*Trigonella foenum-graecum*)	Control of blood glucose Lower blood cholesterol Prevention of CVD	Seed components contain trigonelline, 4-hydroxyisoleucine, and sotolon and coumarins	High content of dietary fiber and pectin may ↓ blood glucose levels as well as ↓ or delay absorption of oral drugs. Coumarin and other constituents could enhance anticoagulant drug activity and ↑ INR and risk of bleeding. Note that not all coumarin derivatives have anticoagulant potential.	Fenugreek has GRAS status in the United States; therefore, it is likely safe when seed preparations are used in amounts commonly found in foods. More evidence is needed to determine the efficacy of fenugreek for lowering of serum cholesterol and triglycerides. Potential side effects include diarrhea, flatulence, and hypoglycemia with large doses. Monitor warfarin levels. Monitor insulin levels.
Ginger (*Zingiber officinale*)	(Possibly) Lower blood pressure	Active constituents of the rhizome and root include gingerol, gingerdione, shogaol, and sesquiterpene and monoterpene volatile oils, depending on form of preparation	Concern that ginger may interact with anticoagulant or antiplatelet herbs and drugs as it may inhibit thromboxane synthetase and ↓ platelet aggregation May also have hypotensive and calcium channel blocking effects	Clinically, it has been shown that ginger could potentiate the antiplatelet effect of nifedipine. Dried ginger has been used for chest pain. The oleoresin of ginger is also used as an ingredient in digestive, laxative, antitussive, antiflatulent, and antacid preparations.
Ginkgo biloba (ginkgo leaf (extract)	Reduce symptoms of peripheral arterial disease	Constituents of ginkgo leaf and its extracts (GBE) include flavonoids and flavone glycosides (ginkgolides and bilobalides), terpenoids, and organic acids	Ginkgolides have antiplatelet activity and are platelet-activating factor receptor antagonists; may have an additive effect with other blood-thinning agents, such as herbs and drugs with anticoagulant or antiplatelet potential. May ↑ INR and risk of bleeding; may also affect bioavailability of other drugs; avoid use with insulin and thiazide	Likely safe when used orally and appropriately Discontinue use before surgery. Avoid in individuals with diabetes. Several cases of cerebral hemorrhage have been reported in those taking prescription anticoagulants; avoid use with warfarin. ACC/AHA Practice Guidelines (2005) note that the effectiveness of *Ginkgo biloba* to improve walking distance for patients with intermittent claudication is marginal and not well established (Level of Evidence: B).

17

Supplement	Reported Uses	Active Ingredient	Potential Interactions	Comments and Suggested Guidelines of Use
Ginseng root, Asian (Panax ginseng)	Acts as an "adaptogen" to enhance energy levels and to relieve stress and eases symptoms of anxiety Antihypertensive Improves control of blood glucose	Ginsenosides and triterpenoid saponins are the main active components derived from the root	Interacts with P-450 enzyme system Potential to interact with anticoagulant and antiplatelet drugs and corticosteroids, calcium channel blockers, digoxin, and methyldopa Interacts with MAO inhibitors, stimulants, and phenelzine sulfate (an antidepressant) May enhance the effect of hypoglycemics	Ginseng has been used for medicinal purposes for more than 2000 years. Safety of long-term (>3 months) use is unknown, but it has been well tolerated in clinical studies. Studies in patients with CVD are lacking. Orally, it appears to have negligible effects on cardiovascular function. Some data suggest that intravenous infusions increase ejection fraction in patients with CHF. Use with caution in individuals with history of CVD or diabetes. Monitor individuals taking warfarin. May interfere with serum digoxin levels by some assay methods Discontinue use before surgery.
Green tea (Camellia sinensis)	Lower blood cholesterol Lower blood pressure Improve cognitive performance Weight loss	Parts used include leaf bud, leaf, and stem Polyphenols (flavanols, such as catechins, flavandiols, flavonoids) and phenolic acids and caffeine	Green tea contains catechins and caffeine as well as vitamin K and thus may interfere with anticoagulant or antiplatelet drugs and antagonize the effect of warfarin. Verapamil has been reported to ↑ plasma caffeine concentrations by 25%.	A green tea health claim for CVD was recently rejected by the FDA. Patients receiving warfarin need to be routinely questioned about their intake of vitamin K–containing foods, beverages, and dietary supplements. Monitor INR in patients who habitually consume green tea and are taking warfarin.
Hawthorn (Crataegus)	Reduce symptoms of mild CHF, ischemic heart disease; reduces the risk of arrhythmias and atherosclerosis	Hawthorn leaf extract (leaves, fruit, and flowers) contains procyanidins, flavonoids, triterpenoids, catechins, and aromatic carboxylic acids.	Has been hypothesized to potentiate the effects of digitalis and have additive effects when combined with beta blockers, calcium channel blockers, and nitrates to ↑ vasodilation	In Germany, hawthorn is prescribed for "mild cardiac insufficiency." It is generally well tolerated and safe for short-term use. Most common side effects are GI upset, fatigue, and dizziness. Recently noted increased risk of death and hospitalization in NYHA stage II or III heart failure patients taking 450 mg twice daily participating in a long-term clinical trial
Horse chestnut seed extracts (Aesculus hippocastanum)	Reduce swelling and discomfort due to chronic venous insufficiency, varicose veins, and phlebitis	Aescin, a triterpene saponin, and aesculin, a glycoside, which is also a hydroxycoumarin	May ↑ effects of anticoagulants and antiplatelet drugs Possibly induces hypoglycemic effects Do not administer with drugs known to cause nephrotoxicity.	Most widely prescribed oral antiedema venous remedy in Germany Treatment for 1 to 3 months may be required before full therapeutic effects are apparent. Side effects are uncommon, but GI irritation and toxic nephropathy may occur. Monitor individuals taking warfarin. Monitor blood glucose levels in diabetics.
Hu zhang (Polygonum cuspidatum)	CVD and lipid lowering	Hu zhang root contains flavonoids, phenolic acids and their derivatives, tannins, stilbenes (resveratrol), and anthraquinones.	Resveratrol has been shown to have antiplatelet effects and therefore could ↑ risk of bleeding. Do not administer with anticoagulant or antiplatelet drugs.	There is limited reliable information available about the effectiveness of Hu zhang. Hu zhang is considered to be one of the richest sources of trans-resveratrol.

Continued

Integrative Medicine in the Prevention of Cardiovascular Disease

17

Supplement	Reported Uses	Active Ingredient	Potential Interactions	Comments and Suggested Guidelines of Use
Jiaogulan (*Gynostemma pentaphyllum*)	Reduce blood cholesterol and blood pressure and improve coronary and cardiovascular functions	Jiaogulan leaves contain triterpene saponins (gypenosides), many of which are similar to ginsenosides found in *Panax ginseng*	Clinical trial data is lacking.	Jiaogulan grows wild in China, and it is a newcomer to TCM. Most of the evidence regarding the pharmacologic effects of jiaogulan comes from preliminary animal or in vitro research. Older studies in humans suggest cholesterol-lowering effects. Newer clinical data suggest an antidiabetic effect.
Kudzu (*Pueraria lobata*)	Lower blood pressure Reduce symptoms of angina pectoris	Kudzu (root, flower, and leaf) contains isoflavones daidzin, daidzein, puerarin, genistin, and genistein	No side effects have been reported in clinical studies. Theoretically, concomitant use with anticoagulant or antiplatelet herbs or drugs might ↑ the risk of bleeding. Dose-dependent Antabuse-like activity with ethanol.	Kudzu has been used medically in Chinese medicine since 200 BC. Kudzu was brought to the southeastern United States in the late 1800s to help prevent soil erosion but has now turned into one of the most invasive species in this region. The kudzu extract puerarin has been used intravenously to treat ischemic stroke.
Lycium (*Lycium chinense*)	Improve circulation and lower blood pressure and blood glucose levels	Lycium (dried berries and root bark) contains beta-sitosterol; the bark also contains kukoamine, which may lower cholesterol; also contains beta carotene, niacin, pyridoxine, and ascorbic acid	Clinical data is lacking.	Lycium is a native Chinese deciduous shrub with bright red berries that has been promoted to increase longevity. Lycium is usually taken orally as a tea. Two case reports suggest interaction with warfarin therapy.
Policosanol	Lower blood cholesterol For peripheral vascular insufficiency and intermittent claudication	Derived from a variety of plant sources and contains a mixture of waxy alcohols	Policosanol may inhibit platelet aggregation, so use caution with anticoagulant and antiplatelet drugs or supplements such as garlic and ginkgo and high doses of vitamin E.	Research for hypercholesterolemia is inconsistent and contradictory. Policosanol appears to be well tolerated; it may cause erythema, migraines, insomnia, irritability, dizziness, upset stomach, and rash. Monitor INR in patients taking warfarin. Discontinue use before surgery.
Schizandra (*Schisandra chinensis*)	Reduce blood pressure and elevated cholesterol	Active constituents in the fruit include lignans (schizandrins, schizandrols, gomisins, schizandrers, schisantherins, wuweizisu) and citral, stigmasterol, and vitamins C and E	Induces cytochrome P-450 2C9 (CYP2C9), possibly altering metabolism of fluvastatin, irbesartan, losartan, and warfarin	It may cause heartburn, acid indigestion, decreased appetite, stomach pain, allergic rashes, and urticaria in some patients.
Selenium	Prevent oxidative stress	Selenomethionine is generally considered to be the best absorbed and used form of selenium	Theoretically, combining selenium with anticoagulant or antiplatelet drugs might ↑ INR and bleeding times through multiple pathways.	Selenium appears to be safe when it is taken short term in amounts below the upper intake level of 400 µg/day. Selenium toxicity can elevate the ST segment and cause T wave changes on EKG characteristic of myocardial infarction. Long-term use has been shown to increase the risk for development of type 2 diabetes and to increase mortality. AHA notes that "antioxidant vitamin supplements or other supplements such as selenium to prevent CVD are not recommended."

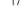

Supplement	Reported Uses	Active Ingredient	Potential Interactions	Comments and Suggested Guidelines of Use
Vitamin E	Prevention of CVD (CHD, stroke)	Family of 8 fat-soluble antioxidants, α-tocopherol most active form	Anticoagulant or antiplatelet drugs and herbal medicines with anticoagulant and antiplatelet potential may ↑ INR. High doses of vitamin E (>800 units/day) can antagonize the effects of vitamin K and ↑ the risk of bleeding.	Relatively nontoxic; safe when used orally in amounts not exceeding the UL of 1000 mg/day Conversion factor: 1 mg = 1.26 IU; RDA of 15 mg = 22 IU (natural form) or 33 IU (synthetic form) Possible ↑ risk of bleeding for those taking anticoagulants or with vitamin K deficiency Possible ↑ risk of hemorrhage in high-risk groups Monitor INR in patients taking warfarin and vitamin E >800 IU daily AHA notes that "antioxidant vitamin supplements or other supplements such as vitamin E to prevent CVD are not recommended"

ACC/AHA, American College of Cardiology/American Heart Association; CAD, coronary artery disease; CHD, coronary heart disease; CHF, congestive heart failure; CVD, cardiovascular disease; EKG, electrocardiogram; FDA, Food and Drug Administration; GI, gastrointestinal; GRAS, generally recognized as safe; HMG-CoA, hydroxymethylglutaryl–coenzyme A reductase; INR, international normalized ratio; MAO, monoamine oxidase; NYHA, New York Heart Association; PVD, peripheral vascular disease; RDA, recommended daily allowance; TCM, traditional Chinese medicine; UL, upper tolerable limit.

REFERENCES

Chavez M, Jordan M, Chavez P: Evidence-based drug–herbal interactions. *Life Sci* 78:2146–2157, 2006.

Costello RB, Leser M, Coates P: Dietary supplements for health maintenance and risk factor reduction. In Bales C, Ritchie C, editors: *Handbook of clinical nutrition and aging*, Totowa, NJ, 2009, Humana Press, pp 553–663.

Hirsch A, Haskal Z, Hertzer N, et al: ACC/AHA 2005 Practice Guidelines for the management of patients with peripheral arterial disease (lower extremity, renal, mesenteric, and abdominal aortic): a collaborative report from the American Association for Vascular Surgery/Society for Vascular Surgery, Society for Cardiovascular Angiography and Interventions, Society for Vascular Medicine and Biology, Society of Interventional Radiology, and the ACC/AHA Task Force on Practice Guidelines (Writing Committee to Develop Guidelines for the Management of Patients With Peripheral Arterial Disease): endorsed by the American Association of Cardiovascular and Pulmonary Rehabilitation; National Heart, Lung, and Blood Institute; Society for Vascular Nursing; TransAtlantic Inter-Society Consensus; and Vascular Disease Foundation. *Circulation* 113:e463, 2006.

Jellin JM, Gregory PJ, Batz F, et al: *Pharmacist's letter/prescriber's letter natural medicines comprehensive database*, ed 10, Stockton, Calif, 2008, Therapeutic Research Faculty.

Lichtenstein AH, Appel LJ, Brands M, et al: Diet and lifestyle recommendations revision 2006: a scientific statement from the American Heart Association Nutrition Committee. *Circulation* 114:82, 2006.

Ulbricht C, Chao W, Costa D, et al: Clinical evidence of herb-drug interactions: a systematic review by the natural standard research collaboration. *Curr Drug Metab* 9:1063, 2008.

Vogel J, Costello RB, Krucoff M: Complementary and alternative approaches to management of patients with heart disease. In Libby P, Bonow RO, Zipes DP, Mann DL, editors: *Braunwald's heart disease: a textbook of cardiovascular medicine*, ed 8, Philadelphia, 2007, Elsevier, pp 1157–1164.

CHAPTER 18

Effects of Alcohol on Cardiovascular Disease Risk

R. Curtis Ellison

KEY POINTS

- Most large prospective cohort studies show that regular, moderate consumers of alcohol have considerably lower risk for development of coronary heart disease and other types of CVD than do abstainers.

- Numerous mechanisms have been demonstrated in basic scientific studies and limited human trials to explain the effects of both alcohol and the polyphenols in some alcoholic beverages on reduction of CVD risk; these include beneficial effects on lipids, coagulation, fibrinolysis, inflammation, glucose metabolism, and endothelial function.

- Evidence is accumulating that moderate drinkers are also at lower risk of other chronic diseases (including diabetes, dementia, and osteoporosis) and have lower all-cause mortality rates than those of nondrinkers.

- In contrast to potential health benefits from moderate drinking, there are many adverse health and societal effects of the abuse of alcohol. Advice to patients regarding alcohol consumption will vary according to their individual characteristics (age, sex, risk factors) but should always be based on scientifically sound and balanced data.

- Any recommendations regarding moderate alcohol consumption for the prevention of CVD for individuals should be based on consultation with the health care provider.

EPIDEMIOLOGIC EVIDENCE RELATING ALCOHOL TO CORONARY HEART DISEASE

Starting in the early 1970s, many scientists began to publish data from prospective studies indicating a lower risk for development of coronary heart disease (CHD) for moderate consumers of alcohol.[1-4] Of hundreds of studies published in the scientific literature during the past few decades, the results have been extremely consistent. Almost uniformly, they have demonstrated that in comparison with nondrinkers, moderate drinkers are less likely to develop CHD.

In a meta-analysis by Corrao and associates[5] based only on high-quality prospective studies, there was a J-shaped curve for the association between alcohol and CHD, with its nadir at about 20 g/day of alcohol, the equivalent of about 1½ U.S. drinks (with 12 g of alcohol, the average amount in a "typical drink"). The relative risk crossed 1.0 (the risk for nondrinkers) between 72 and 89 g of alcohol per day (Fig. 18-1).

A lower risk for CHD and other cardiovascular disease (CVD) among moderate drinkers has been shown in populations with a low intake of alcohol, such as the Chinese,[6] and in those with typically high alcohol intake, as in Scandinavia.[7,8] Data from the latter show that heavy drinking is associated with increases in sudden death.[9] Rimm[10] stated that the evidence to support the hypothesis that the inverse association of alcohol to CHD is causal, and not confounded by healthy lifestyle behaviors, is very strong. This evidence includes the fact that moderate alcohol consumption reduces CHD and mortality in individuals in diverse cultures with varying drinking habits; among subjects with hypertension, diabetes, and existing CHD; and among otherwise healthy individuals.[10] Mukamal and coworkers[11] demonstrated among "very healthy" subjects (who did not smoke, exercised, ate a good diet, and were not obese) that those who drank moderately had a much lower relative risk of CHD (0.38; 95% CI, 0.16-0.89) than that of similar subjects who did not consume any alcohol.

There are notable exceptions to the inverse association between alcohol and coronary artery disease occurrence or mortality in epidemiologic studies. As would be expected, longitudinal studies based primarily on young people tend to have few instances of CVD and may show no protection against CHD.[12] Studies from eastern Europe, where very heavy drinking is the norm, often do not show lower rates of CHD among drinkers. In some studies in which binge drinkers are combined with regular moderate drinkers, lower rates for "moderate" drinking have not been seen.[13,14] Furthermore, if the range considered to be moderate drinking extends to more than three or four typical drinks per day, an inverse association may not be seen among drinkers. The meta-analysis by Corrao and associates[5] demonstrated that essentially all studies show lower CHD for consumers of up to 12.5 g of alcohol per day, but some fail to show lower rates when consumption of up to 25 or 50 g/day is considered the moderate category.

As described by Wannamethee and Shaper,[15] it is essential that ex-drinkers not be included with lifetime abstainers in the nondrinking category, as the former tend to have higher rates of many types of disease that may falsely increase a putative beneficial effect among moderate drinkers. Poikolainen[16] has pointed out the importance of identifying abusive drinkers in a population before attempting to evaluate the association between moderate drinking and CVD. As will be described later, some studies suggest that African Americans may not show a lower risk of CVD from moderate drinking.

LACK OF RANDOMIZED CLINICAL TRIALS OF ALCOHOL CONSUMPTION AND CORONARY HEART DISEASE EVENTS

In lieu of randomized clinical trials of alcohol intake and cardiovascular outcomes, physicians are forced to rely primarily on associations shown in observational

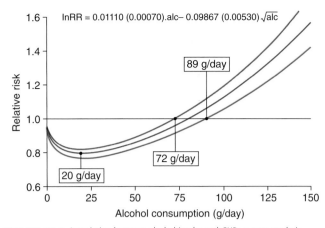

FIGURE 18-1 Association between alcohol intake and CHD: a meta-analysis. Functions (and corresponding 95% CIs) describing the dose-response relationship between alcohol consumption and the relative risk of CHD obtained by pooling from a meta-analysis the 28 cohort studies at which a ≥15 quality score was assigned. The fitted model (with standard errors in parentheses) and three critical exposure levels (nadir point, maximum dose showing statistical evidence of protective effect, and minimum dose showing statistical evidence of harmful effect) are also reported. *(From Corrao G, Rubbiati L, Bagnardi V, et al: Alcohol and coronary heart disease: a meta-analysis.* Addiction *95:1505, 2000. Reprinted with permission.)*

18

studies, experiments of the effects of alcohol on risk factors, and animal experiments. Also, results among subjects in prospective studies who change their drinking habits during follow-up may be informative. Several studies have demonstrated that when former abstainers begin to consume alcohol, their subsequent risk of CVD decreases. Gronbaek and colleagues,[17] in a prospective study of more than 14,000 subjects, showed that moderate drinkers had lower risk of total mortality than nondrinkers or heavy drinkers. Furthermore, based on alcohol assessments 5 years apart, they found that in comparison with stable drinkers, subjects who reduced their drinking from light to none increased their mortality risk (RR = 1.40; 95% CI = 1.00-1.95), and those who went from nondrinking to light drinking reduced their risk (RR = 0.71; 95% CI = 0.44-1.14).[17] In the Health Professionals Study, with repeated alcohol assessments, subjects reporting an increase of ≥10 g/day in alcohol had a decrease in risk of subsequent myocardial infarction (RR = 0.55; CI 0.33-0.91), whereas there was a tendency for a slight increase in risk for subjects decreasing their alcohol intake (RR = 1.10, CI: 0.92, 1.31).[18]

Former abstainers who reported moderate intake in follow-up examinations in the Atherosclerosis Risk in Communities (ARIC) study subsequently had a 38% lower chance for development of CVD than did their persistently nondrinking counterparts.[19] In a large population-based cohort of women in Australia, moderate drinkers showed the best self-reported state of overall health, whereas those who stopped drinking during follow-up (even those with no reported comorbidity) showed a decrease in their ratings of overall health[20]; as in most studies, however, the reasons that the subjects stopped drinking were not known.

DIFFERENCES IN RESPONSE TO ALCOHOL BY GENDER, AGE, AND ETHNICITY

Gender

Women are known to show decreased tolerance to alcohol, which is thought to relate to lower levels of alcohol-clearing enzymes (especially alcohol dehydrogenase), their generally smaller body size, and the greater proportion of their body consisting of fat, which metabolizes alcohol less well than

muscle does. Both the beneficial and adverse effects of alcohol appear at lower dosages for women.[10,21,22] Hence, guidelines generally suggest that moderate drinking for women should be only about half the amount of alcohol for men.[23] From a meta-analysis, Di Castelnuovo and coworkers[24] found that women drinkers showed an increase in mortality over that of nondrinkers above about 2 drinks/day, whereas the increase among men was at about 3½ drinks/day. In the Australia Longitudinal Study on Women's Health, with approximately 12,000 subjects aged 70 years and older, Byles and colleagues[25] found that nondrinkers and women who rarely drink had a significantly higher risk of dying (HR = 1.94; 95% CI, 1.4-2.6) during the survey period than did women who consumed alcoholic beverages at a level of one or two drinks per day; the best general health status and highest levels of physical functioning were among those drinking at this level for 3 to 6 days per week.

Age

Alcohol has been shown to be associated with CHD in the elderly as well as in middle-aged people. In the Cardiovascular Health Study, subjects older than 65 years who consumed 14 or more drinks per week had a risk of incident myocardial infarction or cardiac death about 40% lower than that of abstainers.[26] People tend to drink less as they age,[27,28] and most current recommendations state that individuals older than 65 years should drink less than what is considered moderate for younger people.[23] On the other hand, two analyses comparing the health effects among elderly subjects consuming one or two drinks per day, in comparison with those consuming only one drink per day or less, have not shown higher morbidity or mortality among those consuming more alcohol.[29,30]

Tolvanen and colleagues[31] evaluated 10-year mortality according to alcohol intake among subjects initially aged 60 to 99 years, of whom 50% of men and 40% of women died during follow-up. After adjustment for age, sex, educational level, marital status, chronic diseases, functional ability, and smoking, the relative risk for mortality of frequent drinkers (versus nondrinkers) was 0.6 (95% CI, 0.4, 0.8); for occasional drinkers, 0.7 (0.5, 1.0); and for ex-drinkers, 1.1 (0.8, 1.7).

Ethnicity

Whereas most of the original studies relating alcohol intake to CHD were in Europeans and European Americans, a large number of studies have found essentially the same effects among Asians.[32,33] Data on African Americans are limited, and Sempos and colleagues[34] found no inverse association between alcohol and CVD risk among African Americans. Klatsky and associates,[32] however, found similar inverse associations between alcohol and heart failure in the Kaiser Permanente cohort among whites, Asians, and African Americans. Using data from the Women's Health Initiative, Freiberg and coworkers[35] reported lower total mortality among African American hypertensives who consumed alcohol than among those who did not drink, but a similar relation was not seen among nonhypertensive African Americans.

IMPORTANCE OF PATTERN OF ALCOHOL CONSUMPTION

It has become very clear that the amount of alcohol consumed (within limits) is not as important in terms of health effects as is the pattern of consumption. The two key aspects of pattern are the frequency of drinking and a large number of drinks on a single occasion (binge drinking). Mukamal and coworkers[13] demonstrated among people who had suffered a myocardial infarction that those who drank moderately without binge drinking had 30% fewer deaths, whereas those who reported binge drinking (defined in this study as consuming three or more drinks within 1 to 2 hours) had death rates even higher than those of teetotalers.

Studies of the effects of alcohol intake on CHD, obesity, cognitive function, and other diseases show that more frequent drinkers have the best outcomes; for subjects consuming the same average amount of alcohol during a week, those consuming alcohol every day may have up to 50% lower risk of disease than those consuming the same amount on only 1 or 2 days.[36] In a meta-analysis based on the only six prospective studies in the literature that permitted such an analysis of pattern of drinking and CHD, Bagnardi and coworkers[37] reported that in comparison with not consuming alcohol, regular drinking (even at fairly high levels of consumption) was associated with lower risk of CHD; irregular heavy consumption, or binge drinking, increased the risk.[37] In a population of light to moderate drinkers, alcohol consumption in general was associated with decreased risk of acute myocardial infarction in women, but episodic intoxication was related to a substantial increase in risk.[38]

Cross-cultural prospective studies have shown that simply correlating the average amount of alcohol consumed with CVD outcomes is inadequate.[39] In some cultures, daily drinking is the norm, but in others, alcohol consumption is generally confined to Friday and Saturday nights; whereas benefits are seen in the former, they are absent in the latter.[40] Data are mixed on whether consumption of alcohol in conjunction with food affects the outcome, but elevated risk for hypertension has been reported in one study only for individuals who drink outside of meals.[41] Furthermore, Gorelik and associates[42] found in an intervention study that red wine served with a high-fat meal inhibited the postprandial increase in serum and urinary levels of cytotoxic lipid peroxidation products.

IS IT ALCOHOL OR ASSOCIATED LIFESTYLE FACTORS THAT RESULT IN LOWER RISK FOR CORONARY HEART DISEASE?

Many lifestyle factors are associated with moderate drinking. In all epidemiologic studies, socioeconomic factors are strongly and inversely related to the risk of CHD; better-educated individuals and those with higher income show lower rates of CHD (and most other diseases), presumably because of their more moderate lifestyles. The extent to which residual confounding by such factors may explain the health-protective effects of moderate drinking shown in observational studies has provoked considerable debate.

As a follow-up to concerns from earlier work by Shaper and colleagues,[43] Fillmore and coworkers[44] have described apparent "errors" in prospective studies that call into question their conclusions about an inverse association between alcohol and CHD. One of their arguments is that exposure measures may not be as accurate in prospective cohort studies as in case-control studies, a point not supported by most epidemiologists. In general, there is greater possibility of misclassification of exposure in case-control studies than in follow-up studies, as the former may "introduce a number of subtleties and avenues for bias that are absent in typical cohort studies."[45]

The choice of the referent group in an epidemiologic study is important, and the nondrinker category should not mix ex–heavy drinkers (who usually have higher risks for many diseases) with lifetime abstainers. In a population in which abstinence is rare, choosing very light or occasional drinkers as the referent group may be preferable. A key criticism of existing observational studies of alcohol and CHD relates to the inclusion in some of ex-drinkers in the nondrinking category.[44] This is indeed an important problem, but many recent reports have limited the referent, nondrinking group to lifetime abstainers, and the inverse association between moderate drinking and CHD remains, as described by Rimm and Moats[10] and others.[46]

An approach for dealing with potential residual confounding by social class is to limit analyses to subjects who are very similar in socioeconomic terms, as has been done for nurses,[47] health professionals,[48] and business executives.[49] In each of these groups of subjects, moderate drinking was associated with lower CHD risk. Lee and coworkers[50] evaluated a large variety of measures of lifestyle in seeking to determine if the lower total mortality risk in moderate drinkers is due to the alcohol itself or to associated healthy lifestyle factors. Adjusting for a large number of such factors and using sophisticated analytic techniques, the authors found that moderate drinking (versus not drinking) was still associated with a 38% lower mortality risk.[50] Friesema and colleagues[51] reviewed these relations among subjects in a prospective case-cohort, the Lifestyle and Health Study, consisting of 16,210 men and women between 45 and 70 years of age. The authors concluded that the difference in lifestyle between moderate drinkers and both never drinkers and former drinkers was only a partial explanation of the observed inverse relationships between alcohol intake and CVD and all-cause mortality.[51]

Poikolainen and associates[52] evaluated the effects of a large number of lifestyle factors that were considered to increase the risk of CHD; these included hypertension, increased body mass index (BMI), diabetes, depression, sleep disturbances, smoking, physical inactivity, poor life satisfaction, psychological distress, trait anxiety, independent and dependent life events, longer length of working hours, low levels of job control, job strain, and effort-reward imbalance. Most of these conditions were either the same between lifetime abstainers and light to moderate drinkers or more common among drinkers than among abstainers. Thus, these authors concluded that none of the large number of lifestyle factors evaluated is likely to be the reason that abstainers have higher rates of CHD, which supports the theory that it is the alcohol that is associated with less disease.[52]

Rimm[10] summarized the research data on this topic by stating that results from mechanistic studies provide substantial support for the hypothesis that moderate alcohol intake reduces the risk of CHD and that all beverages containing alcohol have shown beneficial effects. He concluded, "The 'sick-quitter' hypothesis and the concern that moderate drinkers lead a healthier lifestyle may explain a small proportion of the benefit attributed to alcohol in some studies, but recent studies which have removed sick quitters, updated alcohol and covariate information on diet and lifestyle factors, and separately documented benefits of alcohol among healthy and unhealthy populations further add to the evidence that moderate alcohol consumption is causally related to a lower risk of CHD."[10] Sorensen and coworkers[53] stated that because alcohol consumption is so common in most Western cultures, it would be exceedingly difficult to carry out a sufficient number of randomized controlled trials to evaluate adequately the effects of alcohol on CVD outcomes. They pointed out that medical decisions must often be made on the basis of observational studies.[53]

EFFECTS OF ALCOHOL ON SUBJECTS ALREADY DIAGNOSED WITH CORONARY HEART DISEASE

Janszky and coworkers[54] reported results from serial quantitative coronary angiography studies done among middle-aged

BOX 18-1 Mechanisms of Effect of Alcohol and Polyphenols on Cardiovascular Disease

- Improvement of blood lipids (marked increase in HDL, slight decrease in LDL)
- Improvement of coagulation, fibrinolysis
- Improvement of endothelial function
- Activation of genes for fibrinolysis, eNOS
- Improvement of ventricular function
- Reduction of inflammation
- Improvement of glucose metabolism
- Adverse effects on blood pressure, especially for heavier drinking

women at 3 to 6 months and at 3 years after an acute myocardial infarction. They found that moderate alcohol consumption (more than 5 g/day) was protective of coronary atherosclerosis progression. Furthermore, restenosis after stenting has been found to be lower in patients with CHD who continue to consume alcohol.[55] The risk of complications (including death) after an acute myocardial infarction has been shown to be lower for subjects who remain drinkers than for those who abstain.[56,57] Such a protective effect seems to be lost when the subject consumes alcohol as binge-drinking.[13]

BIOLOGIC MECHANISMS FOR CARDIOVASCULAR EFFECTS

Box 18-1 lists some of the key mechanisms by which moderate alcohol consumption, as well as the intake of polyphenols in red wine and other beverages, may lead to a reduction in the risk of CHD and other types of CVD.

Lipids

The first recognized mechanism by which alcohol may prevent CVD relates to induced changes in plasma lipid profile, especially increases in high-density lipoprotein cholesterol (HDL-C) and its subtypes (HDL$_2$, HDL$_3$).[58-61] Numerous observational and experimental studies have confirmed a strong, direct association between alcohol intake and HDL.[8,62,63] Although it was initially believed that only certain HDL subtypes were increased by alcohol (and that those had little effect on CVD risk), alcohol intake has been shown to increase both HDL$_2$ and HDL$_3$, and both play a role in CVD prevention.[64-66] In addition, most studies also show slightly lower LDL concentrations, especially small-particle LDL, and non-HDL lipoprotein levels among moderate drinkers.[67-70] Oxidation of lipids has been shown to be decreased by alcohol or polyphenols in many studies[71-75] but not in all.[76]

Platelet Aggregation and Thrombosis

As described by Booyse and colleagues,[77] other changes in vascular, myocardial, hemostatic, and endothelial cell functions may be equally important in collectively contributing to the reduction of the risk of CVD. These factors appear to result from alcohol, from polyphenols present in some beverages (especially wine), or from a combination of both, resulting in reduced thrombosis.[78]

The early studies of Serge Renaud and his colleagues pointed out the importance of platelet function in the development of atherosclerosis, thrombosis, and CHD.[79] In an

intervention study in humans, Zhang and coworkers[80] showed that alcohol, at physiologically relevant doses, has a dose-dependent inhibitory effect on platelet aggregation. These authors concluded that their findings are consistent with the view that alcohol reduces platelet sensitivity to thrombotic stimuli by inhibition of arachidonic acid release and therefore subsequent thromboxane synthesis. Inhibition of platelet aggregation or function has also been shown by others.[81,82] Ruf[83] suggested that wine has a greater effect on platelet function than alcohol alone does, stating that the polyphenols in wine provide further reduction in prostanoid synthesis from arachidonate and also decrease platelet activity mediated by nitric oxide. Demrow and colleagues[84] demonstrated that polyphenols from both red wine and grape juice favorably affect platelet aggregation.

Many of the effects of alcohol and polyphenols on coagulation are transient effects, and the beneficial effects may last only 24 to 36 hours after someone has consumed alcohol. Furthermore, after heavy alcohol intake, there may be a rebound with increased platelet aggregation if further alcohol is not consumed,[83,85,86] although such rebound may be less after drinking wine than after consuming other beverages.[83] One explanation for the much lower CHD rates in France than in most other countries is that the French have traditionally consumed some alcohol (primarily red wine) with their evening meal every day. Thus, their clotting mechanisms remain in a favorable state all of the time. Unfortunately, many Americans and northern Europeans tend to drink only on the weekend, often consuming a large number of drinks rapidly, a very unhealthy way to drink.

Other Mechanisms

Additional mechanisms for protection of alcohol and polyphenols against CHD and myocardial infarction include decreased myocardial ischemia-reperfusion injury,[87,88] increased endothelial cell–dependent vasorelaxation,[89-92] simultaneous activation of endothelial cell antiapoptotic and proapoptotic pathways,[93] decreased plasma levels of factor VII[94] and fibrinogen,[95] increased fibrinolysis[96-102] and upregulation of fibrinolytic protein gene transcription in cultured human endothelial cells,[103,104] and increased levels of atrial natriuretic peptide.[105]

There is also strong experimental evidence for additional mechanisms by which alcohol and wine polyphenols affect the initiation or progression of atherosclerotic lesions. These include reduced LDL oxidation and aggregation, foam cell formation, and lesion progression[106,107]; inhibition of endothelin 1 synthesis[108]; downregulation of tissue factor gene transcription in cultured human endothelial cells and monocytes[109,110]; and inhibition of smooth muscle cell proliferation.[111,112] Research studies increasingly show a strong protective effect from alcohol and polyphenols against various indices of inflammation.[113,114] Wang and colleagues[115] have shown a U-shaped association between alcohol and high-sensitivity C-reactive protein (hsCRP) levels; a proportional odds model analysis showed an odds ratio for increased hsCRP of 0.32 (95% CI, 0.14-0.74) for consumers of 20 to 70 g/day (about 1½ to almost 6 drinks) in comparison with nondrinkers. Alpert and coworkers[116] found that CRP was lowest in consumers of 5 to 7 drinks/week.

Booyse and coworkers[102] have demonstrated the sequence of molecular events by which endothelial cell expression of tissue plasminogen activator is increased through common activation of p38 MAPK signaling by alcohol as well as by certain wine polyphenols. Gorelik and associates[42] have shown that red wine polyphenols lower levels of postprandial cytotoxic lipid peroxidation products (malondialdehyde) in humans, another possible mechanism for the benefits of the consumption of wine on risk of disease.

In some epidemiologic studies, the combined beneficial effect of alcohol on HDL-C, fibrinogen, and hemoglobin A1c (the last a marker of glycemic control and insulin resistance) can almost entirely explain the reduced CHD risk among moderate drinkers.[95,117]

Hypertension

One cardiovascular risk factor that is generally not associated favorably with alcohol consumption is hypertension, and most studies show an elevation of blood pressure with increasing alcohol intake.[118,119] Some studies[120-122] show that the effect is mainly from heavier drinking and that light alcohol intake has no effect or even a slight lowering of blood pressure. For example, Klatsky and associates[121] found increases in blood pressure only among subjects reporting three or more drinks per day, a finding similar to the association in all groups except African American men in an ARIC report.[119] In the Luebeck Blood Pressure Study in Germany, Keil and associates[123] reported increases in blood pressure for men consuming more than 40 g of alcohol per day (more than three typical drinks) or women reporting more than 20 g/day. Klatsky and associates[124] have shown that hypertension remains a strong risk factor for CVD regardless of alcohol intake, and hypertensives who are heavy drinkers show a substantial decrease in blood pressure when they decrease their intake.[125] Whereas a direct association between alcohol and blood pressure has been confirmed in most studies, important sequelae of hypertension (notably CHD and ischemic stroke) show an inverse association with moderate drinking.

Genetic Risk Factors

There is no question that individuals differ markedly in their response to alcohol consumption, for its beneficial and adverse health effects. Davey Smith[126] has described how "mendelian randomization—the random assortment of genes from parents to offspring that occurs during gamete formation and conception—provides one method for assessing the causal nature of some environmental exposures." Such an approach avoids many of the problems of confounding in observational studies. He concluded that "mendelian randomization provides new opportunities to test causality and demonstrates how investment in the human genome project may contribute to understanding and preventing the adverse effects on human health of modifiable exposures."

At present, however, the association of genes with CHD is poorly understood. The most studied individual genes are those that relate to the metabolism of alcohol, especially those that control alcohol dehydrogenase (ADH) and acetaldehyde dehydrogenase (ALDH). Hines and coworkers[127] showed that moderate drinkers who are homozygous for the slow-oxidizing ADH3 allele had higher HDL levels and a substantially decreased risk of myocardial infarction.[128] However, other studies have failed to show such an association.[129] Jensen and coworkers[130] have found conflicting results across different cohorts in their study relating lipoprotein lipase to CHD.

Current data suggest that there are many genes contributing to the effects of alcohol on the risk of CHD; each tends to play only a small role by itself but a potentially large role in combination with other genes and environmental factors. Furthermore, certain genes seem much more important in certain ethnic groups and cultures than in others. The large number of collaborative genome-wide association studies now being done, with huge numbers of subjects, should help clarify the role that genetic factors play in the potential protection against cardiovascular and other diseases from alcohol use.

Similarly, for cancer, data on genetic factors modifying alcohol's effects are unclear. Druesne-Pecollo and coworkers[131] published an overview of studies on the combined effects of alcohol drinking and polymorphisms in genes for ADH, ALDH, cytochrome P-450 2E1, and methylenetetrahydrofolate reductase on the risk of alcohol-related cancer. They concluded that current data lend support to a role of polymorphisms *ADH1B* and *ALDH2* combined with alcohol consumption in cancer, but other available data are insufficient or inconclusive.

Summary of Mechanisms

Collins and associates[132] have provided a summary of epidemiologic and mechanistic studies demonstrating how alcohol and polyphenols may be cardioprotective (as well as neuroprotective). In Figure 18-2, mechanisms of cardioprotection by both alcohol and resveratrol, one of the polyphenols in red wine that has been studied extensively, are illustrated.

Clinical trials in humans are limited, but Leighton and colleagues[133] have carried out a number of intervention studies looking at the effects of wine on CVD risk factors. Their results show that moderate wine consumption may result in an increase in HDL-C, a decrease in the omega-6/omega-3 ratio, and in some cases a slight increase in triglyceride levels. Observed changes in hemostasis include reduced coagulation and increased fibrinolysis; effects on blood pressure have been inconsistent. They have found a reduction in inflammatory markers and an improvement in endothelial function. These investigators concluded that limitation of consumption to below 30 g of alcohol daily (about 2½ typical U.S. drinks) for men and half that dose for women is necessary to prevent negative changes in cardiovascular risk factors such as hypertension, hypertriglyceridemia, and hyperhomocysteinemia. Other clinical trials have demonstrated improvements in glucose metabolism from the administration of alcohol.[67,134,135] In the future, more such trials as well as genetic studies will help determine the extent to which the beneficial effects of alcohol consumption on CVD risk seen in most observational studies are caused by the alcoholic beverage itself.

EFFECTS OF ALCOHOL ON OTHER TYPES OF CARDIOVASCULAR DISEASE

The third leading cause of death in the United States, and the leading cause of disability, is stroke. It has been shown in many studies that the risk of stroke related to ischemia (atherosclerosis), which is the type of stroke in about 80% of cases in the United States, is reduced by moderate drinking.[136,137] Moreover, Klatsky and associates[138] found that an increase in risk of hemorrhagic stroke from alcohol is seen only in subjects consuming five or more drinks per day. Others have shown that the risk of peripheral artery disease is reduced among moderate drinkers.[139]

For two other cardiovascular conditions, atrial fibrillation and heart failure, recent scientific evidence suggests a lack of harmful effects from moderate alcohol consumption. Ettinger and colleagues[140] described the "holiday heart syndrome" in 1978. This syndrome often includes atrial fibrillation; the syndrome is usually not associated with long-standing heart disease and tends to resolve when alcohol consumption is ceased.[141,142] Nissen and Lemberg[143] stated that even moderate drinking can lead to this syndrome, but others[144,145] have found no effect on the risk of atrial fibrillation for moderate alcohol intake, only for heavy drinking. A recent extensive review of experimental, clinical, and epidemiologic data did not find evidence that alcohol is a factor, certainly not a major factor, in the development of atrial fibrillation.[146]

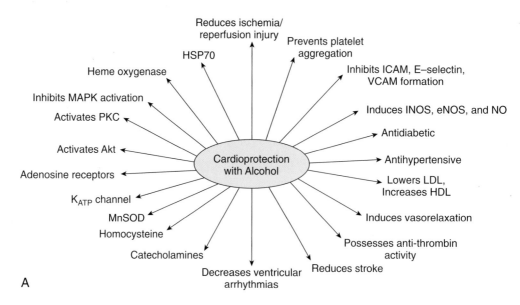

A

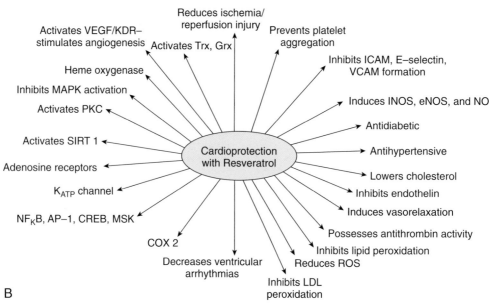

B

FIGURE 18-2 Cardioprotection from alcohol and from resveratrol. **A,** Cardioprotective and molecular targets of alcohol. Cardioprotective targets are shown on the right; the molecular targets are shown on the left. **B,** Cardioprotective and molecular targets of resveratrol. Cardioprotective targets are shown on the right; the molecular targets are shown on the left. *(From Collins MA, Neafsey EJ, Mukamal KJ, et al: Alcohol in moderation, cardioprotection, and neuroprotection: epidemiological considerations and mechanistic studies. Alcohol Clin Exp Res 33:206, 2009. Reprinted with permission.)*

It is known that excessive alcohol intake can result in alcoholic cardiomyopathy, causing heart failure. It was previously believed that heart failure, in general, would be made worse by any alcohol consumption. As reviewed by Djousse and Gaziano,[147] however, most studies have shown that moderate drinkers are at lower risk for development of heart failure.[148-153] For example, in a population of more than 100,000 subjects, Klatsky and associates[151] found that alcohol drinking was inversely related to risk of heart failure related to CHD (e.g., at one or two drinks per day; RR, 0.6; 95% CI, 0.5-0.7), with consistency across subgroups of age, gender, ethnicity, education, smoking status, interval to diagnosis, and presence or absence of baseline heart disease or systemic hypertension. For heart failure not associated with coronary disease, moderate drinking was inversely related only in subjects who had diabetes mellitus.[151]

For patients who already have depressed myocardial function, Cooper and associates[154] showed in the Studies of Left Ventricular Dysfunction (SOLVD) that moderate drinkers had lower subsequent all-cause mortality than abstainers did. In contrast, in the Survival And Ventricular Enlargement (SAVE) trial in subjects after myocardial infarction, Aguilar and coworkers[155] did not show a significant effect of moderate drinking on the development of heart failure or on survival.

EFFECTS OF ALCOHOL ON DIABETES AND METABOLIC SYNDROME

A major risk factor for the development of CVD not discussed before relates to glucose metabolism, especially the development of diabetes or the metabolic syndrome. Not only do data support lower risk for development of these conditions, but for persons with diabetes or the metabolic syndrome, moderate drinking may lower their subsequent risk of CVD.

Development of Diabetes

Stampfer and colleagues[156] reported in 1988 that moderate drinkers in the Nurses' Health Study had a lower risk for development of diabetes than did abstainers; compared with nondrinkers, women consuming 5 to 14.9 g of alcohol per day had an age-adjusted relative risk of diabetes of 0.4 (95% CI, 0.3-0.6); for 15 g or more per day, the relative risk was 0.3 (95% CI, 0.2-0.4). The authors reported that a strong inverse association between alcohol drinking and body weight explained much of the apparent protective effect of alcohol. After simultaneous adjustment for Quetelet index (weight [kg]/height [m]^2), family history of diabetes, total calorie intake, and age, the relative risk of diabetes for consumers of 5 to 14.9 g/day was 0.8 (95% CI, 0.6-1.2), and for women who drank 15+ g/day, the relative risk was 0.6 (95% CI, 0.3-0.9). Reports in the *British Medical Journal* in 1995 from two large prospective studies[157,158] similarly showed a lower risk of diabetes among moderate drinkers. Since then, many epidemiologic studies[159-161] have presented data supporting such an inverse association. Howard and coworkers[162] have provided a good summary of the research on alcohol and diabetes, giving an estimate of 33% to 56% lower incidence of diabetes for consumers of one to three drinks per day. A meta-analysis by Koppes and associates[163] indicated that for a wide range of alcohol intake (from about ½ to more than 3 drinks/day), the relative risk of diabetes for drinkers is about 30% lower than it is for abstainers.

Mechanisms are unclear for the effects of alcohol intake on diabetes. Some studies have shown lower glucose levels and HbA1c.[164] In an intervention trial, Davies and coworkers[165] found among nondiabetic postmenopausal women that the consumption of 30 g/day of alcohol reduced fasting insulin concentration by 19.2%, reduced triglyceride concentration by 10.3%, and increased insulin sensitivity by 7.2% but did not affect plasma glucose levels. Kroenke and associates[166] found that HbA1c was inversely associated with alcohol intake; among overweight women, there was also an inverse association with insulin. Specifically, these investigators found that insulin levels were lowest for drinkers consuming no more than two drinks per day up to three days per week. In a large heterogeneous group of nondiabetic subjects, insulin sensitivity was lower among abstainers than in all categories of drinkers.[167] Adiponectin serum levels were higher in men consuming alcohol on 2+ days/week than in nondrinkers or occasional drinkers; among women, those consuming all levels of alcohol had higher adiponectin concentrations than nondrinkers did.[167]

There have also been a number of clinical trials relating alcohol intake to diabetic mechanisms. Sierksma and coworkers[134] carried out a randomized crossover study of 23 healthy middle-aged men who were given 40 g of ethanol (four glasses of whiskey, versus no alcohol) on a daily basis for 17 days. They found that alcohol increased plasma adiponectin levels by 11% and increased the insulin sensitivity index in an insulin-resistant subgroup by 21%. A randomized crossover trial by Joosten and coworkers[67] showed that moderate alcohol consumption increased insulin sensitivity and *ADIPOQ* expression in postmenopausal women.

Shai and colleagues[135] carried out a randomized trial among 91 formerly abstaining diabetics who were randomly assigned to consume 5 ounces of either sauvignon blanc or merlot at dinner every evening or advised to continue to avoid alcohol. Significantly lower levels of fasting blood glucose concentration during a 3-month intervention period were seen among subjects consuming wine than were seen

for abstainers. The effect of the wine was variable, with beneficial effects primarily among those with more severe disease.

Effects of Alcohol Intake on Cardiovascular Disease Among Diabetics

Valmadrid and coworkers[168] reported that among persons with older-onset diabetes, the relative risk for death from CHD was 0.44 for subjects consuming 2 to 13 g/day and 0.21 for those consuming 14+ g/day, in comparison with nondrinkers. Solomon and colleagues[169] reported from the Nurses' Health Study that the risk for development of CHD among type 2 diabetics who were moderate drinkers was much lower than that for nondrinking diabetic subjects: for <½ drink daily, the relative risk was 0.72, and for ≥½ drink daily, the relative risk was 0.45. In the Physicians' Health Study, increasing levels of alcohol intake were associated with even greater reduction in deaths from CHD among diabetics than among nondiabetic subjects.[170]

A meta-analysis by Koppes and associates[171] indicates that the risk of CHD is 34% to 55% lower among diabetics who are moderate drinkers than in those who consume no alcohol. Among more than 38,000 diabetics observed by the Kaiser Permanente group in California, those who consumed alcohol had evidence of considerably better control of their diabetes than did nondrinkers[172]; the authors concluded that this finding "supports current clinical guidelines for moderate levels of alcohol consumption among diabetes patients."

Alcohol has been shown to affect not only the macrovascular sequelae of diabetes but also the microvascular complications of diabetes. In a report from the EURODIAB Prospective Complications Study, involving the follow-up of 3250 type 1 diabetic patients from 16 different European countries, Beulens and colleagues[173] found a lower occurrence of retinopathy, neuropathy, and nephropathy among those individuals who consumed alcohol moderately in comparison with nondrinkers. The association was strongest among wine drinkers, and to some extent among beer drinkers, but was not seen among those consuming spirits.

In summary, evidence from a large number of prospective epidemiologic studies and limited clinical trials strongly suggests that moderate drinkers are less likely to develop diabetes and its sequelae, especially CHD. Although not all of the mechanisms are known, many studies suggest improved insulin resistance or increased adiponectin levels.

Development of Metabolic Syndrome

The findings relating alcohol to metabolic syndrome show associations with alcohol similar to those for diabetes. In the NHLBI Family Heart Study[174] and in NHANES III,[175] we found evidence that moderate drinking is associated with lower risk of most components of the metabolic syndrome (all components except for hypertension). Fan and coworkers[176] evaluated the association between estimates of lifetime alcohol intake and the metabolic syndrome. They found that subjects who averaged more than one drink per day for women or two drinks per day for men had an increase in their prevalence ratio for metabolic syndrome in comparison with drinkers who did not exceed these limits; nondrinkers were not included in these analyses. In a meta-analysis on alcohol intake and metabolic syndrome, based on data from seven previous studies with a total of 22,000 subjects, Alkerwi and coworkers[177] found that the moderate intake of alcohol (defined as ≤40 g of alcohol per day for men and ≤20 g of alcohol per day for women) was associated with 16% lower risk of metabolic syndrome for men and 25% lower risk for women; no significant effects were seen for heavier drinking.[177]

ALCOHOL AS A COMPONENT OF A HEALTHY LIFESTYLE

18

Alcohol consumption, moderate or otherwise, should not be viewed in isolation but as part of broader social, cultural, and lifestyle issues. We now have good scientific data on which to base our definition of what constitutes a "healthy" diet and lifestyle. The Nurses' Health Study, the Health Professionals Study, and other research have defined a lifestyle that will lead to >70% fewer myocardial infarctions and >90% fewer cases of diabetes. This healthy lifestyle is shown in Box 18-2, based on research by Stampfer,[178] Hu,[179] Mukamal,[11] and others.

Akesson and colleagues,[180] in a large prospective study among middle-aged and older women in Sweden, found that those subjects who met all five components of a healthy lifestyle (defined as following what can be described as a Mediterranean-type diet, not smoking, not being obese, getting regular exercise, and consuming at least 5 g/day of alcohol) had a dramatically reduced risk of having a myocardial infarction. The authors suggested that if all women in their population had such a lifestyle, there would have been 77% fewer cases of CHD.

Khaw and associates,[181] in a large prospective observational study from the United Kingdom, assessed the effects on mortality of four "healthy behaviors": not smoking, being active, having evidence of a high fruit and vegetable intake, and consuming some alcohol but not more than 14 drinks per week (about 9½ typical drinks by U.S. standards). Increasing numbers of these behaviors were associated with lower risk of death from all causes as well as from CVD, cancer, and noncardiovascular causes. The authors calculated that the effect of these four healthy behaviors on total mortality, compared with none of them, is equivalent to a 14-year age difference in mortality risk.

Whereas some suggest that we should focus on the first four components of the healthy lifestyle and not be eager to encourage alcohol use, it has been shown that even among very healthy subjects (i.e., who are lean, eat a healthy diet, are active, and do not smoke), those who also consume a little alcohol have much lower risk of heart disease and death. To address the issue of residual confounding by healthy lifestyle among drinkers, Mukamal and coworkers[182] restricted analyses to 8867 healthy men in the Health Professionals Study who adhered to the first four low-risk behaviors (not including alcohol) and examined the association for alcohol consumption with CHD. In this group of "very healthy" men, there were still 106 incident CHD cases; the men who drank moderately (15.0 to 29.9 g/day) had a relative risk of 0.38 (95% CI, 0.16-0.89) compared with abstainers. This strong inverse association between moderate alcohol consumption and CHD in predominantly healthy individuals adds further evidence to support the hypothesis that the inverse association is causal and not confounded by healthy lifestyle behaviors.[10] On the other hand, a paper with a restrictive definition of "healthy" reported no significant effects of alcohol on risk of CHD among the healthiest subjects.[183]

EFFECTS OF ALCOHOL ON NONCARDIOVASCULAR DISEASES

Before the encouragement of moderate drinking for the possible reduction in the risk of CVD is even considered, the potential effects on other diseases must be taken into account. In addition to CVD, it has long been known that moderate drinkers are at lower risk of gallstones.[184] There are interesting new data relating alcohol intake to obesity, bone mineral density, and dementia. As will be discussed, an increase in the risk of breast cancer from alcohol is of great concern for women, but recent data indicate a lower risk from moderate alcohol intake for certain other cancers.[185-187]

Obesity

An unexpected finding in epidemiologic studies is that obesity is often found to be less common among moderate drinkers than among abstainers. In the prospective Nurses' Health Study,[188] it was found that light to moderate drinking was not associated with weight gain in women (overall, a 16% lower risk for those reporting 15.0 to 29.9 g of alcohol per day versus abstainers). This potentially beneficial effect on weight gain was not seen in African American women or in heavier drinkers. Arif and Rohrer[189] evaluated alcohol intake and BMI among 8236 nonsmoking respondents who participated in the Third National Health and Nutrition Examination Survey. Current drinkers who reported drinking one drink or two drinks per day had 0.46 (95% CI, 0.34-0.62) and 0.59 (95% CI, 0.41-0.86) the odds of obesity, respectively, than did abstainers.

Tolstrup and colleagues[190] found that among men, the odds ratios for having a high BMI among subjects drinking 1 to 3 days/month, 1 day/week, 2 to 4 days/week, 5 or 6 days/week, and 7 days/week were 1.39 (95% CI, 1.36-1.64), 1.17 (1.02-1.34), 1.00 (reference), 0.87 (0.77-0.98), and 0.73 (0.65-0.82), respectively. Similar associations were found for waist circumference, and corresponding results were found for women. These authors concluded that for a given level of total alcohol intake, obesity was inversely associated with drinking frequency, whereas the amount of alcohol intake was positively associated with obesity. Such an association was supported by Breslow and Smothers[191] among 45,896 never-smoking adults in the 1997-2001 National Health Interview Surveys in the United States. As shown in Figure 18-3, from that study, more frequent drinking was associated with lower BMI. On the other hand, given drinking of a certain frequency, the number of drinks per drinking day was directly associated with BMI.

These results suggest that the frequent consumption of small amounts of alcohol is the optimal drinking pattern associated with a lower risk of obesity.

Bone Mineral Density and Hip Fracture

A number of epidemiologic studies have shown that moderate drinkers have less osteoporosis and a lower risk of hip fractures than do abstainers.[192] (This goes against "conventional wisdom," which has always assumed that elderly who drink alcohol may be more unsteady on their feet and at increased risk of falling and sustaining fractures.) Mukamal

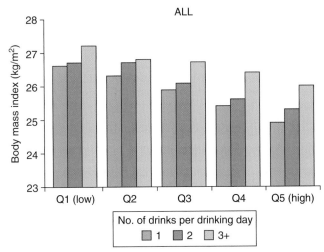

ALL

FIGURE 18-3 Alcohol consumption and BMI by frequency of drinking quintiles and quantity of alcohol. Association between alcohol consumption and BMI in stratified analyses of frequency quintiles within quantity categories, National Health Interview Surveys, 1997-2001. Q, quintile. *(From Breslow RA, Smothers BA: Drinking patterns and body mass index in never smokers: National Health Interview Survey, 1997-2001. Am J Epidemiol 161:368, 2005. Reprinted with permission.)*

and colleagues[193] found that among older adults, moderate alcohol consumption had a U-shaped relationship with risk of hip fracture but a graded positive relationship with bone mineral density at the hip. A meta-analysis by Berg and coworkers[194] involving the review of 33 previous studies supports a reduced risk of hip fracture and higher bone density among men and women who consume small to moderate amounts of alcohol (in comparison with nondrinkers). There is probably a J-shaped curve, with increased risk of fractures among heavier drinkers.

Dementia

Among the most exciting recent scientific findings are that moderate drinkers tend to be less likely to develop Alzheimer disease and other types of dementia. This was reported for wine drinkers in Bordeaux by Orgogozo and colleagues in 1997,[195] and Truelsen and coworkers[196] reported similar protection from wine in Denmark, as did Panza and coworkers[197] in a summary paper.

Britton and coworkers[198] reported from the Whitehall Study in the United Kingdom that there was less cognitive impairment in drinkers for tests of memory (borderline significant), verbal and mathematical reasoning, verbal meaning, and verbal fluency. For men, the risk of dysfunction was lower by about 40% to 50% for drinkers, with the lowest risk at >241 g/week of alcohol, the equivalent of about three drinks per day by U.S. standards. Women drinkers had lower point estimates for most measures, but statistically significant results were seen for verbal and mathematical reasoning (OR = 0.3; CI, 0.2 -0.6) and for verbal fluency (OR = 0.5; CI, 0.3-0.9), both at 49 to 80 g of alcohol per week (the equivalent of about four to seven drinks per week). Lifetime abstaining men and women generally had much greater risk of cognitive dysfunction than did occasional drinkers.

Espeland and colleagues[199] reported from the Women's Health Initiative Memory Study that compared with no intake, intake of one drink or more per day was associated with higher baseline Modified Mini-Mental State Examination scores (*P* < 0.001) and an odds ratio of 0.41 (95% CI, 0.23-0.74) for significant declines in cognitive function. Stampfer and coworkers[200] reported that among women who

were moderate drinkers, compared with nondrinkers, the relative risk of impairment was 0.77 for general cognition (95% CI, 0.67-0.88) and 0.81 on the global cognitive score (95% CI, 0.70-0.93). Zhang and coworkers[201] reported that education modifies the putative effects of alcohol on memory, with better results among those with higher education, probably because of more moderate drinking patterns.

Ganguli and colleagues[202] studied men and women aged 74.4 years at baseline who were observed during 7 years with repeated assessments of cognitive functioning; abstainers showed lower baseline scores and a tendency for more rapid deterioration in cognitive functioning than did drinkers. Solfrizzi and colleagues[203] also found less progression from mild cognitive impairment to dementia for light drinkers in comparison with nondrinkers.

Mehlig and coworkers,[204] in a well-done analysis from a long-term prospective study of women in Sweden, reported that the lifetime risk of dementia was associated differently with wine consumption (a decrease in risk of dementia of 70%) and spirits consumption (an increase in dementia risk of about 50%). The authors concluded that the different associations by type of beverage suggest that the nonalcohol components in wine may be an important factor in lowering the risk of dementia. Whereas the investigators adjusted for the usual risk factors for dementia, including education and social class, there is always the possibility that other lifestyle factors that are different between wine drinkers and spirits drinkers may have influenced the results.

Peters and associates[205] carried out a meta-analysis on alcohol and dementia and concluded that moderate drinkers, especially wine drinkers, were at lower risk than abstainers for development of Alzheimer disease or other dementia. The mechanism for such protection is not known but may relate, among other factors, to prevention of cerebral atherosclerosis or decreased inflammation in brain tissue. Collins and associates[132] have reported additional mechanisms for neuroprotection, as described earlier (under mechanisms of alcohol's effects on CVD).

ADVERSE HEALTH EFFECTS OF DRINKING: ALCOHOL AND CANCER

Most of the adverse health effects associated with alcohol are from drinking too much, too fast, or at an inappropriate time (as just before driving an automobile). Chronic heavy drinking can lead to a number of diseases that are often referred to as alcohol-related diseases, and these include alcoholic cardiomyopathy, cirrhosis of the liver, neurologic diseases, and certain cancers. Of particular concern, however, are some conditions that may relate to even moderate drinking, especially breast cancer in women.

Alcohol-Related Cancers

The strongest association between alcohol drinking and cancer is for upper aerodigestive cancers, usually with an increased risk for a combination of heavy drinking and smoking. Weikert and associates[206] reported that in comparison with drinkers averaging no more than 6 g of alcohol (about ½ drink) per day, squamous upper aerodigestive cancers were increased among both men and women reporting >30 g/day of alcohol (more than about 2½ drinks), with larger increases for heavier-drinking men. Allen and coworkers,[207] in a study based on more than one million women in the United Kingdom, found that for most cancers, the relative risk was lowest among women who reported up to two drinks per week (10 g of alcohol being considered a drink in this study) than among current abstainers, but this study was not able to separate ex-drinkers from lifetime abstainers. Among drinkers, the strongest positive association between increasing alcohol consumption and disease was for upper aerodigestive cancers (mouth, pharynx, esophagus), but this association was seen only among drinkers who were also smokers. In this study, lesser effects were noted for cancers of the rectum and colon.

Most studies show little effect of alcohol drinking on genitourinary tumors[185,208] and an apparent inverse association with renal cell carcinoma.[185,186] Furthermore, moderate drinkers seem to have lower risks of some types of leukemia[187] and non-Hodgkin and other lymphomas.[209,210] In their large study, Allen and coworkers[207] showed among drinkers that an increase in alcohol intake of 10 g/day was associated with lower risks of thyroid cancer (RR = 0.75; 95% CI, 0.61-0.92), renal cell cancer (RR = 0.88; 95% CI, 0.78-0.99), and non-Hodgkin lymphoma (RR = 0.87; 95% CI, 0.81-0.95). Other studies have shown that heavy drinking, but not moderate consumption, may increase the risk of pancreatic cancer.[211] A meta-analysis by Genkinger and colleagues[212] showed a slight positive association with pancreatic cancer risk for alcohol intake of 30 g/day (about 2½ typical drinks) or more versus no alcohol (pooled multivariate relative risk, 1.22; 95% CI, 1.03-1.45).

In an editorial on the association of alcohol intake with Barrett esophagus and esophageal adenocarcinoma, El Serag and Lagergren[213] described three population-based studies that demonstrated no overall effect of alcohol intake on either disease. Instead, these studies showed that the modest intake of wine, but not of other beverages, was associated with a significantly lower risk for both conditions.

Alcohol and Breast Cancer

Particular attention has been focused on the association between alcohol intake and the risk of breast cancer in women. The majority of epidemiologic studies support the findings of Willett and coworkers[214] in 1987 and Longnecker[215] in 1994: breast cancer risk is greater for women who consume alcohol than for abstainers. A notable exception is the Framingham Study, in which the long-term risk of breast cancer was not increased among drinkers in comparison with nondrinkers during a follow-up period of several decades.[216,217] An initial report from the Women's Health Initiative–Observational Study (WHI-OS)[218] describes a slight non–dose-dependent increase in risk of breast cancer for consumers of alcohol. In comparison with no alcohol, the adjusted relative risk for up to 5 g of alcohol per day (less than ½ drink) was 1.10 (95% CI, 0.97-1.24); for 5 to 15 g/day, the relative risk was 1.14 (95% CI, 0.99-1.31); and for >15 g/day, it was 1.13 (95% CI, 0.96-1.32).

In meta-analyses, the estimated increase in risk of breast cancer for the average consumption of one drink per day is usually between 6% and 15%. Stronger associations appear to be more common in hospital-based case-control studies than in cohort studies or community-based case-control studies, in studies published before 1990 than in studies published later, in studies with shorter follow-up periods, and in studies conducted outside of the United States than in U.S. studies.[219]

Some studies show that the increase in risk of breast cancer among women who drink alcohol may be prevented or ameliorated if the women are consuming adequate amounts of folate in the diet,[220,221] but this has not been supported by certain other studies.[218,222] In the WHI-OS, there was no effect of folate intake on the association between alcohol and breast cancer.[218] Other epidemiologic research suggests an increase in breast cancer risk from alcohol intake only among women who are also taking hormone replacement therapy[223,224] or those who binge drink.[225]

Small amounts of alcohol are associated with a larger effect on the risk of CVD and other diseases of aging that are much more common causes of death; CHD deaths are nine times more frequent than breast cancer deaths, and stroke is three or four times more common. Hence, even for a slight increase in the risk of breast cancer for alcohol intake, on average a postmenopausal woman who stops any alcohol intake in an attempt to lower her risk of breast cancer may be increasing her risk of other diseases, and the net effect may be a shorter life span. In any case, advice about alcohol consumption for a postmenopausal woman with strong cardiovascular risk factors will be different from that for a young woman with no cardiovascular risk factors but a very strong family history of breast cancer.

ALCOHOL AND TOTAL MORTALITY

The bottom line is total mortality. Certain religious groups that limit the intake of meat and prohibit the use of alcohol and tobacco tend to have lower mortality rates. For the general population, alcoholics and binge drinkers do not live as long as abstainers, but regular, moderate drinkers live longer than abstainers. In a study of more than 270,000 men by the American Cancer Society,[226] the risk of dying of any cause was 16% lower for those reporting one drink per day than for abstainers. Thun and colleagues[227] evaluated alcohol and mortality among 490,000 Americans; all-cause mortality rates were 21% lower among men and women reporting about one drink daily than among nondrinkers. Doll[228] reported that British physicians who were moderate drinkers had lower total mortality rates than lifetime abstainers.

Di Castelnuovo and colleagues,[24] in a meta-analysis based on more than one million subjects from 56 independent prospective studies, found that the relation between alcohol intake and total mortality is J-shaped, with about 16% reduced risk for light drinkers and increased mortality for heavy drinkers, as shown in Figure 18-4. In the meta-analysis, differences were noted between men and women for the association between alcohol intake and mortality (Fig. 18-5).

As shown in Figure 18-5, the mortality risk for women drinkers exceeded that of nondrinkers at just more than 2 drinks per day, whereas the increase above that of abstainers for men was at about 3½ drinks per day.[24] In subanalyses, the relative risk of drinkers exceeded that of nondrinkers at about 30 g of alcohol per day (the equivalent of about 2½ drinks) in studies in the United States but only at about 65 g/day (or about 5 typical drinks) in studies in Europe. Whereas the reasons for this are not known, they may relate to differences in drinking practices, in that consuming alcohol on a regular basis and with meals is a usual pattern in much of Europe. Among women, the differences between studies in the United States and Europe were less marked.[24]

Contribution of Moderate Drinkers to Alcohol-Related Total Mortality

Some studies claim that moderate drinkers make a large contribution to deaths attributed to alcohol. In a summary of the association of alcohol consumption with mortality in Canada for 2002, Rehm and coworkers[14] showed that when moderate drinking was based on an average weekly consumption of 14 or fewer drinks for men or 7 or fewer drinks for women, the number of deaths "caused" by alcohol exceeded those "prevented" by alcohol, as shown in Figure 18-6A.

However, when subjects classified as moderate drinkers who reported episodes of binge drinking were excluded, there was a marked difference in the number of deaths attributed to alcohol, as shown in Figure 18-6B. Removal of binge drinkers from the moderate category lowered especially the

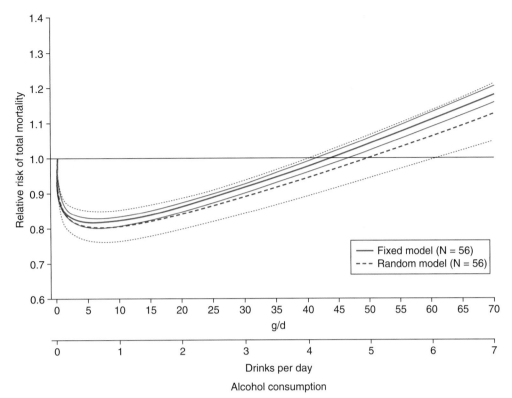

FIGURE 18-4 Alcohol intake and total mortality: a meta-analysis. Relative risk of total mortality (95% CIs) by alcohol intake, extracted from 56 curves using fixed- and random-effects models in a meta-analysis. *(From Di Castelnuovo A, Costanzo S, Bagnardi V, et al: Alcohol dosing and total mortality in men and women: an updated meta-analysis of 34 prospective studies.* Arch Intern Med *166:2437, 2006. Reprinted with permission.)*

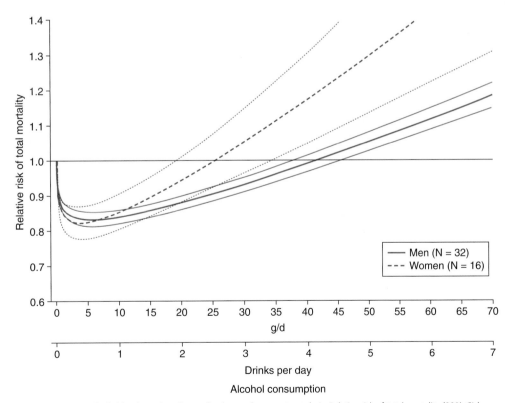

FIGURE 18-5 Alcohol intake and total mortality, by gender: a meta-analysis. Relative risk of total mortality (99% CIs) and alcohol intake in men and women in the United States, Europe, and other countries (Australia, Japan, and China), extracted from adjusted curves in a meta-analysis. *(From Di Castelnuovo A, Costanzo S, Bagnardi V, et al: Alcohol dosing and total mortality in men and women: an updated meta-analysis of 34 prospective studies.* Arch Intern Med *166:2437, 2006. Reprinted with permission.)*

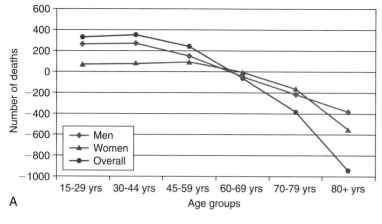

18

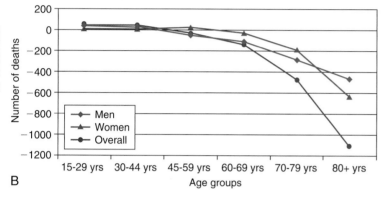

FIGURE 18-6 Number of net deaths attributable to moderate alcohol consumption. **A,** Number of net deaths in Canada in 2002 attributable to persons who reported alcohol intake, on average, placing them in the moderate drinking category, without consideration of binge drinking. Moderate drinking is defined as an average of <40 g/day for men and <20 g/day for women. **B,** Number of net deaths attributable to moderate drinkers who did not report any occasions of binge drinking (such drinkers were excluded from the analysis): sensitivity analysis. *(From Rehm J, Patra J, Taylor B: Harms, benefits, and net effects on mortality of moderate drinking of alcohol among adults in Canada in 2000, Ann Epidemiol 17:S81, 2007. Reprinted with permission.)*

number of excess deaths in younger people. Rehm and coworkers[14] concluded: "If moderate consumption is based on average volume alone, 866 net deaths in 2002 among those younger than 70 years of age were due to moderate consumption of alcohol (1.3% of all the deaths in this age group, consisting of 1653 deaths caused and 787 deaths prevented). When heavy drinking episodes were excluded, the net effect was beneficial (55 prevented deaths, 0.09% of all deaths); the net burden was higher for younger ages and the net benefits for older ages."

Differential Effects of Alcohol on Total Mortality According to Age

The diseases that tend to be "protected against" by moderate drinking occur later in life, among middle-aged and older adults.[14] There are few health benefits of drinking among the young (who, in any case, drink for the social effects of alcohol). Binge drinking, especially among the young, continues to be a serious public health problem around the world. In Germany, deaths caused by alcohol occurred primarily in young people (e.g., from accidents) or middle-aged adults (e.g., from cirrhosis), whereas most of the benefits on mortality were seen among the elderly.[229]

There are an increasing number of reports describing the associations of alcohol use over the life span with health and disease. Powers and Young[20] showed that middle-aged women in Australia who were moderate drinkers (who consumed the equivalent of up to about 10 typical U.S. drinks per week) had the best self-reported state of overall health. Furthermore, those who remained moderate drinkers throughout the study continued to have the highest rating of health and self-reported higher quality of life; those who stopped drinking during follow-up showed a decrease in their ratings of overall health.

ARE THERE DIFFERENCES IN EFFECT BY TYPE OF ALCOHOLIC BEVERAGE?

Most studies show beneficial effects of all types of alcoholic beverages—beer, wine, and spirits—on the risk of CHD and other diseases, but many show more favorable associations among wine drinkers.[230-233] Some studies have found wine drinkers to have a healthier diet overall than drinkers of beer or spirits, which may explain some of the putative additional beneficial effects of wine on health outcomes.[234-237] Still, even with adequate adjustment for diet and other lifestyle factors, many well-done observational studies (especially those among European populations) show significantly lower morbidity and mortality for wine drinkers than for consumers of other beverages. In the prospective ARIC study in the United States, King and associates[19] found that subjects initially reporting no alcohol intake who reported moderate drinking at a later examination had 38% lower risk for a cardiac event during the following 4 years; new wine drinkers had better health outcomes than did new drinkers of other beverages.

Streppel and colleagues[238] have reported that in a long-term follow-up study among men in the Netherlands (until death in most of the subjects), with repeated assessments of alcohol intake, moderate drinkers had lower rates of cardiovascular and all-cause mortality than did abstainers; mortality risks were lower for wine consumers than for consumers of other beverages. Analyses of survival after the age of 50 years from that study, by type of beverage, are shown in Figure 18-7.

As shown in Figure 18-7, the consumption of any type of alcohol (versus not drinking) was associated with somewhat greater survival after the age of 50 years. The median survival after the age of 50 years was several years greater for wine consumers than for nondrinkers and greater than for consumers of other beverages.[238]

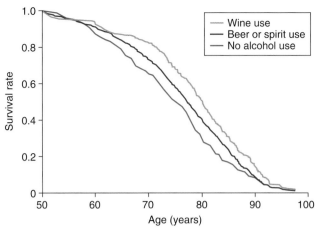

FIGURE 18-7 Survival after the age of 50 years according to long-term alcohol consumption. Survival curves for men with long-term consumption of alcohol from wine, beer, or spirits and for no alcohol consumers within the Zutphen Study. Adjusted for baseline energy intake without energy from alcohol; the number of cigarettes smoked; cigar or pipe smoking; intake of vegetables, fruit, fish, and saturated and *trans* fatty acids; body mass index; prevalence of myocardial infarction, stroke, cancer, and diabetes mellitus; and socioeconomic status. *(From Streppel MT, Ocke MC, Boshuizen HC, et al: Long-term wine consumption is related to cardiovascular mortality and life expectancy independently of moderate alcohol intake: the Zutphen Study.* J Epidemiol Community Health *63:534, 2009. Reprinted with permission.)*

In a large study in Finland among older men of a similar high socioeconomic class (business executives) who were observed during 29 years, those who stated that they preferred wine (rather than beer or spirits) had lower, fully adjusted mortality rates (especially for CVD) and a higher quality of life among survivors compared with subjects reporting the intake of other beverages.[49] These findings from epidemiologic studies are strongly supported by a vast amount of experimental evidence showing that many of the polyphenols in wine have beneficial effects on biologic and genetic mechanisms associated with the development of CHD and other diseases.

CONCLUSION

The scientific data from epidemiologic studies, basic science, and limited clinical trials support a role for moderate alcohol consumption in the prevention of CVD. At the same time, giving advice about alcohol intake must take into consideration that this substance can be a "double-edged sword."[239] We have long known that excesses (in habits, foods, or alcohol) have problems that are inherent not in the activities or substances themselves but in their inappropriate use. For example, in an address to a temperance society in 1842, Abraham Lincoln stated: "It has long been recognized that the problems with alcohol in this country relate not to the use of a bad thing, but to the abuse of a good thing."[240] There are no data showing than encouragement of moderate consumption increases abuse, but it is clear that advice about alcohol should vary according to the characteristics of the individual patient.

As described by Cole,[241] the finest moral rationale for prevention-oriented public health activity should be informing people, and it should not be based on "paternalism" ("we know what is best and will tell you only what you need to know"). We have had examples of sound scientific information relating alcohol intake to CHD that has been sacrificed to be "politically correct."[242]

There are certain people who should not drink at all (including former abusers of drugs or alcohol, people with certain medical conditions, children and adolescents, and people with religious or moral proscriptions against alcohol), and there can never be a general recommendation for everybody to consume alcohol. On the other hand, we should not withhold from our patients and the public scientifically sound and balanced data on alcohol and health. Whereas our current understanding suggests that moderate, sensible drinking can be potentially helpful for prevention of CHD in most adults (those without contraindications) as one component of a healthy lifestyle, any recommendations for its use in the individual should be based on consultation with the health care provider. Given the potential for misuse or abuse, however, major organizations such as the American Heart Association and the American College of Cardiology have not promoted or endorsed general recommendations aimed at the public at large.

REFERENCES

1. Klatsky AL, Friedman GD, Siegelaub AB: Alcohol consumption before myocardial infarction. Results from the Kaiser-Permanente epidemiologic study of myocardial infarction, Ann Intern Med 81:294, 1974.
2. Coate D: Moderate drinking and coronary heart disease mortality: evidence from NHANES I and the NHANES I Follow-up, Am J Public Health 83:888, 1993.
3. Kannel WB, Ellison RC: Alcohol and coronary heart disease: the evidence for a protective effect, Clin Chim Acta 246:59, 1996.
4. Doll R: One for the heart, BMJ 315:1664, 1997.
5. Corrao G, Rubbiati L, Bagnardi V, et al: Alcohol and coronary heart disease: a meta-analysis, Addiction 95:1505, 2000.
6. Lam TH, Chung SF, Janus ED, et al: Smoking, alcohol drinking and non-fatal coronary heart disease in Hong Kong Chinese, Ann Epidemiol 12:560, 2002.
7. Gronbaek M, Becker U, Johansen D et al: Type of alcohol consumed and mortality from all causes, coronary heart disease, and cancer, Ann Intern Med 133:411, 2000.
8. Foerster M, Marques-Vidal P, Gmel G, et al: Alcohol drinking and cardiovascular risk in a population with high mean alcohol consumption, Am J Cardiol 103:361, 2009.
9. Suhonen O, Aromaa A, Reunanen A, Knekt P: Alcohol consumption and sudden coronary death in middle-aged Finnish men, Acta Med Scand 221:335, 1987.
10. Rimm EB, Moats C: Alcohol and coronary heart disease: drinking patterns and mediators of effect, Ann Epidemiol 17:S3, 2007.
11. Mukamal KJ, Chiuve SE, Rimm EB: Alcohol consumption and risk for coronary heart disease in men with healthy lifestyles, Arch Intern Med 166:2145, 2006.
12. Tolstrup J, Gronbaek M: Alcohol and atherosclerosis: recent insights, Curr Atheroscler Rep 9:116, 2007.
13. Mukamal KJ, Maclure M, Muller JE, Mittleman MA: Binge drinking and mortality after acute myocardial infarction, Circulation 112:3839, 2005.
14. Rehm J, Patra J, Taylor B: Harms, benefits, and net effects on mortality of moderate drinking of alcohol among adults in Canada in 2000, Ann Epidemiol 17:S81, 2007.
15. Wannamethee SG, Shaper AG: Lifelong teetotallers, ex-drinkers and drinkers: mortality and the incidence of major coronary heart disease events in middle-aged British men, Int J Epidemiol 26:523, 1997.
16. Poikolainen K: It can be bad for the heart, too—drinking patterns and coronary heart disease, Addiction 93:1757, 1998.
17. Gronbaek M, Johansen D, Becker U, et al: Changes in alcohol intake and mortality: a longitudinal population-based study, Epidemiology 15:222, 2004.
18. Mukamal KJ, Conigrave KM, Mittleman MA, et al: Roles of drinking pattern and type of alcohol consumed in coronary heart disease in men, N Engl J Med 348:109, 2003.
19. King DE, Mainous AG, III, Geesey ME: Adopting moderate alcohol consumption in middle age: subsequent cardiovascular events, Am J Med 121:201, 2008.
20. Powers JR, Young AF: Longitudinal analysis of alcohol consumption and health of middle-aged women in Australia, Addiction 103:424, 2008.
21. Klatsky AL, Udaltsova N: Alcohol drinking and total mortality risk, Ann Epidemiol 17:S63, 2007.
22. Szabo G: Moderate drinking, inflammation, and liver disease, Ann Epidemiol 17:S49, 2007.
23. U.S. Department of Health and Human Services and U.S. Department of Agriculture: Dietary Guidelines for Americans, ed 6, Washington, DC, 2005, U.S. Government Printing Office.
24. Di Castelnuovo A, Costanzo S, Bagnardi V, et al: Alcohol dosing and total mortality in men and women: an updated meta-analysis of 34 prospective studies, Arch Intern Med 166:2437, 2006.
25. Byles J, Young A, Furuya H, Parkinson L: A drink to healthy aging: the association between older women's use of alcohol and their health-related quality of life, J Am Geriatr Soc 54:1341, 2006.
26. Mukamal KJ, Chung H, Jenny NS, et al: Alcohol consumption and risk of coronary heart disease in older adults: the Cardiovascular Health Study, J Am Geriatr Soc 54:30, 2006.
27. Eigenbrodt ML, Mosley TH, Jr, Hutchinson RG, et al: Alcohol consumption with age: a cross-sectional and longitudinal study of the Atherosclerosis Risk in Communities (ARIC) study, 1987-1995, Am J Epidemiol 153:1102, 2001.
28. Zhang Y, Guo X, Saitz R, et al: Secular trends in alcohol consumption over 50 years: the Framingham Study, Am J Med 121:695, 2008.

29. Lang I, Guralnik J, Wallace RB, Melzer D: What level of alcohol consumption is hazardous for older people? Functioning and mortality in U.S. and English national cohorts, *J Am Geriatr Soc* 55:49, 2007.

30. Kirchner JE, Zubritsky C, Cody M, et al: Alcohol consumption among older adults in primary care, *J Gen Intern Med* 22:92, 2007.

31. Tolvanen E, Seppa K, Lintonen T, et al: Old people, alcohol use and mortality. A ten-year prospective study, *Aging Clin Exp Res* 17:426, 2005.

32. Klatsky AL, Chartier D, Udaltsova N, et al: Alcohol drinking and risk of hospitalization for heart failure with and without associated coronary artery disease, *Am J Cardiol* 96:346, 2005.

33. Bazzano LA, Gu D, Reynolds K, et al: Alcohol consumption and risk of coronary heart disease among Chinese men, *Int J Cardiol* 135:78, 2009.

34. Sempos CT, Rehm J, Wu T, et al: Average volume of alcohol consumption and all-cause mortality in African Americans: the NHEFS cohort, *Alcohol Clin Exp Res* 27:88, 2003.

35. Freiberg MS, Chang YF, Kraemer KL, et al: Alcohol consumption, hypertension, and total mortality among women, *Am J Hypertens* 22:1212, 2009.

36. Tolstrup J, Jensen MK, Tjonneland A, et al: Prospective study of alcohol drinking patterns and coronary heart disease in women and men, *BMJ* 332:1244, 2006.

37. Bagnardi V, Zatonski W, Scotti L, et al: Does drinking pattern modify the effect of alcohol on the risk of coronary heart disease? Evidence from a meta-analysis, *J Epidemiol Community Health* 62:615, 2008.

38. Dorn JM, Hovey K, Williams BA, et al: Alcohol drinking pattern and non-fatal myocardial infarction in women, *Addiction* 102:730, 2007.

39. Tunstall-Pedoe H, Kuulasmaa K, Amouyel P, et al: Myocardial infarction and coronary deaths in the World Health Organization MONICA Project. Registration procedures, event rates, and case-fatality rates in 38 populations from 21 countries in four continents, *Circulation* 90:583, 1994.

40. Evans A, Marques-Vidal P, Ducimetiere P, et al: Patterns of alcohol consumption and cardiovascular risk in Northern Ireland and France, *Ann Epidemiol* 17:S75, 2007.

41. Stranges S, Wu T, Dorn JM, et al: Relationship of alcohol drinking pattern to risk of hypertension: a population-based study, *Hypertension* 44:813, 2004.

42. Gorelik S, Ligumsky M, Kohen R, Kanner J: A novel function of red wine polyphenols in humans: prevention of absorption of cytotoxic lipid peroxidation products, *FASEB J* 22:41, 2008.

43. Shaper AG, Wannamethee G, Walker M: Alcohol and mortality in British men: explaining the U-shaped curve [see comments], *Lancet* 2:1267, 1988.

44. Fillmore KM, Stockwell T, Chikritzhs T, et al: Moderate alcohol use and reduced mortality risk: systematic error in prospective studies and new hypotheses, *Ann Epidemiol* 17:S16, 2007.

45. Rothman KJ, Greenland S: Types of epidemiologic studes. In Rothman KJ, Greenland S, editors, *Modern epidemiology*, ed 2. Philadelphia, 1998, Lippicott-Raven, pp 67-78.

46. Conference Panel, Panel Discussion I: Does alcohol consumption prevent cardiovascular disease? *Ann Epidemiol* 5S:S37, 2007.

47. Fuchs CS, Stampfer MJ, Colditz GA, et al: Alcohol consumption and mortality among women, *N Engl J Med* 332:1245, 1995.

48. Rimm EB, Giovannucci EL, Willett WC, et al: Prospective study of alcohol consumption and risk of coronary disease in men [see comments], *Lancet* 338:464, 1991.

49. Strandberg TE, Strandberg AY, Salomaa VV, et al: Alcoholic beverage preference, 29-year mortality, and quality of life in men in old age, *J Gerontol A Biol Sci Med Sci* 62:213, 2007.

50. Lee SJ, Sudore RL, Williams BA, et al: Functional limitations, socioeconomic status, and all-cause mortality in moderate alcohol drinkers, *J Am Geriatr Soc* 57:955, 2009.

51. Friesema IH, Zwietering PJ, Veenstra MY, et al: Alcohol intake and cardiovascular disease and mortality: the role of pre-existing disease, *J Epidemiol Community Health* 61:441, 2007.

52. Poikolainen K, Vahtera J, Virtanen M, et al: Alcohol and coronary heart disease risk—is there an unknown confounder? *Addiction* 100:1150, 2005.

53. Sorensen HT, Lash TL, Rothman KJ: Beyond randomized controlled trials: a critical comparison of trials with nonrandomized studies, *Hepatology* 44:1075, 2006.

54. Janszky I, Mukamal KJ, Orth-Gomer K, et al: Alcohol consumption and coronary atherosclerosis progression—the Stockholm Female Coronary Risk Angiographic Study, *Atherosclerosis* 176:311, 2004.

55. Niroomand F, Hauer O, Tiefenbacher CP, et al: Influence of alcohol consumption on restenosis rate after percutaneous transluminal coronary angioplasty and stent implantation, *Heart* 90:1189, 2004.

56. Mukamal KJ, Maclure M, Muller JE, et al: Prior alcohol consumption and mortality following acute myocardial infarction, *JAMA* 285:1965, 2001.

57. Brugger-Andersen T, Ponitz V, Snapinn S, Dickstein K: Moderate alcohol consumption is associated with reduced long-term cardiovascular risk in patients following a complicated acute myocardial infarction, *Int J Cardiol* 133:229, 2009.

58. Castelli WP, Doyle JT, Gordon T: Alcohol and blood lipids, *Lancet* 2:153, 1977.

59. Suh I, Shaten BJ, Cutler JA, Kuller LH: Alcohol use and mortality from coronary heart disease: the role of high-density lipoprotein cholesterol. The Multiple Risk Factor Intervention Trial Research Group [see comments], *Ann Intern Med* 116:881, 1992.

60. Gaziano JM, Buring JE, Breslow JL: Moderate alcohol intake, increased levels of high-density lipoprotein and its subfractions, and decreased risk of myocardial infarction, *N Engl J Med* 329:1829, 1993.

61. Mukamal KJ, Jensen MK, Gronbaek M, et al: Drinking frequency, mediating biomarkers, and risk of myocardial infarction in women and men, *Circulation* 112:1406, 2005.

62. Ellison RC, Zhang Y, Qureshi MM, et al: Lifestyle determinants of high-density lipoprotein cholesterol: the National Heart, Lung, and Blood Institute Family Heart Study, *Am Heart J* 147:529, 2004.

63. Volcik KA, Ballantyne CM, Fuchs FD, et al: Relationship of alcohol consumption and type of alcoholic beverage consumed with plasma lipid levels: differences between Whites and African Americans of the ARIC study, *Ann Epidemiol* 18:101, 2008.

64. Gaziano JM, Buring JE, Breslow JL, et al: Moderate alcohol intake, increased levels of high-density lipoprotein and its subfractions, and decreased risk of myocardial infarction, *N Engl J Med* 329:1829, 1993.

65. Clevidence BA, Reichman ME, Judd JT, et al: Effects of alcohol consumption on lipoproteins of premenopausal women. A controlled diet study, *Arterioscler Thromb Vasc Biol* 15:179, 1995.

66. Makela SM, Jauhiainen M, Ala-Korpela M, et al: HDL_2 of heavy alcohol drinkers enhances cholesterol efflux from raw macrophages via phospholipid-rich HDL_{2b} particles, *Alcohol Clin Exp Res* 32:991, 2008.

67. Joosten MM, Beulens JW, Kersten S, Hendriks HF: Moderate alcohol consumption increases insulin sensitivity and ADIPOQ expression in postmenopausal women: a randomised, crossover trial, *Diabetologia* 51:1375, 2008.

68. Wakabayashi I: Associations of alcohol drinking and cigarette smoking with serum lipid levels in healthy middle-aged men, *Alcohol Alcohol* 43:274, 2008.

69. Wakabayashi I, Groschner K: Modification of the association between alcohol drinking and non-HDL cholesterol by gender, *Clin Chim Acta* 404:154, 2009.

70. Mukamal KJ, Mackey RH, Kuller LH, et al: Alcohol consumption and lipoprotein subclasses in older adults, *J Clin Endocrinol Metab* 92:2559, 2007.

71. Covas MI, Konstantinidou V, Mysytaki E et al: Postprandial effects of wine consumption on lipids and oxidative stress biomarkers, *Drugs Exp Clin Res* 29:217, 2003.

72. Kerem Z, Chetrit D, Shoseyov O, Regev-Shoshani G: Protection of lipids from oxidation by epicatechin, *trans*-resveratrol, and gallic and caffeic acids in intestinal model systems, *J Agric Food Chem* 54:10288, 2006.

73. Rajdl D, Racek J, Trefil L, Siala K: Effect of white wine consumption on oxidative stress markers and homocysteine levels. *Physiol Res* 56:203-212, 2007.

74. Micallef M, Lexis L, Lewandowski P: Red wine consumption increases antioxidant status and decreases oxidative stress in the circulation of both young and old humans. *Nutr J* 6:27, 2007.

75. Feillet-Coudray C, Sutra T, Fouret G et al: Oxidative stress in rats fed a high-fat high-sucrose diet and preventive effect of polyphenols: Involvement of mitochondrial and NADPH oxidase systems. *Free Radic Biol Med* 46:624-632, 2009.

76. Schroder H, Marrugat J, Fito M, Weinbrenner T, Covas MI: Alcohol consumption is directly associated with circulating oxidized low-density lipoprotein. *Free Radic Biol Med* 40:1474-1481, 2006.

77. Booyse FM, Pan W, Harper VM, et al: Mechanisms by which alcohol and wine polyphenols affect coronary heart disease risk, *Ann Epidemiol* 17:S24, 2007.

78. De Curtis A, Murzilli S, Di Castelnuovo A, et al: Alcohol-free red wine prevents arterial thrombosis in dietary-induced hypercholesterolemic rats: experimental support for the "French paradox," *J Thromb Haemost* 3:346, 2005.

79. Renaud S, de Lorgeril M: Wine, alcohol, platelets, and the French paradox for coronary heart disease [see comments], *Lancet* 339:1523, 1992.

80. Zhang QH, Das K, Siddiqui S, Myers AK: Effects of acute, moderate ethanol consumption on human platelet aggregation in platelet-rich plasma and whole blood, *Alcohol Clin Exp Res* 24:528, 2000.

81. Bucki R, Pastore JJ, Giraud F, et al: Flavonoid inhibition of platelet procoagulant activity and phosphoinositide synthesis, *J Thromb Haemost* 1:1820, 2003.

82. Hubbard AL, Davidson GJ, Patel RH, et al: Host-guest interactions template: the synthesis of a [3]catenane, *Chem Commun (Camb)* 138, 2004.

83. Ruf JC: Alcohol, wine and platelet function, *Biol Res* 37:209, 2004.

84. Demrow HS, Slane PR, Folts JD: Administration of wine and grape juice inhibits in vivo platelet activity and thrombosis in stenosed canine coronary arteries, *Circulation* 91:1182, 1995.

85. Ruf JC, Berger JL, Renaud S: Platelet rebound effect of alcohol withdrawal and wine drinking in rats. Relation to tannins and lipid peroxidation, *Arterioscler Thromb Vasc Biol* 15:140, 1995.

86. Renaud S: Effects of alcohol on platelet functions, *Clin Chim Acta* 246:77, 1996.

87. Miyamae M, Diamond I, Weiner MW, et al: Regular alcohol consumption mimics cardiac preconditioning by protecting against ischemia-reperfusion injury, *Proc Natl Acad Sci U S A* 94:3235, 1997.

88. Guiraud A, de Lorgeril M, Boucher F, et al: Cardioprotective effect of chronic low dose ethanol drinking: insights into the concept of ethanol preconditioning, *J Mol Cell Cardiol* 36:561, 2004.

89. Rendig SV, Symons JD, Longhurst JC, Amsterdam EA: Effects of red wine, alcohol, and quercetin on coronary resistance and conductance arteries, *J Cardiovasc Pharmacol* 38:219, 2001.

90. Flesch M, Schwarz A, Bohm M: Effects of red and white wine on endothelium-dependent vasorelaxation of rat aorta and human coronary arteries, *Am J Physiol* 275:H1183, 1998.

91. Andriambeloson E, Stoclet JC, Andriantsitohaina R: Mechanism of endothelial nitric oxide–dependent vasorelaxation induced by wine polyphenols in rat thoracic aorta, *J Cardiovasc Pharmacol* 33:248, 1999.

92. Rakici O, Kiziltepe U, Coskun B, et al: Effects of resveratrol on vascular tone and endothelial function of human saphenous vein and internal mammary artery, *Int J Cardiol* 105:209, 2005.

93. Liu J, Tian Z, Gao B, Kunos G: Dose-dependent activation of antiapoptotic and pro-apoptotic pathways by ethanol treatment in human vascular endothelial cells: differential involvement of adenosine, *J Biol Chem* 277:20927, 2002.

94. Salem RO, Laposata M: Effects of alcohol on hemostasis, *Am J Clin Pathol* 123(Suppl):S96, 2005.

95. Mukamal KJ, Jensen MK, Gronbaek M, et al: Drinking frequency, mediating biomarkers, and risk of myocardial infarction in women and men, *Circulation* 112:1406, 2005.

96. Ridker PM, Vaughan DE, Stampfer MJ, et al: Association of moderate alcohol consumption and plasma concentration of endogenous tissue-type plasminogen activator [see comments], *JAMA* 272:929, 1994.

97. Hendriks HF, Veenstra J, Velthuis-te Wierik EJ, et al: Effect of moderate dose of alcohol with evening meal on fibrinolytic factors, *BMJ* 308:1003, 1994.

98. Aikens ML, Benza RL, Grenett HE, et al: Ethanol increases surface-localized fibrinolytic activity in cultured endothelial cells, *Alcohol Clin Exp Res* 21:1471, 1997.

99. Booyse FM, Aikens ML, Grenett HE: Endothelial cell fibrinolysis: transcriptional regulation of fibrinolytic protein gene expression (t-PA, u-PA, and PAI-1) by low alcohol, *Alcohol Clin Exp Res* 23:1119, 1999.
100. Abou-Agag LH, Tabengwa EM, Tresnak JA, et al: Ethanol-induced increased surface-localized fibrinolytic activity in cultured human endothelial cells: kinetic analysis, *Alcohol Clin Exp Res* 25:351, 2001.
101. de Lange DW, van de Wiel A: Drink to prevent: review on the cardioprotective mechanisms of alcohol and red wine polyphenols, *Semin Vasc Med* 4:173, 2004.
102. Booyse FM, Pan W, Grenett HE, et al: Mechanism by which alcohol and wine polyphenols affect coronary heart disease risk, *Ann Epidemiol* 17:S24, 2007.
103. Zhao X, Gu Z, Attele AS, Yuan CS: Effects of quercetin on the release of endothelin, prostacyclin and tissue plasminogen activator from human endothelial cells in culture, *J Ethnopharmacol* 67:279, 1999.
104. Abou-Agag LH, Aikens ML, Tabengwa EM, et al: Polyphyenolics increase t-PA and u-PA gene transcription in cultured human endothelial cells, *Alcohol Clin Exp Res* 25:155, 2001.
105. Guillaume P, Jankowski M, Gutkowska J, Gianoulakis C: Effect of chronic moderate ethanol consumption on heart brain natriuretic peptide, *Eur J Pharmacol* 316:49, 1996.
106. Hayek T, Fuhrman B, Vaya J, et al: Reduced progression of atherosclerosis in apolipoprotein E–deficient mice following consumption of red wine, or its polyphenols quercetin or catechin, is associated with reduced susceptibility of LDL to oxidation and aggregation, *Arterioscler Thromb Vasc Biol* 17:2744, 1997.
107. Aviram M, Fuhrman B: Wine flavonoids protect against LDL oxidation and atherosclerosis, *Ann N Y Acad Sci* 957:146, 2002.
108. Corder R, Douthwaite JA, Lees DM, et al: Endothelin-1 synthesis reduced by red wine, *Nature* 414:863, 2001.
109. Di Santo A,, Mezzetti A, Napoleone E, et al: Resveratrol and quercetin down-regulate tissue factor expression by human stimulated vascular cells, *J Thromb Haemost* 1:1089, 2003.
110. Casani L, Segales E, Vilahur G, et al: Moderate daily intake of red wine inhibits mural thrombosis and monocyte tissue factor expression in an experimental porcine model, *Circulation* 110:460, 2004.
111. Iijima K, Yoshizumi M, Hashimoto M, et al: Red wine polyphenols inhibit proliferation of vascular smooth muscle cells and downregulate expression of cyclin A gene, *Circulation* 101:805, 2000.
112. Alcocer F, Whitley D, Salazar-Gonzalez JF, et al: Quercetin inhibits human vascular smooth muscle cell proliferation and migration, *Surgery* 131:198, 2002.
113. Zern TL, Fernandez ML: Cardioprotective effects of dietary polyphenols, *J Nutr* 135:2291, 2005.
114. Avellone G, Di Garbo V, Campisi D, et al: Effects of moderate Sicilian red wine consumption on inflammatory biomarkers of atherosclerosis, *Eur J Clin Nutr* 60:41, 2006.
115. Wang JJ, Tung TH, Yin WH, et al: Effects of moderate alcohol consumption on inflammatory biomarkers, *Acta Cardiol* 63:65, 2008.
116. Albert MA, Glynn RJ, Ridker PM: Alcohol consumption and plasma concentration of C-reactive protein, *Circulation* 107:443, 2003.
117. Djousse L, Lee IM, Buring JE, Gaziano JM: Alcohol consumption and risk of cardiovascular disease and death in women: potential mediating mechanisms, *Circulation* 120:237, 2009.
118. Klatsky AL: Alcohol and hypertension, *Clin Chim Acta* 246:91, 1996.
119. Fuchs FD, Chambless LE, Whelton PK, et al: Alcohol consumption and the incidence of hypertension: the Atherosclerosis Risk in Communities Study, *Hypertension* 37:1242, 2001.
120. Gordon T, Kannel WB: Drinking and its relation to smoking, BP, blood lipids, and uric acid: the Framingham Study, *Arch Intern Med* 143:1366, 1983.
121. Klatsky AL, Friedman GD, Siegelaub AB, Gerard MJ: Alcohol consumption and blood pressure Kaiser-Permanente Multiphasic Health Examination data, *N Engl J Med* 296:1194, 1977.
122. Kimball AW, Friedman LA, Moore RD: Nonlinear modeling of alcohol consumption for analysis of beverage type effects and beverage preference effects, *Am J Epidemiol* 135:1287, 1992.
123. Keil U, Chambless L, Remmers A: Alcohol and blood pressure: results from the Luebeck Blood Pressure Study, *Prev Med* 18:1, 1989.
124. Klatsky AL, Koplik S, Gunderson E, et al: Sequelae of systemic hypertension in alcohol abstainers, light drinkers, and heavy drinkers, *Am J Cardiol* 98:1063, 2006.
125. Klatsky AL, Friedman GD, Armstrong MA: The relationships between alcoholic beverage use and other traits to blood pressure: a new Kaiser Permanente study, *Circulation* 73:628, 1986.
126. Davey Smith G, Ebrahim S: "Mendelian randomization": can genetic epidemiology contribute to understanding environmental determinants of disease? *Int J Epidemiol* 32:1, 2003.
127. Hines LM, Stampfer MJ, Ma J, et al: Genetic variation in alcohol dehydrogenase and the beneficial effect of moderate alcohol consumption on myocardial infarction, *N Engl J Med* 344:549, 2001.
128. Hines LM, Hunter DJ, Stampfer MJ, et al: Alcohol consumption and high-density lipoprotein levels: the effect of ADH1C genotype, gender and menopausal status, *Atherosclerosis* 182:293, 2005.
129. Whitfield JB, O'Brien ME, Nightingale BN, et al: ADH genotype does not modify the effects of alcohol on high-density lipoprotein, *Alcohol Clin Exp Res* 27:509, 2003.
130. Jensen MK, Rimm EB, Rader D, et al: S447X variant of the lipoprotein lipase gene, lipids, and risk of coronary heart disease in 3 prospective cohort studies, *Am Heart J* 157:384, 2009.
131. Druesne-Pecollo N, Tehard B, Mallet Y, et al: Alcohol and genetic polymorphisms: effect on risk of alcohol-related cancer, *Lancet Oncol* 10:173, 2009.
132. Collins MA, Neafsey EJ, Mukamal KJ, et al: Alcohol in moderation, cardioprotection, and neuroprotection: epidemiological considerations and mechanistic studies, *Alcohol Clin Exp Res* 33:206, 2009.
133. Leighton F, Urquiaga I: Changes in cardiovascular risk factors associated with wine consumption in intervention studies in humans, *Ann Epidemiol* 17:S32, 2007.
134. Sierksma A, Patel H, Ouchi N, et al: Effect of moderate alcohol consumption on adiponectin, tumor necrosis factor-alpha, and insulin sensitivity, *Diabetes Care* 27:184, 2004.
135. Shai I, Wainstein J, Harman-Boehm I, et al: Glycemic effects of moderate alcohol intake among patients with type 2 diabetes: a multicenter, randomized, clinical intervention trial, *Diabetes Care* 30:3011, 2007.
136. Truelsen T, Gronbaek M, Schnohr P, Boysen G: Intake of beer, wine, and spirits and risk of stroke: the Copenhagen City Heart Study, *Stroke* 29:2467, 1998.
137. Sacco RL, Elkind M, Boden-Albala B, et al: The protective effect of moderate alcohol consumption on ischemic stroke, *JAMA* 281:53, 1999.
138. Klatsky AL, Armstrong MA, Friedman GD, Sidney S: Alcohol drinking and risk of hemorrhagic stroke, *Neuroepidemiology* 21:115, 2002.
139. Djousse L, Levy D, Murabito JM, et al: Alcohol consumption and risk of intermittent claudication in the Framingham Heart Study, *Circulation* 102:3092, 2000.
140. Ettinger PO, Wu CF, De La Cruz C, Jr, et al: Arrhythmias and the "holiday heart": alcohol-associated cardiac rhythm disorders, *Am Heart J* 95:555, 1978.
141. Menz V, Grimm W, Hoffmann J, Maisch B: Alcohol and rhythm disturbance: the holiday heart syndrome, *Herz* 21:227, 1996.
142. Klatsky AL: Alcohol and cardiovascular diseases: a historical overview, *Ann N Y Acad Sci* 957:7, 2002.
143. Nissen MB, Lemberg L: The "holiday heart" syndrome, *Heart Lung* 13:89, 1984.
144. Djousse L, Levy D, Benjamin EJ, et al: Long-term alcohol consumption and the risk of atrial fibrillation in the Framingham Study, *Am J Cardiol* 93:710, 2004.
145. Mukamal KJ, Tolstrup JS, Friberg J, et al: Alcohol consumption and risk of atrial fibrillation in men and women: the Copenhagen City Heart Study, *Circulation* 112:1736, 2005.
146. Balbao CE, de Paola AA, Fenelon G: Effects of alcohol on atrial fibrillation: myths and truths, *Ther Adv Cardiovasc Dis* 3:53, 2009.
147. Djousse L, Gaziano JM: Alcohol consumption and heart failure: a systematic review, *Curr Atheroscler Rep* 10:117, 2008.
148. Walsh CR, Larson MG, Evans JC, et al: Alcohol consumption and risk for congestive heart failure in the Framingham Heart Study, *Ann Intern Med* 136:181, 2002.
149. Djousse L, Gaziano JM: Alcohol consumption and risk of heart failure in the Physicians' Health Study I, *Circulation* 115:34, 2007.
150. Abramson JL, Williams SA, Krumholz HM, Vaccarino V: Moderate alcohol consumption and risk of heart failure among older persons, *JAMA* 285:1971, 2001.
151. Klatsky AL, Chartier D, Udaltsova N, et al: Alcohol drinking and risk of hospitalization for heart failure with and without associated coronary artery disease, *Am J Cardiol* 96:346, 2005.
152. Bryson CL, Mukamal KJ, Mittleman MA, et al: The association of alcohol consumption and incident heart failure: the Cardiovascular Health Study, *J Am Coll Cardiol* 48:305, 2006.
153. Kloner RA, Rezkalla SH: To drink or not to drink? That is the question, *Circulation* 116:1306, 2007.
154. Cooper HA, Exner DV, Domanski MJ: Light-to-moderate alcohol consumption and prognosis in patients with left ventricular systolic dysfunction, *J Am Coll Cardiol* 35:1753, 2000.
155. Aguilar D, Skali H, Moye LA, et al: Alcohol consumption and prognosis in patients with left ventricular systolic dysfunction after a myocardial infarction, *J Am Coll Cardiol* 43:2015, 2004.
156. Stampfer MJ, Colditz GA, Willett WC, et al: A prospective study of moderate alcohol drinking and risk of diabetes in women, *Am J Epidemiol* 128:549, 1988.
157. Rimm EB, Chan J, Stampfer MJ, et al: Prospective study of cigarette smoking, alcohol use, and the risk of diabetes in men [see comments], *BMJ* 310:555, 1995.
158. Perry IJ, Wannamethee SG, Walker MK, et al: Prospective study of risk factors for development of non–insulin dependent diabetes in middle aged British men, *BMJ* 310:560, 1995.
159. Conigrave KM, Hu BF, Camargo CA, Jr, et al: A prospective study of drinking patterns in relation to risk of type 2 diabetes among men, *Diabetes* 50:2390, 2001.
160. de Vegt F, Dekker JM, Groeneveld WJ, et al: Moderate alcohol consumption is associated with lower risk for incident diabetes and mortality: the Hoorn Study, *Diabetes Res Clin Pract* 57:53, 2002.
161. Wannamethee SG, Camargo CA, Jr, Manson JE, et al: Alcohol drinking patterns and risk of type 2 diabetes mellitus among younger women, *Arch Intern Med* 163:1329, 2003.
162. Howard AA, Arnsten JH, Gourevitch MN: Effect of alcohol consumption on diabetes mellitus: a systematic review, *Ann Intern Med* 140:211, 2004.
163. Koppes LL, Dekker JM, Hendriks HF, et al: Moderate alcohol consumption lowers the risk of type 2 diabetes: a meta-analysis of prospective observational studies, *Diabetes Care* 28:719, 2005.
164. Harding AH, Sargeant LA, Khaw KT, et al: Cross-sectional association between total level and type of alcohol consumption and glycosylated haemoglobin level: the EPIC-Norfolk Study, *Eur J Clin Nutr* 56:882, 2002.
165. Davies MJ, Baer DJ, Judd JT, et al: Effects of moderate alcohol intake on fasting insulin and glucose concentrations and insulin sensitivity in postmenopausal women: a randomized controlled trial, *JAMA* 287:2559, 2002.
166. Kroenke CH, Chu NF, Rifai N, et al: A cross-sectional study of alcohol consumption patterns and biologic markers of glycemic control among 459 women, *Diabetes Care* 26:1971, 2003.
167. Thamer C, Haap M, Fritsche A, et al: Relationship between moderate alcohol consumption and adiponectin and insulin sensitivity in a large heterogeneous population, *Diabetes Care* 27:1240, 2004.
168. Valmadrid CT, Klein R, Moss SE, et al: Alcohol intake and the risk of coronary heart disease mortality in persons with older-onset diabetes mellitus [see comments], *JAMA* 282:239, 1999.
169. Solomon CG, Hu FB, Stampfer MJ, et al: Moderate alcohol consumption and risk of coronary heart disease among women with type 2 diabetes mellitus, *Circulation* 102:494, 2000.

170. Ajani UA, Gaziano JM, Lotufo PA, et al: Alcohol consumption and risk of coronary heart disease by diabetes status, *Circulation* 102:500, 2000.
171. Koppes LL, Dekker JM, Hendriks HF, et al: Meta-analysis of the relationship between alcohol consumption and coronary heart disease and mortality in type 2 diabetic patients, *Diabetologia* 49:648, 2006.
172. Ahmed AT, Karter AJ, Warton EM, et al: The relationship between alcohol consumption and glycemic control among patients with diabetes: the Kaiser Permanente Northern California Diabetes Registry, *J Gen Intern Med* 23:275, 2008.
173. Beulens JW, Kruidhof JS, Grobbee DE, et al: Alcohol consumption and risk of microvascular complications in type 1 diabetes patients: the EURODIAB Prospective Complications Study, *Diabetologia* 51:1631, 2008.
174. Djousse L, Arnett DK, Eckfeldt JH, et al: Alcohol consumption and metabolic syndrome: does the type of beverage matter? *Obes Res* 12:1375, 2004.
175. Freiberg MS, Cabral HJ, Heeren TC, et al: Alcohol consumption and the prevalence of the Metabolic Syndrome in the US.: a cross-sectional analysis of data from the Third National Health and Nutrition Examination Survey, *Diabetes Care* 27:2954, 2004.
176. Fan AZ, Russell M, Naimi T, et al: Patterns of alcohol consumption and the metabolic syndrome, *J Clin Endocrinol Metab* 93:3833, 2008.
177. Alkerwi A, Boutsen M, Vaillant M, et al: Alcohol consumption and the prevalence of metabolic syndrome: a meta-analysis of observational studies, *Atherosclerosis* 204:624, 2009.
178. Stampfer MJ, Hu FB, Manson JE, et al: Primary prevention of coronary heart disease in women through diet and lifestyle, *N Engl J Med* 343:16, 2000.
179. Hu FB, Stampfer MJ, Manson JE, et al: Trends in the incidence of coronary heart disease and changes in diet and lifestyle in women, *N Engl J Med* 343:530, 2000.
180. Akesson A, Weismayer C, Newby PK, Wolk A: Combined effect of low-risk dietary and lifestyle behaviors in primary prevention of myocardial infarction in women, *Arch Intern Med* 167:2122, 2007.
181. Khaw KT, Wareham N, Bingham S, et al: Combined impact of health behaviours and mortality in men and women: the EPIC-Norfolk prospective population study, *PLoS Med* 5:e12, 2008.
182. Mukamal KJ, Chiuve SE, Rimm EB: Alcohol consumption and risk for coronary heart disease in men with healthy lifestyles, *Arch Intern Med* 166:2145, 2006.
183. Britton A, Marmot MG, Shipley M: Who benefits most from the cardioprotective properties of alcohol consumption—health freaks or couch potatoes? *J Epidemiol Community Health* 62:905, 2008.
184. La Vecchia C, Decarli A, Ferraroni M, Negri E: Alcohol drinking and prevalence of self-reported gallstone disease in the 1983 Italian National Health Survey [see comments], *Epidemiology* 5:533, 1994.
185. Sommer F, Klotz T, Schmitz-Drager BJ: Lifestyle issues and genitourinary tumours, *World J Urol* 21:402, 2004.
186. Greving JP, Lee JE, Wolk A, et al: Alcoholic beverages and risk of renal cell cancer, *Br J Cancer* 97:429, 2007.
187. Klatsky AL, Li Y, Baer D, et al: Alcohol consumption and risk of hematologic malignancies, *Ann Epidemiol* 19:746, 2009.
188. Wannamethee SG, Field AE, Colditz GA, Rimm EB: Alcohol intake and 8-year weight gain in women: a prospective study, *Obes Res* 12:1386, 2004.
189. Arif AA, Rohrer JE: Patterns of alcohol drinking and its association with obesity: data from the Third National Health and Nutrition Examination Survey, 1988-1994, *BMC Public Health* 5:126, 2005.
190. Tolstrup JS, Heitmann BL, Tjonneland AM, et al: The relation between drinking pattern and body mass index and waist and hip circumference, *Int J Obes (Lond)* 29:490, 2005.
191. Breslow RA, Smothers BA: Drinking patterns and body mass index in never smokers: National Health Interview Survey, 1997-2001, *Am J Epidemiol* 161:368, 2005.
192. Felson DT, Zhang Y, Hannan MT, et al: Alcohol intake and bone mineral density in elderly men and women. The Framingham Study, *Am J Epidemiol* 142:485, 1995.
193. Mukamal KJ, Robbins JA, Cauley JA, et al: Alcohol consumption, bone density, and hip fracture among older adults: the cardiovascular health study, *Osteoporos Int* 18:593, 2007.
194. Berg KM, Kunins HV, Jackson JL, et al: Association between alcohol consumption and both osteoporotic fracture and bone density, *Am J Med* 121:406, 2008.
195. Orgogozo JM, Dartigues JF, Lafont S, et al: Wine consumption and dementia in the elderly: a prospective community study in the Bordeaux area, *Rev Neurol (Paris)* 153:185, 1997.
196. Truelsen T, Thudium D, Gronbaek M: Amount and type of alcohol and risk of dementia: the Copenhagen City Heart Study, *Neurology* 59:1313, 2002.
197. Panza F, Capurso C, D'Introno A, et al: Alcohol drinking, cognitive functions in older age, predementia, and dementia syndromes, *J Alzheimers Dis* 17:7, 2009.
198. Britton A, Singh-Manoux A, Marmot M: Alcohol consumption and cognitive function in the Whitehall II study, *Am J Epidemiol* 160:240, 2004.
199. Espeland MA, Gu L, Masaki KH, et al: Association between reported alcohol intake and cognition: results from the Women's Health Initiative Memory Study, *Am J Epidemiol* 161:228, 2005.
200. Stampfer MJ, Kang JH, Chen J, et al: Effects of moderate alcohol consumption on cognitive function in women, *N Engl J Med* 352:245, 2005.
201. Zhang Y, Heeren T, Curtis Ellison R: Education modifies the effect of alcohol on memory impairment: the third national health and nutrition examination survey, *Neuroepidemiology* 24:63, 2005.
202. Ganguli M, Vander BJ, Saxton JA, et al: Alcohol consumption and cognitive function in late life: a longitudinal community study, *Neurology* 65:1210, 2005.
203. Solfrizzi V, Capurso C, D'Introno A, et al: Lifestyle-related factors in predementia and dementia syndromes, *Expert Rev Neurother* 8:133, 2008.
204. Mehlig K, Skoog I, Guo X, et al: Alcoholic beverages and incidence of dementia: 34-year follow-up of the prospective population study of women in Goteborg, *Am J Epidemiol* 167:684, 2008.
205. Peters R, Peters J, Warner J, et al: Alcohol, dementia and cognitive decline in the elderly: a systematic review, *Age Ageing* 37:505, 2008.
206. Weikert C, Dietrich T, Boeing H, et al: Lifetime and baseline alcohol intake and risk of cancer of the upper aero-digestive tract in the European Prospective Investigation into Cancer and Nutrition (EPIC) study, *Int J Cancer* 125:406, 2009.
207. Allen NE, Beral V, Casabonne D, et al: Moderate alcohol intake and cancer incidence in women, *J Natl Cancer Inst* 101:296, 2009.
208. Mellemgaard A, Engholm G, McLaughlin JK, Olsen JH: Risk factors for renal cell carcinoma in Denmark. I. Role of socioeconomic status, tobacco use, beverages, and family history, *Cancer Causes Control* 5:105, 1994.
209. Morton LM, Zheng T, Holford TR, et al: Alcohol consumption and risk of non-Hodgkin lymphoma: a pooled analysis, *Lancet Oncol* 6:469, 2005.
210. Besson H, Brennan P, Becker N, et al: Tobacco smoking, alcohol drinking and Hodgkin's lymphoma: a European multi-centre case-control study (Epilymph), *Br J Cancer* 95:378, 2006.
211. Jiao L, Silverman DT, Schairer C, et al: Alcohol use and risk of pancreatic cancer: the NIH-AARP Diet and Health Study, *Am J Epidemiol* 169:1043, 2009.
212. Genkinger JM, Spiegelman D, Anderson KE, et al: Alcohol intake and pancreatic cancer risk: a pooled analysis of fourteen cohort studies, *Cancer Epidemiol Biomarkers Prev* 18:765, 2009.
213. El-Serag HB, Lagergren J: Alcohol drinking and the risk of Barrett's esophagus and esophageal adenocarcinoma, *Gastroenterology* 136:1155, 2009.
214. Willett WC, Stampfer MJ, Colditz GA, et al: Moderate alcohol consumption and the risk of breast cancer, *N Engl J Med* 316:1174, 1987.
215. Longnecker MP: Alcoholic beverage consumption in relation to risk of breast cancer: meta-analysis and review, *Cancer Causes Control* 5:73, 1994.
216. Schatzkin A, Carter CL, Green SB, et al: Is alcohol consumption related to breast cancer? Results from the Framingham Heart Study, *J Natl Cancer Inst* 81:31, 1989.
217. Zhang Y, Kreger BE, Dorgan JF, et al: Alcohol consumption and risk of breast cancer: the Framingham Study revisited, *Am J Epidemiol* 149:93, 1999.
218. Duffy CM, Assaf A, Cyr M, et al: Alcohol and folate intake and breast cancer risk in the WHI Observational Study, *Breast Cancer Res Treat* 116:551, 2009.
219. Ellison RC, Zhang Y, McLennan CE, Rothman KJ: Exploring the relation of alcohol consumption to risk of breast cancer, *Am J Epidemiol* 154:740, 2001.
220. Zhang S, Hunter DJ, Hankinson SE, et al: A prospective study of folate intake and the risk of breast cancer, *JAMA* 281:1632, 1999.
221. Tjonneland A, Christensen J, Olsen A, et al: Folate intake, alcohol and risk of breast cancer among postmenopausal women in Denmark, *Eur J Clin Nutr* 60:280, 2006.
222. Larsson SC, Giovannucci E, Wolk A: Folate and risk of breast cancer: a meta-analysis, *J Natl Cancer Inst* 99:64, 2007.
223. Colditz GA, Stampfer MJ, Willett WC, et al: Prospective study of estrogen replacement therapy and risk of breast cancer in postmenopausal women, *JAMA* 264:2648, 1990.
224. Nielsen NR, Gronbaek M: Interactions between intakes of alcohol and postmenopausal hormones on risk of breast cancer, *Int J Cancer* 122:1109, 2008.
225. Morch LS, Johansen D, Thygesen LC, et al: Alcohol drinking, consumption patterns and breast cancer among Danish nurses: a cohort study, *Eur J Public Health* 17:624, 2007.
226. Boffetta P, Garfinkel L: Alcohol drinking and mortality among men enrolled in an American Cancer Society Prospective Study, *Epidemiology* 1:342, 1990.
227. Thun MJ, Peto R, Lopez AD, et al: Alcohol consumption and mortality among middle-aged and elderly U.S. adults [see comments], *N Engl J Med* 337:1705, 1997.
228. Doll R, Peto R, Boreham J, Sutherland I: Mortality in relation to alcohol consumption: a prospective study among male British doctors, *Int J Epidemiol* 34:199, 2005.
229. Konnopka A, König HH: The health and economic consequences of moderate alcohol consumption in Germany 2002, *Value Health* 12:253, 2009.
230. Gronbaek M, Deis A, Sorensen TI: Mortality associated with moderate intakes of wine, beer, or spirits [letter to editor], *BMJ* 310:1165, 1995.
231. Renaud SC, Gueguen R, Schenker J, d'Houtaud A: Alcohol and mortality in middle-aged men from eastern France, *Epidemiology* 9:184, 1998.
232. Renaud SC, Gueguen R, Siest G, Salamon R: Wine, beer, and mortality in middle-aged men from eastern France, *Arch Intern Med* 159:1865, 1999.
233. Mukamal KJ, Conigrave KM, Mittleman MA, et al: Roles of drinking pattern and type of alcohol consumed in coronary heart disease in men, *N Engl J Med* 348:109, 2003.
234. Ruf JC: Overview of epidemiological studies on wine, health and mortality, *Drugs Exp Clin Res* 29:173, 2003.
235. Theobald H, Bygren LO, Carstensen J, Engfeldt P: A moderate intake of wine is associated with reduced total mortality and reduced mortality from cardiovascular disease, *J Stud Alcohol* 61:652, 2000.
236. Renaud SC, Gueguen R, Conard P, et al: Moderate wine drinkers have lower hypertension-related mortality: a prospective cohort study in French men, *Am J Clin Nutr* 80:621, 2004.
237. Johansen D, Friis K, Skovenborg E, Gronbaek M: Food buying habits of people who buy wine or beer: cross sectional study, *BMJ* 332:519, 2006.
238. Streppel MT, Ocke MC, Boshuizen HC, et al: Long-term wine consumption is related to cardiovascular mortality and life expectancy independently of moderate alcohol intake: the Zutphen Study, *J Epidemiol Community Health* 63:534, 2009.
239. O'Keefe JH, Bybee KA, Lavie CJ: Alcohol and cardiovascular health: the razor-sharp double-edged sword, *J Am Coll Cardiol* 50:1009, 2007.
240. Lincoln A: Talk to Washington Temperance Society of Springfield, Illinois, February 22, 1842, as published in http://www.druglibrary.org/schaffer/lincoln.htm.
241. Cole P: The moral bases for public health interventions, *Epidemiology* 6:78, 1995.
242. Seltzer CC: "Conflicts of interest" and "political science," *J Clin Epidemiol* 50:627, 1997.

CHAPTER 19

Overweight, Obesity, and Cardiovascular Risk

George L. Blackburn, Kristina Spellman, and Samuel Wollner

KEY POINTS

- Obesity is the leading public health crisis of our time. It is a primary target to reduce an avoidable disease burden in the United States.

- Obesity is an independent risk factor for major cardiovascular events, including coronary heart disease, heart failure, and stroke.

- Body mass index is a vital sign for assessment of patients with excess body weight and for stratification of treatments according to the likelihood of underlying disease risk.

- A series of metabolic abnormalities in obesity culminate in a clustering of risk factors for cardiovascular disease and type 2 diabetes mellitus, a condition known as the metabolic syndrome.

- Framingham risk score assessment for cardiovascular disease does not account for obesity. Risk assessment should include body mass index, waist circumference, blood serum biomarkers, and physical fitness.

- Major studies show that lifestyle change leading to weight loss can reduce or reverse risks associated with cardiovascular disease, including sleep apnea, hypertension, type 2 diabetes, and coronary heart disease.

- In patients intractable to lifestyle intervention alone, pharmacotherapy can facilitate weight loss to reduce risk of comorbid conditions. In cases of severe obesity, bariatric surgery is associated with significant weight loss and improvement in diabetes, hypertension, and obstructive sleep apnea.

- Obesity prevention and cardiovascular risk reduction will require a new approach that takes into account the sociopolitical, economic, and environmental forces that interact to create an obesogenic environment.

Obesity is the leading public health crisis of our time. The most recent data from the National Health and Nutrition Examination Survey (NHANES 2005-2006) indicate that the prevalence of obesity (BMI >30 kg/m^2) among adults is 34%[1]; for extreme obesity, the figure is 6%.[2] Minorities are disproportionately affected. Approximately 53% of non-Hispanic African American women and 51% of Mexican American women 40 to 59 years of age are obese compared with an estimated 39% of non-Hispanic white women of the same age.[2] Together, overweight and obesity affect more than 66% of the adult population.[3]

Rates of childhood obesity reflect those for adults. The proportion of 18- to 29-year-olds who were obese in 2004-2006 more than tripled from 8% in 1971-1974 to 24%.[1] NHANES data for the combined years of 2003-2006 indicate that 16.3% of children and adolescents 2 to 19 years of age are obese, defined as at or above the 95th percentile of the 2000 BMI-for-age growth charts; 11.3% of children and adolescents in the same age group are above the 97th percentile, or extremely obese.[4]

Low-income and minority children, like adults, are disproportionately affected.[5] The rates of obesity in Hispanic and non-Hispanic black children are 18.5% and 11.8%, respectively, compared with 12.6% in non-Hispanic white children. Evidence suggests that obesity-associated morbidity may increase with longer duration of the disease,[1,6] adding even more urgency to the need to reverse the trend and to reduce future morbidity.[1]

Modern therapies, such as statins, and lifesaving procedures have reduced the rate of mortality due to heart disease in the United States. There are, however, concerning trends in both nonfatal events and the disability that results from major cardiovascular events.[7] Risk factor levels continue to rise in the United States at alarming rates.[8]

Addressing these risk factors will be the first step in alleviating avoidable burdens on patients and our health care system.[9]

Obesity is an independent risk factor for cardiovascular events in the general population, patients with established cardiovascular disease (CVD), and elderly persons.[10] During the last decade, more than 100 prospective cohort studies and three meta-analyses (with more than 90 prospective studies and 1.1 million participants)[11] have confirmed obesity's central role in the development of CVD.

ETIOLOGY AND PATHOPHYSIOLOGY

Many potential mechanisms have been proposed to explain the association of obesity with cardiovascular events, including increased severity of CVD, systemic inflammation, insulin resistance, neurohormonal activation, and abnormalities in adipokine pathways (Fig. 19-1).[10] Excess weight exacerbates a number of cardiovascular and metabolic risk factors (Box 19-1).[12] Inflammatory adipokines may increase insulin resistance and diabetes,[13] and abnormal lipid metabolism, which is common in those with obesity, can lead to atherosclerotic plaque.[14]

Excess adipose tissue, especially intra-abdominal,[12] predisposes patients to type 2 diabetes, hypertension, dyslipidemia, or the metabolic syndrome largely through increased lipolysis that raises the production of free fatty acids and adipokines. The excess fatty acids interfere with insulin receptor signaling and lead to decreased glucose transport, often referred to as lipotoxicity. They also activate protein kinase C (through increased fatty acyl coenzyme A and diacylglycerols).[13]

Protein kinase C serine phosphorylates insulin receptors, interfering with insulin

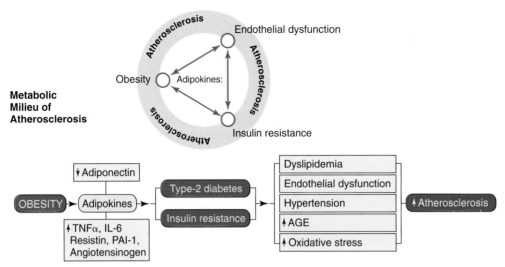

FIGURE 19-1 Adipokines serve as the cellular mediators of metabolic syndrome and endothelial dysfunction. *(From Lau DC, Dhillon B, Yan H, et al: Adipokines: molecular links between obesity and atherosclerosis.* Am J Physiol Heart Circ Physiol *288:H2031, 2005.)*

BOX 19-1 Risk Factors for Atherosclerosis and Vascular Disease Associated with Obesity

- Hypertension
- Dyslipidemia
- Diabetes mellitus (type 2)
- Obstructive sleep apnea
- Hyperinsulinemia, insulin resistance
- Low levels of plasminogen activator inhibitor
- High levels of C-reactive protein
- Hyperviscosity
- Framingham risk score

TABLE 19–1	Criteria for Clinical Diagnosis of the Metabolic Syndrome
3 of 5 Risk Factors	**Defining Level**
Abdominal obesity	Waist circumference* Population- and country-specific definitions
Triglycerides (drug treatment for elevated triglycerides is an alternate indicator†)	≥150 mg/dL
HDL-C (drug treatment for reduced HDL-C is an alternate indicator†)	Men <40 mg/dL Women <50 mg/dL
Blood pressure (antihypertensive drug treatment in a patient with a history of hypertension is an alternate indicator)	≥130/ ≥85 mm Hg
Fasting glucose‡ (drug treatment of elevated glucose is an alternate indicator)	≥100 mg/dL

*It is recommended that the International Diabetes Federation cut points be used for non-Europeans and either the International Diabetes Federation or American Heart Association/National Heart, Lung, and Blood Institute cut points be used for people of European origin until more data are available.

†The most commonly used drugs for elevated triglycerides and reduced high-density lipoprotein cholesterol (HDL-C) are fibrates and nicotinic acid. A patient taking one of these drugs can be presumed to have high triglycerides and low HDL-C. High-dose omega-3 fatty acids presumes high triglycerides.

‡Most patients with type 2 diabetes mellitus will have the metabolic syndrome by the proposed criteria.

signal transduction. Excess free fatty acids also impair phosphoinositide 3-kinase activation in response to insulin, leading to decreased activity of glucose transporter 4 (GLUT4), an important insulin-sensitive glucose transporter in muscle and fat.[13] Growing evidence suggests that insulin resistance in liver, muscle, and adipose tissue is associated with and may be the result of increased proinflammatory cytokines.[15,16]

In an obese state, some adipokines—proteins, such as tumor necrosis factor-α, or cytokines, such as interleukin-6—are elevated. Adipokines inhibit insulin action and contribute to proinflammatory effects, insulin resistance, and endothelial dysfunction. Adiponectin and resistin have recently been associated with incident heart failure.[17]

This series of metabolic abnormalities culminates in a clustering of risk factors for CVD and type 2 diabetes mellitus, a condition known as the metabolic syndrome or prediabetes. The risk factors include raised blood pressure, dyslipidemia (increased triglycerides and lowered high-density lipoprotein cholesterol [HDL-C]), high fasting glucose concentration, and central obesity (Table 19-1).[18] Whereas obesity is an independent risk factor for CVD,[19] the complex interaction between excess body weight, lipid oxidation, and hyperglycemia underlies a strong connection between insulin resistance and risk for CVD. Efforts to prevent CVD must focus strongly on prevention of excess weight gain, insulin resistance, and dyslipidemia.[20]

OBESITY ASSESSMENT AND RISK OF CARDIOVASCULAR DISEASE

To stratify people in different demographic and ethnic groups according to their 10-year risk for coronary heart disease (CHD) events, clinicians use the Framingham risk score.[21] Guidelines recommend use of the Framingham risk score, or a modified version of it, to identify high-risk individuals (10-year risk >20%) who can benefit from aggressive risk reduction measures.[22-24] Although the Framingham risk score is widely used and highly valuable, it does not include

You can calculate BMI as follows

$$BMI = \frac{weight\ (kg)}{height\ squared\ (m^2)}$$

If pounds and inches are used

$$BMI = \frac{weight\ (pounds) \times 703}{height\ squared\ (inches^2)}$$

FIGURE 19-2 Diagnosis of overweight and obese: using body mass index (BMI). *(From* The Practical Guide: identification, evaluation, and treatment of overweight and obesity in adults, *Bethesda, Md, 2000, National Heart, Lung, and Blood Institute, Department of Health and Human Services. NIH publication 00-4084.)*

BOX 19-2 Standard Criteria for Body Mass Index

	BMI, kg/m^2
Underweight	18.5
Healthy weight	18.5-24.9
Overweight	25.0-29.9
Obese	30-39.9
Morbid obesity	≥40

---

measures of obesity or inflammation. This limits its clinical relevance in assessing intermediate risk for CHD.

Body mass index (BMI) is an important screening tool to assess patients with excess body weight and to stratify treatments according to the likelihood of underlying disease risk (Fig. 19-2).[25] BMI is calculated as weight in kilograms divided by height in meters squared (kg/m^2) and categorizes obesity into three classes: class I, BMI of 30 to 34.9; class II, BMI of 35 to 39.9; and class III, BMI ≥40, or extreme obesity (Box 19-2). Across genders and ethnicities, increased BMI is associated with larger comorbidity burden (Fig. 19-3).[26] BMI may provide a better determination of global disease risk than weight alone, but it is of limited diagnostic value in very muscular individuals and those with little muscle mass, such as elderly patients.[25,27]

Waist circumference as a measure of abdominal or central obesity has attracted particular attention because of its inclusion as a prerequisite for the diagnosis of metabolic syndrome.[11,28] It provides important additional prognostic information, especially when an unhealthy level of excessive adiposity is suspected.[25,27] A higher risk for diabetes, dyslipidemia, hypertension, and CVD has been associated with a waist circumference ≥102 cm (≥40 inches) in men and ≥88 cm (35 inches) in women (although the International Diabetes Federation[18] has specified lower cut points of ≥94 cm in men and ≥80 cm in women for European whites and ≥90 cm in men and ≥80 cm in women for certain Asian populations and for those of central or South American ancestry; Table 19-2). A study showed that either BMI or waist circumference independently predicted or was associated with type 2 diabetes.[29]

Unlike in definitions of obesity in adults, the growth curve needs to be taken into account in children.[13] The 2000 growth chart developed by the Centers for Disease Control and Prevention (CDC) is based on national height and weight data for children 2 to 19 years of age. The CDC and the National Heart, Lung, and Blood Institute (NHLBI) have defined obesity

in children as a BMI ≥95% on the 2000 growth chart and overweight as ≥85%. These cutoff points are arbitrary and, unlike adult definitions of overweight and obesity, are not based on health risk data.[13]

In the United States, 23 million adults with no history of CVD are classified as intermediate risk by the Framingham score (a 10-year risk for major CHD events of 10% to 20%).[30] New or emerging risk factors, particularly inflammatory markers and markers of atherosclerotic burden, offer promise as screening tools for these individuals.[24] However, current data from the U.S. Preventive Services Task Force conclude that there is sufficient evidence to recommend the use of high-sensitivity C-reactive protein (hsCRP) among initially intermediate-risk persons.[31] At the discretion of the physician, hsCRP measurements may help direct further evaluation and therapy in primary prevention of CVD.[32]

Childhood Obesity

Childhood obesity has wide-ranging comorbidities with clinical, psychosocial, and economic ramifications.[33] Children who are obese in their preschool years are more likely to be obese in adolescence and adulthood.[34] They are also more likely to develop diabetes, hypertension, hyperlipidemia, asthma, and sleep apnea.[34] Other risk factors for development of CVD and type 2 diabetes in children include a sedentary lifestyle, family history of type 2 diabetes, high low-density lipoprotein cholesterol (LDL-C) levels, hyperinsulinemia, insulin resistance, and high total cholesterol concentration.[35]

With the worldwide epidemic of childhood obesity, disorders once mainly found in adults, such as metabolic syndrome, are occurring in children.[36] The term *pediatric metabolic syndrome* includes a cluster of cardiovascular risk factors, such as insulin resistance, dyslipidemia (including increased triglycerides and decreased HDL-C), hypertension, and obesity. Children with metabolic syndrome have significantly higher BMI and glucose and triglyceride levels and lower HDL-C than do those without the syndrome.[35] Prevalence of the metabolic syndrome in obese children is reported at 30%.[37]

A study of 214 overweight and obese Costa Rican children up to 10 years of age found that obese children had lower mean serum levels of HDL-C and significantly higher mean serum concentrations of insulin, hsCRP, and triglycerides than their overweight peers did. They also had higher insulin resistance.[35]

Maffeis and colleagues[38] tested 1044 Italian children aged 6 to 11 years for blood pressure, serum triacylglycerides, total cholesterol, HDL-C, glucose, insulin, and alanine aminotransferase. The prevalence of high blood pressure in overweight boys and girls was 14.3% and 6.4%, respectively; in obese boys and girls, it was 40.4% and 32.8%, respectively. High blood pressure increased progressively with BMI z-score categories and waist-to-height ratio. Hypertensive children had significantly higher insulin and insulin resistance.

Adult Obesity

Because of its maladaptive effects on various cardiovascular risk factors and its adverse effects on cardiovascular structure and function, obesity has a major impact on cardiovascular diseases, such as heart failure, CHD, sudden cardiac death, and atrial fibrillation.[26,39] A large body of literature shows that obesity can cause and exacerbate many chronic diseases, such as diabetes, hypertension, dyslipidemia, stroke, and obstructive sleep apnea.[40] It more than doubles the risk of heart failure.[41]

Epidemiologic data suggest a linear relationship between BMI and CHD. Jee and coworkers[42] conducted an analysis of

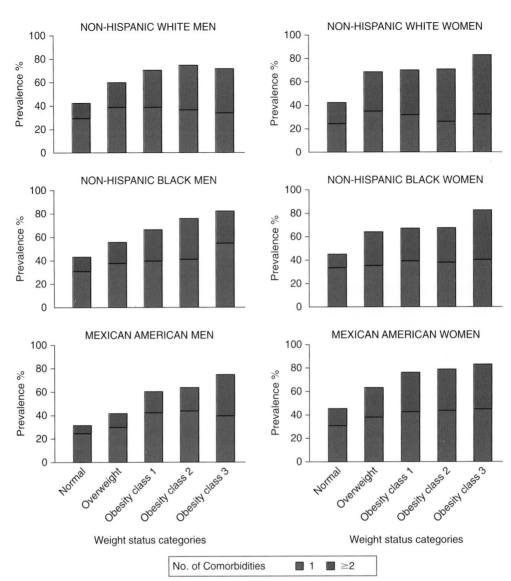

FIGURE 19-3 Prevalence of one and two or more overweight- and obesity-related morbidities by weight status category for sex, race, and ethnic subgroups. *(From Must A, Spadano J, Coakley EH, et al: The disease burden associated with overweight and obesity. JAMA 282:1523, 1999.)*

BMI and CHD incidence among 133,740 participants during 9 years of follow-up. The authors found that after adjustment for age, gender, and smoking status, each unit increase in BMI was associated with a 14% higher risk of incident CHD. Even a normal BMI of 24 to 24.9 was associated with a twofold increased risk of CHD.

A 20-year follow-up analysis of the Nurses' Health Study cohort showed a graded relationship between increasing BMI and incidence of CHD.[43] Compared with normal-weight women, the relative risk of CHD in overweight women was 1.43. For obese women, it was 2.44. In the Women's Health Initiative, overweight and obesity were significantly associated with CHD incidence in both white and black women.[44]

The Framingham Heart Study, which observed more than 5000 individuals for up to 44 years, also reported substantial cardiovascular risk linked to overweight and obesity.[45] One analysis found that overweight and obesity were independently associated with an increased risk for CVD as well as established risk factors, including hypertension, hypercholesterolemia, and type 2 diabetes.[45] A prospective study of more than 17,000 healthy female U.S. nurses with an average age of 50 years found that women who were obese at midlife were 79% less likely to be healthy at the age of 70 years

compared with those who were lean in their 40s and 50s. The odds of being healthy among those who were obese at the age of 18 years and then gained more than 22 pounds by middle age were reduced by 82%.[46]

RISK FACTORS

Visceral Adiposity

Data show that central obesity poses a more significant CVD risk than total obesity and that waist circumference[12] and waist-to-hip ratio, common surrogates for abdominal or central obesity, may be better predictors of atherosclerosis and CVD risk than BMI.[39,47-51] Adipose tissue, especially intra-abdominal visceral fat, has an independent endocrine function that leads to the release of inflammatory adipokines, including tumor necrosis factor-α, interleukin-6, and plasminogen activator inhibitor type 1.[12,52]

Inflammatory adipokines may increase insulin resistance and diabetes in obesity[52] and heighten risk for thrombosis.[12] They may also affect the progression of endothelial dysfunction, further increasing inflammation and the risk for

TABLE 19–2	Current Recommended Waist Circumference Thresholds for Abdominal Obesity by Organization		
		Recommended Waist Circumference Threshold for Abdominal Obesity	
	Organization	Men	Women
Europid	IDF	≥94 cm	≥80 cm
Caucasian	WHO	≥94 cm (increased)	≥80 cm (increased risk)
		≥102 cm (still higher risk)	≥88 cm (still higher risk)
United States	AHA/NHLBI (ATP III)*	≥102 cm	≥88 cm
Canada	Health Canada	≥102 cm	≥88 cm
European	European Cardiovascular Societies	≥102 cm	≥88 cm
Asian (including Japanese)	IDF	≥90 cm	≥80 cm
Asian	WHO	≥90 cm	≥80 cm
Japanese	Japanese Obesity Society	≥85 cm	≥90 cm
China	Cooperative Task Force	≥85 cm	≥80 cm
Middle East, Mediterranean	IDF	≥94 cm	≥80 cm
Sub-Saharan African	IDF	≥94 cm	≥80 cm
Ethnic Central and South American	IDF	≥90 cm	≥80 cm

*Recent AHA/NHLBI guidelines for metabolic syndrome recognize an increased risk for CVD and diabetes at waist circumference thresholds of ≥94 cm in men and ≥80 cm in women and identify these as optional cut points for individuals or populations with increased insulin resistance.

IDF, International Diabetes Federation; AHA/NHLBI, American Heart Association/National Heart, Lung, and Blood Institute; WHO, World Health Organization.

From Alberti KG, Eckel RH, Grundy SM, et al: Harmonizing the metabolic syndrome: a joint interim statement of the International Diabetes Federation Task Force on Epidemiology and Prevention; National Heart, Lung, and Blood Institute; American Heart Association; World Heart Federation; International Atherosclerosis Society; and International Association for the Study of Obesity. *Circulation* 120:1640, 2009.

atherosclerosis.[53] Free fatty acids, produced more readily in the visceral abdominal fat, may decrease insulin sensitivity, impair vascular reactivity, and also increase endothelial dysfunction.[53]

Low Birth Weight

The relationship between low birth weight and increased risk of obesity, hypertension, type 2 diabetes, stroke, and CVD later in life is well documented in epidemiologic studies.[54] These associations remain strong even after adjustment for such lifestyle factors as smoking, physical activity, occupation, dietary habits, and childhood socioeconomic status.[55]

A large number of studies have linked low birth weight to the later development of central adiposity.[55] A landmark cohort study of 300,000 men by Ravelli and coworkers[56] showed that exposure to the Dutch famine of 1944-1945 during the first half of pregnancy resulted in low birth weight associated with significantly higher obesity rates at the age of

19 years. Subsequent research has confirmed the relationship between low birth weight and later development of visceral or central adiposity[55,57] as well as metabolic syndrome[55] and higher blood pressure later in life.[54,58-60] Blood pressure is influenced by size at birth[61,62] as well as by weight gain in childhood.[63] Abnormalities are accompanied by functional changes in the vascular tree, and evidence of early alterations in vascular function has been described in children and adolescents with low birth weight.[61,64]

Hypertension

In 2003-2006, 36% of men and women between the ages of 45 and 54 years had hypertension compared with 65% of men and 80% of women 75 years of age and older.[1] Large differences in blood pressure by ethnic group exist among adults.[65] The National Health Interview Survey found that in 2007, 23% of U.S. adults had been told by a physician or health professional on two or more visits that they had hypertension.[66] The condition in adults is associated with increased risk of myocardial infarction, stroke, and cardiovascular mortality.[67] Hypertension often increases with rising body weight.[68,69] It also affects 1% to 5% of children and adolescents.[70] The condition increases progressively with higher BMI and can be detected in approximately 30% of overweight children (BMI >95th percentile).[71]

In a cross-sectional study of 710 subjects aged 20 to 25 years, Dimkpa and Oij[69] found a significant correlation between BMI and systolic and diastolic blood pressure and resting heart rate after controlling for age and physical activity status. Overweight and obese subjects had a significantly higher risk of hypertension than non-overweight or obese controls did, and the prevalence of hypertension and tachycardia rose with increases in BMI.[69]

Like adults, children and adolescents with severe elevation of blood pressure are at risk of adverse outcomes including cerebrovascular accidents and congestive heart failure.[67] Two autopsy studies in adolescents and young adults found significant relationships between the level of blood pressure and the presence of atherosclerotic lesions in the aorta and coronary arteries.[72,73] Childhood levels of blood pressure are also associated with carotid intima-media thickness,[74] large artery compliance,[75] decreased brachial artery flow-mediated vasodilation,[76] and left ventricular hypertrophy at a level associated with a fourfold greater risk of adverse cardiovascular outcomes in adults.[67] Overweight and high blood pressure are also components of metabolic syndrome, a condition of multiple metabolic risk factors for CVD as well as type 2 diabetes.[11] These outcomes underscore the need to prevent obesity early in life to protect against future life-threatening consequences.[69]

Sleep Apnea

Obstructive sleep apnea is independently associated with increased cardiovascular risk.[77] It has also been linked to insulin resistance and glucose intolerance and is independently associated with impaired glycemic control[77] and type 2 diabetes in patients who report excessive sleepiness.[78] Obstructive sleep apnea is strongly correlated with intra-abdominal fat,[79,80] and serum lipid levels are elevated in patients who have obstructive sleep apnea.[81] Prospective findings from up to 15 years of follow-up data from the Wisconsin Sleep Cohort Study indicate that untreated sleep apnea predicts increases in blood pressure, hypertension, stroke, depression, and mortality.[82]

Obesity causes and exacerbates obstructive sleep apnea,[40,80] and increases in weight have been associated with a rising prevalence of obstructive sleep apnea. Data show a fourfold rise in obstructive sleep apnea with each increase in the standard deviation of BMI.[80] In patients with class II and class III obesity, obstructive sleep apnea is common.[80] Lopez and colleagues[83] found the prevalence of obstructive sleep apnea to be greater than 70% in those with class II and class III obesity and more than 90% in patients with a BMI ≥60.

A population-based prospective cohort study from 1989-2000 found that a 10% weight gain predicted an approximate 32% increase in the apnea-hypopnea index and a sixfold rise in the risk for development of moderate to severe obstructive sleep apnea.[84] The Sleep Heart Health Study showed a similar relationship between BMI and obstructive sleep apnea severity; the odds ratio for moderate to severe obstructive sleep apnea was 1.6 for each standard deviation increment in BMI.[85]

Dyslipidemia

Atherogenic dyslipidemia is associated with an increased risk of CVD, peripheral vascular disease, and stroke.[86,87] The condition is characterized by elevated triglycerides and low plasma levels of HDL-C,[88] often with elevated apolipoprotein B and non–HDL-C. It is prevalent in patients with type 2 diabetes, metabolic syndrome, or established CVD.[89]

Obesity heightens the risk of type 2 diabetes, hypertension, CVD, and dyslipidemia and reduces average life expectancy.[90,91] Metabolic syndrome is closely associated with obesity and a clustering of CVD risk factors, including a dyslipidemia characterized by high levels of triglycerides and LDL-C and low levels of HDL-C, a combination that significantly increases the relative risk of cardiovascular or cerebrovascular events.[92] Triglycerides, HDL-C, and LDL-C, the components of atherogenic dyslipidemia, are interrelated, and each predicts CHD risk.[88]

Individuals with obesity and metabolic syndrome present with increased concentrations of very-low-density lipoprotein (VLDL) particles, increased triglycerides and small-particle LDL, increased LDL particle number, and decreased HDL particle size.[12] These lipoproteins can undergo a process of oxidation that results in the formation of foam cells and enhanced monocyte binding, which leads to the early stages of atherosclerotic plaque. Small-particle LDL has greater atherogenic potential[93] and is more common in individuals with diabetes.[94] As risk indicators, total cholesterol/HDL and LDL/HDL ratios have greater predictive value than isolated parameters used independently, particularly LDL.[93]

Elevated triglyceride concentrations are associated with greater circulating numbers of triglyceride-rich VLDL particles and higher levels of VLDL cholesterol, an environment that alters the metabolism of LDL-C and HDL-C and contributes to atherogenic potential.[93] Atherogenic dyslipidemia, characterized by elevated triglycerides and low levels of HDL-C, often with elevated apolipoprotein B and non–HDL-C, is common in patients with established CVD, type 2 diabetes, or metabolic syndrome and contributes to both macrovascular and microvascular residual risk.[90]

Extensive evidence from large prospective clinical trials involving patients at different levels of risk shows that lipid and lipid protein abnormalities are responsible for residual CVD risk in patients receiving statin therapy.[95] A recent meta-analysis including 90,056 subjects (18,686 with diabetes) from 14 randomized trials reported that for each millimole per liter decrease in LDL-C, statin therapy reduced the risk of major vascular events by 21%. Nonetheless, 14% of patients in the statin group suffered a cardiovascular event compared with 18% randomized to placebo.[96,97]

The importance of dyslipidemia as a major contributor to CVD risk is underscored by the INTERHEART study,[98] a global case-control trial in 52 countries, in which dyslipidemia was responsible for 54% of population attributable risk for myocardial infarction. Extensive evidence supports elevated triglycerides and low HDL-C levels as predictors for CVD, independent of LDL-C.[90] Observational trials, such as the Prospective Cardiovascular Münster (PROCAM) study, have reported a clear prognostic inverse relation between HDL-C levels and coronary artery disease morbidity and mortality, regardless of LDL-C levels.[99] These outcomes reflect the need to identify ways to optimize management of patients with metabolic disorders, such as diabetes, obesity, and dyslipidemia.

Diabetes

CVD affects millions of adults with diabetes and is a major cause of morbidity and mortality. Evidence indicates that the CVD burden among diabetics is increasing. Between 1997 and 2007, those aged 35 years or older with diabetes and a diagnosed CVD condition (i.e., CHD, stroke, or other heart condition) increased from approximately 4 million to almost 6 million.[100] Between 1994 and 2007, there were also unfavorable upward trends in the age-adjusted percentage of obesity in adults with diabetes, an increase from 34.9% to 53.0%.[101] During that same period, the percentage of overweight or obese adults with diabetes increased from 70% to 83%.[102]

Obesity clearly increases the risk for development of type 2 diabetes; inflammatory adipokines may also play a role.[12] Large population studies have confirmed the links between excess weight and the development of insulin resistance and type 2 diabetes.[12] In the Nurses' Health Study, which observed close to 85,000 female nurses, a BMI ≥25 was the single most important factor for the development of type 2 diabetes during a 16-year period.[103]

A 20-year follow-up study of ethnicity, obesity, and risk of type 2 diabetes in a Nurses' Health Study cohort of 78,419 apparently healthy women found that for each 5-unit increment in BMI, the multivariate relative risk of diabetes was 2.36 for Asians, 2.21 for Hispanics, 1.96 for whites, and 1.55 for blacks. For each 5-kg weight gain between the age of 18 years and the year 1980, the risk of diabetes increased by 84% for Asians, 44% for Hispanics, 38% for blacks, and 37% for whites.[104]

A study of 91,246 patients in 27 European countries investigated the impact of adiposity on the frequency of diabetes and CVD. Data showed that waist circumference predicted increased age- and BMI-adjusted risks of CVD and diabetes. In women, odds ratios for CVD per 1 SD increase in waist circumference were 1.28 in northwest Europe, 1.26 in southern Europe, and 1.10 in eastern Europe. Values for diabetes were 1.72, 1.45, and 1.59. Despite regional differences in cardiovascular risk factors and CVD rates, abdominal obesity had a similar impact on the frequency of diabetes across Europe. The authors concluded that increasing abdominal obesity may offset future declines in CVD, even where CVD rates are lower.[105]

Diabetes is a serious weight-related condition in adolescents. The incidence of type 2 diabetes in this age group has increased in tandem with obesity, rising by a factor of more than 10 in the past two decades.[106] This trend in children and adolescents is accelerating in both developed and developing countries.[107] As the prevalence of obesity increases, its health implications are becoming more evident. The earliest alterations are abnormalities in glucose metabolism that can lead to type 2 diabetes.[107]

In adults, the likelihood of the progression of patients with impaired glucose tolerance or impaired fasting glucose to diabetes is 25% during 3 to 5 years.[108] The only longitudinal study published thus far on the natural history of normal and impaired glucose tolerance in children and adolescents showed that children with impaired glucose tolerance who had greater degrees of obesity at baseline and those who continued to gain weight rapidly developed type 2 diabetes.[109] Smaller studies of at-risk populations also suggest a high likelihood of progression to type 2 diabetes.[109] Preliminary data from Canada indicate that adolescents with type 2 diabetes will be at high risk for limb amputation, kidney failure requiring dialysis, and premature death.[106]

The SEARCH for Diabetes in Youth study[110] found significant ethnic variations in the prevalence of type 2 diabetes in children aged 10 to 19 years. The disease accounted for only 6% of all diabetic cases diagnosed in non-Hispanic whites compared with 22% of all diabetic cases diagnosed in Hispanics. In American Indians, type 2 diabetes has overtaken type 1 in prevalence among children, accounting for 72% of all cases of diabetes. Data for this study were obtained largely through chart review and may underestimate the prevalence of type 2 diabetes. As the ethnic diversity of the U.S. population continues to increase, the epidemic of childhood obesity may make pediatric type 2 diabetes a growing public health concern.[13]

EFFECT OF WEIGHT LOSS ON OBESITY COMORBIDITIES

Losing weight has proven benefits on established risk factors for CVD, including diabetes, hypertension, and dyslipidemia (Fig. 19-4).[111] The Look AHEAD (Action for Health in Diabetes) study, a National Institutes of Health–funded clinical trial conducted in 5145 overweight or obese adults with type 2 diabetes, investigated the effectiveness of intentional weight loss in reducing CVD events. At 1 year, participants in the intensive lifestyle intervention group achieved an average weight loss of 8.6% of initial body weight and a 21% improvement in cardiovascular fitness. The intensive lifestyle intervention was associated with an increase from 46% to 73% of participants who met the American Diabetes Association (ADA) goal of A1c <7% and a doubling in the percentage of individuals who met all three of the ADA goals for glycemic control, hypertension, and dyslipidemia.[112]

Weight loss also improves obstructive sleep apnea, strengthening the causal relationship with obesity.[80] In a large, population-based prospective cohort study of 690 people, a 10% weight loss was correlated with a 26% decrease in the apnea-hypopnea index, showing that even minimal weight loss can be beneficial in patients with obstructive sleep apnea.[84] A randomized study of the effect of a low-calorie diet and supervised lifestyle counseling on sleep-disordered breathing produced a 40% decrease in apnea-hypopnea index from baseline. At 3-month follow-up, 61% of the patients in the intervention group were considered cured of sleep apnea compared with 32% in the control group. Changes in apnea-hypopnea index were strongly correlated with changes in weight and waist circumference and were maintained at 1-year follow-up.[113] Data indicate that not only is obesity a risk factor for development of obstructive sleep apnea, it may also be a consequence of obstructive sleep apnea, a finding that emphasizes the importance of treating both disorders.[80]

Previous meta-analyses of clinical trials on the effects of weight reduction on blood pressure show that weight loss is important in the prevention and treatment of hypertension.[114] In the Diabetes Prevention Program, a 2.8-year follow-up found that weight loss was about 5.6 kg in the lifestyle management arm, 2.1 kg in the metformin arm, and 0.1 in the placebo group. There was a small significant decrease of 3.3 mm Hg in systolic blood pressure and a decline of 3.1 mm Hg in diastolic blood pressure in the lifestyle management group, suggesting that at least in the short term, weight loss was associated with some degree of decrease in blood pressure.[115-117]

PREMIER, an NHLBI-sponsored multicenter randomized trial of 810 adults with prehypertension or stage 1 hypertension, compared the effect of advice only with established lifestyle interventions (e.g., weight loss, dietary changes, and increased physical activity) for blood pressure control. The two intervention groups, established lifestyle interventions and established lifestyle interventions plus the DASH diet, reduced estimated 10-year CHD risk by 14% and 12%, respectively.[118] Other investigations have reported a linear association between changes in systolic blood pressure and weight, even with a small amount of weight loss. They have also documented that weight loss is the most important determinant of decreases in systolic blood pressure.[119,120]

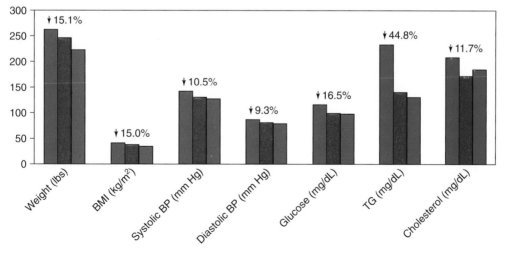

FIGURE 19-4 Effect of moderate weight loss on cardiometabolic risk factors. (From Case CC, Jones PH, Nelson K, et al: Impact of weight loss on the metabolic syndrome. Diabetes Obes Metab 4:407, 2002.)

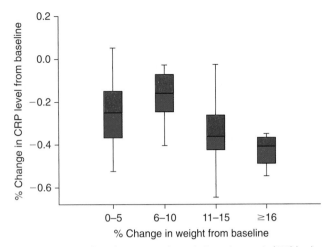

FIGURE 19-5 Box plots of percentage change in C-reactive protein (CRP) level from baseline over categories of percentage change in weight from baseline across all included weight loss interventions. *(From Selvin E, Paynter NP, Erlinger TP: The effect of weight loss on C-reactive protein: a systematic review.* Arch Intern Med *167:31, 2007.)*

19

Weight loss in overweight adolescents is also associated with a decrease in blood pressure[67] as well as with reduced sensitivity of blood pressure to salt and other cardiovascular risk factors, such as dyslipidemia and insulin resistance.[121] In studies that reduce BMI by about 10%, short-term reductions in blood pressure were in the range of 8 to 12 mm Hg. An analysis of 33 weight loss interventions found that for each 1 kg of weight loss, the mean change in CRP level was −0.13 mg/L, suggesting that weight loss is an effective non-pharmacologic strategy for lowering of serum CRP levels (Fig. 19-5).[122] Although difficult, weight loss, if it is successful, is extremely effective.[67,121]

Despite these findings, application of data from observational trials must be carefully considered. Numerous studies have documented an obesity paradox in which overweight and obese individuals with established CVD (including hypertension, heart failure, CHD, and peripheral arterial disease) have a better prognosis compared with patients who are not overweight or obese.[39] Conversely, patients with a healthy weight BMI (18.5 to 24.9 kg/m²) and high body fat are at high risk for cardiometabolic dysregulation, metabolic syndrome, and CVD.

These findings, however, are controversial.[123] Data assessing mortality based on body fat and lean mass rather than on BMI or weight alone have shown that subjects who lose body fat rather than lean mass have a lower mortality.[124] Estimates for all-cause mortality, obesity-related causes of death, and other causes of death showed no statistically significant or systematic differences between BMI and other variables.[125] Although an obesity paradox exists with use of either baseline BMI or baseline percentage fat criteria, studies support the safety and potential long-term benefits of purposeful weight loss in overweight and obese patients with CHD.[39,126]

TREATMENT OPTIONS

Lifestyle Interventions: Diet, Behavioral Modification, and Exercise

A study examined the risk of CHD associated with excess weight in 42,351 men from the Health Professionals Follow-up Study and 76,703 women from the Nurses' Health study. A total of 2771 incident cases of CHD among the men and 2359 among the women were documented during 16 years of follow-up. Overall, the relative risk of CHD associated with a BMI ≥30 compared with a BMI of 18.5 to 22.9 was 2.13 among men and 2.48 among women. The risk of CHD increased with BMI, with and without hypercholesterolemia, hypertension, or diabetes. The authors estimated that more than a third of all incident CHD in U.S. men and women may be attributed to excess weight.[127]

Sedentary lifestyles and poor physical fitness are major contributors to the current obesity and CVD pandemic.[128] Thus, the main treatments of overweight and obesity include dietary changes, increases in physical activity, and other behavioral modifications. Technology-based approaches have also started to emerge.[129] Whichever approach is used, regular activity and appropriate energy intake play critical roles in prevention and management of the negative health consequences of diabetes, obesity, and other cardiovascular diseases.[130]

Nutrition remains a cornerstone of the effort to prevent CVD. Risk for heart disease can be minimized by adopting healthy eating patterns early in life and establishing life-long dietary habits of avoiding excess saturated fat, *trans*-fat, and salt.[131] Dietary changes can also improve CVD risk factors. For prevention of CVD and CVD risk factors, dietary choices that improve the overall quality of the diet are preferred to specific dietary components. The American Heart Association recommends that individuals consume a variety of fruits, vegetables, and grain products, especially whole grains. It also recommends fat-free and low-fat dairy products, legumes, poultry, and lean meats as well as fish, preferably oily fish, at least twice a week.[132] These foods should replace less nutrient dense ones to prevent weight gain associated with additional calorie consumption.

The "whole diet" approach greatly increases the odds of achieving a "prudent diet," characterized by a high intake of vegetables, fruits, legumes, fish, poultry, and whole grains. In a large, 18-year prospective study of 72,113 women, greater adherence to the prudent pattern was related to a lower risk of cardiovascular and total mortality. In contrast, greater adherence to the Western pattern (i.e., high intake of red and processed meat, refined grains, French fries, and sweets and desserts) was linked to a higher risk of CVD, cancer, and total mortality.[133]

The optimal balance of macronutrients for weight loss and weight loss maintenance is a topic of much debate. A 2009 study found that macronutrient composition had a negligible effect on 2-year weight loss outcomes in a cohort of overweight adults.[134] Instead, compliance with calorie restriction and counseling session attendance were strongly correlated with weight loss and, consequently, a reduction in risk for CVD and diabetes. Nevertheless, fat intake should be of particular concern in any lifestyle intervention. Consumption of diets rich in saturated fatty acids is highly correlated with metabolic syndrome and an increased expression of genes involved in inflammation processes in adipose tissue.[135,136] Whereas high-fat, high-protein, low-carbohydrate diets have been associated with short-term improvement in LDL-C, HDL-C, and blood pressure, recent evidence suggests that this diet profile can elevate risk of CVD without altering classic CVD risk factors. Instead, high-fat, high-protein diets can elevate circulating nonesterified fatty acids and suppress endothelial progenitor cell production, thereby increasing arterial plaque buildup (Fig. 19-6).[119,137]

Insulin resistance due to atherogenic dyslipidemia in skeletal muscle may be the primary driving force in the development of the metabolic syndrome.[138] Chronically elevated serum free fatty acids could lead to further metabolic complications and morbidity. The National Cholesterol Education Program's Adult Treatment Panel III report recommendations for diet composition for patients with metabolic

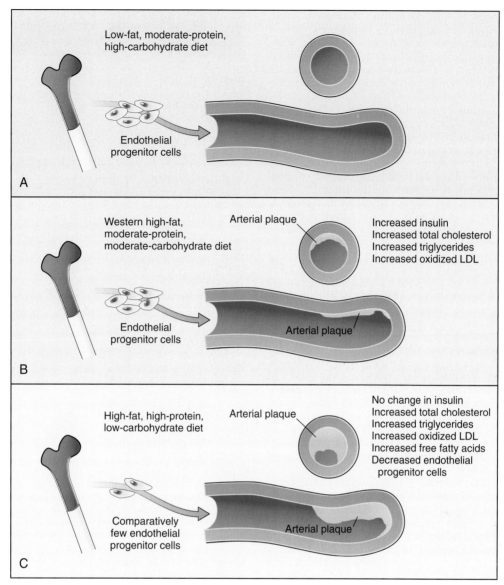

FIGURE 19-6 High-protein, low-carbohydrate diet and atherosclerosis. *(From Smith SR: A look at the low-carbohydrate diet. N Engl J Med 361:2286, 2009.)*

syndrome call for low intake of saturated fats, *trans*-fats, and cholesterol; reduced consumption of simple sugars; and increased intake of fruits, vegetables, and whole grains.[139] Low-fat diets, such as the one used in the Women's Intervention Nutrition Study, have been implemented in the long term to successfully reduce disease risk.[140] In a cohort of patients from the Framingham Offspring Cohort, the consumption of a diet consistent with the principles of the Mediterranean-style diet was associated with protection against metabolic syndrome.[141]

Data also show that replacement of saturated fats with omega-6 polyunsaturated fatty acids can lower risk for heart disease events by 24%.[142] An emphasis on monounsaturated fatty acids in the diet can lead to better inflammatory gene expression profiles, decreases in serum LDL-C concentrations, and an increase in plasma and adipose tissue oleic acid content.[136] *Trans*–fatty acids adversely affect both LDL-C and HDL-C levels and increase the risk for CHD, even at low levels of dietary intake.[143,144] Elimination of exposure to *trans*–fatty acids could have a powerful population impact, potentially protecting 30,000 to 100,000 Americans from death related to heart disease.[143,144]

In general, comprehensive lifestyle modification programs delivered in person induce a loss of approximately 10% of initial weight in 16 to 26 weeks of treatment.[145] Combined with energy restriction, dietary changes can increase weight loss, prevent weight regain, and reduce risk of death related to heart disease.[146] The use of portion-controlled food, which typically involves meal replacement products,[25] has been associated with medically significant weight loss. Energy restriction can, however, have negative consequences if fat-free mass is metabolized along with adipose tissue. Reductions in fat-free mass can reduce basal energy expenditure because of losses in metabolically active lean tissues.[147,148] Therefore, dietary programs that support fat-free mass maintenance and skeletal muscle biogenesis are advisable. Low-protein, calorie-restricted diets are associated with increased loss of fat-free mass.[149] Conversely, higher protein diets can preserve fat-free mass and improve blood lipid profiles.[150]

Behavioral treatment is widely acknowledged as an essential component of effective lifestyle interventions. Traditional behavioral counseling models have assumed that patients and clients will change behavior simply by learning the facts about diet and exercise. There are, however, significant limitations to this counseling strategy.[131] Additional emphasis is needed on ways to implement current guidelines in a contemporary society characterized by wide availability of unhealthy, energy-dense food and stressful lifestyles. In this sense, it may be more important to focus on barriers to implementation before providing specific nutrition counseling.

Self-monitoring, stimulus control, exercise, and cognitive restructuring represent four key components of behavioral modification.[151] Some evidence suggests that the ability to balance the immediate gratification of appetizing, energy-dense foods with their long-term consequences on weight and health may be dependent on the functional capacity of cognitive-emotional processing systems in the brain.[152] These neurocognitive resources may also be critical for maintenance of eating-related goals, cognitive control of eating behavior, and suppression of automatic biases toward food-related stimuli.[152,153]

Group sessions led by registered dietitians or behavioral psychologists are an effective venue for delivery of behavior therapy. These sessions also provide a combination of social support and friendly competition. Web-based programs represent a new frontier for behavioral treatment in obesity medicine as a low-cost and wide-reaching alternative to on-site treatment. Online programs could facilitate ongoing patient-provider contact, a key factor for long-term weight control.[154]

Regular physical activity is an essential component of primary prevention of CVD and obesity.[155] Federal guidelines now recommend exercise for both prevention of disease and improvement of health.[156] Physical activity and exercise both have positive effects on maintenance and promotion of healthy body weight.[146] In the Look AHEAD trial, greater self-reported physical activity was the strongest correlate of weight loss after 1 year.[157]

Most public health guidelines recommend that adults participate in 30 minutes of moderate-intensity physical activity on most days of the week.[158] Aerobic endurance training is effective for improving maximum oxygen uptake and modifying cardiovascular risk factors associated with the development of coronary artery disease.[159] Resistance training, which has long been touted for its strength-enhancing effects, has recently been recognized for its relationship to health and disease risk.[159,160] Moderate- to high-intensity resistance training performed 2 or 3 days per week is associated with improvements in CVD risk factors in the absence of significant weight loss.[146,160,161] The addition of a muscle strengthening exercise program to a weight loss intervention may help conserve fat-free mass and basal energy expenditure and facilitate weight loss maintenance.[162] When it is paired with regular aerobic physical activity, resistance training may represent a feasible exercise intervention to promote healthy body composition and to prevent excess adiposity[163] (Table 19-3).[160] Even among those in the pre-obese range, vigorous physical activity can decrease risk of heart failure.[164]

Guidelines for glycemic control have become controversial. When levels are set too low (e.g., hemoglobin A1c levels as low as 6.5% to 7%), they burden patients with complex treatment programs, hypoglycemia, weight gain, and costs. A review of large randomized trials in patients with type 2 diabetes suggests uncertain benefits and the need for a different approach—one that prioritizes well-being, healthy lifestyles, preventive care, and cardiovascular risk reduction.[165] Important challenges also remain in preventing weight regain after weight loss interventions.[25]

Weight Loss Surgery

Bariatric surgery is associated with significant weight loss and improvement in diabetes, hypertension, and obstructive

| TABLE 19–3 | Comparison of Effects of Aerobic Endurance Training with Strength Training on Health and Fitness Variables |

Variable	Aerobic Exercise	Resistance Exercise
Body composition		
Bone mineral density	↑↑	↑↑
Percentage body fat	↓↓	↓
Lean body mass	0	↑↑
Muscle strength	0↑	↑↑↑
Glucose metabolism		
Insulin response to glucose challenge	↓↓	↓↓
Basal insulin levels	↓	↓
Insulin sensitivity	↑↑	↑↑
Plasma lipids and lipoproteins		
HDL-C	↑0	↑0
LDL-C	↓0	↓0
Triglycerides	↓↓	↓0
Cardiovascular dynamics		
Resting heart rate	↓↓	0
Stroke volume, resting and maximal	↑↑	0
Cardiac output, rest	0	0
Cardiac output, maximal	↑↑	0
Systolic blood pressure at rest	↓0	0
Diastolic blood pressure at rest	↓0	0
Vo₂max	↑↑↑	↑0
Submaximal and maximal endurance time	↑↑↑	↑↑
Submaximal exercise rate-pressure product	↓↓↓	↓↓
Basal metabolic rate	↑0	↑
Health-related quality of life	↑0	↑0

↑, values increase; ↓, values decrease; 0, values remain unchanged; 1 arrow, small effect; 2 arrows, moderate effects; 3 arrows, large effect; HDL-C, high-density lipoprotein cholesterol; LDL-C, low-density lipoprotein cholesterol.

Williams MA, Haskell WL, Ades PA, et al: Resistance exercise in individuals with and without cardiovascular disease: 2007 update: a scientific statement from the American Heart Association Council on Clinical Cardiology and Council on Nutrition, Physical Activity, and Metabolism. *Circulation* 116:572, 2007.

sleep apnea.[166] It remains the most effective tool for the durable reversal of type 2 diabetes.[167] A substantial body of literature shows that it achieves significant long-term weight loss with minimal mortality or complications.[168,169] Studies also indicate that weight loss surgery confers a survival advantage on those who undergo it compared with community controls.[170,171] Landmark findings from the Swedish Obese Subjects study show an estimated 28% reduction in the adjusted overall mortality rate compared with conventionally treated controls.[172] Similar outcomes have been cited in other reports.[168]

Weight loss surgery reduces calorie intake by modifying the anatomy of the gastrointestinal tract through restriction, malabsorption, or a combination of the two techniques.[168] Ensuing changes in the gut-brain axis alter peptides that may regulate appetite and satiety[173] (e.g., ghrelin, glucagon-like peptide, and pancreatic polypeptide). Among several competing approaches for the management of severe obesity, the general trend is toward combined restrictive-malabsorptive procedures, such as gastric bypass and biliopancreatic diversion.[138]

In the United States, laparoscopic Roux-en-Y gastric bypass is the most effective procedure for weight loss and is considered the "gold standard" operation for long-term weight control.[168] It accounts for more than 90% of all bariatric operations. Laparoscopic adjustable gastric banding is the second most commonly performed procedure.[168] Data show that laparoscopic sleeve gastrectomy, which is becoming popular as a stand-alone operation for the treatment of severe obesity and related diseases,[174] is safe and effective, with

19

TABLE 19–4 | **Efficacy and Safety of Weight Loss Medications**

Medication	FDA Approval Year and Intended Use	Action	Weight Loss Pooled Data (placebo corrected)	Length of Treatment	Common Side Effects
Phentermine	1959 Short-term weight loss	Sympathomimetic amine	−3.6 kg	2-24 weeks	Palpitations, tachycardia, elevated blood pressure, gastrointestinal effects
Orlistat	1999 Long-term weight loss	Lipase inhibitor	−2.75 kg	52 weeks	Diarrhea, flatulence, bloating
Sibutramine	1998 Long-term weight loss	Lipase inhibitor	−4.45 kg	52 weeks	Increased blood pressure, increased pulse, dry mouth, insomnia, constipation
Bupropion	1985 Antidepressant; smoking cessation	Weight loss may be due to inhibition of norepinephrine and dopamine uptake	−2.77 kg	24-52 weeks	Dry mouth, diarrhea, constipation, insomnia
Topiramate	1996 Seizure disorder	Weight loss mechanism unknown	−6.5%	24 weeks	Paresthesia, taste aversion
Zonisamide*	2000 Seizure disorder	Weight loss mechanism unknown	−5.0%	16 weeks	Fatigue; small, but insignificant increase in serum creatine
Metformin†	1994 Diabetes mellitus	Insulin sensitizer; suppresses hepatic glucose production	2.0 kg	146 weeks	Gastrointestinal

From Aronne LJ, Wadden T, Isoldi KK, Woodworth KA: When prevention fails: obesity treatment strategies. *Am J Med* 122(Suppl 1):S24, 2009.
*Data obtained from only one trail.
†Data obtained from the Diabetes Prevention Program Trial; individuals with impaired fasting glucose were treated with drug.

results similar to those of gastric bypass.[175] Investigational treatments include intragastric balloon, gastric pacing, and endoluminal interventions.

A recent systematic review[169] summed up the risks and benefits of weight loss surgery. Comorbidities in all groups improved after procedures. Statistically fewer people had metabolic syndrome, and there was higher remission of type 2 diabetes than in nonsurgical groups. In one large cohort study, the incidence of three of six comorbidities assessed 10 years after surgery was significantly reduced compared with conventional treatment. Mortality ranged from none to 10%. Major postoperative adverse events, some necessitating reoperation, included anastomosis leakage, pneumonia, pulmonary embolism, band slippage, and band erosion.

Pharmacotherapy

In a great number of patients who are unable to reduce weight by nonpharmacologic measures, drug therapy can help them reach weight control goals. However, drug treatment should be considered only part of a systematic weight management program that includes dietary and lifestyle changes.[176] *The Practical Guide: Identification, Evaluation, and Treatment of Overweight and Obesity in Adults* recommends pharmacotherapy for patients with cardiometabolic risk and a BMI of 27 to 29.9 or those with a BMI ≥30.[177]

Available pharmacologic options for weight loss that are approved by the Food and Drug Administration (FDA) are limited to anorexiants (e.g., phentermine); orlistat, a lipase inhibitor; and sibutramine, a drug that works by acting on appetite control centers in the brain (Table 19-4).[25,178] Agents approved for other uses, such as antidepressants, have promoted weight loss in preliminary clinical trials. These include bupropion, a drug approved as an antidepressant and smoking cessation aid[179]; topiramate, a therapy approved for migraine prevention and the treatment of seizures[180]; and exenatide, a novel incretin mimetic approved by the FDA for adjunctive therapy to improve glycemic control in patients with type 2

diabetes.[181] Cetilistat, an oral, nonabsorbed synthetic lipase inhibitor, has reached the phase III trial stage of development.[4,182] However, rimonabant, a cannabinoid 1 receptor antagonist that showed efficacy in producing clinically meaningful weight loss, has been withdrawn from the market because of safety concerns.[183]

Emerging data from recently completed and ongoing randomized clinical trials suggest that certain combination drug therapies in development may have greater efficacy than currently available single-drug therapies in terms of weight loss and reduction in risk factors.[179] These drugs include Contrave, a combination of bupropion and the opioid antagonist naltrexone,[184,185] and pramlintide/metreleptin, a novel, integrated neurohormonal approach that combines amylin and leptin.[186]

CONCLUSION

Currently, one third of children and two thirds of adults are overweight or obese; this trend has persisted for the last two decades and shows no sign of abatement.[2,4] Obesity tracks from childhood into adulthood, with serious medical and economic consequences throughout the life course.[187] One recent estimate suggests that if the current trend continues, obesity will account for more than $860 billion or more than 16% of health care expenditures in the United States by 2030.[188] Another projects that by 2035, the prevalence of CHD will increase by a range of 5% to 16%, with more than 100,000 excess cases of CHD attributable to increased adolescent obesity.[189]

To date, most public health strategies to address obesity have focused on efforts targeted to individuals, such as health education and behavioral skills training. However, these have turned out to be largely ineffective and unsustainable.[187] Similarly, the majority of research on obesity prevention has ignored the combined effect of larger societal and political factors in perpetuating the obesity crisis. The lack of success in stopping the spread of obesity underscores the need for a new approach that takes into account the sociopolitical, economic, and environmental forces that interact to create an obesogenic environment.

Individual choice is strongly influenced by the interaction of forces that take place at multiple socioenvironmental levels.[190] These include interpersonal (family, peers, and social networks), community (schools, worksites, and institutions), governmental (local, state, and national policies), and biologic processes (genes, molecular and cellular interactions, and the workings of major organ systems).[190] Change at all of these levels is required to replace unhealthful social norms of diet and physical activity, to increase access to and availability of fresh fruits and vegetables, to provide opportunities for physical activity, and to promote a culture that values and encourages preventive care.[191]

Reliance on free markets and free choice has failed to stem the obesity crisis. Investment in integrated, cross-disciplinary research is required, as are multilevel efforts to address social, economic, and environmental factors that create and sustain the conditions fostering obesity. A multilevel strategy rooted in a socioecologic framework is consistent with the World Health Organization's work on social determinants of health.[192] We already know what needs to be done. The question is whether we have the political will to change policies and practices that undermine public health.

Acknowledgment

The authors acknowledge Rita Buckley for substantive contributions in the research and writing of this article.

REFERENCES

1. Health, United States, 2008 with chartbook, Hyattsville, Md, 2009, National Center for Health Statistics.
2. Ogden CL, Carroll MD, McDowell MA, Flegal KD; Division of Health Nutrition Examination Surveys: *Obesity among adults in the United States—no statistically significant change since 2003-2004, NCHS data brief no. 1*, Hyattsville, Md, 2007, National Center for Health Statistics.
3. Ogden CL, Carroll MD, Curtin LR, et al: Prevalence of overweight and obesity in the United States, 1999-2004. *JAMA* 295:1549, 2006.
4. Ogden CL, Carroll MD, Flegal KM: High body mass index for age among US children and adolescents, 2003-2006. *JAMA* 299:2401, 2008.
5. Wang Y, Beydoun MA: The obesity epidemic in the United States—gender, age, socioeconomic, racial/ethnic, and geographic characteristics: a systematic review and meta-regression analysis. *Epidemiol Rev* 29:6, 2007.
6. Flegal KM, Graubard BI, Williamson DF, Gail MH: Cause-specific excess deaths associated with underweight, overweight, and obesity. *JAMA* 298:2028, 2007.
7. Rosamond W, Flegal K, Furie K, et al: Heart disease and stroke statistics—2008 update: a report from the American Heart Association Statistics Committee and Stroke Statistics Subcommittee. *Circulation* 117:e25, 2008.
8. Ford ES, Li C, Zhao G, et al: Trends in the prevalence of low risk factor burden for cardiovascular disease among United States adults. *Circulation* 120:1181, 2009.
9. van Dam RM, Willett WC: Unmet potential for cardiovascular disease prevention in the United States. *Circulation* 120:1171, 2009.
10. Lau DC, Dhillon B, Yan H, et al: Adipokines: molecular links between obesity and atherosclerosis. *Am J Physiol Heart Circ Physiol* 288:H2031, 2005.
11. Hu FB: *Obesity epidemiology*, New York, 2008, Oxford University Press.
12. Brown WV, Fujioka K, Wilson PW, Woodworth KA: Obesity: why be concerned? *Am J Med* 122(Suppl 1):S4, 2009.
13. McCall A, Raj R: Exercise for prevention of obesity and diabetes in children and adolescents. *Clin Sports Med* 28:393, 2009.
14. Libby P: Vascular biology of atherosclerosis: overview and state of the art. *Am J Cardiol* 91:3A, 2003.
15. Eckel RH, Grundy SM, Zimmet PZ: The metabolic syndrome. *Lancet* 365:1415, 2005.
16. Korner J, Woods SC, Woodworth KA: Regulation of energy homeostasis and health consequences in obesity. *Am J Med* 122(Suppl 1):S12, 2009.
17. Frankel DS, Vasan RS, D'Agostino RB, Sr, et al: Resistin, adiponectin, and risk of heart failure: the Framingham offspring study. *J Am Coll Cardiol* 53:754, 2009.
18. Alberti KG, Eckel RH, Grundy SM, et al: Harmonizing the metabolic syndrome: a joint interim statement of the International Diabetes Federation Task Force on Epidemiology and Prevention; National Heart, Lung, and Blood Institute; American Heart Association; World Heart Federation; International Atherosclerosis Society; and International Association for the Study of Obesity. *Circulation* 120:1640, 2009.
19. Poirier P, Giles TD, Bray GA, et al: Obesity and cardiovascular disease: pathophysiology, evaluation, and effect of weight loss: an update of the 1997 American Heart Association Scientific Statement on Obesity and Heart Disease from the Obesity Committee of the Council on Nutrition, Physical Activity, and Metabolism. *Circulation* 113:898, 2006.
20. Eckel RH, Kahn R, Robertson RM, Rizza RA: Preventing cardiovascular disease and diabetes: a call to action from the American Diabetes Association and the American Heart Association. *Circulation* 113:2943, 2006.
21. D'Agostino RB, Sr, Grundy S, Sullivan LM, Wilson P: Validation of the Framingham coronary heart disease prediction scores: results of a multiple ethnic groups investigation. *JAMA* 286:180, 2001.
22. Third Report of the National Cholesterol Education Program (NCEP) Expert Panel on Detection, Evaluation, and Treatment of High Blood Cholesterol in Adults (Adult Treatment Panel III) final report. *Circulation* 106:3143, 2002.
23. Grundy SM, Cleeman JI, Merz CN, et al: Implications of recent clinical trials for the National Cholesterol Education Program Adult Treatment Panel III guidelines. *Circulation* 110:227, 2004.
24. Helfand M, Buckley DI, Freeman M, et al: Emerging risk factors for coronary heart disease: a summary of systematic reviews conducted for the U.S. Preventive Services Task Force. *Ann Intern Med* 151:496, 2009.
25. Aronne LJ, Wadden T, Isoldi KK, Woodworth KA: When prevention fails: obesity treatment strategies. *Am J Med* 122(Suppl 1):S24, 2009.
26. Must A, Spadano J, Coakley EH, et al: The disease burden associated with overweight and obesity. *JAMA* 282:1523, 1999.
27. The Practical Guide: identification, evaluation, and treatment of overweight and obesity in adults, Bethesda, Md, 2000, National Heart, Lung, and Blood Institute (NHLBI), Department of Health and Human Services. NIH publication 00-4084.
28. Zimmet P, Magliano D, Matsuzawa Y, et al: The metabolic syndrome: a global public health problem and a new definition. *J Atheroscler Thromb* 12:295, 2005.
29. Qiao Q, Nyamdorj R: Is the association of type II diabetes with waist circumference or waist-to-hip ratio stronger than that with body mass index? *Eur J Clin Nutr* 64:30, 2010. Epub 2009 Sep 2.
30. Ford ES, Giles WH, Mokdad AH: The distribution of 10-year risk for coronary heart disease among US adults: findings from the National Health and Nutrition Examination Survey III. *J Am Coll Cardiol* 43:1791, 2004.
31. Buckley DI, Fu R, Freeman M, et al: C-reactive protein as a risk factor for coronary heart disease: a systematic review and meta-analyses for the U.S. Preventive Services Task Force. *Ann Intern Med* 151:483, 2009.
32. U.S. Preventive Services Task Force: Using nontraditional risk factors in coronary heart disease risk assessment: U.S. Preventive Services Task Force Recommendation Statement. *Ann Intern Med* 151:474, 2009.
33. Browne AF, Inge T: How young for bariatric surgery in children? *Semin Pediatr Surg* 18:176, 2009.
34. Centers for Disease Control and Prevention (CDC): Obesity prevalence among low-income, preschool-aged children—United States, 1998-2008. *MMWR Morb Mortal Wkly Rep* 58:769, 2009.
35. Holst-Schumacher I, Nuñez-Rivas H, Monge-Rojas R, Barrantes-Santamaría M: Components of the metabolic syndrome in a sample of overweight and obese Costa Rican schoolchildren. *Food Nutr Bull* 30:161, 2009.
36. D'Adamo E, Santoro N, Caprio S: Metabolic syndrome in pediatrics: old concepts revised, new concepts discussed. *Endocrinol Metab Clin North Am* 38:549, 2009.
37. Körner A, Kratzsch J, Gausche R, et al: Metabolic syndrome in children and adolescents—risk for sleep-disordered breathing and obstructive sleep-apnoea syndrome? *Arch Physiol Biochem* 114:237, 2008.
38. Maffeis C, Banzato C, Brambilla P, et al: Insulin resistance is a risk factor for high blood pressure regardless of body size and fat distribution in obese children. *Nutr Metab Cardiovasc Dis* 20:266, 2010. Epub 2009 Sep 11.
39. Lavie CJ, Milani RV, Artham SM, et al: The obesity paradox, weight loss, and coronary disease. *Am J Med* 122:1106, 2009. Epub 2009 Aug 13.
40. Ness-Abramof R, Apovian CM: Future of obesity prevention and treatment. *Stud Health Technol Inform* 149:386, 2009.
41. European Society of Cardiology: Obesity and diabetes double the risk of heart failure: patients with both conditions very difficult to treat. Science Daily. Available at: http://www.sciencedaily.com/releases/2009/05/090530094510.htm. Accessed October 3, 2009.
42. Jee SH, Pastor-Barriuso R, Appel LJ, et al: Body mass index and incident ischemic heart disease in South Korean men and women. *Am J Epidemiol* 162:42, 2005.
43. Li TY, Rana JS, Manson JE, et al: Obesity as compared with physical activity in predicting risk of coronary heart disease in women. *Circulation* 113:499, 2006.
44. McTigue K, Larson JC, Valoski A, et al: Mortality and cardiac and vascular outcomes in extremely obese women. *JAMA* 296:79, 2006.
45. Wilson PW, D'Agostino RB, Sullivan L, et al: Overweight and obesity as determinants of cardiovascular risk: the Framingham experience. *Arch Intern Med* 162:1867, 2002.
46. Sun Q, Townsend MK, Okereke OI, et al: Adiposity and weight change in mid-life in relation to healthy survival after age 70 in women: prospective cohort study. *BMJ* 339:b3796, 2009. doi: 10.1136/bmj.b3796.
47. de Koning L, Merchant AT, Pogue J, Anand SS: Waist circumference and waist-to-hip ratio as predictors of cardiovascular events: meta-regression analysis of prospective studies. *Eur Heart J* 28:850, 2007.
48. Poirier P: Adiposity and cardiovascular disease: are we using the right definition of obesity? *Eur Heart J* 28:2047, 2007.
49. Romero-Corral A, Lopez-Jimenez F, Sierra-Johnson J, Somers VK: Differentiating between body fat and lean mass—how should we measure obesity? *Nat Clin Pract Endocrinol Metab* 4:322, 2008.
50. Romero-Corral A, Somers VK, Sierra-Johnson J, et al: Diagnostic performance of body mass index to detect obesity in patients with coronary artery disease. *Eur Heart J* 28:2087, 2007.
51. See R, Abdullah SM, McGuire DK, et al: The association of differing measures of overweight and obesity with prevalent atherosclerosis: the Dallas Heart Study. *J Am Coll Cardiol* 50:752, 2007.
52. Bays HE, González-Campoy JM, Bray GA, et al: Pathogenic potential of adipose tissue and metabolic consequences of adipocyte hypertrophy and increased visceral adiposity. *Expert Rev Cardiovasc Ther* 6:343, 2008.

19

53. Caballero AE: Endothelial dysfunction in obesity and insulin resistance: a road to diabetes and heart disease. *Obes Res* 11:1278, 2003.

54. Evensen KA, Steinshamn S, Tjønna AE, et al: Effects of preterm birth and fetal growth retardation on cardiovascular risk factors in young adulthood. *Early Hum Dev* 85:239, 2009.

55. Simmons R: Perinatal programming of obesity. *Semin Perinatol* 32:371, 2008.

56. Ravelli GP, Stein ZA, Susser MW: Obesity in young men after famine exposure in utero and early infancy. *N Engl J Med* 295:349, 1976.

57. Barker DJ: The developmental origins of adult disease. *J Am Coll Nutr* 23(Suppl):588S, 2004.

58. Bonamy AK, Bendito A, Martin H, et al: Preterm birth contributes to increased vascular resistance and higher blood pressure in adolescent girls. *Pediatr Res* 58:845, 2005.

59. Hack M, Schluchter M, Cartar L, Rahman M: Blood pressure among very low birth weight (<1.5 kg) young adults. *Pediatr Res* 58:677, 2005.

60. Johansson S, Iliadou A, Bergvall N, et al: Risk of high blood pressure among young men increases with the degree of immaturity at birth. *Circulation* 112:3430, 2005.

61. Lurbe E, Carvajal E, Torro I, et al: Influence of concurrent obesity and low birth weight on blood pressure phenotype in youth. *Hypertension* 53:912, 2009.

62. Lurbe E, Garcia-Vicent C, Torro I, et al: First-year blood pressure increase steepest in low birthweight newborns. *J Hypertens* 25:81, 2007.

63. Barker DJ, Osmond C, Forsén TJ, et al: Trajectories of growth among children who have coronary events as adults. *N Engl J Med* 353:1802, 2005.

64. Lurbe E, Torro MI, Carvajal E, et al: Birth weight impacts on wave reflections in children and adolescents. *Hypertension* 41(pt 2):646, 2003.

65. Rosner B, Cook N, Portman R, et al: Blood pressure differences by ethnic group among United States children and adolescents. *Hypertension* 54:5028, 2009.

66. Pleis JR, Lucas JW: Summary health statistics for U.S. adults: National Health Interview Survey, 2007. *Vital Health Stat 10* 240:1, 2009.

67. National High Blood Pressure Education Program Working Group on High Blood Pressure in Children and Adolescents: The Fourth Report on the Diagnosis, Evaluation, and Treatment of High Blood Pressure in Children and Adolescents. U.S. Department of Health and Human Services. May 2005. Available at: www.nhlbi.nih.gov/health/prof/heart/hbp/hbp_ped.pdf. Accessed October 3, 2009.

68. Aucott L, Rothnie H, McIntyre L, et al: Long-term weight loss from lifestyle intervention benefits blood pressure? A systematic review. *Hypertension* 54:756, 2009.

69. Dimkpa U, Oji JO: Relationship of body mass index with haemodynamic variables and abnormalities in young adults. *J Hum Hypertens* 24:230, 2010. Epub 2009 Sep 10.

70. Grinsell MM, Norwood VF: At the bottom of the differential diagnosis list: unusual causes of pediatric hypertension. *Pediatr Nephrol* 24:2137, 2009.

71. Sorof J, Daniels S: Obesity hypertension in children: a problem of epidemic proportions. *Hypertension* 40:441, 2002.

72. Berenson GS, Srinivasan SR, Bao W, et al: Association between multiple cardiovascular risk factors and atherosclerosis in children and young adults. The Bogalusa Heart Study. *N Engl J Med* 338:1650, 1998.

73. McGill HC, Jr, McMahan CA, Zieske AW, et al: Effects of nonlipid risk factors on atherosclerosis in youth with a favorable lipoprotein profile. *Circulation* 103:1546, 2001.

74. Davis PH, Dawson JD, Riley WA, Lauer RM: Carotid intimal-medial thickness is related to cardiovascular risk factors measured from childhood through middle age: the Muscatine Study. *Circulation* 104:2815, 2001.

75. Arnett DK, Glasser SP, McVeigh G, et al: Blood pressure and arterial compliance in young adults: the Minnesota Children's Blood Pressure Study. *Am J Hypertens* 14:200, 2001.

76. Knoflach M, Kiechl S, Kind M, et al: Cardiovascular risk factors and atherosclerosis in young males: ARMY study (Atherosclerosis Risk-Factors in Male Youngsters). *Circulation* 108:1064, 2003.

77. Drager LF, Queiroz EL, Lopes HF, et al: Obstructive sleep apnea is highly prevalent and correlates with impaired glycemic control in consecutive patients with the metabolic syndrome. *J Cardiometab Syndr* 4:89, 2009.

78. Ronksley PE, Hemmelgarn BR, Heitman SJ, et al: Obstructive sleep apnoea is associated with diabetes in sleepy subjects. *Thorax* 64:834, 2009.

79. Schäfer H, Pauleit D, Sudhop T, et al: Body fat distribution, serum leptin, and cardiovascular risk factors in men with obstructive sleep apnea. *Chest* 122:829, 2002.

80. Shah N, Roux F: The relationship of obesity and obstructive sleep apnea. *Clin Chest Med* 30:455, 2009.

81. Ip MS, Lam KS, Ho C, et al: Serum leptin and vascular risk factors in obstructive sleep apnea. *Chest* 118:580, 2000.

82. Young T, Palta M, Dempsey J, et al: Burden of sleep apnea: rationale, design, and major findings of the Wisconsin Sleep Cohort study. *WMJ* 108:246, 2009.

83. Lopez PP, Stefan B, Schulman CI, Byers PM: Prevalence of sleep apnea in morbidly obese patients who presented for weight loss surgery evaluation: more evidence for routine screening for obstructive sleep apnea before weight loss surgery. *Am Surg* 74:834, 2008.

84. Peppard PE, Young T, Palta M, et al: Longitudinal study of moderate weight change and sleep-disordered breathing. *JAMA* 284:3015, 2000.

85. Young T, Shahar E, Nieto FJ, et al: Predictors of sleep-disordered breathing in community-dwelling adults: the Sleep Heart Health Study. *Arch Intern Med* 162:893, 2002.

86. Kottler BM, Ferdowsian HR, Barnard ND: Effects of plant-based diets on plasma lipids. *Am J Cardiol* 104:947, 2009.

87. Paraskevas KI, Karatzas G, Pantopoulou A, et al: Targeting dyslipidemia in the metabolic syndrome: an update. *Curr Vasc Pharmacol* 8:450, 2010.

88. Sharma RK, Singh VN, Reddy HK: Thinking beyond low-density lipoprotein cholesterol: strategies to further reduce cardiovascular risk. *Vasc Health Risk Manag* 5:793, 2009.

89. Ginsberg HN, MacCallum PR: The obesity, metabolic syndrome, and type 2 diabetes mellitus pandemic: Part I. Increased cardiovascular disease risk and the importance of atherogenic dyslipidemia in persons with the metabolic syndrome and type 2 diabetes mellitus. *J Cardiometab Syndr* 4:113, 2009.

90. Fruchart JC, Sacks F, Hermans MP, et al: The Residual Risk Reduction Initiative: a call to action to reduce residual vascular risk in patients with dyslipidemia. *Am J Cardiol* 102(Suppl):1K, 2008.

91. Haslam DW, James WP: Obesity. *Lancet* 366:1197, 2005.

92. Sazonov V, Beetsch J, Phatak H, et al: Association between dyslipidemia and vascular events in patients treated with statins: report from the UK General Practice Research Database. *Atherosclerosis* 208:210, 2010. Epub 2009 Sep 20.

93. Millán J, Pintó X, Muñoz A, et al: Lipoprotein ratios: physiological significance and clinical usefulness in cardiovascular prevention. *Vasc Health Risk Manag* 5:757, 2009.

94. Haffner SM; American Diabetes Association: Management of dyslipidemia in adults with diabetes. *Diabetes Care* 26(Suppl 1):S83, 2003.

95. Randomised trial of cholesterol lowering in 4444 patients with coronary heart disease: the Scandinavian Simvastatin Survival Study (4S). *Lancet* 344:1383, 1994.

96. Baigent C, Keech A, Kearney PM, et al: Efficacy and safety of cholesterol-lowering treatment: prospective meta-analysis of data from 90,056 participants in 14 randomised trials of statins. *Lancet* 366:1267, 2005.

97. Cholesterol Treatment Trialists' (CTT) Collaborators; Kearney PM, Blackwell L, Collins R, et al: Efficacy of cholesterol-lowering therapy in 18,686 people with diabetes in 14 randomised trials of statins: a meta-analysis. *Lancet* 371:117, 2008.

98. Yusuf S, Hawken S, Ounpuu S, et al: Effect of potentially modifiable risk factors associated with myocardial infarction in 52 countries (the INTERHEART study): case-control study. *Lancet* 364:937, 2004.

99. Assmann G, Schulte H, Cullen P, Seedorf U: Assessing risk of myocardial infarction and stroke: new data from the Prospective Cardiovascular Münster (PROCAM) study. *Eur J Clin Invest* 37:925, 2007.

100. Centers for Disease Control and Prevention (CDC): Diabetes data & trends. May 12, 2009. Available at: http://www.cdc.gov/diabetes/statistics/cvd/fig1.htm. Accessed October 3, 2009.

101. Centers for Disease Control and Prevention (CDC): Age-adjusted percentage of obesity for adults with diabetes, United States, 1994-2007. July 21, 2009. Available at: http://www.cdc.gov/diabetes/statistics/comp/fig7_obesity.htm. Accessed October 3, 2009.

102. Centers for Disease Control and Prevention (CDC): Data & trends. Age-adjusted percentage of overweight (including obese) for adults with diabetes, United States, 1994-2007. July 21, 2009. Available at: http://www.cdc.gov/diabetes/statistics/comp/fig7_overweight.htm. Accessed October 3, 2009.

103. Hu FB, Manson JE, Stampfer MJ, et al: Diet, lifestyle, and the risk of type 2 diabetes mellitus in women. *N Engl J Med* 345:790, 2001.

104. Shai I, Jiang R, Manson JE, et al: Ethnicity, obesity, and risk of type 2 diabetes in women: a 20-year follow-up study. *Diabetes Care* 29:1585, 2006.

105. Fox KA, Després JP, Richard AJ, et al; IDEA Steering Committee and National Coordinators: Does abdominal obesity have a similar impact on cardiovascular disease and diabetes? A study of 91,246 ambulant patients in 27 European countries. *Eur Heart J* 30:3055, 2009.

106. Ludwig DS: Childhood obesity—the shape of things to come. *N Engl J Med* 357:2325, 2007.

107. Weiss R, Kaufman FR: Metabolic complications of childhood obesity: identifying and mitigating the risk. *Diabetes Care* 31(Suppl 2):S310, 2008.

108. Nathan DM, Davidson MB, DeFronzo RA, et al: Impaired fasting glucose and impaired glucose tolerance: implications for care. *Diabetes Care* 30:753, 2007.

109. Weiss R, Taksali SE, Tamborlane WV, et al: Predictors of changes in glucose tolerance status in obese youth. *Diabetes Care* 28:902, 2005.

110. SEARCH for Diabetes in Youth Study Group; Liese AD, D'Agostino RB, Jr, Hamman RF, et al: The burden of diabetes mellitus among US youth: prevalence estimates from the SEARCH for Diabetes in Youth Study. *Pediatrics* 118:1510, 2006.

111. Case CC, Jones PH, Nelson K, et al: Impact of weight loss on the metabolic syndrome. *Diabetes Obes Metab* 6:407, 2002.

112. Look AHEAD Research Group; Pi-Sunyer X, Blackburn GL, Brancati FL, et al: Reduction in weight and cardiovascular disease risk factors in individuals with type 2 diabetes: one-year results of the look AHEAD trial. *Diabetes Care* 30:1374, 2007.

113. Tuomilehto HP, Seppä JM, Partinen MM, et al: Lifestyle intervention with weight reduction: first-line treatment in mild obstructive sleep apnea. *Am J Respir Crit Care Med* 179:320, 2009.

114. Neter JE, Stam BE, Kok FJ, et al: Influence of weight reduction on blood pressure: a meta-analysis of randomized controlled trials. *Hypertension* 42:878, 2003.

115. Knowler WC, Fowler SE, Hamman RF, et al: 10-year follow-up of diabetes incidence and weight loss in the Diabetes Prevention Program Outcomes Study. *Lancet* 374:1677, 2009.

116. Kuller LH: Weight loss and reduction of blood pressure and hypertension. *Hypertension* 54:700, 2009.

117. Ratner R, Goldberg R, Haffner S, et al: Impact of intensive lifestyle and metformin therapy on cardiovascular disease risk factors in the diabetes prevention program. *Diabetes Care* 28:888, 2005.

118. Maruthur NM, Wang NY, Appel LJ: Lifestyle interventions reduce coronary heart disease risk: results from the PREMIER Trial. *Circulation* 119:2026, 2009.

119. Foo SY, Heller ER, Wykrzykowska J, et al: Vascular effects of a low-carbohydrate high-protein diet. *Proc Natl Acad Sci U S A* 106:15418, 2009.

120. Obarzanek E, Vollmer WM, Lin PH, et al: Effects of individual components of multiple behavior changes: the PREMIER trial. *Am J Health Behav* 31:545, 2007.

121. Williams CL, Hayman LL, Daniels SR, et al: Cardiovascular health in childhood: a statement for health professionals from the Committee on Atherosclerosis, Hypertension, and Obesity in the Young (AHOY) of the Council on Cardiovascular Disease in the Young, American Heart Association. *Circulation* 106:143, 2002.

122. Selvin E, Paynter NP, Erlinger TP: The effect of weight loss on C-reactive protein: a systematic review. *Arch Intern Med* 167:31, 2007.

123. Nilsson PM: Is weight loss beneficial for reduction of morbidity and mortality? What is the controversy about? *Diabetes Care* 21(Suppl 2):S278, 2008.

124. Sørensen TI: Weight loss causes increased mortality: pros. *Obes Rev* 4:3, 2003.

125. Flegal KM, Graubard BI: Estimates of excess deaths associated with body mass index and other anthropometric variables. *Am J Clin Nutr* 89:1213, 2009.
126. Sierra-Johnson J, Romero-Corral A, Somers VK, et al: Prognostic importance of weight loss in patients with coronary heart disease regardless of initial body mass index. *Eur J Cardiovasc Prev Rehabil* 15:336, 2008.
127. Flint AJ, Hu FB, Glynn RJ, et al: Excess weight and the risk of incident coronary heart disease among men and women. *Obesity (Silver Spring)* 18:377, 2010. Epub 2009 Jul 30.
128. Vanhecke TE, Franklin BA, Miller WM, et al: Cardiorespiratory fitness and sedentary lifestyle in the morbidly obese. *Clin Cardiol* 32:121, 2009.
129. Turner-McGrievy GM, Campbell MK, Tate DF, et al: Pounds Off Digitally study: a randomized podcasting weight-loss intervention. *Am J Prev Med* 37:263, 2009.
130. Kerksick C, Thomas A, Campbell B, et al: Effects of a popular exercise and weight loss program on weight loss, body composition, energy expenditure and health in obese women. *Nutr Metab (Lond)* 6:23, 2009.
131. Gidding SS, Lichtenstein AH, Faith MS, et al: Implementing American Heart Association pediatric and adult nutrition guidelines: a scientific statement from the American Heart Association Nutrition Committee of the Council on Nutrition, Physical Activity and Metabolism, Council on Cardiovascular Disease in the Young, Council on Arteriosclerosis, Thrombosis and Vascular Biology, Council on Cardiovascular Nursing, Council on Epidemiology and Prevention, and Council for High Blood Pressure Research. *Circulation* 119:1161, 2009.
132. Lichtenstein AH, Appel LJ, Brands M, et al: Diet and lifestyle recommendations revision 2006: a scientific statement from the American Heart Association Nutrition Committee. *Circulation* 114:82, 2006.
133. Heidemann C, Schulze MB, Franco OH, et al: Dietary patterns and risk of mortality from cardiovascular disease, cancer, and all causes in a prospective cohort of women. *Circulation* 118:230, 2008.
134. Sacks FM, Bray GA, Carey VJ, et al: Comparison of weight-loss diets with different compositions of fat, protein, and carbohydrates. *N Engl J Med* 360:859, 2009.
135. Kennedy A, Martinez K, Chuang CC, et al: Saturated fatty acid–mediated inflammation and insulin resistance in adipose tissue: mechanisms of action and implications. *J Nutr* 139:1, 2009.
136. van Dijk SJ, Feskens EJ, Bos MB, et al: A saturated fatty acid–rich diet induces an obesity-linked proinflammatory gene expression profile in adipose tissue of subjects at risk of metabolic syndrome. *Am J Clin Nutr* 90:1656, 2009.
137. Smith SR: A look at the low-carbohydrate diet. *N Engl J Med* 361:2286, 2009.
138. Petersen KF, Dufour S, Savage DB, et al: The role of skeletal muscle insulin resistance in the pathogenesis of the metabolic syndrome. *Proc Natl Acad Sci U S A* 104:12587, 2007.
139. Grundy SM, Hansen B, Smith SC, Jr, et al: Clinical management of metabolic syndrome: report of the American Heart Association/National Heart, Lung, and Blood Institute/American Diabetes Association conference on scientific issues related to management. *Circulation* 109:551, 2004.
140. Hoy MK, Winters BL, Chlebowski RT, et al: Implementing a low-fat eating plan in the Women's Intervention Nutrition Study. *J Am Diet Assoc* 109:688, 2009.
141. Rumawas ME, Meigs JB, Dwyer JT, et al: Mediterranean-style dietary pattern, reduced risk of metabolic syndrome traits, and incidence in the Framingham Offspring Cohort. *Am J Clin Nutr* 90:1608, 2009.
142. Harris WS, Mozaffarian D, Rimm E, et al: Omega-6 fatty acids and risk for cardiovascular disease: a science advisory from the American Heart Association Nutrition Subcommittee of the Council on Nutrition, Physical Activity, and Metabolism; Council on Cardiovascular Nursing; and Council on Epidemiology and Prevention. *Circulation* 119:902, 2009.
143. Eckel RH, Borra S, Lichtenstein AH, Yin-Piazza SY: Understanding the complexity of trans fatty acid reduction in the American diet: American Heart Association Trans Fat Conference 2006: report of the Trans Fat Conference Planning Group. *Circulation* 115:2231, 2007.
144. Gerberding JL: Safer fats for healthier hearts: the case for eliminating dietary artificial trans fat intake. *Ann Intern Med* 151:137, 2009.
145. Wadden TA, Butryn ML, Wilson C: Lifestyle modification for the management of obesity. *Gastroenterology* 132:2226, 2007.
146. Donnelly JE, Blair SN, Jakicic JM, et al: American College of Sports Medicine Position Stand. Appropriate physical activity intervention strategies for weight loss and prevention of weight regain for adults. *Med Sci Sports Exerc* 41:459, 2009.
147. Leibel RL, Rosenbaum M, Hirsch J: Changes in energy expenditure resulting from altered body weight. *N Engl J Med* 332:621, 1995.
148. Weiss EP, Racette SB, Villareal DT, et al: Lower extremity muscle size and strength and aerobic capacity decrease with caloric restriction but not with exercise-induced weight loss. *J Appl Physiol* 102:634, 2007.
149. Bopp MJ, Houston DK, Lenchik L, et al: Lean mass loss is associated with low protein intake during dietary-induced weight loss in postmenopausal women. *J Am Diet Assoc* 108:1216, 2008.
150. Layman DK, Boileau RA, Erickson DJ, et al: A reduced ratio of dietary carbohydrate to protein improves body composition and blood lipid profiles during weight loss in adult women. *J Nutr* 133:411, 2003.
151. Wadden TA, Butryn ML: Behavioral treatment of obesity. *Endocrinol Metab Clin North Am* 32:981, x, 2003.
152. Alonso-Alonso M, Pascual-Leone A: The right brain hypothesis for obesity. *JAMA* 297:1819, 2007.
153. Appelhans BM: Neurobehavioral inhibition of reward-driven feeding: implications for dieting and obesity. *Obesity (Silver Spring)* 17:640, 2009.
154. Sarwer DB, von Sydow Green A, Vetter ML, Wadden TA: Behavior therapy for obesity: where are we now? *Curr Opin Endocrinol Diabetes Obes* 16:347, 2009.
155. Booth FW, Gordon SE, Carlson CJ, Hamilton MT: Waging war on modern chronic diseases: primary prevention through exercise biology. *J Appl Physiol* 88:774, 2000.
156. Physical activity guidelines for Americans. U.S. Department of Health & Human Services, 2008.
157. Wadden TA, West DS, Neiberg RH, et al: One-year weight losses in the Look AHEAD study: factors associated with success. *Obesity (Silver Spring)* 17:713, 2009.
158. Haskell WL, Lee IM, Pate RR, et al: Physical activity and public health: updated recommendation for adults from the American College of Sports Medicine and the American Heart Association. *Circulation* 116:1081, 2007.
159. Pollock ML, Franklin BA, Balady GJ, et al: AHA Science Advisory. Resistance exercise in individuals with and without cardiovascular disease: benefits, rationale, safety, and prescription: an advisory from the Committee on Exercise, Rehabilitation, and Prevention, Council on Clinical Cardiology, American Heart Association; position paper endorsed by the American College of Sports Medicine. *Circulation* 101:828, 2000.
160. Williams MA, Haskell WL, Ades PA, et al: Resistance exercise in individuals with and without cardiovascular disease: 2007 update: a scientific statement from the American Heart Association Council on Clinical Cardiology and Council on Nutrition, Physical Activity, and Metabolism. *Circulation* 116:572, 2007.
161. Braith RW, Stewart KJ: Resistance exercise training: its role in the prevention of cardiovascular disease. *Circulation* 113:2642, 2006.
162. Hunter GR, Byrne NM, Sirikul B, et al: Resistance training conserves fat-free mass and resting energy expenditure following weight loss. *Obesity (Silver Spring)* 16:1045, 2008.
163. Schmitz KH, Jensen MD, Kugler KC, et al: Strength training for obesity prevention in midlife women. *Int J Obes Relat Metab Disord* 27:326, 2003.
164. Kenchaiah S, Sesso HD, Gaziano JM: Body mass index and vigorous physical activity and the risk of heart failure among men. *Circulation* 119:44, 2009.
165. Montori VM, Fernández-Balsells M: Glycemic control in type 2 diabetes: time for an evidence-based about-face? *Ann Intern Med* 150:803, 2009.
166. Khan NU, Babb JD, Kaul S, et al: A novel complication of bariatric surgery. *Am Heart Hosp J* 7:69, 2009.
167. Dar M, Pories WJ: Bariatric surgery: what is the effect on type 2 diabetes? *Curr Opin Investig Drugs* 10:1078, 2009.
168. Blackburn GL, Hutter MM, Harvey AM, et al: Expert panel on weight loss surgery: executive report update. *Obesity (Silver Spring)* 17:842, 2009.
169. Picot J, Jones J, Colquitt JL, et al: The clinical effectiveness and cost-effectiveness of bariatric (weight loss) surgery for obesity: a systematic review and economic evaluation. *Health Technol Assess* 13:1, 215, iii, 2009.
170. Bray GA: The missing link—lose weight, live longer. *N Engl J Med* 357:818, 2007.
171. Dixon J: Survival advantage with bariatric surgery: report from the 10th International Congress on Obesity. *Surg Obes Relat Dis* 2:585, 2006.
172. Sjöström L, Narbro K, Sjöström CD, et al: Effects of bariatric surgery on mortality in Swedish obese subjects. *N Engl J Med* 357:741, 2007.
173. de Fátima Haueisen Sander Diniz M, de Azeredo Passos VM, Diniz MT: Gut-brain communication: how does it stand after bariatric surgery? *Curr Opin Clin Nutr Metab Care* 9:629, 2006.
174. Todkar JS, Shah SS, Shah PS, Gangwani J: Long-term effects of laparoscopic sleeve gastrectomy in morbidly obese subjects with type 2 diabetes mellitus. *Surg Obes Relat Dis* 6:142, 2010. Epub 2009 Jul 10.
175. Jacobs M, Bisland W, Gomez E, et al: Laparoscopic sleeve gastrectomy: a retrospective review of 1- and 2-year results. *Surg Endosc* 24:781, 2010. Epub 2009 Aug 19.
176. Idelevich E, Kirch W, Schindler C: Current pharmacotherapeutic concepts for the treatment of obesity in adults. *Ther Adv Cardiovasc Dis* 3:75, 2009.
177. National Heart, Lung, and Blood Institute (NHLBI): The Practical Guide: identification, evaluation, and treatment of overweight and obesity in adults. October 2000. Available at: http://www.nhlbi.nih.gov/guidelines/obesity/prctgd_c.pdf. Accessed October 3, 2009.
178. U.S. National Library of Medicine and the National Institutes of Health: Sibutramine. Available at: http://www.nlm.nih.gov/medlineplus/druginfo/meds/a601110.html. Accessed October 12, 2009, 2009.
179. Gadde KM, Xiong GL: Bupropion for weight reduction. *Expert Rev Neurother* 7:17, 2007.
180. Stenlöf K, Rössner S, Vercruysse F, et al: Topiramate in the treatment of obese subjects with drug-naive type 2 diabetes. *Diabetes Obes Metab* 9:360, 2007.
181. Riddle MC, Henry RR, Poon TH, et al: Exenatide elicits sustained glycaemic control and progressive reduction of body weight in patients with type 2 diabetes inadequately controlled by sulphonylureas with or without metformin. *Diabetes Metab Res Rev* 22:483, 2006.
182. Padwal R: Cetilistat, a new lipase inhibitor for the treatment of obesity. *Curr Opin Investig Drugs* 9:414, 2008.
183. Zanella MT, Ribeiro Filho FF: Emerging drugs for obesity therapy. *Arq Bras Endocrinol Metabol* 53:271, 2009.
184. Lee MW, Fujioka K: Naltrexone for the treatment of obesity: review and update. *Expert Opin Pharmacother* 10:1841, 2009.
185. Padwal R: Contrave, a bupropion and naltrexone combination therapy for the potential treatment of obesity. *Curr Opin Investig Drugs* 10:1117, 2009.
186. Ravussin E, Smith SR, Mitchell JA, et al: Enhanced weight loss with pramlintide/metreleptin: an integrated neurohormonal approach to obesity pharmacotherapy. *Obesity (Silver Spring)* 17:1736, 2009.
187. Huang TT, Glass TA: Transforming research strategies for understanding and preventing obesity. *JAMA* 300:1811, 2008.
188. Wang Y, Beydoun MA, Liang L, et al: Will all Americans become overweight or obese? Estimating the progression and cost of the US obesity epidemic. *Obesity (Silver Spring)* 16:2323, 2008.
189. Bibbins-Domingo K, Coxson P, Pletcher MJ, et al: Adolescent overweight and future adult coronary heart disease. *N Engl J Med* 357:2371, 2007.
190. Glass TA, McAtee MJ: Behavioral science at the crossroads in public health: extending horizons, envisioning the future. *Soc Sci Med* 62:1650,2006.
191. F as in fat: how obesity policies are failing America, Washington, DC, 2009, Trust for America's Health.
192. World Health Organization: Social determinants of health. Available at: http://www.who.int/social_determinants/en/. Accessed October 3, 2009.

Tobacco Use, Passive Smoking, and Cardiovascular Disease: Research and Smoking Cessation Interventions

Russell V. Luepker

KEY POINTS

- The smoking of tobacco products increases the risk of cardiovascular diseases, including myocardial infarction, stroke, and peripheral artery disease.

- The continued smoking of tobacco products in patients with cardiovascular disease increases the risk of recurrent events, including sudden death, and smoking cessation reduces this risk.

- Environmental tobacco smoke (secondhand smoke) increases the risk for cardiovascular and other diseases in nonsmokers.

- Cigarette smoking rates among adults and youth have declined in the United States during several decades.

- Effective behavioral and pharmacologic methods are available to help smokers quit.

- Effective educational methods are available to prevent youth from starting to smoke.

- Policies and regulations including smoke-free spaces, limitations on advertising, enforcement of youth access laws, and increased cigarette excise taxes have contributed importantly to reductions in tobacco use.

There are approximately 43 million adult smokers in the United States.[1] It is estimated that 443,000 deaths annually are attributable to cigarette smoking (Fig. 20-1). These deaths are replenished by an estimated 3900 teenagers per day who begin the smoking habit.[2] The economic costs are estimated to be more than $96 billion per year in medical expenses and $97 billion in lost productivity.[3] Worldwide, tobacco is estimated to cause more than 5 million deaths per year.[4] The costs in lost health and in human suffering are incalculable.

The causal links between cigarette smoking and human disease are incontrovertible. Smoking is linked to major cardiovascular diseases including sudden death, acute myocardial infarction, peripheral artery disease, and stroke.[5] Cigarettes are also linked to many cancers and are the prime factor in lung cancer. Smoking is linked to acute and chronic pulmonary diseases including emphysema. There is growing evidence that environmental tobacco smoke, which results in exposure of nonsmokers, poses health risks to that group. Lung cancer, respiratory tract infections, and asthma attacks among those exposed to environmental tobacco smoke are well recognized.[6] More recent evidence finds that environmental tobacco smoke causes heart disease and sudden infant death syndrome.[6] These observations and others have resulted in a widespread call for prevention of tobacco uptake by teens, cessation among smoking adults, and restriction of smoking in the environment. This chapter discusses the scientific evidence relating active and passive tobacco smoking to cardiovascular risk and the benefits of quitting. It also describes the trends in cigarette use. Finally, individual and population intervention strategies for cessation among youth and adults are discussed.

EFFECTS OF CIGARETTE SMOKING ON CARDIOVASCULAR DISEASE

There is a wealth of evidence in the past five decades linking cigarette smoking to the major cardiovascular diseases, including myocardial infarction, sudden death, stroke, and peripheral vascular disease.[5,7] These associations are found across all age, gender, and ethnic groups.

The relationship of coronary heart disease (CHD) mortality to smoking status from the 1959-1965 Cancer Prevention Study is shown in Figure 20-2. CHD increases with age for both men and women; women have lower rates at all ages, and ever-smokers have significantly higher death rates than never-smokers. These differences are greatest in the younger age groups, in which the relative risk of CHD in smokers approaches 8. However, the differences remain into the older years, when relative risks are less but absolute risk is significantly greater. Smoking cessation among adults significantly reduces the risk of CHD and all cardiovascular disease as shown in many populations.[8,9]

Data from the Multiple Risk Factor Intervention Trial (MRFIT) of 316,099 white men also find a graded relationship between number of cigarettes and CHD death.[10] The relative risk for 1 to 25 cigarettes per day is 2.1, rising to 2.9 for daily smoking consumption above 25 cigarettes per day. Similarly, MRFIT found that quitting smoking reduces cardiovascular disease mortality.[11]

In addition to age and gender effects, it is apparent that smoking-related disease also affects all the major ethnic and racial groups in the United States.[1] The ill health effects of smoking cut across national boundaries as demonstrated in the Seven Countries Study of Keys and colleagues.[12]

One of the most disturbing aspects of cigarette smoking is its strong association with sudden, unexpected death, particularly among younger individuals. Although sudden death is common among those with known cardiovascular disease, Escobedo and Caspersen[13] found that only smoking predicted sudden death in those thought to be disease free. Similarly, in both men and women, acute myocardial infarction in younger individuals (younger than 50 years) is strongly associated with cigarette smoking.[14]

332

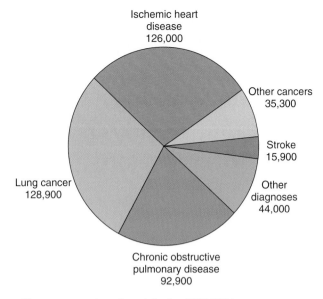

Ischemic heart
disease
126,000

Other cancers
35,300

Stroke
15,900

Other
diagnoses
44,000

Lung cancer
128,900

Chronic obstructive
pulmonary disease
92,900

*Average annual number of deaths, 2000-2004

FIGURE 20-1 About 443,000 U.S. deaths each year are attributable to cigarette smoking. *(Source: cdc.gov.)*

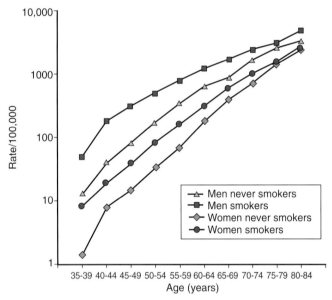

FIGURE 20-2 Coronary heart disease mortality. *(Source: U.S. Department of Health and Human Services: Changes in cigarette-related disease risks and their implication for prevention and control,* Monograph 8, *Rockville, Md, 1997, U.S. Department of Health and Human Services, Public Health Services, National Institutes of Health, National Cancer Institute. NIH publication 97-4213.)*

The interaction of cigarette smoking with other known risk factors is well studied. Some suggest that the effect is additive, whereas others find a multiplicative effect. Cigarette smoking adds to cardiovascular risk associated with lipids, obesity, diabetes mellitus, hypertension, oral contraceptive use, and electrocardiographic abnormalities.[15-17] The additive effects of smoking in relationship to other major risk factors are seen in Figures 20-3 and 20-4 for 10- and 30-year follow-up of men and women aged 25 years at study entry. It is apparent that smoking adds significantly to risk. Smokers who continue in the habit after an acute myocardial infarction have significantly higher rates of recurrent events and death.[18] Individuals who quit smoking reduce that risk of a subsequent event.[18] Smokers also suffer increased rates of

peripheral arterial disease with a relative risk of two to three times[19] and twice the risk of stroke.[20]

The mechanisms by which cigarettes affect cardiovascular diseases have been studied in both animal and human models. Both acute and chronic mechanisms are postulated, and it is likely that both contribute. There is accumulating evidence that smoking plays an important role in the basic atherosclerotic process. This is elegantly confirmed in the PDAY (Pathobiological Determinants of Atherosclerosis in Youth) study.[21] In this study, autopsies were performed on 1443 men and women aged 15 to 34 years who died of external causes, such as auto accidents. Smoking was associated with an excess of fatty streaks and raised lesions in the abdominal aorta in these otherwise healthy individuals.[21] Injury of the arterial endothelium is suggested by some as the mechanism for the atherosclerotic lesions, but other mechanisms are also postulated.[22] Acute effects of smoking are demonstrated by the known short-term vascular effects of nicotine and the rapid improvement in prognosis with smoking cessation.

There are also known associations and interactions of smoking with other recognized elements in the causal chain and biomarkers for cardiovascular disease.[23] For example, many studies find smoking to be inversely associated with high-density lipoprotein cholesterol, the "good cholesterol," whereas some report associations with elevated low-density and very-low-density lipoprotein cholesterol. Smoking has prothrombotic effects, including increasing platelet adhesion, increased fibrinogen, and decreased fibrinolytic activity. All are associated with increased clotting.[24,25] As the interest in atherosclerosis as an inflammatory disease grows, increased leukocyte counts and elevated C-reactive protein support an association.[23]

ENVIRONMENTAL TOBACCO SMOKE

Recently, there is increased emphasis on exposure to environmental tobacco smoke among nonsmokers in the home, workplace, and public settings. This is more hotly debated than individual smoking because it affects those who may not have a choice about being exposed to tobacco smoke. In the 2006 Surgeon General's report *The Health Consequences of Involuntary Exposure to Tobacco Smoke*, cardiovascular disease was clearly implicated along with the demonstrated cancer and respiratory disease effects of environmental tobacco smoke.[6]

A meta-analysis incorporating more home-based studies along with workplace studies (total of 1699 cases) showed an overall increased risk associated with passive smoking (RR = 1.49; 95% CI, 1.29-1.72) and suggested relative risks from workplace exposure similar to those from home-based exposure.[26] In addition, environmental tobacco smoke is associated with sudden infant death syndrome and respiratory diseases in exposed children.[27]

The mechanism by which environmental tobacco smoke affects individuals is still debated, but considerable data are available. It is clear that mainstream smoke, that inhaled by the smoker, differs from sidestream smoke, which is released into the environment immediately.[6,26] Sidestream smoke may be more toxic. It is apparent that nonsmokers who are exposed regularly to cigarette smoke develop a number of physiologic changes. Some studies find that nonsmokers are more sensitive to these changes than those regularly exposed.[28] These include the chronic effects of cigarette smoke, such as lower high-density lipoprotein cholesterol, increased fibrinogen, and platelet abnormalities.[6] It is also apparent that exposed nonsmokers have acute effects including endothelial dysfunction and lower exercise tolerance.[29,30]

These observations are compatible with pathologic cardiovascular effects in nonsmokers exposed to environmental

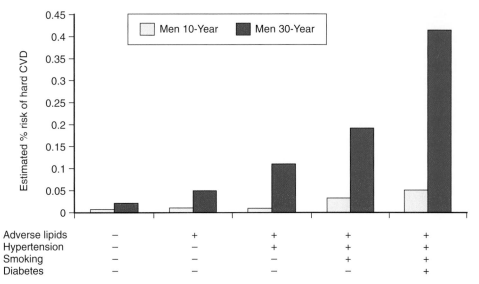

No risk factors profile: Total cholesterol=150 mg/dL; HDL cholesterol=60 mg/dL; untreated SBP=110 mm Hg; nonsmoker; nondiabetic. Adverse lipids: total cholesterol=260 mg/dL; HDL cholesterol=35 mg/dL. Hypertension: SBP=160 mm Hg, untreated.

FIGURE 20-3 The 10-year versus 30-year risk of hard CVD events for 25-year-old men with different risk profiles. *(From Pencina MJ, D'Agostino RB Sr, Larson MG, et al: Predicting the 30-year risk of cardiovascular disease: the Framingham Heart Study. Circulation 119:3078, 2009.)*

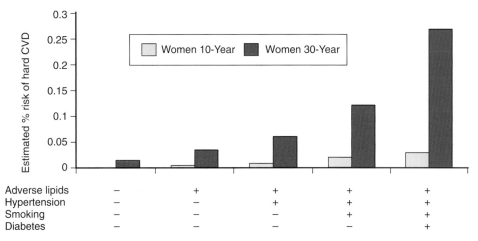

No risk factors profile: Total cholesterol=150 mg/dL; HDL cholesterol=60 mg/dL; untreated SBP=110 mm Hg; nonsmoker; nondiabetic. Adverse lipids: total cholesterol=260 mg/dL; HDL cholesterol=35 mg/dL. Hypertension: SBP=160 mm Hg, untreated.

FIGURE 20-4 The 10-year versus 30-year risk of hard CVD events for 25-year old women with different risk profiles. *(From Pencina MJ, D'Agostino RB Sr, Larson MG, et al: Predicting the 30-year risk of cardiovascular disease: the Framingham Heart Study. Circulation 119:3078, 2009.)*

tobacco smoke. Recent estimates suggest that 23,000 to 70,000 deaths per year from acute myocardial infarction are associated with environmental tobacco smoke exposure.[31] This effect is much larger than that observed for lung cancer. These observations underlie the recent efforts and successes in reducing environmental exposures or secondhand smoke.

PREVALENCE AND TRENDS IN CIGARETTE SMOKING AMONG YOUTH

Cigarette smoking among youth is described in the 1994 Surgeon General's report,[32] and methods of prevention are expanded in the 2000 Surgeon General's report.[33] Most smokers begin this habit in their teenage years. It begins with social pressure based on friends, siblings, and parents who smoke. Youth believe that smoking makes you look more adult and is associated with social success, independence, and rebelliousness, common themes in the teenage years. The environment provides important support through advertising, which reinforces the "coolness" of smoking. The highly effective Joe Camel ads and other media approaches were clearly aimed at and successful with new-onset smokers.[34] The basis of many tobacco lawsuits originated in this marketing practice. The most vulnerable period is in the sixth to eighth grades (ages 12 to 14 years), when much smoking initiation occurs.

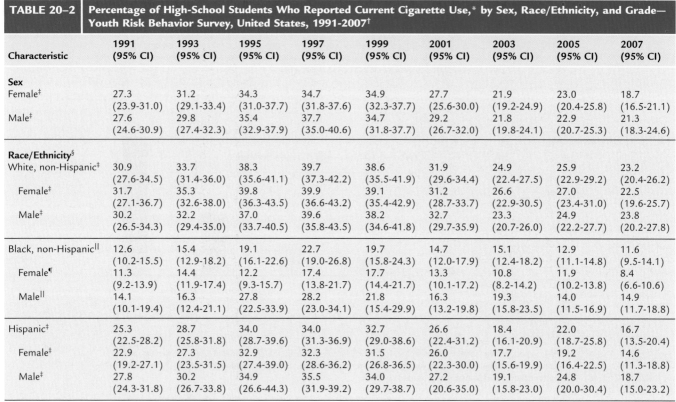

TABLE 20-1 | Percentage of High-School Students Who Reported Lifetime Cigarette Use,* Current Cigarette Use,† and Current Frequent Cigarette Use‡—Youth Risk Behavior Survey, United States, 1991-2007§

Cigarette Use	1991 (95% CI)	1993 (95% CI)	1995 (95% CI)	1997 (95% CI)	1999 (95% CI)	2001 (95% CI)	2003 (95% CI)	2005 (95% CI)	2007 (95% CI)
Lifetime‖	70.1 (67.8-72.3)	69.5 (68.1-70.8)	71.3 (69.5-73.0)	70.2 (68.2-72.1)	70.4 (67.3-73.3)	63.9 (61.6-66.0)	58.4 (55.1-61.6)	54.3 (51.2-57.3)	50.3 (47.2-53.5)
Current¶	27.5 (24.8-30.3)	30.5 (28.6-32.4)	34.8 (32.5-37.2)	36.4 (34.1-38.7)	34.8 (32.3-37.4)	28.5 (26.4-30.6)	21.9 (19.8-24.2)	23.0 (20.7-25.5)	20.0 (17.6-22.6)
Current frequent‖	12.7 (10.6-15.3)	13.8 (12.1-15.5)	16.1 (13.6-19.1)	16.7 (14.8-18.7)	16.8 (14.3-19.6)	13.8 (12.3-15.5)	9.7 (8.3-11.3)	9.4 (7.9-11.0)	8.1 (6.7-9.8)

*Ever tried cigarette smoking, even one or two puffs.

†Smoked cigarettes on at least 1 day during the 30 days before the survey.

‡Smoked cigarettes on 20 or more days during the 30 days before the survey.

§Linear, quadratic, and cubic trend analyses were conducted with a logistic regression model controlling for sex, race/ethnicity, and grade. These prevalence estimates are not standardized by demographic variables.

‖Significant linear and quadratic effects only (P <0.06).

¶Significant linear, quadratic, and cubic effects (P <0.05).

TABLE 20-2 | Percentage of High-School Students Who Reported Current Cigarette Use,* by Sex, Race/Ethnicity, and Grade—Youth Risk Behavior Survey, United States, 1991-2007†

Characteristic	1991 (95% CI)	1993 (95% CI)	1995 (95% CI)	1997 (95% CI)	1999 (95% CI)	2001 (95% CI)	2003 (95% CI)	2005 (95% CI)	2007 (95% CI)
Sex									
Female‡	27.3 (23.9-31.0)	31.2 (29.1-33.4)	34.3 (31.0-37.7)	34.7 (31.8-37.6)	34.9 (32.3-37.7)	27.7 (25.6-30.0)	21.9 (19.2-24.9)	23.0 (20.4-25.8)	18.7 (16.5-21.1)
Male‡	27.6 (24.6-30.9)	29.8 (27.4-32.3)	35.4 (32.9-37.9)	37.7 (35.0-40.6)	34.7 (31.8-37.7)	29.2 (26.7-32.0)	21.8 (19.8-24.1)	22.9 (20.7-25.3)	21.3 (18.3-24.6)
Race/Ethnicity§									
White, non-Hispanic‡	30.9 (27.6-34.5)	33.7 (31.4-36.0)	38.3 (35.6-41.1)	39.7 (37.3-42.2)	38.6 (35.5-41.9)	31.9 (29.6-34.4)	24.9 (22.4-27.5)	25.9 (22.9-29.2)	23.2 (20.4-26.2)
Female‡	31.7 (27.1-36.7)	35.3 (32.6-38.0)	39.8 (36.3-43.5)	39.9 (36.6-43.2)	39.1 (35.4-42.9)	31.2 (28.7-33.7)	26.6 (22.9-30.5)	27.0 (23.4-31.0)	22.5 (19.6-25.7)
Male‡	30.2 (26.5-34.3)	32.2 (29.4-35.0)	37.0 (33.7-40.5)	39.6 (35.8-43.5)	38.2 (34.6-41.8)	32.7 (29.7-35.9)	23.3 (20.7-26.0)	24.9 (22.2-27.7)	23.8 (20.2-27.8)
Black, non-Hispanic‖	12.6 (10.2-15.5)	15.4 (12.9-18.2)	19.1 (16.1-22.6)	22.7 (19.0-26.8)	19.7 (15.8-24.3)	14.7 (12.0-17.9)	15.1 (12.4-18.2)	12.9 (11.1-14.8)	11.6 (9.5-14.1)
Female¶	11.3 (9.2-13.9)	14.4 (11.9-17.4)	12.2 (9.3-15.7)	17.4 (13.8-21.7)	17.7 (14.4-21.7)	13.3 (10.1-17.2)	10.8 (8.2-14.2)	11.9 (10.2-13.8)	8.4 (6.6-10.6)
Male‖	14.1 (10.1-19.4)	16.3 (12.4-21.1)	27.8 (22.5-33.9)	28.2 (23.0-34.1)	21.8 (15.4-29.9)	16.3 (13.2-19.8)	19.3 (15.8-23.5)	14.0 (11.5-16.9)	14.9 (11.7-18.8)
Hispanic‡	25.3 (22.5-28.2)	28.7 (25.8-31.8)	34.0 (28.7-39.6)	34.0 (31.3-36.9)	32.7 (29.0-38.6)	26.6 (22.4-31.2)	18.4 (16.1-20.9)	22.0 (18.7-25.8)	16.7 (13.5-20.4)
Female‡	22.9 (19.2-27.1)	27.3 (23.5-31.5)	32.9 (27.4-39.0)	32.3 (28.6-36.2)	31.5 (26.8-36.5)	26.0 (22.3-30.0)	17.7 (15.6-19.9)	19.2 (16.4-22.5)	14.6 (11.3-18.8)
Male‡	27.8 (24.3-31.8)	30.2 (26.7-33.8)	34.9 (26.6-44.3)	35.5 (31.9-39.2)	34.0 (29.7-38.7)	27.2 (20.6-35.0)	19.1 (15.8-23.0)	24.8 (20.0-30.4)	18.7 (15.0-23.2)

*Smoked cigarettes on at least 1 day during the 30 days before the survey.

†Linear, quadratic, and cubic trend analyses were conducted with a logistic regression model controlling for sex, race/ethnicity, and grade in school. These prevalence estimates are not standardized by demographic variables.

‡Significant linear, quadratic, and cubic effects (P <0.05).

§Numbers for other racial/ethnic groups were too small for meaningful analysis.

‖Significant quadratic and cubic effects only (P <0.05).

¶Significant linear and quadratic effects only (P <0.05).

Early surveys of national trends showed a steady rise in cigarette smoking among youth from 1968 to 1974.[35] During that time, smoking of teenage girls began to exceed that of boys. However, from 1991 to 2007, a national sample of high-school students found a steady fall of smoking rates among this group until 2003, when it leveled (Table 20-1).[36] Importantly, the category never-smoked was increasing. There were also race and ethnicity differences, with non-Hispanic whites more likely to smoke than blacks or Hispanics in 2007 (Table 20-2).[36]

If the long-term health of the nation is to be improved, prevention of cigarette smoking initiation among youth is an essential element.

PREVALENCE AND TRENDS AMONG ADULTS

Cigarette consumption per capita for individuals aged 18 years and older rose steadily from 1900 to the late 1960s.

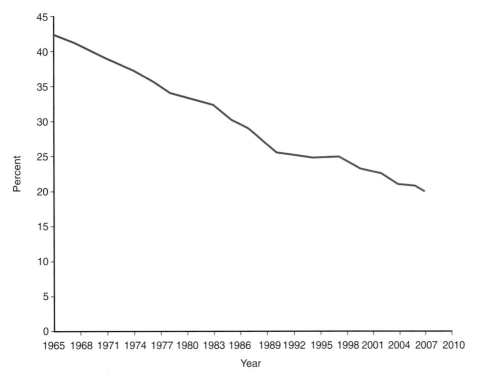

FIGURE 20-5 Trends in current cigarette smoking among adults, United States, 1965-2007. *(Source: cdc.gov.)*

Since that time, it steadily declined through 2007.[37] This pattern is the result of complementary trends including increased levels of smoking cessation and increasing rates of never-smokers. The National Health Interview Survey found that 42.4% of adults smoked in 1965 and 19.8% in 2007 (Fig. 20-5). The proportion of never-smokers in 2008 was 57.6%, with former smokers (21.5%) exceeding current smokers (20.8%) (Fig. 20-6). These national rates confirm a declining number of adult smokers during the past 40 years. Although rates nationally have decreased, there still exists significant variation by region of the country.[38] In 2004, the percentage of adults who smoked ranged from a high of 28.3% in Kentucky to 11.7% in Utah, with an average of 20%.

Whereas cigarette smoking among adults has substantially declined, a sizable portion of the population is still addicted.[37] One of the national health objectives for 2010 is to reduce the prevalence of cigarette smoking among adults to 12% or less. With smoking rates of 19.8% in 2007, that goal may not be met. Prevalence was lowest among Asians (9.6%) and Hispanics (13.3%) and highest among American Indians/Alaska Natives (36.4%). Non-Hispanic whites (21.4%) and blacks (19.8%) were similar. Adults who lived below the poverty level were more likely to smoke (28.8%) than were those at or above this level (20.3%). Persons with graduate or professional post-college degrees were far less likely to smoke (6.2%) than were those with less than a high-school education (33%) or a GED diploma (44%). Smoking prevalence was far lower in those 65 years and older (8.3%) than in the younger age groups.

PREVENTION AND INTERVENTION AMONG YOUTH

School-Based Prevention Programs

Much of the effort in preventing smoking among youth has focused on the school setting. School-based prevention programs generally have been targeted at junior-high

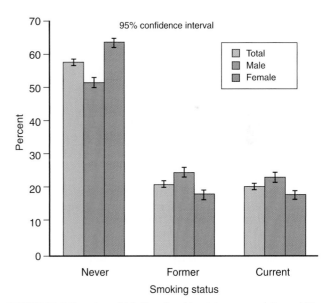

FIGURE 20-6 Percentage distribution of smoking status among adults aged 18 years and older, by sex: United States, January-June 2008. Note: Current smokers were defined as those who smoked more than 100 cigarettes in their lifetime and now smoke every day or some days. The analyses excluded 165 persons (1.3%) with unknown smoking status. *(Based on data collected from January through June in the Sample Adult Core Component of the 2008 National Health Interview Survey. Data are based on household interviews of a sample of the civilian noninstitutionalized population.)*

or middle-school children, when the habit begins. Unfortunately, school-based programming alone may have limited impact in the absence of active parental and community involvement.[32] At one time, it was assumed that simply educating youths about the harmful effects of smoking would be sufficient to prevent them from initiating cigarette use.[39] However, it became apparent that information alone was not sufficient to deter adolescents from beginning to smoke.

Social influence approaches have identified the social environment as a critical determinant of smoking onset. Rather than focusing on long-term disease risk, these interventions have stressed more immediate consequences of smoking, including negative social consequences. Adolescents are seen as often lacking in skills needed to resist peer pressure and other influences that promote smoking.[40] As described in the 1994 Surgeon General's report, the principal messages of successful skills-based interventions focus on the negative short-term social consequences of smoking, on the techniques of tobacco advertising that may be falsely appealing to adolescents, and on the socially salient advantages of being a nonsmoker.

Meta-analyses of school-based smoking prevention programs have indicated that these programs do have an impact on preventing smoking onset.[40-44] Furthermore, social influence approaches appear to be the most effective type of school-based program. On the basis of the results of a meta-analysis, Rooney concluded that the best results were obtained by social influence programs that were delivered to sixth-grade students, included booster sessions, concentrated the program within a short time, and used a peer to present the program.[44a]

Glynn[45] listed essential elements of effective smoking prevention programs based on a consensus panel. These elements were summarized in the 1994 report of the Surgeon General[32] as follows:

1. Classroom sessions should be delivered at least five times per year in each of two years in the sixth through eighth grades.
2. Programs should emphasize the social factors that influence smoking onset, short-term consequences, and refusal skills.
3. Programs should be incorporated into the existing school curricula.
4. Programs should be introduced during the transition from elementary school to junior high or middle school (sixth or seventh grade).
5. Students should be involved in the presentation and delivery of the program (peer teaching).
6. Parental involvement should be sought.
7. Teachers should be adequately trained.
8. Programs should be socially and culturally acceptable to each community.

Although some of these points might appear self-evident (e.g., adequate training of teachers, social and cultural acceptability of programs), they are often overlooked in practice. Furthermore, high-risk populations, including those of low socioeconomic status and some ethnic minorities, present unique challenges as described by Sherman and Primack.[46] These groups require added attention.

Müller-Riemenschneider and colleagues[47] evaluated the long-term effectiveness of smoking prevention programs published from 2001 to 2006. In 35 studies with a follow-up period of 1 to 10 years, they found that most studies reported long-term beneficial effects. They noted that school-based programs alone were least effective but that the addition of community-based and multisectorial approaches to school programs was most effective.

Community-Based Prevention Programs

Several model prevention programs have actively involved parents and the larger community in addition to schools. One example is described by Perry and colleagues[48] in the context of the Minnesota Heart Health Program, a research and demonstration project designed to reduce cardiovascular disease at the community level.[49] Perry and colleagues hypothesized that school-based smoking prevention would be more effective in communities in which multiple complementary

school and community programs were established.[48] Students participated in 5 years of school-based health education including peer-led prevention in a context in which adults were actively involved in community smoking cessation programs, and smoking restrictions were implemented both in schools and in the larger community. Results were very encouraging, with smoking initiation significantly lower among students in the intervention community compared with students in the control community. These differences persisted throughout junior and senior high school. At the end of the twelfth grade, students in the intervention community evidenced 40% lower smoking prevalence than did students in the comparison community; 14.6% of students were weekly smokers at the end of high school compared with 24.1% in the reference community.

Other successful community interventions affecting youth include parental involvement, smoking restrictions (e.g., schools, restaurants), and limitation of access to cigarettes through legal restrictions and increased taxes.[50]

State and Federal Prevention Initiatives

After the successful tobacco lawsuits and increases in cigarette taxes, many states operated comprehensive anti-tobacco programs. A major emphasis of these programs is on prevention of tobacco use in youth. Many of these initiatives include anti-tobacco media campaigns.[51] Florida launched an aggressive media campaign that directly targeted the tobacco industry.[52] After 2 years, current cigarette use dropped from 18.5% to 11.1% among middle-school students and from 27.4% to 22.6% among high-school students.[53]

Flynn and coworkers[54] found that a combination of media intervention and school-based programming fared better than school-based intervention alone. The media campaign included both radio and television spots that were broadcast as paid advertisements over local media. Reported smoking in the past week was 35% less among youth in the school-and-media condition than in the school-only condition (12.8% versus 19.8%).

Restrictions on smoking in public places including schools and on tobacco availability to minors also may reduce smoking prevalence, although findings are inconsistent.[55] All 50 states and the District of Columbia adopted a minimum age of 18 years for the purchase of tobacco, but these laws are variably enforced.

Increased taxation also has an impact on adolescent smoking. Adolescents are more price sensitive than adults are.[56] The impact of significantly higher prices may be even greater in discouraging initiation than in reducing consumption among existing smokers. Furthermore, revenue from these taxes can be dedicated to comprehensive tobacco control programs that will further reduce the onset of smoking in youth.

The Centers for Disease Control published *Best Practices for Comprehensive Tobacco Control Programs* in 1999[57] and updated this report in 2007.[58] This document provides recommendations to the states for establishment of initiatives that include local community programs, chronic disease programs to reduce the burden of tobacco-related diseases, school interventions, enforcement, statewide programs, countermarketing, cessation methods, surveillance and evaluation, and administration and management. Recommended funding levels are given for each of these components. Local community programs can engage young people; school-based interventions can be linked with local community coalitions and statewide counteradvertising; enforcement can reduce access of minors; and statewide initiatives can provide skill, resources, and information for coordinated strategic implementation of community programs.

BOX 20-1 Prevention and Intervention Strategies in Youth

School-based prevention programs
  Social influence approaches show good results.
Community-based prevention programs (may also enhance effects of school-based programs)
State and federal prevention initiatives
  Anti-tobacco media campaigns (may enhance school-based programs)
  Restrictions on tobacco advertising
  Restrictions on tobacco availability to minors
  Restrictions on smoking in public places including schools
  Increased taxation (adolescents may be sensitive to price increases)
Limited work in adolescent cessation
  School-based cessation approaches
  Adolescent cessation in managed care

Cessation Among Youth

Most of the work done with youth has focused on prevention rather than on cessation of smoking. Many of the interventions demonstrated to be effective among adults have not achieved comparable success in adolescent populations.

A review examined the literature on smoking cessation in adolescents.[59] The authors evaluated 34 cessation studies. Program content for these studies was derived from a wide range of theoretical perspectives. Most studies were conducted in school settings that reach less than half of the potential population of adolescent smokers. End of treatment quit rates reported in 12 of the 17 studies averaged 20.7% (range, 0% to 36%); abstinence at follow-up declined to 13%. The most successful programs generally included some type of cognitive-behavioral intervention, such as instruction in coping skills and a focus on the immediate consequences of quitting.

A recently released handbook on cessation for youth, *I Quit! What to Do When You're Sick of Smoking, Chewing, or Dipping,* from the Centers for Disease Control and Prevention, provides helpful tips on quitting tobacco in this group.[60] Strategies for youth are summarized in Box 20-1.

CESSATION INTERVENTIONS AMONG ADULTS

Interventions with adults have focused on cessation rather than on prevention for obvious reasons, but there is a need for prevention in certain groups. Initiation among young adults is relatively common in certain settings, such as in the military. Klesges and colleagues[61] reported that 7% of never-smokers who entered the Air Force and completed basic military training were regular smokers 1 year later. Ethnic differences also have been found in smoking initiation; African Americans tend to initiate later than European Americans.[1] In some other countries, initiation of smoking tends to occur considerably later than in the United States. In China, for example, one cohort study found the mean age for starting smoking to be 22 years.[62] Until recently, it had been widely assumed that those who reached the age of 18 years without cigarettes were very unlikely to initiate smoking as adults. However, the tobacco industry has increasingly targeted advertising and promotion efforts to young adults. In contrast to older adults, smoking prevalence has not been declining in the young adult (18- to 24-year-old) population.

Most of the published work with adults has been limited to individual smokers who have sought assistance in quitting.

Unfortunately, individual smokers who are ready to quit and who seek help represent a very small proportion of the overall smoking population.[63] Furthermore, even among these smokers, absolute long-term outcomes with formal quit smoking programs are disappointing. Intensive multisession group clinics generally produce no more than about 25% abstinence at 1 year.[64] Unaided quit attempts fare substantially less well; of the approximately 17 million smokers in the United States who attempt to quit on their own each year, less than 10% are successful.

Traditionally, interventions have focused on a single assisted quit attempt. A more effective approach may be to view smoking as a chronic disease and to support multiple quit attempts as necessary.[65] More recently, larger scale public health efforts address smoking cessation at the community level and target adults who may not volunteer for treatment or who may not be immediately interested in quitting. For many years, smoking and other tobacco use were seen as essentially learned behaviors. More recently, however, smoking and other tobacco products have been recognized as physically addictive.[66]

Interventions Targeted at Individuals

There has been far more progress in developing effective smoking cessation interventions with adults than with adolescents. A recent clinical practice guideline panel of public and private agencies sponsored by the U.S. Public Health Service reviewed the literature and updated a 2000 report in 2008.[67] An overall conclusion of the panel was that effective smoking cessation treatments are available for adults. Recommendations from this panel are shown in Box 20-2.

Behavioral Treatments

Despite addictive properties of nicotine, behavioral aspects of smoking are still seen as critical cessation tools. The most effective intervention programs, including those using medications, have included behavioral treatment components. A number of specific behavioral components are aversive smoking, intratreatment social support, problem solving/skills training, quit day, extratreatment social support, motivation, weight and diet/nutrition, exercise/fitness, contingency contract, relaxation/breathing, and cigarette fading. Most of these specific treatment components have not been proven effective in isolation but may contribute to an overall multicomponent intervention.

Aversion

Although aversive smoking approaches are effective (and indeed achieve the highest absolute abstinence levels), aversive techniques have largely gone out of favor. These techniques have included rapid smoking[68,69] and oversmoking or satiation.[70] Rapid smoking requires smokers to take very frequent puffs, typically every 6 seconds, for as long as they can tolerate the procedure. Oversmoking requires subjects to dramatically increase (perhaps double) their usual cigarette consumption for an arbitrary period, typically 1 week. Concerns have been expressed about the safety of rapid smoking and oversmoking, particularly in those with prevalent disease.[71] Acceptability of these techniques to smokers has been an additional issue. Other options have included reduced aversion techniques,[72] such as focused smoking (smoking at a regulated but slower rate) and smoke holding (retaining smoke in the mouth and throat while breathing through the nose).

Contingency Contracting

Several studies have required participants to submit monetary deposits that are refunded contingent on maintained

BOX 20-2 Smoking Cessation Clinical Guideline Recommendations for Adults[66]

1. Tobacco dependence is a chronic disease that often requires repeated intervention and multiple attempts to quit. Effective treatments exist, however, that can significantly increase rates of long-term abstinence.
2. It is essential that clinicians and health care delivery systems consistently identify and document tobacco use status and treat every tobacco user seen in a health care setting.
3. Tobacco dependence treatments are effective across a broad range of populations. Clinicians should encourage every patient willing to make a quit attempt to use the counseling treatments and medication recommended.
4. Brief tobacco dependence treatment is effective. Clinicians should offer every patient who uses tobacco at least the brief treatments shown to be effective.
5. Individual, group, and telephone counseling are effective, and their effectiveness increases with treatment intensity. Two components of counseling are especially effective, and clinicians should use these when counseling patients making a quit attempt:
   a. Practical counseling (problem solving/skills training)
   b. Social support delivered as part of treatment
6. Numerous effective medications are available for tobacco dependence, and clinicians should encourage their use by all patients attempting to quit smoking, except when medically contraindicated or with specific populations for which there is insufficient evidence of effectiveness (i.e., pregnant women, smokeless tobacco users, light smokers, and adolescents).
   a. Seven first-line medications (five nicotine and two non-nicotine) reliably increase long-term smoking abstinence rates: bupropion SR, nicotine gum, nicotine inhaler, nicotine lozenge, nicotine nasal spray, nicotine patch, and varenicline.
   b. Clinicians also should consider the use of certain combinations of medications identified as effective.
7. Counseling and medication are effective when used by themselves for treating tobacco dependence. The combination of counseling and medication, however, is more effective than either alone. Thus, clinicians should encourage all individuals making a quit attempt to use both counseling and medication.
8. Telephone quitline counseling is effective with diverse populations and has broad reach. Therefore, clinicians and health care delivery systems should both ensure patient access to quitlines and promote quitline use.
9. If a tobacco user currently is unwilling to make a quit attempt, clinicians should use the motivational treatments shown in the guideline to be effective in increasing future quit attempts.
10. Tobacco dependence treatments are both clinically effective and highly cost-effective relative to interventions for other clinical disorders. Providing coverage for these treatments increases quit rates. Insurers and purchasers should ensure that all insurance plans include the counseling and medication identified as effective as covered benefits.

abstinence.[73,74] Contracts may also call for self-administered rewards for progressively longer periods of abstinence. Typically, contingency contracting has been included as part of multicomponent behavioral programs.

Social Support

Supportive intervention during direct contact with a clinician or in a group (intratreatment social support) increases smoking cessation rates.[67] However, although social support from friends and family is strongly related to successful outcomes in smoking cessation treatments, efforts to systematically enhance natural social support as part of treatment intervention generally have proven unsuccessful.[75]

Relaxation Techniques

Progressive relaxation and deep breathing strategies have been employed for smoking cessation, although rarely in isolation. A major rationale for the use of these procedures is that smoking relapses are very likely to occur during negative emotional states.[76] Relaxation training allows an alternative response for coping with negative emotions or stressful situations and with the stress of quitting smoking and nicotine withdrawal effects. However, there is little evidence to support the efficacy of relaxation training as a stand-alone technique.[77]

Coping Skills

Favorable results have been found for specific training in coping skills. Coping skills include problem solving and methods for management of stress and prevention of relapse. Shiffman[78] found that a combination of cognitive (e.g., mentally reviewing benefits of quitting) and behavioral (e.g., physical activity, leaving a tempting situation) coping responses provided maximum protection against smoking in a potential crisis situation.

Reduced Smoking and Nicotine Fading

Nicotine fading is a nonaversive preparation technique based on the logical premise that withdrawal discomfort might be ameliorated if nicotine consumption is progressively reduced before abstinence. This premise may appear to be in conflict with the results of gradual reduction or cigarette "tapering" procedures. Strategies that have emphasized cutting down the number of cigarettes smoked have been almost uniformly unsuccessful.[79] Smokers typically appear to reach a "stuck point," often at 10 to 12 cigarettes per day.[79] For the typical smoker of approximately a pack per day, compensatory changes in puffing can compensate for reduced numbers of cigarettes at this level. Nicotine fading is an alternative in which smokers switch in a series of progressive steps during several weeks to cigarettes rated lower in tar and nicotine[80] or use commercially available nicotine reduction filters.[81] These procedures have not proved successful in improving smoking cessation outcomes.

Multicomponent Treatment Programs

The most successful behavioral programs have incorporated multiple treatment components. Emphasis has been placed on both initial preparation for quitting and longer term maintenance. Reported long-term abstinence rates for these multicomponent treatment programs have approached 50%.[82]

Hypnosis and Acupuncture

There are numerous approaches to smoking cessation that are not primarily behavioral or pharmacologic. Two commonly advertised methods are hypnosis and acupuncture. Unfortunately, there are few good studies of these methods, and overall results tend to be disappointing. Studies that have compared acupuncture at theoretically correct sites versus "incorrect" or sham sites have generally found no differences in outcome.

Nonprofit and Proprietary Programs

The oldest of the nonprofit programs is the Five-Day Plan sponsored by the Seventh-Day Adventist Church.[83] An estimated 14 million smokers in more than 150 countries have attended Five-Day Plans. This program considers both physical and psychological aspects of cigarette dependence but uses few cognitive-behavioral strategies. Treatment consists of five 90-minute to 2-hour sessions on consecutive days. The Five-Day Plan has been recently revised and renamed the Breathe Free Plan to Stop Smoking, which includes eight sessions during a 3-week period.

Both the American Cancer Society and the American Lung Association offer formal group programs. Lando and associates[84] compared these two programs. Smokers (n = 1041) in three Iowa communities were randomly assigned to American Cancer Society clinics, American Lung Association clinics, or an intensive multicomponent behavioral program derived from laboratory research. Although results initially favored the laboratory program over both nonprofit clinics, by 1-year follow-up, differences between the laboratory program and the American Lung Association program were no longer significant. Sustained abstinence rates at 1 year were 22.2%, 19.0%, and 12.1% for the laboratory, American Lung Association, and American Cancer Society clinics, respectively. The current American Cancer Society Quitline[85] and the American Lung Association smoking cessation programs[86] both offer assistance for those wishing to quit.

A number of commercial programs are available, usually concentrated in larger metropolitan areas. Most programs tend not to be profitable and therefore do not remain active. In evaluating commercial methods, it again appears that the most successful are those that include multicomponent cognitive-behavioral techniques. A number of commercial products (e.g., lozenges, filters) have been introduced as aids to smoking cessation. Currently, none of these products other than nicotine replacement, bupropion (Zyban), and varenicline (Chantix) are recognized as effective.

Self-Help

Simply handing smokers written self-help materials has not been demonstrated to be effective. There is evidence based on a limited number of studies that smoker-initiated calls to telephone hotlines or helplines for cessation counseling or assistance do improve abstinence rates. Although results have been mixed, several studies have found good results for proactive telephone support in which calls are initiated by the helpline rather than by the smoker.[87]

Computer-Tailored Messages

Computer-tailored messages or "expert systems" have the potential to individualize cessation content to the individual smoker. Some encouraging preliminary results have been reported with these types of programs.[88,89]

Pharmacologic Intervention

A number of pharmacologic aids are recognized as effective by the Food and Drug Administration. Most of these aids involve some form of nicotine replacement: nicotine patch, nicotine polacrilex (nicotine gum), nicotine nasal spray, nicotine inhaler, and nicotine lozenge. Each of these products has specific advantages and disadvantages. All may result in dependence in some patients.

The patch is easy to use and needs to be applied only once each day. However, it does not allow flexible dosing (e.g., once the patch is placed on the skin, the delivered dose is not controlled by the patient), and delivery of nicotine is relatively slow. The gum allows more flexible dosing but is somewhat more difficult to use correctly. Most gum users underdose with this medication. Nicotine nasal spray also has the advantage of flexible dosing, plus it provides faster delivery of nicotine. However, many users are bothered by initial eye and nose irritation, and frequent use is necessary

to obtain adequate nicotine levels. The nicotine inhaler allows flexible dosing and at least partially mimics the hand-to-mouth behavior of smoking. The inhaler also has few side effects. A major limitation, however, may be the need to do far more puffing than on a cigarette. For optimal nicotine dosage, many hundreds of puffs may be needed as opposed to perhaps 200 for a regular pack per day smoker. The nicotine lozenge also allows flexible dosing and is easier than nicotine gum for many people to use.

The only Food and Drug Administration–approved non-nicotine medications are bupropion hydrochloride (trade name Zyban) and varenicline (trade name Chantix). Bupropion is available in tablet form. It appears to act on brain chemistry to bring about some of the same effects that nicotine has when people smoke, although its actions are not fully understood. The product is easy to use and can be combined with nicotine replacement. Preliminary evidence suggests that the combination of nicotine patch and bupropion may be more effective than either alone.[90] The main ingredient in bupropion has been available for many years for treatment of depression under the trade name Wellbutrin. However, bupropion works well in smokers with no symptoms of depression. Bupropion is also sold as an antidepressant (Wellbutrin) and has all of the potential side effects of that class of drugs, including suicidality, depression, anxiety, panic attacks, insomnia, and irritability. Monitoring for these symptoms is recommended along with support for cessation. Seizures are a particular problem with doses above 300 mg/day.

Varenicline is also a pill, available through prescription. It works by blocking nicotine receptors in the central nervous system. It should not be used with other quit smoking products. Common side effects are nausea and insomnia, but serious behavioral side effects are also observed. A comparison of varenicline with bupropion and placebo found this agent more effective in smoking cessation at 24 weeks.[91] Varenicline should be stopped if agitation, depression, changes in behavior, or suicidality are observed.

There is evidence that some combinations of medication may be more effective in producing abstinence. A combination of passive dosing (e.g., through nicotine patch) and active dosing (e.g., ad libitum use, such as with nicotine gum) has been demonstrated to be more effective than a single form of dosing in isolation.[92-94]

Clinical Approaches

The many strategies described provide a diverse set of intervention approaches available for clinicians, but there are some proven basic steps summarized as the 5 A's (Box 20-3). These simple actions, aided by intervention strategies, will aid in patients' cessation attempts.

Community and Public Health Approaches

Less than 1% of all smokers have attended formal group or individual treatment programs. Even if half of these smokers achieved permanent abstinence, the overall impact on smoking prevalence would be modest. The need for a

BOX 20-3 Counseling: 5 A's

Ask	Systematically identify all tobacco users at every visit.
Advise	Strongly urge all smokers to quit.
Attempt	Identify smokers willing to try to quit.
Assist	Aid the patient in quitting.
Arrange	Schedule follow-up contact.

Interventions in health systems
    Clinician advice (brief advice significantly increases quitting)
    Pharmacologic treatment
Work site interventions (convenient access to large population of smokers, opportunities to capitalize on social support)
Community programs
    Overall mixed results
    Quit and Win contests widely disseminated
Policy changes

comprehensive public health approach to smoking, which includes community and systems changes in addition to treatment programs of varying types and intensities, is long apparent.[95,96] These approaches are summarized in Box 20-4. There is growing evidence of the success of these programs.[96-99]

Health Care System

Primary care and other clinicians have unique access to the smoking population. At least 70% of smokers see a physician each year. Smokers cite physician advice to quit as an important motivator.[67,100] Brief physician advice alone has been associated with a 30% increase in the probability of quitting.[67] Although absolute abstinence rates were modest, universal application of physician or other clinician advice could have a major public health impact. Combining brief advice with offers of behavioral or pharmacologic treatment could further increase the likelihood of success.

A major issue in health system implementation is lack of reimbursement for smoking cessation services. Curry and colleagues[101] found that use of smoking cessation services varies with the extent of coverage. Full coverage of both behavioral intervention and nicotine replacement therapy led to highest rates of use of smoking cessation services and to the greatest impact on the overall prevalence of smoking.

Work Site Interventions

Work sites provide convenient access to a large population of smokers as well as the opportunity to capitalize on social support in this setting. Some very positive results have been reported for work site interventions, although not all studies have been successful. Jeffery and colleagues[102] found modest but significant reductions in overall work site smoking prevalence with an intervention that provided structured group programs and incentives (e.g., refundable payroll deductions) for quitting. The Working Well Trial conducted in 111 work sites was the largest work site cancer control trial in the United States.[103] Interventions addressed dietary patterns and smoking. Although reductions in tobacco use were in the predicted direction, differences in tobacco use between intervention and control work sites were not significant.

Community Programs

Several major community smoking interventions were offered as part of multicomponent heart disease prevention studies.[49,104,105] The Stanford Five-City project reported significant smoking reductions in the intervention cohort relative to the control, but changes were not found in cross-sectional samples. The Pawtucket Heart Health Program failed to obtain differences in smoking prevalence between an intervention and a comparison city. The Minnesota Heart Health Program found mixed but primarily negative results for smoking intervention. The only evidence of a significant intervention effect was for women in cross-sectional survey data.[106]

Although the overall impact of these community-wide trials on smoking prevalence was disappointing, a useful innovation resulting from these programs was the Quit and Win smoking cessation contest. These contests have been successful at the community level in engaging relatively large proportions of the smoking population. Contests also have engaged large numbers of nonsmokers in support of smokers' quit efforts and have increased community awareness around issues of quitting. Community contests have enrolled as many as 7% of all eligible smokers and have involved many more in reported quit attempts during the contest period.[107] The Quit and Win contest model has been applied in communities in a number of countries around the world and also in national smoking cessation contests in Europe.

A direct successor to these community trials was the COMMIT project, which focused only on smoking.[108,109] In contrast to the earlier studies, COMMIT randomly assigned communities to intervention or control conditions and included sufficient numbers of communities to allow use of the community as the unit of analysis. One community within each of 11 matched community pairs (10 in the United States, 1 in Canada) was randomly assigned to intervention. The initial target of COMMIT was heavy smokers, defined as those who smoked 25 or more cigarettes per day. Intervention channels focused on public education through the media and community-wide events, health care providers, work sites and other organizations, and cessation resources.[108]

No differences were found between intervention and comparison communities in quit rates among heavy smokers. There was a significant intervention effect on quitting in light to moderate smokers.[108] Evaluation of overall smoking prevalence failed to indicate significant differences between intervention and comparison communities, however.[109] Results did indicate significant but overall modest differences between smokers in intervention and comparison communities in receipt of intervention activities.

More promising results have been reported for the American Stop Smoking Intervention Study (ASSIST). ASSIST is the largest tobacco control project ever undertaken in the United States.[110] In this initiative, 17 states funded through ASSIST were compared with 32 others (California, which already had extensive tobacco control activities, was omitted). The primary goal of ASSIST was to reduce smoking prevalence and cigarette consumption among adults in ASSIST states.

ASSIST was designed as a collaborative effort between the National Cancer Institute and the American Cancer Society and was implemented by state health departments. ASSIST targeted those considered at higher risk for smoking, including youth, ethnic minorities, blue-collar workers, unemployed, women, heavy smokers, and smokeless tobacco users. Interventions were delivered to target populations through five channels: community environment, work sites, schools, health care settings, and community groups such as churches and chambers of commerce. Emphasis was primarily on policy and media interventions, with less emphasis on programmatic services. Per capita consumption was almost identical in intervention and comparison states before 1993, when full funding for ASSIST interventions began. By 1996, smokers in the intervention states were consuming approximately 7% fewer cigarettes per capita.[111]

Policy Changes

Perhaps one of the largest impacts on society may be the improvement in health that results from policy changes, such as the passage of smoke-free areas through anti-tobacco legislation or increases in cigarette taxes. An excellent example of this stems from a study of respiratory health before and after recent prohibition began in bars and taverns in

California.[112] In a small study of 53 bartenders in San Francisco, of those with respiratory symptoms at baseline, 59% no longer had symptoms at follow-up; of those with sensory irritations, 78% had resolution of symptoms (both $P < 0.001$). Furthermore, a significant improvement (increase) in mean forced vital capacity (increase of 4.2%) was reported after prohibition, and after cessation, significant improvements in both forced vital capacity (6.8% increase) and mean forced expiratory volume in 1 second (4.5% increase) were reported.

Since these early efforts, based on increased cigarette taxes in California, there have been many policy changes built around smoke-free environments, limiting youth access, and tax increases. Environmental changes include smoke-free buildings, transportation, bars, restaurants, and even outdoor places.[97-99,113-116] Much of the evidence supporting these changes is summarized in an Institute of Medicine report.[117] There is evidence that smoking bans work synergistically with cessation programs.[118] Restricting access of youth to tobacco purchases by enforcing age-related laws is also a successful strategy.[119,120] Finally, increases in tobacco excise taxes have had an effect, especially among younger smokers.[121-124]

CONCLUSION

The evidence linking tobacco use to the incidence of and mortality from cardiovascular diseases is substantial. Approximately a half-million deaths annually are attributed to cigarette smoking, and the economic costs in medical expenses and indirect costs are enormous. Environmental tobacco smoke is also an important culprit, responsible for some 35,000 to 40,000 deaths from heart disease annually. Important interventions among youth include school-based prevention programs, community-based prevention programs, state and federal initiatives, and cessation assistance. For adults, various behavioral treatments, self-help approaches, and pharmacologic therapy are available. Community and public health approaches are invaluable. Physicians and other health care providers need to take greater initiative in reviewing and following up on tobacco use and in informing patients about appropriate community and health care resources for those needing help.

Whereas reductions in adult smoking will have the most immediate benefit in terms of reduced hospitalizations from myocardial infarction and stroke, as well as savings associated with a program reducing smoking prevalence by 1% per year,[125] the key to making future progress is primary prevention of smoking in children and teenagers. The fact that tobacco is dangerous, lethal, and disabling when it is used as directed has resulted in the passage of legislation to have the Food and Drug Administration take steps to regulate its sale and use.[126]

REFERENCES

1. Centers for Disease Control and Prevention: Cigarette smoking among adults—United States, 2007. *MMWR Morb Mortal Wkly Rep* 57:1221, 2008.
2. Centers for Disease Control and Prevention: 2006 national youth tobacco survey and key prevalence indicators. Available at: www.cdc.gov/tobacco/data_statistics/surveys/nyts/pdfs/indicators.pdf.
3. Centers for Disease Control and Prevention: Smoking-attributable mortality, years of potential life lost, and productivity losses—United States, 2000-2004. *MMWR Mortal Wkly Rep* 57:1226, 2008.
4. WHO report on the global tobacco epidemic, 2008, Geneva, 2008, World Health Organization.
5. U.S. Public Health Service: *The health consequences of smoking: cardiovascular disease: a report of the Surgeon General*, Rockville, Md, 1983, U.S. Department of Health and Human Services. DHHS publication (PHS) 84-50204.
6. U.S. Department of Health and Human Services: *The health consequences of involuntary exposure to tobacco smoke: a report of the Surgeon General*, Atlanta, Ga, 2006, U.S. Department of Health and Human Services, Centers for Disease Control and Prevention, National Center for Chronic Disease Prevention and Health Promotion, Office on Smoking and Health.
7. U.S. Department of Health and Human Services: *Changes in cigarette-related disease risks and their implication for prevention and control*, Monograph 8, Rockville, Md, 1997, U.S. Department of Health and Human Services, Public Health Services, National Institutes of Health, National Cancer Institute. NIH publication 97-4213.
8. Kawachi I, Colditz GA, Stampfer MJ, et al: Smoking cessation and time course of decreased risks of coronary heart disease in middle-aged women. *Arch Intern Med* 154:169, 1994.
9. Centers for Disease Control: *The health benefits of smoking cessation: a report of the Surgeon General*, Washington, DC, 1990, Public Health Service, Office on Smoking and Health. DHHS publication (CDC) 90-8416.
10. Neaton JD, Wentworth D; Multiple Risk Factor Intervention Trial Research Group: Serum cholesterol, blood pressure, cigarette smoking, and death from coronary heart disease: overall findings and differences by age for 316,099 white men. *Arch Intern Med* 152:56, 1992.
11. The Multiple Risk Factor Intervention Trial Research Group: Mortality after 16 years for participants randomized to the Multiple Risk Factor Intervention Trial. *Circulation* 94:946, 1996.
12. Keys A, Menotti A, Aravanis C, et al: The seven countries study: 2,289 deaths in 15 years. *Prev Med* 13:141, 1984.
13. Escobedo LG, Caspersen CJ: Risk factors for sudden coronary death in the United States. *Epidemiology* 8:175, 1997.
14. Kannel WB, McGee DL, Castelli WP: Latest perspectives on cigarette smoking and cardiovascular disease: the Framingham Study. *J Cardiac Rehabil* 4:267, 1984.
15. Pooling Project Research Group: Relationship of blood pressure, serum cholesterol, smoking habit, relative weight, and ECG abnormalities to incidence of major coronary events: final report of the Pooling Project. *J Chronic Dis* 31:201, 1978.
16. Suarez L, Barrett-Connor E: Interaction between cigarette smoking and diabetes mellitus in the prediction of death attributed to cardiovascular disease. *Am J Epidemiol* 120:670, 1984.
17. Mishell DR: Use of oral contraceptives in women of older reproductive age. *Am J Obstet Gynecol* 158:1652, 1988.
18. Hermanson B, Omenn GS, Kronmal RA, et al: Beneficial six-year outcome of smoking cessation in older men and women with coronary artery disease: results from the CASS registry. *N Engl J Med* 319:1365, 1988.
19. Hirsch AT, Haskal ZJ, Hertzer NR, et al: ACC/AHA 2005 practice guidelines for the management of patients with peripheral arterial disease (lower extremity, renal, mesenteric, and abdominal aortic). *Circulation* 113:1474, 2006.
20. Ockene IS, Miller NH: Cigarette smoking, cardiovascular disease, and stroke: a statement for healthcare professionals from the American Heart Association. *Circulation* 96:3243, 1997.
21. McGill HC, McMahan CA, Malcom GT, et al; PDAY Research Group: Effects of serum lipoproteins and smoking on atherosclerosis in young men and women. *Arterioscler Thromb Vasc Biol* 17:95, 1997.
22. Fried LP, Moore RD, Pearson TA: Long-term effects of cigarette smoking and moderate alcohol consumption on coronary artery diameter: mechanisms of coronary artery disease independent of atherosclerosis or thrombosis? *Am J Med* 80:37, 1986.
23. U.S. Department of Health and Human Services: *The health consequences of smoking: a report of the Surgeon General*, Atlanta, Ga, 2004, U.S. Department of Health and Human Services, Centers for Disease Control and Prevention, National Center for Chronic Disease Prevention and Health Promotion, Office on Smoking and Health.
24. Meade TW, Imeson J, Stirling Y: Effects of changes in smoking and other characteristics on clotting factors and the risk of ischaemic heart disease. *Lancet* 2:986, 1987.
25. Maouad J, Fernandez F, Barrillon A, et al: Diffuse or segmental narrowing (spasm) of coronary arteries during smoking demonstrated on angiography. *Am J Cardiol* 53:354, 1984.
26. Wells AJ: Heart disease from passive smoking in the workplace. *J Am Coll Cardiol* 31:1, 1998.
27. Kritz H, Schmid P, Sinzinger H: Passive smoking and cardiovascular risk. *Arch Intern Med* 155:1942, 1995.
28. Glantz SA, Parmley WW: Passive smoking and heart disease: mechanisms and risk. *JAMA* 273:1047, 1995.
29. Celermajer DS, Adams MR, Clarkson P, et al: Passive smoking and impaired endothelium-dependent arterial dilation in healthy young adults. *N Engl J Med* 334:150, 1996.
30. Otsuka R, Watanabe H, Hirata K, et al: Acute effects of passive smoking on the coronary circulation in healthy young adults. *JAMA* 286:436, 2001.
31. California Environmental Protection Agency: Proposed identification of environmental tobacco smoke as a toxic air contaminant. 2005. Available at: www.arb.ca.gov/regact/ets2006/ets2006.htm
32. U.S. Department of Health and Human Services: *Preventing tobacco use among young people: a report of the Surgeon General*, Atlanta, Ga, 1994, U.S. Department of Health and Human Services, Public Health Service, Centers for Disease Control and Prevention, National Center for Chronic Disease Prevention and Health Promotion, Office on Smoking and Health.
33. U.S. Department of Health and Human Services: *Reducing tobacco use: a report of the Surgeon General*, Atlanta, Ga, 2000, U.S. Department of Health and Human Services, Centers for Disease Control and Prevention.
34. Wellman RJ, Sugarman DB, DiFranza JR, Winickoff JP: The extent to which tobacco marketing and tobacco use in films contribute to children's use of tobacco. *Arch Pediatr Adolesc Med* 160:1285, 2006.
35. Johnston LD, O'Malley PM, Bachman JG: *National survey results on drug use from the monitoring the future study, 1975-1992, vol 1: secondary school students*, Rockville, Md, 1993, National Institutes on Drug Abuse.
36. Centers for Disease Control and Prevention: Cigarette use among high school students—United States, 1991-2007. *MMWR Morb Mortal Wkly Rep* 57:689, 2008.

37. U.S. Department of Health and Human Services: Trends in current cigarette smoking among high school students and adults, United States, 1965-2007, Centers for Disease Control and Prevention. Available at: cdc.gov/tobacco/data_statistics/tables/trends/cig_smoking/index.htm.

38. Centers for Disease Control and Prevention: State-specific prevalence and trends in adult cigarette smoking—United States, 1998-2007. *MMWR Morb Mortal Wkly Rep* 58:221, 2009.

39. Thompson EL: Smoking education programs 1960-1976. *Am J Public Health* 68:250, 1978.

40. Botvin GJ, Wills TA: Personal and social skills training: cognitive-behavioral approaches to substance abuse prevention. In Bell CS, Battjes R, editors: *Prevention research: deterring drug abuse among children and adolescents*. Monograph No. 63. Bethesda, Md, 1985, U.S. Department of Health and Human Services, Public Health Service, Alcohol, Drug Abuse, and Mental Health Administration, National Institute on Drug Abuse. DHHS publication (ADM) 85-1334.

41. Tobler NS: Meta-analysis of 143 adolescent drug prevention programs: quantitative outcome results of program participants compared to a control or comparison group. *J Drug Issues* 16:537, 1986.

42. Tobler NS: Drug prevention programs can work: research findings. *J Addict Dis* 11:1, 1992.

43. Rundall TG, Bruvold WH: A meta-analysis of school-based smoking and alcohol use prevention programs. *Health Educ Q* 15:317, 1988.

44. Bruvold WH: A meta-analysis of adolescent smoking-prevention programs. *Am J Public Health* 83:872, 1993.

44a. Rooney BL, Murray DM: A meta-analysis of smoking prevention programs after adjustments for errors in the unit of analysis. *Health Educ Q* 23:48, 1996.

45. Glynn TJ: Essential elements of school-based smoking-prevention programs. *J Sch Health* 59:181, 1989.

46. Sherman EJ, Primack BA: What works to prevent adolescent smoking? A systematic review of the National Cancer Institute's research tested programs. *J Sch Health* 79:391, 2009.

47. Müller-Riemenschneider F, Bockelbrink A, Reinhold T, et al: Long-term effectiveness of behavioral intervention to prevent smoking among children and youth. *Tob Control* 17:301, 2008.

48. Perry CL, Kelder SH, Murray DM, et al: Community-wide smoking prevention: long-term outcomes of the Minnesota Heart Health Program and the class of 1989 study. *Am J Public Health* 82:1210, 1992.

49. Luepker RV, Murray DM, Jacobs DR, et al: Community education for cardiovascular disease prevention: risk factor changes in the Minnesota Heart Health Program. *Am J Public Health* 84:1383, 1994.

50. Richardson L, Hemsing N, Greaves L, et al: Preventing smoking in young people: a systematic review of the impact of access interventions. *Int J Environ Res Public Health* 6:1485, 2009.

51. Schar E, Gutierrez K, Murph-Hoefer R, Nelson DE: *Tobacco use prevention media campaigns: lessons learned from youth in nine countries*, Atlanta, Ga, 2006, U.S. Department of Health and Human Services, Centers for Disease Control and Prevention. Available at: www.cdc.gov/tobacco.

52. Sly DF, Heald GR, Ray S: The Florida "truth" anti-tobacco media evaluation: design, first year results, and implications for planning future state media evaluations. *Tob Control* 10:9, 2001.

53. Bauer UE, Johnson TM, Hopkins RS, Brooks RG: Changes in youth cigarette use and intentions following implementation of a tobacco control program: findings from the Florida Youth Tobacco Survey, 1998-2000. *JAMA* 284:723, 2000.

54. Flynn BS, Worden JK, Secker-Walker RH, et al: Prevention of cigarette smoking through mass media intervention and school programs. *Am J Public Health* 82:827, 1992.

55. Rigotti NA, DiFranza JR, YuChiao C, et al: The effect of enforcing tobacco-sales laws on adolescents' access to tobacco and smoking behavior. *N Engl J Med* 337:1044, 1997.

56. Centers for Disease Control and Prevention: *Steady increases in tobacco taxes promote quitting, discourage smoking*, Atlanta, Ga, 2009, U.S. Department of Health and Human Services, Centers for Disease Control and Prevention. Available at: www.cdc.gov/Features/SecondhandSmoke/

57. Centers for Disease Control and Prevention: *Best practices for comprehensive tobacco control programs—August 1999*. Atlanta, Ga, 1999, U.S. Department of Health and Human Services, Centers for Disease Control and Prevention.

58. Centers for Disease Control and Prevention: *Best practices for comprehensive tobacco control programs—2007*. Atlanta, Ga, 2007, U.S. Department of Health and Human Services, Centers for Disease Control and Prevention.

59. Sussman S, Lichtman K, Ritt A, et al: Effects of thirty-four adolescent tobacco use cessation and prevention trials on regular users of tobacco products. *Subst Use Misuse* 34:1469, 1999.

60. Centers for Disease Control and Prevention: *I quit! What to do when you're sick of smoking, chewing, or dipping*, Atlanta, Ga, 2009, U.S. Department of Health and Human Services, Centers for Disease Control and Prevention. Available at: www.cdc.gov/tobacco/quit_smoking/hot_to_quit/iquit/index.htm.

61. Klesges R, Haddock K, Lando H, et al: Efficacy of forced smoking cessation and an adjunctive behavioral treatment on long term smoking rates. *J Consult Clin Psychol* 67:952, 1999.

62. Lam TH, He Y, Li LS, et al: Mortality attributable to cigarette smoking in China. *JAMA* 278:1505, 1997.

63. Lichtenstein E, Glasgow RE: Smoking cessation: what have we learned over the past decade? *J Consult Clin Psychol* 60:518, 1992.

64. U.S. Department of Health and Human Services: *Treating tobacco use and dependence*, Rockville, Md, 2000, U.S. Department of Health and Human Services, Public Health Service, Centers for Disease Control.

65. Lando H, Rolnick S, Klevan D, et al: Telephone support as an adjunct to transdermal nicotine. *Am J Public Health* 87:1670, 1997.

66. U.S. Department of Health and Human Services: *The health consequences of smoking: nicotine addiction: a report of the Surgeon General*, Rockville, Md, 1994, U.S. Department of Health and Human Services, Public Health Service, Centers for Disease Control, Center for Health Promotion and Education, Office on Smoking and Health.

67. U.S. Public Health Service: *Clinical practice guideline: treating tobacco use and dependence: 2008 update*, Washington, DC, 2008, U.S. Department of Health and Human Services.

68. Lichenstein E, Harris DE, Birchler GR, et al: Comparison of rapid smoking, warm, smoky air, and attention placebo in the modification of smoking behavior. *J Consult Clin Psychol* 40:92, 1973.

69. Poole AD, Sanson-Fisher RW, German GA: The rapid-smoking technique: therapeutic effectiveness. *Behav Res Ther* 19:89, 1981.

70. Resnick JH: Effects of stimulus satiation on the overlearned maladaptive response of cigarette smoking. *J Consult Clin Psychol* 32:501, 1968.

71. Hauser R: Rapid smoking as a technique of behavior modification: caution in selection of subjects. *J Consult Clin Psychol* 42:625, 1974.

72. Powell DR, McCann BS: The effects of a multiple treatment program and maintenance procedures on smoking cessation. *Prev Med* 10:94, 1981.

73. Elliott R, Tighe T: Breaking the cigarette habit: effects of a technique involving threatened loss of money. *Psychol Rec* 18:503, 1968.

74. Lando HA: Aversive conditioning and contingency management in the treatment of smoking. *J Consult Clin Psychol* 44:312, 1976.

75. Lichenstein E, Glasgow RE, Abrams DB: Social support in smoking cessation: in search of effective interventions. *Behav Res Ther* 17:607, 1986.

76. Brandon TH, Tiffany ST, Baker TB: The process of smoking relapse. In Tims FM, Leukefeld CG, editors: *Relapse and recovery in drug abuse*, Rockville, Md, 1986, Department of Health and Human Services, Public Health Service, Alcohol, Drug Abuse, and Mental Health Administration, National Institute on Drug Abuse.

77. Hatsukami DK, Lando H: Smoking cessation. In Ott PJ, Tartar RE, Ammerman RT, editors: *Sourcebook on substance abuse: etiology, epidemiology, assessment, and treatment*, Needham Heights, Mass, 1999, Allyn & Bacon.

78. Shiffman S: Relapse following smoking cessation: a situational analysis. *J Consult Clin Psychol* 50:71, 1982.

79. Flaxman J: Quitting smoking now or later: gradual, abrupt, immediate, and delayed quitting. *Behav Res Ther* 9:260, 1978.

80. Foxx RM, Brown RA: A nicotine fading and self-monitoring program to produce cigarette abstinence or controlled smoking. *J Appl Behav Anal* 12:111, 1979.

81. McGovern PG, Lando HA: Reduced nicotine exposure and abstinence outcome in two nicotine fading methods. *Addict Behav* 16:11, 1991.

82. Hall SM, Rugg D, Tunstall C, et al: Preventing relapse to cigarette smoking by behavioral skill training. *J Consult Clin Psychol* 52:372, 1984.

83. McFarland MI: When fire became twenty-five. A silver anniversary of the five-day plan to stop smoking. *Adventist Heritage* 11:57, 1986.

84. Lando H, McGovern P, Barrios F, et al: Comparative evaluation of American Cancer Society and American Lung Association smoking cessation clinics. *Am J Public Health* 80:54, 1990.

85. American Cancer Society quitline. Available at: http://www.cancer.org/docroot/PED/content/PED_10_13X_Guide_for_Quitting_Smoking.asp?from=fast.

86. American Lung Association freedom from smoking. Available at: www.lungusa.org/site/pp.asp?c=dvLUK9O0E&b=33484

87. Zhu S-H, Stretch V, Balabanis M, et al: Telephone counseling for smoking cessation: effects of single-session and multiple-session interventions. *J Consult Clin Psychol* 64:202, 1996.

88. Strecher V: Computer-tailored smoking cessation materials: a review and discussion. *Patient Educ Counsel* 36:107, 1999.

89. Velicer W, Prochaska JO: An expert system intervention for smoking cessation. *Patient Educ Counsel* 36:119, 1999.

90. Hurt RD, Sachs DPL, Glover ED, et al: Comparison of sustained-release bupropion and placebo for smoking cessation. *N Engl J Med* 337:1195, 1997.

91. Gonzales D, Rennard SI, Nides M, et al; Varenicline Phase 3 Study Group: Varenicline, an $\alpha_4\beta_2$ nicotinic acetylcholine receptor partial agonist, vs sustained-release bupropion and placebo for smoking cessation: a randomized controlled trial. *JAMA* 296:47, 2006.

92. Kornitzer M, Bousten M, Thijs J, et al: Efficiency and safety of combined use of nicotine patches and nicotine gum in smoking cessation: a placebo controlled double-blind trial. *Eur Respir J* 6:630s, 1993.

93. Puska P, Korhonen H, Vartiainen E, et al: Combined use of nicotine patch and gum compared with gum alone in smoking cessation: a clinical trial in North Karelia. *Tob Control* 4:231, 1995.

94. Blondal T, Gudmundsson LJ, Olafsdottir I, et al: Nicotine nasal spray with nicotine patch for smoking cessation: randomized trial with six year follow up. *BMJ* 318:285, 1999.

95. Abrams DB, Orleans CT, Niaura RS, et al: Integrating individual and public health perspectives for treatment of tobacco dependence under managed health care: a combined stepped-care and matching model. *Ann Behav Med* 18:290, 1996.

96. Becker DM, Windsor R, Ockene JK, et al: Setting the policy, education, and research agenda to reduce tobacco use. Workshop 1. *Circulation* 88:1381, 1993.

97. Centers for Disease Control and Prevention: Reduced hospitalizations for acute myocardial infarction after implementation of a smoke-free ordinance—City of Pueblo, Colorado, 2002-2006. *MMWR Morb Mortal Wkly Rep* 57:1373, 2009.

98. Juster HR, Loomis BR, Hinman TM, et al: Declines in hospital admissions for acute myocardial infarction in New York State after implementation of a comprehensive smoking ban. *Am J Public Health* 97:2035, 2007.

99. Pell JP, Haw S, Cobbe S, et al: Smoke-free legislation and hospitalizations for acute coronary syndrome. *N Engl J Med* 359:482, 2008.

100. National Cancer Institute: Tobacco and the clinician: interventions for medical and dental practice. *Monogr Natl Cancer Inst* 5:1, 1994, NIH publication 94-3693.

20

101. Curry SJ, Grothaus LC, McAfee T, et al: Use and cost effectiveness of smoking-cessation services under four insurance plans in a health maintenance organization. *N Engl J Med* 339:673, 1998.

102. Jeffery RW, Forster JL, French SA, et al: The Healthy Worker Project: a work-site intervention for weight control and smoking cessation. *Am J Public Health* 83:395, 1993.

103. Sorenson G, Thompson B, Glanz K, et al; Working Well Trial: Work site–based cancer prevention: primary results from the Working Well Trial. *Am J Public Health* 86:39, 1996.

104. Carleton RA, Lasater TM, Assaf AR, et al; Pawtucket Heart Health Program Writing Group: The Pawtucket Heart Health Program: community changes in cardiovascular risk factors and projected disease risk. *Am J Public Health* 85:777, 1995.

105. Farquhar JW, Fortmann SP, Flora JA, et al: Effects of community-wide education on cardiovascular disease risk factors. *JAMA* 264:359, 1990.

106. Lando H, Pechacek TF, Pirie PL, et al: Changes in adult cigarette smoking in the Minnesota Heart Health Program. *Am J Public Health* 85:201, 1995.

107. Pechacek TF, Lando HA, Nothwehr F, et al: Quit and win: a community-wide approach to smoking cessation. *Tob Control* 3:236, 1994.

108. The COMMIT Research Group: Community Intervention Trial for Smoking Cessation (COMMIT): I. Cohort results from a four-year community intervention. *Am J Public Health* 85:183, 1995.

109. The COMMIT Research Group: Community Intervention Trial for Smoking Cessation (COMMIT): II. Changes in adult cigarette smoking prevalence. *Am J Public Health* 85:193, 1995.

110. Manley M, Lynn W, Epps RP, et al: The American Stop Smoking Intervention Study for cancer prevention: an overview. *Tob Control* 6:S5, 1997.

111. Manley MW, Pierce JP, Gilpin EA, et al: Impact of the American Stop Smoking Intervention Study on cigarette consumption. *Tob Control* 6:S12, 1997.

112. Eisner MD, Smith AK, Blanc PD: Bartenders' respiratory health after establishment of smoke-free bars and taverns. *JAMA* 280:1909, 1998.

113. Thomson G, Wilson N, Edwards R: At the frontier of tobacco control: a brief review of public attitudes toward smoke-free outdoor places. *Nicotine Tob Res* 11:584, 2009.

114. Hahn EJ, Rayens MK, Butler KM, et al: Smoke-free laws and adult smoking prevalence. *Prev Med* 47:206, 2008.

115. Pierce JP: Tobacco industry marketing, population-based tobacco control, and smoking behavior. *Am J Prev Med* 33:S327, 2007.

116. Quentin W, Neubauer S, Leidl R, et al: Advertising bans as a means of tobacco control policy: a systematic literature review of time-series analyses. *Int J Public Health* 5:295, 2007.

117. Committee on Secondhand Smoke Exposure and Acute Coronary Events: *Secondhand smoke exposure and cardiovascular effects: making sense of the evidence*, Washington, DC, 2009, Institute of Medicine.

118. Grassi MC, Enea D, Ferketich AK, et al: A smoking ban in public places increases the efficacy of bupropion and counseling on cessation outcomes at 1 year. *Nicotine Tob Res* 11:1114, 2009.

119. Richardson L, Hemsing N, Greaves L, et al: Preventing smoking in young people: a systematic review of the impact of access interventions. *Int J Environ Res Public Health* 6:1485, 2009.

120. Ahmad S, Billimek J: Limiting youth access to tobacco: comparing the long-term health impacts of increasing cigarette excise taxes and raising the legal smoking age to 21 in the United States. *Health Policy* 80:378, 2007.

121. Lee JM: Effect of a large increase in cigarette tax on cigarette consumption: an empirical analysis of cross-sectional survey data. *Public Health* 10:1061, 2008.

122. DeCicca P, McLeod L: Cigarette taxes and older adult smoking: evidence from recent large tax increases. *J Health Econ* 27:918, 2008.

123. Stehr M: The effect of cigarette taxes on smoking among men and women. *Health Econ* 16:1333, 2007.

124. van Baal PHM, Brouwer WBF, Hoogenveen RT, et al: Increasing tobacco taxes: a cheap tool to increase public health. *Health Policy* 82:142, 2007.

125. Lightfoot JM, Glantz SA: Short-term economic and health benefits of smoking cessation: myocardial infarction and stroke. *Circulation* 96:1089, 1997.

126. Senate Passes FDA Tobacco Bill. Historic measure limits ads, packaging; smokeless products affected. *New York Times*, June 12, 2009.

CHAPTER **21**

Diabetes and Cardiovascular Disease

M. Odette Gore, Silvio E. Inzucchi, and Darren K. McGuire

KEY POINTS

- Diabetes mellitus is a major independent risk factor for cardiovascular disease.

- The worldwide prevalence of diabetes is increasing, driven primarily by the rise in type 2 diabetes.

- The pathophysiology of diabetic cardiovascular disease is multifactorial and incompletely understood.

- Lifestyle intervention is fundamental for the prevention of both type 2 diabetes and its cardiovascular complications.

- Glucose control is important for the management of diabetes, but the most appropriate strategies and glucose targets for cardiovascular disease prevention are still uncertain.

- In addition to lifestyle changes, pharmacologic interventions to treat hypertension and dyslipidemia in diabetes are essential for cardiovascular disease prevention.

- The use of antiplatelet interventions to prevent cardiovascular disease is still controversial but recommended in most patients with diabetes.

The incidence and prevalence of diabetes mellitus are on the rise in the United States and globally, almost entirely due to the growing pandemic of type 2 diabetes.[1] Given that diabetes is a major independent risk factor for cardiovascular disease (CVD), in some clinical contexts considered a coronary disease equivalent,[2] the prevention of diabetes and the management of its associated CVD risk factors are of paramount public health importance. This chapter reviews the epidemiology and preventive strategies for diabetes and its associated CVD complications, with special emphasis on type 2 diabetes, which accounts for more than 90% of diabetes cases worldwide.[3,4]

EPIDEMIOLOGY OF DIABETES MELLITUS

Definition

Diabetes mellitus is a group of diseases characterized by insufficient production of insulin or by the failure of the body to appropriately respond to insulin, resulting in hyperglycemia.[3] Vascular complications, the principal clinical risk associated with diabetes, are classified as microvascular (diabetic retinopathy, nephropathy, neuropathy) and macrovascular (ischemic heart disease, cerebrovascular disease, peripheral vascular disease).

Diagnostic Criteria

The World Health Organization and the American Diabetes Association (ADA) criteria for the diagnosis of diabetes have evolved during recent decades, summarized in Table 21-1. A diagnosis of diabetes is usually based on tests repeated on at

least two different days, unless hyperglycemia is unequivocal or the person is symptomatic.[12,13]

Classification

Approximately 90% or more of cases of diabetes mellitus are characterized by relative insulin deficiency with a backdrop of insulin resistance and are classified as type 2 diabetes mellitus.[3,4] The etiology of type 2 diabetes is multifactorial, encompassing genetic, environmental, and behavioral factors, but the exact mechanistic underpinning has not yet been determined; a number of predisposing factors for the development of type 2 diabetes are summarized in Table 21-2.

Type 1 diabetes mellitus results from primary beta-cell loss leading to absolute insulin deficiency, representing less than 10% of cases of diabetes mellitus.[3] The etiology of type 1 diabetes is also multifactorial and poorly understood, although an autoimmune component has been implicated in most cases. Other forms of diabetes not covered in this chapter are gestational diabetes and numerous less common causes (e.g., monogenic defects in insulin production or action; diabetes secondary to other pathologic conditions of the pancreas, such as pancreatitis or tumors; and drugs or chemicals causing beta-cell toxicity).[3]

Incidence and Prevalence of Diabetes Mellitus

World

More than 180 million people worldwide were estimated by the World Health Organization to have diabetes mellitus in 2008,[4] increasing from an estimated 135 million in 1995 and projected to rise to 366 million by

TABLE 21–1	Present and Historical Diagnostic Criteria for Diabetes Mellitus
2010 ADA⁵ (present)	HbA1c >6.5% (The test should be performed in a laboratory using a method that is NGSP certified and standardized to the DCCT assay.) *or* FPG ≥7.0 mmol/L (126 mg/dL) *or* 2-hour PG ≥11.1 mmol/L (200 mg/dL) during OGTT *or* Symptoms of diabetes plus casual PG ≥11.1 mmol/L (200 mg/dL). Casual is defined as any time of day without regard to time since last meal.
2003 ADA⁶	FPG ≥7.0 mmol/L (126 mg/dL) *or* 2-hour PG ≥11.1 mmol/L (200 mg/dL) during OGTT *or* Symptoms of diabetes plus casual PG ≥11.1 mmol/L (200 mg/dL). Casual is defined as any time of day without regard to time since last meal.
1999 WHO⁷ (present)	FPG ≥7.0 mmol/L (126 mg/dL) *or* 2-hour PG ≥11.1 mmol/L (200 mg/dL) during OGTT
1997 ADA⁸	FPG ≥7.0 mmol/L (126 mg/dL)
1985 WHO⁹ 1980 WHO¹⁰ 1979 NDDG¹¹*	FPG ≥7.8 mmol/L (140 mg/dL) *or* 2-hour PG ≥11.1 mmol/L (200 mg/dL) during OGTT

*Before this 1979 NDDG publication, there were no unified diagnostic criteria for diabetes.

ADA, American Diabetes Association; DCCT, Diabetes Control and Complications Trial; FPG, fasting plasma glucose (fasting is defined as no calorie intake for at least 8 hours); NDDG, U.S. National Diabetes Data Group; NGSP, National Glycohemoglobin Standardization Program; OGTT, standardized oral glucose tolerance test, using a glucose load equivalent to 75 g anhydrous glucose dissolved in water; PG, plasma glucose; WHO, World Health Organization.

TABLE 21–2	Selected Factors Predisposing Risk for the Development of Type 2 Diabetes Mellitus

Prediabetes, defined as impaired glucose tolerance (2-hr plasma glucose concentration, 140 mg/dL [7.8 mmol/L] to 199 mg/dL [11.0 mmol/L] during an oral glucose tolerance test) or impaired fasting glucose (fasting plasma glucose concentration, 100 mg/dL [5.6 mmol/L] to 125 mg/dL [6.9 mmol/L])

Overweight (BMI ≥25 kg/m²) and at least one other risk factor:
First-degree relative with diabetes
One or more features of the metabolic syndrome: HDL-C <35 mg/dL (0.90 mmol/L), triglycerides >250 mg/dL (2.82 mmol/L), hypertension (≥140/90 mm Hg or receiving therapy for hypertension)
High-risk population (e.g., African American, Latino or Hispanic, Native American, Asian American, Pacific Islander)
Physical inactivity
Age ≥45 years
Women who were diagnosed with gestational diabetes mellitus or who delivered a baby weighing >4 kg (9 pounds)
Other clinical conditions associated with insulin resistance (e.g., acanthosis nigricans, polycystic ovarian syndrome)

Obesity (BMI ≥30 kg/m²)

Modified from American Diabetes Association: Standards of medical care in diabetes 2009. *Diabetes Care* 32:S13, 2009.

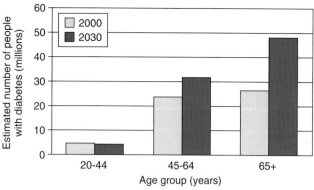

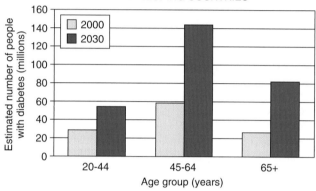

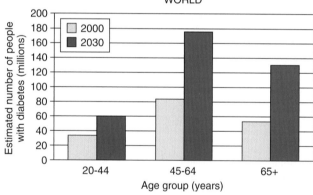

FIGURE 21-1 Estimated number of adults with diabetes by age group, year, and countries for the developed and developing categories and for the world. *(From Wild S, Roglic G, Green A, et al: Global prevalence of diabetes: estimates for the year 2000 and projections for 2030.* Diabetes Care *27:1047, 2004.)*

2030 (Fig. 21-1).¹ This represents a rise in prevalence adjusted for population growth from 2.8% in 2000 projected to 4.4% in 2030.¹ These numbers probably underestimate the burden of diabetes mellitus in the developing world, where only 25% to 30% of cases are diagnosed.¹⁴

United States

The 2007 diabetes mellitus prevalence estimates for the United States included 17.9 million people with diagnosed diabetes and 5.7 million more undiagnosed, representing 7.8% of the U.S. population.¹⁵ The number of Americans with diagnosed diabetes is projected to increase to 29 million by 2050, with less than one third of this increase attributable to population growth.¹⁶ More than 1.6 million new cases of diabetes mellitus were diagnosed in the United States in 2007 alone,¹⁵ representing a marked increase from 625,000 new cases annually in 1990-1992,¹⁷ even with adjustment for total population (incidence rates 5.3 versus 2.4 per 1000 people per year).

Vulnerable Populations

A number of populations are especially vulnerable to development of type 2 diabetes. Older persons, women, and especially elderly women are particularly susceptible (Fig. 21-2).¹ In 2002 in the United States, 1.7% of the population aged 20

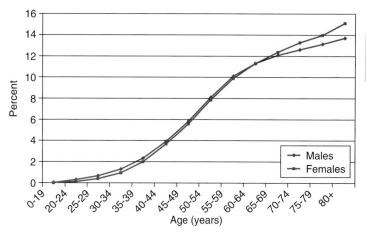

FIGURE 21-2 Global diabetes prevalence by sex and age for 2000. *(From Wild S, Roglic G, Green A, et al: Global prevalence of diabetes: estimates for the year 2000 and projections for 2030. Diabetes Care 27:1047, 2004.)*

to 39 years had diagnosed diabetes compared with 15.1% of those ≥60 years.[18] Diabetes is also more prevalent in certain ethnic groups, including African Americans, Asian Indians, Hispanic or Latino Americans, Native Americans, and Pacific Islanders, among others. For example, the age- and sex-standardized prevalence of diagnosed diabetes reported in NHANES 1999-2002 was almost double in African Americans and Hispanic or Latino Americans compared with non-Hispanic white Americans.[19] The prevalence of diabetes is high but variable in different Native American populations,[20] reaching 40% to 50% in Pima Indians older than 35 years.[21] Somewhat paradoxically, higher socioeconomic status in developing countries and lower socioeconomic status in developed countries have been associated with increased diabetes risk.[22,23]

Whereas type 2 diabetes remains less prevalent in children and adolescents than in any other age group,[24] the trend toward increased obesity and decreased physical activity in youth, especially in industrialized countries, is accompanied by an alarming increase in the incidence and prevalence of pediatric type 2 diabetes,[25] especially among ethnic minorities. For example, the population-based multicenter SEARCH for Diabetes in Youth Study reported that among 1530 youth aged 10 to 19 years with newly diagnosed diabetes, type 2 diabetes accounted for 14.9% of diabetes mellitus cases in non-Hispanic white Americans, 46.1% in Hispanics, 57.8% in African Americans, and 86.2% in Native Americans.[24]

Factors Contributing to the Increasing Incidence and Prevalence of Type 2 Diabetes Mellitus

Obesity

The global prevalence of overweight (body mass index [BMI] ≥25 kg/m² but <30 kg/m²) and obesity (BMI ≥30 kg/m²) continues to increase. The World Health Organization estimates that approximately 1.6 billion adults were overweight and at least 400 million were obese worldwide in 2005 and projects an increase to 2.3 billion overweight and 700 million obese by 2015.[26] The risk of diabetes is proportionally increased with both the severity and duration of obesity, as more people are becoming obese earlier in life and rates of extreme obesity (BMI ≥35 kg/m²) are rising. Beyond BMI, measures of increased abdominal obesity, such as waist circumference and waist-to-hip ratio, are even better predictors of diabetes risk.

Diet

It has been difficult to ascertain the role of dietary factors independent of body weight, but the increased availability of foods high in fat, low in fiber, and with a high glycemic load has been associated with increased risk for type 2 diabetes.[27] Increased consumption of red meats in general and processed meats in particular has also been associated with a higher risk of diabetes. Other dietary factors may also play a role. The rise in diabetes prevalence coincides historically with increasing dietary intake of fructose-rich foods; but in spite of data showing that diets very high in fructose induce insulin resistance and diabetes in laboratory animals, whether high fructose intake plays a role in the pathogenesis of diabetes in humans has not been established.

Sedentary Lifestyle

In spite of recent indications that leisure-time physical activity may be stable or even increasing in the United States, overall levels have declined significantly during the past half-century, and the trend toward an increasingly sedentary lifestyle among Americans continues.[28] Physical inactivity has been associated with an increased risk for development of type 2 diabetes even after adjustment for BMI. Conversely, even modest levels of physical activity intensity and duration are associated with decreased risk. For example, among more than 30,000 women (47% of the Nurses' Health Study cohort) who reported that walking was their sole physical activity, diabetes risk decreased significantly across quintiles of energy expenditure, calculated from walking time and pace.[29] In a high-risk population, the Strong Heart Study of 1651 Native Americans reported an odds ratio for incident diabetes reduced by one third (one fourth after adjustment for BMI) in participants who engaged in even modest amounts of physical activity compared with a control group of no physical activity.[30]

Aging Population

As the incidence and prevalence of type 2 diabetes increase with age, a global trend toward population aging may account for a portion of the increase in diabetes prevalence.[16] Life expectancy at birth in developed countries has increased by approximately 25 years in the twentieth century alone, and even though life expectancy in developing countries has increased at a much slower pace, it is projected that about 80% of the world population older than 60 years will live in developing countries by 2050,[31] with continued aging of the world population projected through the first half of the twenty-first century.

Diagnostic Criteria and Improved Detection

With the thresholds for diagnosis of diabetes becoming more inclusive in recent years and continued improvements in population-based screening, more persons are being diagnosed, with relative increases in the ratio of diagnosed to undiagnosed diabetes.

TYPE 1 DIABETES MELLITUS

Definition

Type 1 diabetes results from absolute insulin deficiency due to autoimmune destruction of the insulin-producing beta cells within the islets of the endocrine pancreas. In addition to the obvious glucose abnormalities, patients with type 1 diabetes are also predisposed to ketoacidosis because of unrestrained lipolysis and ketogenesis when insulin falls to undetectable or nearly undetectable levels. Indeed, the diagnosis is commonly made in this setting, often in the context of a superimposed intervening illness that increases counterregulatory stress hormones, such as epinephrine and cortisol.

The diagnosis of type 1 diabetes is straightforward in a patient with hyperglycemia (defined according to the criteria in Table 21-1) who is both young and lean, especially one presenting with ketosis or catabolic features, such as weight loss. Serologic confirmation with autoantibodies is rarely necessary. Most patients with type 1 diabetes are, however, seropositive for one or more of the following: anti–glutamic acid decarboxylase antibodies, anti–islet cell antibodies 512, and anti-insulin antibodies. When the diagnosis is less clear, such as in an obese child or in a lean older individual, measurement of these serum markers may prove clinically useful.

Type 1 diabetes can be treated only with insulin, and patients are optimally managed with multiple injections per day, involving both basal and prandial components, or continuous subcutaneous insulin infusion (i.e., an insulin pump). Oral agents are essentially ineffective and have no standard role in the therapy for this disease.

Epidemiology

The incidence of type 1 diabetes is low, compared with that of type 2 diabetes, and varies widely between populations, 0.1/100,000 per year in China and Venezuela to approximately 37/100,000 per year in Sardinia and Finland.[32] Although it is typically diagnosed in children, type 1 diabetes may occur at any age; the rapidity of loss of beta cells is inversely proportional to age, with more gradual development in older individuals during many years. The term *latent autoimmune diabetes of adulthood* has gained favor to describe this form, which initially presents with relatively mild hyperglycemia, often successfully treated with oral agents. Over time, however, insulin deficiency dominates the clinical picture, with labile blood glucose control, insulin dependency, and a propensity for ketosis.

Risk Factors

Although it is clearly of autoimmune origin, the underlying cause or causes of type 1 diabetes remain poorly understood. Defined risk factors include certain HLA types, such as DR3 or DR4, and a family history, although the latter is not as potent a factor as it is in type 2 diabetes. For example, children born to men with type 1 diabetes have about a 6% risk for development of the disease. Children born to women with type 1 diabetes have a lower risk, ranging from 1% to 4%, depending on the age of the mother at delivery. Several viruses have also been implicated in the pathogenesis of type 1 diabetes, including mumps, rubella, cytomegalovirus, and coxsackievirus, but they do not appear to be involved in more than a small minority of cases. The possibilities that dietary factors, micronutrient status, and the individual's intestinal flora may play a role in the predisposition to type 1 diabetes are under active investigation.

DIABETES MELLITUS AS RISK FACTOR FOR CARDIOVASCULAR DISEASE

Epidemiology

The World Health Organization estimated that as many as 2.9 million deaths worldwide in the year 2005 could be attributed to diabetes, with more than half of these attributable to CVD.[4] Of the 284,000 deaths attributable to diabetes in the United States in 2007, about two thirds had CVD as the primary cause of death.[33] In spite of a trend for reduced all-cause and cardiovascular mortality in patients with diabetes in the United States during the past half-century, mortality remains approximately twofold higher in those with versus without diabetes (Fig. 21-3).[34]

Diabetic Vascular Disease

Diabetes mellitus is a major risk factor for atherosclerosis, clinically manifested as diabetic macrovascular complications.[35] The risk of ischemic heart disease is twofold to fourfold higher in people with type 2 diabetes compared with those without diabetes, with myocardial infarction (MI) being the number one cause of death. In the Framingham Heart Study between 1976 and 2001, cardiovascular mortality among those with and without diabetes was 6.8 and 2.4 per 1000 person-years, respectively.[34] The risk of MI in patients with diabetes with no history of prior coronary events is, at least in some populations, similar to the risk of MI in patients without diabetes but with prevalent coronary artery disease.[2] For example, in a Finnish population-based study of 1059 patients with type 2 diabetes and 1373 without diabetes aged

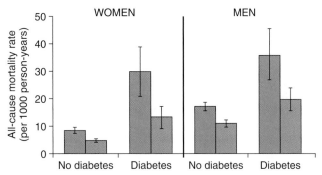

Note: Bars indicate 95% confidence intervals. Rates are adjusted for age in 10-year intervals.

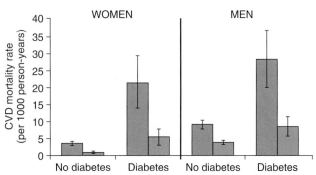

Note: Bars indicate 95% confidence intervals. Rates are adjusted for age in 10-year intervals.

FIGURE 21-3 Age-adjusted all-cause **(top)** and CVD **(bottom)** mortality rates among participants with and without diabetes by sex and time period. Blue bars represent earlier time period (1950 to 1975); red bars represent later time period (1976 to 2001). *(From Preis SR, Hwang SJ, Coady S, et al: Trends in all-cause and cardiovascular disease mortality among women and men with and without diabetes mellitus in the Framingham Heart Study, 1950 to 2005.* Circulation *119:1728, 2009.)*

45 to 64 years, the 7-year incidence of first MI in those with versus without diabetes was 20.2% versus 3.5%, respectively, and the incidence of recurrent MI was 45% and 18.8%, respectively.[36]

This and other similar evidence led the National Cholesterol Education Program (NCEP) Expert Panel to recommend that type 2 diabetes be managed as a coronary heart disease equivalent for the purpose of low-density lipoprotein cholesterol (LDL-C) control.[2] However, more recent data from clinical trial observations, including studies enrolling patients with newly diagnosed diabetes as well as trials of patients with more advanced type 2 diabetes at high CVD risk, suggest that the CVD risk for diabetes is more intermediate, with risk projected during 10 years ranging between 8% and 20%,[37-40] contrasted with the "coronary disease equivalent" risk of >20%/10 years.

Type 1 diabetes is also associated with significantly increased cardiovascular risk, especially in younger patients. Data from the Diabetes U.K. Cohort, an observational study of 23,751 patients diagnosed with type 1 diabetes in Great Britain, showed that mortality from ischemic heart disease in men and women older than 40 years with type 1 diabetes is increased 4-fold and 7-fold, respectively, compared with the general population; in those younger than 40 years, the risk increase is 9-fold for men and >40-fold for women.[41] The Pittsburgh Epidemiology of Diabetes Complications Study, a single-center observational study of 906 patients with type 1 diabetes,[42] demonstrated ~15% incidence of CVD after 30 years in this relatively young cohort (median age at onset, 8.5 years).

Having type 2 diabetes doubles one's risk of stroke, even after adjustments for other risk factors (hypertension, dyslipidemia),[43] and increases by 15-fold the risk of lower extremity amputation due to peripheral arterial disease.[44] These risks have also been demonstrated in type 1 diabetes, the earlier onset of which results in significantly higher relative risk in younger age groups. For example, the risk of cerebrovascular mortality in the Diabetes U.K. Cohort was increased by approximately twofold in patients with type 1 diabetes 60 years and older compared with participants without diabetes but by more than fivefold and sevenfold, respectively, in men and women aged 20 to 39 years.[45] Finally, atherosclerotic events such as MI and stroke are associated with higher short- and long-term mortality, higher rate of recurrence, and worse overall prognosis in the context of diabetes.[35]

Hypertension

Approximately 70% of patients with type 2 diabetes have hypertension (more than double the prevalence in the general population),[46] which further increases their CVD risk. For example, an observational analysis of 3642 patients with type 2 diabetes enrolled in the United Kingdom Prospective Diabetes Study (UKPDS) demonstrated a positive adjusted correlation between mean systolic blood pressure and the risk of MI, stroke, and heart failure (Fig. 21-4).[47] Hypertension is also an independent risk factor for chronic kidney disease,[48] which in turn may exacerbate CVD risk, resulting in a vicious circle.[49]

Heart Failure

People with type 2 diabetes have a twofold to fivefold increased risk of congestive heart failure (CHF) compared with those without diabetes and have worse outcomes once CHF has developed.[50] Diabetes increases the incidence of CHF following the entire spectrum of acute coronary syndromes[51] and remains an independent predictor of CHF even after adjustment for the increased prevalence of ischemic heart disease among patients with diabetes.[52] The increased CHF observed in diabetes is multifactorial and includes more prevalent systolic and diastolic dysfunction due to both

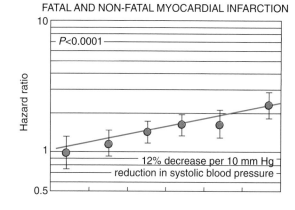

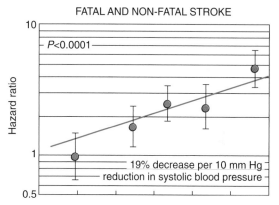

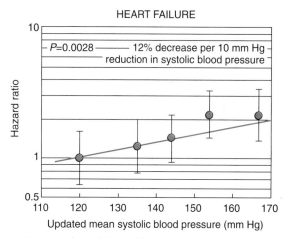

FIGURE 21-4 Hazard rates (95% confidence intervals as floating absolute risks) as estimate of association between category of updated mean systolic blood pressure and myocardial infarction, stroke, and heart failure, with log linear scales. Reference category (hazard ratio 1.0) is systolic blood pressure <120 mm Hg for myocardial infarction and <130 mm Hg for stroke and heart failure; *P* value reflects contribution of systolic blood pressure to multivariate model. Data adjusted for age at diagnosis of diabetes, ethnic group, smoking status, presence of albuminuria, hemoglobin A1c, high- and low-density lipoprotein cholesterol, and triglyceride. (*Modified from Adler AI, Stratton IM, Neil HA, et al: Association of systolic blood pressure with macrovascular and microvascular complications of type 2 diabetes [UKPDS 36]: prospective observational study. BMJ 321:412, 2000.*)

circulatory impairments and derangements of myocardial metabolism (diabetic cardiomyopathy).[53]

Sex and Ethnic Differences

Available data suggest that relative cardiovascular risk is higher in women compared with men with type 1 or type 2 diabetes and that diabetes reduces the sex differences in CVD incidence that otherwise exist in the nondiabetic population.[34,41,54] For example, type 2 diabetes in the Framingham Heart Study increased the risk of CVD mortality by 3.5- to 5-fold in women and 2- to 3-fold in men.[34]

The risk for diabetic complications is also not uniform across ethnic groups. Data from an observational study of 62,432 diabetic patients showed that African Americans, Asians, and Hispanics have a relatively lower risk of MI than that of whites (adjusted hazard ratio [HR], 0.56, 0.68, and 0.68, respectively). Asians and Hispanics have a lower risk of stroke and CHF than that of both whites and African Americans (HR, 0.76 and 0.72, stroke; 0.70 and 0.61, CHF).[55] In Pima Indians, despite a very high overall prevalence of diabetes, the incidence of fatal coronary heart disease is comparatively low.[56]

Potential Mechanistic Links Between Diabetes Mellitus and Cardiovascular Disease

Diabetic Macrovascular Disease

The complex mechanistic interrelationships between type 2 diabetes and atherosclerosis have been the focus of extensive and ongoing investigation. A detailed review of this field is beyond the scope of this chapter, but a number of published review articles provide excellent summaries of the present knowledge in this area.[35,57,58] Among the principal vascular perturbations associated with type 2 diabetes is increased endothelial dysfunction, driven largely by dysregulated nitric oxide biology, indirect and direct vascular effects of advanced glycation end products, direct adverse effects of increased circulating nonesterified free fatty acids, and increased systemic inflammation and aberrant leukocyte-endothelial interactions, among others.[57,59]

Compounding the direct vascular effects of diabetes are a number of perturbations in the proteo-fibrinolytic system and platelet biology yielding a constitutive prothrombotic milieu.[35,57,60] These abnormalities include increased circulating tissue factor, factor VII, von Willebrand factor, and plasminogen activator inhibitor 1, with decreased levels of antithrombin III and protein C. In addition, disturbances of platelet activation, aggregation, morphology, and life span have been well described, further contributing to increased thrombotic potential as well as acceleration of atherosclerosis.[61]

Finally, diabetic dyslipidemia is a major contributor to the pathogenesis and progression of atherosclerosis.[62-64] Diabetic dyslipidemia is a constellation of metabolically interconnected lipid and lipoprotein abnormalities, including increased plasma triglycerides, decreased high-density lipoprotein (HDL), and a modest increase in low-density lipoproteins (LDL), with larger proportions of atherogenic LDL such as small dense LDL and oxidized LDL. Decreased HDL impairs reverse cholesterol transport (the movement of cholesterol from peripheral tissues to the liver) and reduces the anti-inflammatory and antioxidant effects of HDL in the circulation.[65] Elevated levels of apolipoprotein B–containing lipoproteins, such as LDL and triglyceride-rich very-low-density lipoproteins (VLDL), and increased remnant lipoproteins (produced by the hydrolysis of VLDL and chylomicrons) directly promote atherosclerosis.[63]

Diabetic Cardiomyopathy

Several pathophysiologic processes, individually or in combination, have been proposed to contribute to the pathogenesis of diabetic cardiomyopathy and CHF.[53] Principal among these processes are abnormal insulin action at the level of the cardiac myocyte coupled with increased circulating free fatty acids, resulting in aberrant myocardial metabolism with accumulation of free fatty acids and triglycerides, and the generation of reactive oxygen species and toxic lipid metabolites, termed cardiac lipotoxicity.

In addition, diabetes is associated with impaired myocellular metabolic substrate switching, deleteriously perturbing the balance between free fatty acid and glucose metabolism under periods of stress such as ischemia, with increased free fatty acid metabolism increasing myocardial oxygen consumption. Hyperglycemia may exacerbate these effects by inhibiting free fatty acid oxidation, with excess intracellular glucose resulting in nonenzymatic protein glycation, formation of intracellular and extracellular advanced glycation end products, and resultant adverse mechanical and metabolic consequences.

PREVENTION OF TYPE 2 DIABETES MELLITUS

The first line of defense against diabetic CVD is prevention of diabetes. The identification of modifiable risk factors and populations at increased risk for development of type 2 diabetes has made diabetes prevention or delay theoretically feasible. Preventive measures should specifically target people at high risk (see Table 21-2) but could also be applied to the general population.[66]

Lifestyle Modification

Weight Loss

A combined intervention consisting of diet, physical activity, and weight loss reduces diabetes risk, as summarized in Figure 21-5. The Finnish Diabetes Prevention Study included 522 overweight subjects with impaired glucose tolerance randomized to either usual care or intensive lifestyle intervention (aimed at reduction of total intake of fat to <30% and saturated fat to <10% of energy consumed, increase in the intake of fiber to >15 g per 1000 kcal, moderate exercise for at least 30 minutes per day, and at least 5% weight reduction).[67] After a median follow-up of 4 years, the relative risk of diabetes was reduced by 58% in the intervention group, with sustained benefit observed up to 3 years after the study.[68]

The U.S. Diabetes Prevention Program randomized 3234 people with impaired glucose tolerance or impaired fasting glucose to placebo control, metformin, or an intensive

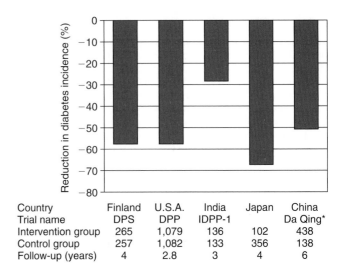

Country	Finland	U.S.A.	India	Japan	China
Trial name	DPS	DPP	IDPP-1		Da Qing*
Intervention group	265	1,079	136	102	438
Control group	257	1,082	133	356	138
Follow-up (years)	4	2.8	3	4	6

FIGURE 21-5 Summary of the effect of lifestyle intervention (diet, exercise, weight loss) on diabetes incidence in randomized controlled trials (*the Da Qing study was cluster randomized). For each study, the difference between groups was statistically significant. DPP, U.S. Diabetes Prevention Program; DPS, Finnish Diabetes Prevention Study; IDPP-1, Indian Diabetes Prevention Program.[67,69-71,73]

lifestyle modification program aimed at a minimum of 150 minutes of exercise per week, low-fat diet, and 7% weight loss. The incidence of diabetes was reduced by 58% in the lifestyle modification group and by 31% in the metformin group after an average follow-up of 2.8 years.[69]

In other high-risk populations, the Indian Diabetes Prevention Program reported a 28.5% reduction in progression to diabetes with lifestyle modification (diet and exercise) for 3 years in Asian Indians with impaired glucose tolerance,[70] and a randomized trial of Japanese men with impaired glucose tolerance observed for 4 years reported a 67.4% reduction in the risk of diabetes with diet, exercise, and sustained weight loss.[71] The cluster-randomized (by clinic rather than by participant) Chinese Da Qing study found that at-risk individuals in the combined intervention groups (diet, exercise, and diet plus exercise) had a 51% lower incidence of diabetes compared with the control group during 6 years of active intervention and a 43% lower incidence during a 20-year period including 14 years of post-trial follow-up.[72,73] Despite the variability in risk reduction across these studies, each has demonstrated that a combination of diet, physical activity, and weight loss significantly reduces or delays the development of type 2 diabetes, with several showing sustained effects. On the basis of the available evidence, the ADA recommends reduced intake of dietary calories and fat, regular moderate-intensity physical activity (≥150 min/week), and sustained weight loss (≥7% of body weight) for diabetes prevention in people at risk.[74]

Independent of weight effects, dietary composition also plays a role in type 2 diabetes risk. Overall, diets high in red and processed meats and saturated fats have been associated with increased risk for type 2 diabetes, and conversely, low–saturated fat, high-fiber diets containing whole grains, fruits, vegetables, and fish have been associated with reduced risk of type 2 diabetes.[67,69,75] The dietary composition recommended by the ADA for diabetes prevention includes reduced intake of fat, increased dietary fiber (14 g fiber per 1000 kcal), and whole grains (at least half of grain intake), and foods with low glycemic index (generally less processed) are encouraged.[74]

Physical Activity and Exercise

Even though physical activity (overall) and exercise (planned and structured leisure-time physical activity) may have only a modest effect on weight if they are not accompanied by dietary measures,[76] increasing physical activity, which directly improves insulin sensitivity in skeletal muscle,[77] may be beneficial for diabetes prevention independent of weight loss. Prospective cohort studies of 21,271 American men aged 40 to 84 years participating in the Physicians' Health Study and of 7735 British men aged 40 to 59 years, all free of diabetes at baseline, showed that individuals who engaged in moderate levels of physical activity had a significantly lower risk for diabetes compared with those who were physically inactive, even after adjustment for age and BMI.[78,79]

Similarly, data from the Nurses' Health Study (70,102 nondiabetic women aged 40 to 65 years observed for 8 years) showed that higher quintiles of physical activity were associated with decreased diabetes risk, and the trend remained significant after adjustment for BMI.[29]

On the basis of the available evidence, regular physical activity (at least 30 min/day on most days or 150 min/week as recommended by the ADA) is important for diabetes prevention. It should be recommended to individuals at risk in addition to other weight loss strategies.[74,80]

Treatment of Obesity

When lifestyle modification alone fails to reduce body weight in obese patients, pharmacologic or surgical intervention

may be considered. Orlistat is a gastric and pancreatic lipase inhibitor that reduces fat absorption by ~30%. In a 4-year trial of 3305 obese patients randomized to lifestyle changes plus either orlistat or placebo, orlistat was associated with a greater weight loss (5.8 kg versus 3.0 kg) and a lower incidence of diabetes (9.0% versus 6.2%; 37.3% relative risk reduction).[81]

Bariatric surgery, which modifies the gastrointestinal tract anatomy through a variety of techniques to reduce calorie intake and to affect weight loss, has also been shown to have myriad beneficial effects on measures of glucose and lipid metabolism, including reducing the risk of diabetes.[82] In addition to weight reduction, bariatric procedures are associated with beneficial effects on the secretion of nutrient-responsive gut hormones, including incretins, ghrelin, and peptide YY, that may improve insulin responsiveness independent of weight loss.[82]

Several studies support the use of bariatric surgery as an effective strategy for weight loss in severely obese patients. The prospective controlled nonrandomized Swedish Obese Subjects trial reported mean weight reductions of 25% for the Roux-en-Y procedure and 13% to 16% for the restrictive procedures at 10 years after intervention, compared with a trend for further weight gain in the control group (nonsurgical, nonstandardized obesity management).[83] The incidence of diabetes at 2 and 10 years was 1% and 7%, respectively, in the overall bariatric surgery group, compared with 8% and 24%, respectively, in the control group, with suggestions of modest long-term mortality benefit.[84,85] However, the potential benefits of bariatric surgery should be carefully weighed against its significant risk for perioperative complications (including early death) and long-term gastrointestinal and nutritional adverse effects.

Drug Therapy for Prevention of Diabetes Mellitus

Metformin

The most compelling evidence for pharmacologic prevention of diabetes comes from a study of 2155 individuals with impaired glucose tolerance randomized to either metformin or placebo in the Diabetes Prevention Program. After a mean follow-up of 2.8 years, the incidence of diabetes was 4.8% in the metformin group versus 7.8% in the placebo group, representing a 31% relative risk reduction.[69] Notably, however, metformin was indistinguishable from placebo in participants older than 60 years as well as in those whose fasting glucose concentration was <110 mg/dL and in those whose BMI was <35 kg/m^2.

To determine whether the effect of metformin was transient ("masking" of diabetes) or sustained (true prevention), 1274 participants who had not developed diabetes by the end of the Diabetes Prevention Program were subjected to an oral glucose tolerance test 1 to 2 weeks after the discontinuation of study medication. There was an increased incidence of diabetes in the metformin group during this washout period (indicating that masking did occur in those cases), but when the washout data were included in the overall analysis, the diabetes risk reduction with metformin remained significant at 25%.[86]

On the basis of these observations, metformin is the only drug recommended by the ADA to be considered for diabetes prevention. It is specifically recommended for high-risk patients with both impaired fasting glucose and impaired glucose tolerance who are younger than 60 years, have a BMI >35 kg/m^2, and have other diabetes risk factors (HbA1c >6.0%, hypertension, low HDL-C, high triglycerides, family history).[12]

The Study To Prevent Non–Insulin-Dependent Diabetes Mellitus (STOP-NIDDM) randomized 1429 participants with impaired glucose tolerance to either acarbose or placebo. After a mean follow-up of 39 months, the cumulative incidence of diabetes was 32% in the acarbose group and 42% in the placebo group, representing a 25% relative risk reduction.[87] However, the incidence of diabetes during 3 months of single-blind post-trial follow-up on placebo was 45% higher in the former acarbose group, suggesting a significant masking component.

Another drug in this class, voglibose, was studied in a randomized trial of 1780 Japanese subjects at high risk for diabetes and was found to reduce the incidence of diabetes by 40% after a short mean follow-up of 48 weeks.[88] This trial was stopped early because of apparent benefit, which is controversial and could in fact overestimate the effects of the active medication.[89] Of note, agents in this class have significant gastrointestinal side effects that limit their broad appeal.

Thiazolidinediones

By virtue of their insulin-sensitizing effects through activation of the nuclear receptor peroxisome proliferator-activated receptor γ (PPARγ) that regulates gene transcription, the thiazolidinediones (TZDs), including rosiglitazone and pioglitazone, target the principal pathologic underpinning of type 2 diabetes. In addition, over longer duration, the achieved insulin sensitization may improve beta-cell preservation, which could plausibly enhance their effects on prevention or delay of progression to diabetes.[90] Thus, the TZDs appear promising in this regard, with supportive data deriving from a number of randomized controlled trials enrolling patients at exaggerated diabetes risk, including Hispanic women with gestational diabetes,[90] and large trials of subjects with impaired fasting glucose or impaired glucose tolerance (Fig. 21-6).[91,92] The magnitude of the treatment effects in these trials was large, ranging from 55% to 81% relative risk reduction for diabetes, but commensurate with the risk reduction achieved by lifestyle intervention described before.

Despite the robust effects observed across the TZD drug class and across trials, however, neither of the two currently available TZDs has a product label indication for this purpose,

and they are not recommended for diabetes prevention in society guidelines.[12] The absence of recommendation stems from a number of considerations, including ongoing concerns about adverse effects such as increased heart failure and fracture risk as well as the current expense of these drugs. In addition, data are discordant regarding the effects of these drugs on atherosclerotic disease risk,[93] and none of the diabetes prevention trials was designed or powered to assess effects on macrovascular or microvascular disease endpoints. On the basis of these considerations, TZDs are not presently recommended for prevention of type 2 diabetes.

MANAGEMENT OF HYPERGLYCEMIA TO PREVENT CARDIOVASCULAR DISEASE

Glucose and Cardiovascular Disease Risk: Epidemiology

Extensive epidemiologic evidence has linked measures of hyperglycemia, including fasting plasma glucose, random plasma glucose, 2-hour post-challenge plasma glucose, and HbA1c, with increased overall and CVD mortality,[94,95] with associations extending well into what is considered the normal range for glucose. One large meta-analysis by Levitan and coworkers[96] of 38 investigations found that overall, those with the highest measures of glucose experience approximately one third more CVD events than those with the lowest (RR, 1.36; 95% CI, 1.23-1.52). This relationship persisted even when diabetic subjects were excluded from the analysis (RR, 1.26; 95% CI, 1.11-1.43) (Fig. 21-7). Adjustment for CVD risk factors attenuated the relationship to some degree (RR, 1.19; 95% CI, 1.07-1.32). A second and separate meta-analysis by Selvin and colleagues[97] of 13 observational studies of diabetic patients (N = 9123) found a pooled relative risk for CVD of 1.18 in type 2 diabetes (95% CI, 1.10-1.26) and 1.15 in type 1 diabetes (95% CI, 0.92-1.43) for each 1% increase in HbA1c.

In a more recent analysis using NHANES III data from 19,025 adult participants (baseline survey in 1988-1994 with follow-up through 2000), Saydah and coworkers[98] found that higher levels of HbA1c were associated with increased mortality, including that due to heart disease. After adjustment for other CVD risk factors, the hazard ratio for adults with HbA1c ≥8% versus <6% was 2.59 (95% CI, 1.88-3.56) and 3.38 (95% CI, 1.98-5.77) for all-cause and cardiovascular mortality, respectively. The comparative hazard ratios for adults with a diagnosis of diabetes were 1.68 (1.03-2.74) and 2.48 (1.09-5.64), respectively. However, in this analysis, among those without diagnosed diabetes, no significant association between either all-cause or cardiovascular mortality and HbA1c category was found.

Within the context of a clinical trial, the largest epidemiologic analysis comes from the UKPDS, involving 5102 patients with newly diagnosed type 2 diabetes. In line with the estimates of Selvin and colleagues, Stratton and collaborators[99] have shown that each 1% reduction in HbA1c was associated with a 14% reduction in MI events. Of note, however, the graded association between HbA1c and microvascular endpoints was far steeper than that for MI (Fig. 21-8).

Overview of Current Antihyperglycemic Drug Classes

A variety of both oral and injectable antihyperglycemic agents are used for blood glucose control in patients with type 2 diabetes. In general, these include drugs that stimulate insulin release, improve the body's response to insulin, or delay carbohydrate absorption. In those patients not responding adequately to these agents, typically used in combination,

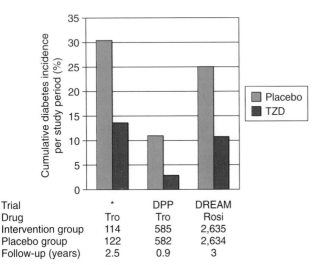

Trial	*	DPP	DREAM
Drug	Tro	Tro	Rosi
Intervention group	114	585	2,635
Placebo group	122	582	2,634
Follow-up (years)	2.5	0.9	3

FIGURE 21-6 Summary of the effect of thiazolidinedione (TZD) treatment on diabetes incidence in randomized controlled trials. For each study, the difference between groups was statistically significant. *Hispanic women with previous gestational diabetes; DPP, U.S. Diabetes Prevention Program; DREAM, Diabetes Reduction Assessment with Ramipril and Rosiglitazone Medication; Rosi, rosiglitazone; Tro, troglitazone.[90-92]

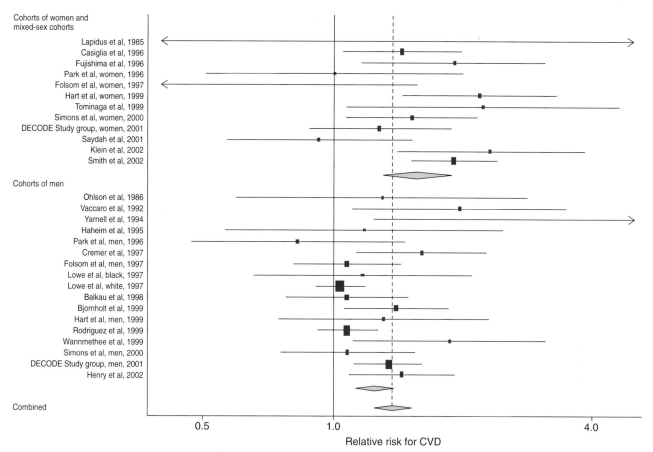

FIGURE 21-7 Relative risks for CVD comparing the highest with the lowest glycemia categories stratified by sex. Size of the solid squares is inversely proportional to the variance of the study estimate. Arrows represent error bars that continue beyond the scale of the figure, and diamonds represent the random-effects pooled relative risk and 95% confidence interval overall and for analyses by sex. The dashed line is drawn at the overall pooled estimate. *(Modified from Levitan EB, Song Y, Ford ES, et al: Is nondiabetic hyperglycemia a risk factor for cardiovascular disease? A meta-analysis of prospective studies.* Arch Intern Med *164:2147, 2004.)*

insulin therapy may be used, although patients usually do not require the highly intensive programs needed in those with type 1 diabetes.

There are now 11 individual drug categories approved for glucose lowering in patients with type 2 diabetes in the United States. Their mechanisms of action, potency, advantages, and disadvantages are summarized in Table 21-3.

The sulfonylurea drug class is the oldest, in use since the 1950s. Their main side effect is hypoglycemia, which activates an adrenergic response and therefore can be potentially deleterious to the cardiovascular system. Direct negative effects on the heart from these agents have also been proposed because the receptor they activate, the sulfonylurea receptor, is expressed in cardiomyocytes, and activation causes closure of ATP-dependent potassium channels (K_{ATP}). Because K_{ATP} closure in myocytes during ischemia may impair preconditioning, sulfonylureas may theoretically exacerbate cardiac injury. Although several animal models have suggested such an effect, the degree to which the drugs bind to K_{ATP} channels in the heart is much less than in pancreatic beta cells, and there are no convincing human data to suggest harm. Sulfonylureas are therefore widely considered to be safe in diabetic patients, including those with coronary artery disease, although this remains consensus opinion in the absence of rigorous data from clinical outcomes trials. Logically, however, these drugs should not be used in the setting of acute coronary syndromes.

Metformin, a biguanide, reduces glucose primarily by attenuating hepatic glucose output, probably by activation of the enzyme AMP kinase. In the UKPDS randomized trial, the risk of MI was reduced by 39% ($P = 0.01$) with metformin compared with those receiving conventional care (diet alone).[100] Such an effect was not convincingly demonstrated in the group assigned to sulfonylureas or insulin (relative risk reduction, 16%; $P = 0.052$).[101] On the basis of these data, paired with a low hypoglycemia risk, modest weight loss, high tolerability with few adverse effects, and low cost, metformin is widely favored as initial monotherapy in most patients with type 2 diabetes. Whereas the use of metformin is cautioned for patients with decompensated heart failure and contraindicated in patients with advanced renal disease because of concern for lactic acidosis, the aggregate data suggest that this risk is quite small or possibly even nonexistent.[102]

The TZDs (pioglitazone, rosiglitazone) activate PPARγ and improve insulin sensitivity by increasing glucose uptake by peripheral tissues, mainly skeletal muscle. They also augment lipogenesis by inducing differentiation of preadipocytes. Their use is associated with a glucose-lowering effectiveness on the same order as that seen with sulfonylureas and metformin and is not associated with hypoglycemia. Pioglitazone, but probably not rosiglitazone, also has beneficial lipid effects, including a 10% to 15% increase in HDL-C and a commensurate decrease in triglycerides.[103,104] Unfortunately, TZDs are associated with weight gain and fluid retention as well as increased fracture risk in women. The fluid retention is associated with incident or worsening heart failure.[105] The incidence of peripheral edema in TZD-treated patients is

21

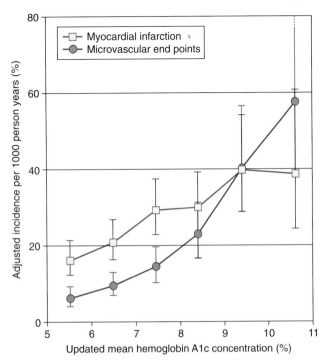

FIGURE 21-8 Incidence rates and 95% confidence intervals for myocardial infarction and microvascular complications by category of updated mean hemoglobin A1c concentration, adjusted for age, sex, and ethnic group, expressed for white men aged 50 to 54 years at diagnosis and with mean duration of diabetes of 10 years. *(From Stratton IM, Adler AI, Neil HA, et al: Association of glycaemia with macrovascular and microvascular complications of type 2 diabetes [UKPDS 35]: prospective observational study. BMJ 321:405, 2000.)*

approximately 5% to 10%, more so when they are used in conjunction with insulin. The risk of heart failure is approximately 1%, also higher in insulin-treated patients. The relative risk of heart failure in patients taking TZDs is approximately 1.7 compared with a non-TZD regimen, with higher reported risk increase with rosiglitazone than with pioglitazone.[106,107]

There is little cardiovascular information available for the other antihyperglycemic therapies presently marketed for diabetes. There are very few data with the newer incretin-based therapies, such as the glucagon-like peptide 1 (GLP-1) agonists and the dipeptidyl peptidase 4 inhibitors. There is great interest in the potential cardiovascular benefit of GLP-1 agonists (e.g., exenatide) because these agents result in substantial weight loss in some patients, with the early demonstration of associated improvement in various cardiovascular risk factors. Studies suggesting a benefit on ventricular function in heart failure and after acute coronary events are very preliminary.[108]

Of note, regulatory agencies around the globe have recently begun requiring clinical trial assessment of the CVD effects of diabetes drugs under development, with a requirement to demonstrate a nominal degree of cardiovascular safety before drug approval.[109,110]

Type 2 Diabetes Mellitus

UKPDS

The UKPDS demonstrated microvascular risk reduction from more intensive glycemic control (relative risk reduction, 21% to 34%) in 5102 patients with newly diagnosed type 2 diabetes.[101] Patients were randomized to treatment with sulfonylurea or insulin as first-line therapy compared with diet alone. During a mean follow-up of 10 years, mean HbA1c was 7.0%

in actively treated patients versus 7.9% in the control group, but the effect on macrovascular outcomes (nonfatal and fatal MI and sudden death) did not reach statistical significance (16% risk reduction; P = 0.052). In a randomized substudy (N = 753) of the UKPDS, initial monotherapy in overweight patients (>120% of ideal body weight) with metformin resulted in improved macrovascular outcomes, an outcome not observed within the main trial (see earlier).

From the UKPDS came the original notion that glucose control, although apparently important for microangiopathy, had more obscure effect on CVD complications. Given the metformin findings, it also raised concerns about whether the method by which glucose is lowered may play some role in altering this disease's cardiovascular risk equation.

Long-term post-trial follow-up of the UKPDS cohort has demonstrated cardiovascular benefit from previous intensive glucose control. Despite a loss in the HbA1c differences between the groups, during 10 years of post-trial monitoring, the patients previously intensively treated with sulfonylurea or insulin experienced relative risk reductions for any diabetes-related endpoint (9%; P = 0.04) and microvascular disease (24%; P = 0.001), whereas decreases in the relative risk for MI (15%; P = 0.01) and all-cause mortality (21%; P = 0.01) eventually emerged.[39] In the overweight metformin-treated patients, corresponding reductions in any diabetes-related endpoint (21%; P = 0.01), MI (33%; P = 0.005), and all-cause mortality (27%; P = 0.002) were observed. These important results demonstrate a "glycemic memory" concept whereby the effects of intensive treatment continued beyond the randomization phase of the study, eventually resulting in beneficial macrovascular outcome differences.

ACCORD, ADVANCE, VADT

More recently, three randomized clinical trials (ACCORD,[37] ADVANCE,[40] and VADT[38]) formally tested the cardiovascular effect of more versus less intensive glucose control (HbA1c target of 6% to 6.5% versus 7% to 9.0%) during a period of 3 to 5 years, all three failing to demonstrate significant benefit (Table 21-4). In the ACCORD trial, cardiovascular mortality was actually *increased* in the intensive group, although the explanation for this phenomenon remains enigmatic. Hypoglycemia was more common in patients who died in both intensive and standard control groups, but post hoc analyses have not been able to demonstrate a causative relationship. Notably, more than three of four intensively treated patients received insulin during the course of the trial, and the majority of patients were prescribed at least three oral agents simultaneously. Whether such polypharmacy may have played a role in the study results is also not clear.

In post hoc analyses from both ACCORD and ADVANCE, the subgroup of patients without preexisting vascular complications actually showed a benefit from more intensive management, experiencing fewer cardiovascular events. In ADVANCE, the primary endpoint, which was a composite of both microvascular and macrovascular events, was modestly reduced in the intensive arm, although this was driven solely by improved intermediate markers of renal disease (relative risk reduction, 21%; P = 0.006). In a post hoc analysis from the VADT, intensive glycemic control appeared to confer a CVD benefit in patients with duration of diabetes <12 years but had a neutral or even adverse effect in patients with longer duration of the disease. Post hoc exploratory data from the VADT also suggested that an episode of severe hypoglycemia within 90 days was a strong predictor of CVD events and CVD mortality. Importantly, none of these trials addressed the question of whether more intensive glycemic management may have macrovascular benefits if it is applied and maintained for longer than 5 years or if it is initiated at the time of diagnosis before vascular complications have become established. An even more recent post hoc analysis suggests

| TABLE 21–3 | Pharmacologic Therapy for Type 2 Diabetes Mellitus |

Drug Class	Examples	Underlying Mechanism	Main Metabolic Effects	↓A1c	Advantages	Disadvantages
Sulfonylureas	Glyburide Glipizide Glimepiride	Closes K_{ATP} channels	↑ Pancreatic insulin secretion	~1%-2%	Microvascular risk	Hypoglycemia Weight gain Ischemic preconditioning (?) Beta-cell exhaustion
Glinides	Repaglinide Nateglinide	Closes K_{ATP} channels	↑ Pancreatic insulin secretion	~1%-1.5%	More physiologic than sulfonylureas ↓ Postprandial glucose	Hypoglycemia Weight gain Ischemic preconditioning (?) Beta-cell exhaustion Dosing frequency
Biguanides	Metformin	Activates AMP kinase	↓ Hepatic glucose production	~1%-2%	No hypoglycemia Weight loss ↓ CVD events	Gastrointestinal side effects (diarrhea) Lactic acidosis Multiple contraindications to consider
Thiazolidinediones	Rosiglitazone Pioglitazone	Activates PPARγ	↑ Peripheral insulin sensitivity	~1%-1.5%	No hypoglycemia Beta-cell preservation ↓ CVD events (?) (pio) ↑ HDL-C ↓ Triglycerides ↓ Blood pressure	Weight gain Edema, heart failure Bone fractures (women) ↑ LDL-C (↑ particle size) Rosiglitazone controversy in coronary heart disease
α-Glucosidase Inhibitors	Acarbose Miglitol	Blocks small intestine α-glucosidase	↓ Intestinal carbohydrate absorption	~0.5%-1%	No hypoglycemia Nonsystemic ↓ Postprandial glucose ↓ CVD events (?)	Gastrointestinal side effects (flatulence) Dosing frequency
Glucagon-like peptide 1 (GLP-1) agonists	Exenatide	Activates GLP-1 receptors	↑ Pancreatic insulin secretion ↓ Pancreatic glucagon secretion Delays gastric emptying ↑ Satiety	~1%	Weight loss No hypoglycemia Beta-cell preservation ↓ Postprandial glucose Cardiovascular benefits (?)	Gastrointestinal side effects (nausea, vomiting) Pancreatitis (?) Injectable
Amylinomimetics	Pramlintide	Activates amylin receptors	↓ Pancreatic glucagon secretion Delays gastric emptying ↑ Satiety	~0.5%	Weight loss ↓ Postprandial glucose	Gastrointestinal side effects (nausea, vomiting) Dosing frequency Injectable
Dipeptidyl peptidase (DPP) 4 inhibitors	Sitagliptin Vildagliptin Saxagliptin	Inhibits DPP-4 ↑ Endogenous incretin levels	↑ Pancreatic insulin secretion ↓ Pancreatic glucagon secretion	~0.6%-0.8%	No hypoglycemia	Urticaria, angioedema, pancreatitis (?)
Bile acid sequestrants	Colesevelam	Binds bile acid cholesterol	?	~0.5%	No hypoglycemia ↓ LDL-C	Gastrointestinal side effects (constipation) ↑ Triglycerides Dosing frequency
Dopaminergic receptor 2 (D_2) agonists	Bromocriptine	Activates dopaminergic receptors	Modulates hypothalamic circadian organization ↓ Hepatic glucose production	~0.5%	No hypoglycemia	Gastrointestinal side effects (nausea) Dizziness
Insulin	Human NPH Human regular Glargine, detemir Lispro Aspart Glulisine Premixed (various types)	Activates insulin receptors	↑ Peripheral glucose disposal ↓ Hepatic glucose production ↓ Proteolysis ↓ Lipolysis ↓ Ketogenesis	No limit	↓ Microvascular risk Universal effectiveness	Hypoglycemia Weight gain Injectable Training requirements "Stigma"

TABLE 21–4 | Baseline Characteristics and Main Results from Three Large Randomized Cardiovascular Trials in Patients with Type 2 Diabetes Mellitus

	ACCORD[37]		ADVANCE[40]		VADT[38]	
N	10,251		11,140		1791	
Age (mean, years)	62		66		60	
BMI (mean, kg/m²)	32		28		31	
Follow-up (mean, years)	3.5		5		5.6	
HbA1c target	<6.0% vs. 7.0%-7.9%		≤6.5% vs. "standard"		<6% vs. 8%-9%	
Baseline HbA1c (mean)	8.3%		7.5%		9.4%	
Endpoint HbA1c (mean)	Intensive 6.4%	Standard 7.5%	Intensive 6.43%	Standard 7.0%	Intensive 6.9%	Standard 8.4%
Severe hypoglycemic events	Intensive 10.5%	Standard 3.5%	Intensive 2.7%	Standard 1.5%	Intensive 8.5%	Standard 2.1%
Weight change	Intensive +3.5 kg	Standard +0.4 kg	Intensive −0.1 kg	Standard −1.0 kg	Intensive +8.1%	Standard +4.1%
Major macrovascular or microvascular event	Not reported		0.9 (0.82-0.98); $P = 0.01$		0.88 (0.74-1.05); $P = 0.14$	
Nonfatal MI or stroke, cardiovascular death	HR, 0.9 (0.78-1.04); $P = 0.16$		0.94 (0.84-1.06); $P = 0.32$		Not reported	
All-cause mortality	HR, 1.22 (1.01-1.46); $P = 0.04$		0.93 (0.83-1.06); $P = 0.28$		1.07 (0.81-1.42); $P = 0.62$	
Nonfatal MI	HR, 0.76 (0.62-0.92); $P = 0.004$		0.98 (0.77-1.22); $P = NS$		0.82 (0.59-1.14); $P = 0.24$	

unsuccessful intensive glycemic control (the failure to respond to the intervention) was linked to the increased cardiovascular disease mortality seen in the intensive group.[110a]

A rational synthesis of the data has led the ADA to maintain its general treatment target of HbA1c <7%, primarily to minimize microvascular disease risk.[12,111] The data in support of this target for macrovascular risk reduction are uneven at best, and there is little evidence to support any lower target from a CVD standpoint. In fact, the ADA statements have considered that a less stringent target may be reasonable for diabetic patients with a history of severe hypoglycemia, advanced complications, or comorbid conditions or for those who are difficult to control or who have had diabetes for many years. Importantly, as described later, meticulous attention to other cardiovascular risk factors, such as lipids and blood pressure, has a much more prominent role than glucose lowering in this realm.

Thiazolidinedione Studies: PROactive, RECORD

Because of the well-recognized association between insulin resistance and CVD, the development of an insulin-sensitizing class of medications was initially met with great hope that these agents could not only lower glucose but also directly reduce CVD complications. Indeed, preliminary in vitro and animal investigations suggested a potent antiatherosclerotic effect of the TZDs, results that were subsequently confirmed in humans by use of surrogate endpoints, such as coronary and carotid atherosclerosis as measured by ultrasound as well as intracoronary stent restenosis.[112,113] However, it has been more challenging to confirm an actual benefit on cardiovascular events.

In the Prospective Evaluation of Pioglitazone and Macrovascular Events (PROactive), 5238 patients with type 2 diabetes and established macrovascular disease were assigned to pioglitazone versus placebo, added to their prior antihyperglycemic regimen.[103] The primary endpoint, a broad CVD composite, occurred in similar numbers of those assigned to active therapy versus placebo (21% versus 23.5%; HR, 0.90; 95% CI, 0.80-1.02). In analysis of the main secondary

composite endpoint of mortality, MI, and stroke, however, a significant benefit was apparent in patients receiving pioglitazone (12.3% versus 14.3%; HR, 0.84; 95% CI, 0.72-0.98) (Fig. 21-9). This apparent benefit was to some degree attenuated by an increased risk of heart failure hospitalizations in active therapy patients (5.7% versus 4.1%), although no commensurate increase in heart failure mortality was observed.[105] Pioglitazone compared with placebo was also associated with improvements in several CVD risk factors, including HbA1c, blood pressure, HDL-C, and triglycerides, that could individually or aggregately contribute to the observed effects on atherosclerotic disease endpoints. A direct effect of pioglitazone on atherosclerosis is further supported by results from two randomized active-controlled trials using ultrasound assessments of carotid and coronary arteries; favorable effects of pioglitazone compared with glimepiride on these imaging intermediates were demonstrated in both trials.[112,113] In spite of these results, it is not yet possible to ascribe the proposed antiatherosclerotic effect of pioglitazone to a *direct* effect at the level of the vasculature or, for that matter, to a reduction in insulin resistance. Notwithstanding, in retrospect, the positive findings from PROactive stand alone to some degree, in light of the ACCORD, ADVANCE, and VADT results. They also indicate that the theory that improving insulin sensitivity may decrease cardiovascular events remains worthy of further study.

The other TZD, rosiglitazone, has had an even more controversial history. In 2007, a widely publicized meta-analysis suggested that rosiglitazone was associated with an *increase* in MI risk (HR, 1.43; 95% CI, 1.03-1.98) and a trend toward increased cardiovascular mortality (HR, 1.64; 95% CI, 0.98-2.74).[114] Subsequently, in the RECORD trial involving 4447 patients with type 2 diabetes in whom rosiglitazone was added to either metformin or a sulfonylurea, compared with patients receiving both traditional agents, the hazard ratio for the primary composite CVD endpoint was 0.99 (0.85-1.16).[115] On the basis of these data, the effect of rosiglitazone on ischemic heart disease risk remains uncertain. In 2010, given the uncertain CVD safety of rosiglitazone, U.S. and European

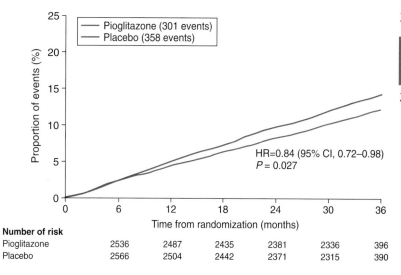

FIGURE 21-9 Kaplan-Meier curve of time to the main secondary endpoint, death from any cause, nonfatal myocardial infarction (excluding silent myocardial infarction), or stroke, from the PROactive randomized trial of pioglitazone versus placebo in 5238 patients with diabetes and cardiovascular disease. *(From Dormandy JA, Charbonnel B, Eckland DJ, et al: Secondary prevention of macrovascular events in patients with type 2 diabetes in the PROactive Study [PROspective pioglitAzone Clinical Trial In macroVascular Events]: a randomised controlled trial. Lancet 366:1279, 2005.)*

regulatory agencies acted to suspend rosiglitazone from the European market and severely restrict its use in the United States. The disparate CVD outcomes with rosiglitazone and pioglitazone could in part be explained by the differential effects these two TZDs have on lipid metabolism.[104]

The BARI 2D study demonstrated no benefit on CVD events in a group of 2368 coronary artery disease patients with type 2 diabetes from a glucose-lowering strategy that emphasized insulin sensitization (metformin or TZD) versus one that focused on insulin provision (sulfonylurea or insulin).[116] However, the results of this study cannot be considered conclusive because the TZD in this study was rosiglitazone, and there was a fair degree of crossover therapy in both groups, especially in those randomized to the insulin sensitizers. BARI 2D also explored prompt versus deferred revascularization in a 2 × 2 factorial design. From post hoc analyses, in those patients assigned to prompt revascularization, the insulin sensitizer strategy was associated with a trend toward a lower rate of major cardiovascular events (20.3% versus 25.2%; P = 0.059). This appeared to be driven mainly by a strong trend in the strata undergoing coronary artery bypass grafting (18.7% versus 26%; P = 0.066).

Societal Guidelines for Antihyperglycemic Therapy

As noted before, the ADA continues to recommend that patients with diabetes have their HbA1c controlled to <7%. This professional organization does not advise a specific method to lower glucose, appreciating the fact that individualization is important. Specifically, older patients with overt CVD did not benefit from the more stringent glycemic policies in ACCORD, ADVANCE, and VADT and may be at increased risk from hypoglycemia or polypharmacy. Accordingly, less rigid targets may be appropriate for this group. A consensus statement sponsored by the ADA and the European Association for the Study of Diabetes was published in 2004 and revised in 2007 and again in 2009.[117] The current cardinal recommendations from this group include the initiation of metformin as foundation therapy in all patients, proceeding expeditiously to combination therapy once glycemic goals are no longer being attained, including consideration of the early use of insulin. The proposed algorithm is shown in simplified form in Figure 21-10.

These recommendations are not considered to be official positions by the organizations, and there remains a significant variability in practice, especially regarding which drug to add after metformin monotherapy. The American Association of Clinical Endocrinologists has proposed a "road map" for the treatment of type 2 diabetes. This is, generally speaking, more inclusive of some of the newer therapies (Fig. 21-11).[118]

In all, the simplest regimen that is effective in lowering glucose, that is acceptable to the patient, and that minimizes side effects, especially hypoglycemia, is likely to be the best program for an individual patient. From a CVD standpoint, the early use of metformin is most justifiable. The precise form of antihyperglycemic therapy beyond metformin remains arguable. The central points to consider are the risk of heart failure with TZDs, the possible CVD risk with rosiglitazone and CVD benefits of pioglitazone, the risk of hypoglycemia with both insulin and insulin secretagogues, and the potential emerging benefit in the form of weight reduction from the newer GLP-1–based therapies.[105,108]

Vascular Complications of Type 1 Diabetes Mellitus and Their Relationship to Glucose Control

Type 1 diabetes mellitus is associated with both microvascular and macrovascular complications, with a clear relation to quality of glucose control achieved. The Diabetes Control and Complications Trial (DCCT) assessed the effect of tighter versus conventional glucose management with insulin therapy in 1441 patients with type 1 diabetes, mean age ~27 years, for a mean of 6.5 years.[119] It compared the more stringent strategy of three or four insulin injections per day or an insulin pump and monitoring of blood glucose concentration at least four times daily with conventional treatment of one or two injections per day and just daily monitoring. The glycemic goals in the intensive group included a preprandial blood glucose concentration of 70 to 120 mg/dL, postprandial blood glucose concentration of <180 mg/dL, and HbA1c level of <6.05%. In the conventional group, there were no specific glycemic targets, the prime goal being to avoid symptomatic hyperglycemia and hypoglycemia. The mean HbA1c level at the end of the trial in those randomized to intensive therapy was 7.4% compared with 9.1% in the conventional therapy group.

The relative risk for the development or progression of microvascular complications (retinopathy, nephropathy, or neuropathy) was reduced by 54% to 63% in the more tightly managed cohort (Figs. 21-12 to 21-14). Cardiovascular events, however, were few in these relatively young patients. Whereas there were less cardiovascular and peripheral vascular events in intensively treated individuals, the results did not achieve statistical significance (0.5 versus 0.8 events per 100 patient-years; relative risk reduction, 41%; 95% CI, −10% to 65%).

At the conclusion of the trial, the DCCT patients continued to be observed in the nonrandomized, uncontrolled

2009 ADA / EASD Proposed Consensus Algorithm

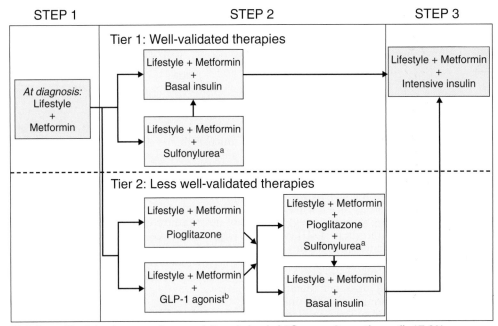

Reinforce lifestyle changes at every visit and check A1C every 3 months until < 7.0%, then at least every 6 months thereafter. Change interventions whenever A1C ≥ 7.0%.

[a]Sulfonylureas other than glibenclamide (glyburide) or chlorpropamide.
[b]Insufficient clinical use to be confident regarding safety.

FIGURE 21-10 Algorithm for the metabolic management of type 2 diabetes. The **tier 1 algorithm** represents the best established and most effective and cost-effective therapeutic strategy for achieving the target glycemic goals. **Step 1,** Lifestyle interventions should be initiated as the first step in treating new-onset type 2 diabetes, and should be reinforced at every visit. Metformin is recommended as the initial pharmacological therapy, in the absence of specific contraindications, for its effect on glycemia, absence of weight gain or hypoglycemia, generally low level of side effects, high level of acceptance, and relatively low cost. **Step 2,** If lifestyle intervention and the maximal tolerated dose of metformin fail to achieve or sustain the glycemic goals (or if metformin is contraindicated or not tolerated), another medication should be added within 2-3 months of the initiation of therapy or at any time when the target A1c level is not achieved. The second medication recommended is either insulin or a sulfonylurea, with insulin usually reserved for patients with an A1c >8.5% or with symptoms secondary to hyperglycemia. **Step 3,** If lifestyle, metformin, and sulfonylurea or basal insulin do not result in achievement of target glycemia, the next recommended step is initiation or intensification of insulin therapy (with discontinuation of insulin secretagogues). The **tier 2 algorithm** may be considered in selected clinical settings. Specifically, when hypoglycemia is particularly undesirable (e.g., in patients who have hazardous jobs), the addition of exenatide or pioglitazone may be considered. Rosiglitazone is not recommended. If promotion of weight loss is a major consideration and the A1c level is close to target (<8.0%), exenatide is an option. If these interventions are not effective in achieving target A1c, or are not tolerated, addition of a sulfonylurea could be considered. Alternatively, the tier 2 interventions should be stopped and basal insulin started. *(Modified from Nathan DM, Buse JB, Davidson MB, et al: Medical management of hyperglycemia in type 2 diabetes: a consensus algorithm for the initiation and adjustment of therapy: a consensus statement of the American Diabetes Association and the European Association for the Study of Diabetes. Diabetologia 52:17, 2009.)*

AACE Road Map for Glycemic Control in Treatment-Naive T2DM Patients

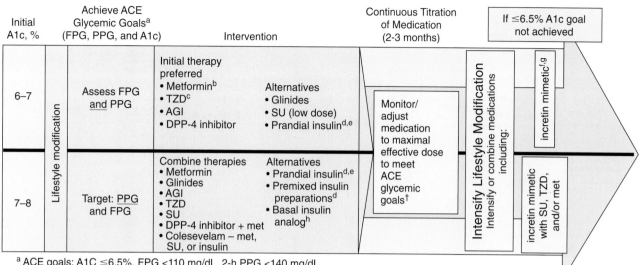

a ACE goals: A1C ≤6.5%, FPG <110 mg/dL, 2-h PPG <140 mg/dL
b Preffered first agent in most patients
c According to the FDA, rosiglitazone not recommended with insulin
d Analog preparations preferred
e Rapid-acting insulin analog (available as lispro, aspart, and glulisine) or regular insulin
f Indicated for patients not at goal despite SU and/or metformin or TZD; incretin mimetic is not indicated with insulin
g Available as exenatide
h Available as glargine and detemir

FIGURE 21-11 The American Association of Clinical Endocrinologists has proposed this road map for the pharmacologic management of hyperglycemia in patients with type 2 diabetes.[118] It is generally more inclusive than other guidelines and is unique insofar as it advises a different approach based on the initial HbA1c level.

Epidemiology of Diabetes and Its Complications (EDIC) study.[120] All patients were offered intensive management, although the meticulous follow-up by the study investigators and coordinators could no longer be provided. Not surprisingly, within 1 year, the HbA1c distinction between the two groups had disappeared. After 11 years, the mean HbA1c level in the original intensive group had risen to 7.9%, whereas it had fallen in the original conventional cohort to 7.8%.

Importantly, despite what appeared to be similar glucose control for most of the follow-up period, differences in microvascular complications persisted, and to some degree, cardiovascular complications appeared to continue to diverge. Ultimately, there were 46 total CVD events in 31 patients in the intensive group and 98 events in 52 patients in the conventional group, for a relative risk reduction of 42% (95% CI, 9%-63%; $P = 0.02$) (Fig. 21-15).[121] The composite risk of cardiovascular mortality, nonfatal myocardial infarction, or stroke was decreased by 57% (95% CI, 12%-7%; $P = 0.02$). Notably, other cardiovascular risk factors, including blood pressure, lipids, and BMI, were similar between the groups. One exception was the degree of albuminuria, which was persistently elevated in the conventional cohort (116 versus 54 mg/24 hr) and proved to be an independent predictor of cardiovascular risk.

This persistence of benefit for microvascular complications and the emergence of apparent benefit for macrovascular complications has been termed the legacy effect. Although it is not yet fully explained biologically, this term suggests a vascular benefit from any sustained period of good glycemic control in previous years. It is not yet known whether patients with type 1 diabetes may incur further benefit from even tighter glycemic control, such as the near-normalization of

blood glucose concentration. In light of recent trial results in type 2 diabetes (see earlier), this would seem unlikely, however, especially because patients with type 1 diabetes are even more prone to hypoglycemia and its sequelae.

Global CVD risk prevention strategies beyond glucose control in patients with type 1 diabetes mirror those interventions used in type 2 diabetes, as discussed next, although there have been no large, randomized clinical trials addressing other specific comorbidities in this group of patients.

GLOBAL MANAGEMENT OF TYPE 2 DIABETES MELLITUS FOR THE PREVENTION OF CARDIOVASCULAR DISEASE

Therapeutic Lifestyle Intervention

Lifestyle intervention is the cornerstone of CVD prevention in type 2 diabetes. The general principles of lifestyle intervention summarized earlier in this chapter for type 2 diabetes prevention are also applicable for the management of diagnosed type 2 diabetes. The goals of lifestyle intervention to prevent cardiovascular complications in patients with type 2 diabetes are improved glycemic control, reduced dyslipidemia and hypertension, and smoking cessation.

Weight Loss

Sustained moderate weight loss is recommended by the ADA in all patients with diabetes who are overweight or obese.[12] Moderate weight loss has been shown to reduce insulin resistance, dyslipidemia, and blood pressure.[2,67,69-71,73,74] Although overweight and obesity were associated with lower mortality

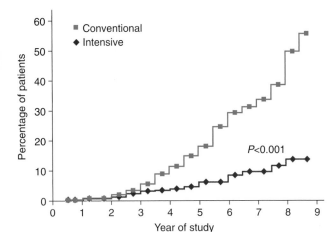

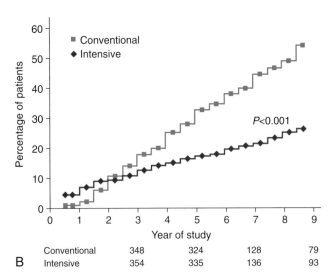

FIGURE 21-12 Microvascular complications in the Diabetes Complications and Control Trial, intensive versus conventional groups. In the primary prevention **(A)** and secondary intervention **(B)** cohorts, intensive therapy reduced the adjusted mean risk of the onset of retinopathy by 76% (*P* < 0.001) and 54% (*P* < 0.001), respectively, compared with conventional therapy. The numbers of patients in each therapy group who were evaluated at years 3, 5, 7, and 9 are shown below the graphs. *(From The Diabetes Control and Complications Trial Research Group: The effect of intensive treatment of diabetes on the development and progression of long-term complications in insulin-dependent diabetes mellitus. N Engl J Med 329:977, 1993.)*

(the so-called obesity paradox) in some studies of patients with established CVD, current evidence supports the role of moderate weight loss in CVD prevention in overweight or obese individuals.[122]

The ongoing Look AHEAD (Action for Health in Diabetes) multicenter prospective trial has randomized 5145 overweight or obese patients with type 2 diabetes (mean BMI, 36.0 kg/m^2) to intensive lifestyle intervention (diet and exercise) or control (support and education), aiming to examine the long-term effects of lifestyle intervention on the incidence of major CVD events.[123] The study is scheduled to conclude in 2012, but the 1-year interim results have already shown that intensive lifestyle intervention led to an average 8.6% weight reduction, compared with 0.7% in the control group, and was associated with significant improvement in glycemic control and cardiovascular risk factors (Table 21-5).[123]

Continued intervention and follow-up will determine whether these effects are sustained in the long term and are associated with reduced incidence of CVD events. As

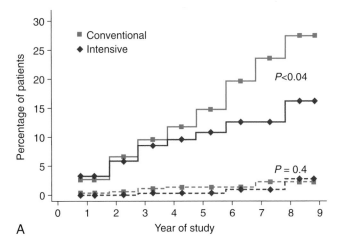

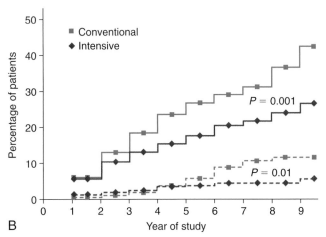

FIGURE 21-13 Microvascular complications in the Diabetes Complications and Control Trial, intensive versus conventional groups. In the primary prevention cohort **(A)**, intensive therapy reduced the adjusted mean risk of microalbuminuria by 34% (*P* < 0.04), *(solid lines)*. In the secondary intervention cohort **(B)**, intensive therapy reduced the risks of macroalbuminuria by 56% (*P* = 0.01) *(dashed lines)* and microalbuminuria by 43% (*P* = 0.001) *(solid lines). (From The Diabetes Control and Complications Trial Research Group: The effect of intensive treatment of diabetes on the development and progression of long-term complications in insulin-dependent diabetes mellitus. N Engl J Med 329:977, 1993.)*

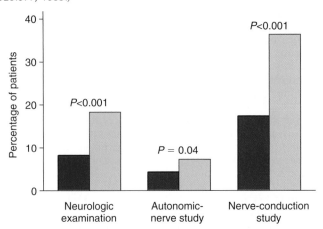

FIGURE 21-14 Microvascular complications in the Diabetes Complications and Control Trial, intensive versus conventional groups. Prevalence of abnormal clinical neurologic examination, autonomic nerve studies, and nerve conduction studies at 5 years between intensive (purple bars) and conventional (blue bars) treatment groups. *(From The Diabetes Control and Complications Trial Research Group: The effect of intensive treatment of diabetes on the development and progression of long-term complications in insulin-dependent diabetes mellitus. N Engl J Med 329:977, 1993.)*

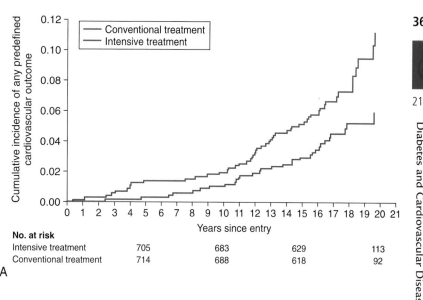

FIGURE 21-15 Intensive diabetes treatment and cardiovascular disease in patients with type 1 diabetes—observations from the Diabetes Control and Complications Trial/Epidemiology of Diabetes Interventions and Complications (DCCT/EDIC) study. Cumulative incidence of the first of any of the predefined cardiovascular disease outcomes **(A)** and of the first occurrence of nonfatal myocardial infarction, stroke, or death from cardiovascular disease **(B)**. Compared with conventional treatment, intensive treatment reduced the risk of any predefined cardiovascular disease outcome by 42% (95% CI, 9%-63%; *P* = 0.02) **(A)** and reduced the risk of the first occurrence of nonfatal myocardial infarction, stroke, or death from cardiovascular disease by 57% (95% CI, 12%-79%; *P* = 0.02) **(B)**. *(From Nathan DM, Cleary PA, Backlund JY, et al: Intensive diabetes treatment and cardiovascular disease in patients with type 1 diabetes. N Engl J Med 353:2643, 2005.)*

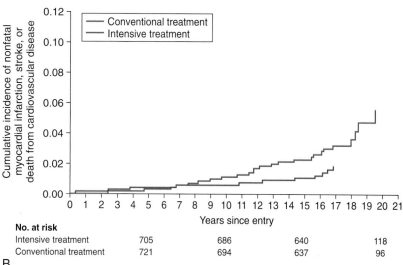

discussed before, when lifestyle intervention and pharmacologic therapy fail to provide adequate control of diabetes in patients with severe obesity (BMI ≥35 kg/m²) and type 2 diabetes, bariatric surgery may be recommended and has been demonstrated to commonly resolve diabetes.[12,82] However, the long-term effect of bariatric surgery on diabetic CVD complications has not been adequately studied in randomized controlled trials.

Healthy Food Choices

In addition to the benefits of controlling calorie intake, certain food choices may help prevent CVD in patients with type 2 diabetes.[12,74] To prevent or to delay atherosclerosis, the ADA recommends that people with diabetes minimize their intake of saturated fat (<7% of total calories), cholesterol (<200 mg/day), and *trans*-fats and encourages the consumption of two or more servings of fish per week (not commercially fried) to provide omega-3 fatty acids. Diets high in fruits, vegetables, whole grains, and nuts and low in red meats, processed sweets, and sugar-containing beverages may also contribute to CVD risk reduction. Reduced intake of sodium lowers blood pressure (<2300 mg sodium per day) and may also be beneficial for patients with symptomatic CHF (<2000 mg sodium per day). Finally, moderate consumption of ethanol (less than one drink per day for women and two for men) may reduce CVD risk in patients with diabetes.

Physical Activity and Exercise

In addition to playing an important role in weight reduction and weight control, regular physical activity in patients with diabetes may independently lower the risk of cardiovascular complications. In several large cohorts of diabetic patients, higher levels of physical activity or aerobic fitness were associated with lower incidence of cardiovascular events and lower cardiovascular mortality, even with adjustment for glycemic control, BMI, and other risk factors.[124]

The ADA recommends that people with diabetes perform at least 150 min/week of moderate-intensity aerobic physical activity (50% to 70% of maximum heart rate) as well as resistance training at least three times/week.[12] Exercise programs should be tailored to individual patients, depending on age, prior levels of physical activity, risk of ischemic heart disease, and coexisting conditions.

Smoking Cessation

There is overwhelming evidence from both cross-sectional and prospective studies that smokers with diabetes have a higher risk of complications (both microvascular and macrovascular) and death compared with nonsmokers.[125] Diabetes and smoking act synergistically to increase cardiovascular risk, and the cardiovascular benefits of smoking cessation, especially in this high-risk population, cannot be overstated.

TABLE 21–5	Changes in Measures of Diabetes Control, Blood Pressure Control, Measures of Lipid/Lipoproteins Control, Albumin-to-Creatinine Ratio, and Prevalence of Metabolic Syndrome Among Participants in the Look AHEAD Trial at Year 1: Mean or Percent (Standard Error)		
Measure	**Intensive Lifestyle Intervention** **N = 2496**	**Diabetes Support and Education** **N = 2463**	**P Value**
Use of Diabetes Medicines (%)			
Baseline	86.5 (0.7)	86.5 (0.7)	0.93*
Year 1	78.6 (0.8)	88.7 (0.6)	<0.001*
Change	−7.8 (0.6)	2.2 (0.5)	<0.001[†]
Fasting Glucose (mg/dL)			
Baseline	151.9 (0.9)	153.6 (0.9)	0.21[‡]
Year 1	130.4 (0.8)	146.4 (0.9)	<0.001[‡]
Change	−21.5 (0.9)	−7.2 (0.9)	<0.001[‡]
Hemoglobin A1c (%)			
Baseline	7.25 (0.02)	7.29 (0.02)	0.26[‡]
Year 1	6.61 (0.02)	7.15 (0.02)	<0.001[‡]
Difference	−0.64 (0.02)	−0.14 (0.02)	<0.001[‡]
Use of Antihypertensive Medicines (%)			
Baseline	75.3 (0.9)	73.7 (0.9)	0.23*
Year 1	75.2 (0.9)	75.9 (0.9)	0.54*
Change	−0.1 (0.6)	2.2 (0.6)	0.02[†]
Systolic Blood Pressure (mm Hg)			
Baseline	128.2 (0.4)	129.4 (0.3)	0.01[‡]
Year 1	121.4 (0.4)	126.6 (0.4)	<0.001[‡]
Change	−6.8 (0.4)	−2.8 (0.3)	<0.001[‡]
Diastolic Blood Pressure (mm Hg)			
Baseline	69.9 (0.2)	70.4 (0.2)	0.11[‡]
Year 1	67.0 (0.2)	68.6 (0.2)	<0.001[‡]
Change	−3.0 (0.2)	−1.8 (0.2)	<0.001[‡]
Use of Lipid-Lowering Medicines (%)			
Baseline	49.4 (1.0)	48.4 (1.0)	0.52*
Year 1	53.0 (1.0)	57.8 (1.0)	<0.001*
Change	3.7 (0.8)	9.4 (0.8)	<0.001[†]
LDL-C (mg/dL)			
Baseline	112.2 (0.4)	112.4 (0.6)	0.78[‡]
Year 1	107.0 (0.6)	106.7 (0.7)	0.74[‡]
Change	−5.2 (0.6)	−5.7 (0.6)	0.49[‡]
HDL-C (mg/dL)			
Baseline	43.5 (0.2)	43.6 (0.2)	0.80[‡]
Year 1	46.9 (0.3)	44.9 (0.2)	<0.001[‡]
Change	3.4 (0.2)	1.4 (0.1)	<0.001[‡]
Triglycerides (mg/dL)			
Baseline	182.8 (2.3)	180.0 (2.4)	0.38[‡]
Year 1	152.5 (1.8)	165.4 (1.9)	<0.001[‡]
Change	−30.3 (2.0)	−14.6 (1.8)	<0.001[‡]
Albumin-To-Creatinine Ratio >30.0 μg/mg (%)			
Baseline	16.4 (0.7)	16.9 (0.8)	0.69[‡]
Year 1	12.5 (0.7)	15.4 (0.7)	0.005[‡]
Change	−3.9 (0.6)	−1.5 (0.6)	0.002[‡]
Metabolic Syndrome (%)			
Baseline	93.6 (0.5)	94.4 (0.5)	0.23[‡]
Year 1	78.9 (0.8)	87.3 (0.7)	<0.001[‡]
Change	−14.7 (0.8)	−7.1 (0.7)	<0.001[‡]

*Logistic regression with adjustment for clinical site.
[†]Mantel-Haenszel test with adjustment for clinical site.
[‡]Analysis of covariance with adjustment for clinical site.

Hypertension

Hypertension affects approximately 70% of patients with diabetes[46] and is more common in the elderly, in men, and in African Americans as well as in those with longer duration of diabetes, poorer glucose control, and concomitant proteinuria. Hypertension adversely affects both microvascular and macrovascular disease risk and has been estimated to account for between 35% and 40% of the incremental CVD risk associated with diabetes.

Treatment of Hypertension in Patients with Diabetes Mellitus

The keystone of cardiovascular risk prevention remains lifestyle change, and this most certainly applies to the prevention and treatment of hypertension. Frequent modest-intensity aerobic exercise, alcohol and sodium moderation, and weight reduction all markedly contribute to improved blood pressure. Numerous classes of antihypertensive therapies have been proven safe and effective for the treatment of hypertension in patients with diabetes on the basis of assessment of clinical outcomes in randomized trials by subanalyses of diabetes cohorts and also in trials exclusively studying patients with diabetes. A number of randomized trials have proven the efficacy of several classes of antihypertensive medications in this context, including angiotensin-converting enzyme (ACE) inhibitors, angiotensin receptor blockers (ARBs), calcium channel blockers, thiazide diuretics, and beta blockers.[126]

Angiotensin-Converting Enzyme Inhibitors. Patients with diabetes and hypertension derive particular benefit from ACE inhibitors.[126] Observations of treatment effects among patients with diabetes participating in long-term primary and secondary cardiovascular risk prevention randomized trials with ACE inhibitors underscore the important clinical benefit of this class of drugs,[127-132] supporting their recommendation as the first-line antihypertensive treatment of most patients with diabetes.[133] ACE inhibitors are also renoprotective, in both type 1 and type 2 diabetes.[134]

Angiotensin Receptor Blockers. Whereas the evidence base for ARBs is not as robust as that for the ACE inhibitors with regard to effects on CVD outcomes, the aggregate data support consideration of ARBs as an alternative treatment option in those patients intolerant of ACE inhibitors because of cough, rash, or angioedema.[126,133] ARBs may also be preferred for renoprotection in type 2 diabetes by a stronger evidence base from large randomized trials of patients with type 2 diabetes and impaired kidney function, such as IDNT and RENAAL.[135,136] The ONTARGET randomized trial comparing ramipril versus telmisartan versus the combination of the two demonstrated comparable efficacy between telmisartan and ramipril, but it did not demonstrate incremental CVD benefits with the two drugs combined and in that setting increased adverse effects and intolerance.[137] Therefore, the combination of ACE inhibitors and ARBs is not routinely recommended.

Dihydropyridine Calcium Channel Blockers. Dihydropyridine calcium channel blockers are well tolerated and effective at lowering blood pressure. Analyses of diabetes subsets of randomized clinical trials have suggested CVD clinical benefits of similar or greater magnitude compared with those observed in the nondiabetic cohorts, including the evaluations of nitrendipine, nisoldipine, and amlodipine.[126] In active controlled comparisons, amlodipine has been proven superior to hydrochlorothiazide when it is added to a background of benazepril therapy,[138] but in direct randomized comparisons of calcium channel blockers (fosinopril versus amlodipine,[139] enalapril versus nisoldipine[140]), ACE inhibitors had superior efficacy on CVD outcomes.

Thiazide Diuretics. Thiazide diuretic medications adversely affect glucose metabolism and have been associated with increased risk for incident diabetes. However, despite these glycometabolic effects, thiazides have been proven effective at modifying cardiovascular risk among patients with diabetes and impaired fasting glucose concentration, even in the setting of trials in which the thiazide was associated with increased diabetes incidence (e.g., ALLHAT).[141] The clinical efficacy of thiazide diuretics among patients with diabetes is supported by the results of subanalyses of the diabetic patients participating in the Systolic Hypertension in the Elderly Program (SHEP) trial, in which chlorthalidone was compared with placebo in patients aged >60 years with isolated systolic hypertension.[142]

In these analyses, the magnitude of treatment effect in the diabetes group was twice as large compared with those without diabetes at study entry. In the ALLHAT trial, the CVD effect of chlorthalidone was quantitatively similar to effects observed with amlodipine and lisinopril[127]; and in the ADVANCE trial of high-risk diabetic patients that included the thiazide diuretic indapamide plus perindopril versus placebo, the combination treatment proved superior for CVD outcomes.[130] Despite their possible effects on glucose metabolism, thiazide diuretics should be considered among the evidence-based second-line antihypertensive agents in diabetic patients, given their well-documented effects on blood pressure and CVD events. They are particularly suited in combination regimens with ACE inhibitors or ARBs, most of which are now available in fixed-dose combination formulations.

Beta Blockers. For decades, common opinion was that beta blockers should be contraindicated for the treatment of patients with diabetes on the basis of concerns about adverse effects on glucose, insulin, and lipid metabolism, similar to observations with thiazide diuretics discussed before, as well as the masking of symptoms of hypoglycemia. Although these concerns persist, data from the UKPDS demonstrated superiority of the beta blocker atenolol compared with placebo with regard to diabetes-related clinical outcomes among diabetic patients without prior CVD, with treatment effects comparable to those observed with captopril.[131]

Subsequent trials, however, have demonstrated both increased incidence of diabetes compared with nondiuretic antihypertensive therapies and slightly less efficacy at reducing major adverse CVD events compared with treatment with ACE inhibitors or calcium channel blockers.[143] In this context, metabolic differences between the beta blockers may be of importance, such as the superiority of carvedilol over atenolol or metoprolol demonstrated in randomized head-to-head comparisons of glucose and lipid effects; the clinical relevance of these observations remains to be defined.[144,145]

Despite the accumulated clinical outcomes evidence, there continues to be some resistance across the broad clinical community to use of beta blockers in patients with diabetes. However, whereas ACE inhibitors, calcium channel blockers, and thiazide diuretics appear to have some advantages over beta blockers, both metabolic and with regard to clinical outcomes, because achievement of aggressive blood pressure targets for patients with diabetes commonly will require three or four medications, beta blockers remain a therapeutic option in this setting. These agents should be considered part of the antihypertensive regimen in any diabetic patient with coexisting coronary artery disease, especially if MI has already occurred, and in the setting of systolic heart failure.

Therapeutic Targets

Given the incremental CVD risk associated with hypertension in diabetes and the clearly demonstrated graded association between magnitude of blood pressure reduction and CVD clinical risk reduction, patients with diabetes have been identified as a special population warranting more aggressive than usual blood pressure control. Targets for patients with diabetes of <130/80 mm Hg have been endorsed by a number of professional guidelines.[12,133,146] These recommendations, based largely on epidemiologic data, have been supported by observations of more recent randomized clinical trials. In the Hypertension Optimal Treatment trial, participants with elevated diastolic blood pressure were randomized to treatment to three different targets: ≤90 mm Hg, ≤85 mm Hg, and ≤80 mm Hg.

Whereas the overall trial failed to demonstrate significant differences by intensity of blood pressure treatment, a post hoc analysis of the subset of patients with diabetes exhibited a significant intensity-dependent reduction in CVD, including a 50% relative risk reduction for major adverse CVD events in the group with the lowest compared with the highest diastolic blood pressure target.[147] Likewise, the average blood pressure achieved in the diabetic subset of HOPE (139/77) and in the ADVANCE trials (136/73) provides further direct support for the safety and efficacy of such intensified blood pressure targets in the high-risk population of patients with diabetes. However, in the ACCORD randomized clinical trial, in which more than 10,000 patients with diabetes at increased CVD risk were randomized to systolic blood pressure goals of <120 mm Hg versus <140 mg Hg, more intensive blood pressure control did not significantly reduce the combined risk of fatal or nonfatal CVD events.[147a]

Angiotensin-Converting Enzyme Inhibition
Independent of Hypertension

The reduction of CVD risk among patients with diabetes treated with ACE inhibitors appears to extend beyond hypertension, with both microvascular and macrovascular benefits consistently greater in magnitude than that predicted on the basis of the differences in blood pressure achieved.[126] These observations suggest pleiotropic benefits of ACE inhibition, including but not limited to favorable effects on glucose metabolism and insulin resistance.[148] This discordance between expected and observed effects of ACE inhibitors was first demonstrated in the Heart Outcomes Prevention Evaluation (HOPE) trial,[132] which randomized patients with normal ventricular function and either diabetes with at least one additional risk factor or prevalent CVD to ramipril or placebo, independent of blood pressure at study entry.

The results from HOPE demonstrated that treatment with ramipril titrated to 10 mg daily was associated with a 25% relative reduction in the long-term risk of major adverse cardiovascular events and also reduced renal complications among the large subset of patients with diabetes enrolled in that trial, despite just achieving a mean difference in blood pressure between the groups of only 3 mm Hg. These observations have subsequently been supported by results in the diabetes subset of the European trial on reduction of cardiac events with perindopril in patients with stable coronary artery disease (EUROPA) comparing perindopril versus placebo in a cohort with a high prevalence of diabetes and in the ADVANCE trial comparing perindopril-indapamide combination versus placebo in patients with type 2 diabetes. ACE inhibitor–based regimens reduced CVD risk, with only modest differences in blood pressure achieved between the groups (approximately 5 to 6 mm Hg). In aggregate, the data reported to date support consideration of ACE inhibitor use in all patients with diabetes at increased CVD risk, such as those aged ≥40 years and those with CVD occurring at an earlier age, as recommended by contemporary professional guidelines.[12]

Summary of Hypertension Management

Given the high prevalence and adverse microvascular and CVD consequences of hypertension in the diabetes population, aggressive control of blood pressure should be among the principal therapeutic objectives in the management of this high-risk population of patients. Aggressive blood pressure management should have a target of <130/80 mm Hg

and, in addition to intensive lifestyle counseling, can use an arsenal of at least five classes of evidence-based medications for CVD risk modification. ACE inhibitors should be considered first-line therapy (and ARBs for those intolerant of ACE inhibitors), independent of blood pressure, for all diabetic patients aged >55 years with additional cardiac risk factors or younger if prevalent CVD is present, especially in the context of their incremental benefit on renal outcomes.

Dyslipidemia

Dyslipidemia is common among patients with type 2 diabetes, especially in the majority of patients with significant insulin resistance, most commonly manifested as a characteristic pattern consisting of elevated triglyceride levels, decreased HDL levels, and only modest elevations of LDL but with an increased proportion of small, dense LDL particles.[62,64] The cornerstone for treatment of this dyslipidemia remains lifestyle interventions as described before, and lipid disturbances are also favorably affected by intensification of glucose control to contemporary targets.

Several pharmacologic agents are especially effective at modifying this spectrum of abnormalities, including niacin and fibric acid derivatives, but the net CVD clinical effects of these interventions remain uncertain. In contrast, the statin drugs have a robust CVD clinical outcomes data basis in the setting of diabetes and are the primary drugs advocated for use in patients with diabetes. Fish oil preparations also have an evidence basis for favorable effects on CVD risk, although clearly much weaker than that for statins, and can also be considered, given their beneficial effects on triglycerides. Several ongoing trials should help clarify the role of these agents alone and in combination with statins in the management of diabetic dyslipidemia.

Pharmacologic Treatment of LDL-C

Despite the fact that marked elevations of LDL are not characteristic of diabetes dyslipidemia, statin medications have been firmly established as the primary lipid drug therapy to affect CVD risk modification. This is due to some degree to the propensity for patients with diabetes to have small, dense LDL particles, resulting in a much higher concentration of particles for any given mass of circulating LDL. This is reflected by increased LDL particle number and increased apolipoprotein B concentrations.

Prospective studies have demonstrated a strong, independent relationship between LDL particle size or concentration and the risk of coronary artery disease.[149,150] This is thought to be attributable to increased atherogenic propensity for the small, dense LDL particles by virtue of their ability to more readily cross into the arterial wall; and once there, they are more prone to oxidation to initiate and to propagate the atheromatous process, to induce endothelial dysfunction, and to increase thromboxane formation.[151] On the basis of these observations and the demonstrated efficacy of the approach, LDL-C remains the principal therapeutic target in patients with diabetes.

The most convincing evidence for the efficacy of statins for primary CVD risk prevention in the setting of diabetes derives primarily from two randomized trials,[152,153] supported by a meta-analysis of statin use in diabetes.[154] In the Heart Protection Study (HPS) comparing simvastatin 40 mg daily versus placebo among a population of patients at increased CVD risk but not meeting contemporary indications for statin therapy, 5963 patients with diabetes were enrolled, including 67% without prior CVD and 41% with an LDL level below 116 mg/dL at study entry.[153] In the overall diabetes subset, simvastatin was associated with a 22% (P < 0.0001) relative reduction in the first occurrence of a major coronary event, stroke, or revascularization and a 20% reduction in coronary mortality ($P = 0.02$). Furthermore, in the cohort of 2912 diabetes subjects without prior CVD, major adverse CVD events were decreased by 33% ($P = 0.0003$) with simvastatin.

In the Collaborative Atorvastatin Diabetes Study (CARDS),[152] 2838 patients with type 2 diabetes and at least one other cardiovascular risk factor but without clinical indication for statin therapy were randomized to atorvastatin 10 mg versus placebo. In this cohort with an average baseline LDL level of 120 mg/dL, atorvastatin treatment resulted in a 37% ($P = 0.001$) relative reduction in major cardiovascular events, prompting early termination of the study. In summary, these data support the recommendation that patients with diabetes at sufficient risk for cardiovascular events should be considered for statin therapy regardless of baseline cholesterol levels, underpinning the most recent guideline recommendations for statin use in all patients with diabetes aged >40 years or younger with prevalent CVD,[12] and with an aggressive LDL target of <70 mg/dL to be considered.[155]

A number of other approved therapies for dyslipidemia favorably affect LDL concentrations, including ezetimibe, bile acid binders, fibric acids, and niacin. However, none of these alternative agents affects LDL as potently as the statin medications do, and as mentioned before, none has yet been proven through rigorous randomized trial assessment to consistently benefit CVD risk and outcomes. On that basis, these should be considered alternatives or possibly add-on therapies for those patients with diabetes intolerant of statins or unable to achieve therapeutic targets with statin monotherapy.

Pharmacologic Treatment of Triglycerides and HDL

Elevation of triglyceride levels is a key component of diabetic dyslipidemia, and epidemiologic observations have consistently demonstrated a robust independent association between high triglyceride levels and adverse CVD outcomes. Similarly, another hallmark feature of dyslipidemia associated with insulin resistance and diabetes is low HDL-C concentration, and across epidemiologic studies, low HDL concentration is among the strongest and most consistent predictors of adverse CVD risk. However, results from randomized trials assessing the effects on CVD risk of various therapeutic strategies targeted at treating high triglyceride and low HDL levels have been discordant and have largely failed to prove the therapeutic concept.

Omega-3 Fatty Acids. Long-chain omega-3 fatty acids (fish oil) lower triglyceride levels on average by 50 to 75 mg/dL, dependent to some degree on baseline abnormality and dose of fish oil, with up to 30% reduction when doses of 4 g/day are used. Fish oil has minimal effects on HDL and total cholesterol, modestly raises LDL, and despite early concerns to the contrary, has no discernible effects on glycemic parameters in patients with diabetes.[156] Complementing these net effects on lipid parameters, data from randomized clinical outcomes trials including notable representation of patients with diabetes have consistently demonstrated improved cardiovascular clinical outcomes.[157,158]

Randomized clinical trials assessing the effects of these agents on cardiovascular outcomes in patients with diabetes are lacking. The most robust evidence to date is derived from a subanalysis of the Japan EPA Intervention Study (JELIS) of 4565 patients with impaired fasting glucose or diabetes, demonstrating a 22% risk reduction ($P = 0.048$) for major adverse CVD events with eicosapentaenoic acid treatment at 1.8 g daily.[159] Presently, a large-scale randomized trial is under way, the Outcome Reduction with Initial Glargine Intervention (ORIGIN) trial, that is assessing the CVD effects of fish oil versus placebo in a population of ~10,000 patients with impaired fasting glucose, impaired glucose tolerance, or early type 2 diabetes, including but not limited to those receiving background statin therapy.

Fibric Acid Derivatives. Fibric acid derivatives (fibrates) are prime candidates for the treatment of diabetic dyslipidemia by virtue of their favorable effects on a number of the characteristic perturbations. Fibrates lower triglyceride levels and modestly increase HDL concentration by inhibiting VLDL production and activating lipoprotein lipase, which increases catabolism of triglyceride-rich lipoproteins.[160] Despite these lipid effects, results from randomized clinical trials have been mixed and have largely failed to prove the cardiovascular benefit anticipated on the basis of the triglyceride and HDL effects.

In the Veterans Affairs High-Density Lipoprotein Intervention Trial (VA-HIT), 2531 subjects with a history of coronary artery disease and low HDL levels (≤40 mg/dL) were randomized to treatment with gemfibrozil 1200 mg daily versus placebo.[161] In a post hoc subgroup analysis of 391 participants with diabetes, gemfibrozil was associated with a 32% ($P = 0.004$) risk reduction in cardiovascular events, with a 41% ($P = 0.02$) reduction in death attributable to coronary artery disease.[162] Key limitations of extrapolating the VA-HIT observations to contemporary practice include the small number of diabetes subjects enrolled, the exclusion of statin use during the trial, the exclusive enrollment of men, and the present awareness of adverse drug interactions of gemfibrozil with statins, especially simvastatin.

Subsequently, three large-scale randomized trials of fibrates in high-risk CVD cohorts have failed to demonstrate superiority of fibrates versus placebo. In the Bezafibrate Infarction Prevention (BIP) trial, 3090 patients with coronary artery disease and low HDL concentration were enrolled, including 309 with diabetes, and randomized to treatment with bezafibrate 400 mg daily versus placebo.[163] After 6.2 years of average follow-up, bezafibrate failed to significantly reduce the risk of sudden death or MI compared with placebo (13.6% versus 15.0%; $P = 0.26$); exploratory post hoc analyses suggested benefit in subjects with triglyceride levels >200 mg/dL as well as in patients with the metabolic syndrome, which should be interpreted as hypothesis-generating observations requiring confirmation.[163,164]

In the Fenofibrate Intervention and Event Lowering in Diabetes (FIELD) trial,[165] 9795 patients with type 2 diabetes not taking a statin at study entry were randomized to micronized fenofibrate 200 mg daily versus placebo. Despite an average of 5 years of follow-up and acquisition of 544 primary outcome events, fenofibrate failed to significantly reduce fatal and nonfatal MI risk (5.9% versus 5.2%; $P = 0.16$). This less than anticipated benefit was in part attributed to a significantly greater drop-in rate for nonstudy lipid-lowering drugs, predominantly statins, in the placebo group (17%) compared with the fenofibrate group (8%; $P < 0.0001$). The ACCORD trial also failed to demonstrate a CVD benefit of fenofibrate versus placebo in patients with type 2 diabetes at increased CVD risk who had residual elevation of triglycerides after achieving target LDL concentrations with statin therapy.[164a]

In summary, randomized clinical outcome assessment of fibrates has failed to demonstrate clear CVD clinical benefit in the context of contemporary prevalent use of statin medications, with many results trending in the right direction but interpretation and generalizability substantially confounded by issues of concomitant statin use, both in the trials and in clinical practice. In addition, one fibrate, gemfibrozil, is known to increase circulating statin levels (especially simvastatin) when it is used in combination and may increase the risk of statin-associated toxicities.

Niacin. Niacin is particularly attractive for treatment of diabetic dyslipidemia as it increases HDL levels up to 35% and also reduces triglyceride levels 15% to 20%, reduces LDL concentration 10% to 15%, and increases LDL particle size.[166] Despite these consistently favorable lipid effects on the lipoprotein spectrum of diabetic dyslipidemia, clinical outcomes

21

data for this class of drugs remain lacking. In addition, clinical use is often confounded by the common side effect of flushing, which has been mitigated but not eliminated by the development of sustained-release preparations of niacin. Niacin is also known to exacerbate insulin resistance, which may result in increasing glucose levels in patients with type 2 diabetes.

The only large-scale randomized trial reported to date assessing the CVD effect of monotherapy with niacin is the Coronary Drug Project (CDP),[18] which randomized 1119 men with prior CVD to treatment with immediate-release niacin and compared CVD outcomes with placebo treatment in 2789 patients. Niacin therapy was associated with a modest 17% ($P < 0.05$) reduction in coronary death or nonfatal MI after 6 years and, after an extended 15-year post-trial follow-up period, a 16% ($P < 0.005$) reduction in all-cause mortality.[167] However, interpretation of the CDP trial results is challenging, given an extreme rate of study drug noncompliance in the niacin arm and comparisons of CVD events partitioned over six randomized treatment arms, only one of which included niacin.

Similar limitations of compliance and power apply to the accumulated data set regarding the CVD effects of niacin, largely limited by small studies and challenges of trial execution with excessive dropout among subjects taking niacin. In addition, there has been limited power to assess effects unique to patients with diabetes because of the relatively low numbers enrolled.

In addition to the uncertainties about the CVD efficacy of niacin monotherapy, few data are available regarding the incremental efficacy and safety of niacin added to statins. In the HDL-Atherosclerosis Treatment Study (HATS),[168] 160 patients with low HDL concentration and obstructive coronary disease were randomized to a combination of simvastatin and niacin, simvastatin-niacin and antioxidant therapy, antioxidant therapy alone, or placebo. Compared with placebo, simvastatin-niacin was associated with regression of coronary plaque and, on the basis of only 12 versus 1 major adverse CVD events, statistically superior clinical outcomes; these effects were eliminated in the group also treated with antioxidants, suggesting an adverse treatment interaction. Given the very small sample size, however, the validity of these observations is notably uncertain.

To more rigorously assess the CVD effects of niacin added to statin therapy, a large ongoing study sponsored by the National Heart, Lung, and Blood Institute, the Atherothrombosis Intervention in Metabolic Syndrome with Low HDL/High Triglycerides and Impact on Global Health Outcomes (AIM-HIGH), is comparing the effects of niacin added to simvastatin versus simvastatin alone on CVD outcomes in a randomized controlled trial of ~3300 patients with prevalent CVD, type 2 diabetes, and metabolic syndrome.

Therapeutic Targets

The key therapeutic target underpinning any treatment of diabetic dyslipidemia remains lifestyle intervention focused on optimization of medical nutrition therapy, weight control, and the habituation of adequate physical activity. The first-line pharmacologic therapy for diabetic dyslipidemia is the statin medications, as reflected in the most recent update of the NCEP Adult Treatment Panel (ATP III)[155] and supported by other professional society guidelines.[12,133,169] Whereas some minor differences in recommended lipid management strategies exist across the guidelines, those formulated by the ADA updated annually are the most current,[12] recommending statin therapy for all patients with diabetes aged >40 years or younger in the setting of either prevalent CVD or the presence of CVD risk factors other than diabetes.

The recommended LDL therapeutic targets are as follows: LDL <100 mg/dL in the absence of underlying CVD; LDL <70 mg/dL in the setting of prevalent CVD; and, at maximal tolerated statin dose, at least 30% to 40% reduction from baseline LDL concentration. Importantly, none of these recommendations for statin prescription is based on the baseline LDL level; instead, they are driven by the underlying CVD risk burden. The updated NCEP ATP III guidelines regard diabetes as a coronary disease equivalent and advocate an "optional" LDL goal of <70 mg/dL in all patients with diabetes that is independent of underlying CVD prevalence or risk estimate.[155]

Beyond LDL interventions, as reviewed in this section, little evidence is available to guide decision making with regard to other lipid targets. For the treatment of patients who have persistently elevated triglyceride levels (>200 mg/dL) after achieving therapeutic LDL targets, a consensus opinion across guidelines advocates that the principal secondary lipid target should be non-HDL (i.e., non-HDL = total cholesterol − HDL), with target levels 30 mg/dL higher than the individual patient's corresponding LDL target. This can be achieved by intensifying lifestyle intervention or statin prescription or by the addition of a second drug, such as fish oil, niacin, or a fibrate (but not gemfibrozil). As summarized in the ADA guidance, however, the net safety and efficacy of add-on drug therapy remain poorly understood, with a noted increase in the risk for liver and muscle side effects. Despite the intuitive appeal of treating to triglyceride or HDL targets, such strategies lack a solid evidence base.

Antiplatelet Therapies

Insulin resistance and type 2 diabetes are associated with myriad abnormalities in platelet structure, life span, activation, and aggregation, yielding a prothrombotic state.[60,61] This is compounded by secondary platelet effects of other coagulation factor abnormalities associated with diabetes, such as increased circulating levels of fibrinogen, thromboxane, plasminogen activator inhibitor 1, and von Willebrand factor, which contribute to platelet activation and aggregation.[170] On that basis, the CVD effects of antiplatelet therapies have been of great interest for the treatment of patients with diabetes.

Aspirin. Whereas the evidence basis for the use of aspirin to reduce CVD risk in the setting of prevalent CVD is well established,[171] the role of aspirin for primary CVD risk prevention is much less well defined.[172] This is especially true in the setting of diabetes, for which the data are substantially limited by relatively few diabetic patients studied to date. Analyses from the diabetes subsets of reported clinical trials suggest an attenuation of aspirin benefit among patients with diabetes, as demonstrated in the Antithrombotic Trialists' meta-analysis of antiplatelet therapy (predominantly aspirin) comprising a patient mix of primary and secondary CVD risk and including assessment of almost 5000 patients with diabetes.[171] That analysis revealed a significant relative odds reduction with antiplatelet therapy of 22% in the overall cohort but only a trend of 7% reduction in the subset with diabetes that was not statistically significant.

The Hypertension Optimal Treatment (HOT) randomized clinical trial evaluated the efficacy of aspirin 75 mg daily versus placebo on CVD event risk reduction among patients with hypertension, including 1501 (8%) with diabetes.[147] After a mean follow-up of 3.8 years, aspirin was associated with a 36% relative reduction in risk for MI and a 15% relative reduction in major cardiovascular events in the overall trial. The authors qualitatively commented that the results among the diabetes subset were similar, although no data were presented for these analyses.

Subsequently, the results from three randomized clinical trials of aspirin in the setting of primary CVD prevention have challenged the utility of routine aspirin use for primary CVD prevention in diabetes. The Primary Prevention Project

(PPP) randomized trial assessed the CVD effects of 75 mg of aspirin daily versus placebo and included 1031 (23%) patients with diabetes.[173] Treatment with aspirin was associated with a nonsignificant trend of 10% relative risk reduction for death, MI, and cerebrovascular accident, contrasted with a significant 41% reduction observed in the nondiabetic group. However, because of early termination of the trial due to efficacy in the overall trial, only 42 primary events were evaluable within the diabetes subanalysis, thus markedly limiting statistical power and validity of this observation.

In the Prevention of Progression of Arterial Disease and Diabetes (POPADAD) trial,[174] 1276 patients aged >40 years with type 1 or type 2 diabetes but without CVD were randomized to treatment with aspirin 100 mg daily versus placebo, with a median follow-up of 6.7 years. In the assessment of 233 primary outcome events of death, MI, cerebrovascular accident, and amputation, no benefit of aspirin was observed (116 versus 117 events; relative risk reduction, 0.98; 95% CI, 0.76-1.26). Again, statistical power in this study was modest, and the study was further limited by 50% withdrawal rate of study subjects by 5 years.

The Japanese Primary Prevention of Atherosclerosis with Aspirin for Diabetes (JPAD) trial randomized 2539 patients with type 2 diabetes to aspirin 81 to 100 mg daily versus placebo, with follow-up for a median of 4.4 years, accumulating 154 primary events of cardiovascular death, MI, cerebrovascular accident, and peripheral arterial disease.[175] Treatment with aspirin was associated with a trend toward a 20% hazard reduction that did not achieve statistical significance (HR = 0.80; 95% CI, 0.58-1.10; $P = 0.16$).

In the context of this uncertainty in the setting of primary CVD risk prevention in diabetes, two large-scale randomized clinical trials are under way. A Study of Cardiovascular Events in Diabetes (ASCEND) is designed to enroll 10,000 patients with type 1 or type 2 diabetes without CVD in a double-blind, placebo-controlled trial with a factorial randomization to treatment with (1) 100 mg aspirin daily versus placebo and (2) omega-3 fatty acid 1 g daily versus placebo, with a primary endpoint of major adverse cardiovascular events (http://www.ctsu.ox.ac.uk/ascend/). The Aspirin and Simvastatin Combination for Cardiovascular Events Prevention Trial in Diabetes (ACCEPT-D) plans to enroll 4700 patients with type 1 or type 2 diabetes to receive 100 mg aspirin plus simvastatin versus simvastatin alone in a prospective, open-label, blinded endpoint evaluation (PROBE) design trial to assess the cardiovascular efficacy of aspirin in primary prevention for patients with diabetes treated with statins.[176]

In addition to uncertainty overall about the utility of aspirin in primary prevention populations with diabetes, additional uncertainty remains about the most appropriate dose of aspirin to prevent CVD in diabetes; most contemporary guidelines recommend doses of 75 to 162 mg/day.[12,133,177,178] However, all such aspirin dosing recommendations in the setting of type 2 diabetes are acknowledged to derive primarily from expert opinion, as randomized comparative data guiding the choice of daily aspirin dose for patients with type 2 diabetes are effectively nonexistent. It remains possible that higher doses of aspirin may be more effective in type 2 diabetes, as suggested by results from the Early Treatment Diabetic Retinopathy Study (ETDRS) randomized trial that demonstrated superior CVD outcomes with 650 mg daily of aspirin versus placebo among patients with type 1 and type 2 diabetes,[179] a concept that requires confirmation before clinical application.

Other Antiplatelet Therapies. Based on the platelet abnormalities of type 2 diabetes and the ongoing uncertainty with regard to aspirin described before, the possibility remains that the more potent antiplatelet agents or agents targeting novel therapeutic targets may be especially beneficial in diabetes. Support for this concept derives from several published reports from acute coronary syndrome studies, demonstrating incremental efficacy of parenteral glycoprotein IIb/IIIa antagonists[180] and of both presently available thienopyridine antiplatelet agents, clopidogrel and prasugrel.[181,182] These concepts remain unproven in the setting of primary CVD risk prevention and are the focus of numerous ongoing research programs.

In summary, despite the uncertainties deriving from the accumulated data, the routine use of aspirin at doses ranging from 75 to 162 mg daily remains widely recommended by contemporary guidelines for primary CVD risk prevention for most adult patients with diabetes, including those aged >40 years or younger with additional CVD risk factors.[12,133,183] The strength of such recommendations is variable across guidelines, ranging from Level I indication (i.e., should be recommended)[12,133] to Level IIb[183]; most guidelines acknowledge that these recommendations remain expert opinion, citing a level of evidence of C. Until further evidence becomes available, it remains reasonable to consider daily aspirin therapy for patients with diabetes, especially those with other markers of increased CVD risk.

CONCLUSION

Diabetes mellitus is common and increasing globally, driven primarily by the ever-increasing prevalence of type 2 diabetes. The management of this at-risk population begins with attempts to prevent diabetes in the first place, and once it is present, continues with efforts to mitigate the associated clinical risk, which is primarily CVD. Lifestyle intervention remains the cornerstone of such management; when it is applied effectively, it potently prevents diabetes and its myriad associated CVD risk factors.

Glucose control strategies, although effective for microvascular disease risk intervention, remain unproven with regard to CVD risk reduction, with ongoing uncertainty about the most appropriate strategies and glucose targets. Beyond glucose, interventions broadly demonstrated to favorably affect CVD in the general population are especially effective for patients with diabetes, including intensive blood pressure and LDL management added to lifestyle interventions.

REFERENCES

1. Wild S, Roglic G, Green A, et al: Global prevalence of diabetes: estimates for the year 2000 and projections for 2030. *Diabetes Care* 27:1047, 2004.
2. National Cholesterol Education Program (NCEP) Expert Panel on Detection, Evaluation, and Treatment of High Blood Cholesterol in Adults (Adult Treatment Panel III): Third Report of the National Cholesterol Education Program (NCEP) Expert Panel on Detection, Evaluation, and Treatment of High Blood Cholesterol in Adults (Adult Treatment Panel III) Final Report. *Circulation* 106:3143, 2002.
3. American Diabetes Association: Diagnosis and Classification of Diabetes Mellitus. *Diabetes Care* 32:S62, 2009.
4. World Health Organization: *Diabetes, fact sheet N° 312*, 2008.
5. International Expert Committee report on the role of the A1c assay in the diagnosis of diabetes. *Diabetes Care* 32:1327, 2009.
6. The Expert Committee on the Diagnosis and Classification of Diabetes Mellitus: Report of the Expert Committee on the Diagnosis and Classification of Diabetes Mellitus. *Diabetes Care* 26(Suppl 1):S5, 2003.
7. World Health Organization: *Definition, diagnosis and classification of diabetes mellitus and its complications: report of a WHO Consultation. Part 1. Diagnosis and classification of diabetes mellitus*, Geneva, 1999, World Health Organization.
8. The Expert Committee on the Diagnosis and Classification of Diabetes Mellitus: Report of the Expert Committee on the Diagnosis and Classification of Diabetes Mellitus. *Diabetes Care* 20:1183, 1997.
9. World Health Organization: *Diabetes mellitus: report of a WHO study group*, Geneva, 1985, World Health Organization. Tech. Rep. Ser. 727.
10. World Health Organization: *Second report of the expert committee on diabetes mellitus*, Geneva, 1980, World Health Organization. Tech. Rep. Ser. 646.
11. National Diabetes Data Group: Classification and diagnosis of diabetes mellitus and other categories of glucose intolerance. *Diabetes* 28:1039, 1979.

12. American Diabetes Association: Standards of medical care in diabetes 2009. *Diabetes Care* 32:S13, 2009.

13. World Health Organization: *Definition and diagnosis of diabetes mellitus and intermediate hyperglycemia: report of a WHO/IDF consultation*, Geneva, Switzerland, 2006, WHO Document Production Services.

14. Gu D, Reynolds K, Duan X, et al: Prevalence of diabetes and impaired fasting glucose in the Chinese adult population: International Collaborative Study of Cardiovascular Disease in Asia (InterASIA). *Diabetologia* 46:1190, 2003.

15. National Diabetes Information Clearinghouse, National Institute of Diabetes and Digestive and Kidney Diseases, National Institutes of Health: *National diabetes statistics, 2007*, Bethesda, Md, 2008, U.S. Department of Health and Human Services, National Institutes of Health. NIH publication 08-3892.

16. Boyle JP, Honeycutt AA, Narayan KM, et al: Projection of diabetes burden through 2050: impact of changing demography and disease prevalence in the U.S.. *Diabetes Care* 24:1936, 2001.

17. National Diabetes Data Group: *Diabetes in America*, ed 2, Bethesda, Md, 1995, National Institutes of Health, National Institute of Diabetes and Digestive and Kidney Diseases. NIH publication 95-1468.

18. The Coronary Drug Project Investigators: Clofibrate and niacin in coronary heart disease. *JAMA* 231:360, 1975.

19. Cowie CC, Rust KF, Byrd-Holt DD, et al: Prevalence of diabetes and impaired fasting glucose in adults in the U.S. population: National Health and Nutrition Examination Survey 1999-2002. *Diabetes Care* 29:1263, 2006.

20. Carter J, Horowitz R, Wilson R, et al: Tribal differences in diabetes: prevalence among American Indians in New Mexico. *Public Health Rep* 104:665, 1989.

21. Knowler WC, Bennett PH, Hamman RF, et al: Diabetes incidence and prevalence in Pima Indians: a 19-fold greater incidence than in Rochester, Minnesota. *Am J Epidemiol* 108:497, 1978.

22. Drewnowski A: Obesity, diets, and social inequalities. *Nutr Rev* 67(Suppl 1):S36, 2009.

23. Mohan V, Shanthirani S, Deepa R, et al: Intra-urban differences in the prevalence of the metabolic syndrome in southern India—the Chennai Urban Population Study (CUPS No. 4). *Diabet Med* 18:280, 2001.

24. Dabelea D, Bell RA, D'Agostino RB, Jr, et al: Incidence of diabetes in youth in the United States. *JAMA* 297:2716, 2007.

25. Rosenbloom AL, Joe JR, Young RS, et al: Emerging epidemic of type 2 diabetes in youth. *Diabetes Care* 22:345, 1999.

26. World Health Organization: *Obesity and overweight, fact sheet N° 311*, 2006.

27. van Dam RM, Rimm EB, Willett WC, et al: Dietary patterns and risk for type 2 diabetes mellitus in U.S. men. *Ann Intern Med* 136:201, 2002.

28. Brownson RC, Boehmer TK, Luke DA: Declining rates of physical activity in the United States: what are the contributors? *Annu Rev Public Health* 26:421, 2005.

29. Hu FB, Sigal RJ, Rich-Edwards JW, et al: Walking compared with vigorous physical activity and risk of type 2 diabetes in women: a prospective study. *JAMA* 282:1433, 1999.

30. Fretts AM, Howard BV, Kriska AM, et al: Physical activity and incident diabetes in American Indians: the Strong Heart Study. *Am J Epidemiol* 170:632, 2009.

31. Butler RN: Population aging and health. *BMJ* 315:1082, 1997.

32. Karvonen M, Viik-Kajander M, Moltchanova E, et al: Incidence of childhood type 1 diabetes worldwide. Diabetes Mondiale (DiaMond) Project Group. *Diabetes Care* 23:1516, 2000.

33. American Diabetes Association: Economic costs of diabetes in the U.S. in 2007. *Diabetes Care* 31:596, 2008.

34. Preis SR, Hwang SJ, Coady S, et al: Trends in all-cause and cardiovascular disease mortality among women and men with and without diabetes mellitus in the Framingham Heart Study, 1950 to 2005. *Circulation* 119:1728, 2009.

35. Beckman JA, Creager MA, Libby P: Diabetes and atherosclerosis: epidemiology, pathophysiology, and management. *JAMA* 287:2570, 2002.

36. Haffner SM, Lehto S, Ronnemaa T, et al: Mortality from coronary heart disease in subjects with type 2 diabetes and in nondiabetic subjects with and without prior myocardial infarction. *N Engl J Med* 339:229, 1998.

37. The Action to Control Cardiovascular Risk in Diabetes Study Group: Effects of intensive glucose lowering in type 2 diabetes. *N Engl J Med* 358:2545, 2008.

38. Duckworth W, Abraira C, Moritz T, et al: Glucose control and vascular complications in veterans with type 2 diabetes. *N Engl J Med* 360:129, 2009.

39. Holman RR, Paul SK, Bethel MA, et al: 10-year follow-up of intensive glucose control in type 2 diabetes. *N Engl J Med* 359:1577, 2008.

40. Patel A, MacMahon S, Chalmers J, et al: Intensive blood glucose control and vascular outcomes in patients with type 2 diabetes. *N Engl J Med* 358:2560, 2008.

41. Laing SP, Swerdlow AJ, Slater SD, et al: Mortality from heart disease in a cohort of 23,000 patients with insulin-treated diabetes. *Diabetologia* 46:760, 2003.

42. Pambianco G, Costacou T, Ellis D, et al: The 30-year natural history of type 1 diabetes complications: the Pittsburgh Epidemiology of Diabetes Complications Study experience. *Diabetes* 55:1463, 2006.

43. Burchfiel CM, Curb JD, Rodriguez BL, et al: Glucose intolerance and 22-year stroke incidence. The Honolulu Heart Program. *Stroke* 25:951, 1994.

44. Most RS, Sinnock P: The epidemiology of lower extremity amputations in diabetic individuals. *Diabetes Care* 6:87, 1983.

45. Laing SP, Swerdlow AJ, Carpenter LM, et al: Mortality from cerebrovascular disease in a cohort of 23,000 patients with insulin-treated diabetes. *Stroke* 34:418, 2003.

46. Geiss LS, Rolka DB, Engelgau MM: Elevated blood pressure among U.S. adults with diabetes, 1988-1994. *Am J Prev Med* 22:42, 2002.

47. Adler AI, Stratton IM, Neil HA, et al: Association of systolic blood pressure with macrovascular and microvascular complications of type 2 diabetes (UKPDS 36): prospective observational study. *BMJ* 321:412, 2000.

48. Ravera M, Re M, Deferrari L, et al: Importance of blood pressure control in chronic kidney disease. *J Am Soc Nephrol* 17:S98, 2006.

49. Weiner DE, Tabatabai S, Tighiouart H, et al: Cardiovascular outcomes and all-cause mortality: exploring the interaction between CKD and cardiovascular disease. *Am J Kidney Dis* 48:392, 2006.

50. Baliga V, Sapsford R: Diabetes mellitus and heart failure—an overview of epidemiology and management. *Diab Vasc Dis Res* 6:164, 2009.

51. McGuire DK, Emanuelsson H, Granger CB, et al: Influence of diabetes mellitus on clinical outcomes across the spectrum of acute coronary syndromes. Findings from the GUSTO-IIb study. GUSTO IIb Investigators. *Eur Heart J* 21:1750, 2000.

52. Stone PH, Muller JE, Hartwell T, et al: The effect of diabetes mellitus on prognosis and serial left ventricular function after acute myocardial infarction: contribution of both coronary disease and diastolic left ventricular dysfunction to the adverse prognosis. The MILIS Study Group. *J Am Coll Cardiol* 14:49, 1989.

53. Saunders J, Mathewkutty S, Drazner MH, et al: Cardiomyopathy in type 2 diabetes: update on pathophysiological mechanisms. *Herz* 33:184, 2008.

54. Sowers JR: Diabetes mellitus and cardiovascular disease in women. *Arch Intern Med* 158:617, 1998.

55. Karter AJ, Ferrara A, Liu JY, et al: Ethnic disparities in diabetic complications in an insured population. *JAMA* 287:2519, 2002.

56. Nelson RG, Sievers ML, Knowler WC, et al: Low incidence of fatal coronary heart disease in Pima Indians despite high prevalence of non–insulin-dependent diabetes. *Circulation* 81:987, 1990.

57. Creager MA, Luscher TF, Cosentino F, et al: Diabetes and vascular disease: pathophysiology, clinical consequences, and medical therapy: part I. *Circulation* 108:1527, 2003.

58. Orasanu G, Plutzky J: The pathologic continuum of diabetic vascular disease. *J Am Coll Cardiol* 53:S35, 2009.

59. Goldin A, Beckman JA, Schmidt AM, et al: Advanced glycation end products: sparking the development of diabetic vascular injury. *Circulation* 114:597, 2006.

60. Natarajan A, Zaman AG, Marshall SM: Platelet hyperactivity in type 2 diabetes: role of antiplatelet agents. *Diab Vasc Dis Res* 5:138, 2008.

61. Mathewkutty S, McGuire DK: Platelet perturbations in diabetes: implications for cardiovascular disease risk and treatment. *Expert Rev Cardiovasc Ther* 7:541, 2009.

62. Adiels M, Olofsson SO, Taskinen MR, et al: Diabetic dyslipidaemia. *Curr Opin Lipidol* 17:238, 2006.

63. Carmena R, Duriez P, Fruchart JC: Atherogenic lipoprotein particles in atherosclerosis. *Circulation* 109:III2, 2004.

64. Garg A, Grundy SM: Diabetic dyslipidemia and its therapy. *Diabetes Rev* 5:425, 1997.

65. Barter PJ, Nicholls S, Rye KA, et al: Antiinflammatory properties of HDL. *Circ Res* 95:764, 2004.

66. Alberti KG, Zimmet P, Shaw J: International Diabetes Federation: a consensus on type 2 diabetes prevention. *Diabet Med* 24:451, 2007.

67. Tuomilehto J, Lindstrom J, Eriksson JG, et al: Prevention of type 2 diabetes mellitus by changes in lifestyle among subjects with impaired glucose tolerance. *N Engl J Med* 344:1343, 2001.

68. Lindstrom J, Ilanne-Parikka P, Peltonen M, et al: Sustained reduction in the incidence of type 2 diabetes by lifestyle intervention: follow-up of the Finnish Diabetes Prevention Study. *Lancet* 368:1673, 2006.

69. Knowler WC, Barrett-Connor E, Fowler SE, et al: Reduction in the incidence of type 2 diabetes with lifestyle intervention or metformin. *N Engl J Med* 346:393, 2002.

70. Ramachandran A, Snehalatha C, Mary S, et al: The Indian Diabetes Prevention Programme shows that lifestyle modification and metformin prevent type 2 diabetes in Asian Indian subjects with impaired glucose tolerance (IDPP-1). *Diabetologia* 49:289, 2006.

71. Kosaka K, Noda M, Kuzuya T: Prevention of type 2 diabetes by lifestyle intervention: a Japanese trial in IGT males. *Diabetes Res Clin Pract* 67:152, 2005.

72. Li G, Zhang P, Wang J, et al: The long-term effect of lifestyle interventions to prevent diabetes in the China Da Qing Diabetes Prevention Study: a 20-year follow-up study. *Lancet* 371:1783, 2008.

73. Pan XR, Li GW, Hu YH, et al: Effects of diet and exercise in preventing NIDDM in people with impaired glucose tolerance. The Da Qing IGT and Diabetes Study. *Diabetes Care* 20:537, 1997.

74. Bantle JP, Wylie-Rosett J, Albright AL, et al: Nutrition recommendations and interventions for diabetes: a position statement of the American Diabetes Association. *Diabetes Care* 31(Suppl 1):S61, 2008.

75. Roumen C, Blaak EE, Corpeleijn E: Lifestyle intervention for prevention of diabetes: determinants of success for future implementation. *Nutr Rev* 67:132, 2009.

76. Franz MJ, Bantle JP, Beebe CA, et al: Evidence-based nutrition principles and recommendations for the treatment and prevention of diabetes and related complications. *Diabetes Care* 25:148, 2002.

77. Perseghin G, Price TB, Petersen KF, et al: Increased glucose transport-phosphorylation and muscle glycogen synthesis after exercise training in insulin-resistant subjects. *N Engl J Med* 335:1357, 1996.

78. Manson JE, Nathan DM, Krolewski AS, et al: A prospective study of exercise and incidence of diabetes among US male physicians. *JAMA* 268:63, 1992.

79. Perry IJ, Wannamethee SG, Walker MK, et al: Prospective study of risk factors for development of non–insulin dependent diabetes in middle aged British men. *BMJ* 310:560, 1995.

80. American Diabetes Association: Diabetes mellitus and exercise. *Diabetes Care* 23(Suppl 1):S50, 2000.

81. Torgerson JS, Hauptman J, Boldrin MN, et al: XENical in the prevention of diabetes in obese subjects (XENDOS) study: a randomized study of orlistat as an adjunct to lifestyle changes for the prevention of type 2 diabetes in obese patients. *Diabetes Care* 27:155, 2004.

82. Vetter ML, Cardillo S, Rickels MR, et al: Narrative review: effect of bariatric surgery on type 2 diabetes mellitus. *Ann Intern Med* 150:94, 2009.

83. Sjostrom L, Lindroos AK, Peltonen M, et al: Lifestyle, diabetes, and cardiovascular risk factors 10 years after bariatric surgery. *N Engl J Med* 351:2683, 2004.

84. Adams TD, Gress RE, Smith SC, et al: Long-term mortality after gastric bypass surgery. *N Engl J Med* 357:753, 2007.

85. Sjostrom L, Narbro K, Sjostrom CD, et al: Effects of bariatric surgery on mortality in Swedish obese subjects. *N Engl J Med* 357:741, 2007.

86. The Diabetes Prevention Program Research Group: Effects of withdrawal from metformin on the development of diabetes in the diabetes prevention program. *Diabetes Care* 26:977, 2003.

87. Chiasson JL, Josse RG, Gomis R, et al: Acarbose for prevention of type 2 diabetes mellitus: the STOP-NIDDM randomised trial. *Lancet* 359:2072, 2002.

88. Kawamori R, Tajima N, Iwamoto Y, et al: Voglibose for prevention of type 2 diabetes mellitus: a randomised, double-blind trial in Japanese individuals with impaired glucose tolerance. *Lancet* 373:1607, 2009.

89. Bassler D, Montori VM, Briel M, et al: Early stopping of randomized clinical trials for overt efficacy is problematic. *J Clin Epidemiol* 61:2416, 2008.

90. Buchanan TA, Xiang AH, Peters RK, et al: Preservation of pancreatic beta-cell function and prevention of type 2 diabetes by pharmacological treatment of insulin resistance in high-risk Hispanic women. *Diabetes* 51:2796, 2002.

91. Gerstein HC, Yusuf S, Bosch J, et al: Effect of rosiglitazone on the frequency of diabetes in patients with impaired glucose tolerance or impaired fasting glucose: a randomised controlled trial. *Lancet* 368:1096, 2006.

92. Knowler WC, Hamman RF, Edelstein SL, et al: Prevention of type 2 diabetes with troglitazone in the Diabetes Prevention Program. *Diabetes* 54:1150, 2005.

93. Rohatgi A, McGuire DK: Effects of the thiazolidinedione medications on micro- and macrovascular complications in patients with diabetes—update 2008. *Cardiovasc Drugs Ther* 22:233, 2008.

94. The DECODE study group: Glucose tolerance and mortality: comparison of WHO and American Diabetes Association diagnostic criteria. *Lancet* 354:617, 1999.

95. Saydah SH, Loria CM, Eberhardt MS, et al: Subclinical states of glucose intolerance and risk of death in the U.S. *Diabetes Care* 24:447, 2001.

96. Levitan EB, Song Y, Ford ES, et al: Is nondiabetic hyperglycemia a risk factor for cardiovascular disease? A meta-analysis of prospective studies. *Arch Intern Med* 164:2147, 2004.

97. Selvin E, Marinopoulos S, Berkenblit G, et al: Meta-analysis: glycosylated hemoglobin and cardiovascular disease in diabetes mellitus. *Ann Intern Med* 141:421, 2004.

98. Saydah S, Tao M, Imperatore G, et al: GHb level and subsequent mortality among adults in the U.S. *Diabetes Care* 32:1440, 2009.

99. Stratton IM, Adler AI, Neil HA, et al: Association of glycaemia with macrovascular and microvascular complications of type 2 diabetes (UKPDS 35): prospective observational study. *BMJ* 321:405, 2000.

100. UK Prospective Diabetes Study (UKPDS) Group: Effect of intensive blood-glucose control with metformin on complications in overweight patients with type 2 diabetes (UKPDS 34). *Lancet* 352:854, 1998.

101. UK Prospective Diabetes Study (UKPDS) Group: Intensive blood-glucose control with sulphonylureas or insulin compared with conventional treatment and risk of complications in patients with type 2 diabetes (UKPDS 33). *Lancet* 352:837, 1998.

102. Misbin RI: The phantom of lactic acidosis due to metformin in patients with diabetes. *Diabetes Care* 27:1791, 2004.

103. Dormandy JA, Charbonnel B, Eckland DJ, et al: Secondary prevention of macrovascular events in patients with type 2 diabetes in the PROactive Study (PROspective pioglitAzone Clinical Trial In macroVascular Events): a randomised controlled trial. *Lancet* 366:1279, 2005.

104. Goldberg RB, Kendall DM, Deeg MA, et al: A comparison of lipid and glycemic effects of pioglitazone and rosiglitazone in patients with type 2 diabetes and dyslipidemia. *Diabetes Care* 28:1547, 2005.

105. McGuire DK, Inzucchi SE: New drugs for the treatment of diabetes mellitus: part I: thiazolidinediones and their evolving cardiovascular implications. *Circulation* 117:440, 2008.

106. Juurlink DN, Gomes T, Lipscombe LL, et al: Adverse cardiovascular events during treatment with pioglitazone and rosiglitazone: population based cohort study. *BMJ* 339:b2942, 2009.

107. Lago RM, Singh PP, Nesto RW: Congestive heart failure and cardiovascular death in patients with prediabetes and type 2 diabetes given thiazolidinediones: a meta-analysis of randomised clinical trials. *Lancet* 370:1129, 2007.

108. Inzucchi SE, McGuire DK: New drugs for the treatment of diabetes: part II: incretin-based therapy and beyond. *Circulation* 117:574, 2008.

109. Gore MO, McGuire DK: Cardiovascular disease and type 2 diabetes mellitus: regulating glucose and regulating drugs. *Curr Cardiol Rep* 11:258, 2009.

110. U.S. Food and Drug Administration: Guidance for industry: diabetes mellitus—evaluating cardiovascular risk in new antidiabetic therapies to treat type 2 diabetes. Available at: www.fda.gov/downloads/Drugs/GuidanceComplianceRegulatoryInformation/Guidances/ucm071627.pdf. Accessed August 3, 2009.

110a. Riddle MC, Ambrosius WT, Brillon DJ, et al: Epidemiologic relationships between A1c and all-cause mortality during a median 3.4-year follow-up of glycemic treatment in the ACCORD trial. *Diabetes Care* 33:983, 2010.

111. Skyler JS, Bergenstal R, Bonow RO, et al: Intensive glycemic control and the prevention of cardiovascular events: implications of the ACCORD, ADVANCE, and VA Diabetes Trials: a position statement of the American Diabetes Association and a Scientific Statement of the American College of Cardiology Foundation and the American Heart Association. *J Am Coll Cardiol* 53:298, 2009.

112. Mazzone T, Meyer PM, Feinstein SB, et al: Effect of pioglitazone compared with glimepiride on carotid intima-media thickness in type 2 diabetes: a randomized trial. *JAMA* 296:2572, 2006.

113. Nissen SE, Nicholls SJ, Wolski K, et al: Comparison of pioglitazone vs glimepiride on progression of coronary atherosclerosis in patients with type 2 diabetes: the PERISCOPE randomized controlled trial. *JAMA* 299:1561, 2008.

114. Nissen SE, Wolski K: Effect of rosiglitazone on the risk of myocardial infarction and death from cardiovascular causes. *N Engl J Med* 356:2457, 2007.

115. Home PD, Pocock SJ, Beck-Nielsen H, et al: Rosiglitazone evaluated for cardiovascular outcomes in oral agent combination therapy for type 2 diabetes (RECORD): a multicentre, randomised, open-label trial. *Lancet* 373:2125, 2009.

116. Frye RL, August P, Brooks MM, et al: A randomized trial of therapies for type 2 diabetes and coronary artery disease. *N Engl J Med* 360:2503, 2009.

117. Nathan DM, Buse JB, Davidson MB, et al: Medical management of hyperglycemia in type 2 diabetes: a consensus algorithm for the initiation and adjustment of therapy: a consensus statement of the American Diabetes Association and the European Association for the Study of Diabetes. *Diabetes Care* 32:193, 2009.

118. Lebovitz HE, Austin MM, Blonde L, et al: ACE/AACE consensus conference on the implementation of outpatient management of diabetes mellitus: consensus conference recommendations. *Endocr Pract* 12(Suppl 1):6, 2006.

119. The Diabetes Control and Complications Trial Research Group: The effect of intensive treatment of diabetes on the development and progression of long-term complications in insulin-dependent diabetes mellitus. *N Engl J Med* 329:977, 1993.

120. The Diabetes Control and Complications Trial/Epidemiology of Diabetes Interventions and Complications (DCCT/EDIC) Study Research Group: Intensive diabetes treatment and cardiovascular disease in patients with type 1 diabetes. *N Engl J Med* 353:2643, 2005.

121. Nathan DM, Cleary PA, Backlund JY, et al: Intensive diabetes treatment and cardiovascular disease in patients with type 1 diabetes. *N Engl J Med* 353:2643, 2005.

122. Lavie CJ, Milani RV, Ventura HO: Obesity and cardiovascular disease: risk factor, paradox, and impact of weight loss. *J Am Coll Cardiol* 53:1925, 2009.

123. Pi-Sunyer X, Blackburn G, Brancati FL, et al: Reduction in weight and cardiovascular disease risk factors in individuals with type 2 diabetes: one-year results of the Look AHEAD trial. *Diabetes Care* 30:1374, 2007.

124. Sigal RJ, Kenny GP, Wasserman DH, et al: Physical activity/exercise and type 2 diabetes: a consensus statement from the American Diabetes Association. *Diabetes Care* 29:1433, 2006.

125. Haire-Joshu D, Glasgow RE, Tibbs TL: Smoking and diabetes. *Diabetes Care* 22:1887, 1999.

126. Turnbull F, Neal B, Algert C, et al: Effects of different blood pressure–lowering regimens on major cardiovascular events in individuals with and without diabetes mellitus: results of prospectively designed overviews of randomized trials. *Arch Intern Med* 165:1410, 2005.

127. The ALLHAT Officers and Coordinators for the ALLHAT Collaborative Research Group: Major outcomes in high-risk hypertensive patients randomized to angiotensin-converting enzyme inhibitor or calcium channel blocker vs diuretic: the Antihypertensive and Lipid-Lowering Treatment to Prevent Heart Attack Trial (ALLHAT). *JAMA* 288:2981, 2002.

128. Fox KM: Efficacy of perindopril in reduction of cardiovascular events among patients with stable coronary artery disease: randomised, double-blind, placebo-controlled, multicentre trial (the EUROPA study). *Lancet* 362:782, 2003.

129. Heart Outcomes Prevention Evaluation Study Investigators: Effects of ramipril on cardiovascular and microvascular outcomes in people with diabetes mellitus: results of the HOPE study and MICRO-HOPE substudy. *Lancet* 355:253, 2000.

130. Patel A, MacMahon S, Chalmers J, et al: Effects of a fixed combination of perindopril and indapamide on macrovascular and microvascular outcomes in patients with type 2 diabetes mellitus (the ADVANCE trial): a randomised controlled trial. *Lancet* 370:829, 2007.

131. UK Prospective Diabetes Study (UKPDS) Group: Tight blood pressure control and risk of macrovascular and microvascular complications in type 2 diabetes: UKPDS 38. *BMJ* 317:703, 1998.

132. Yusuf S, Sleight P, Pogue J, et al: Effects of an angiotensin-converting-enzyme inhibitor, ramipril, on cardiovascular events in high-risk patients. The Heart Outcomes Prevention Evaluation Study Investigators. *N Engl J Med* 342:145, 2000.

133. Buse JB, Ginsberg HN, Bakris GL, et al: Primary prevention of cardiovascular diseases in people with diabetes mellitus: a scientific statement from the American Heart Association and the American Diabetes Association. *Circulation* 115:114, 2007.

134. National Kidney Foundation: KDOQI Clinical Practice Guidelines and Clinical Practice Recommendations for Diabetes and Chronic Kidney Disease. *Am J Kidney Dis* 49:S12, 2007.

135. Brenner BM, Cooper ME, de Zeeuw D, et al: Effects of losartan on renal and cardiovascular outcomes in patients with type 2 diabetes and nephropathy. *N Engl J Med* 345:861, 2001.

136. Lewis EJ, Hunsicker LG, Clarke WR, et al: Renoprotective effect of the angiotensin-receptor antagonist irbesartan in patients with nephropathy due to type 2 diabetes. *N Engl J Med* 345:851, 2001.

137. Yusuf S, Teo KK, Pogue J, et al: Telmisartan, ramipril, or both in patients at high risk for vascular events. *N Engl J Med* 358:1547, 2008.

138. Jamerson K, Weber MA, Bakris GL, et al: Benazepril plus amlodipine or hydrochlorothiazide for hypertension in high-risk patients. *N Engl J Med* 359:2417, 2008.

139. Tatti P, Pahor M, Byington RP, et al: Outcome results of the Fosinopril Versus Amlodipine Cardiovascular Events Randomized Trial (FACET) in patients with hypertension and NIDDM. *Diabetes Care* 21:597, 1998.

140. Estacio RO, Jeffers BW, Hiatt WR, et al: The effect of nisoldipine as compared with enalapril on cardiovascular outcomes in patients with non–insulin-dependent diabetes and hypertension. *N Engl J Med* 338:645, 1998.

141. Barzilay JI, Davis BR, Cutler JA, et al: Fasting glucose levels and incident diabetes mellitus in older nondiabetic adults randomized to receive 3 different classes of antihypertensive treatment: a report from the Antihypertensive and Lipid-Lowering Treatment to Prevent Heart Attack Trial (ALLHAT). *Arch Intern Med* 166:2191, 2006.

142. Curb JD, Pressel SL, Cutler JA, et al: Effect of diuretic-based antihypertensive treatment on cardiovascular disease risk in older diabetic patients with isolated systolic hypertension. Systolic Hypertension in the Elderly Program Cooperative Research Group. *JAMA* 276:1886, 1996.

143. Bangalore S, Parkar S, Grossman E, et al: A meta-analysis of 94,492 patients with hypertension treated with beta blockers to determine the risk of new-onset diabetes mellitus. *Am J Cardiol* 100:1254, 2007.

144. Bakris GL, Fonseca V, Katholi RE, et al: Metabolic effects of carvedilol vs metoprolol in patients with type 2 diabetes mellitus and hypertension: a randomized controlled trial. *JAMA* 292:2227, 2004.

145. Giugliano D, Acampora R, Marfella R, et al: Metabolic and cardiovascular effects of carvedilol and atenolol in non–insulin-dependent diabetes mellitus and hypertension. A randomized, controlled trial. *Ann Intern Med* 126:955, 1997.

146. Chobanian AV, Bakris GL, Black HR, et al: The Seventh Report of the Joint National Committee on Prevention, Detection, Evaluation, and Treatment of High Blood Pressure: the JNC 7 report. *JAMA* 289:2560, 2003.

147. Hansson L, Zanchetti A, Carruthers SG, et al: Effects of intensive blood-pressure lowering and low-dose aspirin in patients with hypertension: principal results of the Hypertension Optimal Treatment (HOT) randomised trial. HOT Study Group. *Lancet* 351:1755, 1998.

147a. Cushman WC, Evans GW, Byington RP, et al: Effects of intensive blood-pressure control in type 2 diabetes mellitus. *N Engl J Med* 362(17):1575, 2010.

148. McGuire DK, Winterfield JR, Rytlewski JA, et al: Blocking the renin-angiotensin-aldosterone system to prevent diabetes mellitus. *Diab Vasc Dis Res* 5:59, 2008.

149. Gardner CD, Fortmann SP, Krauss RM: Association of small low-density lipoprotein particles with the incidence of coronary artery disease in men and women. *JAMA* 276:875, 1996.

150. Lamarche B, Tchernof A, Moorjani S, et al: Small, dense low-density lipoprotein particles as a predictor of the risk of ischemic heart disease in men. Prospective results from the Quebec Cardiovascular Study. *Circulation* 95:69, 1997.

151. Sattar N, Petrie JR, Jaap AJ: The atherogenic lipoprotein phenotype and vascular endothelial dysfunction. *Atherosclerosis* 138:229, 1998.

152. Colhoun HM, Betteridge DJ, Durrington PN, et al: Primary prevention of cardiovascular disease with atorvastatin in type 2 diabetes in the Collaborative Atorvastatin Diabetes Study (CARDS): multicentre randomised placebo-controlled trial. *Lancet* 364:685, 2004.

153. Collins R, Armitage J, Parish S, et al: MRC/BHF Heart Protection Study of cholesterol-lowering with simvastatin in 5963 people with diabetes: a randomised placebo-controlled trial. *Lancet* 361:2005, 2003.

154. Kearney PM, Blackwell L, Collins R, et al: Efficacy of cholesterol-lowering therapy in 18,686 people with diabetes in 14 randomised trials of statins: a meta-analysis. *Lancet* 371:117, 2008.

155. Grundy SM, Cleeman JI, Merz CN, et al: Implications of recent clinical trials for the National Cholesterol Education Program Adult Treatment Panel III guidelines. *Circulation* 110:227, 2004.

156. Montori VM, Farmer A, Wollan PC, et al: Fish oil supplementation in type 2 diabetes: a quantitative systematic review. *Diabetes Care* 23:1407, 2000.

157. Gruppo Italiano per lo Studio della Sopravvivenza nell'Infarto Miocardico: Dietary supplementation with n-3 polyunsaturated fatty acids and vitamin E after myocardial infarction: results of the GISSI-Prevenzione trial. *Lancet* 354:447, 1999.

158. Yokoyama M, Origasa H, Matsuzaki M, et al: Effects of eicosapentaenoic acid on major coronary events in hypercholesterolaemic patients (JELIS): a randomised open-label, blinded endpoint analysis. *Lancet* 369:1090, 2007.

159. Oikawa S, Yokoyama M, Origasa H, et al: Suppressive effect of EPA on the incidence of coronary events in hypercholesterolemia with impaired glucose metabolism: subanalysis of the Japan EPA Lipid Intervention Study (JELIS). *Atherosclerosis* 206:535, 2009.

160. Staels B, Dallongeville J, Auwerx J, et al: Mechanism of action of fibrates on lipid and lipoprotein metabolism. *Circulation* 98:2088, 1998.

161. Rubins HB, Robins SJ, Collins D, et al: Gemfibrozil for the secondary prevention of coronary heart disease in men with low levels of high-density lipoprotein cholesterol. Veterans Affairs High-Density Lipoprotein Cholesterol Intervention Trial Study Group. *N Engl J Med* 341:410, 1999.

162. Rubins HB, Robins SJ, Collins D, et al: Diabetes, plasma insulin, and cardiovascular disease: subgroup analysis from the Department of Veterans Affairs high-density lipoprotein intervention trial (VA-HIT). *Arch Intern Med* 162:2597, 2002.

163. The Bezafibrate Infarction Prevention (BIP) study group: Secondary prevention by raising HDL cholesterol and reducing triglycerides in patients with coronary artery disease: the Bezafibrate Infarction Prevention (BIP) study. *Circulation* 102:21, 2000.

164. Tenenbaum A, Motro M, Fisman EZ, et al: Bezafibrate for the secondary prevention of myocardial infarction in patients with metabolic syndrome. *Arch Intern Med* 165:1154, 2005.

164a. Ginsberg HN, Elam MB, Lovato LC, et al: Effects of combination lipid therapy in type 2 diabetes mellitus. *N Engl J Med* 362:1563, 2010.

165. Keech A, Simes RJ, Barter P, et al: Effects of long-term fenofibrate therapy on cardiovascular events in 9795 people with type 2 diabetes mellitus (the FIELD study): randomised controlled trial. *Lancet* 366:1849, 2005.

166. Pan J, Lin M, Kesala RL, et al: Niacin treatment of the atherogenic lipid profile and Lp(a) in diabetes. *Diabetes Obes Metab* 4:255, 2002.

167. Canner PL, Furberg CD, Terrin ML, et al: Benefits of niacin by glycemic status in patients with healed myocardial infarction (from the Coronary Drug Project). *Am J Cardiol* 95:254, 2005.

168. Brown BG, Zhao XQ, Chait A, et al: Simvastatin and niacin, antioxidant vitamins, or the combination for the prevention of coronary disease. *N Engl J Med* 345:1583, 2001.

169. Snow V, Aronson MD, Hornbake ER, et al: Lipid control in the management of type 2 diabetes mellitus: a clinical practice guideline from the American College of Physicians. *Ann Intern Med* 140:644, 2004.

170. Juhan-Vague I, Alessi MC, Mavri A, et al: Plasminogen activator inhibitor-1, inflammation, obesity, insulin resistance and vascular risk. *J Thromb Haemost* 1:1575, 2003.

171. Antithrombotic Trialists' Collaboration: Collaborative meta-analysis of randomised trials of antiplatelet therapy for prevention of death, myocardial infarction, and stroke in high risk patients. *BMJ* 324:71, 2002.

172. Baigent C, Blackwell L, Collins R, et al: Aspirin in the primary and secondary prevention of vascular disease: collaborative meta-analysis of individual participant data from randomised trials. *Lancet* 373:1849, 2009.

173. Sacco M, Pellegrini F, Roncaglioni MC, et al: Primary prevention of cardiovascular events with low-dose aspirin and vitamin E in type 2 diabetic patients: results of the Primary Prevention Project (PPP) trial. *Diabetes Care* 26:3264, 2003.

174. Belch J, MacCuish A, Campbell I, et al: The prevention of progression of arterial disease and diabetes (POPADAD) trial: factorial randomised placebo controlled trial of aspirin and antioxidants in patients with diabetes and asymptomatic peripheral arterial disease. *BMJ* 337:a1840, 2008.

175. Ogawa H, Nakayama M, Morimoto T, et al: Low-dose aspirin for primary prevention of atherosclerotic events in patients with type 2 diabetes: a randomized controlled trial. *JAMA* 300:2134, 2008.

176. De Berardis G, Sacco M, Evangelista V, et al: Aspirin and Simvastatin Combination for Cardiovascular Events Prevention Trial in Diabetes (ACCEPT-D): design of a randomized study of the efficacy of low-dose aspirin in the prevention of cardiovascular events in subjects with diabetes mellitus treated with statins. *Trials* 8:21, 2007.

177. Colwell JA: Aspirin therapy in diabetes. *Diabetes Care* 27(Suppl 1):S72, 2004.

178. Smith SC, Jr, Allen J, Blair SN, et al: AHA/ACC guidelines for secondary prevention for patients with coronary and other atherosclerotic vascular disease: 2006 update: endorsed by the National Heart, Lung, and Blood Institute. *Circulation* 113:2363, 2006.

179. ETDRS Investigators: Aspirin effects on mortality and morbidity in patients with diabetes mellitus. Early Treatment Diabetic Retinopathy Study report 14. *JAMA* 268:1292, 1992.

180. Roffi M, Chew DP, Mukherjee D, et al: Platelet glycoprotein IIb/IIIa inhibitors reduce mortality in diabetic patients with non-ST-segment-elevation acute coronary syndromes. *Circulation* 104:2767, 2001.

181. Bhatt DL, Marso SP, Hirsch AT, et al: Amplified benefit of clopidogrel versus aspirin in patients with diabetes mellitus. *Am J Cardiol* 90:625, 2002.

182. Wiviott SD, Braunwald E, Angiolillo DJ, et al: Greater clinical benefit of more intensive oral antiplatelet therapy with prasugrel in patients with diabetes mellitus in the trial to assess improvement in therapeutic outcomes by optimizing platelet inhibition with prasugrel—Thrombolysis in Myocardial Infarction 38. *Circulation* 118:1626, 2008.

183. Ryden L, Standl E, Bartnik M, et al: Guidelines on diabetes, pre-diabetes, and cardiovascular diseases: executive summary. The Task Force on Diabetes and Cardiovascular Diseases of the European Society of Cardiology (ESC) and of the European Association for the Study of Diabetes (EASD). *Eur Heart J* 28:88, 2007.

CHAPTER 22

Metabolic Syndrome and Cardiovascular Disease

Shaista Malik and Nathan D. Wong

KEY POINTS

- The metabolic syndrome is a constellation of risk factors that even in the absence of diabetes precedes development of cardiovascular disease.

- Visceral obesity and ensuing insulin resistance have been proposed as central features of the pathophysiology of metabolic syndrome.

- The definitions of metabolic syndrome have evolved over time and include visceral obesity, dyslipidemia, hypertension, and hyperglycemia.

- The prevalence of metabolic syndrome is approximately 34% among U.S. adults and is growing.

- Initial evaluation of coronary heart disease risk in metabolic syndrome subjects without diabetes involves global risk estimation by Framingham or other algorithms for risk prediction.

- Novel risk factors such as high-sensitivity C-reactive protein as well as subclinical atherosclerosis (from carotid ultrasound, computed tomography, or ankle-brachial index) can refine the estimation of cardiovascular disease risk.

- The treatment of metabolic syndrome centers around lifestyle modification, supplemented with appropriate pharmacologic management, when indicated, for dyslipidemia, hypertension, and hyperglycemia.

The metabolic syndrome is a clustering of risk factors including visceral obesity, dyslipidemia, hypertension, and hyperglycemia, each an important risk factor for development of diabetes and cardiovascular disease (CVD). The constellation of these risk factors was initially described by Reaven as syndrome X and included insulin resistance, hyperglycemia, hypertension, low high-density lipoprotein cholesterol (HDL-C), and high very-low-density lipoprotein triglycerides.[1] Cross-sectional surveys indicate that in the United States, one third of adults and an alarming proportion of youth have the metabolic syndrome.[2,3]

Although there have been advances in understanding of the pathophysiology, epidemiology, and prognostic implications of the metabolic syndrome and treatment strategies for it, uncertainties persist about whether metabolic syndrome has utility beyond its individual components. Focus on the metabolic syndrome ensures that attention is drawn clearly to the risk of CVD at all levels of the health care system. In particular, the metabolic syndrome criteria with the basic screening tool of waist measurement allow a relatively simple stepwise approach with particular attention to early detection of those at risk so that intervention can start. Although the metabolic syndrome may influence choice of drug therapies, its presence essentially denotes the need to emphasize lifestyle management in clinical practice. In this chapter, we outline the historical perspective, pathophysiology, and evolving definitions of the metabolic syndrome; its significance as a tool for cardiovascular risk assessment; and therapeutic options.

HISTORICAL PERSPECTIVE

As early as 1923, Kylin, a Swedish physician, described the clustering of cardiovascular risk factors, such as hypertension, obesity, and gout.[4] More recently, in 1988, Reaven linked insulin resistance to hyperglycemia and hypertension and called this clustering "syndrome X." In time, syndrome X took on the name metabolic syndrome and similar synonyms, such as the insulin resistance syndrome and the cardiometabolic syndrome. The American Association of Clinical Endocrinologists in 2001 promoted the recognition of the metabolic syndrome as a diagnostic entity with its own ICD-9 code. This action gave physicians the ability to diagnose and to manage the syndrome as its own entity rather than as component diagnoses. Moreover, in the same year, the Third Adult Treatment Panel of the National Cholesterol Education Program promoted the utility of easily determined criteria for defining the metabolic syndrome, which remain the most widely used criteria in the United States.[5] Similar criteria were proposed shortly thereafter by the International Diabetes Federation, except that they focused on abdominal obesity to be one of the three criteria required for diagnosis of the metabolic syndrome.[6]

Then, in a joint statement, the American Diabetes Association and the European Association for the Study of Diabetes (ADA-EASD) questioned the value of diagnosis of the syndrome.[7] The main concerns that the ADA-EASD joint statement outlined included ambiguous or incomplete criteria for the diagnosis of the metabolic syndrome, uncertain role of insulin resistance as the cause of the syndrome, CVD risk attributable to the metabolic syndrome possibly not being greater than that attributable to individual components of the syndrome, and treatment of the metabolic syndrome not being different from treatment of component features.

In contrast, the position of the American Heart Association and the National Heart, Lung, and Blood Institute is that "... recognition of the syndrome in clinical practice is encouraged for the identification of a multiple-risk-factor condition and to promote lifestyle therapies that will reduce all of the metabolic risk factors simultaneously."[8]

These differing position statements are essentially matters of perspective.[9,10] In reviewing previous literature on the metabolic syndrome, Blaha and Elasy found that some papers used the metabolic syndrome as a study exposure (the clinical epidemiologic perspective) and that others used it as an outcome (the pathophysiologic perspective). In their analysis, they found that the ADA-EASD position statement aligns with the pathophysiologic perspective and that the basis for most of the expressed concerns is the imprecise definition of the syndrome and incomplete understanding of its pathophysiology. By contrast, the American Heart Association position statement aligns itself with the clinical epidemiologic perspective and finds the recognition of features of the metabolic syndrome of substantial clinical use in the identification of patients at high risk for atherosclerotic events.

PATHOPHYSIOLOGY

Insulin resistance was proposed by Reaven to play the causative role in the pathophysiology of metabolic syndrome. It is certainly closely related to several of the components of the metabolic syndrome, and several metabolic pathways linking insulin resistance to the other factors, such as dyslipidemia and hypertension, have been proposed.[11,12] Insulin is a hormone that facilitates glucose uptake in adipocytes, hepatocytes, and skeletal muscle (Fig. 22-1). It also regulates hepatic glucose production and lipolysis. Insulin resistance has been defined as a condition of decreased responsiveness of target tissues to normal levels of circulating insulin, resulting in hyperinsulinemia.

Insulin resistance arises from both genetic and acquired defects. A major contributor to the development of insulin resistance is an overabundance of circulating free fatty acids, released from an expanded adipose tissue mass. Free fatty acids reduce insulin sensitivity in muscle by inhibiting insulin-mediated glucose uptake. Increased levels of circulating glucose increase pancreatic insulin secretion, resulting in hyperinsulinemia. In the liver, free fatty acids increase the production of glucose, triglycerides, and secretion of very-low-density lipoproteins. The consequence is the reduction in glucose transformation to glycogen and increased lipid accumulation in triglycerides.

Multiple mechanisms have been proposed to explain the link between hypertension and insulin resistance. Hyperinsulinemia is associated with adrenergic overactivity, leading to increased cardiac output and urinary catecholamine excretion.[13] Insulin also has an antinatriuretic effect, causing sodium retention and plasma volume expansion. Increased sympathetic activity also stimulates the renin-angiotensin system (RAS). There is also an effect of insulin resistance on endothelial function. The elevation in free fatty acids and tumor necrosis factor-α (TNF-α) and the decrease in adiponectin adversely affect endothelial function and promote atherogenesis.[14,15]

More recently, it has been suggested that low-grade inflammation underlies or exacerbates the syndrome. The excess adipose tissue observed in the metabolic syndrome results in overproduction of the inflammatory cytokines TNF-α, interleukin-6, and C-reactive protein (CRP).[16]

DEFINING METABOLIC SYNDROME

During the past decade, several different definitions of metabolic syndrome have been proposed and used (Table 22-1). This has led to confusion and lack of comparability between studies. The first attempt to define metabolic syndrome was by a World Health Organization (WHO) diabetes group in 1998, which proposed a working definition that could be modified as more information became available.[17,18] Most of the criteria in the WHO definition were based on Reaven's

suggestions for syndrome X with the addition of obesity and microalbuminuria. The essential components of metabolic syndrome were considered to be glucose intolerance, impaired glucose tolerance or diabetes, and insulin resistance together with two or more of the following: raised arterial pressure, raised triglycerides, or low levels of HDL-C; central obesity or body mass index (BMI) >30 kg/m^2; and microalbuminuria (see Table 22-1). Other possible components of the syndrome, such as hyperuricemia, coagulation disorders, and raised circulating levels of plasminogen activator inhibitor 1 (PAI-1), were mentioned but not added as necessary components of the syndrome. The European Group for the Study of Insulin Resistance then produced a modification of the WHO criteria excluding people with diabetes and requiring hyperinsulinemia to be present.[19]

In 2001, the U.S. National Cholesterol Education Program (NCEP) Adult Treatment Panel III (ATP III) recognized the existence of the metabolic syndrome as a major contributor to cardiovascular risk.[5] A strong emphasis of the definition was on recognition of people at high risk for CVD in addition to the conventional risk factors of low-density lipoprotein cholesterol (LDL-C), smoking, and family history. They produced a set of criteria in which people had to meet three of the five criteria that were similar to those of the WHO group but also showed some significant differences. Specifically, these criteria included increased waist circumference, elevated blood pressure, impaired fasting glucose, increased triglycerides, and low HDL-C. Central adiposity was represented by waist circumference. Also, HDL-C and raised triglycerides could count separately. Blood pressure was also slightly lower for the ATP III definition (130/85 mm Hg or higher) than for the WHO criteria, and NCEP ATP III restricted glucose to the fasting state and included known diabetes. It was generally agreed that the NCEP ATP III definition was simpler for use in clinical practice.

The International Diabetes Federation (IDF) believed there was a strong need for one practical definition that would be useful in any country for the identification of people at high risk for diabetes and CVD.[6] Central obesity, as assessed by waist circumference, was agreed as essential because of the strength of the evidence linking waist circumference with CVD and the other metabolic syndrome components; its inclusion as a required component meant that this could be used as an initial screening, followed by evaluation of the other components only if it is increased. The waist circumference cutoff selected was lower than the NCEP ATP III recommendations (above 94 cm in men and 80 cm in women), and ethnic-specific waist circumference cutoffs have been incorporated into the definition, including lower cutoffs in Asians/South Asians of 90 cm in men and 80 cm in women. These cutpoints are also recommended for those of Central and South American ancestry. The levels of the other variables were as described by ATP III, except that the revised cut point from the American Diabetes Association for impaired fasting glucose (100 mg/dL) was used. The consensus group also recommended additional criteria that should be part of further research into metabolic syndrome, including tomographic assessment of visceral adiposity and liver fat, biomarkers of adipose tissue (adiponectin, leptin), apolipoprotein B, LDL particle size, formal measurement of insulin resistance and an oral glucose tolerance test, endothelial dysfunction, urinary albumin, inflammatory markers (CRP, TNF-α, interleukin-6), and thrombotic markers (PAI-1, fibrinogen).

Most recently, the NCEP ATP III definition has undergone a revision in the American Heart Association/National Heart, Lung, and Blood Institute scientific statement on the diagnosis and management of the metabolic syndrome[20] (see Table 22-1). Many of these revisions bring ATP III in line with the IDF recommendations. Given the recent American Diabetes Association revision of the lower cut point of impaired fasting

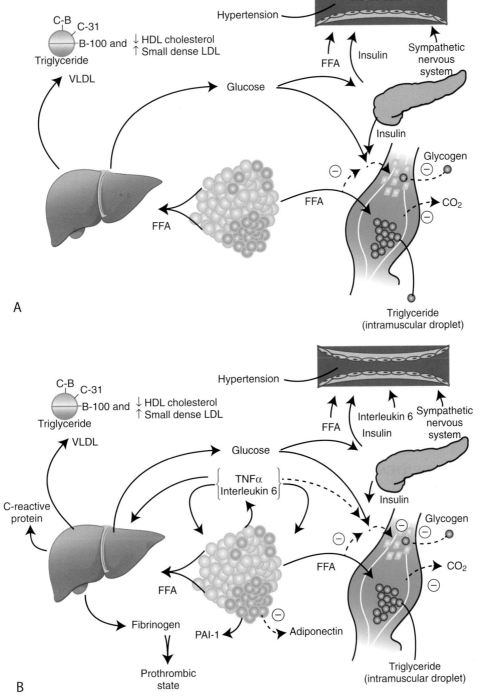

FIGURE 22-1 Pathophysiology of the metabolic syndrome (insulin resistance). **A,** Free fatty acids (FFA) are released in abundance from an expanded adipose tissue mass. In the liver, FFA increase production of glucose, triglycerides, and secretion of very-low-density lipoproteins (VLDL). Associated lipid and lipoprotein abnormalities include reductions in high-density lipoprotein (HDL) cholesterol and an increased density of low-density lipoproteins (LDL). FFA also reduce insulin sensitivity in muscle by inhibiting insulin-mediated glucose uptake. Associated defects include a reduction in glucose partitioning to glycogen and increased lipid accumulation in triglyceride (TG). Increases in circulating glucose and to some extent FFA increase pancreatic insulin secretion, resulting in hyperinsulinemia. Hyperinsulinemia may result in enhanced sodium reabsorption and increased sympathetic nervous system activity and contribute to the hypertension, as might increased levels of circulating FFA. **B,** Superimposed and contributory to the insulin resistance produced by excessive FFA is the paracrine and endocrine effect of the proinflammatory state. Produced by a variety of cells in adipose tissue including adipocytes and monocyte-derived macrophages, the enhanced secretion of interleukin-6 and tumor necrosis factor-α (TNF-α), among others, results in more insulin resistance and lipolysis of adipose tissue triglyceride stores to circulating FFA. Interleukin-6 and other cytokines also are increased in the circulation and may enhance hepatic glucose production, the production of VLDL by the liver, and insulin resistance in muscle. Cytokines and FFA also increase the production of fibrinogen and plasminogen activator inhibitor 1 (PAI-1) by the liver that complements the overproduction of PAI-1 by adipose tissue. This results in a prothrombotic state. Reductions in the production of the anti-inflammatory and insulin-sensitizing cytokine adiponectin are also associated with the metabolic syndrome and may contribute to the pathophysiology of the syndrome. *(Modified from Eckel RH, Grundy SM, Zimmet PZ: The metabolic syndrome.* Lancet *365:1415, 2005.)*

TABLE 22-1	**Comparison of Definitions of Metabolic Syndrome**		
WHO (1999)	**EGIR (1999)**	**NCEP ATP III (2001), AHA/ NHLBI (2005)**	**IDF (2005)**
Diabetes or impaired fasting glycemia or impaired glucose tolerance or insulin resistance (euglycemic clamp: glucose uptake in lowest 25%, hyperinsulinemia) Plus two or more of the following: Obesity: BMI >30 or waist-to-hip ratio of >0.9 for men and >0.85 for women Dyslipidemia: elevated triglycerides ≥150 mg/dL (≥1.7 mmol/L) or HDL <35 mg/dL (0.9 mmol/L) for men or <39 mg/dL (1.0 mmol/L) for women Hypertension: blood pressure ≥140/90 mm Hg Microalbuminuria: albumin excretion >20 μg/min	Insulin resistance, hyperinsulinemia: top 25% of fasting insulin values from nondiabetic population Plus two or more of the following: Central obesity: waist circumference ≥94 cm (man) or ≥80 cm (woman) Dyslipidemia: triglycerides >2.0 mmol/L (178 mg/dL) or HDL cholesterol <1.0 mmol/L (39 mg/dL) Hypertension: blood pressure ≥140/90 mm Hg or on antihypertensive Fasting plasma glucose ≥6.1 mmol/L (110 mg/dL) but no diabetes	Three or more of the following: Central obesity: waist circumference >102 cm (40 inches) in men, >88 cm (35 inches) in women Hypertriglyceridemia: triglycerides ≥1.7 mmol/L (150 mg/dL) or *medication for elevated triglycerides Low HDL-C: <1.03 mmol/L (40 mg/dL) for men, <1.29 mmol/L (50 mg/dL) for women, *or medication for low HDL-C Hypertension: blood pressure ≥130/85 mm Hg or on *antihypertensive medication *Fasting plasma glucose ≥5.6 mmol/L (100 mg/dL) or on medication for hyperglycemia	Central obesity (ethnicity specific), defined by waist circumference: Europids: ≥94 cm (37 inches) in men and ≥80 cm (31.5 inches) in women Asians/South Asians: ≥90 cm in men or ≥80 cm in women Plus two or more of the following: Hypertriglyceridemia: triglycerides ≥1.7 mmol/L (150 mg/dL) Low HDL-C: <1.03 mmol/L (40 mg/dL) for men, <1.29 mmol/L (50 mg/dL) for women Hypertension: blood pressure ≥130/85 mm Hg or on antihypertensive medication Fasting plasma glucose ≥5.6 mmol/L (100 mg/dL)

*Revisions incorporated by the American Heart Association/National Heart, Lung, and Blood Institute (AHA/NHLBI) definition (2005). EGIR, European Group for the Study of Insulin Resistance; IDF, International Diabetes Federation; NCEP ATP III, National Cholesterol Education Program Adult Treatment Panel III; WHO, World Health Organization.

glucose to 100 mg/dL, this lower cut point has now been adopted in the revised definition. In addition, the criteria for elevated blood pressure, elevated triglycerides, and low HDL-C now also include medication for these conditions. The statement also comments on possible ethnic differences and that lower waist values may be adopted in certain ethnic groups, such as those recommended by the IDF.

PREVALENCE AND EPIDEMIOLOGY

The most recent data from the National Health and Nutrition Examination Survey (NHANES) 2003-2006 show a prevalence of metabolic syndrome of 34% among U.S. adults by the NCEP ATP III guidelines criteria.[21] This estimate is identical to that with use of data from NHANES 1999-2002, which showed a prevalence (age adjusted) of metabolic syndrome of 34.4% among men and 34.5% among women by NCEP definition, with higher estimates of 40.7% and 37.1%, respectively, by the IDF definition[22] (Fig. 22-2). Earlier data among U.S. adults show a substantially lower prevalence of approximately 25% in U.S. adults examined in 1988-1994,[23] with increases in prevalence from 1988-1994 to 1999-2000 noted to be most dramatic among women (increase of 23.5% during this period) and attributable mainly to increases in high blood pressure, waist circumference, and hypertriglyceridemia.[24]

Wide variations in prevalence of metabolic syndrome are observed across ethnic groups within the United States and worldwide but depend on the definition used. Despite attempts in recent years to reach an agreement on the definition of the metabolic syndrome, comparison of prevalences published for different populations is difficult because studies often differ with respect to the study design, the sample selection, the year that a study was conducted, the precise definition of the metabolic syndrome used, and the age and sex distribution of the population itself. Despite these obstacles, Cameron and associates[25] reported on the prevalence of the NCEP ATP III definition of the metabolic syndrome among various populations around the world (Fig. 22-3). Looking at those studies that include a population sample aged 20 to 25 years and older, the prevalence varies from 8% (India) to 24% (United States) in men and from 7% (France) to 46% (India) in women.

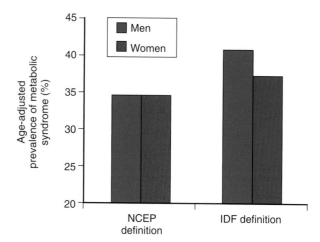

FIGURE 22-2 Prevalence of metabolic syndrome by National Cholesterol Education Program (NCEP) and International Diabetes Federation (IDF) definitions, U.S. adults, National Health and Nutrition Examination Survey 1999-2002. *(Modified from Ford ES: Prevalence of the metabolic syndrome defined by the International Diabetes Federation among adults in the U.S. Diabetes Care 28:2745, 2005.)*

In a large United Kingdom study, South Asians had the highest prevalence of metabolic syndrome (29% in men and 32% in women by the NCEP definition) and European women the lowest (14%).[26] In a large study involving 11 European cohorts, prevalence with use of a modified WHO definition was slightly higher in men (15.7%) than in women (14.2%).[27] Also, in Greek adults, age-adjusted prevalences of metabolic syndrome were 24.5% by the NCEP ATP III definition versus 43.4% by the IDF definition.[28] Lower prevalence rates were recently noted by the ATP III definition among 2100 Italian adults: 18% in women and 15% in men.[29]

Ethnic-specific data among U.S. adults have shown metabolic syndrome to be most prevalent among Mexican Americans; among African Americans, in particular men, prevalence was lower than in whites[22] (Fig. 22-4). From the Mexico City Diabetes Study, prevalence estimates from 1997-1999 show 39.9% of men and 59.9% of women to have the metabolic

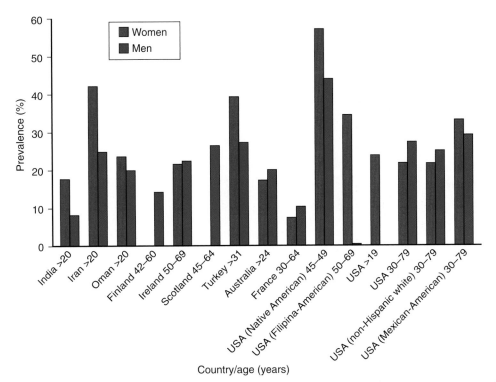

FIGURE 22-3 Worldwide prevalence of metabolic syndrome by NCEP ATP III definition. *(Modified from Cameron AJ, Shaw JE, Zimmet PZ: The metabolic syndrome: prevalence in worldwide populations.* Endocrinol Metab Clin North Am *33:351, 2004.)*

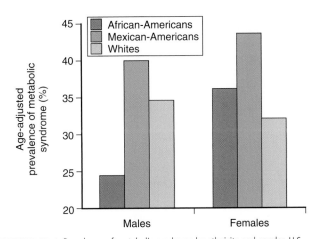

FIGURE 22-4 Prevalence of metabolic syndrome by ethnicity and gender, U.S. adults, National Health and Nutrition Examination Survey 1999-2002. *(Modified from Ford ES: Prevalence of the metabolic syndrome defined by the International Diabetes Federation among adults in the U.S.* Diabetes Care *28:2745, 2005.)*

syndrome, representing little change from 1990-1992 among men (38.9%) but a decrease in women from that period (65.4%). Increases in prevalence were attributed to those with elevated waist circumference, elevated fasting glucose value, and low levels of HDL-C.[30] These data, however, contrast with a nationwide study in Mexico involving 2158 men and women aged 20 to 69 years, in which the age-adjusted prevalence of metabolic syndrome was noted to be 13.6% by WHO criteria and 26.6% by the NCEP ATP III definition (and 9.2% and 21.4%, respectively, among those without diabetes).[31]

Among Asian populations, lower prevalences of metabolic syndrome are generally noted. For example, among Hong Kong Chinese, prevalence was 9.6% by the NCEP definition and 13.4% by the WHO definition,[32] but in another study of

Hong Kong Chinese, prevalences were greater: 16.7% by the NCEP definition but 21.2% with incorporation of lower waist circumference criteria recommended for Asians by the WHO (>80 cm for men and >90 cm for women).[33] In 1230 Korean adults aged 30 to 79 years, the prevalence by WHO criteria was 21.8% in men and 19.4% in women; however, this increased to 34.2% of men and 38.7% of women with use of the modified NCEP definition.[34] Japanese and Mongolian adults had prevalences of only 6% and 12%, respectively, by ATP III criteria; however, these estimates did not factor in lower IDF-recommended waist circumference cut points for Asians.[35]

Among U.S. adolescents aged 12 to 19 years from the NHANES 2001-2006 survey, a prevalence of metabolic syndrome of 8.6% overall (10.8% in males and 6.1% in females) has been recently reported,[36] a clear increase from an overall prevalence of 6.4% in 1999-2000 and 4.2% in 1988-1992.[37] In a school-based cross-sectional study of 1513 black, white, and Hispanic teens, the overall prevalence of NCEP-defined metabolic syndrome was 4.2%, and that of WHO-defined metabolic syndrome was 8.4%; among obese teens, this increased to 19.5% and 38.9%, respectively. Moreover, non-white teens were more likely to have metabolic syndrome defined by WHO criteria.[38] A recent review on the prevalence of metabolic syndrome in children and adolescents found ranges from 1.2% to 22.6%, with rates of up to 60% observed in the overweight and obese, in 36 studies from general population and community-based sampling.[39]

CARDIOVASCULAR RISK IN PERSONS WITH THE METABOLIC SYNDROME

Prediction of Diabetes

Recent analysis of data from the Prospective Study of Pravastatin in the Elderly at Risk (PROSPER) study and the British

Regional Heart Study (BRHS) found a strong association of metabolic syndrome with the incidence of type 2 diabetes.[40] Metabolic syndrome predicted an increased risk of diabetes in PROSPER participants (HR = 4.41; 95% CI, 3.33-5.84), and an even stronger association was observed in BRHS participants (HR = 7.47; 4.90-11.46). Similarly, data from the San Antonio Heart Study (n = 2559) showed that the metabolic syndrome predicted diabetes beyond glucose intolerance alone.[41]

Prediction of Cardiovascular Events and Mortality

The risk of CVD has been well studied and documented in persons with diabetes; in fact, diabetes is considered to be a coronary heart disease (CHD) risk equivalent according to the NCEP ATP III guidelines.[5] The East-West study showed that in the absence of prior myocardial infarction, persons with diabetes have a risk of future cardiovascular mortality similar to that of persons with a prior myocardial infarction without diabetes. The presence of both diabetes and prior myocardial infarction is associated with an even higher risk of cardiovascular mortality.[42] In our study involving up to 12 years of follow-up of 6255 adults from NHANES 1988-1994 we demonstrated total mortality to be similar among persons with diabetes but without preexisting CVD and those with CVD without diabetes[43] (Fig. 22-5).

The combination of diabetes and metabolic syndrome is associated with a much higher prevalence of CHD, and even those with metabolic syndrome in the absence of diabetes have a higher prevalence of CHD than do those with diabetes who do not have the metabolic syndrome.[44] Conversely, among those with preexisting atherosclerotic vascular disease, metabolic syndrome is highly prevalent. Among a cross-sectional survey of 1117 patients with CHD, cerebrovascular disease, peripheral vascular disease, or abdominal aortic aneurysm, an overall prevalence of metabolic syndrome was noted to be 46%; it was 58% in those with peripheral vascular disease, 41% in those with CHD, 43% in those with CVD, and 47% in those with abdominal aortic aneurysm. Moreover, age did not have an impact on these prevalences.[45]

We recently demonstrated in the U.S. population of men and women a twofold greater risk of mortality from CHD and CVD in persons with metabolic syndrome; even those with metabolic syndrome but without diabetes and those with only one or two metabolic syndrome risk factors were at an increased risk of death from CHD and CVD. Increased risks associated with metabolic syndrome held similarly for men and women. Moreover, those with diabetes had a risk of future mortality similar to that of those with preexisting CVD. Those with both diabetes and preexisting CVD had the highest risk.[43] These observations are consistent with other reports documenting the prognostic importance of the metabolic syndrome; among 6447 men in the West of Scotland study, it predicted both incident diabetes (HR, 3.50; 95% CI, 2.51-4.90) and CHD events (HR = 1.30; 95% CI, 1.00-1.67)[46]; and among 1209 Finnish men observed for 11.4 years, it predicted increased CVD mortality (2.6- to 4.2-fold increased risk, depending on definition used) and total mortality (1.9- to 3.3-fold increased risk, depending on definition used).[47]

More recently, Jeppesen and colleagues[48] presented analysis of data from a large Danish population-based study of 2493 men and women and used both insulin resistance and metabolic syndrome as predictors of incident CVD. They reported that both insulin resistance and metabolic syndrome were independent predictors; the relative risk for CVD was 1.49 (95% CI = 1.07-2.07) for insulin resistance as quantified by homeostasis model assessment (HOMA-IR) and 1.56 for NCEP-defined metabolic syndrome (95% CI = 1.12-2.17).

Other U.S. population-based studies have also demonstrated a relation of metabolic syndrome to cardiovascular event risk. In the Framingham Offspring Study, Rutter and coworkers[49] showed an age-, sex-, and CRP-adjusted hazard ratio for metabolic syndrome of 1.8 (95% CI = 1.4-2.5) for prediction of incident CVD events during 7 years. Moreover, among 12,089 black and white middle-aged individuals in

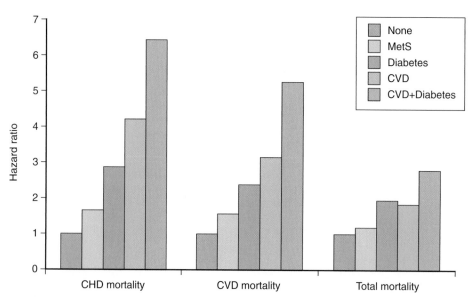

FIGURE 22-5 Cardiovascular disease and total mortality in U.S. men and women aged 30 to 74 years: age-, gender-, and risk factor–adjusted Cox regression, NHANES II follow-up (n = 6255). In comparison to those without metabolic syndrome, diabetes, or CVD, metabolic syndrome: P < 0.05 for CHD mortality and P < 0.01 for CVD mortality; diabetes, CVD, and CVD plus diabetes: P < 0.001 for CHD, CVD, and total mortality. CHD, coronary heart disease; CVD, cardiovascular disease; MetS, metabolic syndrome. (*Modified from Malik S, Wong ND, Franklin SS, et al: Impact of the metabolic syndrome on mortality from coronary heart disease, cardiovascular disease, and all causes in United States adults.* Circulation 110:1239, 2004.)

the Atherosclerosis Risk in Communities (ARIC) study, in which metabolic syndrome was found prevalent in 23% of those without diabetes or prevalent CVD at baseline, during an average 11 years of follow-up, those with versus without metabolic syndrome were 1.5 to 2 times more likely to develop CHD in risk factor–adjusted analyses. However, metabolic syndrome did not improve risk prediction beyond that achieved by the Framingham risk score.[50]

In 2175 elderly subjects in the Cardiovascular Health Study, metabolic syndrome defined by the ATP III but not by the WHO criteria was associated with a significant 38% increased risk (HR, 1.38; 95% CI = 1.06-1.79) of coronary or cerebrovascular events.[51] In the San Antonio Heart Study, among 2815 subjects aged 24 to 64 years, the NCEP metabolic syndrome definition predicted all-cause mortality (multivariable hazard ratio = 1.47; 95% CI = 1.13-1.92), but the WHO metabolic syndrome definition did not; among those without diabetes or prior CVD, the NCEP metabolic syndrome definition predicted only cardiovascular mortality (HR, 2.01; 95% CI = 1.13-3.57); there was evidence also for stronger relations of metabolic syndrome with cardiovascular mortality in women compared with men.[52] Among a large, primarily healthy cohort of 19,223 men who received a clinical examination and fitness examination, adjusted relative risks for all-cause and cardiovascular mortality were 1.29 (1.05-1.57) and 1.89 (1.36-2.60), respectively, among those with versus without metabolic syndrome.[53] Additional adjustment for cardiorespiratory fitness, however, resulted in associations being no longer significant. Also, among 10,950 men in the Multiple Risk Factor Intervention Trial (MRFIT), modified NCEP-defined metabolic syndrome was associated with increased hazard ratios during a median of 18.4 years of follow-up for total mortality (1.21 [1.13-1.29]), CVD mortality (1.49 [1.35-1.64]), and CHD mortality (1.52 [1.34-1.70]), with elevated blood glucose and low HDL-C being the factors most predictive of CVD mortality among those men with metabolic syndrome.[54]

In a meta-analysis of risks for all-cause mortality, CVD, and diabetes, Ford[55] noted that among studies that used the exact NCEP definition of the metabolic syndrome, relative risks (and 95% confidence intervals) associated with the metabolic syndrome were 1.27 (0.90-1.78) for all-cause mortality, 1.65 (1.38-1.99) for CVD, and 2.99 (1.96-4.57) for diabetes. For the WHO definition, corresponding estimates were 1.37 (1.09-1.74), 1.93 (1.39-2.67), and 2.60 (1.55-4.38). The authors concluded population attributable fractions of the metabolic syndrome to be 6% to 7% for all-cause mortality, 12% to 17% for CVD, and 30% to 52% for diabetes.

The association between metabolic syndrome and CVD events may be attenuated in certain population subgroups. A study by Sattar and coworkers[56] fueled the controversy over the importance of metabolic syndrome for determination of vascular risk. A nonsignificant relationship was observed between metabolic syndrome and incident CVD in an elderly cohort from the PROSPER study (HR, 1.07; 95% CI = 0.86-1.32), and a weak association was observed in a similar cohort from the BRHS study (HR, 1.27; 1.04-1.56). In another study looking at the predictive value of metabolic syndrome in the elderly, Mozaffarian and colleagues[57] used data from the Cardiovascular Health Study and examined data from 4258 U.S. adults. Although those with metabolic syndrome had a 22% higher mortality risk (RR, 1.22; 95% CI, 1.11-1.34), in looking at the population attributable risk fraction [PAR %], higher proportions of death were attributable to elevated fasting glucose and hypertension (PAR, 22.2%) than to metabolic syndrome (PAR, 6.3%). This study reinforces the concept that there is limited short-term risk assessment value in using metabolic syndrome. In general, the metabolic syndrome may help identify younger cohorts who face a high long-term cardiovascular risk.

Finally, a large meta-analysis of the risk of incident cardiovascular events and death associated with metabolic syndrome analyzed data from 37 studies and 172,573 individuals. Metabolic syndrome in this analysis had a much stronger association with cardiovascular events and death, with a relative risk of 1.78 (95% CI = 1.58-2.00) (Fig. 22-6). This relationship was stronger in women and remained significant after adjustment for traditional cardiovascular risk factors.[58]

Prediction of Stroke

Metabolic syndrome is also related to the risk of stroke. Among 14,284 subjects with CHD, 26% of whom had the metabolic syndrome, those with metabolic syndrome but without diabetes had a 1.49-fold greater odds for ischemic stroke or transient ischemic attacks (95% CI, 1.20-1.84), whereas those with diabetes had a 2.29-fold increased odds (95% CI, 1.88-2.78); risks were higher in women than in men.[59] Case-control studies have also recently reported on the association of metabolic syndrome with stroke. In a Japanese study, among 197 stroke survivors and 356 matched controls, metabolic syndrome was associated with a significant 3.1-fold greater odds of stroke.[60] In another case-control study in Greece involving 163 stroke survivors aged 70 years and older and 166 controls, in risk factor–adjusted analyses, metabolic syndrome was associated with a 2.6-fold greater odds of stroke.[61]

Metabolic Syndrome Risks Among Subjects with Known Cardiovascular Disease

Among subjects with established CVD, the metabolic syndrome is also associated with future CVD event risk. Among subjects with acute coronary syndromes within the Myocardial Ischemia Reduction with Aggressive Cholesterol Lowering (MIRACL) trial, 38% of patients met the criteria for metabolic syndrome; those with metabolic syndrome had a hazard ratio of 1.49 (95% CI, 1.24-1.79) for the primary endpoint of death, nonfatal myocardial infarction, cardiac arrest, or recurrent unstable myocardial ischemia.[62] Within the GISSI-Prevenzione trial, among 11,232 patients with a prior myocardial infarction, those with metabolic syndrome had a 29% greater risk of death and 23% greater risk of major cardiovascular events; these risks were amplified in diabetic patients (68% and 47%, respectively).[63] Finally, of interest are data from the Scandinavian Simvastatin Survival Study (4S) showing, among 3933 nondiabetic subjects with known CHD, those with the metabolic syndrome to have at least as great (if not greater) reduction in the risk of total mortality (RR, 0.54), coronary mortality (RR, 0.39), or major coronary artery disease events (RR, 0.59) as those without the metabolic syndrome (0.72, 0.62, and 0.71, respectively).[64]

Global Risk Assessment of Metabolic Syndrome

To best target treatment strategies, adequate assessment of risk for CVD is needed in persons with metabolic syndrome. Initial evaluation of risk can be determined by Framingham risk scores,[65] given the significant heterogeneity in estimated risk of persons with metabolic syndrome. In a study applying Framingham global risk algorithms to the U.S. population with metabolic syndrome, 38.5% were classified as low risk (<6% 10-year risk of CHD), 8.5% were classified as moderate risk (6% to 10% 10-year risk of CHD), 15.8% were classified as moderately high risk (10% to 20% 10-year risk of CHD), and 37.3% were classified as high risk (>20% 10-year risk of CHD, or preexisting CVD or diabetes).[66]

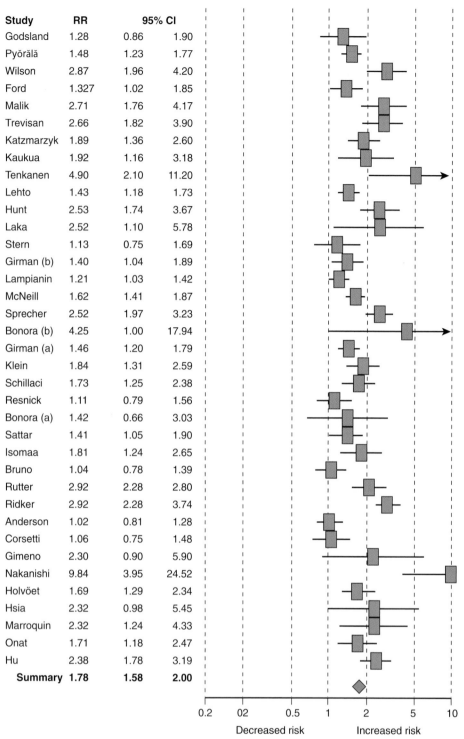

FIGURE 22-6 Relative risks and 95% confidence intervals for metabolic syndrome and incident cardiovascular events and death. Studies are listed in chronologic order by the year in which their cohorts were created (except for the last study listed, which includes multiple cohorts). Results are for available analyses of incident cardiovascular disease and death and may differ from the results of the total study populations. Boxes represent the relative risk, and lines represent the 95% confidence interval for studies. The diamond represents the pooled relative risk, and its width represents its 95% confidence interval. *(Modified from Gami AS, Witt BJ, Howard DE, et al: Metabolic syndrome and risk of incident cardiovascular events and death.* J Am Coll Cardiol *49:403, 2007.)*

Older persons or those who are smokers or have increased total cholesterol or increased LDL-C levels, even if only minimal elevations of defined metabolic syndrome risk factors are present, may be at intermediate or higher risk of CHD. However, an important limitation of Framingham risk or other global risk algorithms is that they often do not include critical metabolic syndrome risk factors such as fasting glucose concentration or elevated triglycerides, which, although possibly not providing additive predictive value in a *general* population, could be critically important in stratifying risk in those with metabolic syndrome. Therefore, in situations in which a calculated global risk score results in a borderline figure (e.g., 18% to 19% 10-year risk), the presence of significant metabolic risk factors not included in the global risk algorithm may warrant the individual to be stratified to a higher risk stratum (e.g., >20% or CHD risk equivalent status in this case). The scientific statement on the clinical management of the metabolic syndrome released by the American Heart Association and National Heart, Lung, and Blood Institute noted, however, that the Framingham algorithms do capture most of the risk for CVD in persons with the metabolic syndrome and that adding obesity, triglyceride levels, and fasting glucose concentration does not appear to increase the power of prediction.[67]

For those with diabetes, the United Kingdom Prospective Diabetes Study (UKPDS) in 2001 developed a risk engine based on data from 4540 male and female patients with diabetes to predict the risk of new CHD events. Unlike previously published equations, this model is diabetes specific and incorporates glycemia, systolic blood pressure, and lipid levels in addition to age, sex, ethnic group, smoking status, and time since diagnosis of diabetes.[68] Recent reports have examined the performance of this risk engine in relation to the Joint British Societies (JBS) risk calculator[69] and the earlier version of the Framingham risk equations that incorporated diabetes status.[70] Among 700 patients with type 2 diabetes, the UKPDS risk calculator identified a higher mean 10-year CHD risk (21.5%) than the JBS risk calculator did (18.3%).[71]

The more recent report compared the ability of the UKPDS risk engine and the Framingham risk equation to predict events that actually occurred among 428 subjects with newly diagnosed type 2 diabetes observed for a median of 4.2 years. The Framingham risk equations significantly underestimated the overall number of cardiovascular events by 33% and coronary events by 32%, compared with a lower and nonsignificant underestimation of coronary artery disease events of 13% by the UKPDS risk engine, although both similarly performed in terms of discrimination and calibration for a 15% 10-year CHD risk threshold.[72] Another risk calculator was derived from the Prospective Cardiovascular Münster (PROCAM) study. In another study, adjustment of the PROCAM estimated global risk to include BMI or waist circumference corresponded very well with observed cardiovascular event rates.[73]

Utility of Novel Biomarkers for Additional Risk Assessment in the Metabolic Syndrome

Once global risk assessment is done, additional information about the CHD risk for a given individual can be made with information obtained from novel biomarkers. For example, there has been interest in whether the addition of such risk factors as high-sensitivity CRP (hsCRP), fibrinogen, and small dense LDL will further add to prediction of risk in persons with metabolic syndrome. It has been shown that hsCRP levels add predictive value for CVD risk among individuals with metabolic syndrome. In the Nurses' Health Study,

among persons with metabolic syndrome, age-adjusted incidence rates of future CVD events of 3.4 and 5.0 per 1000 person-years were demonstrated for those with hsCRP levels of 3 mg/L or more and levels of less than 3 mg/L, respectively, with additive effects of higher hsCRP levels also observed for those with four or five metabolic syndrome risk factors. Framingham investigators recently reported hsCRP levels to provide additive value over metabolic syndrome in predicting CVD events.[74] In addition, the authors have reported that in the NHANES 1999-2000 sample, those with increased hsCRP levels and metabolic syndrome had a similar odds of CVD as those with diabetes and low hsCRP levels, and those with diabetes and high hsCRP levels had the highest odds of CVD.[75]

Importantly, the JUPITER trial has shown that screening for hsCRP can identify within the primary prevention setting a subset of patients (those with elevated hsCRP levels) most likely to benefit from preventive therapy with a statin. Both patients with and without metabolic syndrome, all of whom had hsCRP levels >2 mg/L, benefited from treatment.[76] Disputing the relative importance of hsCRP, a recent comprehensive meta-analysis from the Emerging Risk Factors Collaboration examined data from 54 studies and 160,309 participants and found that statistical adjustment for conventional cardiovascular risk factors resulted in attenuation of the linear relationship between hsCRP concentration and CHD, stroke, and other vascular mortality.[77] The role of other novel risk markers, such as fibrinogen, interleukin (IL-1, IL-6), and adiponectin levels, in providing additive risk stratification in persons with metabolic syndrome needs to be examined and documented before any recommendations can be made.

Screening for Subclinical Atherosclerosis

Evaluation of subclinical atherosclerosis may have important implications for persons with metabolic syndrome, given the uncertainty of risk assessment on the basis of global risk assessment alone. Given recent recommendations to target atherosclerosis screening for those with intermediate global risk of CHD[78,79] whereby those found to have clinically significant atherosclerosis could have their risk level stratified upward (e.g., reclassification of an intermediate-risk individual as high risk), such screening may have implications for refining risk assessment in many persons with metabolic syndrome. Although such screening in persons with diabetes could also offer improved risk stratification, as diabetes is considered a CHD risk equivalent and aggressive treatment guidelines already exist for those with diabetes, such evaluation is not normally recommended for those with diabetes.

Ingelsson and colleagues[80] evaluated the incidence of CVD associated with metabolic syndrome and diabetes according to the presence or absence of subclinical disease, which was categorized on the basis of any abnormalities on carotid ultrasound or ankle-brachial blood pressure, left ventricular hypertrophy on echocardiography or electrocardiography, or abnormal urinary albumin, with data from the Framingham Offspring Study. The authors found that participants who had metabolic syndrome and exhibited subclinical disease had a risk of CVD that was 2.5-fold higher (HR, 2.67; 95% CI, 1.62-4.41) than that of those without metabolic syndrome or subclinical disease. The association of metabolic syndrome and CVD was attenuated in those without subclinical disease (HR, 1.59; 95% CI, 0.87-2.90).

Carotid Ultrasound

Intima-media thickness (IMT) of carotid arteries, as assessed noninvasively by carotid ultrasonography, is also a useful measure of preclinical atherosclerosis. Carotid IMT has been found to predict future risk of myocardial infarction and stroke, and a change in carotid IMT has been validated as a vascular marker for the progression of atherosclerosis.[81] Specifically, studies in patients with the metabolic syndrome have demonstrated that carotid IMT abnormalities exist in patients with this syndrome and predict risk of CHD. Among 313 postmenopausal women, metabolic syndrome conferred an approximate threefold adjusted odds of subclinical carotid atherosclerosis, as measured by carotid IMT.[82] In these women, the metabolic syndrome but not BMI was associated with increased carotid IMT. Obesity had no independent effect, suggesting that metabolic abnormalities mediate the risk of subclinical atherosclerosis. Prospective data also show increased carotid IMT in those with metabolic syndrome. Bonera and associates[83] reported that 51% of people with metabolic syndrome aged 40 to 79 years developed carotid plaque in 5-year follow-up.

An increasing number of metabolic syndrome risk factors have also been shown to predict the progression of carotid IMT in elderly women during a 12-year period.[84] In this prospective study, the more metabolic syndrome risk factors that developed during the 12-year period, the greater was the increase in mean carotid IMT. Incident metabolic syndrome was a stronger predictor of subclinical atherosclerosis than were individual components of the syndrome. Metabolic syndrome was associated with progression of carotid IMT even after the Framingham risk score was accounted for. Finally, a cross-sectional analysis of 14,502 patients in the ARIC study demonstrated that the metabolic syndrome is associated with increased average carotid IMT.[85] In addition, in a separate investigation of 14,502 black and white subjects in the ARIC study comparing those with versus those without metabolic syndrome, both prevalence of CHD (7.4% versus 3.6%) and average carotid IMT were significantly greater in those with versus those without metabolic syndrome.[86] Finally, even among nondiabetic young subjects from the Bogalusa Heart Study (n = 507), composite carotid IMT increased significantly with the number of metabolic syndrome components present, and metabolic syndrome predicted composite carotid IMT 75th percentile or higher by receiver operator characteristics curves.[87]

Whereas the evidence relating metabolic syndrome to carotid IMT is strong, there remains debate as to whether carotid IMT can be used as a surrogate for assessment of the effects of therapy. Although some prevention trials with lipid-lowering medications that used carotid IMT as a surrogate endpoint have shown that retardation in the progression of carotid IMT is accompanied by a reduction of clinical cardiovascular endpoints,[88,89] others have not shown this.

Coronary Artery Calcification

The presence and extent of coronary artery calcification (CAC) strongly correlate with the overall magnitude of coronary atherosclerosis plaque burden and with the development of subsequent coronary events.[90,91] The authors have previously demonstrated the presence of metabolic syndrome to be independently associated with an increased likelihood of CAC (compared with those without metabolic syndrome) and those with diabetes to have the highest likelihood of CAC.[92] Moreover, the prevalence of calcium among women with metabolic syndrome was as high as in those with diabetes. Metabolic syndrome without diabetes was independently associated with an increased likelihood of CAC. Similarly, the National Heart, Lung, and Blood Institute Family Heart Study has demonstrated metabolic syndrome to be independently associated with an increased likelihood of CAC and abdominal aortic calcification in both men and women after adjustment for other risk factors.[93]

The Dallas Heart Study assessed the association between metabolic syndrome, diabetes mellitus, and subclinical atherosclerosis defined as CAC or abdominal aortic plaque detected by magnetic resonance imaging. Among 2735 participants, the prevalence of CAC was increased from those with neither metabolic syndrome nor diabetes (16.6%) to metabolic syndrome only (24%), to diabetes only (30.2%), to those with both metabolic syndrome and diabetes (44.7%). After adjustment, metabolic syndrome and diabetes were each independently associated with CAC.[94] Analysis of abdominal aortic plaque showed similar results, with highest prevalence of subclinical atherosclerosis in those with both diabetes and metabolic syndrome.

In addition to having independent effects of other traditional risk factors, metabolic syndrome has a synergistic effect. A cross-sectional study examining the combined effect of high LDL-C and metabolic syndrome on CAC found that CAC in asymptomatic men with moderate or high LDL-C was magnified in persons with metabolic syndrome.[95] LDL-C was more strongly associated with subclinical atherosclerosis when subjects had metabolic syndrome.

Not only metabolic syndrome but high-normal fasting blood glucose concentration has been shown to have increased levels of subclinical atherosclerosis. In one study, high-normal fasting blood glucose concentration was found to be associated with increased CAC in asymptomatic nondiabetic men.[96] The authors found that high-normal fasting blood glucose concentration was associated with CAC independent of metabolic syndrome. In another study, these authors found an association of metabolic syndrome with CAC in asymptomatic men independent of the Framingham risk score.[97] Metabolic syndrome was present in 24% of the study participants. The prevalence of CAC increased with increasing number of metabolic syndrome risk factors. The presence of metabolic syndrome increased the risk of any CAC by almost twofold.

Computed Tomographic Angiography

Recent advances in contrast-enhanced computed tomographic angiography allow the direct visualization of calcified and noncalcified plaque. There are now some data showing that assessment of plaque by this method strongly correlates with cardiovascular events.[98] Using data from the ROMICAT study, Butler and colleagues recently showed that those with metabolic syndrome have a higher prevalence of coronary plaque than do those without metabolic syndrome.[99] The presence of any, calcified, and noncalcified plaque was higher in patients with than without metabolic syndrome (91%, 74%, and 77% versus 46%, 45%, and 40% of coronary segments with plaque, respectively). Metabolic syndrome was independently associated with both the presence and extent of overall plaque after adjustment for the Framingham risk score (odds ratio, 6.7). However, given the current radiation dose from computed tomographic angiography, routine use in asymptomatic patients should be avoided.

Ankle-Brachial Index and Peripheral Arterial Disease

A low ankle-brachial index has been previously shown to strongly predict morbidity and mortality in persons without known CVD.[100,101] There are limited data on the association of ankle-brachial index with metabolic syndrome. The study population of this cross-sectional survey consisted of 502 patients recently diagnosed with CHD, 236 with stroke, 218 with peripheral arterial disease, and 89 with abdominal aortic aneurysm. The prevalence of the metabolic syndrome in the study population was 45%. In patients with peripheral arterial disease, this was 57%; in CHD patients, 40%; in stroke patients, 43%; and in patients with abdominal aortic aneurysm, 45%. Patients with the metabolic syndrome more often had a decreased ankle-brachial index (14% versus 10%; $P = 0.06$).[102]

Myocardial Perfusion and Imaging of Inflammation

In addition to direct (multidetector computed tomographic angiography) and indirect (CAC) assessment of coronary plaque, coronary perfusion has also been shown to vary with metabolic syndrome. Some initial observations in this regard include the finding that among persons with metabolic abnormalities (metabolic syndrome or diabetes), there is an increased likelihood of myocardial ischemia, as assessed by nuclear single-photon emission computed tomography (SPECT), at intermediate levels of CAC (e.g., 100 to 399), similar to that of those without such abnormalities who have higher levels of CAC (e.g., >400).[103] Also, the number of metabolic syndrome abnormalities increases the amount of ischemic area on stress SPECT.[104]

In addition to perfusion imaging, we can now assess degree of inflammation in different vascular beds. Fluorodeoxyglucose (FDG) positron emission tomography can measure inflammation within the aorta and carotid arteries. Interscan plaque FDG variability during 2 weeks was very low, with high intraclass correlation (0.79-0.92) and intraobserver agreement high across most territories, suggesting its usefulness as a noninvasive plaque imaging technique for use in drug intervention studies.[105] A study showed that FDG uptake was significantly associated with waist circumference, HDL-C, HOMA insulin resistance, hsCRP, and a number of metabolic syndrome components ($P < 0.05$ to $P < 0.001$).[106]

Other Subclinical Disease Measures

Others have also examined the relation of metabolic syndrome to other measures of subclinical atherosclerosis. In a random sample of 1153 French adults aged 35 to 65 years, the presence of metabolic syndrome was independently associated with the number of carotid and femoral plaques, carotid IMT, and pulse wave velocity, with odds ratios ranging from 1.8 to 2.15 by use of the NCEP definition and 1.48 to 1.97 with the WHO definition.[107] A recently published investigation from the ARIC study demonstrated a stepwise gradient in echocardiographic left ventricular mass by increasing number of metabolic syndrome disorders (none, any, two, or all three risk factors) in both men and women.[108] Moreover, among overweight hypertensive patients, those with versus without metabolic syndrome had significantly greater left ventricular mass even after control for age, gender, and blood pressure.[109] Finally, in a study of 607 adults with normal left ventricular function assessed by echocardiography, whereas left ventricular ejection fraction was similar among normals, those with one or two metabolic syndrome criteria (pre–metabolic syndrome), and those with metabolic syndrome, there were progressive increases in left ventricular mass and decreases in tissue Doppler imaging of diastolic function.[110] Others, however, have demonstrated that there is greater impairment of global left ventricular function in patients with versus without metabolic syndrome based on an index of myocardial performance.[111]

MANAGEMENT OF METABOLIC SYNDROME

The treatment goal for metabolic syndrome is to prevent future development of type 2 diabetes and diabetes-related cardiovascular complications. Lifestyle modification is the mainstay therapy for metabolic syndrome. The NCEP ATP III included metabolic syndrome within its lipid management guidelines to reinforce lifestyle therapies, including weight reduction, antiatherogenic diet, and increased physical activity. The treatment approach focuses on glycemic control and control of cardiovascular risk factors, mainly hypertension and hyperlipidemia. Although most persons (>75%) with metabolic syndrome (exclusive of diabetes) have increased

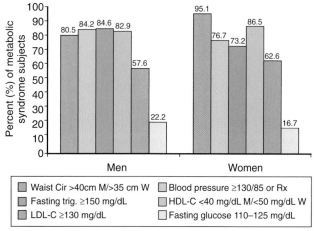

FIGURE 22-7 Prevalence of metabolic syndrome risk factors among U.S. adults with metabolic syndrome (but without diabetes), National Health and Nutrition Examination Survey 1988-1994. *(Modified from Wong ND, Pio JR, Franklin SS, et al: Preventing coronary events by optimal control of blood pressure and lipids in patients with the metabolic syndrome.* Am J Cardiol *91:1421, 2003.)*

waist circumference, blood pressure, and triglyceride levels and depressed HDL-C concentration, 58% of men and 63% of women with metabolic syndrome also have levels of LDL-C of 130 mg/dL (3.4 mmol/L) or higher[112] (Fig. 22-7). The potential benefits from optimal control of lipids and blood pressure, in particular, can be significant. We have additionally shown (by statistically controlling lipids and blood pressure with Framingham risk algorithms) that approximately 80% of coronary artery disease events could potentially be prevented by control of blood pressure, LDL-C, and HDL-C to optimal levels in persons with the metabolic syndrome without diabetes (Fig. 22-8).[112]

Mounting evidence suggests that lifestyle modification with weight loss and increased physical activity is beneficial, although specific studies in metabolic syndrome are needed. There are suggestions from the Finnish Diabetes Prevention Study that individuals with metabolic syndrome show less development of diabetes with lifestyle advice.[113] In many people, however, pharmacologic intervention will be needed. Long-term studies will help establish whether existing or newer agents, such as agonists for the peroxisome proliferator-activated (PPAR) α and γ receptors or cannabinoid 1 receptor blockers, could be of specific benefit.

Lifestyle Modification

Intensive lifestyle modification is the mainstay of treatment in low-risk patients. The most recent (2005) American Heart Association/National Heart, Lung, and Blood Institute statement[20] on the diagnosis and management of metabolic syndrome noted specific lifestyle-related therapeutic targets to include abdominal obesity, physical inactivity, and diet (Table 22-2). For abdominal obesity, a goal of reducing body weight by 7% to 10% during the first year, with continued weight loss to achieve a BMI <25 kg/m[2], is noted. In addition, regular moderate-intensity physical activity of at least 30minutes and preferably 60 minutes a day at least 5 days per week is recommended. Dietary recommendations focus in particular on reducing intakes of saturated fat, *trans*-fat, and cholesterol.

No single diet is currently recommended for patients with the metabolic syndrome, although evidence suggests a lower prevalence of metabolic syndrome with dietary patterns rich in fruit, vegetables, whole grains, dairy products,

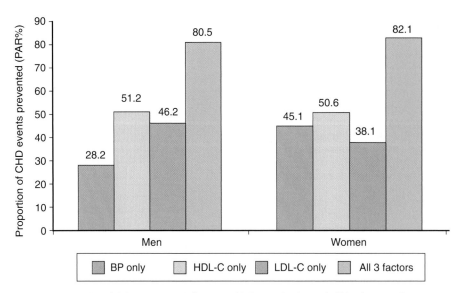

FIGURE 22-8 Proportion of CHD events potentially preventable from optimal control of blood pressure (to <120 mm Hg/<80 mm Hg), LDL-C (to <100 mg/dL), and HDL-C (to >60 mg/dL) in men and women. *(Modified from Wong ND, Pio JR, Franklin SS, et al: Preventing coronary events by optimal control of blood pressure and lipids in patients with the metabolic syndrome.* Am J Cardiol 91:1421, 2003.)

and unsaturated fats. The literature favors diets that are lower in carbohydrates and higher in healthy unsaturated fats and protein, compared with traditional high-carbohydrate and low-fat diets, to treat obesity, to reduce triglycerides, and to increase HDL-C. Diets that foster adherence, such as those modeled after the Mediterranean diet, not only improve risk factors but also reduce coronary mortality after myocardial infarction.[114] For example, recent evidence indicates that a Mediterranean-style diet reduces the prevalence of the metabolic syndrome while improving endothelial function.[115] Moreover, a Mediterranean diet is associated with increasing longevity[116] and improved survival after myocardial infarction.[117]

In a study using data from NHANES III, participants diagnosed with metabolic syndrome had a lower consumption of fruit, vegetables, and antioxidants than did those without metabolic syndrome.[118] The Coronary Artery Risk Development in Young Adults (CARDIA) study showed that consumption of dairy products was associated with a significantly reduced risk of metabolic syndrome.[119] The Framingham Offspring Study showed that whole-grain and cereal fiber intakes were associated with reduced risk of metabolic syndrome.[120] Importantly, both the US Diabetes Prevention Program[121] and the Finnish Diabetes Prevention Study[122] showed a 58% lower risk for the development of new onset diabetes in prediabetic individuals resulting from prescribed weight reduction and physical activity.

Lifestyle and behavior modification can be difficult. O'Malley and coworkers[123] examined the effect of case management on the development of the metabolic syndrome. In a randomized control trial with 450 patients, they were able to demonstrate greater improvement in motivation to change behavior and lower prevalence of metabolic syndrome in 6 months after intervention with a cardiovascular case management program.

In severely obese patients in whom lifestyle measures are not sufficient to adequately address the problem, pharmacologic therapy for weight loss (see Chapter 19) can be recommended as an adjunct. Finally, laparoscopic weight reduction surgery for the sole purpose of treating metabolic syndrome, although not recommended, has been shown in studies that had follow-up after this procedure to result in reversal of metabolic syndrome in 80%[124] to 96%[125] of patients.

Pharmacologic Treatment

When lifestyle modification fails and in high-risk patients, medications that target individual risk factors are recommended (e.g., antihypertensives, lipid-lowering drugs, hypoglycemic drugs, antiplatelet drugs, and weight loss drugs). Specific therapeutic targets recommended by the American Heart Association/National Heart, Lung, and Blood Institute statement[20] on metabolic syndrome focus on atherogenic dyslipidemia, elevated blood pressure, elevated glucose, and prothrombotic and proinflammatory states (Table 22-3).

Dyslipidemia

For atherogenic dyslipidemia, LDL-C remains the primary target of therapy. Goals are consistent with the NCEP guidelines, namely, <100 mg/dL in high-risk patients (with an option for <70 mg/dL), <130 mg/dL in moderately high risk subjects (with an option for <100 mg/dL), <130 mg/dL in moderate-risk patients, and <160 mg/dL in lower-risk patients. In addition, non–HDL-C is a secondary target for therapy when triglycerides are 200 mg/dL or greater; goals are 30 mg/dL higher than the respective LDL-C targets. HDL-C remains a tertiary target of therapy; lifestyle or pharmacologic therapy is recommended to raise HDL-C levels <40 mg/dL in men or <50 mg/dL in women (see Table 22-3).

Treatment of dyslipidemia associated with metabolic syndrome with fibrates or niacin, especially in combination with statins, has been shown to be effective in addressing elevated triglycerides and low HDL-C, which are highly prevalent in persons with metabolic syndrome. Post hoc analysis of several of the fibrate studies shows that those with metabolic syndrome derive a disproportionately large reduction in cardiovascular events with treatment by these agents.[126] A meta-analysis of the Familial Atherosclerosis Treatment Study (FATS), the HDL-Atherosclerosis Treatment Study (HATS), and the Armed Forces Regression Study (AFREGS) showed that patients with metabolic syndrome had 50% more rapid coronary stenosis progression than did those without metabolic syndrome and that combination of lowering LDL-C plus increasing HDL-C resulted in added benefit.[127] Combination therapy with a statin and fibrate or niacin resulted in a 54% decrease in cardiovascular events in those with metabolic

TABLE 22–2 | **Treatment of Lifestyle Risk Factors for Long-Term Prevention of Atherosclerotic Cardiovascular Disease or Prevention and Treatment of Type 2 Diabetes**

Therapeutic Target and Goals of Therapy	Therapeutic Recommendations
Abdominal Obesity Goal: Reduce total body weight by 7%-10% during first year of therapy. Continue weight loss thereafter to extent possible, with goal to ultimately achieve desirable weight (BMI <25 kg/m²)	Consistently encourage weight maintenance or reduction through appropriate balance of physical activity, calorie intake, and formal behavioral programs when indicated to maintain or to achieve waist circumference of <40 inches in men and <35 inches in women. Aim initially at slow reduction of 7% to 10% from baseline weight. Even small amounts of weight loss are associated with significant health benefits.
Physical Inactivity Goal: Regular moderate-intensity physical activity; at least 30 min of continuous/intermittent (preferably 60 min) 5 days/wk, but preferably daily	In patients with established CVD, assess risk with detailed physical activity history or exercise test to guide prescription. Encourage 30-60 min moderate-intensity aerobic activity (e.g., brisk walking), preferably daily, supplemented by increase in daily lifestyle activities (e.g., pedometer step tracking, walking breaks at work, gardening, household work). Higher exercise times can be achieved by accumulating exercise throughout day. Encourage resistance training 2 days/wk. Advise medically supervised programs for high-risk patients (e.g., recent acute coronary syndrome or revascularization, congestive heart failure).
Atherogenic Diet Goal: Reduced intakes of saturated fat, *trans*-fat, cholesterol	Recommendations: Saturated fat <7% of total calories; reduce *trans*-fat; dietary cholesterol <200 mg/day; total fat 25%-35% of total calories. Most dietary fat should be unsaturated; simple sugars should be limited.

Modified from Grundy SM: Metabolic syndrome scientific statement by the American Heart Association and the National Heart, Lung, and Blood Institute. *Arterioscler Thromb Vasc Biol* 25:2243, 2005.

syndrome; each 10% decrease in LDL-C or 10% increase in HDL-C was associated with an 11% or 22% event risk reduction, respectively. The evidence supports treatment of dyslipidemia associated with metabolic syndrome, beyond statin therapy for LDL-C, to include fibrates or niacin, used in combination with statins to incrementally improve HDL-C and triglycerides in addition to LDL-C. The safety of combination lipid therapy is better established, with fenofibrate lacking the well-known strong interaction of statins with gemfibrozil.

Elevated Glucose Concentration

The goal is to delay progression to type 2 diabetes for patients with impaired fasting glucose or to reduce the HbA1c to <7.0% if the patient is diabetic (although recent guidelines have suggested less stringent guidelines for those with long-standing diabetes or diabetes complicated by other comorbidities including CVD). Weight reduction and increased physical activity remain the primary intervention for persons with impaired fasting glucose, and in those with diabetes, pharmacotherapy should be supplemented as needed to reach HbA1c goals (see Table 22-3).

Metformin, a biguanide, improves insulin sensitivity and decreases hepatic glucose output. The Diabetes Prevention Program demonstrated that metformin is effective at slowing onset of diabetes in those with impaired glucose tolerance, but participants taking metformin in the Diabetes Prevention Program trial did not have significant resolution of metabolic syndrome compared with those taking placebo.[128] Studies done with rimonabant (which was marketed for only a brief period in Europe and never came to market in the United States) did show approximately one third of participants taking the drug for 1 year to have resolution of metabolic syndrome.[129-131] The goals for cardiovascular risk factor control are similar to those for patients with diabetes.

Currently, only metformin is recommended as an option for therapy in persons with impaired fasting glucose; there are no such recommendations for thiazolidinediones or other antidiabetic agents at present.[132,133] Drugs that could potentially target insulin resistance include weight loss drugs, PPARα agonists (fibrates), and PPARγ agonists (thiazolidinediones).

In persons with diabetes, fibrates and thiazolidinediones have also been shown to have benefits. In the recent PROACTIVE clinical trial, although the primary composite endpoint was not reduced significantly in those receiving pioglitazone, the principal secondary endpoint of myocardial infarction, stroke, or CVD death was significantly reduced in the group receiving pioglitazone.[134] Also, in the Fenofibrate Intervention and Event Lowering in Diabetes (FIELD) study, although the effect of fenofibrate on the primary study endpoint of CHD events in the entire trial was not significant, there was a reduction in CVD events in those with low HDL-C, high triglycerides, or hypertension.[135] The thiazolidinediones lessen insulin resistance and modestly improve various metabolic risk factors. Moreover, the thiazolidinedione rosiglitazone in the Diabetes Reduction Assessment with Ramipril and Rosiglitazone Medication (DREAM) trial and the thiazolidinedione pioglitazone in the ACT-NOW study, administered to subjects with prediabetes, showed significant reductions in the onset of diabetes.[136,137]

Elevated Blood Pressure

Blood pressure goals call for a reduction of blood pressure to at least <140/90 mm Hg (or <130/80 mm Hg if diabetes is present); and if blood pressure is at or above 120/80 mm Hg, lifestyle modification is initiated or maintained by weight control, increased physical activity, alcohol moderation, and sodium restriction. Pharmacologic therapy should be supplemented as needed when blood pressure is ≥140/90 mm Hg (see Table 22-3), although more recent guidelines call for lower targets of <130/80 mm Hg in persons at intermediate or higher risk with multiple risk factors whose 10-year risk of CHD exceeds 10% (many metabolic syndrome patients fit this criterion).[138] A recently recognized effect of angiotensin-converting enzyme inhibitors and angiotensin receptor blockers is a consistent reduction in the incidence of new-onset diabetes among patients with essential hypertension. Thus, pharmacologic blockade of the RAS, in addition to having proven benefits in reducing cardiovascular events and reducing progression of renal disease, may also be able to prevent the development of diabetes. Elucidation of the mechanisms by which these drugs prevent or delay diabetes might open the door to new therapeutic strategies.

TABLE 22–3 | Therapy for Metabolic Risk Factors for Prevention of Atherosclerotic Cardiovascular Disease or Treatment of Type 2 Diabetes

Therapeutic Target and Goals of Therapy	Therapeutic Recommendations
Atherogenic Dyslipidemia Primary target: LDL-C Reduce LDL-C levels to ATP III goals (see Therapeutic Recommendations).	For elevated LDL-C: Give priority to reduction of LDL-C over other lipid parameters. Achieve LDL-C goals based on patient's risk category. LDL-C goals for different risk categories: High risk*: <100 mg/dL (optional <70 mg/dL for very-high-risk patients[†]) Moderately high risk[‡]: <130 mg/dL (optional <100 mg/dL) Moderate risk[§]: <130 mg/dL Lower risk[||]: <160 mg/dL
Secondary target: non-HDL-C If TG ≥200 mg/dL, reduce non-HDL-C to ATP III goals (after attaining LDL-C goals; see Therapeutic Recommendations).	If TG ≥200 mg/dL, goal for non-HDL-C for each risk category is 30 mg/dL higher than for LDL-C. If TG ≥200 mg/dL after achieving LDL-C goal, consider additional therapies to attain non-HDL-C goal.
Tertiary target: HDL-C If HDL-C <40 mg/dL in men or <50 mg/dL in women after attaining non-HDL-C goal, raise HDL-C to extent possible with standard therapies for atherogenic dyslipidemia.	For reduced HDL-C: If HDL-C is low after achieving non-HDL-C, either lifestyle therapy can be intensified or drug therapy can be used for raising HDL-C levels, depending on patient's risk category.
Elevated BP Reduce BP to at least achieve BP of <140/90 mm Hg (or <130/80 mm Hg if diabetes is present). Reduce BP further to extent possible through lifestyle changes.	For BP ≥120/80 mm Hg: Initiate or maintain lifestyle modification by weight control, increased physical activity, alcohol moderation, sodium reduction, and emphasis on increased consumption of fresh fruits, vegetables, and low-fat dairy products in all patients with metabolic syndrome. For BP ≥140/90 mm Hg (or ≥130/80 mm Hg if diabetes is present), add BP medication as needed to achieve goal BP.
Elevated Glucose For IFG, delay progression to type 2 diabetes mellitus. For diabetes, hemoglobin A1c <7%.	For IFG, encourage weight reduction and increased physical activity. For type 2 diabetes, lifestyle therapy and pharmacotherapy, if necessary, should be used to achieve near-normal HbA1c (<7%). Modify other risk factors and behaviors (e.g., abdominal obesity, physical inactivity, elevated BP, lipid abnormalities).
Prothrombotic State Reduce thrombotic and fibrinolytic risk factors	For high-risk patients, initiate and continue low-dose aspirin therapy; in patients with ASCVD, consider clopidogrel if aspirin is contraindicated. For moderately high risk patients, consider low-dose aspirin prophylaxis.
Proinflammatory state	Recommendations: No specific therapies beyond lifestyle therapies

*High-risk patients have established atherosclerotic CVD, diabetes, or 10-year risk for CHD >20%. For cerebrovascular disease, high-risk conditions include transient ischemic attack or stroke of carotid origin or >50% carotid stenosis.

†Very-high-risk patients are likely to have major CVD events during next few years; diagnosis depends on clinical assessment. Factors that may confer very high risk include recent acute coronary syndromes, established CHD plus multiple major risk factors (especially diabetes), severe and poorly controlled risk factors (especially continued cigarette smoking), and metabolic syndrome.

‡Moderately high risk patients have 10-year risk for CHD of 10% to 20%. Factors favoring therapeutic option of non-HDL-C <100 mg/dL are those that can elevate patients to upper range of moderately high risk: multiple major risk factors, severe and poorly controlled risk factors (especially continued cigarette smoking), metabolic syndrome, and documented advanced subclinical atherosclerotic disease (e.g., coronary calcium or carotid intima-media thickness >75th percentile for age and sex).

§Moderate-risk patients have ≥2 major risk factors and 10-year risk <10%.

||Lower-risk patients have 0-1 major risk factor and 10-year risk <10%.

ASCVD, atherosclerotic cardiovascular disease; BP, blood pressure; CHD, coronary heart disease; IFG, impaired fasting glucose; TG, triglycerides.

Modified from Grundy SM: Metabolic syndrome scientific statement by the American Heart Association and the National Heart, Lung, and Blood Institute. *Arterioscler Thromb Vasc Biol* 25:2243, 2005.

Two large clinical trials, the Heart Outcomes Prevention Evaluation (HOPE) study (ramipril) and Losartan Intervention For Endpoint (LIFE) reduction in hypertension study (losartan), have demonstrated the benefit of blocking the RAS with either an angiotensin-converting enzyme inhibitor or angiotensin receptor blocker and the improvement in insulin sensitivity.[139,140] Other clinical studies have shown that inhibition of the RAS with either angiotensin-converting enzyme inhibitors or angiotensin receptor blockers results in increasing levels of adiponectin, which is associated with improved insulin sensitivity.[141]

A prospective long-term randomized trial assessed the effectiveness of an angiotensin receptor blocker in reducing the incidence of diabetes among those with metabolic syndrome. Results from the DREAM trial concluded that among persons with impaired fasting glucose levels or impaired glucose tolerance, the use of ramipril (compared with placebo) did not significantly reduce the incidence of diabetes or death but did improve normoglycemia.[136]

Prothrombotic and Proinflammatory States

To reduce thrombotic risk, low-dose aspirin therapy is initiated or continued in moderately high risk (e.g., when 10-year risk of CHD is 10% or greater) or high-risk patients; and in those with CVD, clopidogrel is considered if aspirin is contraindicated. For proinflammatory states, there are no specific recommended therapies beyond lifestyle modifications, however (see Table 22-2).

CONCLUSION

The metabolic syndrome is associated with an increased risk for development of diabetes, CHD, and CVD. Whereas diabetes is frequently regarded as a CHD risk equivalent, a wide spectrum of risk for CHD is present in persons with metabolic syndrome (but without diabetes), necessitating careful assessment of cardiovascular risk. Although initial global risk assessment can use Framingham or other risk algorithms, consideration should be given to stratification of risk by the presence and extent of other metabolic syndrome risk factors, novel risk markers, and measures of subclinical atherosclerosis.

Health care providers should regularly assess for the presence of multiple risk factors as well as metabolic syndrome at regular intervals in each patient. Identification of the metabolic syndrome as a clinical condition will also accustom physicians to simultaneous treatment of multiple risk factors (particularly abdominal obesity, dyslipidemia, and elevated blood pressure), instead of the traditional model of treatment of risk factors in isolation. Most important, intensified efforts at lifestyle therapies, including effective dietary and physical activity counseling by trained individuals who can provide the necessary guidance and follow-up, are needed and crucial if significant strides are to be made in reducing the prevalence of metabolic syndrome and its future diabetic and cardiovascular complications.

REFERENCES

1. Reaven G: Role of insulin resistance in human disease. *Diabetes* 37:1595, 1988.
2. Ford ES, Giles WH, Mokdad AH: Increasing prevalence of the metabolic syndrome among U.S. adults. *Diabetes Care* 27:2444, 2004.
3. Goodman E, Daniels SR, Morrison JA, et al: Contrasting prevalence of and demographic disparities in the World Health Organization and National Cholesterol Education Program Adult Treatment Panel III definitions of metabolic syndrome among adolescents. *J Pediatr* 145:445, 2004.
4. Kylin E: Studien über das Hypertonie-Hyperglykämie-Hyperurikämiesyndrom. *Zentralbl Innere Medizin* 44:105, 1923.
5. Expert Panel on Detection, Evaluation, and Treatment of High Blood Cholesterol in Adults: Executive Summary of the third report of the National Cholesterol Education Program (NCEP) Expert Panel on Detection, Evaluation, and Treatment of High Blood Cholesterol in Adults (ATP III). *JAMA* 285:2486, 2001.
6. Alberti KG, Zimmet P, Shaw J; IDF Epidemiology Task Force Consensus Group: The metabolic syndrome—a new worldwide definition. *Lancet* 366:1059, 2005.
7. Kahn R, Buse J, Ferrannini E, et al: The metabolic syndrome: time for a critical appraisal: joint statement from the American Diabetes Association and the European Association for the Study of Diabetes. *Diabetes Care* 28:2289, 2005.
8. Grundy SM: Metabolic syndrome scientific statement by the American Heart Association and the National Heart, Lung, and Blood Institute. *Arterioscler Thromb Vasc Biol* 25:2243, 2005.
9. Brietzke SA: Controversy in diagnosis and management of the metabolic syndrome. *Med Clin North Am* 91:1041, 2007.
10. Blaha M, Elasy TA: Clinical use of the metabolic syndrome: why the confusion? *Clin Diabetes* 24:125, 2006.
11. Reaven G: The metabolic syndrome or the insulin resistance syndrome? Different names, different concepts, and different goals. *Endocrinol Metab Clin North Am* 33:283, 2004.
12. Eckel RH, Grundy SM, Zimmet PZ: The metabolic syndrome. *Lancet* 365:1415, 2005.
13. Ferrannini E: Is insulin resistance the cause of the metabolic syndrome? *Ann Med* 38:42, 2006.
14. Steinberg HO, Baron AD: Vascular function, insulin resistance, and fatty acids. *Diabetologia* 45:623, 2002.
15. Reaven GM: Role of insulin resistance in human disease. *Diabetes* 37:1595, 1988.
16. Trayhurn P, Wood IS: Adipokines: inflammation and the pleiotropic role of white adipose tissue. *Br J Nutr* 92:347, 2004.
17. Alberti KG, Zimmet PZ: Definition, diagnosis and classification of diabetes mellitus and its complications. Part 1: diagnosis and classification of diabetes mellitus. Provisional report of a WHO Consultation. *Diabet Med* 15:539, 1998.
18. World Health Organization: *Definition, diagnosis and classification of diabetes mellitus and its complications. Part 1: diagnosis and classification of diabetes mellitus*, Geneva, 1999, Department of Noncommunicable Disease Surveillance. WHO/NCD/NCS/99.2.
19. Del Prato S, Maran A, Beck-Nielsen H, on behalf of EGIR: The plurimetabolic syndrome in the European population: the experience of the European Group for the Study of Insulin Resistance. In Crepaldi G, Tiengo A, Del Prato S, editors: *Insulin resistance, metabolic diseases and diabetic complications*, New York, 1999, Elsevier Science, pp 25-30.
20. Grundy SM, Cleeman JI, Daniels SR, et al: Diagnosis and management of the metabolic syndrome. An American Heart Association/National Heart, Lung and Blood Institute Scientific Statement. *Circulation* 112:2735, 2005.
21. Ervin RB: *Prevalence of metabolic syndrome among adults 20 years of age and over, by sex, age, race and ethnicity, and body mass index: United States, 2003-2006*, National health statistics reports, no 13, Hyattsville, Md, 2009, National Center for Health Statistics.
22. Ford ES: Prevalence of the metabolic syndrome defined by the International Diabetes Federation among adults in the U.S. *Diabetes Care* 28:2745, 2005.
23. Ford ES, Giles WH, Dietz WH: Prevalence of the metabolic syndrome in U.S. adults. *JAMA* 287:356, 2002.
24. Ford ES, Giles WH, Mokdad AH: Increasing prevalence of the metabolic syndrome among U.S. adults. *Diabetes Care* 27:2444, 2004.
25. Cameron AJ, Shaw JE, Zimmet PZ: The metabolic syndrome: prevalence in worldwide populations. *Endocrinol Metab Clin North Am* 33:351, 2004.
26. Tillin T, Forhouhi N, Johnston DG, et al: Metabolic syndrome and coronary heart disease in South Asians, African-Caribbeans and white Europeans: a UK population-based cross-sectional study. *Dibetologia* 48:649, 2005.
27. Hu G, Qiao Q, Tuomilehto J, et al: Prevalence of the metabolic syndrome and its relation to all-cause and cardiovascular mortality in nondiabetic European men and women. *Arch Intern Med* 164:1066, 2004.
28. Athyros VG, Ganotakis ES, Elisaf M, Mikhailidis DP: The prevalence of the metabolic syndrome using the National Cholesterol Education Program and International Diabetes Federation definitions. *Curr Med Res Opin* 21:1157, 2005.
29. Miccoli R, Bianchi C, Odoguardi L, et al: Prevalence of the metabolic syndrome among Italian adults according to the ATP III definition. *Nutr Metab Cardiovasc Dis* 15:250, 2005.
30. Lorenzo C, Williams K, Gonzalez-Villalpando C, Haffner SM: The prevalence of the metabolic syndrome did not increase in Mexico City between 1990-1992 and 1997-1999 despite more central obesity. *Diabetes Care* 28:2480, 2005.
31. Aguilar S, Salinas CA, Rojas R, et al: High prevalence of metabolic syndrome in Mexico. *Arch Med Res* 35:76, 2004.
32. Ko GT, Cockram CS, Chow CC, et al: High prevalence of metabolic syndrome in Hong Kong Chinese—comparison of three diagnostic criteria. *Diabetes Res Clin Pract* 69:160, 2005.
33. Thomas GN, Ho SY, Janus ED, et al: The US National Cholesterol Education Program Adult Treatment Panel III (NCEP ATP III) prevalence of the metabolic syndrome in a Chinese population. *Diabetes Res Clin Pract* 67:251, 2005.
34. Choi SH, Ahgn CW, Cha BS, et al: The prevalence of the metabolic syndrome in Korean adults. *Yonsei Med J* 46:198, 2005.
35. Enkhmaa ZB, Shiwaku K, Anuurad E: Prevalence of the metabolic syndrome using the Third Report of the National Cholesterol Education Program Expert Panel on Detection, Evaluation, and Treatment of High Blood Cholesterol in Adults (ATP III) and the modified ATP III definitions for Japanese and Mongolians. *Clin Chim Acta* 352:105, 2005.
36. Johnson WD, Kroon JJ, Greenway FL, et al: Prevalence of risk factors for metabolic syndrome in adolescents: National Health and Nutrition Examination Survey (NHANES) 2001-2006. *Arch Pediatr Adolesc Med* 163:371, 2009.
37. Molnar D: The prevalence of the metabolic syndrome and type 2 diabetes mellitus in children and adolescents. *Int J Obes Relat Metab Disord* 28(Suppl 3):S70, 2004.
38. Goodman E, Daniels SR, Morrison JA, et al: Contrasting prevalence of and demographic disparities in the World Health Organization and National Cholesterol Education Program Adult Treatment Panel III definitions of metabolic syndrome among adolescents. *J Pediatr* 145:445, 2004.
39. Tailor AM, Peeters PH, Norat T, et al: An update on the prevalence of metabolic syndrome in children and adolescents. *Int J Pediatr Obes* 5:202, 2010.
40. Sattar N, McConnachie A, Shaper GA, et al: Can metabolic syndrome usefully predict cardiovascular disease and diabetes? Outcome data from two prospective studies. *Lancet* 371:1927, 2008.
41. Lorenzo C, Williams K, Hunt KJ, Haffner SM: The National Cholesterol Education Program–Adult Treatment Panel III, International Diabetes Federation, and World Health Organization definitions of the metabolic syndrome as predictors of incident cardiovascular disease and diabetes. *Diabetes Care* 30:8, 2007.
42. Haffner SM, Lehto S, Ronnemaa T, et al: Mortality from coronary heart disease in subjects with type 2 diabetes and in nondiabetic subjects with and without prior myocardial infarction. *N Engl J Med* 339:229, 1998.
43. Malik S, Wong ND, Franklin SS, et al: Impact of the metabolic syndrome on mortality from coronary heart disease, cardiovascular disease, and all causes in United States adults. *Circulation* 110:1239, 2004.
44. Alexander CM, Landsman PB, Teutsch SM, Haffner SM: NCEP-defined metabolic syndrome, diabetes, and prevalence of coronary heart disease among NHANES III participants age 50 years and older. *Diabetes* 52:1210, 2003.
45. Gorter PM, Olijhoek JK, van der Graaf Y, et al; SMART Study Group: Prevalence of the metabolic syndrome in patients with coronary heart disease, cerebrovascular disease, peripheral arterial disease, or abdominal aortic aneurysm. *Atherosclerosis* 173:363, 2004.
46. Sattar N, Gaw A, Scherbakova O, et al: Metabolic syndrome with and without C-reactive protein as a predictor of coronary heart disease and diabetes in the West of Scotland Coronary Prevention Study. *Circulation* 108:414, 2003.
47. Lakka HM, Laaksonen DE, Lakka TA, et al: The metabolic syndrome and total and cardiovascular mortality in middle-aged men. *JAMA* 288:2709, 2002.
48. Jeppesen J, Hansen TW, Rasmussen S, et al: Insulin resistance, the metabolic syndrome, and risk of incident cardiovascular disease. *J Am Coll Cardiol* 49:2112, 2007.
49. Rutter MK, Meigs JB, Sullivan LM, et al: C-reactive protein, the metabolic syndrome, and prediction of cardiovascular events in the Framingham Offspring Study. *Circulation* 110:380, 2004.
50. McNeill AM, Rosamond WD, Girman CJ, et al: The metabolic syndrome and 11-year incident cardiovascular disease in the atherosclerosis risk in communities study. *Diabetes Care* 28:385, 2005.
51. Scuteri A, Najjar SS, Morrell CH, Lakatta EG: The metabolic syndrome in older individuals: prevalence and prediction of cardiovascular events: the Cardiovascular Health Study. *Diabetes Care* 28:82, 2005.
52. Hunt KJ, Resendez RG, Williams K, et al; San Antonio Heart Study: National Cholesterol Education Program versus World Health Organization metabolic syndrome in relation to all-cause and cardiovascular mortality in the San Antonio Heart Study. *Circulation* 110:1251, 2004.

53. Katzmarzyk PT, Church TS, Blair SN: Cardiorespiratory fitness attenuates the effects of the metabolic syndrome on all-cause and cardiovascular disease mortality. *Arch Intern Med* 164:1092, 2004.
54. Eberly LE, Prineas R, Cohen JD, et al: Metabolic syndrome: risk factor distribution and 18-year mortality in the Multiple Risk Factor Intervention Trial. *Diabetes Care* 29:123, 2006.
55. Ford ES: Risks for all-cause mortality, cardiovascular disease, and diabetes associated with the metabolic syndrome: summary of the evidence. *Diabetes Care* 28:1769, 2005.
56. Sattar N, McConnachie A, Shaper A, et al: Can metabolic syndrome usefully predict cardiovascular disease and diabetes? Outcome data from two prospective studies. *Lancet* 371:1927, 2008.
57. Mozaffarian D, Kamineni A, Prineas RJ, Siscovick DS: Metabolic syndrome and mortality in older adults: the Cardiovascular Health Study. *Arch Intern Med* 168:969, 2008.
58. Gami AS, Witt BJ, Howard DE, et al: Metabolic syndrome and risk of incident cardiovascular events and death. *J Am Coll Cardiol* 49:403, 2007.
59. Koren-Morag N, Goldbourt U, Tanne D: Relation between the metabolic syndrome and ischemic stroke or transient ischemic attack: a prospective cohort study in patients with atherosclerotic cardiovascular disease. *Stroke* 36:1366, 2005.
60. Kawamoto R, Tomita H, Oka Y, Kodama A: Metabolic syndrome as a predictor of ischemic stroke in elderly persons. *Intern Med* 44:922, 2005.
61. Milionis JH, Rizos E, Goudevenos J, et al: Components of the metabolic syndrome and risk for first-ever acute ischemic nonembolic stroke in elderly subjects. *Stroke* 36:1372, 2005.
62. Schwartz GG, Olsson AG, Szarek M, Sasiela WJ: Relation of characteristics of metabolic syndrome to short-term prognosis and effects of intensive statin therapy after acute coronary syndrome: an analysis of the Myocardial Ischemia Reduction with Aggressive Cholesterol Lowering (MIRACL) trial. *Diabetes Care* 28:2508, 2005.
63. Levantesi G, Macchia A, Marfisi R, et al: Metabolic syndrome and risk of cardiovascular events after myocardial infarction. *J Am Coll Cardiol* 46:277, 2005.
64. Pyorala K, Ballantyne CM, Gumbiner B, et al: Reduction of cardiovascular events by simvastatin in nondiabetic coronary heart disease patients with and without the metabolic syndrome: subgroup analysis of the Scandinavian Simvastatin Survival Study (4S). *Diabetes Care* 27:1735, 2004.
65. Third report of the National Cholesterol Education Program (NCEP) expert panel on the detection, evaluation, and treatment of high blood cholesterol in adults (Adult Treatment Panel III): final report. *Circulation* 106:3143, 2002.
66. Hoang KC, Ghandehari H, Lopez VA, et al: Global coronary heart disease risk assessment of individuals with metabolic syndrome in the U.S.. *Diabetes Care* 31:1405, 2008.
67. Grundy SM, Cleeman JI, Daniels SR, et al: Diagnosis and management of the metabolic syndrome: an American Heart Association/National Heart, Lung, and Blood Institute Scientific Statement. *Circulation* 112:2735, 2005.
68. Stevens RJ, Kothari V, Adler AI, et al; on behalf of the United Kingdom Prospective Diabetes Study (UKPDS) Group: The UKPDS risk engine: a model for the risk of coronary heart disease in type II diabetes (UKPDS 56). *Clin Sci* 101:671, 2001.
69. Song SH, Brown PM: Coronary heart disease risk assessment in diabetes mellitus: comparison of UKPDS risk engine with Framingham risk assessment function and its clinical implications. *Diabet Med* 21:238, 2004.
70. Guzder RN, Gatling W, Mullee MA, et al: Prognostic value of the Framingham cardiovascular risk equation and the UKPDS risk engine for coronary heart disease in newly diagnosed type 2 diabetes: results from a United Kingdom study. *Diabet Med* 22:554, 2005.
71. International Diabetes Federation: Worldwide definition of the metabolic syndrome. Available at: http://www.idf.org/webdata/docs/IDF_Meta-syndrome_definition.pdf. Accessed November 10, 2009.
72. Guzder RN, Gatling W, Mullee MA, et al: Prognostic value of the Framingham cardiovascular risk equation and the UKPDS risk engine for coronary heart disease in newly diagnosed type 2 diabetes: results from a United Kingdom study. *Diabet Med* 22:554, 2005.
73. Assmann G, Schulte H, Seedorf U: Cardiovascular risk assessment in the metabolic syndrome: results from the Prospective Cardiovascular Munster (PROCAM) study. *Int J Obes* 32:S11, 2008.
74. Rutter MK, Meigs JB, Sullivan LM, et al: C-reactive protein, the metabolic syndrome, and prediction of cardiovascular events in the Framingham Offspring study. *Circulation* 110:380, 2004.
75. Malik S, Wong ND, Frankin SS, et al: Cardiovascular disease in US persons with metabolic syndrome, diabetes, and elevated C-reactive protein. *Diabetes Care* 28:690, 2005.
76. Ridker PM, Danielson E, Fonseca FA: Rosuvastatin to prevent vascular events in men and women with elevated C-reactive protein. *N Engl J Med* 21:2195, 2008.
77. The Emerging Risk Factors Collaboration: C-reactive protein concentration and risk of coronary heart disease, stroke, and mortality: an individual participant meta-analysis. *Lancet* 375:132, 2010.
78. Wilson PW, Smith SC, Blumenthal RS, et al: 34th Bethesda Conference: Task force #4—How do we select patients for atherosclerosis imaging? *J Am Coll Cardiol* 41:1898, 2003.
79. Greenland P, Bonow RO, Brundage BH, et al: ACCF/AHA 2007 clinical expert consensus document on coronary artery calcium scoring by computed tomography in global cardiovascular risk assessment and in evaluation of patients with chest pain. *J Am Coll Cardiol* 49:378, 2007.
80. Ingelsson E, Sullivan LM, Murabito JM, et al: Prevalence and prognostic impact of subclinical cardiovascular disease in individuals with the metabolic syndrome and diabetes. *Diabetes* 56:1718, 2007.
81. Bots ML, Grobbee DE: Intima media thickness as a surrogate marker for generalized atherosclerosis. *Cardiovasc Drugs Ther* 16:341, 2002.
82. Montalcini T, Gorgone G, Gazzaruso C, et al: Carotid atherosclerosis associated to metabolic syndrome but not BMI in healthy menopausal women. *Diabetes Res Clin Pract* 76:378, 2007.
83. Bonora E, Kiechl S, Willeit J, et al: Carotid atherosclerosis and coronary heart disease in the metabolic syndrome: prospective data from the Bruneck study. *Diabetes Care* 26:1251, 2003.
84. Hassinen M, Komulainen P, Lakka TA, et al: Metabolic syndrome and the progression of carotid intima-media thickness in elderly women. *Arch Intern Med* 166:444, 2006.
85. McNeill AM, Rosamond WD, Girman CJ, et al: Prevalence of coronary heart disease and carotid arterial thickening in patients with the metabolic syndrome (the ARIC study). *Am J Cardiol* 94:1249, 2004.
86. McNeill AM, Rosamond WD, Girman CJ, et al: The metabolic syndrome and 11-year risk of incident cardiovascular disease in the atherosclerosis risk in communities study. *Diabetes Care* 28:385, 2003.
87. Tzou WS, Douglas PS, Srinivasan SR: Increased subclinical atherosclerosis in young adults with metabolic syndrome: the Bogalusa Heart Study. *J Am Coll Cardiol* 46:457, 2005.
88. Salonen R, Nyyssonen K, Porkkala E, et al: Kuopio Atherosclerosis Prevention Study (KAPS): a population-based primary prevention trial of the effect of LDL lowering on atherosclerotic progression in carotid and femoral arteries. *Circulation* 92:1758, 1995.
89. Furberg CD, Adams HP, Applegate WB, et al: Effect of lovastatin on early carotid atherosclerosis and cardiovascular events. Asymptomatic Carotid Artery Progression Study (ACAPS) Research Group. *Circulation* 90:1679, 1994.
90. Arad Y, Spadaro LA, Goodman K, et al: Prediction of coronary events with electron-beam computed tomography. *J Am Coll Cardiol* 36:1253, 2000.
91. Raggi P, Callister TQ, Cooil B, et al: Identification of patients at increased risk of first unheralded acute myocardial infarction by electron-beam computed tomography. *Circulation* 101:850, 2000.
92. Wong ND, Sciammarella MG, Polk D: The metabolic syndrome, diabetes, and subclinical atherosclerosis assessed by coronary calcium. *J Am Coll Cardiol* 41:1547, 2003.
93. Kullo IJ, Cassidy AE, Peyser PA, et al: Association between metabolic syndrome and subclinical coronary atherosclerosis in asymptomatic adults. *Am J Cardiol* 94:1554, 2004.
94. Chen K, Lindsey JB, Khera A, et al: Independent associations between metabolic syndrome, diabetes mellitus and atherosclerosis: observations from the Dallas Heart Study. *Diab Vasc Dis Res* 5:96, 2008.
95. Campbell CY, Nasir K, Sarwar A, et al: Combined effect of high low-density lipoprotein cholesterol and metabolic syndrome on subclinical coronary atherosclerosis in white men without clinical evidence of myocardial ischemia. *Am J Cardiol* 100:840, 2007.
96. Nasir K, Santos RD, Tufail K, et al: High-normal fasting blood glucose in non-diabetic range is associated with increased coronary artery calcium burden in asymptomatic men. *Atherosclerosis* 195:e155, 2007.
97. Santos RD, Nasir K, Tufail K, et al: Metabolic syndrome is associated with coronary artery calcium in asymptomatic white Brazilian men considered low-risk by Framingham Risk Score. *Prev Cardiol* 10:141, 2007.
98. Pundziute G, Schuijf JD, Jukema JW, et al: Prognostic value of multislice computed tomography coronary angiography in patients with known or suspected coronary artery disease. *J Am Coll Cardiol* 49:62, 2007.
99. Butler J, Mooyaart EA, Dannemann N, et al: Relation of the metabolic syndrome to quantity of coronary atherosclerotic plaque. *Am J Cardiol* 8:1127, 2008.
100. Criqui MH, Langer Rd, Fronek A, et al: Mortality over a period of 10 years in patients with peripheral arterial disease. *N Engl J Med* 326:381, 1992.
101. Neuman AB, Sutton-Tyrrell K, et al: Morbidity and mortality in hypertensive adults with a low ankle/arm blood pressure index. *JAMA* 270:487, 1993.
102. Olijhoek JK, van der Graaf Y, Banga JD, et al: The metabolic syndrome is associated with advanced vascular damage in patients with coronary heart disease, stroke, peripheral arterial disease or abdominal aortic aneurysm. *Eur Heart J* 25:342, 2004.
103. Wong ND, Rozanski AR, Gransar H, et al: Metabolic syndrome increases the likelihood of inducible myocardial ischemia among patients with subclinical atherosclerosis. *Diabetes Care* 28:1445, 2005.
104. Shaw LJ, Berman DS, Hendel RC, et al: Cardiovascular disease risk stratification with stress single-photon emission computed tomography technetium-99m tetrofosmin imaging in patients with the metabolic syndrome and diabetes mellitus. *Am J Cardiol* 97:1538, 2006.
105. Rudd JH, Myers KS, Bansilal S: ^{18}Fluorodeoxyglucose positron emission tomography imaging of atherosclerotic plaque inflammation is highly reproducible: implications for atherosclerosis therapy trials. *J Am Coll Cardiol* 9:892, 2007.
106. Tahara N, Kai H, Yamagishi S, et al: Vascular inflammation evaluated by [^{18}F]-fluorodeoxyglucose positron emission tomography is associated with the metabolic syndrome. *J Am Coll Cardiol* 49:1533, 2007.
107. Ahluwalia N, Drouet L, Ruidavets JB, et al: Metabolic syndrome is associated with markers of subclinical atherosclerosis in a French population-based sample. *Atherosclerosis* 186:345, 2006.
108. Burchfiel CM, Skelton TN, Andrew ME: Metabolic syndrome and echocardiographic left ventricular mass in blacks: the Atherosclerosis Risk in Communities (ARIC) study. *Circulation* 112:819, 2006.
109. Mule G, Nardi E, Cottone S, et al: Impact of metabolic syndrome on left ventricular mass in overweight and obese hypertensive subjects. *Int J Cardiol* 121:267, 2007.
110. de las Fuentes L, Brown AL, Mathews SJ, et al: Metabolic syndrome is associated with abnormal left ventricular diastolic function independent of left ventricular mass. *Int J Cardiol* 28:553, 2007.
111. Turhan H, Yasar AS, Yagmur J, et al: The impact of metabolic syndrome on left ventricular function: evaluated by using the index of myocardial performance. *Int J Cardiol* 132:382, 2009.
112. Wong ND, Pio JR, Franklin SS, et al: Preventing coronary events by optimal control of blood pressure and lipids in patients with the metabolic syndrome. *Am J Cardiol* 91:1421, 2003.
113. Lindström J, Louheranta A, Mannelin M, et al: The Finnish Diabetes Prevention Study (DPS): Lifestyle intervention and 3-year results on diet and physical activity. *Diabetes Care* 26:3230, 2003.

114. de Lorgeril M, Renaud S, Mamelle N, et al: Mediterranean alpha-linolenic acid–rich diet in secondary prevention of coronary heart disease. *Lancet* 343:1454, 1994.

115. Esposito K, Marfella R, Ciotola M, et al: Effect of a Mediterranean-style diet on endothelial dysfunction and markers of vascular inflammation in the metabolic syndrome: a randomized trial. *JAMA* 292:1440, 2004.

116. Trichopoulou A, Orfanos P, Norat T, et al: Modified Mediterranean diet and survival: EPIC-elderly prospective cohort study. *BMJ* 330:991, 2005.

117. Trichopoulou A, Bamia C, Trichopoulos D: Mediterranean diet and survival among patients with coronary heart disease in Greece. *Arch Intern Med* 165:929, 2005.

118. Ford ES, Mokdad AH, Giles WH, et al: The metabolic syndrome and antioxidant concentrations: findings from the third National Health and Nutrition Examination Survey. *Diabetes* 52:2346, 2003.

119. Pereira MA, Jacobs DR, Jr, Van Horn L, et al: Dairy consumption, obesity, and the insulin resistance syndrome in young adults: the CARDIA study. *JAMA* 287:2081, 2002.

120. McKeown NM, Meigs JB, Liu S, et al: Carbohydrate nutrition, insulin resistance, and the prevalence of metabolic syndrome in the Framingham Offspring Cohort. *Diabetes Care* 27:538, 2004.

121. Knowler WC, Barrett-Conner E, Fowler SE, et al; for the Diabetes Prevention Program Reasearch Group: Reduction in the incidence of type 2 diabetes with lifestyle intervention or metformin. *N Engl J Med* 346:393, 2002.

122. Tuomilehto J, Lindstrom J, Eriksson JG, et al; for the Finnish Diabetes Prevention Study Group: Prevention of type 2 diabetes mellitus by changes in lifestyle among subjects with impaired glucose tolerance. *N Engl J Med* 344:1343, 2001.

123. O'Malley PG, Kowalczyk C, Bindeman J, Taylor AJ: The impact of cardiovascular risk factor case management on the metabolic syndrome in a primary prevention population: results from a randomized control trial. *J Cardiometab Syndr* 1:6, 2006.

124. Mattar SG, Velcu LM, Rabinovitz M, et al: Surgically-induced weight loss significantly improves non-alcoholic fatty liver disease and the metabolic syndrome. *Ann Surg* 242:610, 2005.

125. Lee WJ, Huang MT, Wang W, et al: Effects of obesity surgery on the metabolic syndrome. *Arch Surg* 139:1088, 2004.

126. Barter PJ, Rye KA: Is there a role for fibrates in the management of dyslipidemia in the metabolic syndrome? *Arterioscler Thromb Vasc Biol* 28:39, 2008.

127. Zhao XQ, Krasuski RA, Baer J, et al: Effects of combination lipid therapy on coronary stenosis progression and clinical cardiovascular events in coronary disease patients with metabolic syndrome: a combined analysis of the Familial Atherosclerosis Treatment Study (FATS), the HDL-Atherosclerosis Treatment Study (HATS), and the Armed Forces Regression Study (AFREGS). *Am J Cardiol* 104:1457, 2009.

128. Orchard TJ, Tempros M, Goldberg R, et al: The effect of metformin and intensive lifestyle intervention on the metabolic syndrome: the Diabetes Prevention Program randomized trial. *Ann Intern Med* 142:611, 2005.

129. Van Gaal LF, Rissanen AM, Scheen AJ, et al; for the RIO-Europe Study Group: Effects of the cannabinoid-1 receptor blocker rimonabant on weight reduction and cardiovascular risk factors in overweight patients: 1-year experience from the RIO-Europe study. *Lancet* 365:1389, 2005.

130. Després J-P, Golay A, Sjöström L; for the Rimonabant in Obesity–Lipids Study Group: Effects of rimonabant on metabolic risk factors in overweight patients with dyslipidemia. *N Engl J Med* 353:2121, 2005.

131. Pi-Sunyer FX, Aronne LJ, Heshmati HM, et al; for the RIO-North America Study Group: Effect of rimonabant, a cannabinoid-1 receptor blocker, on weight and cardiometabolic risk factors in overweight or obese patients: RIO-North America: a randomized controlled trial. *JAMA* 295:761, 2006.

132. American Diabetes Association: Standards of medical care in diabetes—2009. *Diabetes Care* 32:S13, 2009.

133. Nathan DM, Davidson MB, DeFronzo RA, et al: Impaired fasting glucose and impaired glucose tolerance: implications for care. *Diabetes Care* 30:753, 2007.

134. Dormandy JA, Charbonnel B, Eckland DJ, et al; PROactive investigators: Secondary prevention of macrovascular events in patients with type 2 diabetes in the PROactive study. *Lancet* 366:1279, 2005.

135. Scott R, O'Brien R, Fulcher G, et al: Effect of fenofibrate treatment on cardiovascular disease risk in 9,795 individuals with type 2 diabetes and various components of the metabolic syndrome: the Fenofibrate Intervention and Event Lowering in Diabetes (FIELD) study. *Diabetes Care* 32:493, 2009.

136. The DREAM Trial Investigators: Effect of ramipril on the incidence of diabetes. *N Engl J Med* 355:1551, 2006.

137. Defronzo RA, Banerji M, Bray GA, et al: Actos Now for the prevention of diabetes (ACT NOW) study. *BMC Endocr Disord* 9:17, 2009.

138. Rosendorff C, Black HR, Cannon CP, et al: Treatment of hypertension in the prevention and management of ischemic heart disease; a scientific statement from the American Heart Association Council for High Blood Pressure Research and the Councils on Clinical Cardiology and Epidemiology and Prevention. *Circulation* 115:2761, 2007.

139. Yusuf S, Sleight P, Pogue J, et al: Effects of an angiotensin-converting enzyme inhibitor, ramipril, on cardiovascular event in high-risk patients. The heart outcomes prevention evaluation study investigators. *N Engl J Med* 342:145, 2000.

140. Dahlof B, Devereux RB, Kjeldsen SE, et al: Cardiovascular morbidity and mortality in the losartan intervention for endpoint reduction in hypertension study (LIFE): a randomized trial against atenolol. *Lancet* 359:995, 2002.

141. Furuhashi M, Ura N, Higashiura K, et al: Blockade of the renin-angiotensin system increases adiponectin concentrations in patients with essential hypertension. *Hypertension* 42:76, 2003.

Special Populations

CHAPTER **2 3**

Role of Ethnicity in Cardiovascular Disease: Lessons Learned from MESA and Other Population-Based Studies

Karol E. Watson and Ashkan Afshin

CARDIOVASCULAR DISEASE IN RACIAL AND ETHNIC MINORITIES: OVERVIEW AND PERSPECTIVES

Cardiovascular disease (CVD) is the leading cause of death in the United States and worldwide.[1] In 2001, heart disease accounted for approximately 29% of deaths among U.S. residents; 17% of those deaths occurred among persons aged <65 years.[2] From 1996 to 2006, death rates from CVD have decreased 29%; however, the decline has not been uniform for all populations.[3] It is well documented that cardiovascular morbidity and mortality rates differ among diverse racial and ethnic groups in the United States.[4]

Recent data from the Centers for Disease Control and Prevention reveal that African Americans have earlier and higher mortality rates from coronary heart disease (CHD) than those of whites, American Indian/Alaska Natives, Asian/Pacific Islanders, or Hispanics[4] (Fig. 23-1). Ethnic differences in the prevalence of complex diseases such as atherosclerosis are undoubtedly multifactorial. It is clear that there are social, environmental, biologic, genetic, and probably other determinants leading to the disparities in CHD.

Whereas earlier articles have explored many of these factors, ongoing large population-based and cohort studies are lending valuable insight. One of these studies, the Multi-Ethnic Study of Atherosclerosis (MESA), is adding important insights into

CVD among various ethnic groups in the United States. MESA was initiated in July 2000 to investigate the prevalence, correlates, and progression of subclinical CVD in a population-based sample of 6814 men and women aged 45 to 84 years. The cohort was selected from six United States field centers and is approximately 38% white, 28% African American, 23% Hispanic, and 11% Asian (primarily of Chinese descent). Baseline measurements taken included measurement of coronary calcium by computed tomography, measurement of ventricular mass and function by cardiac magnetic resonance imaging, measurement of flow-mediated brachial artery endothelial vasodilation, carotid intima-media wall thickness, and measurement of peripheral vascular disease by ankle and brachial blood pressures. Assessments of demographic measures, standard CVD risk factors, sociodemographic factors, life habits, and psychosocial factors were also made. Blood samples were assayed for blood chemistries, lipids, inflammatory markers, and DNA.

The MESA cohort has been observed since 2000 for identification and characterization of CVD events, including acute myocardial infarction and other CHD, stroke, peripheral arterial disease, heart failure, therapeutic interventions for CVD, and mortality. Thus, MESA and other epidemiologic studies will lend invaluable insights into the role of race and ethnicity in CVD.

This chapter summarizes currently available data on ethnic differences in CVD,

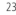

23

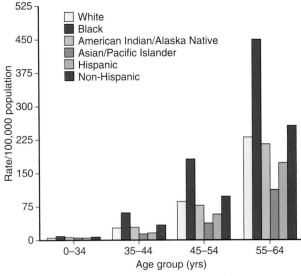

FIGURE 23-1 The 2001 CHD mortality rates among persons <65 years from different racial and ethnic groups. African Americans (blue bar) have higher CHD rates compared with all other groups. *(From Centers for Disease Control and Prevention [CDC]: Disparities in premature deaths from heart disease—50 States and the District of Columbia, 2001. MMWR Morb Mortal Wkly Rep 53:121, 2004.)*

cardiac risk factors, vascular biology, genetic factors, and socioeconomic determinants of atherosclerosis, but it is important to keep in mind that ethnic populations are far from homogeneous with respect to many genetic and biologic traits.[5] Nonetheless, investigation into variations among ethnic groups can be an important key to understanding the causes of complex genetic conditions like atherosclerosis. Such investigations can also lead to important research into pathophysiology and treatment, thus improving outcomes for all populations.

EPIDEMIOLOGY OF CARDIOVASCULAR RISK FACTORS AMONG RACIAL AND ETHNIC POPULATIONS IN THE UNITED STATES

Considerable information has been gathered about cardiovascular risk factors in ethnic populations. The major cardiac risk factors are the same in all ethnic and racial groups in the United States and worldwide; however, the demographics and relative weight attributed to each factor may differ. Among African Americans, for example, some of the excess CHD may be accounted for by the excess prevalence of known complicating risk factors, such as hypertension, left ventricular hypertrophy, and diabetes mellitus. Differences in other risk factors, such as plasma lipoprotein profiles, may not completely explain disparities but may lend insight into ethnic differences in the biology of atherosclerosis.

Hypertension

Worldwide, hypertension is known to account for considerable cardiovascular risk.[6] The INTERHEART trial highlighted this risk.[7] In the INTERHEART study, a standardized case-control study that screened all patients admitted to the coronary care unit or equivalent cardiology ward for a first myocardial infarction at 262 participating centers in 52 countries throughout Africa, Asia, Australia, Europe, the Middle East, and North and South America, hypertension was thought to account for 23.4% of the population-attributed risk for a myocardial infarction.

Compared with all other ethnic groups in the United States, hypertension in African Americans is more common, begins earlier, is more severe, and causes more target organ damage.[8-12] Relative to hypertensive whites, African Americans with hypertension demonstrate delayed sodium excretion, plasma volume expansion, lower plasma renin activity, elevated intracellular sodium concentration, and altered numbers and activities of sodium transporters (Na^+-H^+ antiporter, Na^+,K^+-ATPase, and Na^+-K^+-Cl^- cotransporter).[13,14] Many of these differences may have a genetic basis.

To possibly explain the greater prevalence and severity of hypertension in African Americans, several candidate genes have been explored. Genes encoding components of epithelial sodium channels,[15] the renin-angiotensin-aldosterone system,[16-18] alpha- and beta-adrenergic receptors,[19,20] endothelin,[21,22] kallikrein,[23] natriuretic peptides,[24] and the nitric oxide pathway[25] have been investigated. To date, few convincing genetic explanations for ethnic differences have emerged.

Hypertension in part increases CHD risk by predisposing to left ventricular hypertrophy.[26] Left ventricular hypertrophy increases cardiac risk up to fourfold and is more common in African Americans, even after adjustment for blood pressure. The mechanisms by which left ventricular hypertrophy increases risk are poorly understood but likely include predisposition to ischemia and arrhythmias.[26]

The MESA has given us valuable insight into the prevalence, treatment, and control of hypertension in the United States. Whereas most prior studies investigating the association between ethnicity and hypertension in the United States focused on differences between African Americans and whites and did not include other racial and ethnic groups such as Chinese or Hispanics, a paper by Kramer and colleagues[27] used MESA data to examine the association between ethnicity and hypertension and hypertension treatment among white, African American, Chinese, and Hispanic ethnic groups. These authors found that the prevalence of hypertension, defined as systolic blood pressure ≤140 mm Hg and/or diastolic blood pressure ≤90 mm Hg or self-reported treatment for hypertension, was significantly higher in African Americans compared with whites (60% versus 38%; $P < 0.0001$), whereas prevalence in Hispanic (42%) and Chinese participants (39%) did not differ significantly from that in whites. After adjustment for age, body mass index (BMI), prevalence of diabetes mellitus, and smoking, African American ethnicity (OR, 2.21; 95% CI, 1.91-2.56) and Chinese ethnicity (OR, 1.30; 95% CI, 1.07-1.56) were significantly associated with hypertension compared with whites. They further found that among hypertensive MESA participants, the percentage of treated but uncontrolled hypertension in whites (24%) was significantly lower than that in African Americans (35%; $P < 0.0001$), Chinese (33%; $P = 0.003$), and Hispanics (32%; $P = 0.0005$), but only African American race and ethnicity remained significantly associated with treated but uncontrolled hypertension after control for socioeconomic factors (OR, 1.35; 95% CI, 1.07-1.71).

Dyslipidemia

The epidemiologic relationship between serum cholesterol levels and the risk of CHD is well documented.[28-32] Across cultures, cholesterol is linearly related to CHD mortality, and despite differences in the prevalence of CHD between various populations, the relative increase in CHD mortality rates for a given cholesterol increase is remarkably consistent.[32] There is a complex interplay between genetic and environmental factors that influences the expression of lipoprotein levels in individuals and between groups of people, and differences in plasma lipoprotein levels have been reported between various ethnic groups.

African Americans have one of the highest CHD event rates of any ethnic or racial group in the United States.[33,34] Despite this fact, epidemiologic studies have consistently shown that plasma lipoprotein concentrations appear more favorable in African Americans than in white Americans.[35-38]

African Americans have been shown to have higher high-density lipoprotein cholesterol (HDL-C) levels than white populations. This is likely due, at least in part, to the lower activity of hepatic lipase in African Americans.[39] Hepatic lipase is an enzyme involved in HDL-C catabolism; thus, the lower the hepatic lipase activity, the higher the HDL-C level. Hepatic lipase activity has been found to be lower in African American men than in white men by Vega and colleagues,[39] in part because of increased prevalence of a hepatic lipase allele (514T) that is associated with reduced hepatic lipase activity.

Two other polymorphisms that cause amino acid substitutions in hepatic lipase (N193S and L334F) have since been found that are also associated with lower hepatic lipase activity and are also much more common in African Americans than in whites.[40] This higher HDL-C level, however, may not protect African Americans from CHD, as one might expect. In an analysis of the Veterans Affairs HDL Intervention Trial (VA-HIT), Rubins and colleagues[41] found that the African American participants, all of whom had CHD, had low-density lipoprotein cholesterol (LDL-C) levels similar to those of the white men with CHD in the study but substantially higher HDL-C levels. Furthermore, compared with whites, African Americans have been found to have similar or slightly lower total cholesterol levels, lower LDL-C levels, and lower triglyceride levels,[42,43] thus giving African Americans what would appear to be a more favorable lipoprotein profile.

Small, dense LDL-C particles are associated with an atherogenic lipoprotein phenotype that increases risk of myocardial infarction up to three times.[44] In a study by Kral and colleagues,[45] racial differences in the prevalence of small, dense LDL-C were studied. They investigated 159 African American and 477 white siblings of persons with premature CHD (CHD occurring at <60 years). Multiple logistic regression analysis demonstrated that white race ($P = 0.009$), triglyceride level ($P = 0.0001$), and diabetes ($P = 0.02$) were independent predictors of the likelihood of having small, dense LDL-C particles. White individuals had more small, dense LDL-C particles than African Americans did despite comparable levels of total cholesterol and LDL-C.

Lipoprotein(a) is structurally similar to LDL-C, with an additional disulfide-linked glycoprotein termed apolipoprotein(a).[46] Apolipoprotein(a) shares extensive structural homology with plasminogen but varies in size, which is due to the variation in the number of kringle 4–like domains (type 2 repeats) of plasminogen. Because of the size heterogeneity, apolipoprotein(a) exhibits a genetic size polymorphism with apparent molecular masses of isoforms ranging from 300 to 800 kDa.[47,48]

There are considerable differences in the mean of plasma lipoprotein(a) concentrations between different populations and ethnic groups.[49] Many although not all epidemiologic and case-control studies have shown that when lipoprotein(a) is present in high level in the plasma, it is an independent risk factor for CHD.[50-52] In addition to high lipoprotein(a) levels, the presence of small apolipoprotein(a) isoforms (with fewer kringle 4 type 2 repeats) has been associated with CHD in whites.[53,54] Interestingly, although mean lipoprotein(a) levels are more than twice as high in African Americans as in whites, some studies have failed to establish a significant association between elevated lipoprotein(a) levels and CHD among African Americans.[55,56] The reason for this may be that the majority of whites with high lipoprotein(a) levels possess at least one small apolipoprotein(a) isoform; however, the majority of African Americans with high lipoprotein(a) levels have no small apolipoprotein(a) isoforms.[57,58]

The major Hispanic subgroups are Mexican Americans, Central and South Americans, Puerto Ricans, and Cuban Americans, with Mexican Americans making up the largest single Hispanic group.[59] Native Mexicans have lipids characterized by low HDL-C and elevated triglyceride levels.[60] In a survey done in 417 Mexican cities, information on lipid levels was obtained for 15,607 subjects, 20 to 69 years of age. Mean total cholesterol concentration in this cohort was 185 mg/dL; mean triglyceride level was 212 mg/dL; mean HDL-C level was 40 mg/dL; and mean LDL-C concentration was 118 mg/dL. The most prevalent lipoprotein abnormality in this cohort was low HDL-C (HDL-C levels below 35 mg/dL), which occurred in 46% of men and 29% of women.

Hypertriglyceridemia (triglyceride levels ≥200 mg/dL) was the second most prevalent abnormality, occurring in 24.3% of participants, with severe hypertriglyceridemia (≥1000 mg/dL) being observed in 0.42% of this population. Half of the subjects with hypertriglyceridemia had a mixed dyslipidemia with low HDL-C levels as well. Insulin resistance was found to be prevalent in this population, being found in 59% of the subjects. Thus, the prevalence of dyslipidemia in urban Mexican adults is very high, with much of this likely due to insulin resistance.

This pattern of dyslipidemia has also been seen in Mexican American adults and children living in the United States.[61] When Hispanics of different ancestry are studied, similar results are seen as well. Bermudez and colleagues[62] studied 490 Hispanics of Caribbean origin (Puerto Rico and the Dominican Republic) and 163 non-Hispanic whites. They found that concentrations of total cholesterol, HDL-C, and apolipoprotein A-I were significantly lower among Hispanic women than among non-Hispanic white women. Although LDL-C concentrations are not higher in Hispanics, there appears to be a higher incidence of small, dense LDL-C.

In the Insulin Resistance Atherosclerosis Study, Hispanics not only had lower HDL-C and higher triglyceride levels than non-Hispanic whites did but also a smaller LDL-C particle size.[63] In regard to lipoprotein(a), available data suggest somewhat higher values in Hispanics compared with non-Hispanic whites. In a study by Chiu and associates,[64] 390 non-Hispanic whites and 214 Hispanics from San Luis Valley, Colorado, were studied. Mean (±SD) and median lipoprotein(a) levels were 9.6 ± 12.5 mg/dL and 3.8 mg/dL, respectively, in non-Hispanic whites and 12.1 ± 15.6 mg/dL and 4.9 mg/dL, respectively, in Hispanics.

Asian Indians are known to be at increased risk for CHD.[65] Rates of coronary artery disease in young Asian Indians younger than 40 years are 3 to 10 times higher than those in other populations, and some of this increased risk may be conferred by dyslipidemia. The typical lipid profile of Asian Indians living in Western societies is characterized by hypertriglyceridemia, low levels of HDL-C, and high levels of small, dense LDL-C.[66] In a study by Hoogeveen and colleagues,[67] Asian Indian subjects living in India and Asian Indians living in the United States were examined. Asian Indians living in the United States had higher plasma levels of triglyceride, total cholesterol, and LDL-C as well as lower HDL-C levels than did Asian Indians in India. Much of the dyslipidemia in Asian Indians also may at least in part be due to the greater prevalence of insulin resistance observed in this population.[68]

Small, dense LDL-C is also found more commonly in Asian Indians than in whites. In a study of 78 subjects, the prevalence of small, dense LDL-C was significantly higher in Asian Indians compared with white subjects (44% versus 21%; $P < 0.05$).[69] In this study, the increased prevalence of small, dense LDL-C type appeared to be due to the increased triglycerides.

TABLE 23–1	Relative Changes in Plasma Lipoprotein Concentrations in Various Ethnic Groups in the United States Compared with American Whites					
Ethnic Group	Total Cholesterol	LDL	% Small, Dense LDL	HDL	Triglyceride	Lipoprotein(a)
African American	⇓	⇓	⇓	⇑	⇓	⇑⇑⇑
Hispanic	⇔	⇓	⇑	⇓	⇑	⇑
Asian Indian	⇔	⇔	⇑	⇓	⇑	⇑

⇔, similar values; ⇑, higher values; ⇓, lower values.

23

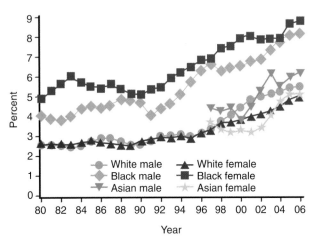

FIGURE 23-2 Age-adjusted percentage of civilian, noninstitutionalized population with diagnosed diabetes, by race and sex, United States, 1980-2006. Data show that blacks are disproportionately affected by diabetes. From 1980 through 2006, the age-adjusted prevalence of diagnosed diabetes increased among all sex-race groups examined. From 1980 through 2006, the age-adjusted prevalence of diagnosed diabetes was higher among blacks than whites and highest among black females. During this period, age-adjusted prevalence increased 116% among white males, 81% among white females, 100% among black males, and 69% among black females. Among Asians, the age-adjusted prevalence increased 42% among males and 38% among females from 1997 through 2006. *(Data source: Centers for Disease Control and Prevention, National Center for Health Statistics, Division of Health Interview Statistics, data from the National Health Interview Survey. U.S. Bureau of the Census, census of the population and population estimates. Data computed by the Division of Diabetes Translation, National Center for Chronic Disease Prevention and Health Promotion, Centers for Disease Control and Prevention.)*

Higher serum lipoprotein(a) concentrations have also been reported in Asian Indians. In a study of young Asian Indian patients (younger than 45 years) who had suffered a myocardial infarction, the mean lipoprotein(a) level was 22.3 ± 5.4 mg/dL in patients and 9.3 ± 22.6 mg/dL in controls.[67,70]

These data on ethnic differences in lipoprotein levels are summarized in Table 23-1. Of course, these general trends are based on population studies, and lipoprotein levels in a given individual may depart significantly. Nonetheless, knowledge of ethnic trends in plasma lipoprotein levels is useful for prognosis and treatment of CHD.

Insulin Resistance and Diabetes Mellitus

Type 2 diabetes varies considerably more by race and ethnicity as shown in Figure 23-2. The highest rates in the United States are seen in African Americans, Hispanic Americans, American Indians, and Asian/Pacific Islanders.

In the Atherosclerosis Risk in Communities (ARIC) study, the incidence of diabetes was 2.4-fold greater in African American women and 1.5-fold greater in African American men than in their white counterparts.[71] Excess adipose tissue accounted for almost half of the increased risk in African American women but little of the excess risk in African American men. African Americans with diabetes also have an increased risk of target organ damage,[72,73] and several studies have documented a higher prevalence of insulin resistance in African Americans, even after correction for obesity and lifestyle factors.[74]

In 2000, of the 30 million Hispanic Americans, about 2 million had been diagnosed with diabetes.[75] Hispanic Americans are about twice as likely to have diabetes as are non-Hispanic whites of similar age. Diabetes is particularly common among middle-aged and older Hispanic Americans. For those aged 50 years or older, about 25% to 30% have either diagnosed or undiagnosed diabetes.[75] Diabetes is twice as common in Mexican American and Puerto Rican adults as in non-Hispanic whites. The prevalence of diabetes in Cuban Americans is lower, but it is still higher than that of non-Hispanic whites.[75]

Asian Americans are a diverse population composed of individuals of Chinese, Filipino, Asian Indian, Vietnamese, Korean, and Japanese descent and others with Asian ancestry, such as Pacific Islanders.[76] Studies suggest that Asians are more likely to develop diabetes than are whites, even when they are less obese. For example, in the Honolulu Heart Study, the prevalence of physician-diagnosed plus newly diagnosed diabetes was 40% in Japanese American men older than 70 years[77] compared with 19.2% in white men aged 75 years or older from the third National Health and Nutrition Examination Survey (NHANES III).[78]

Excess weight, particularly central obesity, is recognized to be a major determinant of diabetes risk in all populations. Regardless of which measure of excess weight is used, the prevalence of diabetes is consistently higher among Asians than among whites at any given level of obesity.[78] Because of this known heterogeneity of relationship between central obesity (waist circumference) and insulin resistance, race- and ethnic-specific cut points have been developed. Race-specific cut points for waist circumference in relation to insulin resistance risk are shown in Table 23-2.

It is clear that both genetic and environmental risk factors play critical roles in the development of type 2 diabetes; however, despite strong evidence of heritability, there has been little success in identification of specific genes. Numerous candidate genes have been investigated, and although some gene variants have been found that confer increased risk of type 2 diabetes,[79,80] many others have not been verified. No genes that explain genetic differences have been established. Because of the considerable cardiovascular risk conferred by diabetes, further studies exploring ethnic differences are essential to reduce disparities.

Inflammation

It is now recognized that atherosclerosis is an inflammatory disease.[81] Chronic, subclinical inflammation appears to be one pathophysiologic mechanism explaining the increased risk of atherosclerotic disease regardless of the amount of

Table 23–2	Recommended Waist Circumference Thresholds for the Definition of Abdominal Obesity by Race-Ethnicity		
		Recommended Waist Circumference Threshold for Abdominal Obesity	
Population	Organization	Men	Women
United States	AHA/NHLBI (ATP III)	≥102 cm	≥88 cm
Europid	IDF	≥94 cm	≥80 cm
Middle East, Mediterranean	IDF	≥94 cm	≥80 cm
Sub-Saharan African	IDF	≥94 cm	≥80 cm
Ethnic Central and South American	IDF	≥90 cm	≥80 cm
Asian	IDF	≥90 cm	≥80 cm

AHA/NHLBI (ATP III), American Heart Association/National Heart, Lung and Blood Institute (Adult Treatment Panel III); IDF, International Diabetes Federation.

obstruction produced by that coronary disease. In the inflammatory model of atherosclerosis, it is the degree of inflammation, not the degree of obstruction, that causes acute coronary syndromes and increased CHD mortality.

Cytokines are key mediators of the inflammatory response and have been implicated in the development of atherosclerosis. Studies have shown that African Americans are more likely than white Americans to carry allelic variants demonstrated to increase production of inflammatory cytokines.[82]

There is now accumulating evidence that markers of subclinical inflammation may indeed predict future CHD events. One of the most studied markers is C-reactive protein (CRP),[84] and with use of a highly sensitive assay (hsCRP), elevation of hsCRP has been found to be associated with several major CHD risk factors and with unadjusted and age-adjusted projections of 10-year CHD risk in both men and women.[83,84]

Levels of hsCRP have been shown to vary by race and ethnicity.[85] In one study, with use of the NHANES data base, CRP levels were found to be highest among non-Hispanic black men and Mexican American women. According to multiple logistic regression analysis, cigarette smoking and increased age, BMI, and systolic blood pressure in men and BMI and diabetes in women were strongly associated with a greater likelihood of CRP levels ≥1.0 mg/dL ($P < 0.001$).

Whereas hsCRP levels have been shown to be related to cardiovascular risk factors, public health approaches to modification of hsCRP levels have been less well studied. One study,[86] however, addressed physical fitness and its relation to hsCRP by ethnicity. LaMonte and colleagues hypothesized that physical fitness might protect against high levels of hsCRP. They analyzed data from a subset of 44 African American women, 45 Native American women, and 46 white women who were part of the Cross-Cultural Activity Participation Study (CAPS) in the mid-1990s.

In CAPS, physical fitness was determined by exercise on a treadmill while both speed and incline were increased, and the women continued on the treadmill until they reached their point of exhaustion. Each woman's treadmill time was adjusted for her age, and women in each of the three ethnic groups were divided into three levels of fitness (low, moderate, and high) on the basis of their treadmill tests. The researchers assessed CRP levels by race, fitness, obesity, and waist size. They found that CRP levels were 4.3 mg/L in African American women, 2.5 mg/L in Native American women, and 2.3 mg/L in white women. They also found that women with low fitness had significantly higher CRP levels

(4.3 mg/L) than did those in the moderate (2.6 mg/L) and high (2.3 mg/L) fitness categories. They also reported that CRP was significantly elevated in women with the highest BMI. Women with BMI values from 18.5 to 24.9 had hsCRP levels of 1.9 mg/L, whereas overweight and obese women had hsCRP levels of 4.2 mg/L. Finally, they found that women whose waists measured more than 35 inches had CRP concentrations of 4.2 mg/L, whereas those with waist circumference of less than 35 inches had CRP levels of 2.5 mg/L. These data provide evidence of a key mechanism through which chronic stressors may accelerate atherosclerosis and may have important implications for certain racial and ethnic populations.

Obesity

Obesity is the most important cause of preventable death and the second leading cause of premature death in the United States. About 300,000 excess deaths are linked to obesity and its complications annually. Excessive adiposity is a major cause of hypertension, dyslipidemia, and type 2 diabetes mellitus.[87] These clinical risk factors are known to be the primary precursors of CVD, and the obesity epidemic has the potential to reduce further gains in the U.S. life expectancy,[88] largely through an effect on cardiovascular risk and mortality.[89] As the prevalence of obesity and overweight in the United States increases, the CVD consequences may also be concurrently increasing.

The prevalence of obesity doubled in U.S. adults between 1980 and 2004.[90,91] Although data from 2005 to 2006 have shown no statistically significant increase in the prevalence of obesity since 2004, more than one third of U.S. adults are now obese.[92] According to NHANES data, the increase in prevalence of overweight and obesity has been similar across racial and ethnic groups in both men and women during the past three decades; however, there are racial differences in the prevalence of obesity as well as racial differences in the prevalence of health complications associated with obesity.[93,94]

Data from Behavioral Risk Factor Surveillance System surveys conducted during 2006-2008 show that African American women had the greatest prevalence of obesity (39.2%), followed by African American men (31.6%), Hispanic women (29.4%), Hispanic men (27.8%), non-Hispanic white men (25.4%), and non-Hispanic white women (21.8%). According to these data, African Americans (35.7%) had 51% greater prevalence of obesity, and Hispanics (28.7%) had 21% greater prevalence, compared with non-Hispanic whites (23.7%). Other studies also have shown that the prevalence of obesity among Asian Americans has been much lower than the national average, but differences between different Asian groups are considerable, and the highest prevalence of obesity has been reported among native Hawaiians and Samoans.[95]

Despite obesity's disproportionately high prevalence in African Americans and Hispanic Americans,[96] studies suggest that its adverse impact on cardiovascular risk and mortality may be reduced in some minority populations.[97,98] For example, even though African Americans have a higher prevalence of hypertension, diabetes, and hypercholesterolemia[99] than white Americans do, evidence suggests that the relationship of BMI to most CVD risk factors is steeper in whites, suggesting a stronger influence of obesity on risk factor levels in whites than in African Americans. Prior studies have suggested that for a given BMI category, rates of CVD death among African Americans are lower compared with whites.[100-103]

This observation indicates that even with higher rates of risk factors in African Americans, risk factors are more strongly associated with increasing BMI in whites. These paradoxical observations might be explained by the higher rates of type 2 diabetes mellitus, hypertension, elevated LDL-C, and low HDL among African Americans than among whites in the normal weight group. Moreover, although the relative associations between BMI and cardiometabolic risk factors are stronger in whites than in African Americans, there is a strong association between increasing BMI and cardiometabolic risk factors in both groups.

Smoking

Smoking is an independent risk factor for CVD. There are a number of ways that smoking contributes to the pathogenesis of CVD. Smoking impairs lipoprotein metabolism, increases blood thrombogenicity,[104] reduces the distensibility of blood vessel walls,[105] and induces proinflammatory state.[106,107] Smokers have higher serum levels of cholesterol and lower plasma concentrations of HDL-C. Also, cigarette smoking is associated with higher plasma concentrations of triglyceride.

According to the 2008 National Health Interview Survey, approximately 20.5% of adults are current smokers.[108] Data from national surveys indicate broad disparities in cigarette smoking by race or ethnicity. Native Americans and Alaskan natives have the highest smoking prevalence (36.4%), followed by whites (21.4%), African Americans (25), Hispanics (19.8%), and Asians (13.3%).[109] There are also large differences by ethnicity in receiving advice from providers to quit smoking. African Americans and Hispanics are significantly less likely to be offered assistance with cessation.

Nationally, only 21% of Hispanics report receiving regular care from a racially concordant physician, compared with 88% of whites and 23% of blacks.[110] The lower frequency of smoking cessation advice among Hispanics and African American reflects disparities in health care providers' perceptions of the need for or effectiveness of cessation advice in this ethnic subgroup.

Moreover, interest in quitting and attempts to quit differ in ethnic groups. Only 62% of Hispanic smokers reported wanting to quit compared with 71% of whites, 68% of African Americans, and 70% of Native Americans. The percentage of smokers who quit also varies sharply by ethnic group, with the highest level of success among whites (51%) and the lowest for African Americans (37%).[111]

RISK CALCULATION AMONG ETHNIC GROUPS

Prediction of cardiovascular risk is a cornerstone of CVD prevention and treatment. The most commonly used risk prediction algorithm comes from the Framingham Heart Study, which has developed multivariable mathematical functions that assign weights to major CHD risk factors such as sex, age, blood pressure, total cholesterol, LDL-C, HDL-C, smoking status, and diabetes status.[112-115] The Framingham risk prediction algorithm is used to predict the risk a person free of CVD has for development of CHD within a certain period. One of the concerns about this algorithm, however, is that the Framingham Heart Study consists primarily of white middle-class individuals; thus, there is concern as to whether this algorithm can be generalized to populations of different racial and ethnic groups.

To test the validity of the Framingham CHD prediction functions in diverse populations, the National Heart, Lung, and Blood Institute organized a workshop for this purpose. Sex-specific CHD functions were derived from Framingham data for prediction of coronary death and myocardial infarction. These functions were applied to six prospectively studied, ethnically diverse cohorts (n = 23,424) including whites, African Americans, Native Americans, Japanese American men, and Hispanic men: the ARIC study

(1987-1988), Physicians' Health Study (1982), Honolulu Heart Program (1980-1982), Puerto Rico Heart Health Program (1965-1968), Strong Heart Study (1989-1991), and Cardiovascular Health Study (1989-1990).

The performance or ability to accurately predict CHD risk of the Framingham functions was compared with the performance of risk functions developed specifically from the individual cohorts' data. Comparisons included evaluation of the equality of relative risks for standard CHD risk factors, discrimination, and calibration. This workshop found that for white men and women and for black men and women, the Framingham functions performed reasonably well for prediction of CHD events within 5 years of follow-up. Among Japanese American and Hispanic men and Native American women, the Framingham functions systematically overestimated the risk of 5-year CHD events; but after recalibration, taking into account different prevalences of risk factors and underlying rates for development of CHD, the Framingham functions worked well in these populations.[116]

To reduce some of the limitations of risk assessment in different populations, investigators have considered adding data to the Framingham algorithm. In one study, investigators used data from the ARIC study and then validated their model in a second cohort, the NHANES linked to the National Death Index.[117] They assessed the effect of measures of socioeconomic status (SES), specifically having <12 years of education or low income, on model discrimination and calibration when added to the Framingham risk score in a prospective cohort. They found that based on Framingham risk score alone, persons of higher and lower SES had a predicted CHD risk of 3.7% and 3.9%, respectively, compared with the observed risks of 3.2% and 5.6%. When they added SES to the model, predicted risk estimates improved to 3.1% and 5.2% for those with higher and lower SES, closely mirroring the actual observed outcomes. Inclusion of SES in the model resulted in upgrading of risk classification for 15.1% of low-SES participants (95% CI, 13.9-29.4%).[117]

Other investigators have advocated addition of measures of subclinical atherosclerosis to the Framingham algorithm to minimize ethnic discrepancies. One subclinical atherosclerosis measure of interest is measurement of coronary calcium. Several studies evaluating the prognostic accuracy of the measurement of coronary calcium by computed tomography have shown that coronary calcification is predictive of coronary events independently of standard risk factors or risk factor scores.[118-121]

Data from several studies, including MESA, have determined that coronary calcium prevalence differs by race and ethnicity. In MESA, coronary calcification was measured in 6814 white, black, Hispanic, and Chinese men and women aged 45 to 84 years with no clinical CVD.[122] After multiple adjustments, compared with whites, the relative risks for having coronary calcification were 0.78 (95% CI, 0.74 to 0.82) in blacks, 0.85 (95% CI, 0.79 to 0.91) in Hispanics, and 0.92 (95% CI, 0.85 to 0.99) in Chinese.

Further data from MESA suggest that despite different prevalence, the predictive value of coronary calcium in various ethnic groups remains.[123] Participants in MESA were observed for a median of 3.8 years, during which time there were 162 coronary events, of which 89 were major events (myocardial infarction or death from CHD). In comparison with participants with no coronary calcium, the adjusted risk of a coronary event was 7.7-fold greater among participants with coronary calcium scores between 101 and 300 and 9.7-fold greater among participants with scores above 300 ($P < 0.001$ for both comparisons). Among the four racial and ethnic groups, a doubling of the calcium score increased the risk of a major coronary event by 15% to 35% and the risk of any coronary event by 18% to 39%.

HEALTH CARE USE

Racial and ethnic minority populations in the United States bear disproportionate burden of death and disability related to CVD.[124] The degree of racial and ethnic variations in burden of CVD goes beyond that which can be explained by risk factor variation alone. This discrepancy is thought to be partially attributable to differentials in cardiovascular care.

Disparities in cardiovascular health care across the racial and ethnic groups are well documented. Limited access to care, delays in seeking cardiac care,[125] limited health literacy and education,[126-128] mistrust of the health care system by patients of color,[129,130] inadequate cultural competency of providers,[131,132] provider stereotyping of communities of color,[133] and racism of providers[134] are likely contributors to disparities in cardiovascular care.

Financial barriers are much more likely in African American and Hispanic cardiac patients. Data from the Kaiser Family Foundation reports show that one third of Hispanics and 21% of African Americans are uninsured compared with 13% of whites, and these groups are less likely to receive preventive care.[135,136] African Americans and Hispanics are also 10% to 40% less likely to receive outpatient secondary prevention therapies for CVD.[137] Furthermore, African Americans and Hispanics appear to receive cardiovascular care at health care organizations that perform a lower volume of procedures and have higher risk-adjusted mortality after coronary artery bypass graft surgery[138] and acute myocardial infarction.[139] Mortality and morbidity gaps between ethnic groups widen further in studies that look at long-term cardiovascular outcomes after hospitalizations or procedures.[140,141]

ETHNIC-SPECIFIC TREATMENT ISSUES

Are Certain Groups More or Less Sensitive to Certain Therapies?

Physicians have known for some time that patients of different races respond differently to a variety of cardiovascular medications. A classic example is the lesser blood pressure–lowering effect of angiotensin-converting enzyme inhibitors in African American compared with white patients,[142] but several other examples exist as well.[143,144] In discussing issues of race and ethnicity, however, it is crucial to remember that humans are essentially the same, with as great or greater variation within self-defined racial groups as across groups.[5] In fact, race and ethnicity are poor proxies for genetic variation but can potentially lend insight into differences in response to therapy, side effects related to therapy, or novel therapeutics altogether.

The issue of race-specific treatments was brought to the forefront in 2005 with the Food and Drug Administration (FDA) approval of the first cardiovascular therapeutic that was approved for a specific racial group.[145] Hydralazine–isosorbide dinitrate is a combination pill containing two commonly available vasodilators, hydralazine and isosorbide dinitrate, that had been studied more than 20 years earlier as a potential treatment of heart failure.[146,147] Whereas earlier trials had shown this combination to be less effective than angiotensin-converting enzyme inhibition for treatment of patients with heart failure, a beneficial effect of this combination was noted in African American patients. Thus, a further study, the African-American Heart Failure Trial (A-HeFT), was initiated.[148]

This trial enrolled only African American patients who were randomized to a fixed-dose combination of isosorbide and hydralazine (target daily dose, 120 mg and 225 mg, respectively) or placebo added to their existing medications. Follow-up was planned for 18 months, but the study was stopped early (mean duration of follow-up, 10 months) because of excess mortality in the placebo group (54 deaths in the placebo group versus 32 deaths in the active therapy group, for a 43% relative risk reduction). On the basis of these impressive findings, an FDA advisory panel recommended on June 16, 2005, that BiDiL be approved specifically for the treatment of heart failure in self-defined African American patients, the group enrolled in the A-HeFT trial.

The race-specific FDA approval of Bidil was not based on a known genetic or physiologic difference between the races; rather, it reflected the population in which the study was performed. In fact, there is good reason to believe that BiDil would also be effective in non–African American patients. The case of BiDil is unique in medicine, and in the future, it is likely that race and ethnicity will be used less often than true indices of genetic variation.

CONCLUSION

Excess CVD and stroke morbidity and mortality are seen among various ethnic groups. This excess burden of disease is partially explained by variations in extent or implications of risk factors, but other elements such as genetic, socioeconomic, and cultural factors are also important yet poorly understood. Better understanding of the multitude of factors contributing to disparities in cardiovascular outcomes is essential to the reduction of these disparities in addition to the improvement of cardiovascular health for all.

REFERENCES

1. American Heart Association: *Heart disease and stroke statistics—2008 update*, Dallas, Texas, 2008, American Heart Association.
2. Arias E, Anderson RN, Hsiang-Ching K, et al: *Deaths: final data for 2001*, National vital statistics reports, vol 52, no 3, Hyattsville, Md, 2003, U.S. Department of Health and Human Services.
3. Cooper R, Cutler J, Desvigne-Nickens P, et al: Trends and disparities in coronary heart disease, stroke, and other cardiovascular diseases in the United States: findings of the National Conference on Cardiovascular Disease Prevention. *Circulation* 102:3137, 2000.
4. Centers for Disease Control and Prevention (CDC): Disparities in premature deaths from heart disease—50 States and the District of Columbia, 2001. *MMWR Morb Mortal Wkly Rep* 53:121, 2004.
5. Royal CD, Dunston GM: Changing the paradigm from "race" to human genome variation. *Nat Genet* 36(Suppl):S5, 2004.
6. Chockalingam A: World Hypertension Day and global awareness. *Can J Cardiol* 24:441, 2008.
7. Yusuf S, Hawken S: Ounpuu Sl; on behalf of the INTERHEART Study Investigators: Effect of potentially modifiable risk factors associated with myocardial infarction in 52 countries (the INTERHEART study): case-control study. *Lancet* 364:937, 2004.
8. Kaplan NM: Ethnic aspects of hypertension. *Lancet* 344:450, 1994.
9. Saunders E: Hypertension in African-Americans. *Circulation* 83:1465, 1991.
10. Cooper RS, Liao Y, Rotimi C: Is hypertension more severe among US blacks, or is severe hypertension more common? *Ann Epidemiol* 6:173, 1996.
11. Jamerson KA: Geographical aspects of hypertension. Prevalence of complications and response to different treatments of hypertension in African Americans and white Americans in the US. *Clin Exp Hypertens* 15:979, 1993.
12. Rahman M, Douglas JG, Wright JT, Jr: Pathophysiology and treatment implications of hypertension in the African-American population. *Endocrinol Metab Clin North Am* 26:125, 1997.
13. Weinberger MH: Hypertension in African Americans: the role of sodium chloride and extracellular fluid volume. *Semin Nephrol* 16:110, 1996.
14. Baker EH, Dong YB, Sagnella GA, et al: Association of hypertension with T594M mutation in beta subunit of epithelial sodium channels in black people resident in London. *Lancet* 351:188, 1998.
15. Rutledge DR, Browe CS, Ross EA: Frequencies of the angiotensinogen gene and angiotensin I converting enzyme (ACE) gene polymorphisms in African Americans. *Biochem Mol Biol Int* 34:1271, 1994.
16. Rotimi C, Puras A, Cooper R, et al: Polymorphisms of renin-angiotensin genes among Nigerians, Jamaicans, and African Americans. *Hypertension* 27(pt 2):591, 1996.
17. Fisher ND, Gleason RE, Moore TJ, et al: Regulation of aldosterone secretion in hypertensive blacks. *Hypertension* 23:179, 1994.
18. Lockette W, Ghosh S, Farrow S, et al: Alpha$_2$-adrenergic receptor gene polymorphism and hypertension in blacks. *Am J Hypertens* 8(pt 1):390, 1995.
19. Kotanko P, Binder A, Tasker J, et al: Essential hypertension in African Caribbeans associates with a variant of the β$_2$-adrenoceptor. *Hypertension* 30:773, 1997.
20. Ergul S, Parish CD, Puett D, Ergul A: Racial differences in plasma endothelin-1 concentrations in individuals with essential hypertension. *Hypertension* 28:652, 1996.

21. Ergul A, Tackett RL, Puett D: Distribution of endothelin receptors in saphenous veins of African Americans: implications of racial differences. *J Cardiovasc Pharmacol* 34:327, 1999.

22. Song Q, Chao J, Chao L: DNA polymorphisms in the 5′ flanking region of the human tissue kallikrein gene. *Hum Genet* 99:727, 1997.

23. Barley J, Carter ND, Cruickshank JK, et al: Renin and atrial natriuretic peptide restriction fragment length polymorphisms: association with ethnicity and blood pressure. *J Hypertens* 9:993, 1991.

24. Deng AY, Rapp JP: Locus for the inducible, but not a constitutive, nitric oxide synthase cosegregates with BP in the Dahl salt-sensitive rat. *J Clin Invest* 95:2170, 1995.

25. Tin LL, Beevers DG, Lip GY: Hypertension, left ventricular hypertrophy, and sudden death. *Curr Cardiol Rep* 4:449, 2002.

26. Benjamin EJ, Levy D: Why is left ventricular hypertrophy so predictive of morbidity and mortality? *Am J Med Sci* 317:168, 1999.

27. Kramer H, Han C, Post W, et al: Racial/ethnic differences in hypertension and hypertension treatment and control in the multi-ethnic study of atherosclerosis (MESA). *Am J Hypertens* 17:963, 2004.

28. Zemel PC, Sowers JR: Relation between lipids and atherosclerosis: epidemiologic evidence and clinical implications. *Am J Cardiol* 66:7I, 1990.

29. Executive summary of the third report of the National Cholesterol Education Program (NCEP) Expert Panel on Detection, Evaluation, and Treatment of High Blood Cholesterol in Adults (Adult Treatment Panel III). *JAMA* 285:2486, 2001.

30. Stamler J, Daviglus ML, Garside DB, et al: Relationship of baseline serum cholesterol levels in 3 large cohorts of younger men to long-term coronary, cardiovascular, and all-cause mortality and to longevity. *JAMA* 284:311, 2000.

31. Neaton JD, Blackburn H, Jacobs D, et al: Serum cholesterol level and mortality findings for men screened in the Multiple Risk Factor Intervention Trial. Multiple Risk Factor Intervention Trial Research Group. *Arch Intern Med* 152:1490, 1992.

32. Kromhout D: Serum cholesterol in cross-cultural perspective. The Seven Countries Study. *Acta Cardiol* 54:155, 1999.

33. Crook ED, Clark BL, Bradford ST, et al: From 1960s Evans County Georgia to present-day Jackson, Mississippi: an exploration of the evolution of cardiovascular disease in African Americans. *Am J Med Sci* 325:307, 2003.

34. Clark LT, Ferdinand KC, Flack JM, et al: Coronary heart disease in African Americans. *Heart Dis* 3:97-108, 2001.

35. Tyroler HA, Glueck CJ, Christensen B, Kwiterovich PO, Jr: Plasma high-density lipoprotein cholesterol comparisons in black and white populations. The Lipid Research Clinics Program Prevalence Study. *Circulation* 62:99-107, 1980.

36. Sprafka JM, Norsted SW, Folsom AR, et al: Life-style factors do not explain racial differences in high-density lipoprotein cholesterol: the Minnesota Heart Survey. *Epidemiology* 3:156, 1992.

37. Webber LS, Srinivasan SR, Wattigney WA, Berenson GS: Tracking of serum lipids and lipoproteins from childhood to adulthood. The Bogalusa Heart Study. *Am J Epidemiol* 133:884, 1991.

38. Brown SA, Hutchinson R, Morrisett J, et al: Plasma lipid, lipoprotein cholesterol, and apoprotein distributions in selected US communities. The Atherosclerosis Risk in Communities (ARIC) Study. *Arterioscler Thromb* 13:1139, 1993.

39. Vega GL, Clark LT, Tang A, et al: Hepatic lipase activity is lower in African American than in white American men: effects of 5′ flanking polymorphism in the hepatic lipase gene. *J Lipid Res* 39:228, 1998.

40. Nie L, Niu S, Vega GL, et al: Three polymorphisms associated with low hepatic lipase activity are common in African Americans. *J Lipid Res* 39:1900, 1998.

41. Rubins HB, Robins SJ, Collins D, et al: Distribution of lipids in 8,500 men with coronary artery disease. Department of Veterans Affairs HDL-C Intervention Trial Study Group. *Am J Cardiol* 75:1196, 1995.

42. Metcalf PA, Sharrett AR, Folsom AR, et al: African American–white differences in lipids, lipoproteins, and apolipoproteins, by educational attainment, among middle-aged adults: the Atherosclerosis Risk in Communities Study. *Am J Epidemiol* 148:750, 1998.

43. Donahue RP, Jacobs DR, Jr, Sidney S, et al: Distribution of lipoproteins and apolipoproteins in young adults: the CARDIA Study. *Arteriosclerosis* 9:656, 1989.

44. O'Brien R: Biological importance of low-density-lipoprotein subfractions. *J Cardiovasc Risk* 1:207, 1994.

45. Kral BG, Becker LC, Yook RM, et al: Racial differences in low-density lipoprotein particle size in families at high risk for premature coronary heart disease. *Ethn Dis* 11:325, 2001.

46. Uterman G: The mysteries of lipoprotein(a). *Science* 246:904, 1989.

47. Gunther MF, Catherin AR, Angelo MS: Heterogeneity of human lipoprotein(a). *J Biol Chem* 259:11470, 1984.

48. Para HG, Luyey I, Buramoue C, et al: Black-white differences in serum lipoprotein(a) levels. *Clin Chim Acta* 167:27, 1987.

49. Scanu AM: Lipoprotein(a): a genetic risk factor for premature coronary heart disease. *JAMA* 267:3326, 1992.

50. Marcovina SM, Koschinsky ML: Lipoprotein(a) as a risk factor for coronary artery disease. *Am J Cardiol* 82:57U, 1998.

51. Rim L, Ali B, Slim BA, Bechir Z: Lipoprotein(a): a new risk factor for coronary artery disease. *Tunis Med* 78:648, 2000.

52. Ridker PM: An epidemiologic reassessment of lipoprotein(a) and atherothrombotic risk. *Trends Cardiovasc Med* 5:225, 1995.

53. Wild SH, Fortmann SP, Marcovina SM: A prospective case-control study of lipoprotein(a) levels and apo(a) size and risk of coronary heart disease in Stanford Five-City Project participants. *Arterioscler Thromb Vasc Biol* 17:239, 1997.

54. Sandholzer C, Saha N, Kark JD, et al: Apo(a) isoforms predict risk for coronary heart disease: a study in six populations. *Arterioscler Thromb* 12:1214, 1992.

55. Moliterno DJ, Jokinen EV, Miserez AR, et al: No association between plasma lipoprotein(a) concentrations and the presence or absence of coronary atherosclerosis in African-Americans. *Arterioscler Thromb Vasc Biol* 15:850, 1995.

56. Sorrentino MJ, Vielhauer C, Eisenbart JD, et al: Plasma lipoprotein(a) protein concentration and coronary artery disease in black patients compared with white patients. *Am J Med* 93:658, 1992.

57. Marcovina SM, Albers JJ, Wijsman E, et al: Differences in Lp(a) concentrations and apo(a) polymorphs between black and white Americans. *J Lipid Res* 37:2569, 1996.

58. Paultre F, Pearson TA, Weil HF, et al: High levels of Lp(a) with a small apo(a) isoform are associated with coronary artery disease in African American and white men. *Arterioscler Thromb Vasc Biol* 20:2619, 2000.

59. Statistical tables for the Hispanic Origin population, *Current Population Survey, March 1994*, Washington, DC, 1995, Bureau of the Census.

60. Aguilar-Salinas CA, Olaiz G, Valles V, et al: High prevalence of low HDL-C cholesterol concentrations and mixed hyperlipidemia in a Mexican nationwide survey. *J Lipid Res* 42:298, 2001.

61. Reaven P, Nader PR, Berry C, Hoy T: Cardiovascular disease insulin risk in Mexican-American and Anglo-American children and mothers. *Pediatrics* 101:E12, 1998.

62. Bermudez OI, Velez-Carrasco W, Schaefer EJ, Tucker KL: Dietary and plasma lipid, lipoprotein, and apolipoprotein profiles among elderly Hispanics and non-Hispanics and their association with diabetes. *Am J Clin Nutr* 76:1214, 2002.

63. Haffner SM, D'Agostino R, Jr, Goff D, et al: LDL-C size in African Americans, Hispanics, and non-Hispanic whites: the insulin resistance atherosclerosis study. *Arterioscler Thromb Vasc Biol* 19:2234, 1999.

64. Chiu L, Hamman RF, Kamboh MI: Apolipoprotein A polymorphisms and plasma lipoprotein(a) concentrations in non-Hispanic Whites and Hispanics. *Hum Biol* 72:821, 2000.

65. Enas EA, Mehta J: Malignant coronary artery disease in young Asian Indians: thoughts on pathogenesis, prevention and therapy. *Clin Cardiol* 18:131, 1995.

66. Miller GJ, Kotecha S, Wilkinson WH, et al: Dietary and other characteristics relevant for coronary heart disease in men of Indian, West Indian and European descent in London. *Atherosclerosis* 70:63, 1988.

67. Hoogeveen RC, Gambhir JK, Gambhir DS, et al: Evaluation of Lp[a] and other independent risk factors for CHD in Asian Indians and their USA counterparts. *J Lipid Res* 42:631, 2001.

68. Cruickshank JK, Cooper J, Burnett M, et al: Ethnic differences in fasting plasma C-peptide and insulin in relation to glucose tolerance and blood pressure. *Lancet* 338:842, 1991.

69. Kulkarni KR, Markovitz JH, Nanda NC, Segrest JP: Increased prevalence of smaller and denser LDL-C particles in Asian Indians. *Arterioscler Thromb Vasc Biol* 19:2749, 1999.

70. Isser HS, Puri VK, Narain VS, et al: Lipoprotein (a) and lipid levels in young patients with myocardial infarction and their first-degree relatives. *Indian Heart J* 53:463, 2001.

71. Brancati FL, Kao WH, Folsom AR, et al: Incident type 2 diabetes mellitus in African American and white adults: the Atherosclerosis Risk in Communities Study. *JAMA* 283:2253, 2000.

72. Goldschmid MG, Domin WS, Ziemer DC, et al: Diabetes in urban African-Americans. II. High prevalence of microalbuminuria and nephropathy in African-Americans with diabetes. *Diabetes Care* 18:955, 1995.

73. Arfken CL, Salicrup AE, Meuer SM, et al: Retinopathy in African Americans and whites with insulin-dependent diabetes mellitus. *Arch Intern Med* 154:2597, 1994.

74. Falkner B: Insulin resistance in African Americans. *Kidney Int Suppl* 83:S27, 2003.

75. National Diabetes Information Clearinghouse: National diabetes statistics. NIH publication 02-3892. 2002. Fact sheet. Available at: www.niddk.nih.gov/health/diabetes/pubs/dmstats/dmstats.htm.

76. U. S. Census Bureau Population Estimates Program: Profiles of general demographic characteristics: national summary: 2000 census of population and housing, 2001. Available from http://www2.census.gov/census_2000/datasets/demographic_profile/0_National_Summary/2khus.pdf.

77. Rodriguez BL, Curb JD, Burchfiel CM, et al: Impaired glucose tolerance, diabetes, and cardiovascular disease risk factor profiles in the elderly: the Honolulu Heart Program. *Diabetes Care* 19:587, 1996

78. Harris MI, Flegal KM, Cowie CC, et al: Prevalence of diabetes, impaired fasting glucose, and impaired glucose tolerance in U. S. adults: the Third National Health and Nutrition Examination Survey, 1988-1994. *Diabetes Care* 21:518, 1998.

79. Altshuler D, Hirschhorn JN, Klannemark M, et al: The common PPAR Pro12Ala polymorphism is associated with decreased risk of type 2 diabetes. *Nat Genet* 26:76, 2000.

80. Malecki MT, Jhala US, Antonellis A, et al: Mutations in NEUROD1 are associated with the development of type 2 diabetes mellitus. *Nat Genet* 23:323, 1999.

81. Ross R: Atherosclerosis: an inflammatory disease. *N Engl J Med* 340:115, 1999.

82. Ness RB, Haggerty CL, Harger G, Ferrell R: Differential distribution of allelic variants in cytokine genes among African Americans and White Americans. *Am J Epidemiol* 160:1033, 2004.

83. Ridker PM: High-sensitivity C-reactive protein: potential adjunct for global risk assessment in the primary prevention of cardiovascular disease. *Circulation* 103:1813, 2001.

84. Ridker PM, Glynn RJ, Hennekens CH: C-reactive protein adds to the predictive value of total and HDL cholesterol in determining risk of first myocardial infarction. *Circulation* 97:2007, 1998.

85. Wong ND, Pio J, Valencia R, Thakal G: Distribution of C-reactive protein and its relation to risk factors and coronary heart disease risk estimation in the National Health and Nutrition Examination Survey (NHANES) III. *Prev Cardiol* 4:109, 2001.

86. LaMonte MJ, Durstine JL, Yanowitz FG, et al: Cardiorespiratory fitness and C-reactive protein among a tri-ethnic sample of women. *Circulation* 106:403, 2002.

87. Clinical Guidelines on the Identification, Evaluation, and Treatment of Overweight and Obesity in Adults—The Evidence Report. National Institutes of Health. *Obes Res* 6(Suppl 2):51S, 1998.

88. Olshansky SJ, Passaro DJ, Hershow RC, et al: A potential decline in life expectancy in the United States in the 21st century. *N Engl J Med* 352:1138, 2005.

89. Flegal KM, Graubard BI, Williamson DF, Gail MH: Excess deaths associated with underweight, overweight, and obesity. *JAMA* 293:1861, 2005.

90. Ogden CL, Carroll MD, Curtin LR, et al: Prevalence of overweight and obesity in the United States, 1999-2004. *JAMA* 295:1549, 2006.

91. Flegal KM, Carroll MD, Ogden CL, Johnson CL: Prevalence and trends in obesity among US adults, 1999-2000. *JAMA* 288:1723, 2002.

92. Ogden CL, Carroll MD, McDowell MA, Flegal KM: *Obesity among adults in the United States—no change since since 2003-2004*, NCHS Data Brief no. 1, Hyattsville, Md, 2007, National Center for Health Statistics.

93. Cossrow N, Falkner B: Race/ethnic issues in obesity and obesity-related comorbidities. *J Clin Endocrinol Metab* 89:2590, 2004.

94. Racette SB, Deusinger SS, Deusinger RH: Obesity: overview of prevalence, etiology, and treatment. *Phys Ther* 83:276, 2003.

95. Davis J, Busch J, Hammatt Z, et al: The relationship between ethnicity and obesity in Asian and Pacific Islander populations: a literature review. *Ethn Dis* 14:111, 2004.

96. Mokdad AH, Marks JS, Stroup DF, Gerberding JL: Actual causes of death in the United States, 2000. *JAMA* 291:1238, 2004.

97. Folsom AR, Stevens J, Schreiner PJ, McGovern PG: Body mass index, waist/hip ratio, and coronary heart disease incidence in African Americans and whites. Atherosclerosis Risk in Communities Study Investigators. *Am J Epidemiol* 148:1187, 1998.

98. Stevens J, Plankey MW, Williamson DF, et al: The body mass index–mortality relationship in white and African American women. *Obes Res* 6:268, 1998.

99. Taylor HA, Jr, Coady SA, Levy D, et al: Relationships of BMI to cardiovascular risk factors differ by ethnicity. *Obesity (Silver Spring)* 18:1638, 2010.

100. Bacha F, Saad R, Gungor N, et al: Obesity, regional fat distribution, and syndrome X in obese black versus white adolescents: race differential in diabetogenic and atherogenic risk factors. *J Clin Endocrinol Metab* 88:2534, 2003.

101. Brown CD, Higgins M, Donato KA, et al: Body mass index and the prevalence of hypertension and dyslipidemia. *Obes Res* 8:605, 2000.

102. Carnethon MR, Lynch EB, Dyer AR, et al: Comparison of risk factors for cardiovascular mortality in black and white adults. *Arch Intern Med* 166:1196, 2006.

103. Carpenter MA, Crow R, Steffes M, et al: Laboratory, reading center, and coordinating center data management methods in the Jackson Heart Study. *Am J Med Sci* 328:131, 2004.

104. Hung J, Lam JY, Lacoste L, Letchacovski G: Cigarette smoking acutely increases platelet thrombus formation in patients with coronary artery disease taking aspirin. *Circulation* 92:2432, 1995.

105. Libby P, Ridker PM, Maseri A: Inflammation and atherosclerosis. *Circulation* 105:1135, 2002.

106. van der Vaart H, Postma DS, Timens W, ten Hacken NH: Acute effects of cigarette smoke on inflammation and oxidative stress: a review. *Thorax* 59:713, 2004.

107. Bazzano LA, He J, Muntner P, et al: Relationship between cigarette smoking and novel risk factors for cardiovascular disease in the United States. *Ann Intern Med* 138:891, 2003.

108. Heyman KM, Barnes PM, Schiller JS: *Early release of selected estimates based on data from the 2008 National Health Interview Survey*, Hyattsville, Md, 2009, National Center for Health Statistics.

109. Centers for Disease Control and Prevention: Cigarette smoking among adults—United States, 2007. *MMWR Morb Mortal Wkly Rep* 57:1221, 2008.

110. Saha S, Komaromy M, Koepsell TD, Bindman AB: Patient-physician racial concordance and the perceived quality and use of health care. *Arch Intern Med* 159:997, 1999.

111. Trosclair A, Husten C, Pederson L, Dhillon I: Cigarette smoking among adults—United States, 2000. *MMWR Morb Mortal Wkly Rep* 51:642, 2002.

112. Kannel WB, McGee D, Gordon T: A general cardiovascular risk profile: the Framingham Study. *Am J Cardiol* 38:46, 1976.

113. Gordon T, Kannel WB: Multiple risk functions for predicting coronary heart disease: the concept, accuracy, and application. *Am Heart J* 103:1031, 1982.

114. Anderson M, Wilson PW, Odell PM, Kannel WB: An updated coronary risk profile: a statement for health professionals. *Circulation* 83:356, 1991.

115. Wilson PWF, D'Agostino RB, Levy D, et al: Prediction of coronary heart disease using risk factor categories. *Circulation* 97:1837, 1998.

116. D'Agostino RB, Sr, Grundy S, Sullivan LM, Wilson P, CHD Risk Prediction Group: Validation of the Framingham coronary heart disease prediction scores: results of a multiple ethnic groups investigation. *JAMA* 286:180, 2001.

117. Fiscella K, Tancred D, Franks P: Adding socioeconomic status to Framingham scoring to reduce disparities in coronary risk assessment. *Am Heart J* 157:988, 2009.

118. Greenland P, LaBree L, Azen SP, et al: Coronary artery calcium score combined with Framingham score for risk prediction in asymptomatic individuals [erratum in *JAMA* 291:563, 2004]. *JAMA* 291:210, 2004.

119. Arad Y, Goodman K, Roth M, et al: Coronary calcification, coronary disease risk factors, C-reactive protein, and atherosclerotic cardiovascular disease events: the St. Francis Heart Study. *J Am Coll Cardiol* 46:158, 2005.

120. O'Malley PG, Taylor AJ, Jackson JL, et al: Prognostic value of coronary electron-beam computed tomography for coronary heart disease events in asymptomatic populations. *Am J Cardiol* 85:945, 2000.

121. Raggi P, Callister TQ, Shaw LJ: Progression of coronary artery calcium and risk of first myocardial infarction in patients receiving cholesterol-lowering therapy. *Arterioscler Thromb Vasc Biol* 24:1272, 2004.

122. Bild DE, Detrano R, Peterson D, et al: Ethnic differences in coronary calcification: the Multi-Ethnic Study of Atherosclerosis (MESA). *Circulation* 111:1313, 2005.

123. Detrano R, Guerci AD, Carr JJ, et al: Coronary calcium as a predictor of coronary events in four racial or ethnic groups. *N Engl J Med* 358:1336, 2008.

124. Eliminating racial and ethnic health disparities, Centers for Disease Control and Prevention, Office of Minority Health & Health Disparities. Available at: http://www.cdc.gov/omhd/about/disparities.htm.

125. Moser DK, Kimble LP, Alberts MJ, et al: Reducing delay in seeking treatment by patients with acute coronary syndrome and stroke: a scientific statement from the American Heart Association Council on cardiovascular nursing and stroke council. *Circulation* 114:168, 2006.

126. Daumit GL, Hermann JA, Coresh J, Powe NR: Use of cardiovascular procedures among black persons and white persons: a 7-year nationwide study in patients with renal disease. *Ann Intern Med* 130:173, 1999.

127. Fiscella K, Franks P: Should years of schooling be used to guide treatment of coronary risk factors? *Ann Family Med* 2:469, 2004.

128. Sudore RL, Mehta KM, Simonsick EM, et al: Limited literacy in older people and disparities in health and healthcare access. *J Am Geriatr Soc* 54:770, 2006.

129. Ranjit N, Diez-Roux AV, Shea S, et al: Psychosocial factors and inflammation in the multi-ethnic study of atherosclerosis. *Arch Intern Med* 167:174, 2007.

130. Jacobs EA, Rolle I, Ferrans CE, et al: Understanding African Americans' views of the trustworthiness of physicians. *J Gen Intern Med* 21:642, 2006.

131. Fisher T, Burnet DL, Huang ES, et al: Cultural leverage: interventions utilizing culture to narrow racial disparities in health care. *Med Care Res Rev* 64(Suppl):243S, 2007.

132. Taylor SL, Lurie N: The role of culturally competent communication in reducing ethnic and racial healthcare disparities. *Am J Managed Care* 10(spec no):SP1, 2004.

133. van Ryn M, Burgess D, Malat J, Griffin J: Physicians' perceptions of patients' social and behavioral characteristics and race disparities in treatment recommendations for men with coronary artery disease. *Am J Public Health* 96:351, 2006.

134. Fiscella K, Williams DR: Health disparities based on socioeconomic inequities: implications for urban health care. *Acad Med* 79:1139, 2004.

135. Key facts about Americans without health insurance, Menlo Park, Calif, Kaiser Family Foundation. Available at: http://www.kff.org.

136. Access to care for the uninsured: an update, Menlo Park, Calif, Kaiser Family Foundation. Available at: http://www.kff.org.

137. Rahimi AR, Spertus JA, Reid KJ, et al: Financial barriers to health care and outcomes after acute myocardial infarction. *JAMA* 297:1063, 2007.

138. Trivedi AN, Sequist TD, Ayanian JZ: Impact of hospital volume on racial disparities in cardiovascular procedure mortality. *J Am Coll Cardiol* 47:417, 2006.

139. Skinner J, Chandra A, Staiger D, et al: Mortality after acute myocardial infarction in hospitals that disproportionately treat black patients. *Circulation* 112:2634, 2005.

140. Bhandari VK, Kushel M, Price L, Schillinger D: Racial disparities in outcomes of inpatient stroke rehabilitation. *Arch Phys Med Rehabil* 86:2081, 2005.

141. Horner RD, Swanson JW, Bosworth HB, Matchar DB: Effects of race and poverty on the process and outcome of inpatient rehabilitation services among stroke patients. *Stroke* 34:1027, 2003.

142. Exner DV, Dries DL, Domanski MJ, Cohn JN: Lesser response to angiotensin-converting-enzyme inhibitor therapy in black as compared with white patients with left ventricular dysfunction. *N Engl J Med* 344:1351, 2001.

143. Yancy CW, Fowler MB, Colucci WS, et al: Race and the response to adrenergic blockade with carvedilol in patients with chronic heart failure. *N Engl J Med* 344:1358, 2001.

144. Wood AJ: Racial differences in the response to drugs—pointers to genetic differences. *N Engl J Med* 344:1394, 2001.

145. Proceedings of the U.S. Food and Drug Administration Center for Drug Evaluation and Research, Cardiovascular and Renal Drugs Advisory Committee [transcript], June 16, 2005. Available at: http://www.fda.gov/ohrms/dockets/ac/05/transcripts/2005-4183T1.pdf.

146. Cohn JN, Archibald DG, Ziesche S, et al: Effect of vasodilator therapy on mortality in chronic congestive heart failure. Results of a Veterans Administration Cooperative Study. *N Engl J Med* 314:1547, 1986.

147. Cohn JN, Johnson G, Ziesche S, et al: A comparison of enalapril with hydralazine-isosorbide dinitrate in the treatment of chronic congestive heart failure. *N Engl J Med* 325:303, 1991.

148. Taylor AL, Ziesche S, Yancy C, et al; African-American Heart Failure Trial Investigators: Combination of isosorbide dinitrate and hydralazine in blacks with heart failure. *N Engl J Med* 351:2049, 2004. Epub 2004 Nov 8.

CHAPTER 24

Prevention of Ischemic Heart Disease in Women

Raza H. Orakzai, Chrisandra L. Shufelt, Leslee J. Shaw, and
C. Noel Bairey Merz

KEY POINTS

- Cardiovascular disease is the leading cause of death among women in the United States.

- Women receive fewer preventive recommendations, such as lipid-lowering therapy, aspirin, and lifestyle advice, than do men with similar Framingham risk scores.

- The Framingham risk score and the Reynolds score can be used to estimate CVD risk in women.

- Dyslipidemia treatment recommendations are similar between women and men. Clinical trials demonstrate the efficacy and safety of statin dyslipidemia therapy, including more intensive treatments, for protection against major cardiovascular events in women.

- Blood pressure and diabetes treatment recommendations do not differ between women and men. Impaired glucose tolerance during pregnancy is a risk factor for future CVD in women.

- The use of aspirin for women aged 55 to 79 years is recommended when the potential benefit of a reduction in ischemic strokes outweighs the potential harm of an increase in gastrointestinal hemorrhage.

- Women should accumulate a minimum of 30 minutes of moderate-intensity physical activity (e.g., brisk walking) daily.

- Women should consume a diet rich in fruits and vegetables, whole-grain high-fiber foods, and fish at least twice a week, with limited intake of saturated fat (<7% to 10%) and cholesterol (<300 mg/ day); alcohol intake should be

limited to no more than one drink per day; sodium intake should be limited to <2.3 g/ day; and consumption of *trans*–fatty acids should be as low as possible.

- Hormone therapy used for contraception, management of menopause symptoms, or other clinically indicated conditions should not be used for CVD prevention.

Cardiovascular disease (CVD), the leading cause of death among women regardless of race or ethnicity, accounts for more than 500,000 deaths in the United States each year.[1] This amounts to more deaths from CVD than from lung cancer, chronic obstructive lung disease, and breast cancer combined.[2] In many countries including the United States, more women than men die of CVD every year, a fact largely unknown by physicians and lay public.[2,3] Typically, women cite cancer, specifically breast cancer, as a major threat to their health. Nevertheless, the annual mortality of women from CVD is twice that for all cancers combined, and almost one in two women will die of CVD compared with one in 30 of breast cancer.[4,5] Paradoxical sex differences are observed in which women have less anatomically obstructive coronary artery disease (CAD) and relatively preserved left ventricular function yet higher rates of myocardial ischemia and mortality compared with similarly aged men.[6-9] Accordingly, the term *ischemic heart disease* (IHD) is more appropriate for a discussion specific to women, rather than CAD or coronary heart disease (CHD). Data from the National Heart, Lung, and Blood Institute (NHLBI)–sponsored Women's Ischemia Syndrome Evaluation (WISE) and related studies implicate adverse coronary

This work was supported by contracts from the National Heart, Lung, and Blood Institute, N01-HV-68161, N01-HV-68162, N01-HV-68163, N01-HV-68164, R01 HL090957-01A1, R03 AG032631-01; a GCRC grant MO1-RR00425 from the National Center for Research Resources; and grants from the Gustavus and Louise Pfeiffer Research Foundation (Danville, NJ), the Women's Guild of Cedars-Sinai Medical Center (Los Angeles, Calif), the Edythe L. Broad Women's Heart Research Fellowship, Cedars-Sinai Medical Center (Los Angeles, Calif), and the Barbra Streisand Women's Cardiovascular Research and Education Program, Cedars-Sinai Medical Center (Los Angeles, Calif).

reactivity,[10] microvascular dysfunction,[11] and plaque erosion or distal microembolization[12,13] as contributory to female-specific IHD pathophysiology. Thus, knowledge beyond an anatomic description of obstructive CAD may provide important clues to IHD risk detection and treatment for women.

AWARENESS

In a survey conducted by the American Heart Association (AHA) in 2003, only 13% of U.S. women (7% in 1997) perceived heart disease as a major health risk.[14] Black and Hispanic women are less likely than white women to be aware that heart disease is the primary cause of death in women. Only about one third of women recall discussing heart disease risk with their physicians.[15] Women receive fewer preventive recommendations, such as lipid-lowering therapy, aspirin, and lifestyle advice, than do men with similar Framingham risk scores.[3,16]

Despite the availability of numerous preventive and therapeutic options, women often do not take steps to modify their cardiac risk factors; low awareness is likely to contribute to this. Although mortality from IHD has declined gradually among men since 1979 (by 30% to 50%), mortality from IHD in women has increased during the same period.[2] A greater proportion of women (52%) than men (42%) with myocardial infarction (MI) die of sudden cardiac death before reaching the hospital; two thirds of women who suffer MI never completely recover.[2] Since the late 1970s, hospital discharges from heart failure among women have increased at a markedly faster rate than among men.[2] Thus, an understanding of even subtle differences between men and women in development and progression of IHD and in the use of proven therapies and response to therapy could have a significant impact on improving outcomes. Even modest preventive measures can have an enormous impact. It is projected that a reduction in death rate due to chronic diseases by just 2% during one decade would prevent 36 million deaths.[17]

It has long been recognized that the first presentation with IHD occurs on average 10 years later among women than among men, commonly after menopause. Although IHD, in general, is manifested earlier in less developed countries, the approximate 8- to 10-year age gap in time at onset between men and women remains universal (Fig. 24-1). The INTER-HEART study, a large cohort study of more than 52,000 individuals with MI, has demonstrated that the age gap between the sexes is consistent across various socioeconomic, climatic, and cultural environments.[18] However, lifetime IHD risk for women is essentially equivalent to that of men.[19] Menopause is associated with a threefold increase in risk, although it is unclear if this is simply attributable to age.[20] It

has been widely speculated that the observed sex-related age difference reflects premenopausal protection afforded by circulating estrogen; however, younger premenopausal women face a twofold increase in MI-related mortality compared with age-matched men (Fig. 24-2).[21] The role that endogenous and exogenous reproductive hormones play in IHD remains poorly understood.

Women are underrepresented in IHD prevention studies. Equal inclusion of women in large cardiovascular trials is now mandated by the NHLBI.[22] In practice, women are less likely to receive preventive therapy, possibly because of a lack of perceived sex-specific benefit resulting from studies predominantly conducted in men. Notably, evidence-based guidelines for CVD prevention in women were published by the AHA in 2004 and later updated in 2007.[5,14,23]

RISK STRATIFICATION

The 2007 AHA update recommends a scheme for a general risk stratification approach to the female patient that classifies her as at high risk, at risk, or at optimal risk (Table 24-1). The 2007 AHA update focuses on the high average lifetime risk for CVD, which approaches one in two women. Conversely, the Framingham risk score focuses on a relatively narrow period of 10-year risk of CHD death or MI that does not adequately reflect the long-term or lifetime risk of women. The limitations of risk stratification with the Framingham risk score in diverse populations of women are well recognized. These include the lack of inclusion of family history, obesity, metabolic syndrome, and physical inactivity; inaccurate estimation of risk in nonwhite populations; and the preponderance of low risk scores in women despite a high prevalence of subclinical disease.[24]

A Framingham risk score >20% can identify a woman at high risk, but a lower Framingham risk score is insufficient to ensure that an individual woman is at low lifetime risk. The Reynolds risk score, derived from almost 25,000 participants in the Women's Health Study, was recently suggested as a superior alternative risk score for women,[25] although validation and translation into clinical practice are needed.[26] The Reynolds score incorporates novel risk markers, including high-sensitivity C-reactive protein (hsCRP) and a family

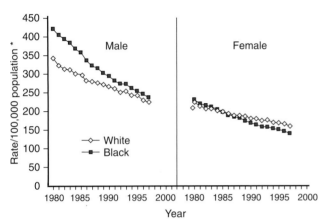

FIGURE 24-1 Death rates for coronary heart disease by sex and race in the United States from 1980 through 1997. *Rates are age adjusted to the 2000 standard. (From Cooper R, Cutler J, Desvigne-Nickens P, et al: Trends and disparities in coronary heart disease, stroke, and other cardiovascular diseases in the United States: findings of the national conference on cardiovascular disease prevention. Circulation 102:3137, 2000.)

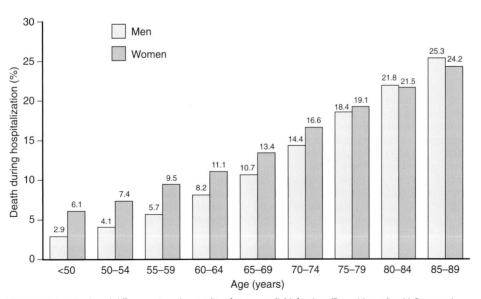

FIGURE 24-2 Sex-based differences in early mortality after myocardial infarction. (From Vaccarino V, Parsons L, Every NR, et al: Sex-based differences in early mortality after myocardial infarction. National Registry of Myocardial Infarction 2 Participants. N Engl J Med 341:217, 1999.)

TABLE 24–1	Classification of Cardiovascular Disease Risk in Women
Risk Status	**Criteria**
High risk	Established coronary heart disease Cerebrovascular disease Peripheral arterial disease Abdominal aortic aneurysm End-stage or chronic renal disease Diabetes mellitus 10-year Framingham global risk >20%*

At risk	≥1 major risk factors for CVD, including
	  Cigarette smoking
	  Poor diet
	  Physical inactivity
	  Obesity, especially central adiposity
	  Family history of premature CVD (CVD at <55
	    years of age in male relative and <65 years of
	    age in female relative)
	  Hypertension
	  Dyslipidemia
	  Evidence of subclinical vascular disease (e.g.,
	    coronary calcification)
	  Metabolic syndrome
	  Poor exercise capacity on treadmill test and/or
	    abnormal heart rate recovery after stopping
	    exercise

Optimal risk	Framingham global risk <10% and a healthy lifestyle, with no risk factors

*Or at high risk on the basis of another population-adapted tool used to assess global risk.

From Mosca L, Banka CL, Benjamin EJ, et al: Evidence-based guidelines for cardiovascular disease prevention in women: 2007 update. *Circulation* 115:1481, 2007.

history of CAD, that may aid in unique detection of risk in women. It also has the advantage of including cerebrovascular events as an outcome; this point is important because of the higher frequency of stroke in women compared with men. Application of the Reynolds risk score reclassified 40% to 50% of women with an intermediate Framingham risk score into higher or lower risk categories.[27]

D'Agostino and colleagues[28] proposed a sex-specific multivariable risk factor algorithm that can be used to assess general CVD risk and risk of individual cardiovascular events (coronary, cerebrovascular, and peripheral arterial disease and heart failure). The authors used Cox proportional hazards regression to evaluate the risk for development of a first cardiovascular event in 8491 Framingham study participants (mean age, 49 years; 4522 women) who attended a routine examination between 30 and 74 years of age and were free of CVD. Sex-specific multivariable risk functions ("general CVD" algorithms) were derived that incorporated age, total and high-density lipoprotein cholesterol, systolic blood pressure, treatment of hypertension, smoking, and diabetes status. During 12 years of follow-up, 1174 participants (456 women) developed a first cardiovascular event. The general CVD algorithm demonstrated good discrimination (C-statistic, 0.763 [men] and 0.793 [women]) and calibration.

There is considerable evidence that elevated levels of total cholesterol (TC) and low-density lipoprotein cholesterol (LDL-C) increase IHD risk in women,[4,29] although these relationships are less prominent in elderly women compared with younger women.[4,30] In contrast, low levels of high-density lipoprotein cholesterol (HDL-C) and elevated levels of triglyceride (TG) impart comparable risk in young and elderly women.[4,30] Despite this evidence, men are more likely to have their lipid levels measured, and abnormal values are generally treated more aggressively than in women.[4,31] In women

enrolled in the HERS study (1993), all of whom had established CHD, 91% failed to meet the National Cholesterol Education Program (NCEP) Adult Treatment Panel (ATP II, 1993) LDL-C goal of <100 mg/dL.[32] In a trial in patients with stable IHD, 31% of men and only 12% of women reached LDL-C of <100 mg/dL.[33] In the WISE study, which enrolled women with chest pain and myocardial ischemia documented on noninvasive testing between 1996 and 2003, only 24% met their LDL-C goals.[34] These studies document less aggressive treatment of dyslipidemia in high-risk women, including those with documented IHD, compared with men.[4,5,29]

RISK FACTORS AND RISK REDUCTION INTERVENTIONS

Age

Age is one of the most powerful risk factors for the development of IHD and accompanying clinical events. IHD events including MI lag 10 to 15 years in women compared with men. As men age, they continue to have a linear increase in IHD incidence, particularly during the fifth and sixth decades, whereas women have an almost exponential increase in IHD incidence after the age of 60 years,[35] although population-adjusted curves suggest that this may be due to survivor effects. One in eight women between the ages of 45 and 64 years has evidence of CAD, which increases to one in three after the age of 65 years.[36] With more women living to elderly ages, a majority of IHD victims are not surprisingly now women. It is for these reasons that NCEP ATP III has different age cutoffs for sex; at or above 55 years is the age considered a risk factor for women compared with 45 years for men.

Family History

It is well established that CVD has a hereditary component. However, few prospective studies have evaluated the relationship between family history and future IHD events in women. Retrospective review of much larger data bases of women (e.g., the Nurses' Health Study) has demonstrated conflicting results. In women with a family history of MI before the age of 60 years, the age-adjusted relative risk was 2.8 for nonfatal MI and 5.0 for fatal cardiovascular events.[37] With adjustment for other cardiovascular risk factors, family history remained an independent risk factor for CVD. NCEP ATP III defines family history of premature CHD before the age of 65 years for women and before the age of 55 years for men.[38] Although family history of premature CHD signifies high risk, risk remains elevated when the definition is broadened to include older first-degree relatives.

Dyslipidemia

More than half of the women in the United States have a TC level >200 mg/dL, and 36% have LDL-C concentration >130 mg/dL.[2] Notably, only 13% of women have HDL-C concentration <40 mg/dL (compared with 23% of Americans overall); the higher threshold of <50 mg/dL is used for women. The relative risk for IHD events associated with elevation of various lipid variables was determined in a nested case-control study from the Nurses' Health Study. Among 32,826 healthy women, the multivariable relative risks (adjusted for hsCRP, homocysteine, and other traditional cardiac risk factors) for the highest quintiles of lipid variables were as follows: apolipoprotein B: RR, 4.1 (2-8.3); low levels of HDL-C: RR, 2.6 (1.4-5); LDL-C: RR, 3.1 (1.7-5.8); and TG: RR, 1.9 (1-3.9).[39] Adverse changes in lipid profile accompany menopause.[40] Perimenopausal TG levels are the

TABLE 24–2 | **Major Lipid-Lowering Trials Using Statin Therapy for Coronary Heart Disease (CHD) Prevention**

Study	Patients (n)	Women, n (%)	Prevention Category	Drug	Year	Risk Reduction in Major CHD Events in Women (%)
4S[43]	4444	827 (19)	Secondary	Simvastatin	1994	35
CARE[44]	4159	576 (14)	Secondary	Pravastatin	1996	46
LIPID[45]	9014	1516 (17)	Secondary	Pravastatin	1998	11
AFCAPS/TexCAPS[46]	6605	997 (15)	Primary	Lovastatin	1998	46
PROSPER[47]	5804	3000 (52)	Both	Pravastatin	2002	NS benefit for women
HPS[48]	20,536	5082 (25)	Primary	Simvastatin	2002	19
ALLHAT-LLT[49]	10,355	5051 (49)	Primary (hypertension) 14% CHD	Pravastatin	2002	Sex-specific data not reported; NS in total cohort
GREACE[50]	1600	344 (21)	Secondary	Atorvastatin	2002	54
ASCOT-LLA[51]	10,305	1942 (19)	Primary (hypertension)	Atorvastatin	2003	NS benefit for women

NS, Not significant.

From Lavie CJ, Wenger NK: Special patient populations: women and elderly. In Ballantyne CM, editor: *Clinical lipidology*, Philadelphia, 2009, Saunders/Elsevier, p 465.

most erratic but follow roughly the same pattern of increased TC and LDL-C on average by ~10% from levels 6 months before menopause. Menopause can influence HDL-C less dramatically, with mild declines noted.

Dyslipidemia is strongly predictive of IHD risk in older women. Women in the Framingham study with TC >265 mg/dL were at two to three times greater risk for experiencing an IHD event compared with women with TC <205 mg/dL. Overall, a 1% increase in TC translated to a 2% increase in IHD incidence.[41] Elevated TG levels and low HDL-C levels are more closely associated with the risk of IHD in women, especially in those at least 65 years old. Lower levels of HDL-C are associated with an increased risk of IHD in the Lipid Research Clinics Follow-up Study. HDL-C was second to age in predicting IHD risk. The ratio of TC and HDL-C was a more accurate marker of IHD risk than either level alone. The NCEP guidelines call for measurement of TC as well as of HDL-C as part of the initial cholesterol screening after the age of 20 years. The TC/HDL-C ratio is typically lower in women than in men through middle age but then increases and parallels that of men by 75 years of age. After the age of 55 years, elevated TC and TC/HDL-C ratio significantly increase IHD risk.

The protective role of lipid-lowering therapy in women, especially with the 3-hydroxy-3-methylglutaryl coenzyme A reductase inhibitors (i.e., statins), is well established by numerous randomized clinical trials noting consistent reductions in CVD risk ranging from 11% to 54%[4,42-51] (Table 24-2). Although the representation of women in most trials is relatively low (averaging <20% of the population), a positive trend for benefit was consistent across all trials. Importantly, the protective effect of statins based on these trials appeared equivalent to or greater than that observed for men. The reduction in risk of major cardiovascular events in women ranged from 11% in the Long-term Intervention with Pravastatin Ischaemic Disease (LIPID) study[45] to 54% in the Greek Atorvastatin and Coronary-heart-disease Evaluation (GREACE) trial.[50] There was no significant effect in the subgroup of women in the Prospective Study of Pravastatin in the Elderly at Risk (PROSPER)[47] or in the lipid-lowering arm of the Anglo-Scandinavian Cardiac Outcomes Trial (ASCOT).[51] There was no significant effect in the total cohort (men or women) in the lipid-lowering arm of the Antihypertensive and Lipid-Lowering Treatment to Prevent Heart Attack Trial (ALLHAT)[49]; however, Treating to New Targets (TNT), a trial of high-dose (80 mg) versus low-dose (10 mg) atorvastatin, showed equal protection against major cardiovascular events

with more intensive therapy in women, statistically similar to that of men, without a sex difference in serious adverse events. There was modestly higher frequency of discontinuation of statins (10% versus 6.5%) and liver function test abnormalities (2.5% versus 1%) in women than in men.[52] Likewise, in patients with acute coronary syndromes (n = 4162 patients, 22% women), more intensive lipid treatment with atorvastatin 80 mg versus pravastatin 40 mg also yielded similar benefits for women and men.[53]

In aggregate, these trials demonstrate the efficacy and safety of statin therapy, including more intensive treatments, for protection against major cardiovascular events in women. In addition to significant reductions of LDL-C and moderate improvements in HDL-C and TG, other potential beneficial effects of statins include improvements in endothelial function, plaque stabilization, anti-inflammatory effects, and antiplatelet effects, among others. Higher risk patients, such as secondary prevention, offer the best short-term efficacy targets. Whereas it has been argued that treatment of dyslipidemic young women is not cost-effective, recent prevention guidelines focused on longer term lifetime risk question this rationale.[5,25,27] In addition, women carry a high short-term mortality rate associated with first IHD events (more than twice that for men), providing further support for consideration of statin therapy for both primary and secondary prevention of IHD in women (Table 24-3).

On the basis of a number of trials in high-risk subjects,[53,54] the 2004 revision of the NCEP ATP III guidelines introduced a new LDL-C goal of <70 mg/dL for patients at very high risk, which includes women with established CVD and multiple other cardiovascular risk factors.[55] A meta-analysis of primary prevention trials (excluding the recent JUPITER trial)[56] concluded that pharmacologic lipid lowering, primarily with statins, does not reduce mortality or events in women without known CVD.[57] Caution, however, is warranted in the interpretation of this finding because of the relatively small number of cardiovascular events and the relatively young age of the female enrollees. As young women have a lower absolute risk than that of men in a limited observational period, it is conceivable that the number needed to treat is significantly higher for women than for men. As statins primarily affect LDL-C reduction, one can speculate whether targeting of HDL-C or TGs may be more promising in women compared with men. The documented benefits of lipid-lowering therapy in high-risk women, on the other hand, are convincing and robust. It is therefore important to implement aggressive pharmacotherapy to new lipid targets in high-risk women.[58]

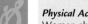

TABLE 24–3 | **Guidelines for Prevention of Cardiovascular Disease in Women: Clinical Recommendations**

Lifestyle Interventions
Cigarette Smoking
Women should not smoke and should avoid environmental tobacco smoke. Provide counseling, nicotine replacement, and other pharmacotherapy as indicated in conjunction with a behavioral program or formal smoking cessation program *(Class I, Level B)*.

Physical Activity
Women should accumulate a minimum of 30 minutes of moderate-intensity physical activity (e.g., brisk walking) on most and preferably all days of the week *(Class I, Level B)*.
Women who need to lose weight or sustain weight loss should accumulate a minimum of 60 to 90 minutes of moderate-intensity physical activity (e.g., brisk walking) on most and preferably all days of the week *(Class I, Level C)*.

Rehabilitation
A comprehensive risk reduction regimen, such as cardiovascular or stroke rehabilitation or a physician-guided home- or community-based exercise training program, should be recommended to women with a recent acute coronary syndrome or coronary intervention, new-onset or chronic angina, recent cerebrovascular event, peripheral arterial disease *(Class I, Level A)*, or current/prior symptoms of heart failure and LVEF <40% *(Class I, Level B)*.

Dietary Intake
Women should consume a diet rich in fruits and vegetables; choose whole-grain, high-fiber foods; consume fish, especially oily fish,* at least twice a week; limit intake of saturated fat to <10% of energy and if possible to <7%, cholesterol to <300 mg/day, alcohol intake to no more than 1 drink per day,† and sodium intake to <2.3 g/day (approximately 1 tsp salt). Consumption of *trans*–fatty acids should be as low as possible (e.g., <1% of energy) *(Class I, Level B)*.

Weight Maintenance or Reduction
Women should maintain or lose weight through an appropriate balance of physical activity, calorie intake, and formal behavioral programs when indicated to maintain or to achieve a BMI between 18.5 and 24.9 kg/m² and a waist circumference ≤35 inches *(Class I, Level B)*.

Omega-3 Fatty Acids
As an adjunct to diet, omega-3 fatty acids in capsule form (approximately 850 to 1000 mg of EPA and DHA) may be considered in women with CHD, and higher doses (2 to 4 g) may be used for treatment of women with high triglyceride levels *(Class IIb, Level B)*.

Depression
Consider screening women with CHD for depression and refer or treat when indicated *(Class IIa, Level B)*.

Major Risk Factor Interventions
Blood Pressure—Optimal Level and Lifestyle
Encourage an optimal blood pressure of <120/80 mm Hg through lifestyle approaches such as weight control, increased physical activity, alcohol moderation, sodium restriction, and increased consumption of fresh fruits and vegetables and low-fat dairy products *(Class I, Level B)*.

Blood Pressure—Pharmacotherapy
Pharmacotherapy is indicated when blood pressure is ≥140/90 mm Hg or at an even lower blood pressure in the setting of chronic kidney disease or diabetes (≥130/80 mm Hg). Thiazide diuretics should be part of the drug regimen for most patients unless contraindicated or if there are compelling indications for other agents in specific vascular diseases. Initial treatment of high-risk women‡ should be with beta blockers and/or ACE inhibitors or ARBs, with addition of other drugs such as thiazides as needed to achieve goal blood pressure *(Class I, Level A)*.

Lipid and Lipoprotein Levels—Optimal Levels and Lifestyle
The following levels of lipids and lipoproteins in women should be encouraged through lifestyle approaches: LDL-C <100 mg/dL, HDL-C >50 mg/dL, triglycerides <150 mg/dL, and non–HDL-C (total cholesterol minus HDL cholesterol) <130 mg/dL *(Class I, Level B)*. If a woman is at high risk‡ or has hypercholesterolemia, intake of saturated fat should be <7% and cholesterol intake <200 mg/day *(Class I, Level B)*.

Lipids—Pharmacotherapy for LDL Lowering, High-Risk Women
Use LDL-C–lowering drug therapy simultaneously with lifestyle therapy in women with CHD to achieve an LDL-C <100 mg/dL *(Class I, Level A)* and similarly in women with other atherosclerotic CVD or diabetes mellitus or 10-year absolute risk >20% *(Class I, Level B)*.
A reduction to <70 mg/dL is reasonable in very-high-risk women§ with CHD and may require an LDL-lowering drug combination *(Class IIa, Level B)*.

Lipids—Pharmacotherapy for LDL Lowering, Other At-Risk Women
Use LDL-C–lowering therapy if LDL-C level is ≥130 mg/dL with lifestyle therapy and there are multiple risk factors and 10-year absolute risk 10% to 20% *(Class I, Level B)*.
Use LDL-C–lowering therapy if LDL-C level is ≥160 mg/dL with lifestyle therapy and multiple risk factors even if 10-year absolute risk is <10% *(Class I, Level B)*.
Use LDL-C–lowering therapy if LDL ≥190 mg/dL regardless of the presence or absence of other risk factors or CVD on lifestyle therapy *(Class I, Level B)*.

Lipids—Pharmacotherapy for Low HDL or Elevated Non-HDL, High-Risk Women
Use niacin‖ or fibrate therapy when HDL-C is low or non–HDL-C is elevated in high-risk women‡ after LDL-C goal is reached *(Class IIa, Level B)*.

Lipids—Pharmacotherapy for Low HDL or Elevated Non-HDL, Other At-Risk Women
Consider niacin‖ or fibrate therapy when HDL-C is low or non–HDL-C is elevated after LDL-C goal is reached in women with multiple risk factors and a 10-year absolute risk 10% to 20% *(Class IIb, Level B)*.

Diabetes Mellitus
Lifestyle and pharmacotherapy should be used as indicated in women with diabetes *(Class I, Level B)* to achieve HbA1c <7% if this can be accomplished without significant hypoglycemia *(Class I, Level C)*.

Preventive Drug Interventions

Aspirin, High Risk

Aspirin therapy (75 to 325 mg/day)[¶] should be used in high-risk[‡] women unless contraindicated (*Class I, Level A*).
If a high-risk[‡] woman is intolerant of aspirin therapy, clopidogrel should be substituted (*Class I, Level B*).

Aspirin—Other At-Risk or Healthy Women

In women ≥65 years of age, consider aspirin therapy (81 mg daily or 100 mg every other day) if blood pressure is controlled and benefit for ischemic stroke and MI prevention is likely to outweigh risk of gastrointestinal bleeding and hemorrhagic stroke (*Class IIa, Level B*) and in women <65 years of age when benefit for ischemic stroke prevention is likely to outweigh adverse effects of therapy (*Class IIb, Level B*).

Beta Blockers

Beta blockers should be used indefinitely in all women after MI, acute coronary syndrome, or left ventricular dysfunction with or without heart failure symptoms, unless contraindicated (*Class I, Level A*).

ACE Inhibitors/ARBs

ACE inhibitors should be used (unless contraindicated) in women after MI and in those with clinical evidence of heart failure or LVEF ≤40% or with diabetes mellitus (*Class I, Level A*). In women after MI and in those with clinical evidence of heart failure or LVEF ≤40% or with diabetes mellitus who are intolerant of ACE inhibitors, ARBs should be used instead (*Class I, Level B*).

Aldosterone Blockade

Use aldosterone blockade after MI in women who do not have significant renal dysfunction or hyperkalemia who are already receiving therapeutic doses of an ACE inhibitor and beta blocker and have LVEF ≤40% with symptomatic heart failure (*Class I, Level B*).

ACE, angiotensin-converting enzyme; ARB, angiotensin receptor blocker; BMI, body mass index; CHD, coronary heart disease; CVD, cardiovascular disease; DHA, docosahexaenoic acid; EPA, eicosapentaenoic acid; HDL-C, high-density lipoprotein cholesterol; LDL-C, low-density lipoprotein cholesterol; LVEF, left ventricular ejection fraction; MI, myocardial infarction.

*Pregnant and lactating women should avoid eating fish potentially high in methylmercury (e.g., shark, swordfish, king mackerel, or tile fish) and should eat up to 12 oz/wk of a variety of fish and shellfish low in mercury and check the Environmental Protection Agency and the U.S. Food and Drug Administration's websites for updates and local advisories about safety of local catch.

[†]A drink equivalent is equal to a 12-oz bottle of beer, a 5-oz glass of wine, or a 1.5-oz shot of 80-proof spirit.

[‡]Criteria for high risk include established CHD, cerebrovascular disease, peripheral arterial disease, abdominal aortic aneurysm, end-stage or chronic renal disease, diabetes mellitus, and 10-year Framingham risk >20%.

[§]Criteria for very high risk include established CVD plus any of the following: multiple major risk factors, severe and poorly controlled risk factors, diabetes mellitus.

[||]Dietary supplement niacin should not be used as a substitute for prescription niacin.

[¶]After percutaneous intervention with stent placement or coronary artery bypass grafting within previous year and in women with noncoronary forms of CVD, use current guidelines for aspirin and clopidogrel.

From Mosca L, Banka CL, Benjamin EJ, et al: Evidence-based guidelines for cardiovascular disease prevention in women: 2007 update. *Circulation* 115:1481, 2007.

A 2003 national survey highlighted that women remain undertreated compared with men and that significantly fewer high-risk women achieved their LDL-C goal compared with men.[59]

From the recent JUPITER trial, 17,802 apparently healthy men and women with LDL-C levels of <130 mg/dL and hsCRP levels of >2.0 mg/L were randomized to 20 mg of rosuvastatin daily versus placebo.[56] The trial was stopped early after a median follow-up of 1.9 years, with rosuvastatin reducing LDL-C levels by 50% and hsCRP levels by 37%. Rosuvastatin significantly reduced the primary endpoint, a composite of nonfatal MI, nonfatal stroke, hospitalization for unstable angina, revascularization, and CVD death, by 44% compared with individuals treated with placebo. This reduction was observed across nearly all of the endpoints, including a 55% reduction in nonfatal MI, a 48% reduction in the risk of nonfatal stroke, and a 47% reduction in the risk of "hard" cardiac events (a composite of MI, stroke, and CVD death). Consistent effects were observed in all subgroups including women. Among the 6801 women (38%) included in JUPITER, rosuvastatin significantly reduced the primary composite end point by 46%, a magnitude similar to that observed in men.

Women are often concerned about stroke more than MI. Data from statin trials such as JUPITER, which showed a 48% reduction in the risk of nonfatal stroke with rosuvastatin, might help physicians provide a more convincing argument for women who may be reluctant about taking statins, especially if familial risk of stroke is great relative to that of MI.

Smoking

Cigarette smoking is the most preventable IHD risk factor in women and men and increases the risk of MI in women relatively greater than in men.[60,61] More than 60% of MIs in women younger than 50 years are attributable to smoking, as are 21% of all deaths from IHD. For women smokers, a dose-dependent relationship between consumption and risk has been described.[62,63] Rosenberg and colleagues[62] cited an increased risk of nonfatal MI from 2.4 in women who smoke 15 to 24 cigarettes/day to 7 for those who smoke >25 cigarettes/day. In addition, smoking increases the IHD risk when other cardiac risk factors are present or when oral contraceptive pills are being taken. Women not taking oral contraceptive pills who smoke >25 cigarettes/day have a 4.8-fold relative risk of nonfatal MI compared with a 23-fold relative risk in female smokers taking oral contraceptives.

In the United States, fewer women than men currently smoke, and the prevalence of smoking among women has declined during the past three decades. However, tobacco use has decreased more dramatically in men than in women. More worrisome is the increased prevalence of female adolescents who are smoking. Compared with male smokers, women more often smoke to relieve stress, anger, boredom, or depression. Women are more likely than men to cite smoking as a strategy for weight loss, and they more often give weight gain as a major reason for relapsing.[64] All women benefit from smoking cessation, regardless of age at cessation, which should provide a tremendous incentive for elderly smokers to quit. In the Nurses' Health Study, women who stopped smoking experienced an immediate benefit as well as a further long-term decline in IHD risk to levels comparable to those of women who never smoked.[65] Total mortality risk among former smokers decreases nearly to that of never-smokers within 10 to 14 years of cessation.[66] The risk of an index MI in women declines soon after the cessation of smoking and is largely dissipated after 2 to 3 years.[67]

Compared with men, women find it more difficult to quit smoking with and without treatment and are also more likely to relapse. Simple encouragement to stop smoking should be part of every follow-up encounter with an active smoker. In women who are unable to quit without assistance, use of nicotine replacement and other pharmacotherapy (e.g., bupropion, varenicline) in conjunction with behavioral therapy or a formal smoking cessation program is warranted.

Physical Inactivity

Sedentary lifestyle is a common risk factor for IHD in women and men. Data from the National Center for Health Statistics indicate that 39% of white women and 57% of women of color do not exercise regularly.[68] Rates of physical inactivity are highest among poor women. Increased levels of physical activity are associated with lower blood pressure, lower cholesterol levels, improved glucose metabolism, higher bone density, and improved mental health variables. Physical inactivity contributes to obesity and is an independent risk factor for MI.[69] Even modest exercise has been strongly associated with risk reduction in observational studies. Investigators in the Nurses' Health Study[70] found that 30 to 45 minutes of walking three times weekly reduces the risk of MI by 50% in women across the ages. Exercise has also been found to reduce the risk of type 2 diabetes mellitus, even in obese women and those with a family history of diabetes.[71]

Physical activity has an even more beneficial role in women after MI or coronary artery bypass surgery. However, despite improved health outcomes associated with cardiac rehabilitation, fewer women than men enroll. A variety of reasons, including referral bias, difficulty with transportation, and elder and child care responsibilities, often prevent women from participating in cardiac rehabilitation programs. According to the 2007 prevention guidelines for women, women should accumulate a minimum of 30 minutes of moderate-intensity physical activity (e.g., brisk walking) daily (Class I recommendation) (see Table 24-3).

Diet

In the Nurses' Health Study, the dietary score, based on intake of cereal fiber, marine-3 fatty acids, folate, glycemic load, and ratio of polyunsaturated to saturated fat, acted as an independent factor for IHD.[69] A second report from the Nurses' Health Study evaluated the relationship between diet and cardiovascular events during 1980-1994 in 85,941 apparently healthy women. Improvement in dietary score consisting of reduced consumption of red meat, trans-fats, and high-fat products during the study was associated with a significant 16% decline in IHD incidence.[72] Current recommendations suggest that women should consume a diet rich in fruits and vegetables, whole-grain high-fiber foods, and fish at least twice a week, with limited intake of saturated fat (<7% to 10%) and cholesterol (<300 mg/day). Alcohol intake should be limited to no more than one drink per day and sodium intake to <2.3 g/day. Consumption of trans–fatty acids should be as low as possible (see Table 24-3). Nutrition intervention trials have demonstrated reductions in CVD and mortality,[73-75] although sex-stratified trial results are typically not available.

Obesity

Between 1988 and 1991, the Third National Health and Nutrition Examination Survey (NHANES III) reported that one third of U.S. adults (35% of the women and 31% of the men) were overweight.[76,77] Obesity was defined by a body mass index (BMI) of 27.8 kg/m^2 in men and 27.3 kg/m^2 in women (120% of desirable weight). Obesity is associated with glucose intolerance (or pre–diabetes mellitus), hypertension, and hypercholesterolemia and is also considered an independent risk factor for IHD.[76,78,79] In the Nurses' Health Study, obesity was strongly associated with an increased incidence of cardiovascular events even after control for older age and smoking.[78] Women who were >30% of ideal body weight had an increased risk ratio of 3.3 for nonfatal MI and IHD death. Recent data suggest that regional fat distribution, particularly a waist-to-hip ratio of >0.88 (android body type), may be more of an accurate marker for chronic ischemic IHD risk than obesity. Several studies have reported an increased risk of MI and IHD or CVD death in women with increased truncal adiposity even after adjustment of other cardiac risk factors.[80,81]

Data from the Framingham study indicate a doubling in the incidence of diabetes for both sexes during the past 30 years; most of this increase occurred in individuals with a BMI of 30 kg/m^2 and above.[82] The Coronary Artery Risk Development in Young Adults (CARDIA) study illustrated that young adults who maintained a stable BMI over time had minimal progression of risk factors and lower incidence of metabolic syndrome, regardless of baseline BMI. However, among 1358 men and 1321 women, only 16.3% maintained a stable BMI, and 73.9% had an increased BMI.[83] The increasing prevalence of obesity and diabetes in the population, despite a reduction of dietary fat intake during the past decades, highlights the importance of dietary recommendations for exercise and carbohydrate and fat intake. The Nurses' Health Study reported a positive association between dietary glycemic load and IHD in women, which was even more pronounced in overweight and obese women.[84] Thus, reducing the glycemic load in the diet should be as much of a priority as replacing saturated fats by unsaturated fats. Avoidance of refined sugars and restriction of sugar-sweetened beverages may particularly help reduce dietary glycemic load.[85] A diet high in fruits and vegetables may reduce the risk of diabetes; however, high consumption of fruit juices may be associated with an increased diabetes hazard among women.[86]

Diabetes and the Metabolic Syndrome

Diabetes is a relatively greater risk factor in women than in men, increasing IHD risk by threefold to sevenfold in diabetic women compared with a twofold to threefold increase in risk for diabetic men.[23] Furthermore, the risk of IHD death is higher in diabetic women than in diabetic men.[87] Whereas angiographic CAD is generally more prevalent in men than in women, diabetes eliminates this difference by increasing risk disproportionately in women. Large-scale prospective studies, including the Framingham study and the Nurses' Health Study, report diabetes mellitus as an independent risk factor; diabetic women were six to seven times more likely to experience nonfatal MI and CVD death. In addition, the risk of CVD morbidity and mortality in women with diabetes is minimally affected by the duration of diabetes, and a significant risk for cardiovascular events is still noted in patients with diabetes of less than 4 years in duration.[41]

Diabetic women have not experienced a decrease in IHD mortality during the past three decades compared with their male counterparts.[88] In fact, there was an increase in IHD mortality in the subgroup of diabetic women.[89] As diabetes is considered a CHD risk equivalent by the NCEP, all diabetic women are classified as high or very high risk. A history of diabetes in women was associated with a 37% increased IHD-related mortality.[90] Diabetes appears to have a greater adverse effect on TG, HDL-C, and LDL-C concentrations in diabetic women than in diabetic men.[91]

Milder forms of glucose intolerance and asymptomatic hyperglycemia may still place women at risk for IHD events. Type 2 diabetes or milder forms of glucose intolerance tend to cluster in women with visceral obesity, hypertension, and dyslipidemia.[92] This clinical pattern confers a much higher IHD risk in diabetic women, depending on the accompanying risk factor profile. Because other risk factors, such as hypertension, smoking, and obesity, act synergistically with diabetes, control of these other risk factors attenuates the risk of MI in diabetic women.

According to the American Diabetes Association, diabetes screening should be considered for women and men older than 45 years and repeated every 3 years, if results are normal.[93] Women with a history of gestational diabetes or polycystic ovarian syndrome should be screened earlier. History of gestational diabetes doubles the risk of diabetes within 4 months post partum, and it remains a lifelong risk factor for the development of diabetes, which is largely risk of type 2 diabetes.[94] Fasting plasma glucose levels of ≥121 mg/dL during pregnancy increase the risk for diabetes in the early puerperium by 21-fold.[95] Expert panels recommend fasting glucose testing or oral glucose tolerance tests 6 to 12 weeks post partum, then every 1 to 2 years in women with gestational diabetes. To prevent the development of diabetes in high-risk women, pre-pregnancy weight should be reached within 6 to 12 months post partum, and physical activity should be recommended.

Furthermore, it is reasonable to screen for diabetes earlier if obesity, hypertension, and dyslipidemia are present because these characteristics frequently co-occur as the metabolic syndrome. The prevalence of metabolic syndrome is similar for both sexes after adjustment for age. A hallmark of the metabolic syndrome is insulin resistance, defined as impaired fasting glucose (100 to 125 mg/dL), which is considered to be a prediabetic state. For women in the Framingham study, impaired fasting glucose was associated with increased IHD risk to a similar degree as established diabetes, a finding that was not seen in the men.[96]

Clinical trials demonstrate the value of risk factor management in diabetics. The Collaborative Atorvastatin Diabetes Study (CARDS) trial, which used atorvastatin 10 mg every day versus placebo in more than 3000 diabetic patients, was terminated early because of a 37% risk reduction with the statin.[97] In the Diabetes Control and Complications Trial, type 1 diabetics receiving conventional therapy observed for 6.5 years had fewer microvascular and neurologic complications with no impact on major cardiovascular events[98]; however, in the follow-up trial, Epidemiology of Diabetes Interventions and Complications (EDIC),[99] a 42% risk reduction for any cardiovascular event and 57% reduction for major cardiovascular events (including fatal or nonfatal MI or stroke) was observed in the intensively treated subjects. In addition, the PROspective pioglitAzone Clinical Trial in macroVascular Events (PROactive)[100] study of 5238 type 2 diabetics, which randomized patients to the PPARγ agonist pioglitazone or placebo, produced a nonsignificant reduction in the primary endpoint (all-cause mortality, nonfatal MI, stroke, leg amputation, and cardiovascular or leg revascularization). There was, however, a significant 20% reduction in the secondary endpoint of all-cause mortality, nonfatal MI, and stroke. Finally, the Diabetes Prevention Program demonstrated efficacy with both lifestyle interventions and metformin; high-risk individuals who exercised to goal had the lowest development of diabetes, whereas the addition of metformin significantly reduced diabetes development by 31% in those

receiving the drug.[101] Overall, these intervention trial results aimed at CVD risk in diabetes and metabolic syndrome subjects are not available stratified by sex.

Hypertension

The overall prevalence of hypertension is higher among women than among men, although it varies by age. Until the age of 45 years, the prevalence of hypertension is higher in men than in women. In older individuals, hypertension is more prevalent in women, with a much higher prevalence in women aged 65 years and older.[102] Hypertension is two to three times more common in women taking oral contraceptives.[103] Of note, incidence rates for black individuals are approximately twice the rates for white women and men across the ages.[104]

The association of hypertension and IHD has been reported in many prospective studies in both men and women. Hypertension is also the leading risk factor for congestive heart failure. The Systolic Hypertension in the Elderly Program evaluated pharmacologic intervention with a thiazide diuretic in the treatment of systolic hypertension. This study included a study population of 57% women and demonstrated reductions in stroke and IHD incidence by 36% and 25%, respectively.[105] A second trial tested the benefit of beta blockers and thiazide diuretics in decreasing target organ damage from hypertension and demonstrated similar risk reduction in women and men; however, in absolute terms, the benefit in women was seen primarily for stroke, whereas in men, treatment prevented as many IHD events as strokes.[106]

Blood pressure treatment recommendations, based on the Seventh Report of the Joint National Committee on the Prevention, Detection, and Treatment of High Blood Pressure (JNC 7), do not differ between women and men.[103] An optimal blood pressure of below 120/80 mm Hg should be encouraged through lifestyle modifications, such as weight control, physical activity, alcohol moderation, sodium restriction, and increased consumption of fruits and vegetables and low-fat dairy products (see Table 24-3). Pharmacotherapy is indicated if the blood pressure remains higher than 140/90 mm Hg or 130/80 mm Hg in women with diabetes or chronic kidney disease. Once medications are initiated, thiazide diuretics should be part of the regimen unless contraindicated or if another drug has a compelling indication and achieves sufficient blood pressure control.[49] Thiazide diuretics have a favorable effect on calcium excretion and thus may be especially appropriate for use in women who are at risk for osteoporosis. Despite similar treatment rates throughout different age groups, hypertension control is especially poor in older women, with only 29% of hypertensive women aged 70 to 79 years reaching their blood pressure target.[107]

Although some studies have shown that the treatment of hypertension among women conferred relatively less benefit against cardiac events compared with antihypertensive treatment among men,[106,108-111] the national guidelines recommend the same approach for treatment of hypertensive men and women. A recent publication based on data from the National Nutrition and Health Examination Survey 1999-2004 showed that hypertensive women are significantly more likely to be treated than are men but less likely to have achieved blood pressure control.[112]

Novel Risk Factors

Traditional risk factors and the Framingham risk score underestimate IHD risk in women,[113-118] and novel risk markers may improve risk detection.[11,119-121] Women have, on average, higher hsCRP measures compared with men, a sex difference apparent at the time of puberty.[122] This difference in inflammatory markers is consistent with the higher frequency of inflammation-mediated autoimmune diseases, such as rheumatoid arthritis and systemic lupus erythematosus, observed in women compared with men[123] and suggests a more prominent role for inflammation in IHD in women. The relative risk of IHD events increases proportionally with rising levels of hsCRP and acts synergistically with other risk factors to accelerate IHD risk in women.[120,124-128] A number of inflammatory markers, including hsCRP, are related to other IHD risk markers, such as the metabolic syndrome, type 2 diabetes, and heart failure.[126,129-130] The use of multiple biomarkers appears to improve IHD risk assessment in women.[131-133]

Antiplatelet Therapy

An overview of randomized trials from the Antiplatelet Trialists' Collaboration found that aspirin (75 to 162 mg/day) was beneficial in women for secondary prevention of IHD.[134] Among patients with an acute coronary syndrome, aspirin should be part of preventive management for women and men.

Although the benefits of aspirin therapy in reducing the risk of MI, stroke, and vascular death among men and women with preexisting CVD are well established,[134-136] the role of aspirin in primary prevention in women is less established, primarily because of a lack of inclusion of women in clinical trials. Aspirin has proven benefit and is recommended for all women at high risk without contraindications and for select at-risk women[5] (see Table 24-3). Previously, there were few data on the use of aspirin for primary prevention of IHD in women. Earlier recommendations were based on extrapolation from large studies primarily done in men demonstrating a reduction in risk for MI but not stroke in men of middle age or older at intermediate or high risk. Investigators in the Nurses' Health Study observed a decreased risk of first MI and death in women who took one to six aspirins per week.[137] In the Hypertension Optimal Treatment (HOT) study, men (53%) and women (47%) were randomized to receive 75 mg of aspirin per day or placebo, in addition to hypertension treatment. The HOT study showed an association between aspirin use and reductions in major CVD and MI.[138]

A sex-specific meta-analysis conducted by Berger and coworkers[139] found that aspirin therapy reduced cardiovascular events by 12% in a group of 51,342 women and by 14% in a group of 44,114 men. Aspirin therapy reduced MI by 32% in men and had no significant impact on stroke; it had no significant impact on MI in women but reduced stroke by 17%. The decrease in stroke in women was due to reductions in ischemic stroke out of proportion to a small increase in hemorrhagic stroke. There was no significant effect on CVD mortality for either sex. Whereas the study found that aspirin therapy was effective in lowering the occurrence of cardiovascular events, the differences found between men and women suggest differences in mechanisms of benefit.

The use of aspirin for primary prevention in women was evaluated in the Women's Health Study[140] with the same dosing strategy as in the Physicians' Health Study (100 mg every other day), which had shown a striking reduction in the risk of index MI among 22,071 healthy men.[141] In the Women's Health Study (n = 39,876 women aged 45 years or older), aspirin lowered the risk of stroke by 17%, including a 24% reduction in the risk of ischemic stroke with a nonsignificant increase in the risk of hemorrhagic stroke, with no reduction in fatal or nonfatal MI except for those older than 65 years. Importantly, there was a significant increase (40%) in gastrointestinal bleeding. Thus, a woman who is at risk is treated differently from those at high risk with regard to platelet inhibition. All high-risk women should be prescribed a daily aspirin (75 to 325 mg) unless it is contraindicated. If the woman is aspirin intolerant, clopidogrel should be used (see Table 24-3). Women classified as at risk who are younger

than 65 years should not take aspirin for primary MI prevention but may consider it when the benefit of stroke prevention outweighs the increased bleeding risk associated with aspirin. In women at risk aged 65 years or older, daily aspirin reduces MI and stroke significantly; however, there was an almost comparable occurrence of gastrointestinal bleeding. Therefore, weighing of the individual risk of gastrointestinal or cerebral hemorrhage versus benefit in preventing ischemic stroke is preferred in at-risk women of all ages because aspirin has no effect on cardiovascular mortality.[139] Aspirin resistance was found to be four times more prevalent in women than in men in a study by Dorsch and coworkers,[142] although the validity of this phenomenon remains unknown.

The U.S. Preventive Services Task Force (USPSTF) recommends the use of aspirin for women aged 55 to 79 years when the potential benefit of a reduction in ischemic stroke outweighs the potential harm of an increase in gastrointestinal hemorrhage.[143] The USPSTF concluded that the current evidence is insufficient to assess the balance of benefits and harms of aspirin for CVD prevention in men and women 80 years or older. The USPSTF recommended against the use of aspirin for stroke prevention in women younger than 55 years and for MI prevention in men younger than 45 years.

REPRODUCTIVE HORMONES

Postmenopausal Hormone Therapy

Until the mid-1990s, our knowledge of IHD risk and postmenopausal hormone therapy was based on observational trials that consistently reported a 40% to 50% reduction in CVD.[144] In addition, no difference was observed between the observational trials using estrogen alone and those using estrogen and progesterone.[145] In 1998, the results from the Heart and Estrogen/Progestin Replacement Study (HERS), a secondary prevention randomized trial designed to address whether estrogen and progestin would reduce IHD events in postmenopausal women with known CHD, called the role of hormone therapy into question.[146] More than 2700 women were randomized to receive conjugated equine estrogen and medroxyprogesterone or placebo and prospectively observed for the primary outcome of nonfatal MI and death. The average age of the study participants was 67 years; 19% were diabetic, and 13% were current smokers. During a follow-up period of 4.1 years, no group outcome differences were found, despite a decrease in TC and LDL-C and an increase in HDL-C in the active treatment group. In a post hoc analysis, there was a statistically significant 52% increase in MI in the active treatment group during the first year.[146] In the follow-up HERS II trial, more than 90% of the original HERS participants were observed for 3 additional years; no evidence of cardioprotective benefit was seen with longer duration of follow-up.[147]

Subsequent to the HERS trial, many other trials with different hormone replacement formulations and delivery routes also found no significant difference in IHD.[146,148-153] The Estrogen Replacement and Atherosclerosis (ERA) trial was an invasive angiographic study in which 309 women with CAD (defined as stenosis >30%) underwent coronary angiography at entry and exit. All participants were randomized to conjugated equine estrogen and medroxyprogesterone or placebo and observed for an average of 3.2 years. The results revealed no change in luminal diameter and no change in atherosclerotic lesion extent between the two groups.[148]

The Estrogen and Prevention of Atherosclerosis Trial (EPAT)[154] was a double-blind, placebo-controlled trial in 199 women with no IHD but elevated LDL-C (≥130 mg/dL) to determine if estrogen reduced the progression of subclinical atherosclerosis by use of carotid intima-media thickness. Women (mean age, 62 years) were randomized to 17β-estradiol

(1 mg/day) or placebo plus lipid-lowering therapy with LDL-C >160 mg/dL and observed for 2 years. Results demonstrated that the estradiol treatment group had greater carotid intima-media thickness regression compared with placebo ($P = 0.046$), and among those not receiving statin medication, the difference was even larger ($P = 0.002$). No difference was seen between estradiol and placebo groups for the women receiving lipid-lowering therapy. These findings suggest that among younger menopausal women without established atherosclerosis, estradiol may be of benefit, although of a lesser magnitude compared with lipid-lowering therapy.

The Women's Health Initiative (WHI), a prospective randomized double-blind placebo-controlled trial of more than 27,000 healthy women aged 50 to 79 years, assessed the risks and benefits of hormone therapy with respect to CVD, stroke, breast and colorectal cancer, and osteoporotic fractures.[155,156] There were two parallel clinical trials: estrogen-progestin and estrogen-only compared with placebo, based on a woman's hysterectomy status. A total of 16,608 women were randomized to receive conjugated equine estrogen 0.625 mg plus medroxyprogesterone 2.5 mg or placebo, and 10,739 women with a prior hysterectomy were randomized to receive conjugated equine estrogen 0.625 mg or placebo in the estrogen-only study. The primary outcome of the trial was nonfatal MI or CHD death. The duration of the follow-up for WHI was planned for 8.5 years; however, the estrogen-progestin study was stopped after 5.2 years because of a global adverse event outcome that included an increased incidence of breast cancer. For IHD events, there was no significant difference in adjusted nonfatal MI and IHD deaths between the randomized groups (HR, 1.24; 95% CI, 0.97-1.60).[155] The estrogen-alone trial continued but was also subsequently stopped early after 6.8 years of follow-up because of an increased risk of stroke. In the estrogen-alone trial, there was no increase in IHD risk (HR, 0.91; 95% CI, 0.75-1.12).[156]

A post hoc analysis of WHI revealed fewer IHD events when postmenopausal hormone therapy was initiated closer to menopause.[157] Although this analysis was not statistically significant, it was not prospectively designed or powered to test this question. Nevertheless, the use of hormones closer to the time of menopause (<10 years) evidenced a lower risk of IHD compared with those who began therapy farther from menopause (>20 years) for both the estrogen-only and estrogen-progestin trials. The results of this analysis have provided the rationale for what has come to be termed the timing hypothesis (the timing of hormone therapy initiation closer to menopause may be cardioprotective, whereas initiation later may be adverse).

In an additional substudy within the WHI, 1064 women from the estrogen-only trial aged 50 to 59 years at study enrollment underwent coronary artery calcium scans.[158] The average age of the women was 64 years, and mean duration of follow-up was 7.4 years. Women who had been randomized to conjugated equine estrogen 0.625 mg had a significantly lower mean coronary calcium score of 83.1 compared with those taking placebo, 123.1 ($P = 0.02$). Women with at least 80% medication compliance were found to have 60% lower odds of more extensive coronary artery calcium ($P = 0.004$). These results are also supportive of the hypothesis that hormone therapy initiated during the menopause transition (i.e., between 50 and 59 years old) may play a role in reducing the atherosclerotic plaque burden, although this hypothesis has not yet been directly tested in humans.

There are differences between the WHI clinical trial and observational reports that may account for variability between the study results. Patients with menopausal symptoms were excluded in the WHI, whereas in observational studies such as the Nurses' Health Study, they were predominant. In the WHI, only 16% of study participants were within 5 years of their last menses, with the average being 12 years, compared with the observational studies in which enrollment was largely within 5 years of menses.[159] Another way to examine these data is to evaluate differences in average age between the trials and observational data. The average age in the WHI was 63 years; in observational studies, the age range at enrollment was 30 to 55 years. Finally, the average BMI was 29 in the WHI, with nearly one third being obese, placing these women at relatively higher IHD risk compared with those in the Nurses' Health study, in which the average BMI was 25. All of these factors may have contributed to variable findings between the trials and observational reports.

Two clinical trials are under way to address the timing of hormone therapy initiation. Both studies are addressing whether starting of hormone therapy closer to menopause elicits a cardioprotective effect. In the Early versus Late Intervention Trial with Estradiol (ELITE), 504 women within 6 years (the early cohort) or more than 10 years since menopause (the late cohort) will be randomized to receive estradiol or placebo. In the 3-year follow-up period, outcome measures of this trial will include carotid intima-media thickness.[160] The Kronos Early Estrogen Prevention Study (KEEPS) is a multicenter, randomized study during a 5-year period in which 720 women within 3 years of their final menstrual period will be randomized to pill and transdermal patch hormone therapy versus placebo; it also uses carotid intima-media thickness as an outcome in addition to other variables.[161]

Reproductive Hormones and Premenopausal Women

Estrogen administration, in animal models, directly prevents atherosclerosis.[162] In the cardiovascular system, when estrogen receptors are activated on endothelial and myocardial cells, it has been shown to have antioxidant effects and improved endothelial cell injury recovery.[162] In specific pathways, these receptors modulate a rapid vasodilatory response through nitric oxide and also have long-term effects by increasing endothelial cell growth and inhibiting smooth muscle cell proliferation. Estrogen reduces LDL-C oxidation and binding, reduces platelet aggregation, and increases cyclooxygenase 2 activity.[162] There is relatively less known about cardiovascular actions of progesterone and progestins, and there appear to be differential effects dependent on whether preexistent atherosclerosis is present (Fig. 24-3).

IHD risk is elevated in premenopausal women with the disruption of ovulatory cycling, indicated by estrogen deficiency and hypothalamic dysfunction,[6] or irregular menstrual cycling.[163] Animal studies also demonstrated that relative estrogen deficiency is associated with atherosclerosis. These studies demonstrated that hypoestrogenemia in female monkeys is associated with loss of normal coronary artery dilation or even constriction in response to an endothelial stimulus.[164-166]

In the WISE study, 95 premenopausal women were evaluated for hypothalamic hypoestrogenemia, defined as estradiol <184 pmol/L (50 pg/mL), follicle-stimulating hormone <10 IU/L, and luteinizing hormone <10 IU/L. Premenopausal women with significant angiographic CAD had significantly lower blood levels of estradiol, bioavailable estradiol, and follicle-stimulating hormone (all P <0.05), consistent with ovulatory dysfunction, compared with women without angiographic CAD. Hypothalamic hypoestrogenemia was significantly more prevalent among the women with CAD than among those without CAD (69% versus 29%, respectively; $P = 0.01$). These findings suggest that low estrogen levels due to disruption of ovarian function may be an IHD risk factor for premenopausal women.

Reproductive events in a woman's life are associated with changes in metabolic and cardiovascular function, such as blood lipids, blood pressure, and blood glucose. Despite these

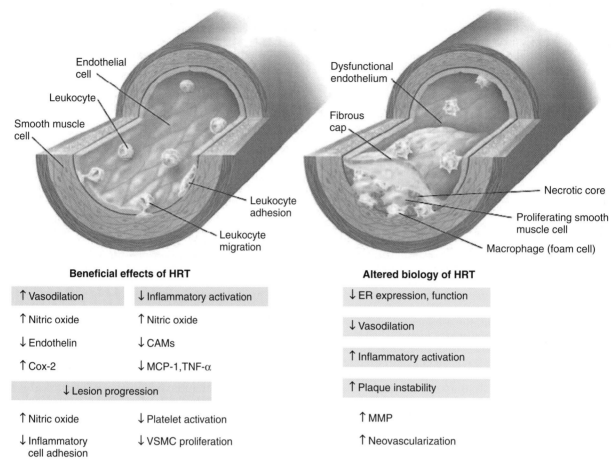

Early atherogenesis

Endothelial cell

Leukocyte

Smooth muscle cell

Leukocyte adhesion

Leukocyte migration

Established atherosclerosis

Dysfunctional endothelium

Fibrous cap

Necrotic core

Proliferating smooth muscle cell

Macrophage (foam cell)

Beneficial effects of HRT

↑ Vasodilation	↓ Inflammatory activation
↑ Nitric oxide	↑ Nitric oxide
↓ Endothelin	↓ CAMs
↑ Cox-2	↓ MCP-1,TNF-α

↓ Lesion progression	
↑ Nitric oxide	↓ Platelet activation
↓ Inflammatory cell adhesion	↓ VSMC proliferation

↓ LDL oxidation/binding

Altered biology of HRT

↓ ER expression, function

↓ Vasodilation

↑ Inflammatory activation

↑ Plaque instability

↑ MMP

↑ Neovascularization

FIGURE 24-3 The beneficial and thrombogenic effects of estrogen. CAMs, cell adhesion molecules; Cox-2, cyclooxygenase 2; ER, estrogen receptor; HRT, hormone replacement therapy; LDL, low-density lipoprotein; MCP-1, monocyte chemoattractant protein 1; MMP, matrix metalloproteinase; TNF-α, tumor necrosis factor-α; VSMC, vascular smooth muscle cell. *(From Ouyang P, Michos ED, Karas RH: Hormone replacement therapy and the cardiovascular system: lessons learned and unanswered questions. J Am Coll Cardiol 47:1741, 2006.)*

transient changes, a large prospective study in 1987 found no important association between variables such as age at menarche, age at first birth, and parity and IHD, whereas established risk factors showed the expected relationships.[63] Another analysis of two prospective studies, however, concluded that six or more pregnancies is associated with a small but consistent increase in the risk of IHD and CVD.[167]

Polycystic ovary syndrome (PCOS) is prevalent in 10% to 13% of women and is linked with a clustering of risk factors, incident type 2 diabetes mellitus,[168] and adverse IHD events in the postmenopausal period.[169] The cardiometabolic syndrome is a clustering of risk factors including at least three of the following: insulin resistance, dyslipidemia (elevated TGs, low HDL-C), hypertension, or abdominal obesity; it is frequently associated with alterations in endogenous estrogens and androgens in women.[163,170,171]

In the NHLBI-sponsored WISE study of 390 postmenopausal women with features of PCOS, 104 had clinical features of PCOS as defined by biochemical evidence of hyperandrogenemia and history of irregular menses. Cumulative 5-year cardiovascular event–free survival was 79% for PCOS women (Fig. 24-4; n = 104) versus 89% for women without PCOS (n = 286; *P* = 0.006). PCOS women with

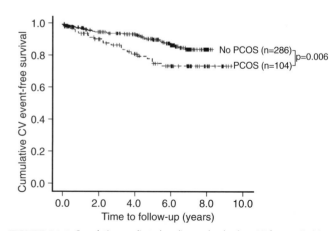

FIGURE 24-4 Cumulative unadjusted cardiovascular death or MI-free survival in postmenopausal women with or without clinical features of PCOS. *(From Shaw LJ, Bairey Merz CN, Azziz R, et al: Postmenopausal women with a history of irregular menses and elevated androgen measurements at high risk for worsening cardiovascular event-free survival: results from the National Institutes of Health–National Heart, Lung, and Blood Institute sponsored Women's Ischemia Syndrome Evaluation. J Clin Endocrinol Metab 93:1276, 2008.)*

elevated hsCRP had a 12.2-fold higher risk of CVD death or nonfatal MI compared with non-PCOS women and lower levels of hsCRP. PCOS status remained a significant predictor ($P < 0.01$) in prognostic models including diabetes, waist circumference, hypertension, and angiographic CAD as covariates. These data suggest that recognition of clinical features of PCOS in postmenopausal women may facilitate an opportunity for early risk factor intervention for the prevention of IHD.

Contraceptive Hormone Therapy

Contraceptive hormones, most commonly known as the pill, were first introduced in the 1960s to provide high hormonal blood levels that suppress ovulation, implantation, and therefore pregnancy. Contemporary oral contraceptives are considered low dose compared with first generations but remain fairly high in estrogen doses compared with menopausal hormone replacement therapy, which typically contains one tenth the dose of oral contraceptives. In addition, oral contraceptives have a synthetic form of progestin, which ranges from the older potent androgenic progestins to newer generation progestins that are aldosterone antagonists with antiandrogenic and diuretic properties.[172] The hormones in oral contraceptives affect the cardiovascular system indirectly through their impact on CAD risk factors, such as the lipid profile, blood pressure, thrombosis, vasomotion, and arrhythmogenesis.

Lipid Effects

Changes and the amount of alteration in the lipid profile are dose dependent but also vary according to the delivery route. For example, transdermal contraceptive hormone delivery is relatively less potent than oral because it bypasses first metabolism in the liver.[162] Oral contraceptives cause hepatic apolipoprotein upregulation through the genomic pathway, which alters the lipid profiles.[162,173,174] Estrogen passes through the lipid membrane and binds receptors located in the nucleus, which either activates or suppresses gene transcription. Low-dose oral contraceptives of combined estrogen-progestin formulations have demonstrated reductions in HDL-C and small increases in LDL-C and TGs compared with higher dose oral contraceptives.[175,176]

Blood Pressure

Normotensive women taking oral contraceptives have an increase in blood pressure with use up to 7 to 8 mm Hg.[177,178] More recently, the use of oral contraceptives with newer generation progestins (drospirenone) with antimineralocorticoid diuretic effect has been associated with lower blood pressure (a decrease ranging up to 4 mm Hg in systolic blood pressure) and lower body weight.[179-181] Whereas these results are suggestive of a possible cardioprotective effect, more work is needed.

Thrombosis

Oral contraceptives have an increased risk of venous thromboembolism and prothrombotic risk through the mechanism of increasing prothrombin and decreasing antithrombin III.[182] Compared with nonusers, users of oral contraceptive formulations with less than 50 µg estrogen have a fourfold higher risk of venous thromboembolism (95% CI, 2.77-4.00).[183] Third-generation (desogestrel or gestodene) progestins are twice as likely to provoke a nonfatal venous thromboembolism compared with second-generation (levonorgestrel) progestins, adjusting for smoking and BMI.[184]

Coronary Vasomotion

Cyclical circulating levels of endogenous and exogenous estrogen have been associated with migraine headaches,

Raynaud phenomenon, and Prinzmetal angina.[185,186] Animal and human studies demonstrate that low endogenous estrogen levels can exacerbate endothelial dysfunction, and exogenous estrogen replacement has been shown to eliminate this effect.[166,187-189] Primate studies have also shown an adverse coronary vasoconstrictive effect with medroxyprogesterone that was not apparent with progesterone.[190,191] Long-term studies in humans are needed because it is unknown if reproductive hormones play a role in maintaining or improving coronary or peripheral endothelial function in humans.

Arrhythmogenesis

Drug-induced QT interval prolongation and drug-induced arrhythmias are relatively more prevalent in women and contribute to a lifelong higher risk of sudden cardiac death associated with electrocardiographic QT prolongation compared with men.[192] Although data are conflicting, hormone therapy with estrogen alone usually produces a prolongation of the QT interval, and estrogen plus progesterone has no significant effects on QT interval but reduces QT dispersion.[193,194] To date, studies have not been directed at the impact of oral contraceptives and mechanisms of arrhythmogenesis.

Figure 24-5 depicts the known mechanisms whereby contraceptive hormones affect the cardiovascular system, including effects on atherosclerosis, thrombosis, vasomotion, and arrhythmogenesis.[181] Table 24-4 lists the prescribing guidelines for hormonal contraceptives in women with elevated cardiovascular risk.

Selective Estrogen Receptor Modulators

Depending on the tissue, selective estrogen receptor modulators (SERMs) have both estrogen agonist and antagonist properties. The SERMs available in the United States and Canada are raloxifene used for prevention and treatment of osteoporosis and breast cancer prevention, tamoxifen used to prevent recurrence of estrogen receptor–positive breast cancer, and toremifene used for advanced breast cancer.

SERMs have been found to have favorable changes in regard to the lipid profiles. Raloxifene lowers TC and LDL-C; however, it does not change HDL-C or TGs.[195] In addition, raloxifene does not raise hsCRP, in contrast to hormone replacement therapy; raloxifene also reduces homocysteine levels.[196]

Raloxifene is the most studied SERM with respect to the cardiovascular system. The Multiple Outcomes of Raloxifene Evaluation (MORE) trial was a 4-year follow-up study designed to determine the effect of raloxifene versus placebo on bone density in postmenopausal women with osteoporosis. Although this trial was designed to evaluate fracture risk, the incidence of major cardiovascular events (MI, coronary bypass surgery, percutaneous angioplasty, or stroke) was also reported. No significant differences in these events were observed between raloxifene doses (60 mg or 120 mg) and placebo.[195] In a subset of women with higher risk defined as prior cardiovascular event, revascularization procedure, or multiple risk factors, raloxifene was found to have a 40% significantly reduced event rate compared with placebo.[195]

A subset of the MORE trial was observed for an additional 4 years in the Continuing Outcomes Relevant to Evista (CORE) trial to evaluate raloxifene and invasive breast cancer risk.[197,198] The combined 8-year incidence of major cardiovascular events was similar between the raloxifene group and placebo (5.5% versus 4.7%, respectively). In addition, no difference was found between treatment and placebo when IHD and stroke events were analyzed separately.

The Raloxifene Use for The Heart (RUTH) trial was the first trial designed to evaluate raloxifene and the effect on cardiovascular events as a primary outcome.[199] This trial enrolled 10,101 postmenopausal women with known CHD or

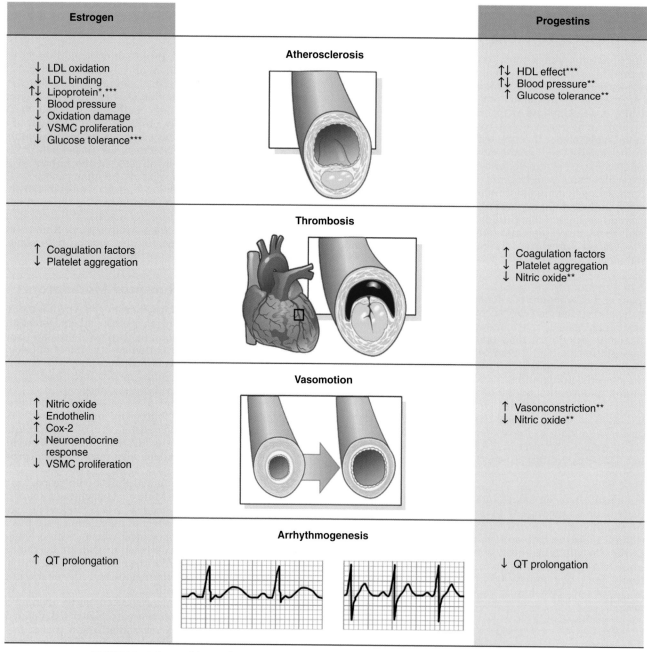

FIGURE 24-5 Impact of hormonal contraception on mechanisms of cardiovascular disease. Cox-2, cyclooxygenase 2; HDL, high-density lipoprotein; LDL, low-density lipoprotein; VSMC, vascular smooth muscle cell. *Dependent on delivery route of estrogen. **Dependent on type of progestin. ***Dependent on the dose of estrogen. *(From Shufelt CL, Bairey Merz CN: Contraceptive hormone use and cardiovascular disease. J Am Coll Cardiol 53:221, 2009.)*

TABLE 24–4	Summary of Hormonal Contraceptive Prescribing Guidelines for Women with Elevated Cardiovascular Risk
Hypertension	Well-controlled blood pressure in women <35 years of age and otherwise healthy, nonsmoking → trial of oral contraceptives. Monitor blood pressure and if controlled after starting, oral contraceptives may be continued. If blood pressure not well controlled, alternative methods such as progestin-only pills or intrauterine device (IUD) may be started.
Dyslipidemia	LDL-C >160 mg/dL or multiple cardiac risk factors → alternative nonhormonal contraceptive methods, such as an IUD.
Diabetes	Diabetes type 1 or 2, oral contraceptive is appropriate for use *only* in otherwise healthy nonsmokers <35 years of age. Otherwise, progestin-only or IUD may be started.
Smoking	Smoking and >35 years of age → alternative nonhormonal contraceptive methods, such as an IUD. Smokers <35 years of age are not addressed.
Obesity	Obesity (BMI >30 kg/m^2) → alternative nonhormonal contraceptive methods such as progestin-only contraception or IUD. Obesity is thought to be an independent risk factor for venous thromboembolism.
Women older than 35 years	Healthy, nonsmoking women → oral contraceptives with <50 µg ethinyl estradiol remain safer than pregnancy and can be continued until 50 to 55 years of age or until menopause after reviewing risks and benefits.

From Shufelt CL, Bairey Merz CN: Contraceptive hormone use and cardiovascular disease. *J Am Coll Cardiol* 53:221, 2009.

risk factors for a median follow-up of 5.6 years and found that raloxifene did not reduce cardiovascular event risk (death from coronary causes, nonfatal MI, or hospitalization from acute MI).[200] In a post hoc analysis, women <60 years old had significantly less cardiovascular events when randomized to raloxifene versus placebo (HR, 0.59; 95% CI, 0.41 to 0.83; *P* = 0.003).[200] These findings suggest, similar to the animal, observational, and clinical trial data, that there may be a CVD benefit with hormonal therapy at younger ages.

GUIDELINES FOR PREVENTION OF CARDIOVASCULAR DISEASE IN WOMEN

The 2007 AHA update recommends an integrated scheme for a general risk stratification approach to the female patient that classifies her as at high risk, at risk, or at optimal risk, focused on the high average lifetime risk for CVD, approaching one in two women. The guidelines recommend aggressive risk factor modification through lifestyle modification and pharmacotherapy consistent with the ATP III guidelines, including smoking cessation, exercise, weight reduction, and a diet rich in fruits and vegetables. The guidelines also emphasize the importance of aggressive control of blood pressure and lipids through lifestyle modification and pharmacotherapy. Aspirin therapy is recommended in high-risk women if there are no contraindications. Aspirin therapy is also recommended for women ≥65 years, if blood pressure is controlled and benefit for ischemic stroke and MI prevention is likely to outweigh the risk of gastrointestinal bleeding and hemorrhagic stroke, and for women <65 years when benefit for ischemic stroke prevention is likely to outweigh adverse

TABLE 24–5	Class III Interventions (Not Useful/Effective and May Be Harmful) for Cardiovascular Disease or Myocardial Infarction Prevention in Women

Menopausal Therapy
Hormone therapy and selective estrogen receptor modulators (SERMs) should not be used for the primary or secondary prevention of CVD (*Class III, Level A*).

Antioxidant Supplements
Antioxidant vitamin supplements (e.g., vitamin E, vitamin C, and beta carotene) should not be used for the primary or secondary prevention of CVD (*Class III, Level A*).

Folic Acid*
Folic acid, with or without B$_6$ and B$_{12}$ supplementation, should not be used for the primary or secondary prevention of CVD (*Class III, Level A*).

Aspirin for Myocardial Infarction in Women <65 Years of Age†
Routine use of aspirin in healthy women <65 years of age is not recommended to prevent myocardial infarction (*Class III, Level B*).

*Folic acid supplementation should be used in the childbearing years to prevent neural tube defects.
†For recommendation for aspirin to prevent CVD in women ≥65 years of age or stroke in women <65 years of age, see Table 24-3.
From Mosca L, Banka CL, Benjamin EJ, et al: Evidence-based guidelines for cardiovascular disease prevention in women: 2007 update. *Circulation* 115:1481, 2007.

effects of therapy. Beta blockers are recommended in women after MI, acute coronary syndrome, or left ventricular dysfunction with or without heart failure symptoms. Similarly, angiotensin-converting enzyme inhibitors are recommended in women after MI and in those with heart failure, left ventricular dysfunction, or diabetes mellitus. Hormone therapy, antioxidants, and vitamins should not be used for primary or secondary prevention in women (Table 24-5).

CONCLUSION

CVD is the leading cause of death among women in the United States, and women receive fewer preventive recommendations, such as lipid-lowering therapy, aspirin, and lifestyle advice, than do men with similar Framingham risk scores. Both the Framingham risk score and the Reynolds score can be used to estimate CVD risk in women. Treatment of dyslipidemia, hypertension, and diabetes is similar between women and men. The use of aspirin for women aged 55 to 79 years is recommended when the potential benefit of a reduction in ischemic strokes outweighs the potential harm of an increase in gastrointestinal hemorrhage. Lifestyle is an important component of prevention of IHD; women should accumulate a minimum of 30 minutes of moderate-intensity physical activity (e.g., brisk walking) daily, consume a heart-healthy diet, and avoid smoking or passive smoke. Hormone therapy used for contraception, management of menopause symptoms, or other clinically indicated conditions should not be used for CVD prevention. Sex-specific guidelines exist for women for the prevention of CVD and should be used by health care providers.

REFERENCES

1. World Heart Federation: Go red for women. Available at: http://www.worldheart.org/awareness-women.php. Accessed June 11, 2009.
2. Thom T, Haase N, Rosamond W, et al: Heart disease and stroke statistics—2006 update: a report from the American Heart Association Statistics Committee and Stroke Statistics Subcommittee. *Circulation* 113:e85, 2006.

3. Mosca L, Linfante AH, Benjamin EJ, et al: National study of physician awareness and adherence to cardiovascular disease prevention guidelines. *Circulation* 111:499, 2005.
4. Wenger NK: Lipid abnormalities in women: data for risk, data for management. *Cardiol Rev* 14:276, 2006.
5. Mosca L, Banka CL, Benjamin EJ, et al: Evidence-based guidelines for cardiovascular disease prevention in women: 2007 update. *Circulation* 115:1481, 2007.
6. Bairey Merz CN, Johnson BD, Sharaf BL, et al: Hypoestrogenemia of hypothalamic origin and coronary artery disease in premenopausal women: a report from the NHLBI-sponsored WISE study. *J Am Coll Cardiol* 41:413, 2003.
7. Moriel M, Rozanski A, Klein J, et al: The limited efficacy of exercise radionuclide ventriculography in assessing prognosis of women with coronary artery disease. *Am J Cardiol* 76:1030, 1995.
8. Shaw LJ, Olson MB, Kip K, et al: The value of estimated functional capacity in estimating outcome: results from the NHBLI-Sponsored Women's Ischemia Syndrome Evaluation (WISE) Study. *J Am Coll Cardiol* 47(Suppl):S36, 2006.
9. Shaw LJ, Shaw RE, Merz CN, et al: Impact of ethnicity and gender differences on angiographic coronary artery disease prevalence and in-hospital mortality in the American College of Cardiology–National Cardiovascular Data Registry. *Circulation* 117:1787, 2008.
10. von Mering GO, Arant CB, Wessel TR, et al: Abnormal coronary vasomotion as a prognostic indicator of cardiovascular events in women: results from the National Heart, Lung, and Blood Institute–sponsored Women's Ischemia Syndrome Evaluation (WISE). *Circulation* 109:722, 2004.
11. Wong TY, Klein R, Sharrett AR, et al: Retinal arteriolar narrowing and risk of coronary heart disease in men and women. The Atherosclerosis Risk in Communities Study. *JAMA* 287:1153, 2002.
12. Burke AP, Farb A, Malcom GT, et al: Effect of risk factors on the mechanism of acute thrombosis and sudden coronary death in women. *Circulation* 97:2110, 1998.
13. Burke AP, Virmani R, Galis Z, et al: 34th Bethesda Conference: Task force #2—What is the pathologic basis for new atherosclerosis imaging techniques? *J Am Coll Cardiol* 41:1874, 2003.
14. Mosca L, Appel LJ, Benjamin EJ, et al: Evidence-based guidelines for cardiovascular disease prevention in women. *Circulation* 109:672, 2004.
15. Mosca L, Ferris A, Fabunmi R, et al: Tracking women's awareness of heart disease: an American Heart Association national study. *Circulation* 109:573, 2004.
16. Abuful A, Gidron Y, Henkin Y: Physicians' attitudes toward preventive therapy for coronary artery disease: is there a gender bias? *Clin Cardiol* 28:389, 2005.
17. Strong K, et al: Preventing chronic diseases: how many lives can we save? *Lancet* 366:1578, 2005.
18. Yusuf S, Hawken S, Ounpuu S, et al: Effect of potentially modifiable risk factors associated with myocardial infarction in 52 countries (the INTERHEART study): case-control study. *Lancet* 364:937, 2004.
19. World Health Organization: World Health Statistics 2007. Available at: www.who.int/cardiovascular_dieases/resources/atlas/en/index.html.
20. Kannel WB, Wilson PW: Risk factors that attenuate the female coronary disease advantage. *Arch Intern Med* 155:57, 1995.
21. Vaccarino V, Parsons L, Every NR, et al: Sex-based differences in early mortality after myocardial infarction. National Registry of Myocardial Infarction 2 Participants. *N Engl J Med* 341:217, 1999.
22. Harris DJ, Douglas PS: Enrollment of women in cardiovascular clinical trials funded by the National Heart, Lung, and Blood Institute. *N Engl J Med* 343:475, 2000.
23. Mosca L, Grundy SM, Judelson D, et al: Guide to Preventive Cardiology for Women. AHA/ACC Scientific Statement Consensus panel statement. *Circulation* 99:2480, 1999.
24. Sibley C, Blumenthal RS, Merz CN, Mosca L: Limitations of current cardiovascular disease risk assessment strategies in women, *J Womens Health (Larchmt)* 15:54, 2006.
25. Ridker PM, Buring JE, Rifai N, Cook NR: Development and validation of improved algorithms for the assessment of global cardiovascular risk in women: the Reynolds Risk Score. *JAMA* 297:611, 2007.
26. Wenger NK: The Reynolds Risk Score: improved accuracy for cardiovascular risk prediction in women? *Nat Clin Pract Cardiovasc Med* 4:366, 2007.
27. Blumenthal RS, Michos ED, Nasir K: Further improvements in CHD risk prediction for women. *JAMA* 297:641, 2007.
28. D'Agostino RB, Sr, Vasan RS, Pencina MJ, et al: General cardiovascular risk profile for use in primary care: the Framingham Heart Study. *Circulation* 117:743, 2008.
29. Lavie CJ: Assessment and treatment of lipids in elderly persons. *Am J Geriatr Cardiol* 13(Suppl 1):2, 2004.
30. Wenger NK: Dyslipidemia as a risk factor at elderly age. *Am J Geriatr Cardiol* 13(Suppl 1):4, 2004.
31. Kim C, Hofer TP, Kerr EA: Review of evidence and explanations for suboptimal screening and treatment of dyslipidemia in women. A conceptual model. *J Gen Intern Med* 18:854, 2003.
32. Schrott HG, Bittner V, Vittinghoff E, et al: Adherence to National Cholesterol Education Program Treatment goals in postmenopausal women with heart disease. The Heart and Estrogen/Progestin Replacement Study (HERS). The HERS Research Group. *JAMA* 277:1281, 1997.
33. Miller M, Byington R, Hunninghake D, et al: Sex bias and underutilization of lipid-lowering therapy in patients with coronary artery disease at academic medical centers in the United States and Canada. Prospective Randomized Evaluation of the Vascular Effects of Norvasc Trial (PREVENT) Investigators. *Arch Intern Med* 160:343, 2000.
34. Bittner V, Olson M, Kelsey SF, et al: Effect of coronary angiography on use of lipid-lowering agents in women: a report from the Women's Ischemia Syndrome Evaluation (WISE) study. For the WISE Investigators. *Am J Cardiol* 85:1083, 2000.
35. Wenger NK, Speroff L, Packard B: Cardiovascular health and disease in women. *N Engl J Med* 329:247, 1993.
36. Wenger NK: Coronary heart disease: an older woman's major health risk. *BMJ* 315:1085, 1997.
37. Colditz GA, Stampfer MJ, Willett WC, et al: A prospective study of parental history of myocardial infarction and coronary heart disease in women. *Am J Epidemiol* 123:48, 1986.
38. Executive Summary of the Third Report of the National Cholesterol Education Program (NCEP) Expert Panel on Detection, Evaluation, and Treatment of High Blood Cholesterol in Adults (Adult Treatment Panel III). *JAMA* 285:2486, 2001.
39. Shai I, Rimm EB, Hankinson SE, et al: Multivariate assessment of lipid parameters as predictors of coronary heart disease among postmenopausal women: potential implications for clinical guidelines. *Circulation* 110:2824, 2004.
40. Jensen J, Nilas L, Christiansen C: Influence of menopause on serum lipids and lipoproteins. *Maturitas* 12:321, 1990.
41. Kuhn FE, Rackley CE: Coronary artery disease in women. Risk factors, evaluation, treatment, and prevention. *Arch Intern Med* 153:2626, 1993.
42. Wenger N: Lipid abnormalities recognition and management. In Wenger N, Collins P, editors: *Women and heart disease*, ed 2, New York, 2005, Taylor & Francis, pp 53-63.
43. Miettinen TA, Pyörälä K, Olsson AG, et al: Cholesterol-lowering therapy in women and elderly patients with myocardial infarction or angina pectoris: findings from the Scandinavian Simvastatin Survival Study (4S). *Circulation* 96:4211, 1997.
44. Lewis SJ, Sacks FM, Mitchell JS, et al: Effect of pravastatin on cardiovascular events in women after myocardial infarction: the cholesterol and recurrent events (CARE) trial. *J Am Coll Cardiol* 32:140, 1998.
45. Prevention of cardiovascular events and death with pravastatin in patients with coronary heart disease and a broad range of initial cholesterol levels. The Long-Term Intervention with Pravastatin in Ischaemic Disease (LIPID) Study Group. *N Engl J Med* 339:1349, 1998.
46. Downs JR, Clearfield M, Weis S, et al: Primary prevention of acute coronary events with lovastatin in men and women with average cholesterol levels: results of AFCAPS/TexCAPS. Air Force/Texas Coronary Atherosclerosis Prevention Study. *JAMA* 279:1615, 1998.
47. Shepherd J, Blauw GJ, Murphy MB, et al: Pravastatin in elderly individuals at risk of vascular disease (PROSPER): a randomised controlled trial. *Lancet* 360:1623, 2002.
48. MRC/BHF Heart Protection Study of cholesterol lowering with simvastatin in 20,536 high-risk individuals: a randomised placebo-controlled trial. *Lancet* 360:7, 2002.
49. Major outcomes in moderately hypercholesterolemic, hypertensive patients randomized to pravastatin vs usual care: The Antihypertensive and Lipid-Lowering Treatment to Prevent Heart Attack Trial (ALLHAT-LLT). *JAMA* 288:2998, 2002.
50. Athyros VG, Papageorgiou AA, Mercouris BR, et al: Treatment with atorvastatin to the National Cholesterol Educational Program goal versus " "usual' care in secondary coronary heart disease prevention. The GREek Atorvastatin and Coronary-heart-disease Evaluation (GREACE) study. *Curr Med Res Opin* 18:220, 2002.
51. Sever PS, Dahlöf B, Poulter NR, et al: Prevention of coronary and stroke events with atorvastatin in hypertensive patients who have average or lower-than-average cholesterol concentrations, in the Anglo-Scandinavian Cardiac Outcomes Trial–Lipid Lowering Arm (ASCOT-LLA): a multicentre randomised controlled trial. *Lancet* 361:1149, 2003.
52. Wenger NK, Lewis SJ, Welty FK, et al: Effect of 80 mg versus 10 mg of atorvastatin in women and men with stable coronary heart disease. TNT steering Committee and Investigators. *Circulation* 112(suppl II):II-819, 2005.
53. Cannon CP, Braunwald E, McCabe CH, et al: Intensive versus moderate lipid lowering with statins after acute coronary syndromes. *N Engl J Med* 350:1495, 2004.
54. LaRosa JC, Grundy SM, Waters DD, et al: Intensive lipid lowering with atorvastatin in patients with stable coronary disease. *N Engl J Med* 352:1425, 2005.
55. Grundy SM, Cleeman JI, Merz CN, et al: Implications of recent clinical trials for the National Cholesterol Education Program Adult Treatment Panel III guidelines. *Circulation* 110:227, 2004.
56. Ridker PM, Danielson E, Fonseca FA, et al: Rosuvastatin to prevent vascular events in men and women with elevated C-reactive protein. *N Engl J Med* 359:2195, 2008.
57. Walsh JM, Pignone M: Drug treatment of hyperlipidemia in women. *JAMA* 291:2243, 2004.
58. Wenger NK, Lewis SJ, Welty FK, et al: Beneficial effects of aggressive low-density lipoprotein cholesterol lowering in women with stable coronary heart disease in the Treating to New Targets (TNT) study. *Heart* 94:434, 2008.
59. Ansell BJ, Fonarow GC, Maki KC, et al: Reduced treatment success in lipid management among women with coronary heart disease or risk equivalents: results of a national survey. *Am Heart J* 152:976, 2006.
60. Colditz GA, Bonita R, Stampfer MJ, et al: Cigarette smoking and risk of stroke in middle-aged women. *N Engl J Med* 318:937, 1988.
61. Willett WC, Green A, Stampfer MJ, et al: Relative and absolute excess risks of coronary heart disease among women who smoke cigarettes. *N Engl J Med* 317:1303, 1987.
62. Rosenberg L, Kaufman DW, Helmrich SP, et al: Myocardial infarction and cigarette smoking in women younger than 50 years of age. *JAMA* 253:2965, 1985.
63. Colditz GA, Willett WC, Stampfer MJ, et al: Menopause and the risk of coronary heart disease in women. *N Engl J Med* 316:1105, 1987.
64. Sorensen G, Pechacek TF: Attitudes toward smoking cessation among men and women. *J Behav Med* 10:129, 1987.
65. Kawachi I, Colditz GA, Stampfer MJ, et al: Smoking cessation and time course of decreased risks of coronary heart disease in middle-aged women. *Arch Intern Med* 154:169, 1994.
66. Kawachi I, Colditz GA, Stampfer MJ, et al: Smoking cessation in relation to total mortality rates in women. A prospective cohort study. *Ann Intern Med* 119:992, 1993.
67. Rosenberg L, Palmer JR, Shapiro S: Decline in the risk of myocardial infarction among women who stop smoking. *N Engl J Med* 322:213, 1990.
68. National Center for Health Statistics: Prevalence of sedentary leisure-time behavior among adults in the United States. Available at: http://www.cdc.gov/nchs/products/pubs/pubd/hestats/3and4/sedentary.htm. Accessed June 11, 2009.
69. Stampfer MJ, Hu FB, Manson JE, et al: Primary prevention of coronary heart disease in women through diet and lifestyle. *N Engl J Med* 343:16, 2000.
70. Colditz GA, Coakley E: Weight, weight gain, activity, and major illnesses: the Nurses' Health Study. *Int J Sports Med* 18(Suppl 3):S162, 1997.
71. Manson JE, Rimm EB, Stampfer MJ, et al: Physical activity and incidence of non–insulin-dependent diabetes mellitus in women. *Lancet* 338:774, 1991.

72. Hu FB, Stampfer MJ, Manson JE, et al: Trends in the incidence of coronary heart disease and changes in diet and lifestyle in women. *N Engl J Med* 343:530, 2000.

73. de Lorgeril M, Salen P: The Mediterranean diet in secondary prevention of coronary heart disease. *Clin Invest Med* 29:154, 2006.

74. Burr ML, Fehily AM, Gilbert JF, et al: Effects of changes in fat, fish, and fibre intakes on death and myocardial reinfarction: diet and reinfarction trial (DART). *Lancet* 2:757, 1989.

75. Singh RB, Niaz AM, Ghosh S, et al: Randomized, controlled trial of antioxidant vitamins and cardioprotective diet on hyperlipidemia, oxidative stress, and development of experimental atherosclerosis: the diet and antioxidant trial on atherosclerosis (DATA). *Cardiovasc Drugs Ther* 9:763, 1995.

76. Kuczmarski RJ, Flegal KM, Campbell SM, Johnson CL: Increasing prevalence of overweight among US adults. The National Health and Nutrition Examination Surveys, 1960 to 1991. *JAMA* 272:205, 1994.

77. Ogden CL, Carroll MD, Curtin LR, et al: Prevalence of overweight and obesity in the United States, 1999-2004. *JAMA* 295:1549, 2006.

78. Manson JE, Colditz GA, Stampfer MJ, et al: A prospective study of obesity and risk of coronary heart disease in women. *N Engl J Med* 322:882, 1990.

79. Rexrode KM, Carey VJ, Hennekens CH, et al: Abdominal adiposity and coronary heart disease in women. *JAMA* 280:1843, 1998.

80. Eaker ED, Chesebro JH, Sacks FM, et al: Cardiovascular disease in women. *Circulation* 88(pt 1):1999, 1993.

81. Folsom AR, Stevens J, Schreiner PJ, McGovern PG: Body mass index, waist/hip ratio, and coronary heart disease incidence in African Americans and whites. Atherosclerosis Risk in Communities Study Investigators. *Am J Epidemiol* 148:1187, 1998.

82. Fox CS, Pencina MJ, Meigs JB, et al: Trends in the incidence of type 2 diabetes mellitus from the 1970s to the 1990s: the Framingham Heart Study. *Circulation* 113:2914, 2006.

83. Lloyd-Jones DM, Liu K, Colangelo LA, et al: Consistently stable or decreased body mass index in young adulthood and longitudinal changes in metabolic syndrome components: the Coronary Artery Risk Development in Young Adults Study. *Circulation* 115:1004, 2007.

84. Liu S, Willett WC, Stampfer MJ, et al: A prospective study of dietary glycemic load, carbohydrate intake, and risk of coronary heart disease in US women. *Am J Clin Nutr* 71:1455, 2000.

85. Hu FB: Diet and cardiovascular disease prevention: the need for a paradigm shift. *J Am Coll Cardiol* 50:22, 2007.

86. Bazzano LA, Li TY, Joshipura KJ, Hu FB: Intake of fruit, vegetables, and fruit juices and risk of diabetes in women. *Diabetes Care* 31:1311, 2008.

87. Huxley R, Barzi F, Woodward M: Excess risk of fatal coronary heart disease associated with diabetes in men and women: meta-analysis of 37 prospective cohort studies. *BMJ* 332:73, 2006.

88. Gregg EW, Gu Q, Cheng YJ, et al: Mortality trends in men and women with diabetes, 1971 to 2000. *Ann Intern Med* 147:149, 2007.

89. Gu K, Cowie CC, Harris MI: Diabetes and decline in heart disease mortality in US adults. *JAMA* 281:1291, 1999.

90. Hu G, Jousilahti P, Qiao Q, et al: The gender-specific impact of diabetes and myocardial infarction at baseline and during follow-up on mortality from all causes and coronary heart disease. *J Am Coll Cardiol* 45:1413, 2005.

91. Walden CE, Knopp RH, Wahl PW, et al: Sex differences in the effect of diabetes mellitus on lipoprotein triglyceride and cholesterol concentrations. *N Engl J Med* 311:953, 1984.

92. Reaven GM, Chen YD: Insulin resistance, its consequences, and coronary heart disease. Must we choose one culprit? *Circulation* 93:1780, 1996.

93. American Diabetes Association: Clinical practice recommendations 2002. *Diabetes Care* 25(Suppl 1):S1, 2002.

94. Ratner RE: Prevention of type 2 diabetes in women with previous gestational diabetes. *Diabetes Care* 30(Suppl 2):S242, 2007.

95. Schaefer-Graf UM, Buchanan TA, Xiang AH, et al: Clinical predictors for a high risk for the development of diabetes mellitus in the early puerperium in women with recent gestational diabetes mellitus. *Am J Obstet Gynecol* 186:751, 2002.

96. Levitzky YS, Pencina MJ, D'Agostino RB, et al: Impact of impaired fasting glucose on cardiovascular disease: the Framingham Heart Study. *J Am Coll Cardiol* 51:264, 2008.

97. Colhoun HM, Betteridge DJ, Durrington PN, et al: Primary prevention of cardiovascular disease with atorvastatin in type 2 diabetes in the Collaborative Atorvastatin Diabetes Study (CARDS): multicentre randomised placebo-controlled trial. *Lancet* 364:685, 2004.

98. The effect of intensive treatment of diabetes on the development and progression of long-term complications in insulin-dependent diabetes mellitus. The Diabetes Control and Complications Trial Research Group. *N Engl J Med* 329:977, 1993.

99. Nathan DM, Cleary PA, Backlund JY, et al: Intensive diabetes treatment and cardiovascular disease in patients with type 1 diabetes. *N Engl J Med* 353:2643, 2005.

100. Dormandy JA, Charbonnel B, Eckland DJ, et al: Secondary prevention of macrovascular events in patients with type 2 diabetes in the PROactive Study (PROspective pioglitAzone Clinical Trial In macroVascular Events): a randomised controlled trial. *Lancet* 366:1279, 2005.

101. Gaede P, Vedel P, Larsen N, et al: Multifactorial intervention and cardiovascular disease in patients with type 2 diabetes. *N Engl J Med* 348:383, 2003.

102. Centers for Disease Control and Prevention, National Center for Health Statistics: Health data for all ages. Available at: www.cdc.gov/nchs/health_data_for_all_ages. htm. Accessed June 11, 2009.

103. Chobanian AV, Bakris GL, Black HR, et al: The Seventh Report of the Joint National Committee on Prevention, Detection, Evaluation, and Treatment of High Blood Pressure: the JNC 7 report. *JAMA* 289:2560, 2003.

104. Cornoni-Huntley J, LaCroix AZ, Havlik RJ: Race and sex differentials in the impact of hypertension in the United States. The National Health and Nutrition Examination Survey I Epidemiologic Follow-up Study. *Arch Intern Med* 149:780, 1989.

105. Prevention of stroke by antihypertensive drug treatment in older persons with isolated systolic hypertension. Final results of the Systolic Hypertension in the Elderly Program (SHEP). SHEP Cooperative Research Group. *JAMA* 265:3255, 1991.

106. Gueyffier F, Boutitie F, Boissel JP, et al: Effect of antihypertensive drug treatment on cardiovascular outcomes in women and men. A meta-analysis of individual patient data from randomized, controlled trials. The INDANA Investigators. *Ann Intern Med* 126:761, 1997.

107. Wassertheil-Smoller S, Anderson G, Psaty BM, et al: Hypertension and its treatment in postmenopausal women: baseline data from the Women's Health Initiative. *Hypertension* 36:780, 2000.

108. Kaplan NM: The treatment of hypertension in women. *Arch Intern Med* 155:563, 1995.

109. Reynolds E, Baron RB: Hypertension in women and the elderly. Some puzzling and some expected findings of treatment studies. *Postgrad Med* 100:58, 67, 1996.

110. Safar ME, Smulyan H: Hypertension in women. *Am J Hypertens* 17:82, 2004.

111. Oparil S, Miller AP: Gender and blood pressure. *J Clin Hypertens (Greenwich)* 7:300, 2005.

112. Gu Q, Burt VL, Paulose-Ram R, Dillon CF: Gender differences in hypertension treatment, drug utilization patterns, and blood pressure control among US adults with hypertension: data from the National Health and Nutrition Examination Survey 1999-2004. *Am J Hypertens* 21:789, 2008.

113. Hecht HS, Superko HR: Electron beam tomography and National Cholesterol Education Program guidelines in asymptomatic women. *J Am Coll Cardiol* 37:1506, 2001.

114. Pasternak RC, Abrams J, Greenland P, et al: 34th Bethesda Conference: Task force #1—Identification of coronary heart disease risk: is there a detection gap? *J Am Coll Cardiol* 41:1863, 2003.

115. Shaw LJ, Lewis JF, Hlatky MA, et al: Women's Ischemic Syndrome Evaluation: current status and future research directions: report of the National Heart, Lung and Blood Institute workshop: October 2-4, 2002: Section 5: gender-related risk factors for ischemic heart disease. *Circulation* 109:e56, 2004.

116. Michos ED, Nasir K, Braunstein JB, et al: Framingham risk equation underestimates subclinical atherosclerosis risk in asymptomatic women. *Atherosclerosis* 184:201, 2006.

117. Lakoski SG, Greenland P, Wong ND, et al: Coronary artery calcium scores and risk for cardiovascular events in women classified as "low risk" based on Framingham risk score: the multi-ethnic study of atherosclerosis (MESA). *Arch Intern Med* 167:2437, 2007.

118. Nasir K, Michos ED, Blumenthal RS, Raggi P: Detection of high-risk young adults and women by coronary calcium and National Cholesterol Education Program Panel III guidelines. *J Am Coll Cardiol* 46:1931, 2005.

119. Wong TY, Hubbard LD, Klein R, et al: Retinal microvascular abnormalities and blood pressure in older people: the Cardiovascular Health Study. *Br J Ophthalmol* 86:1007, 2002.

120. Cook NR, Buring JE, Ridker PM: The effect of including C-reactive protein in cardiovascular risk prediction models for women. *Ann Intern Med* 145:21, 2006.

121. Raggi P, Shaw LJ, Berman DS, Callister TQ: Gender-based differences in the prognostic value of coronary calcification. *J Womens Health (Larchmt)* 13:273, 2004.

122. Wong ND, Pio J, Valencia R, Thakal G: Distribution of C-reactive protein and its relation to risk factors and coronary heart disease risk estimation in the National Health and Nutrition Examination Survey (NHANES) III. *Prev Cardiol* 4:109, 2001.

123. Bessant R, Hingorani A, Patel L, et al: Risk of coronary heart disease and stroke in a large British cohort of patients with systemic lupus erythematosus. *Rheumatology (Oxford)* 43:924, 2004.

124. Ridker PM, Buring JE, Cook NR, Rifai N: C-reactive protein, the metabolic syndrome, and risk of incident cardiovascular events: an 8-year follow-up of 14 719 initially healthy American women. *Circulation* 107:391, 2003.

125. Johnson BD, Kip KE, Marroquin OC, et al: Serum amyloid A as a predictor of coronary artery disease and cardiovascular outcome in women: the National Heart, Lung, and Blood Institute–Sponsored Women's Ischemia Syndrome Evaluation (WISE). *Circulation* 109:726, 2004.

126. Marroquin OC, Kip KE, Kelley DE, et al: Metabolic syndrome modifies the cardiovascular risk associated with angiographic coronary artery disease in women: a report from the Women's Ischemia Syndrome Evaluation. *Circulation* 109:714, 2004.

127. Ridker PM, Rifai N, Rose L, et al: Comparison of C-reactive protein and low-density lipoprotein cholesterol levels in the prediction of first cardiovascular events. *N Engl J Med* 347:1557, 2002.

128. Ridker PM, Buring JE, Shih J, et al: Prospective study of C-reactive protein and the risk of future cardiovascular events among apparently healthy women. *Circulation* 98:731, 1998.

129. Kuller LH, Tracy RP: The role of inflammation in cardiovascular disease. *Arterioscler Thromb Vasc Biol* 20:901, 2000.

130. Tracy RP: Inflammation in cardiovascular disease: cart, horse or both—revisited. *Arterioscler Thromb Vasc Biol* 22:1514, 2002.

131. Kip KE, Marroquin OC, Kelley DE, et al: Clinical importance of obesity versus the metabolic syndrome in cardiovascular risk in women: a report from the Women's Ischemia Syndrome Evaluation (WISE) study. *Circulation* 109:706, 2004.

132. Zethelius B, Berglund L, Sundström J, et al: Use of multiple biomarkers to improve the prediction of death from cardiovascular causes. *N Engl J Med* 358:2107, 2008.

133. Arant CB, Wessel TR, Ridker PM, et al: Multimarker approach predicts adverse cardiovascular events in women evaluated for suspected ischemia: results from the National Heart, Lung, and Blood Institute–sponsored Women's Ischemia Syndrome Evaluation. *Clin Cardiol* 32:244, 2009.

134. Collaborative meta-analysis of randomised trials of antiplatelet therapy for prevention of death, myocardial infarction, and stroke in high risk patients. *BMJ* 324:71, 2002.

135. Collaborative overview of randomised trials of antiplatelet therapy—I: prevention of death, myocardial infarction, and stroke by prolonged antiplatelet therapy in various categories of patients. Antiplatelet Trialists' Collaboration. *BMJ* 308:81, 1994.

136. Patrono C, Coller B, FitzGerald GA, et al: Platelet-active drugs: the relationships among dose, effectiveness, and side-effects: the Seventh ACCP Conference on Antithrombotic and Thrombolytic Therapy. *Chest* 126(Suppl):234S, 2004.

137. Manson JE, Stampfer MJ, Colditz GA, et al: A prospective study of aspirin use and primary prevention of cardiovascular disease in women. *JAMA* 266:521, 1991.

138. Hansson L, Zanchetti A, Carruthers SG, et al: Effects of intensive blood-pressure lowering and low-dose aspirin in patients with hypertension: principal results of the Hypertension Optimal Treatment (HOT) randomised trial. HOT Study Group. *Lancet* 351:1755, 1998.
139. Berger JS, Roncaglioni MC, Avanzini F, et al: Aspirin for the primary prevention of cardiovascular events in women and men: a sex-specific meta-analysis of randomized controlled trials. *JAMA* 295:306, 2006.
140. Ridker PM, Cook NR, Lee IM, et al: A randomized trial of low-dose aspirin in the primary prevention of cardiovascular disease in women. *N Engl J Med* 352:1293, 2005.
141. Final report on the aspirin component of the ongoing Physicians' Health Study. Steering Committee of the Physicians' Health Study Research Group. *N Engl J Med* 321:129, 1989.
142. Dorsch MP, Lee JS, Lynch DR, et al: Aspirin resistance in patients with stable coronary artery disease with and without a history of myocardial infarction. *Ann Pharmacother* 41:737, 2007.
143. Aspirin for the prevention of cardiovascular disease: U.S. Preventive Services Task Force recommendation statement. *Ann Intern Med* 150:396, 2009.
144. Grodstein F, Stampfer MJ, Manson JE, et al: Postmenopausal estrogen and progestin use and the risk of cardiovascular disease. *N Engl J Med* 335:453, 1996.
145. Falkeborn M, Persson I, Adami HO, et al: The risk of acute myocardial infarction after oestrogen and oestrogen-progestogen replacement. *Br J Obstet Gynaecol* 99:821, 1992.
146. Hulley S, Grady D, Bush T, et al: Randomized trial of estrogen plus progestin for secondary prevention of coronary heart disease in postmenopausal women. Heart and Estrogen/progestin Replacement Study (HERS) Research Group. *JAMA* 280:605, 1998.
147. Grady D, Herrington D, Bittner V, et al: Cardiovascular disease outcomes during 6.8 years of hormone therapy: Heart and Estrogen/progestin Replacement Study follow-up (HERS II). *JAMA* 288:49, 2002.
148. Herrington DM, Reboussin DM, Brosnihan KB, et al: Effects of estrogen replacement on the progression of coronary-artery atherosclerosis. *N Engl J Med* 343:522, 2000.
149. Viscoli CM, Brass LM, Kernan WN, et al: A clinical trial of estrogen-replacement therapy after ischemic stroke. *N Engl J Med* 345:1243, 2001.
150. Waters DD, Alderman EL, Hsia J, et al: Effects of hormone replacement therapy and antioxidant vitamin supplements on coronary atherosclerosis in postmenopausal women: a randomized controlled trial. *JAMA* 288:2432, 2002.
151. Cherry N, Gilmour K, Hannaford P, et al: Oestrogen therapy for prevention of reinfarction in postmenopausal women: a randomised placebo controlled trial. *Lancet* 360:2001, 2002.
152. Clarke SC, Kelleher J, Lloyd-Jones H, et al: A study of hormone replacement therapy in postmenopausal women with ischaemic heart disease: the Papworth HRT atherosclerosis study. *BJOG* 109:1056, 2002.
153. Hodis HN, Mack WJ, Azen SP, et al: Hormone therapy and the progression of coronary-artery atherosclerosis in postmenopausal women. *N Engl J Med* 349:535, 2003.
154. Hodis HN, Mack WJ, Lobo RA, et al: Estrogen in the prevention of atherosclerosis. A randomized, double-blind, placebo-controlled trial. *Ann Intern Med* 135:939, 2001.
155. Manson JE, Hsia J, Johnson KC, et al: Estrogen plus progestin and the risk of coronary heart disease. *N Engl J Med* 349:523, 2003.
156. Anderson GL, Limacher M, Assaf AR, et al: Effects of conjugated equine estrogen in postmenopausal women with hysterectomy: the Women's Health Initiative randomized controlled trial. *JAMA* 291:1701, 2004.
157. Rossouw JE, Prentice RL, Manson JE, et al: Postmenopausal hormone therapy and risk of cardiovascular disease by age and years since menopause. *JAMA* 297:1465, 2007.
158. Manson JE, Allison MA, Rossouw JE, et al: Estrogen therapy and coronary-artery calcification. *N Engl J Med* 356:2591, 2007.
159. Hodis HN, Mack WJ: Postmenopausal hormone therapy and cardiovascular disease in perspective. *Clin Obstet Gynecol* 51:564, 2008.
160. ELITE: Early versus late intervention trial with estradiol (NCT00114517). Available at: http://www.clinicaltrials.gov. Accessed July 7, 2009.
161. Harman SM, Brinton EA, Cedars M, et al: KEEPS: The Kronos Early Estrogen Prevention Study. *Climacteric* 8:3, 2005.
162. Mendelsohn ME, Karas RH: The protective effects of estrogen on the cardiovascular system. *N Engl J Med* 340:1801, 1999.
163. Tannenbaum C, Barrett-Connor E, Laughlin GA, Platt RW: A longitudinal study of dehydroepiandrosterone sulphate (DHEAS) change in older men and women: the Rancho Bernardo Study. *Eur J Endocrinol* 151:717, 2004.
164. Kaplan JR, Adams MR, Clarkson TB, Koritnik DR: Psychosocial influences on female "protection" among cynomolgus macaques. *Atherosclerosis* 53:283, 1984.
165. Kaplan JR, Manuck SB, Anthony MS, Clarkson TB: Premenopausal social status and hormone exposure predict postmenopausal atherosclerosis in female monkeys. *Obstet Gynecol* 99:381, 2002.
166. Williams JK, Adams MR, Klopfenstein HS: Estrogen modulates responses of atherosclerotic coronary arteries. *Circulation* 81:1680, 1990.
167. Ness RB, Harris T, Cobb J, et al: Number of pregnancies and the subsequent risk of cardiovascular disease. *N Engl J Med* 328:1528, 1993.
168. Ding EL, Song Y, Malik VS, Liu S: Sex differences of endogenous sex hormones and risk of type 2 diabetes: a systematic review and meta-analysis. *JAMA* 295:1288, 2006.
169. Shaw LJ, Bairey Merz CN, Azziz R, et al: Postmenopausal women with a history of irregular menses and elevated androgen measurements at high risk for worsening cardiovascular event-free survival: results from the National Institutes of Health–National Heart, Lung, and Blood Institute sponsored Women's Ischemia Syndrome Evaluation. *J Clin Endocrinol Metab* 93:1276, 2008.
170. Spencer EA, Pirie KL, Stevens RJ, et al; Million Women Study Collaborators: Diabetes and modifiable risk factors for cardiovascular disease: the prospective Million Women Study. *Eur J Epidemiol* 23:793, 2008.
171. Zambon S, Zanoni S, Romanato G, et al: Metabolic syndrome and all-cause and cardiovascular mortality in an Italian elderly population: the Progetto Veneto Anziani (Pro.V.A.) Study. *Diabetes Care* 32:153, 2009.
172. Krattenmacher R: Drospirenone: pharmacology and pharmacokinetics of a unique progestogen. *Contraception* 62:29, 2000.
173. Jones DR, Schmidt RJ, Pickard RT, et al: Estrogen receptor–mediated repression of human hepatic lipase gene transcription. *J Lipid Res* 43:383, 2002.
174. Sitruk-Ware RL, Menard J, Rad M, et al: Comparison of the impact of vaginal and oral administration of combined hormonal contraceptives on hepatic proteins sensitive to estrogen. *Contraception* 75:430, 2007.
175. Endrikat J, Klipping C, Cronin M, et al: An open label, comparative study of the effects of a dose-reduced oral contraceptive containing 20 μg ethinyl estradiol and 100 μg levonorgestrel on hemostatic, lipids, and carbohydrate metabolism variables. *Contraception* 65:215, 2002.
176. Skouby SO, Endrikat J, Düsterberg B, et al: A 1-year randomized study to evaluate the effects of a dose reduction in oral contraceptives on lipids and carbohydrate metabolism: 20 μg ethinyl estradiol combined with 100 μg levonorgestrel. *Contraception* 71:111, 2005.
177. Chasan-Taber L, Willett WC, Manson JE, et al: Prospective study of oral contraceptives and hypertension among women in the United States. *Circulation* 94:483, 1996.
178. Narkiewicz K, Graniero GR, D'Este D, et al: Ambulatory blood pressure in mild hypertensive women taking oral contraceptives. A case-control study. *Am J Hypertens* 8:249, 1995.
179. Suthipongse W, Taneepanichskul S: An open-label randomized comparative study of oral contraceptives between medications containing 3 mg drospirenone/30 μg ethinylestradiol and 150 μg levonogestrel/30 μg ethinylestradiol in Thai women. *Contraception* 69:23, 2004.
180. Oelkers W, Foidart JM, Dombrovicz N, et al: Effects of a new oral contraceptive containing an antimineralocorticoid progestogen, drospirenone, on the renin-aldosterone system, body weight, blood pressure, glucose tolerance, and lipid metabolism. *J Clin Endocrinol Metab* 80:1816, 1995.
181. Shufelt CL, Bairey Merz CN: Contraceptive hormone use and cardiovascular disease. *J Am Coll Cardiol* 53:221, 2009.
182. Ouyang P, Michos ED, Karas RH: Hormone replacement therapy and the cardiovascular system: lessons learned and unanswered questions. *J Am Coll Cardiol* 47:1741, 2006.
183. Sidney S, Petitti DB, Soff GA, et al: Venous thromboembolic disease in users of low-estrogen combined estrogen-progestin oral contraceptives. *Contraception* 70:3, 2004.
184. Jick H, Jick SS, Gurewich V, et al: Risk of idiopathic cardiovascular death and nonfatal venous thromboembolism in women using oral contraceptives with differing progestagen components. *Lancet* 346:1589, 1995.
185. Lafitte C, Even C, Henry-Lebras F, et al: Migraine and angina pectoris by coronary artery spasm. *Headache* 36:332, 1996.
186. Williams JK, Shively CA, Clarkson TB: Determinants of coronary artery reactivity in premenopausal female cynomolgus monkeys with diet-induced atherosclerosis. *Circulation* 90:983, 1994.
187. Reis SE, Gloth ST, Blumenthal RS, et al: Ethinyl estradiol acutely attenuates abnormal coronary vasomotor responses to acetylcholine in postmenopausal women. *Circulation* 89:52, 1994.
188. Gilligan DM, Quyyumi AA, Cannon RO, 3rd: Effects of physiological levels of estrogen on coronary vasomotor function in postmenopausal women. *Circulation* 89:2545, 1994.
189. Herrington DM, Werbel BL, Riley WA, et al: Individual and combined effects of estrogen/progestin therapy and lovastatin on lipids and flow-mediated vasodilation in postmenopausal women with coronary artery disease. *J Am Coll Cardiol* 33:2030, 1999.
190. Hermsmeyer RK, Mishra RG, Pavcnik D, et al: Prevention of coronary hyperreactivity in preatherogenic menopausal rhesus monkeys by transdermal progesterone. *Arterioscler Thromb Vasc Biol* 24:955, 2004.
191. Mishra RG, Hermsmeyer RK, Miyagawa K, et al: Medroxyprogesterone acetate and dihydrotestosterone induce coronary hyperreactivity in intact male rhesus monkeys. *J Clin Endocrinol Metab* 90:3706, 2005.
192. Drici MD, Burklow TR, Haridasse V, et al: Sex hormones prolong the QT interval and downregulate potassium channel expression in the rabbit heart. *Circulation* 94:1471, 1996.
193. Cheng J: Evidences of the gender-related differences in cardiac repolarization and the underlying mechanisms in different animal species and human. *Fundam Clin Pharmacol* 20:1, 2006.
194. Kurokawa J, Tamagawa M, Harada N, et al: Acute effects of oestrogen on the guinea pig and human I_{Kr} channels and drug-induced prolongation of cardiac repolarization. *J Physiol* 586(pt 12):2961, 2008.
195. Barrett-Connor E, Grady D, Sashegyi A, et al: Raloxifene and cardiovascular events in osteoporotic postmenopausal women: four-year results from the MORE (Multiple Outcomes of Raloxifene Evaluation) randomized trial. *JAMA* 287:847, 2002.
196. Walsh BW, Paul S, Wild RA, et al: The effects of hormone replacement therapy and raloxifene on C-reactive protein and homocysteine in healthy postmenopausal women: a randomized, controlled trial. *J Clin Endocrinol Metab* 85:214, 2000.
197. Martino S, Cauley JA, Barrett-Connor E, et al: Continuing outcomes relevant to Evista: breast cancer incidence in postmenopausal osteoporotic women in a randomized trial of raloxifene. *J Natl Cancer Inst* 96:1751, 2004.
198. Ensrud K, Genazzani AR, Geiger MJ, et al: Effect of raloxifene on cardiovascular adverse events in postmenopausal women with osteoporosis. *Am J Cardiol* 97:520, 2006.
199. Barrett-Connor E, Mosca L, Collins P, et al: Effects of raloxifene on cardiovascular events and breast cancer in postmenopausal women. *N Engl J Med* 355:125, 2006.
200. Collins P, Mosca L, Geiger MJ, et al: Effects of the selective estrogen receptor modulator raloxifene on coronary outcomes in the Raloxifene Use for The Heart trial: results of subgroup analyses by age and other factors. *Circulation* 119:922, 2009.

CHAPTER **2 5**

Cardiovascular Aging: The Next Frontier in Cardiovascular Prevention

Samer S. Najjar, Edward G. Lakatta, and Gary Gerstenblith

KEY POINTS

- The incidence and prevalence of most cardiovascular diseases increase with advancing age.

- Age is the dominant risk factor for cardiovascular diseases, but age has traditionally been viewed as a nonmodifiable risk factor.

- Physiologic aging of the cardiovascular system is associated with myriad structural and functional alterations in the heart and in the blood vessels, which are themselves risk factors for cardiovascular diseases and thus may help explain the "risky" aspects of aging.

- The hallmarks of arterial aging include thickening and stiffening of the walls of the central arteries and endothelial dysfunction.

- Cardiac aging includes structural alterations in the heart, deficits in reserve functions, alterations in calcium regulation, and increased generation of reactive oxygen species during stress.

- Clinical interventions to retard cardiovascular aging include lifestyle changes (e.g., exercise, smoking cessation) and pharmacologic interventions (e.g., renin-angiotensin-aldosterone antagonists, antihypertensive medications, statins).

- Future studies should examine whether interventions aimed at retarding cardiovascular aging can have a positive impact on the adverse cardiovascular effects of accelerated cardiovascular aging and attenuate the impact of age as the dominant risk factor for cardiovascular diseases. Importantly, this should help alter our view of aging from an immutable risk factor to one that is amenable to modification and prevention.

The epidemic of cardiovascular diseases has taken on a global dimension and is no longer restricted to Western societies. Cardiovascular diseases now represent more than 30% of all deaths worldwide, and by the year 2020, they are expected to surpass infectious diseases as the leading cause of mortality and disability. According to the *World Health Report,*[1] cardiovascular diseases were responsible for 15 million annual deaths worldwide, of which 9 million were in developing countries and 2 million in economies in transition. This situation is expected to worsen as the world population in both industrialized and developing countries is aging. For example, in the United States, 35 million people are older than 65 years, and the number of older Americans is expected to double by the year 2030. In many developing countries, the older population is progressively becoming more predominant as life expectancy increases.

The clinical and economic implications of this demographic shift are staggering because age is the most potent individual risk factor for cardiovascular diseases, especially in individuals older than 50 years.[2] Both the incidence and prevalence of hypertension, coronary artery disease, congestive heart failure, and stroke increase exponentially with age. In older community-dwelling healthy volunteers, the incidence of silent coronary atherosclerosis, assessed by combined electrocardiographic treadmill stress testing and thallium perfusion imaging, increases dramatically with age.[3]

Age influences not only the incidence and prevalence of coronary atherosclerosis but also the severity and prognosis of this disease. In survivors of a myocardial infarction, age is an independent predictor of short- and long-term morbidity, mortality, and disability, even after adjustment for the infarct size and location, the number of diseased vessels, and the extent of coronary artery disease.[4] Similar considerations pertain to the impact of age on other cardiovascular diseases, such as hypertension, congestive heart failure, and stroke.

In spite of the fact that age is the dominant risk factor for cardiovascular diseases, most of the research efforts on prevention of these diseases have ignored age and have focused instead on development of interventions that target "traditional" cardiovascular risk factors (such as hypertension and hyperlipidemia) or identification of newer risk markers. This is because age has usually been viewed as an unmodifiable risk factor and therefore one that is not amenable to prevention or treatment. However, this concept has recently been challenged by an emerging school of thought, which proposes that aging can indeed be construed as a modifiable risk factor.[5]

The key paradigm shift is that the components of aging associated with cardiovascular disease risk should no longer be simplistically attributed to an increased time of exposure to other established cardiovascular risk factors. Instead, the risky components of aging need to be recognized as accelerated or dysregulated age-associated alterations in the cardiovascular system, at the molecular, enzymatic, biochemical, cellular, histologic, and organismal levels. In this chapter, we review some of these alterations, at both the microscopic and clinical levels, with a view toward illustrating the overlapping features of aging with some cardiovascular diseases and risk factors. We provide an integrated view of the risky components of cardiovascular aging and of age-disease interactions, which are in dire need of targeted preventive and therapeutic strategies.

EPIDEMIOLOGY OF CARDIOVASCULAR DISEASES IN OLDER INDIVIDUALS

The incidence and prevalence of most cardiovascular diseases increase with advancing age in both sexes.[6] For example, the incidence of heart failure in the Framingham Heart Study (1980-2003) per 1000 person-years was 9.2 and 4.7 in men and women between the ages of 65 and 74 years, 22.3 and 14.8 in men and women between the ages of 75 and 84 years, and 41.9 and 32.7 in men and women older than 85 years. The prevalence of heart failure according to NHANES (2003-2006) was 2% and 1% in men and women between the ages of 40 and 59 years, 9% and 5% in men and women between the ages of 60 and 79 years, and 15% and 12% in men and women older than 80 years.

The prevalence of hypertension (defined as systolic blood pressure higher than 140 mm Hg or diastolic blood pressure higher than 90 mm Hg) in NHANES (2003-2006) was 39% and 38% in men and women between the ages of 45 and 54 years, about 54% in men and women between the ages of 55 and 64 years, 65% and 71% in men and women between the ages of 65 and 74 years, and 65% and 77% in men and women older than 75 years.

The incidence of stroke in ARIC (1987-2001) per 1000 person-years was 2.4 for white men and women between the ages of 45 and 54 years and 9.7 and 7.2 for black men and women in the same age range. These numbers increased to 6.1 and 4.8 for white men and women between the ages of 55 and 64 years and 13.1 and 10.0 for black men and women in this age range. The incidence of stroke increased to 12.1 and 9.8 in white men and women between the ages of 65 and 74 years and to 16.2 and 15 in black men and women in this age range. The prevalence of stroke in NHANES (2003-2006) was 1% and 6% in men and women between the ages of 40 and 59 years, 7% in men and women between the ages of 60 and 79 years, and 15% and 13% in men and women older than 80 years.

Last, the prevalence of coronary heart disease in NHANES (2003-2006) was 7% in both men and women between the ages of 40 and 59 years, 25% and 17% in men and women between the ages of 60 and 79 years, and 37% and 23% in men and women older than 80 years.

Importantly, age also influences the prognosis after a cardiovascular event, such that within 1 year after a myocardial infarction, the rate of death is 8% and 12% in white men and women between the ages of 40 and 69 years and 14% and 11% in black men and women in this age range. This rate increases to 27% and 32% of white men and women older than 70 years and to 26% and 28% of black men and women in this age range. Similarly, the risk of heart failure 5 years after a myocardial infarction increases with age. It is 7% and 12% in men and women between the ages of 40 and 69 years and 22% and 25% in men and women older than 70 years.

AGING OF CENTRAL ARTERIES IN APPARENTLY HEALTHY HUMANS

The large central arteries had originally been construed as pipes that simply allowed blood to flow from the heart to distal organs and thus were originally dubbed "conduit" arteries. Changes in their mechanical properties with aging were considered to result largely from passive wear and tear in response to the unrelenting stress and strain incurred with each heartbeat throughout life. However, recent insights into

TABLE 25–1	Arterial Remodeling with Aging Across Species			
	Humans >65 years	Aging Monkeys 15-20 years	Rats 24-30 months	Rabbits 2-6 years
Luminal dilation	+	+	+	+
↑ Stiffness	+	+	+	+
Endothelial dysfunction	+	+	+	+
Diffuse intimal thickening	+	+	+	+
Collagen degradation	+	+	+	+
Collagen deposition	+	+	+	+
VSMC number	+	+	+	+
Macrophages	+	–	+	+
T cells	+	–	–	–
↑ Local angiotensin II–ACE	+	+	+	+
MMP dysregulation	+	+	+	?
↑ MCP-1/CCR2	+	+	+	+
↑ ICAM	+	+	+	?
↑ TGF-β	+	+	+	+
↑ NADPH oxidase	+	+	+	+
↓ VEGF	+	?	?	+
↓ Nitric oxide bioavailability	+	+	+	+

?, information unknown. ACE, angiotensin-converting enzyme; ICAM, intercellular adhesion molecule; MCP-1, monocyte chemotactic protein 1; MMP, matrix metalloproteinase; TGF-β, transforming growth factor-β; VEGF, vascular endothelial growth factor; VSMC, vascular smooth muscle cell.

the multiple signaling mechanisms that modulate their ability to adapt, repair, and remodel and that govern their structural and functional properties have left us marveling at these dynamic organs, which play pivotal roles in regulating pulsatile flow and modulating vascular impedance. The age-associated changes in central arterial structure and function in primates and in apparently healthy humans are summarized in Table 25-1.[1] Some of these features are discussed in the following sections.

Overall cardiovascular structure and function vary dramatically among older individuals.[7] Identification of cardiovascular structural and functional changes that reflect an "aging process" is a formidable task. Neither functional differences among individuals in cross-sectional studies nor changes over time within a given individual in longitudinal studies are necessarily manifestations of an aging process. Rather, interactions among aging, disease, and lifestyle must be considered in interpreting age-associated changes in cardiovascular structure and function as measured in various studies.[8]

Lumen Diameter

Cross-sectional studies show that on average, the central aorta dilates with age, leading to an increase in lumen size[9] (Fig. 25-1A). Studies found an inverse and independent

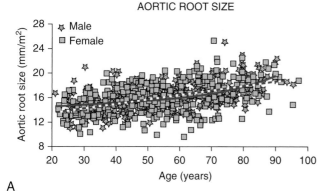

AORTIC ROOT SIZE

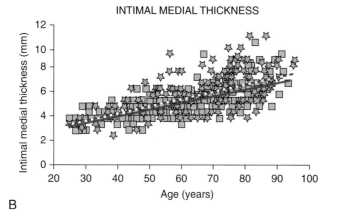

A

INTIMAL MEDIAL THICKNESS

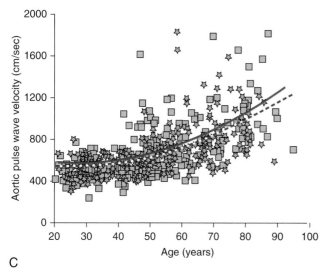

B

C

FIGURE 25-1 Age-associated changes in arterial structure and function in men (blue stars) and women (red squares) in the Baltimore Longitudinal Study of Aging. Best fit regression lines (quadratic or linear) are shown for men (solid lines) and women (dotted lines). **A,** Aortic root size (measured by M-mode echocardiography) indexed to body surface area. **B,** Common carotid intima-medial thickness (measured by B-mode ultrasonography). **C,** Carotid-femoral pulse wave velocity (an index of central arterial stiffness).

association between aortic root diameter and pulse pressure, suggesting that luminal size may play a role in the pathogenesis of systolic hypertension.[10] This provocative concept awaits the results of longitudinal studies to clarify the significance of the cross-sectional relationship between aortic root diameter and pulse pressure, which could have important implications for putative future therapies to delay or to prevent systolic hypertension, the dominant form of hypertension in older individuals.

Wall Thickness

Aging is also associated with thickening of the walls of the central arteries (Fig. 25-1B). Intima-media thickness rises nearly threefold between the third and ninth decades of life, an increase that is mainly attributable to an increase in intimal thickness.[11] The age-associated intima-media thickening is often ascribed to atherosclerosis, and intima-media thickness is often equated with subclinical atherosclerosis. This is because a growing body of literature has shown that traditional cardiovascular risk factors and prevalent cardiovascular diseases are associated with intima-media thickening and that intima-media thickening is a potent and independent predictor of adverse cardiovascular events. However, intima-media thickness is only modestly correlated with the extent and severity of coronary artery disease,[12] and it can be influenced by factors other than atherosclerosis (e.g., aging, hypertension).

For example, intima-media thickening increases with advancing age in animal models that are devoid of atherosclerosis,[13] thus indicating that these age-associated alterations are due to the aging process and not to superimposed atherosclerosis. This thickening is due to myriad age-associated biochemical, cellular, and morphologic changes in the arterial wall, which are modulated by the same factors that have been implicated in the genesis of various cardiovascular diseases.[14] Thus, intima-media thickening should not be construed as synonymous with "subclinical atherosclerosis," particularly in the absence of plaques. Nonetheless, it remains a useful marker of subclinical vascular disease.[15]

Wall Remodeling

Although we have discussed arterial wall thickness and luminal diameter separately, arteries undergo a remodeling process, in response to hemodynamic and metabolic stimuli, that can be better characterized by an index that combines the diameter, wall thickness, and vascular mass variables than by each of these variables individually. For example, in the carotid artery, three remodeling patterns that deviate from normal can be described[16]: (1) concentric remodeling, due to a smaller lumen in the setting of a normal vascular mass; (2) vascular hypertrophy, due to an increase in vascular mass, which results from wall thickening, in the setting of a normal lumen size; and (3) eccentric hypertrophy, due to an increase in vascular mass in the setting of a dilated lumen. In a study of normotensive and untreated hypertensive Taiwanese subjects, these geometric patterns yielded prognostic information, with the two hypertrophic groups being associated with an increased risk of cardiovascular events.[17] This underscores the importance of integrating the markers of arterial aging to better appreciate their clinical utility.

Arterial Stiffness

One of the hallmarks of central arterial aging is an age-associated increase in stiffness (Fig. 25-1C). Central arterial stiffness can be assessed by several invasive and noninvasive indexes. Recently, carotid-femoral pulse wave velocity has been anointed the "gold standard" for the noninvasive assessment of central arterial stiffness.[18] Pulse wave velocity has been shown to be an independent predictor of morbidity and mortality in healthy subjects and in individuals with various levels of cardiovascular risk. It is likely that arterial stiffness is not only a risk marker for cardiovascular diseases but also a risk factor for these diseases. Indeed, increased central arterial stiffness leads to an increase in the load (afterload) on the left ventricle, leading to increased hypertrophy and increased oxygen consumption. Furthermore, increased stiffness is associated with a decrease in diastolic blood pressure, which could compromise coronary blood flow, which occurs predominantly in diastole.

The age-associated increase in stiffness has traditionally been attributed to the fraying and breakdown of elastin due to the lifelong repeated cycles of distention and recoil of the central aorta as well as the increased deposition and covalent cross-linking of collagen molecules. It is now recognized that arterial stiffening can be modulated by several factors including lifestyle considerations (e.g., salt intake, exercise, weight loss),[19] signaling pathways (e.g., nitric oxide),[20] inflammation, and genetics.[21] Interventions to prevent or to delay arterial stiffening have predominantly focused on pharmacologic antihypertensive therapies. However, these strategies are aimed at lowering blood pressure, whereby the reduction in stiffness is a secondary effect due to reverse remodeling of the arterial wall in response to the lower pressures.

Because arterial stiffness is a potent predictor of mortality and morbidity, independent of blood pressure, a more direct approach that would target the stiffening process is desirable. However, there is a dearth of interventions at present that have attempted this, with the one notable exception being the advanced glycation end products cross-link breaker Alagebrium (ALT-711). This compound cleaves the covalent cross-link bonds that form between adjacent collagen fibrils in the medial layer of the arterial wall and that contribute to increasing the tensile strength of the collagen molecules. Alagebrium has been shown to reduce arterial stiffness in rodents and in nonhuman primates.

In humans with systolic hypertension and increased arterial stiffness, a randomized, double-blind, placebo-controlled study showed that treatment with Alagebrium for 8 weeks resulted in a significant decrease in arterial stiffness, without an apparent disproportionate decline in mean arterial pressure, systemic vascular resistance, heart rate, or cardiac output.[22] Although a multicenter, randomized, double-blind, placebo-controlled clinical trial failed to show an effect of Alagebrium on blood pressure,[23] the primary effect of this compound should be a reduction in stiffness, and a reduction in stiffness may not necessarily translate into a reduction in blood pressure (at least in the short or intermediate term) because the lowering in stiffness could be accompanied by an increase in stroke volume (lower afterload on the heart), which could potentially offset the effects of a lower stiffness on blood pressure. Unfortunately, these hemodynamic features were not assessed in the aforementioned clinical study.

In contrast to the central elastic arteries, the stiffness of the muscular arteries (e.g., brachial and femoral arteries) does not increase with age. Thus, the manifestations of arterial aging may vary among the different vascular beds, reflecting differences in the structural compositions of the arteries and perhaps differences in the age-associated signaling cascades that modulate the arterial properties or differences in the response to these signals across the arterial tree.

Reflected Waves

The increased load that is imposed on the heart by increasing stiffness is due not only to an increase in characteristic impedance (intrinsic stiffness of the vessel) but also to an increase in central systolic blood pressure. The latter is due, in part, to a shift in the return of reflected waves to an earlier time during systole, which leads to an increase in central pressure augmentation and thus to a higher central systolic blood pressure and a higher central pulse pressure. It is now appreciated that the timing and amplitude of reflected waves are governed both by arterial stiffness and by properties of the distal reflecting sites (usually areas of impedance mismatch). These reflected waves play an important role in influencing the central to peripheral pressure augmentation across the arterial tree.[24] Even though peripheral systolic pressure and pulse pressure increase with age, the central to peripheral pressure amplification decreases with age.

Central Blood Pressure

Recent methodologic advances have made it possible to noninvasively estimate central blood pressures with relative ease. This is fueling a growing clinical interest in assessing central blood pressures. The Conduit Artery Functional Endpoint (CAFÉ) study showed that the combination of the calcium channel blocker amlodipine with or without the angiotensin-converting enzyme (ACE) inhibitor perindopril in the treatment of hypertension achieved a greater reduction in central blood pressure than the beta blocker atenolol with or without a diuretic, even though the peripheral blood pressures were not significantly different between the two groups.[25] CAFÉ was a substudy of the Anglo-Scandinavian Cardiac Outcomes Trial (ASCOT), which showed that patients in the amlodipine-perindopril arm had better clinical outcomes than those in the atenolol-diuretic arm.[26]

The findings from CAFÉ suggest that the lower central blood pressures achieved with amlodipine-perindopril may explain, in part, the differences in outcomes between the two groups. The usefulness and feasibility of integrating measurements of central arterial blood pressures into routine medical practice are areas of intense ongoing research. As a first step, studies have established that central pressures are independent predictors of outcomes[27] and may be even better predictors of cardiovascular mortality than peripheral blood pressures.[28]

Increased central arterial stiffness is associated with an increase in central systolic blood pressure and a decrease in diastolic blood pressure, resulting in a widening of the pulse pressure. This is a likely explanation of the age-associated changes in blood pressures, whereby systolic blood pressure continues to increase with advancing age, whereas diastolic blood pressure increases until the fifth decade, then levels off and starts to decrease after the age of 60 years.[29] Numerous clinical and epidemiologic studies in several different populations with varying prevalence of cardiovascular diseases have demonstrated that pulse pressure is an important predictor of adverse outcomes, often more potent than systolic or diastolic blood pressures. However, the clinical role of pulse pressure has remained limited to a few clinical conditions (e.g., advanced heart failure, severe aortic regurgitation), although it could serve as an easily obtainable surrogate marker of stiffness.

Arterial-Ventricular Coupling

In addition to the age-associated alterations in arterial properties, advancing age is also associated with alterations in left ventricular (LV) structure and function. Importantly, the left ventricle and the central arteries have bidirectional constant interactions. One useful index of this interaction, termed arterial-ventricular coupling, can be assessed by the ratio of effective arterial elastance (Ea), a measure of the net arterial load exerted on the left ventricle, to LV end-systolic elastance (ELV), a load-independent measure of LV chamber performance.[30] Ea increases with advancing age, predominantly because of the age-associated increase in arterial stiffness, as peripheral vascular resistance and heart rate (the other main determinants of Ea) do not significantly change with age.[31]

ELV also increases with advancing age. Interestingly, even though Ea and ELV both increase with advancing age, their ratio, Ea/ELV, remains relatively unchanged across the age spectrum in men,[32] suggesting that the increases in Ea and ELV are matched. This tight coupling is thought to allow the cardiovascular system to optimize energetic efficiency. In contrast, in healthy women, Ea/ELV declines slightly with advancing age,[31] which is due to a disproportionate age-associated increase in ELV compared with the age-associated increase in Ea. This suggests that in women, but not in men, aging exerts a greater impact on ventricular than arterial properties.

Therapies that improve the coupling of ventricular and vascular elastances are likely to improve cardiac function and exercise tolerance in healthy subjects. This concept is supported by two studies in healthy older subjects. Administration of the direct vasodilator sodium nitroprusside caused reductions in reflected waves (manifested as a reduction in preload), resulting in reduced cardiac volumes and higher ejection fraction at rest and during maximal exercise compared with placebo therapy.[33] Administration of intravenous verapamil reduced noninvasive indexes of arterial and ventricular systolic stiffness and improved exercise tolerance and oxygen consumption before reaching the anaerobic threshold.

Aging of Endothelial Cells

An important feature of arterial aging is age-associated compromise in endothelial function. In humans, the function of endothelial cells in central arteries has not been directly assessed. Nonetheless, endothelial function has been assessed in the brachial artery, where measurement of vasoreactivity by both agonist- and flow-mediated techniques has shown that it declines with advancing age.[34]

Endothelial cells play a pivotal role in modulating myriad arterial structural and functional properties, including vascular tone, vascular permeability, angiogenesis, production of extracellular matrix proteins and of growth factors, neurohormonal signaling (nitric oxide, renin-angiotensin-aldosterone system, sympathetic nervous system), and response to inflammation. The critical role of endothelial cells in several cardiovascular diseases is increasingly being appreciated. For example, endothelial dysfunction has been described in patients with hypertension and, interestingly, in the normotensive offspring of hypertensive individuals,[35] suggesting that endothelial dysfunction may precede the development of clinical hypertension. Endothelial dysfunction has also been implicated in the pathogenesis of atherosclerosis and is one of the earliest pathologic manifestations of this disease. Interestingly, arterial regions with low shear stress are particularly vulnerable to the development of atherosclerosis, and vascular wall shear stress is an important modulator of endothelial cell morphology and endothelial cell metabolic and synthetic functions. Endothelial dysfunction, in both the coronary and peripheral arterial beds, has been shown to be an independent predictor of future cardiovascular events.

Endothelial dysfunction can also be induced by loss of telomere function. Telomeres are DNA-protein complexes that form the ends of chromosomes, and they shorten with each replicative cycle, which is why they have been proposed to be possible indicators of biologic aging. Interestingly, inhibition of telomere shortening can suppress the age-associated endothelial dysfunction.[36]

Vascular cell senescence is increasingly recognized as an important feature of arterial aging. Thus, there is growing interest in and excitement at the promises held by regenerative therapies. Endothelial cells play a pivotal role in angiogenesis, the process through which new vessels grow from existing microvasculature. However, studies in animal models of aging indicate that angiogenesis is impaired with advancing age. Endothelial progenitor cells offer the prospects of putatively replenishing or replacing senescent endothelial cells. However, both the number[37] and activity[38] of

endothelial progenitor cells appear to be reduced with aging, suggesting an age-associated impairment in regenerative and repair capacities, which, experimentally, can be reversed with growth hormone–mediated increase in insulin-like growth factor 1 (IGF-1) levels.[39]

Plasminogen Activator Inhibitor 1

Thrombotic cardiovascular diseases increase in incidence in the elderly, a tendency dependent on the age-related changes in vascular and hemostatic systems that include platelets, coagulation, and fibrinolytic factors as well as in the endothelium. The hypercoagulability of and advanced sclerotic changes in the vascular wall may contribute to the increased incidence of thrombosis in the elderly. One of the important key genes for aging-associated thrombosis is plasminogen activator inhibitor 1 (PAI-1), a principal inhibitor of fibrinolysis.

The expression of PAI-1 not only is elevated in the elderly but also is significantly induced in a variety of pathologic conditions associated with the process of aging. These conditions include obesity, insulin resistance, emotional stress, immune responses, and vascular sclerosis and remodeling. Several cytokines and hormones, including tumor necrosis factor-α (TNF-α), transforming growth factor-β (TGF-β), angiotensin II, and insulin, positively regulate the gene expression of PAI-1.

The recent epidemic of obesity with aging in industrialized societies may heighten the risk for thrombotic cardiovascular disease because adipose tissue is a primary source of PAI-1 and cytokines. Emotional or psychosocial stress and inflammation also cause the elevated expression of PAI-1 in an age-specific pattern. Thus, PAI-1 could play a key role in the progression of cardiovascular aging by promoting thrombosis and vascular (athero)sclerosis. Further studies on the genetic mechanism of aging-associated PAI-1 induction will be necessary to define the basis for cardiovascular aging in relation to thrombosis.

CARDIAC AGING

The preceding section focused on age-associated changes in the vasculature. Aging is also associated with structural and functional changes in the heart.

Cardiac Aging in Humans

With advancing age, the walls of the left ventricle increase in thickness, largely because of an increase in ventricular myocyte size and an increase in vascular impedance, and this helps moderate the increase in LV wall tension. Modest increases in collagen levels also occur with aging.

A unified interpretation of identified cardiac changes that accompany advancing age in otherwise healthy persons suggests that at least in part, these are adaptive, occurring in response to arterial changes that occur with aging (Fig. 25-2).[9] Prolonged contraction of the thickened LV wall maintains a normal ejection time in the presence of the late augmentation of aortic impedance. This preserves the systolic cardiac pumping function at rest. One disadvantage of prolonged contraction is that at the time of the mitral valve opening, myocardial relaxation is relatively more incomplete in older than in younger individuals and causes the early LV filling rate to be reduced in older individuals.

Structural changes and functional heterogeneity occurring within the left ventricle with aging may also contribute to this reduction in peak LV filling rate. However, concomitant adaptations—left atrial enlargement and an enhanced atrial contribution to ventricular filling—compensate for the

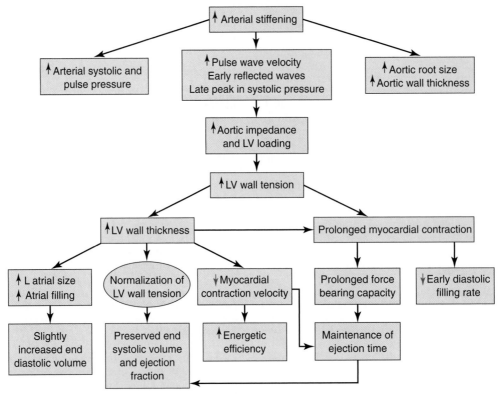

FIGURE 25-2 Arterial and cardiac changes that occur with aging in healthy humans.

reduced early filling and prevent a reduction of the end-diastolic volume. Age-associated changes in the tissue levels of or responses to growth factors (catecholamines, angiotensin II, endothelin, TGF-β, or fibroblast growth factor) that influence myocardial or vascular cells or their extracellular matrices (see later) may also have a role in the schema depicted in Figure 25-2.

Biologic sex is a well-recognized factor in the physiology and pathophysiology of the cardiovascular system, including the aging heart (reviewed in references 40 and 41). Postmortem morphometric assessments in nonfailing human hearts have shown extensive age-related myocyte loss and hypertrophy of the surviving myocytes in male hearts but preserved ventricular myocardial mass and average cell diameter and volume in aging female hearts. These sex differences may stem, in part, from differences in the replicative potential of cardiac myocytes. Analysis of gene expression differences by sex and age in samples of the left ventricle from patients with dilated cardiomyopathy has identified more than 1800 genes displaying sexual dimorphism in the heart. A significant number of these genes were highly represented in gene ontology pathways involved in ion transport and G protein–coupled receptor signaling.[42]

Cardiovascular Reserve

Impaired heart rate acceleration and impaired augmentation of blood ejection from the left ventricle, accompanied by an acute modest increase in LV end-diastolic volume, are the most dramatic changes in cardiac reserve capacity that occur with aging in healthy, community-dwelling persons (Table 25-2). Mechanisms that underlie the age-associated reduction in maximum ejection fraction are multifactorial and include a reduction in intrinsic myocardial contractility, an increase in vascular afterload, and arterial-ventricular load mismatching.

Ventricular load is the opposition to myocardial contraction and the ejection of blood; afterload is the component of load that pertains to the time after excitation, as opposed to preload, before excitation. Although these age-associated changes in cardiovascular reserve are insufficient to produce clinical heart failure, they do affect its clinical presentation, that is, the threshold for symptoms and signs, or the severity and prognosis of heart failure secondary to any level of disease burden (e.g., chronic hypertension that causes either systolic or diastolic heart failure).

A sizeable component of the age-associated deficit in cardiovascular reserve is composed of diminished effectiveness of the autonomic modulation of heart rate, LV contractility, and arterial afterload. The essence of sympathetic modulation of the cardiovascular system is to ensure that the heart beats faster; to ensure that it retains a small size, by reducing the diastolic filling period, reducing LV afterload; to augment myocardial contractility and relaxation; and to redistribute blood to working muscles and to skin to dissipate heat. Each of the deficient components of cardiovascular regulation with aging, that is, heart rate (and thus filling time), afterload (both cardiac and vascular), myocardial contractility, and redistribution of blood flow, exhibits a deficient sympathetic modulation.

Multiple lines of evidence support the idea that the efficiency of postsynaptic beta-adrenergic signaling declines with aging.[9] One line of evidence stems from the observation that cardiovascular responses to beta-adrenergic agonist infusions at rest decrease with age. A second type of evidence for a diminished efficacy of postsynaptic beta-adrenergic receptor signaling is that acute beta-adrenergic receptor blockade changes the exercise hemodynamic profile of younger persons to make it resemble that of older individuals. Significant beta blockade–induced LV dilation occurs only in younger subjects (Fig. 25-3A). The heart rate reduction during exercise in the presence of acute beta-adrenergic blockade is greater in

TABLE 25–2	Exhaustive Upright Exercise: Changes in Aerobic Capacity and Cardiac Regulation Between the Ages of 20 and 80 Years in Healthy Men and Women
Oxygen consumption	↓ (50%)
(A-V)O$_2$	↓ (25%)
Cardiac index	↓ (25%)
Heart rate	↓ (25%)
Stroke volume	No change
Preload	
EDV	↑ (30%)
Afterload	↑
Vascular (PVR)	↑ (30%)
Cardiac (ESV)	↑ (275%)
Cardiac (EDV)	↑ (30%)
Contractility	↓ (60%)
Ejection fraction	↓ (15%)
Plasma catecholamines	↑
Cardiac and vascular responses to beta-adrenergic stimulation	↓

EDV, end-diastolic volume; ESV, end-systolic volume; PVR, peripheral vascular resistance.

younger versus older subjects (Fig. 25-3B), as are the age-associated deficits in LV early diastolic filling rate, both at rest and during exercise (Fig. 25-3C). It has also been observed in older dogs that the age-associated increase in aortic impedance during exercise is abolished by acute beta-adrenergic blockade.

Apparent deficits in sympathetic modulation of cardiac and arterial functions with aging occur in the presence of exaggerated neurotransmitter levels. Plasma levels of norepinephrine and epinephrine, during any perturbation from the supine basal state, increase to a greater extent in older compared with younger healthy humans. The age-associated increase in plasma levels of norepinephrine results from an increased spillover into the circulation and, to a lesser extent, reduced plasma clearance. The degree of norepinephrine spillover into the circulation differs among body organs; increased spillover occurs within the heart. Deficient norepinephrine reuptake at nerve endings is a primary mechanism for increased spillover during acute graded exercise. During prolonged exercise, however, diminished neurotransmitter reuptake might also be associated with depletion and reduced release and spillover. Cardiac muscarinic receptor density and function are also diminished with increasing age and might contribute to the decrease in baroreflex activity observed in aged subjects.[43]

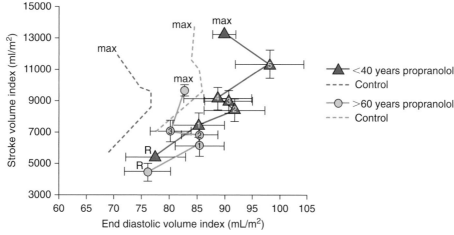

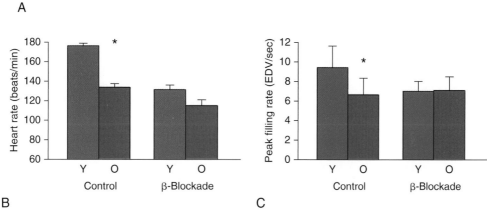

FIGURE 25-3 Cardiovascular reserve in the presence and absence of a beta-adrenergic blocker.

TABLE 25–3 | **Myocardial Changes with Adult Aging in Rodents**

Structural Change	Functional Change	Ionic, Biophysical, and Biochemical Mechanisms	Molecular Mechanisms
↑ Myocyte size	Prolonged contraction	Prolonged cytosolic Ca^{2+} transient	
↓ Myocyte number		↓ SR Ca^{2+} pumping rate ↓ Pump site density ↓ I_{Ca} inactivation ↓ I_{To} density	↓ SR Ca^{2+} pump mRNA No change in calsequestrin mRNA ↑ Na^+/Ca^+ exchanger mRNA
	Prolonged action potential		
	Diminished contraction velocity	↓ α-MHC protein ↑ β-MHC protein ↓ Myosin ATPase activity ↓ RXRβ1 and γ mRNA ↓ RXRβ1 and γ protein ↓ Thyroid receptor protein	↓ α-MHC mRNA ↑ β-MHC mRNA No change in actin mRNA ↓ RXRβ1 and γ mRNA
	Diminished beta-adrenergic contractile response	↓ Coupling beta-adrenergic receptor–acyclase No change in G_i activation No change in BARK activity ↓ TNI phospholamban ↓ Phospholamban phosphorylation ↓ I_{Ca} augmentation ↓ Ca_i transient augmentation ↑ Enkephalin peptides ↑ Proenkephalin mRNA	↓ Beta$_1$-adrenergic receptor mRNA No change in BARK mRNA
↑ Matrix connective tissue	↑ Myocardial stiffness	↑ Hydroxyline proline content ↑ Activity of myocardial RAS ↑ Atrial natriuretic peptide	↑ Collagen mRNA ↑ Fibronectin mRNA ↑ AT_1R mRNA ↑ Atrial natriuretic peptide mRNA ↑ Induction of immediate-early genes
	↓ Growth response ↓ Heat shock response		↓ Activation of HSF

AT_1R, angiotensin AT_1 receptor; BARK, beta-adrenergic receptor kinase; Ca_i, intracellular calcium concentrations; G_i, inhibitory G protein; HSF, heat shock factor; I_{ca}, calcium influx; MHC, myosin heavy chain; mRNA, messenger RNA; RAS, renin-angiotensin system; RXR, retinoid X receptor; SR, sarcoplasmic reticulum; TNI, troponin I.

Cardiac Aging in Animal Models

Cardiac Structure

Cellular and molecular mechanisms implicated in age-associated changes in myocardial structure and function have been largely studied in rodents. Some underlying mechanisms that drive age-related cardiac remodeling are listed in Table 25-3. The altered cardiac structural phenotype that evolves with aging in rodents includes an increase in LV mass due to an enlargement of myocyte size and focal proliferation of the matrix in which the myocytes reside, which may be linked to an altered cardiac fibroblast number or function. The number of cardiac myocytes becomes reduced because of necrosis and apoptosis, with necrosis predominating.

Putative stimuli for cardiac cell enlargement with aging in rodents include an age-associated increase in vascular load due to arterial stiffening and stretching of cells caused by dropout of neighboring myocytes.[44] Stretch of cardiac myocytes and fibroblasts initiates growth factor signaling (e.g., angiotensin II/TGF-ß), which, in addition to modulating cell growth and matrix production, leads to apoptosis. In mouse heart, activation of the calcineurin-NFAT pathway increases with age.[45] The expression of atrial natriuretic[46] and opioid peptides, molecules that are usually produced in response to chronic stress, is increased in the senescent rodent heart.

There is evidence that transcriptional events associated with hypertrophic stressors become altered with advancing age; for example, the nuclear binding activity of the transcription factor nuclear factor-κB is increased and that of another transcription factor, Sp1, is diminished. A proteomic comparison study[47] discovered 117 proteins to be differentially expressed in the aged left ventricle. An increase in oxidative stress is also implicated in age-related cardiac remodeling,[48] and aging is indeed well recognized to be associated with

increased production of reactive oxygen species (ROS) in many different tissues.[49]

Angiotensin II Signaling

Many experimental studies have shown that increased activation of the renin-angiotensin-aldosterone system (RAAS) is a prominent feature of age-related cardiac remodeling that may account for many of the phenotypic changes observed.[8,50]

It is increasingly appreciated that RAAS activation may itself be a significant driver of increased oxidative stress. Notably, NADPH oxidase family members are activated by angiotensin II, aldosterone, endothelin 1, cytokines (e.g., TNF-α), growth factors (e.g., TGF-β, platelet-derived growth factor), and mechanical forces.[51]

The regulated production of small amounts of ROS in response to such stimuli appears to be ideally designed for involvement in redox signaling pathways, and an involvement of NADPH oxidases in such signaling has indeed been demonstrated in many studies.[51] Experimental studies have confirmed that NADPH oxidase–derived ROS play important roles in the pathogenesis of cardiovascular pathologic processes such as endothelial dysfunction, atherosclerosis, diabetic vasculopathy, RAAS-related hypertension, and ischemic vascular remodeling. Recently, it has also been shown that NADPH oxidase activation is involved in several types of cardiac remodeling, including angiotensin II–induced cardiac hypertrophy, aldosterone-induced cardiac fibrosis, and cardiac remodeling after myocardial infarction.[52-54] In addition, increased myocardial NADPH oxidase activity is found in human heart failure.[55,56]

In male Fischer 344 cross brown Norway rats aged 2 months (young rats), 8 months (young adult rats), or 30 months (old rats), age-associated increases in blood pressure, cardiomyocyte area, coronary artery remodeling, and cardiac fibrosis were associated with increased myocardial NADPH oxidase activity, which was attributable to the Nox2 isoform. These changes were accompanied by increased expression of connective tissue growth factor and TGF-β1 and by a significant activation of matrix metalloproteinase 2 (MMP-2) and MT1-MMP, a membrane-bound activator of MMP-2.

The changes in old rats were replicated in 8-month-old rats that were chronically treated with angiotensin II for 28 days. Other cytokines that could be involved in the process include TNF-α, which is implicated in aging-related disease possibly by an upregulation of MMP levels.[57] TNF-α is also a known activator of NADPH oxidase, and its possible involvement in aging-related cardiac remodeling merits investigation.

Because NADPH oxidases are activated by multiple factors, including angiotensin II, aldosterone, endothelin 1, and cytokines, it is arguable that they may be a suitable therapeutic target for the prevention of aging-related cardiac remodeling in addition to targeting of the individual agonists (such as the RAAS) that activate the oxidase.

Calcium Regulation

Age-altered myocardial Ca^{2+} cycling is closely related to coordinated changes in levels of sarcoplasmic reticulum (SR) Ca^{2+}-handling proteins or their function. In aged hearts, selective downregulation of sarcoendoplasmic reticulum calcium-ATPase (SERCA) protein levels, decreased phospholamban phosphorylation (which might be reflected in the desensitized adenylyl cyclase response), and increased levels of Na$^+$/Ca^{2+} exchanger could lead to the reduction in SR Ca^{2+} load. It is also suggested that the aged heart uses the compensatory increase in the L-type Ca^{2+} currents and the significant prolongation of action potential duration to preserve SR loading and to keep the amplitude of intracellular Ca^{2+} transients and contractions in the old ventricle similar to those of the young organism.[58]

Cardiac myocyte Ca^{2+} cycling is modulated by beta-adrenergic receptor stimulation. The well-documented age-associated reduction in the postsynaptic response of myocardial cells to beta-adrenergic receptor stimulation appears to be the result of multiple changes in the molecular and biochemical steps that couple the receptor to postreceptor effectors. The major limiting modification of acute beta-adrenergic receptor signaling with advancing age in rodents appears to be at the coupling of the beta-adrenergic receptor to adenylyl cyclase through the G$_s$ protein and changes in adenylyl cyclase protein. This leads to a reduction in the ability to sufficiently augment cell cyclic adenosine monophosphate and to activate protein kinase A to drive the phosphorylation of key proteins that are required to augment cardiac contractility. In contrast, the apparent desensitization of beta-adrenergic receptor signaling with aging does not appear to be mediated by increased beta-adrenergic receptor kinase or increased G$_i$ activity.

The age-associated reduction in beta-adrenergic receptor signaling may, in part, also be related to upregulation of opioid peptide receptor signaling because of the significant antagonistic effects between stimulation of opioid peptide receptor and beta-adrenergic receptor–mediated positive contractile response.[59]

Remarkably, the available examinations of cardiac excitation-contraction coupling in rodents of both sexes[60] or females show only a lack of age-related changes in the configuration of the Ca^{2+} transient in myocytes from female hearts. The somewhat unexpected findings in aged female myocytes include (1) an apparent increase in the SR Ca^{2+} content, (2) the lack of the effect of the increase in the SR Ca^{2+} content on the configuration of the Ca^{2+} transients and contraction, and (3) a reduction of fractional SR Ca^{2+} release, in the presence of unchanged I$_{Ca,L}$. Nevertheless, these results provide

an initial direct demonstration of sexually dimorphic changes in cardiac excitation-contraction coupling associated with normal adult aging.

Calcium Regulation During Acute Stress. Aging-associated major changes in heart structure and function place the aged heart constantly "on the edge" and at risk, including the loss of its adaptive response to stress. Acute excess myocardial Ca^{2+} loading leads to dysregulation of Ca^{2+} homeostasis, impaired diastolic and systolic function, arrhythmias, and cell death.[61] The cell Ca^{2+} load is determined by membrane structure and permeability characteristics, the intensity of stimuli that modulate Ca^{2+} influx or efflux by their impact on regulatory function of proteins within membranes, and ROS, which affect both membrane structure and function.

Excessive cytosolic Ca^{2+} loading occurs during physiologic and pharmacologic scenarios that increase Ca^{2+} influx (e.g., neurotransmitters, postischemic reperfusion, or oxidative stress).[62] In hearts or myocytes from the older heart, enhanced Ca^{2+} influx, impaired relaxation, and increased diastolic tone occur during pacing at an increased frequency.[63] This is a "downside" of the aforementioned age-associated adaptation that occurs within the cells of senescent heart (and also of young animals chronically exposed to arterial pressure overload). The amounts and ratios of each class of proteins involved in cell ion homeostasis, the lipid milieu of membranes in which these proteins reside (e.g., types and amounts of long-chain polyunsaturated fatty acids), and the threshold requirement to produce ROS and ROS-derived alkenes all change with aging and reduce the threshold for acute Ca^{2+} overload that occurs within the older heart.

Increased Mitochondrial ROS Generation in the Aged Heart During Acute Stress

Mitochondria possess a unique Ca^{2+} transport machinery, regulate metabolism under partial control by Ca^{2+},[64] and may themselves contribute to cell Ca^{2+} homeostasis. Mitochondrial production of ROS in the heart and mitochondrial dysfunction associated with reperfusion appear to increase with age.[65,66] Thus, mitochondria appear to play a central role in the reduced Ca^{2+} tolerance observed in aged animals.

Like the rest of the cell, mitochondria undergo aging-related changes that may enhance their sensitivity and compromise their response to stress (such as ischemia) but can also result in the loss of the ability to trigger cardioprotective mechanisms. These changes can obviously have deleterious effects on the fate of the mitochondrion, cell, and organism. Compared with young adult myocardium, the senescent myocardium is more sensitive to ischemia,[67] suggesting that protective pathways existing in adult myocardium are modified or impaired by aging.

Repetitive ischemia is an endogenous cardioprotective mechanism, and this protection is reduced in the older heart. This may relate to diminished heat shock protein HSP-70 expression. Nitric oxide, produced by endothelial nitric oxide synthase (eNOS) or inducible nitric oxide synthase (iNOS), plays a role in cardioprotection. However, iNOS and eNOS expression and activity are modified in senescent myocardium.[68] Changes in protein kinase C translocation have been described in aged myocardium,[69] leading to certain age-associated changes in the specific sites targeted by each protein kinase C isoform.

Several studies indicate that reperfusion that follows ischemia generates ROS and that exogenous application of ROS to cells causes Ca^{2+} overload, ATP depletion, and rigor (i.e., cellular stiffening caused by interlocking of actin and myosin).[62] Although multiple enzymes including NADPH oxidase at the plasma membrane and cyclooxygenases and xanthine oxidase in the cytoplasm also contribute to the overall oxidative burden, mitochondria contribute the majority of ROS generation as a byproduct of electron transfer and oxidative phosphorylation.

The permeability transition pore (PTP) is a nonselective, high-conductance channel in the mitochondrial inner membrane that causes the loss of the proton motive force in the respiratory chain and the failure to generate ATP. ROS generated within mitochondria play a role in causing the occurrence of mitochondrial membrane permeability transition (MPT). The release of mitochondrial contents into the cytosol resulting from the MPT induction can lead to high $[Ca_i]$ and to the generation of additional ROS, whereby necrosis and apoptosis are initiated and cell death ensues. Studies have discovered a phenomenon referred to as ROS-induced ROS release,[70] that is, the initial or "trigger" ROS generated by mitochondria in response to laser excitation of fluorescent mitochondrial membrane label leads to an amplification of ROS production by the mitochondria themselves.

This amplification is associated with induction of the MPT and collapse of the mitochondrial membrane potential, which renders the mitochondrial membrane permeable to bulk movement of ions, larger molecules, and water between the cytosol and the mitochondrial matrix. Cells from senescent hearts have a substantially lower threshold for the generation of ROS-induced ROS release and less likelihood of the MPT. ROS, such as the hydroxyl radical (OH), are highly reactive and generally short-lived species. Therefore, they might be expected to cause damage at or near the site of their formation.

Mitochondrial ROS lead to mitochondrial DNA damage and dysfunction in a feed-forward manner, causing functional cellular and organ declines. Protein carbonyls and oxidative damage are increased in mitochondrial extracts of the aged mouse heart, and mitochondrial DNA point mutation and deletion frequencies increase approximately threefold.[45] Mitochondrial damage in mouse hearts is manifested by disrupted cristae and vacuolation (loss of electron density) and is accompanied by an increase in mtDNA copy number and by increased mitochondrial transcription factor A, nuclear respiratory factors, and PPARγ coactivator 1α (PGC-1α).[45] Life span is prolonged by more than 15% in mice with catalase overexpression targeted to the mitochondria, and these mice do not exhibit an age-associated change in LV mass or myocardial dysfunction. Furthermore, catalase overexpression results in significant reductions in mitochondrial oxidative damage, mtDNA mutation deletion frequencies, mitochondrial protein carbonyls, and activation of mitochondrial biogenesis.[45]

Reduction in Membrane Polyunsaturated Fatty Acids

Membrane polyunsaturated fatty acids (PUFAs) undergo lipid peroxidation by ROS, producing various aldehydes, alkenals, and hydroxyalkenals, such as malonaldehyde and 4-hydroxy-2-nonenal (HNE).[71] HNE, potentially the most reactive of these compounds, is formed by superoxide reactions with membrane omega-6 PUFAs and reacts with protein sulfhydryl groups to induce altered protein conformation.[71] Because the mitochondrial respiratory chain represents a major subcellular source of ROS during reperfusion of ischemic myocardium, and because ischemia-reperfusion has been associated with decreased rates of NADH-linked, ADP-dependent respiration, mitochondrial membranes are likely targets of lipid peroxidation and HNE-mediated enzymatic dysfunction. The concentration of HNE is increased in the reperfused postischemic myocardium.[72]

In contrast to many ROS species, HNE is rather long-lived and can therefore diffuse from the site of its origin in membranes to affect potential targets distant from the initial site of ROS production.[71] Thus, if membrane bilayer PUFAs are converted to lipid hydroperoxides, then lipid peroxidation may be viewed as an "amplifier" for the initial ROS.

Furthermore, the reactive aldehydes generated in this process may well act as "toxic second messengers" of the complex chain reactions that follow ROS production.[71] Ischemic HNE modification of mitochondrial proteins occurs exclusively in hearts isolated from senescent rats, but it has not been established whether ROS-induced peroxidation of mitochondrial membranes leading to the production of HNE is related to the amplification of ROS and "mitochondrial catastrophe."

Studies show that exposure of intact cardiac mitochondria to HNE leads to decreased NADH-linked respiration, partly due to HNE-dependent inactivation of α-ketoglutarate dehydrogenase and pyruvate dehydrogenase. These enzymes contain lipoic acid residues that are prime targets for HNE. An age-associated inactivation of α-ketoglutarate dehydrogenase during reperfusion has been identified.[73]

PUFAs differ with respect to their susceptibility to lipid peroxidation. Indeed, omega-6 rather than omega-3 PUFAs appear to be preferred targets of ROS-induced peroxidation that produces HNE. Thus, the increase in omega-6/omega-3 PUFA that occurs with aging may be a mechanism for increased HNE production after ischemia-reperfusion, but this effect can be markedly attenuated by an omega-3 PUFA-rich diet. Notably, an omega-3 PUFA-rich diet also prevents the age-linked decrement of the mitochondria-specific membrane phospholipid cardiolipin, a crucial cofactor for cytochrome-*c* oxidase and adenine nucleotide translocase (ANT) activity.[74]

ANT may participate in the formation of a nonspecific membrane pore through a Ca^{2+}-mediated, cyclophilin D–dependent conformational change in ANT.[75] Cyclophilin D binding to ANT increases after oxidative stress that enhances the Ca^{2+}-dependent formation of the PTP, which induces MPT. Adenine nucleotides located in the mitochondrial matrix bind to ANT and decrease the sensitivity of the PTP to Ca^{2+}, but this effect is antagonized by modification of specific thiol groups on ANT—by oxidative stress products such as HNE or by thiol reagents such as carboxyatractyloside—to the extent that MPT induction may be enhanced.[75]

Reduced Chronic Adaptive Capacity of the Older Heart

Many of the multiple changes in cardiac structure, excitation, myofilament activation, contraction mechanisms, Ca^{2+} dysregulation, deficient beta-adrenergic receptor signaling, and altered gene expression of proteins involved in excitation-contraction coupling that occur with aging (see Table 25-2) also occur in the hypertrophied myocardium of younger animals with experimentally induced chronic hypertension[76] and in failing animal or human hearts, in which they have been construed as an adaptive response to a chronic increase in LV loading. When chronic mechanical stresses that evoke substantial myocardial hypertrophy (e.g., pressure or volume overload) are imposed on the older heart, the response in many instances is reduced.

Transcription factors that influence expression of a number of genes become altered in abundance during aging and may contribute to the pattern of gene expression observed in the hearts of senescent rodents and may also dictate the limits of adaptive responses to the imposition of additional chronic stress. The acute induction of both immediate-early genes and later responding genes that are expressed during the hypertrophic response is blunted in hearts of aged rats after aortic constriction.[77] Similarly, the acute induction of HSP-70 genes in response to either ischemia or heat shock is reduced in hearts of senescent rats.[78] A similar loss of adaptive capacity is observed in younger rats that have used a part of their reserve capacity before a growth factor challenge.[79]

Premature development of heart failure or death in males compared with matching females has been documented in rat models of pressure overload and myocardial infarction.[41] Sexually dimorphic cardiac phenotypes have also been discovered in some studies in genetically engineered mice.[41,40] In general, transgenic models of heart failure present a more rapid onset or a greater severity of cardiac dysfunction in male versus female hearts. For instance, mice with cardiac-specific overexpression of TNF-α exhibit heart failure and increased mortality that is markedly higher in young males than in females (~50% and 4%, respectively, by 20 weeks of age).[80]

At 12 weeks of age, female mice displayed LV hypertrophy without dilation and only a small reduction of basal LV fractional shortening and response to isoproterenol; male mice showed a large LV dilation, reduced fractional shortening relative to both wild-type littermates and transgenic females, and minimal response to isoproterenol.[81] Cardiac myocyte hypertrophy was similar in male and female transgenic mice. Compared with wild-type mice, myocytes from female TNF-α transgenic mice displayed a slower decline of the Ca²⁺ transient but similar amplitudes of Ca²⁺ transients and contractions and the inotropic response to isoproterenol. In contrast, the amplitude and the rate of decline of Ca²⁺ transients and contractions and the response to isoproterenol were significantly reduced in myocytes from male transgenic TNF-α mice.[81]

Myocyte Progenitors in the Aging Heart

Observations in humans and animals suggest that myocyte maturation and aging are characterized by loss of replicative potential, telomeric shortening, and expression of the senescence-associated protein/cell cycle inhibitor $p16_{INK4a}$.[82-84] Telomeric shortening in precursor cells leads to generation of progeny that rapidly acquire the senescent phenotype. The activity of telomerase, an enzyme present only during cell replication, was decreased 31% in aging male rat myocytes but increased 72% in female counterparts.[85] Thus, understanding of the biology of cardiac precursor cells, including factors enhancing the activation of the precursor cell pool, their mobilization, and translocation, may facilitate the development of novel strategies to prevent or to reverse the diminished adaptive capacity to increases in pressure and volume loads (and perhaps heart failure) in the old population. This involves progressive increase in the size of the cell (up to a critical volume beyond which myocyte hypertrophy is no longer possible); deficits in the electrical, Ca²⁺ cycling, and mechanical properties; and cell death.

Cardiac myocytes with senescent and nonsenescent phenotypes already coexist at young age.[86] However, aging limits the growth and differentiation potential of precursor cells, thus interfering not only with their ability to sustain physiologic cell turnover but also with their capacity to adapt to increases in pressure and volume loads.[87,88]

The loss of precursor cell function with aging is mediated partly by an imbalance between factors enhancing oxidative stress, telomere attrition, and death and factors promoting growth, migration, and survival. Recent findings suggest a preeminent position of IGF-1 among factors that interfere with cardiac cellular senescence. Specifically, cardiac-restricted overexpression of IGF-1 in transgenic mice has been shown to delay the aging myopathy and the manifestations of heart failure[89] and to restore SERCA-2a expression and rescue age-associated impairment of cardiac myocyte contractile function.[90] This effect was also partly mimicked by short-term in vitro treatment with recombinant IGF-1.[90] Furthermore, intramyocardial delivery of IGF-1 improved senescent heart phenotype in male Fischer 344 rats,[83] including increased proliferation of functionally competent precursor cells and diminished angiotensin II–induced apoptosis. Myocardial regeneration mediated by precursor cell activation attenuated ventricular dilation and the decrease in the ratio of ventricular mass to chamber volume, resulting in

INTERVENTIONS TO RETARD CARDIOVASCULAR AGING

Despite the fact that age is the dominant risk factor for hypertension and atherosclerotic disease, most prior clinical studies in older individuals focused on evaluating and implementing interventions that targeted "traditional" risk factors (e.g., hypertension and elevated lipids), in part because age-associated vascular changes were not identified and in part due to the view that whatever changes were present could not be prevented or treated. During the past 10 years, however, there has been considerable progress in understanding the vascular changes associated with age and how they may be modified. Some of these interventions are currently used only for those with demonstrated disease or "abnormal" blood pressure or lipid levels. Preclinical and some small clinical trials suggest, however, that they may be beneficial in retarding or ameliorating age-associated altered vascular properties before the development of hypertension or clinically evident vascular disease. This section discusses those currently available interventions that may modify these processes.

Exercise and Vascular Risk Factors

Physical conditioning status is strongly associated with cardiovascular events and mortality.[91] It is probable that one responsible mechanism is an impact on the age-associated vascular changes that contribute to the marked increase in hypertension and atherosclerosis with advanced age.

One of the most important of these is an increase in central vascular stiffness.[92] Studies in middle-aged and the relatively "younger" older groups indicate that aerobic exercise can favorably affect central vascular stiffness. Tanaka and associates[93] employed both cross-sectional and intervention studies to assess the impact of physical conditioning status, and changes in status, on central arterial compliance using carotid B-mode ultrasonography and applanation tonometry in men without disease as assessed by history, examination, laboratory studies, electrocardiography, and, in those older than 40 years, exercise testing.

In the cross-sectional study, central arterial compliance was approximately 40% higher in the endurance-trained (participation in vigorous aerobic exercise ≥5 times/week) than in the sedentary or recreationally active (light to moderate exercise ≥3 times/week) older groups. The best correlate of arterial compliance in all groups was maximal oxygen consumption ($r = 0.44$ to 0.45), probably the best index of physical conditioning status. The exercise intervention was performed in 20 previously sedentary men during 3 months. It consisted primarily of walking, an average of 5 days/week for 42 minutes/day, at 73% of maximal heart rate. Although maximal oxygen consumption did not change with this regimen, there was a 25% increase in central arterial compliance, to a level not significantly different from that in the endurance-trained men in the cross-sectional study. Thus, a relatively short and modest exercise program can significantly affect the important age-associated increase in central vascular stiffness.

Similar observational, cross-sectional study results using less direct measures of stiffness are reported in both men and women.[94,95] In addition to affecting systolic and pulse pressures, vascular compliance also interacts with ventricular stiffness and contractility to affect cardiac output. One proposed index of this ventricular-arterial coupling, or interaction, is the beat-to-beat relationship between LV end-diastolic pressure and stroke volume as modified by respiratory-induced changes in intrathoracic pressure.[96]

In a study examining the impact of physical fitness on this relationship, the index was significantly higher, indicating improved coupling, in Master athletes (mean age, 68 ± 3 years) than it was in older sedentary individuals; in an intervention study, a 1-year period of endurance training in nine individuals showed a trend to improved coupling with the exercise intervention.[97] The benefits of aerobic exercise are less apparent in octogenarians.[98] In one study of 22 men and women (mean age, 82 ± 4 years), 9 months of training at higher than 80% of peak heart rate did not change arterial stiffness as assessed by carotid applanation tonometry.

Potential responsible mechanisms include mechanical distention-induced modification of collagen cross-linking and vascular smooth muscle relaxation due to enhanced nitric oxide signaling or decreased sympathetic tone. In addition to the favorable influences on systolic blood pressure associated with decreased stiffness (less of a change in pressure for any given ejected stroke volume), chronic physical activity also likely enhances baroreceptor-mediated parasympathetic cardiac stimuli,[99] which may maintain vascular homeostasis during hypervolemic and hypovolemic stresses as well as decrease the likelihood of adverse cardiac arrhythmias.

The type of exercise training may, however, influence the effect on central vascular stiffness.[98] In contrast to aerobic exercise, and although it has not been examined in older adults, one intervention study in young men[100] and another in young women[101] demonstrated that high-intensity resistance training significantly increased arterial stiffness, an effect that was reversed after a deconditioning period.[100] A third intervention study using a more conventional resistance protocol, again in a young population, showed no effect.[102]

Another important age-related vascular change is a decrease in endothelial function,[103,104] believed to be related to several factors, most importantly decreased nitric oxide bioavailability, accompanied by decreased prostacyclin and increased endothelin 1, systemic angiotensin II, and sympathetic vasoconstrictors. The clinical consequences are believed to include increased development and progression of atherosclerosis and inappropriate vasoconstriction, which may result in acute coronary syndromes.

Cross-sectional observational studies as well as intervention studies in previously sedentary middle-aged and older men indicate that aerobic exercise training can prevent and reverse, respectively, age associated declines in endothelial function.[105,106] Several mechanisms are likely to be involved. The initiating event is most likely increased shear stress resulting from the increased pulse pressure during exercise.[107] This leads to an acute increase in nitric oxide but also to chronic changes that increase nitric oxide bioavailability, including increased eNOS gene expression, reduced oxidative stress, and decreased production and increased scavenging of free radicals.[84,108]

Sustained increases in nitric oxide associated with long-term exercise training may result in favorable arterial remodeling, resulting in decreased shear stress for any given exercise-induced increase in stroke volume. The importance of shear stress is indicated by studies reporting that exercise of large muscle groups results in improved endothelial function in distant arteries (e.g., improved forearm endothelial function after leg exercise), whereas exercise of small muscle groups (e.g., one forearm) does not have remote effects. The extent of endothelial function improvement with exercise training is directly related to the extent of preexisting dysfunction, suggesting that even healthy older individuals would benefit. In general, benefits are evident as early as 4 to 8 weeks after the initiation of training and are lost within several weeks after cessation of an exercise program.

There are additional potential although less investigated favorable effects of exercise on vascular risk in older individuals. In one study,[109] a 3-month aerobic exercise program decreased endothelin 1–mediated vasoconstriction in 15 older men, mean age 62 ± 2 years; and in another, endothelial-mediated tissue-type plasminogen activator in human forearms was increased by 55% in 10 men, mean age 60 ± 2 years, after 3 months of aerobic exercise.[110] Physical activity is also associated with improved mood in adults with depression, a risk factor for vascular disease.[111] The relationships among changes in physical activity, increased mood, decreased anxiety, and vascular function and structure, however, have not been examined.

In summary, habitual exercise and periods as short as weeks to months of exercise training are associated with significant improvement in vascular structure and function, at least in the "younger" group of older individuals (i.e., in the seventh decade). Despite these favorable effects, these changes are not uniform; for example, there appears to be no benefit in terms of endothelial progenitor cell number in healthy older individuals[112] or in terms of carotid intima-media thickness. In addition, the majority of the exercise studies were performed in men, and it is unclear whether similar benefits occur in women. Importantly, the clinical relevance of the findings is unclear; although stiffness and the other studied vascular parameters are associated with important cardiovascular outcomes, it is unclear whether exercise-induced changes in these variables actually change these outcomes. Finally, the effects of different types, duration, and intensity of exercise on vascular function require additional study, as do the mechanisms for the beneficial effects.

Specific activity recommendations are tailored to the individual on the basis of comorbid conditions and baseline fitness levels, which may limit the type and duration of exercise. Because of this variability, a subjective intensity of exercise is recommended by the American College of Sports Medicine and the American Heart Association concerning the initiation, type, and intensity of physical activity in older Americans.[113] Thus, moderate-intensity aerobic physical activity is recommended for a minimum of 30 minutes a day, 5 days each week; or vigorous-intensity aerobic activity is recommended for 20 minutes a day, 3 days each week. Moderate is defined as 5 or 6 and vigorous as 7 or 8 on a 10-point scale; sitting is 0. Moderate activity produces "noticeable increases" in heart rate and breathing, and vigorous-intensity activity produces large increases in heart rate and breathing. Resistance or muscle strengthening activities should be performed on two more nonconsecutive days per week with a weight that allows 10 to 15 repetitions for each major muscle group. The level of effort should be 5 to 8, where 0 is no movement and 10 is maximal effort. Additional goals include exercises directed to maintenance and strengthening of flexibility and balance.

Estrogen and Vascular Risk Factors

Premenopausal women experience significantly less atherosclerotic disease than do men, premature menopause is associated with increased vascular risk, and observational studies indicate that estrogen use is associated with decreased vascular risk. The effects of estrogen on coronary endothelial function in postmenopausal women[114] and in numerous preclinical models and studies[115] suggest significant benefits. These include stimulation of eNOS in vascular endothelial cells,[116] improved mitochondrial function and decreased oxidative stress in vascular endothelium,[117] reduced angiotensin II–induced free radical production in vascular smooth muscle cells, and stimulation of endothelial progenitor cell production[118] and the catalytic subunit of human telomerase.[71] All of these correlate well with endothelial cell senescence and aging, and the favorable impact of estrogen on them would suggest a significant clinical benefit.

Nevertheless, the Women's Health Initiative, the most recent and largely regarded as definitive study of estrogen in postmenopausal women with prior hysterectomy, demonstrated no benefit on the primary composite endpoint of nonfatal myocardial infarction or death and an increase in stroke and pulmonary embolism.[119] Although it was concluded that estrogen should not be used for primary or secondary prevention in postmenopausal women, as is presently recommended, studies of the potential benefits of this therapeutic approach still continue. Therapy was started in the Women's Health Initiative study an average of 10 years after menopause, when significant changes in the vascular substrate had already occurred.

The preclinical studies all suggest a preventive effect of estrogen, rather than a reversal of preexisting abnormalities, arguing that estrogen administration during the perimenopausal or early postmenopausal period should be studied. Furthermore, polymorphisms of the estrogen receptor are known to significantly alter the vascular response to estrogen administration[120] and cardiovascular disease risk, suggesting that genome-based estrogen therapy may be beneficial. In addition, new selective estrogen receptor modulators may provide greater vascular benefit and less vascular risk than current estrogen preparations.

Testosterone and Vascular Risk Factors

There is considerable epidemiologic evidence that androgen deficiency in older men is associated with increased cardiovascular mortality and atherosclerotic risk factors.[121,122] The most important of these risk factors are the components of the metabolic syndrome, including increased waist-to-hip ratio, insulin resistance, and hypertension, but they also include increased total and low-density lipoprotein cholesterol and carotid intima-media thickness and decreased flow-mediated dilation.

Androgen deprivation therapy in men with prostate cancer is associated with hypertension, insulin resistance, and vascular stiffening. Small studies in hypogonadal older men indicate that androgen treatment can increase both flow-mediated and nitroglycerin-mediated brachial artery vasodilation, decrease systolic and diastolic blood pressures, improve lipid profiles, and reduce inflammatory cytokines. The extent to which these may be mediated, in part, by their favorable effect on body composition, including increased lean body and muscle mass and decreased visceral and total body adiposity, is not known.

Despite these small studies as well as strong basic and preclinical plausibility for a beneficial effect of androgen-based therapies in patients with increased cardiovascular risk and low testosterone levels, there are relatively few placebo-controlled randomized trials. The conduct of such trials is limited by several factors. Testosterone may be associated with increased risk for prostate hypertrophy and acceleration of subclinical prostate cancer.

Oral therapies may be associated with liver toxicity and injectable forms with discomfort and inconvenience. In this regard, selective androgen receptor modulators may be a desirable alternative. These may be taken orally without liver toxicity and in animal models demonstrate positive effects of androgen therapy while eliminating some negative effects. As any treatment would be most effective in those with hypogonadism, the determination of whether an individual patient is hypogonadal is not straightforward. Despite the significant age-associated decrease in mean testosterone levels, there is considerable individual variability. In this regard, administration of androgen therapy to those with normal levels may result in no benefit and unwanted side effects, whereas administration of placebo to those with low testosterone is not ethical. Free and bioavailable rather than total testosterone levels may most clearly correlate with any androgen-mediated benefit and risk.

HMG-CoA Reductase Inhibitors

The beneficial effects of statin therapy on cardiovascular events in older subsets of randomized trials are similar to those in the younger groups.[123,124] In the Heart Protection Study subset of more than 5800 individuals 70 years or older who were randomized to placebo or simvastatin, the occurrence of nonfatal myocardial infarction, coronary death, stroke, or revascularization was significantly lower in the group randomized to statin (23.6%) than in the group randomized to placebo (28.7%) during the 5-year study period.

The pleiotropic effects of statins, however, are remarkably suited to inhibit the adverse consequences of aging on the vascular substrate that predispose to the development, progression, and clinical manifestations of atherosclerosis. These include increased nitric oxide bioavailability, anti-inflammatory effects, improved endothelium-dependent vasoreactivity, reversal of vascular endothelial growth factor–induced endothelial cell hyperpermeability,[125] and probable stabilization of vulnerable atherosclerotic plaques. One of the most important aspects of the vascular substrate that is altered with age concerns endothelial progenitor cells, which affect vascular function, integrity, and, most important, repair.

The effects of statins on endothelial progenitor cell number, function, and survival have been extensively studied. Statins increase endothelial progenitor cell numbers by increasing bone marrow hematopoietic stem cells and inducing endothelial progenitor cell differentiation through the phosphatidylinositol 3-kinase/Akt pathway, improve progenitor cell functional capacity,[126] and enhance endothelial progenitor cell survival and prevent telomere erosion in the presence of oxidative stress.[127] Considering the impact of age as a risk factor for vascular disease and the benefits of statins on the responsible mechanisms, randomized trials examining the impact of statins on age changes in vascular substrate and relating them to subclinical and clinical manifestations of atherosclerosis appear warranted.

Renin-Angiotensin-Aldosterone Inhibition

The importance of hypertension as a risk factor for vascular disease and mortality[128] and the benefits of antihypertensive therapy[129,130] in the older population are well documented. In fact, the benefit of intervention is at least as great in the older population as it is in the younger and middle-aged groups.

A randomized study compared treatment systolic pressure goals of less than 140 mm Hg versus 130 mm Hg in more than 1100 nondiabetic individuals with a systolic pressure of 150 mm Hg or higher.[131] In the subset of patients older than 70 years, the odds ratio of experiencing the primary outcome (development of left ventricular hypertrophy, a potent predictor of cardiovascular events) in the lower versus the higher systolic pressure goal group was 0.49, whereas that for the entire study cohort was 0.61.

In addition to arteriolar changes, which increase peripheral resistance, changes in the central vasculature associated with aging (e.g., fibrosis, inflammation, and media thickening) may predispose to atherosclerosis and vascular events,[7] some of which may be particularly related to increased angiotensin II activity. As such, these changes offer additional targets that, if successfully treated, may decrease event rates over and above those achieved with blood pressure lowering alone.

25

Although nearly all antihypertensive therapies can lower blood pressure in older individuals, those that inhibit the RAAS may also ameliorate these age-specific changes. Thus, ACE inhibition decreases measures of central vascular stiffness in human studies, in part independent of blood pressure reduction,[25,132] as well as TNF-α, a mediator of inflammation.[133] Angiotensin receptor blockade also has favorable effects on indices of central vascular stiffness, including pulse wave velocity and aortic augmentation index, as well as the media-to-lumen ratio measured from biopsy specimens.[134]

Although ACE inhibitors and angiotensin receptor blockers have different sites of action, and the reduction in arterial stiffness is significantly greater when the combination is used,[135] a large randomized study (ONTARGET) demonstrated adverse clinical outcomes with the combination compared with the individual agents.[136] In this trial, there was a 9% increase in the primary outcome (dialysis, doubling of creatinine, or death) and a 24% increase in dialysis or creatinine doubling in the patients randomized to ramipril and telmisartan compared with those randomized to ramipril alone.

Aldosterone antagonists are useful in the management of blood pressure in individuals with primary hyperaldosteronism who will not undergo surgery; in many patients with resistant hypertension, defined as inability to achieve blood pressure goal despite the use of three antihypertensives; and in those with hypertension and hypokalemia.[137] Older individuals may be more likely to experience hyperkalemia and therefore require closer monitoring, and sex hormone–related side effects can be largely avoided with the use of eplerenone, a more selective agent.

Apart from the diuretic effect, aldosterone antagonists have additional benefits that may ameliorate age-associated vascular changes. Aldosterone increases vascular inflammation, perivascular fibrosis,[138] and vascular expression of the angiotensin type 1 receptor. In addition, wall stiffness in individuals with primary hyperaldosteronism is greater than what would be expected on the basis of blood pressure alone.[139] Treatment with aldosterone antagonists prevents the age-associated increase in arterial stiffness and fibrosis in old, normotensive rats by altering vascular collagen and elastin. In patients, aldosterone antagonism decreases pulse wave velocity and augmentation index measures of central vascular stiffness,[140] and in a separate study, it decreased stiffness in gluteal subcutaneous resistance vessels as well as several circulating inflammatory mediators.[141] Thus, inhibition of the RAAS not only lowers blood pressure and improves outcomes in older individuals with hypertension but also ameliorates those age-associated vascular changes that predispose to the development of hypertension and atherosclerosis. The risks associated with relying on surrogate markers alone, however, are well illustrated by the results of the ONTARGET study, which demonstrates again the importance of obtaining meaningful clinical outcomes before any general recommendations concerning antiaging strategies can be advised and implemented.

Smoking

Although the proportion of older individuals who smoke is lower than that of the rest of the population, 10.8% of men and 8.4% of women older than 65 years do so.[142] There is consistent evidence that cigarette use is associated with an increased risk of adverse cardiovascular outcomes in all age groups. In a prospective data analysis of more than 1 million adults, the relative risk for ischemic heart disease, cardiovascular disease, and mortality was increased above that of those who never smoked by approximately 1.5-fold in the subset of those who were older than 65 years.[143] The potential mechanisms are multifactorial, including increased ROS, altered autonomic tone, platelet activation, increased arterial stiffness, and probably many of the toxins in the product itself.[144] These would affect several of the changes associated with the mechanisms underlying increased atherosclerotic risk associated with vascular aging. Exposure to cigarette smoke impairs endothelial function as assessed by flow-dependent brachial artery vasodilation, increases elaboration of vascular endothelial growth factor (one response to vascular injury), decreases nitric oxide production, and decreases endothelial progenitor cell function as assessed by chemotaxis.[145] Some of these vascular effects are reversed with cigarette cessation,[146] and cessation is associated with decreased risk for cardiovascular events as well.[147] Cigarette cessation should be encouraged for all populations of patients.

Considerations in Older Individuals

The increased prevalence of atherosclerotic risk factors, disease, and complications once an event has occurred emphasizes the importance of risk factor identification and aggressive, appropriate intervention in the older population. Primary and secondary prevention strategies do not differ between the older and younger populations at risk for or with cardiovascular disease. As noted before, similar or more significant clinical benefits (because of the increased absolute risk) accrue with lipid- and blood pressure–lowering therapies, at least up until 80 years of age. Cigarette cessation and other lifestyle factors, particularly maintaining physical activity, are valuable from cardiovascular and multiple other health perspectives.

However, age changes in body composition and in renal and hepatic function and the increased likelihood of comorbidities and concomitant medications may influence the type of therapy selected, the intensity of the regimen, the dose of the agent, and the dosing interval. Age is associated with increased bleeding risk with antiplatelet and anticoagulation therapies. Low doses, attempts to avoid combining of antiplatelet agents, and careful monitoring are all more important in the older age groups. Advanced age is often associated with a decrease in lean muscle and an increase in fat body mass. Renal function as defined by formulas for creatinine clearance includes age as one variable.

Age is associated with a decrease in hepatic clearance of drugs as well, particularly those metabolized through the cytochrome P-450 pathway. Older individuals may also be more likely to experience side effects, such as constipation, urinary retention, postural hypotension, and cognitive changes, because of preexisting impairments or concomitant medications. Excellent resources are available, including those from the Food and Drug Administration, regarding drug selection, dosing, and interactions in all age groups.

CLINICAL IMPLICATIONS OF CARDIOVASCULAR AGING

Our present understanding of the age-associated alterations in cardiac and arterial structure and function at both the cellular and molecular levels provides valuable clues that may assist in the development of effective therapies to prevent, to delay, or to attenuate the cardiovascular changes that accompany aging. Many of these age-associated changes are being increasingly recognized as risk factors for cardiovascular diseases. In spite of the interest in the physiology of the age-associated changes in cardiovascular structure and function, cardiovascular aging has remained, for the most part, outside of mainstream clinical medicine. This is because the pathophysiologic implications of these changes are largely underappreciated and are not well disseminated in the medical community. In fact, age has traditionally been considered a

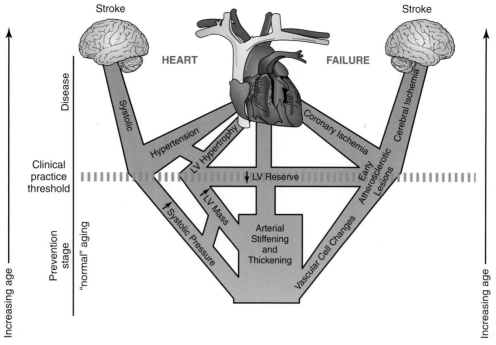

FIGURE 25-4 Aging: the major risk factor for cardiovascular morbidity and mortality.

nonmodifiable risk factor. Because many of the age-associated alterations in cardiovascular structure and function, at both the cellular and molecular levels, are specific risk factors for cardiovascular diseases (see Table 25-3), there is an urgency to incorporate cardiovascular aging into clinical medicine.

One way to conceptualize why the clinical manifestations and the prognosis of these diseases worsen with age is that in older individuals, the specific pathophysiologic mechanisms that cause clinical disorders are superimposed on heart and vascular substrates that are modified by aging (Fig. 25-4). Imagine that age increases as one moves from the lower to the upper part of Figure 25-4 and that the line bisecting the top and bottom parts represents the clinical practice "threshold" for disease recognition. Thus, entities above the line are presently classified as "diseases" and lead to heart and brain failure.

The vascular and cardiac changes presently thought to occur as a result of the "normal aging process" (i.e., those addressed in the previous sections) are depicted below the line. These age-associated changes in cardiac and vascular properties alter the substrate on which cardiovascular disease is superimposed in several ways. First, they lower the extent of disease severity required to cross the threshold that results in clinically significant signs and symptoms. For example, a mild degree of ischemia-induced relaxation abnormalities that may be asymptomatic in a younger individual may cause dyspnea in an older individual, who, by virtue of age alone, has preexisting slowed and delayed early diastolic relaxation.

Age-associated changes may also alter the manifestations and presentation of common cardiac diseases. This usually occurs in patients with acute infarction, in whom the diagnosis is delayed because of atypical symptoms resulting in increased time to onset of therapy. Age-associated changes, including those in beta-adrenergic responsiveness and in vascular stiffness, also influence the response to and therefore the selection of different therapeutic interventions in older individuals with cardiovascular disease.

In one sense, those processes below the line in Figure 25-4 ought not to be considered to reflect normal aging. Rather, they might be construed as specific risk factors for the diseases that they relate to and thus might be targets of interventions designed to decrease the occurrence or manifestations of cardiovascular disease at later ages. Such a strategy would thus advocate treatment of normal aging. Additional studies of the specific risks of each normal age-associated change are required.

CONCLUSION

Aging is the dominant risk factor for cardiovascular diseases. However, aging should no longer be viewed as an immutable risk factor. A steady stream of incremental knowledge, derived from both animal and human studies, has established that several of the aging-associated changes in the heart and in the walls of the central arteries are themselves potent and independent risk factors for cardiovascular diseases. This suggests that these age-associated alterations in arterial and cardiac structure and function could represent the link that explains, at least in part, the risky component of aging.

Policy makers, researchers, and clinicians should intensify their efforts toward identification of novel pathways that could be targeted for interventions aiming at retardation or attenuation of these age-associated alterations, particularly in individuals in whom these alterations are accelerated. Future studies would then examine whether these strategies (i.e., those targeting cardiovascular aging) can have a salutary impact on the adverse cardiovascular effects of accelerated cardiovascular aging. As such, cardiovascular aging is a promising frontier in preventive cardiology that is ripe for and in dire need of attention.

Acknowledgment

The authors would like to thank Ruth Sadler for expert editing assistance.

1. *The World Health Report 1997—conquering, suffering, enriching humanity,* Geneva, 1997, World Health Organization.
2. Wilson PW, D'Agostino RB, Levy D, et al: Prediction of coronary heart disease using risk factor categories. *Circulation* 97:1837, 1998.
3. Fleg JL, Gerstenblith G, Zonderman AB, et al: Prevalence and prognostic significance of exercise-induced silent myocardial ischemia detected by thallium scintigraphy and electrocardiography in asymptomatic volunteers. *Circulation* 81:428, 1990.
4. Maggioni AP, Maseri A, Fresco C, et al: Age-related increase in mortality among patients with first myocardial infarctions treated with thrombolysis. The Investigators of the Gruppo Italiano per lo Studio della Sopravvivenza nell'Infarto Miocardico (GISSI-2). *N Engl J Med* 329:1442, 1993.
5. Najjar SS, Scuteri A, Lakatta EG: Arterial aging: is it an immutable cardiovascular risk factor? *Hypertension* 46:454, 2005.
6. Lloyd-Jones D, Adams RJ, Brown TM, et al: Heart disease and stroke statistics—2010 Update. *Circulation* 121:e46, 2010.
7. Lakatta EG: Arterial and cardiac aging: major shareholders in cardiovascular disease enterprises. Part III: cellular and molecular clues to heart and arterial aging. *Circulation* 107:490, 2003.
8. Lakatta EG, Levy D: Arterial and cardiac aging: major shareholders in cardiovascular disease enterprises. Part I: aging arteries: a "set up" for vascular disease. *Circulation* 107:139, 2003.
9. Lakatta EG: Cardiovascular regulatory mechanisms in advanced age. *Physiol Rev* 73:413, 1993.
10. Farasat SM, Morrell CH, Scuteri A, et al: Pulse pressure is inversely related to aortic root diameter implications for the pathogenesis of systolic hypertension. *Hypertension* 51:196, 2008.
11. Virmani R, Avolio AP, Mergner WJ, et al: Effect of aging on aortic morphology in populations with high and low prevalence of hypertension and atherosclerosis. Comparison between occidental and Chinese communities. *Am J Pathol* 139:1119, 1991.
12. Adams MR, Nakagomi A, Keech A, et al: Carotid intima-media thickness is only weakly correlated with the extent and severity of coronary artery disease. *Circulation* 92:2127, 1995.
13. Asai K, Kudej RK, Shen YT, et al: Peripheral vascular endothelial dysfunction and apoptosis in old monkeys. *Arterioscler Thromb Vasc Biol* 20:1493, 2000.
14. Lakatta EG, Wang M, Najjar SS: Arterial aging and subclinical arterial disease are fundamentally intertwined at macroscopic and molecular levels. *Med Clin North Am* 93:583, 2009.
15. Najjar SS: IMT as a risk marker: the plot thickens. *J Am Soc Echocardiogr* 22:505, 2009.
16. Scuteri A, Chen CH, Yin FC, et al: Functional correlates of central arterial geometric phenotypes. *Hypertension* 38:1471, 2001.
17. Scuteri A, Manolio TA, Marino EK, et al: Prevalence of specific variant carotid geometric patterns and incidence of cardiovascular events in older persons. The Cardiovascular Health Study (CHS E-131). *J Am Coll Cardiol* 43:187, 2004.
18. Laurent S, Cockcroft J, Van Bortel L, et al: Expert consensus document on arterial stiffness: methodological issues and clinical applications. *Eur Heart J* 27:2588, 2006.
19. Wildman RP, Farhat GN, Patel AS, et al: Weight change is associated with change in arterial stiffness among healthy young adults. *Hypertension* 45:187, 2005.
20. Wilkinson IB, Franklin SS, Cockcroft JR: Nitric oxide and the regulation of large artery stiffness: from physiology to pharmacology. *Hypertension* 44:1126, 2004.
21. Tarasov KV, Sanna S, Scuteri A, et al: COL4A1 is associated with arterial stiffness by genome-wide association scan. *Circ Cardiovasc Genet* 2:151, 2009.
22. Kass DA, Shapiro EP, Kawaguchi M, et al: Improved arterial compliance by a novel advanced glycation end-product crosslink breaker. *Circulation* 104:1464, 2001.
23. Bakris GL, Bank AJ, Kass DA, et al: Advanced glycation end-product cross-link breakers. A novel approach to cardiovascular pathologies related to the aging process. *Am J Hypertens* 17:23S, 2004.
24. Avolio AP, Van Bortel LM, Boutouyrie P, et al: Role of pulse pressure amplification in arterial hypertension: experts' opinion and review of the data. *Hypertension* 54:375, 2009.
25. Williams B, Lacy PS, Thom SM, et al: Differential impact of blood pressure–lowering drugs on central aortic pressure and clinical outcomes: principal results of the Conduit Artery Function Evaluation (CAFE) study. *Circulation* 113:1213, 2006.
26. Sever PS, Dahlof B, Poulter NR, et al: Prevention of coronary and stroke events with atorvastatin in hypertensive patients who have average or lower-than-average cholesterol concentrations, in the Anglo-Scandinavian Cardiac Outcomes Trial–Lipid Lowering Arm (ASCOT-LLA): a multicentre randomised controlled trial. *Lancet* 361:1149, 2003.
27. Roman MJ, Devereux RB, Kizer JR, et al: High central pulse pressure is independently associated with adverse cardiovascular outcome: the Strong Heart Study. *J Am Coll Cardiol* 54:1730, 2009.
28. Wang KL, Cheng HM, Sung SH, et al: Wave reflection and arterial stiffness in the prediction of 15-year all-cause and cardiovascular mortalities: a community-based study. *Hypertension* 55:799, 2010.
29. Franklin SS, Gustin Wt, Wong ND, et al: Hemodynamic patterns of age-related changes in blood pressure. The Framingham Heart Study. *Circulation* 96:308, 1997.
30. Chantler PD, Lakatta EG, Najjar SS: Arterial-ventricular coupling: mechanistic insights into cardiovascular performance at rest and during exercise. *J Appl Physiol* 105:1342, 2008.
31. Redfield MM, Jacobsen SJ, Borlaug BA, et al: Age- and gender-related ventricular-vascular stiffening: a community-based study. *Circulation* 112:2254, 2005.
32. Najjar SS, Schulman SP, Gerstenblith G, et al: Age and gender affect ventricular-vascular coupling during aerobic exercise. *J Am Coll Cardiol* 44:611, 2004.
33. Nussbacher A, Gerstenblith G, O'Connor F, et al: Hemodynamic effects of unloading the old heart. *Am J Physiol* 277:H1863, 1999.
34. Gerhard M, Roddy MA, Creager SJ, Creager MA: Aging progressively impairs endothelium-dependent vasodilation in forearm resistance vessels of humans. *Hypertension* 27:849, 1996.
35. Taddei S, Virdis A, Mattei P, et al: Defective l-arginine–nitric oxide pathway in offspring of essential hypertensive patients. *Circulation* 94:1298, 1996.
36. Minamino T, Miyauchi H, Yoshida T, et al: Endothelial cell senescence in human atherosclerosis: role of telomere in endothelial dysfunction. *Circulation* 105:1541, 2002.
37. Rauscher FM, Goldschmidt-Clermont PJ, Davis BH, et al: Aging, progenitor cell exhaustion, and atherosclerosis. *Circulation* 108:457, 2003.
38. Conboy IM, Conboy MJ, Wagers AJ, et al: Rejuvenation of aged progenitor cells by exposure to a young systemic environment. *Nature* 433:760, 2005.
39. Thum T, Hoeber S, Froese S, et al: Age-dependent impairment of endothelial progenitor cells is corrected by growth-hormone-mediated increase of insulin-like growth-factor-1. *Circ Res* 100:434, 2007.
40. Leinwand LA: Sex is a potent modifier of the cardiovascular system. *J Clin Invest* 112:302, 2003.
41. Konhilas JP, Leinwand LA: The effects of biological sex and diet on the development of heart failure. *Circulation* 116:2747, 2007.
42. Fermin DR, Barac A, Lee S, et al: Sex and age dimorphism of myocardial gene expression in nonischemic human heart failure. *Circ Cardiovasc Genet* 1:117, 2008.
43. Brodde OE, Konschak U, Becker K, et al: Cardiac muscarinic receptors decrease with age. In vitro and in vivo studies. *J Clin Invest* 101:471, 1998.
44. Lakatta EG: Cardiovascular aging research: the next horizons. *J Am Geriatr Soc* 47:613, 1999.
45. Dai DF, Santana LF, Vermulst M, et al: Overexpression of catalase targeted to mitochondria attenuates murine cardiac aging. *Circulation* 119:2789, 2009.
46. Younes A, Boluyt MO, O'Neill L, et al: Age-associated increase in rat ventricular ANP gene expression correlates with cardiac hypertrophy. *Am J Physiol* 38:H1003, 1995.
47. Grant JE, Bradshaw AD, Schwacke JH, et al: Quantification of protein expression changes in the aging left ventricle of *Rattus norvegicus*. *J Proteome Res* 8:4252, 2009.
48. Benigni A, Corna D, Zoja C, et al: Disruption of the Ang II type I receptor promotes longevity in mice. *J Clin Invest* 119:524, 2009.
49. Finkel T, Holbrook NJ: Oxidants, oxidative stress and the biology of ageing. *Nature* 408:239, 2000.
50. Lakatta EG, Levy D: Arterial and cardiac aging: major shareholders in cardiovascular disease enterprises. Part II: the aging heart in health: links to heart disease. *Circulation* 107:346, 2003.
51. Bedard K, Krause KH: The NOX family of ROS-generating NADPH oxidases: physiology and pathophysiology. *Physiol Rev* 87:245, 2007.
52. Grieve DJ, Byrne JA, Siva A, et al: Involvement of the nicotinamide adenosine dinucleotide phosphate oxidase isoform Nox2 in cardiac contractile dysfunction occurring in response to pressure overload. *J Am Coll Cardiol* 47:817, 2006.
53. Johar S, Cave AC, Narayanapanicker A, et al: Aldosterone mediates angiotensin II–induced interstitial cardiac fibrosis via a Nox2-containing NADPH oxidase. *FASEB J* 20:1546, 2006.
54. Looi YH, Grieve DJ, Siva A, et al: Involvement of Nox2 NADPH oxidase in adverse cardiac remodeling after myocardial infarction. *Hypertension* 51:319, 2008.
55. Dworakowski R, Walker S, Momin A, et al: NADPH oxidase–derived reactive oxygen species in the regulation of endothelial phenotype. *J Am Coll Cardiol* 51:1349, 2008.
56. Maack C, Kartes T, Kilter H, et al: Oxygen free radical release in human failing myocardium is associated with increased activity of rac1-GTPase and represents a target for statin treatment. *Circulation* 108:1567, 2003.
57. Csiszar A, Labinskyy N, Smith K, et al: Vasculoprotective effects of anti–tumor necrosis factor-alpha treatment in aging. *Am J Pathol* 170:388, 2007.
58. Janczewski AM, Spurgeon HA, Lakatta EG: Action potential prolongation in cardiac myocytes of old rats is an adaptation to sustain youthful intracellular Ca^{2+} regulation. *J Mol Cell Cardiol* 34:641, 2002.
59. Pepe S, Xiao RP, Hohl C, et al: "Cross-talk" between opioid peptide and adrenergic receptor signaling in isolated rat heart. *Circulation* 95:2122, 1997.
60. Grandy SA, Howlett SE: Cardiac excitation-contraction coupling is altered in myocytes from aged male mice but not in cells from aged female mice. *Am J Physiol* 291:H2362, 2006.
61. Lakatta EG: Functional implications of spontaneous sarcoplasmic reticulum Ca^{2+} release in the heart. *Cardiovasc Res* 26:193, 1992.
62. Lakatta EG, Sollott SJ, Pepe S: The old heart: operating on the edge. In Bock G, Goode J, editors: *Ageing vulnerability: causes and interventions,* New York, 2001, Wiley, pp 172-201. Novartis Foundation Symposium 235.
63. Tate CA, Taffet GE, Hudson EK, et al: Enhanced calcium uptake of cardiac sarcoplasmic reticulum in exercise-trained old rats. *Am J Physiol* 258:H431, 1990.
64. Hansford RG, Zorov D: Role of mitochondrial calcium transport in the control of substrate oxidation. *Mol Cell Biochem* 184:359, 1998.
65. Pepe S, Tsuchiya N, Lakatta EG, Hansford RG: PUFA and aging modulate cardiac mitochondrial membrane lipid composition and Ca^{2+} activation of PDH. *Am J Physiol* 276:H149, 1999.
66. Sohal R, Arnold L, Sohal B: Age-related changes in antioxidant enzymes and prooxidant generation in tissues of the rat with special reference to parameters in two insect species. *Free Radic Biol Med* 10:495, 1990.
67. Tani M, Suganuma Y, Hasegawa H, et al: Decrease in ischemic tolerance with aging in isolated perfused Fischer 344 rat hearts: relation to increases in intracellular Na^{+} after ischemia. *J Mol Cell Cardiol* 29:3081, 1997.
68. Chou TC, Yen MH, Li CY, Ding YA: Alterations of nitric oxide synthase expression with aging and hypertension in rats. *Hypertension* 31:643, 1998.
69. Korzick DH, Holiman DA, Boluyt MO, et al: Diminished $alpha_1$-adrenergic–mediated contraction and translocation of PKC in senescent rat heart. *Am J Physiol Heart Circ Physiol* 281:H581, 2001.

70. Zorov DB, Filburn CR, Klotz LO, et al: Reactive oxygen species (ROS)–induced ROS release: a new phenomenon accompanying induction of the mitochondrial permeability transition in cardiac myocytes. *J Exp Med* 192:1001, 2000.
71. Farsetti A, Crasselli A, Bacchetti S, et al: The telomerase tale in vascular aging: regulation by estrogen and nitric oxide signaling. *J Appl Physiol* 106:333, 2009.
72. Blasig I, Grune T, Schonheit K, et al: 4-Hydroxynonenal, a novel indicator of lipid peroxidation for reperfusion injury of the myocardium. *Am J Physiol* 269:H14, 1995.
73. Lucas, D, Szweda L: Declines in mitochondrial respiration during cardiac reperfusion: age-dependent inactivation of α-ketoglutarate dehydrogenase. *Proc Natl Acad Sci U S A* 96:6689, 1999.
74. Paradies G, Ruggiero FM, Petrosillo G, et al: Effect of aging and acetyl-L-carnitine on the activity of cytochrome oxidase and adenine nucleotide translocase in rat heart mitochondria. *FEBS Lett* 350:213, 1994.
75. Halstrup A, Kerr P, Javador S, Woodfield K: Elucidating the molecular mechanism of the permeability transition pore and its role in reperfusion injury in the heart. *Biochim Biophys Acta* 1366:79, 1998.
76. Yin FC, Spurgeon HA, Weisfeldt ML, Lakatta EG: Mechanical properties of myocardium from hypertrophied rat hearts. A comparison between hypertrophy induced by senescence and by aortic banding. *Circ Res* 46:292, 1980.
77. Shida M, Isoyama S: Effects of age on c-fos and c-myc gene expression in response to hemodynamic stress in isolated, perfused rat hearts. *J Mol Cell Cardiol* 25:1025, 1993.
78. Boluyt MO, Lakatta EG: Cardiovascular aging in health. In Altschuld RA, Haworth RA, editors: *Heart metabolism in failure*, Greenwich, Conn, 1998, JAI Press, pp 257-303.
79. Shunkert H, Weinberg E, Bruckschlegel G, et al: Alteration of growth responses in established cardiac pressure overload hypertrophy in rats with aortic banding. *J Clin Invest* 96:2768, 1995.
80. Kadokami T, McTiernan CF, Kubota T, et al: Sex-related survival differences in murine cardiomyopathy are associated with differences in TNF-receptor expression. *J Clin Invest* 106:589, 2000.
81. Janczewski AM, Kadokami T, Lemster B, et al: Morphological and functional changes in cardiac myocytes isolated from mice overexpressing TNF-α. *Am J Physiol* 284:H960, 2003.
82. Chimenti C, Kajstura J, Torella D, et al: Senescence and death of primitive cells and myocytes leads to premature cardiac aging and heart failure. *Circ Res* 93:604, 2003.
83. Gonzalez A, Rota M, Nurzynska D, et al: Activation of cardiac progenitor cells reverses the failing heart senescent phenotype and prolongs lifespan. *Circ Res* 102:597, 2008.
84. Seals DR, DeSouza CA, Donato AJ, Tanaka H: Habitual exercise and arterial aging. *J Appl Physiol* 105:1323, 2008.
85. Leri A, Malhotra A, Liew CC, et al: Telomerase activity in rat cardiac myocytes is age and gender dependent. *J Mol Cell Cardiol* 32:385, 2000.
86. Rota M, Hosoda T, De Angelis A, et al: The young mouse heart is composed of myocytes heterogeneous in age and function. *Circ Res* 101:387, 2007.
87. Anversa P, Rota M, Urbanek K, et al: Myocardial aging—a stem cell problem. *Basic Res Cardiol* 100:482, 2005.
88. Kajstura J, Urbanek K, Rota M, et al: Cardiac stem cells and myocardial disease. *J Mol Cell Cardiol* 45:505, 2008.
89. Torella D, Rota M, Nurzynska D, et al: Cardiac stem cell and myocyte aging, heart failure, and insulin-like growth factor-1 overexpression. *Circ Res* 94:514, 2004.
90. Li Q, Wu S, Li SY, et al: Cardiac-specific overexpression of insulin-like growth factor 1 attenuates aging-associated cardiac diastolic contractile dysfunction and protein damage. *Am J Physiol* 292:H1398, 2007.
91. Blair SN, Kohl HW, Paffenbarger RS, et al: Physical fitness and all-cause mortality: a prospective study of men and women. *JAMA* 262:2395, 1989.
92. Avolio AP, Fa-Quan D, Wei-Qiang L, et al: Effects of aging on arterial distensibility in populations with high and low prevalence of hypertension: comparison between urban and rural communities in China. *Circulation* 71:202, 1985.
93. Tanaka H, Dinenno FA, Monahan KD, et al: Aging, habitual exercise, and dynamic arterial compliance. *Circulation* 102:1270, 2000.
94. Tanaka H, DeSouza CA, Seals DR: Absence of age-related increases in central arterial stiffness in physically active women. *Arterioscler Thromb Vasc Biol* 18:127, 1998.
95. Vaitkevicius PV, Fleg JL, Engel JH, et al: Effects of age and aerobic capacity on arterial stiffness in healthy adults. *Circulation* 88:1456, 1993.
96. Shibata S, Hastings JL, Prasad A, et al: "Dynamic" Starling mechanism: effects of ageing and physical fitness on ventricular-arterial coupling. *J Physiol* 586:1951, 2008.
97. Shi X, Schaller FA, Tierney N, et al: Physically active lifestyle enhances vagal-cardiac function but not central autonomic neural interaction in elderly humans. *Exp Biol Med* 233:209, 2008.
98. Spina RJ, Meyer TE, Peterson LR: Absence of left ventricular and arterial adaptations to exercise in octogenarians. *J Appl Physiol* 97:1654, 2004.
99. Braith RW, Stewart KJ: Resistance exercise training. Its role in the prevention of cardiovascular disease. *Circulation* 113:2642, 2006.
100. Miyachi M, Kawano H, Sugawara J, et al: Unfavorable effects of resistance training on central arterial compliance. A randomized intervention study. *Circulation* 110:2858, 2004.
101. Cortez-Cooper MY, DeVan AE, Anton MM, et al: Effects of high intensity resistance training on arterial stiffness and wave reflection in women. *Am J Hypertens* 18:930, 2005.
102. Rakobowchuk M, McGowan CL, de Groot PC, et al: Effect of whole body resistance training on arterial compliance in young men. *Exp Physiol* 90:645, 2005.
103. Brades RP, Fleming I, Busse R: Endothelial aging. *Cardiovasc Res* 66:286, 2005.
104. Taddei S, Virdis A, Mattei P, et al: Aging and endothelial function in normotensive subjects and patients with essential hypertension. *Circulation* 91:1981, 1995.
105. Black MA, Green DJ, Cable NT: Exercise prevents age-related decline in nitric-oxide mediated vasodilator function in cutaneous microvessels. *J Physiol* 586:3511, 2008.
106. DeSouza CA, Shapiro LF, Clevenger CM, et al: Regular aerobic exercise prevents and restores age-related declines in endothelium-dependent vasodilation in healthy men. *Circulation* 102:1351, 2000.
107. Laughlin MH, Newcomer SC, Bender SB: Importance of hemodynamic forces as signals for exercise-induced changes in endothelial cell phenotype. *J Appl Physiol* 104:588, 2008.
108. Green DJ, Maiorana A, O'Driscoll G, Taylor R: Effect of exercise training on endothelium-derived nitric oxide function in humans. *J Physiol* 561:1, 2004.
109. Van Guilder GP, Westby CM, Greiner JJ, et al: Endothelin-1 vasoconstrictor tone increases with age in healthy men but can be reduced by regular aerobic exercise. *Hypertension* 50:403, 2007.
110. Smith DT, Hoetzer GL, Greiner JJ, et al: Effects of aging and regular aerobic exercise on endothelial fibrinolytic capacity in humans. *J Physiol* 546:289, 2003.
111. Brosse AL, Sheets ES, Lett HS, Blumenthal JA: Exercise and the treatment of clinical depression in adults. Recent findings and future directions. *Sports Med* 32:741, 2002.
112. Thijsssen DHJ, Vos JB, Verseyden C, et al: Hematopoietic stem cells and endothelial progenitor cells in healthy men: effect of aging and training. *Aging Cell* 5:495, 2006.
113. Nelson ME, Rajeski WJ, Blair SN, et al: Physical activity and public health in older adults. Recommendations from the American College of Sports Medicine and the American Heart Association. *Circulation* 116:1094, 2007.
114. Reis SE, Gloth ST, Blumenthal RS, et al: Ethinyl estradiol acutely attenuates abnormal coronary vasomotor responses to acetylcholine in postmenopausal women. *Circulation* 89:52, 1994.
115. Miller VM, Duckles SP: Vascular actions of estrogen: functional implications. *Pharmacol Rev* 60:210, 2008.
116. Moriarity K, Kim KH, Bender JR: Minireview: estrogen receptor–mediated rapid signaling. *Endocrinology* 147:5557, 2006.
117. Stirone C, Duckles SP, Krause DN, Procaccio V: Estrogen increases mitochondrial efficiency and reduces oxidative stress in cerebral blood vessels. *Mol Pharmacol* 68:959, 2005.
118. Strehlow K, Werner N, Berweiler J, et al: Estrogen increases bone marrow–derived endothelial progenitor cell production and diminishes neointima formation. *Circulation* 107:3059, 2003.
119. Anderson GL, Limacher M, Assad AR, et al; Women's Health Initiative Steering Committee: Effects of conjugated equine estrogen in postmenopausal women with hysterectomy: the Women's Health Initiative randomized controlled trial. *JAMA* 291:1701, 2004.
120. Hayashi T, Maeda S, Iemitsu M, et al: Sex differences in the relationship between estrogen receptor alpha gene polymorphisms and arterial stiffness in older humans. *Am J Hypertens* 20:650, 2007.
121. Traish AM, Saad F, Feeley RJ, Guays A: The dark side of testosterone deficiency: III. Cardiovascular disease. *J Androl* 30:477, 2009.
122. Vitale C, Mendelsohn ME, Rosano GMC: Gender differences in the cardiovascular effect of sex hormones. *Nat Rev Cardiol* 6:532, 2009.
123. Heart Protection Study Collaborative Group: MRC/BHF Heart Protection Study of cholesterol lowering with simvastatin in 20,536 high-risk individuals: a randomised placebo-controlled trial. *Lancet* 360:7, 2002.
124. Wenger NK, Lewis SJ, Herrington DM, et al: Treating to New Targets Study Steering Committee and Investigators: Outcomes of using high- or low-dose atorvastatin in patients 65 years of age or older with stable coronary heart disease. *Ann Intern Med* 147:1, 2007.
125. Zeng L, Xu H, Chew TL, et al: HMG-CoA reductase inhibition modulates VEGF-induced endothelial cell hyperpermeability by preventing RhoA activation and myosin regulatory light chain phosphorylation. *FASEB J* 19:1845, 2005.
126. Spyridopoulos I, Haendeler J, Urbich C, et al: Statins enhance migratory capacity by upregulation of the telomere repeat-binding factor TRF2 in endothelial progenitor cells. *Circulation* 110:3136, 2004.
127. Satoh M, Minami Y, Takahashi Y, et al: Effect of intensive lipid-lowering therapy on telomere erosion in endothelial progenitor cells obtained from patients with coronary artery disease. *Clin Sci (London)* 116:827, 2009.
128. Prospective Studies Collaboration: Age-specific relevance of usual blood pressure to vascular mortality: a meta-analysis of individual data for one million adults in 61 prospective studies. *Lancet* 360:1903, 2002.
129. Gueyffier F, Bulpitt C, Boissel JP, et al: Antihypertensive drugs in very old people: a subgroup meta-analysis of randomized controlled trials. *Lancet* 353:793, 1999.
130. SHEP Cooperative Research Group: Prevention of stroke by antihypertensive drug treatment in older persons with isolated systolic hypertension. Final results of the Systolic Hypertension in the Elderly Program (SHEP). *JAMA* 265:3255, 1991.
131. Verdecchia P, Staessen JjA, Angeli F, et al: Usual versus tight control of systolic blood pressure in non-diabetic patients with hypertension (Cardio-Sis): an open-label randomized trial. *Lancet* 374:525, 2009.
132. Mallareddy M, Parikh CR, Peixoto AJ: Effect of angiotensin-converting enzyme inhibitors on arterial stiffness in hypertension: systematic review and meta-analysis. *J Clin Hypertens* 8:398, 2006.
133. Ceconi C, Fox KM, Remme WJ, et al: ACE inhibition with perindopril and endothelial function. Results of a substudy of the EUROPA study. *Cardiovasc Res* 73:237, 2007.
134. Schriffrin EL, Park JB, Intengan HD: Correction of arterial structure and endothelial function in human essential hypertension by the angiotensin receptor antagonist losartan. *Circulation* 101:1653, 2000.
135. Mahmud A, Feely J: Reduction in arterial stiffness with angiotensin II antagonist is comparable with an additive to ACE inhibition. *Am J Hypertens* 15:321, 2002.
136. Yusuf S, Teo KK, Pogue J; ONTARGET Investigators: Telmisartan, ramipril, or both in patients at high risk for vascular events. *N Engl J Med* 358:1547, 2008.
137. Jansen PM, Danser AH, Imholz BP, van den Meiracker AH: Aldosterone-receptor antagonism in hypertension. *J Hypertens* 27:680, 2009.
138. Brown NJ: Aldosterone and vascular inflammation. *Hypertension* 51:161, 2008.
139. Strauch B, Petrak O, Wichterie D, et al: Increased arterial wall stiffness in primary aldosteronism in comparison with essential hypertension. *Am J Hypertens* 19:909, 2006.

432

140. Mahmud A, Feely J: Aldosterone-to-renin ratio, arterial stiffness, and the response to aldosterone antagonism in essential hypertension. *Am J Hypertens* 18:50, 2005.

141. Savoia C, Touz RM, Amin F, Schiffrin EL: Selective mineralocorticoid receptor blocker eplerenone reduces resistance artery stiffness in hypertensive patients. *Hypertension* 51:432, 2008.

142. Centers for Disease Control and Prevention (CDC): Cigarette smoking among adults and trends in smoking cessation—United States, 2008. *MMWR Morb Mortal Wkly Rep* 58:1227, 2009.

143. Pope CA, Burnett RT, Krewski D, et al: Cardiovascular mortality and exposure to airborne fine particular matter and cigarette smoke. *Circulation* 120:941, 2009.

144. Barnoya J, Glantz SA: Cardiovascular effects of secondhand smoke. *Circulation* 111:2684, 2005.

145. Heiss C, Amabile N, Lee AC, et al: Brief secondhand smoke exposure depresses endothelial progenitor cells activity and endothelial function. *J Am Coll Cardiol* 51:1760, 2008.

146. Kondo T, Hayashi M, Takeshita K, et al: Smoking cessation rapidly increases circulating progenitor cells in peripheral blood in chronic smokers. *Arterioscler Thromb Vasc Biol* 24:1442, 2004.

147. Juster HR, Loomis BR, Hinman TM, et al: Declines in hospital admissions for acute myocardial infarction in New York state after implementation of a comprehensive smoking ban. *Am J Public Health* 97:2035, 2007.

25

Diagnostic Testing to Help Improve Risk Prediction

CHAPTER **26**

Concepts of Screening for Cardiovascular Risk Factors and Disease

Donald M. Lloyd-Jones

KEY POINTS

- Screening involves the routine testing of asymptomatic individuals for the purpose of detecting the presence of a condition or a disease. The ultimate goal of screening is to identify the disease or condition of interest in an early phase, when intervention may be more effective in reducing subsequent morbidity or mortality.

- A number of metrics are available to assess the performance of screening tests, including sensitivity, specificity, predictive values, model fit characteristics, discrimination measures, and risk reclassification.

- Unlike with cancer, screening for CVD has typically involved screening for risk factors, for which there is solid evidence of utility, rather than for CVD itself.

- Current CVD clinical practice guidelines recommend screening for global cardiovascular risk by use of multivariable risk equations to assist in decision making regarding the intensity of prevention strategies.

- Use of imaging modalities to screen for subclinical CVD is an area of intense research interest. Current guidelines do not recommend routine screening for atherosclerosis in asymptomatic individuals, but accumulating evidence may help define a role for these screening tests, perhaps in refining risk stratification among those at intermediate risk for CVD events by traditional risk factor levels.

Screening involves the routine evaluation or testing of asymptomatic individuals for the purpose of detecting the presence of a condition or a disease. The ultimate goal of screening is generally to identify the disease or condition of interest in an early, or latent, phase, when intervention may be more effective in reducing subsequent morbidity or mortality. Historically, many of the concepts that have been used to define the utility of screening tests (sensitivity, specificity, predictive values) in patients and populations arose from the assessment of tests designed to detect medical conditions with a clear pathologic diagnosis, such as cancer. In recent years, these classical measures of diagnostic utility and many novel metrics have been employed as screening increasingly is used for preclinical conditions in the causal pathways for clinical disease and for prognosis, rather than merely for diagnosis. In the realm of cardiovascular disease (CVD), screening is a topic of significant import and heated debate, given the high incidence of disease across the life span, the substantial burden of morbidity and mortality, and the potentially high costs of screening tests and therapies. This is especially true in the current health care and economic environment. Thus, understanding of the basic concepts related to screening for CVD is of paramount importance. A review of the conceptual framework for screening tests and the means for evaluating their utility will serve as background for a discussion of the relative merits of screening for CVD risk factors (traditional and novel), global cardiovascular risk, and subclinical atherosclerosis.

CONCEPTS IN SCREENING

Criteria for Screening

In 1968, the World Health Organization[1] defined criteria for screening for disease in medicine. As shown in Box 26-1, these criteria indicate that screening for disease should be considered when the disease has a significant impact (in terms of prevalence or severity), has an adverse natural history

BOX 26-1 World Health Organization Criteria for Screening

The condition sought should be an important health problem for the individual and community.

There should be an accepted treatment or useful intervention for patients with the disease.

The natural history of the disease should be adequately understood.

There should be a latent or early symptomatic stage.

There should be a suitable and acceptable screening test or examination.

Facilities for diagnosis and treatment should be available.

There should be an agreed policy on whom to treat as patients.

Treatment started at an early stage should be of more benefit than treatment started later.

The cost should be economically balanced in relation to possible expenditure on medical care as a whole.

Case finding should be a continuing process and not a once and for all project.

Modified with permission from Wilson JMG, Jungner G: Principles and practice of screening for disease. *WHO Chronicle* 22:473, 1968.

that is well understood, and is treatable or modifiable during its asymptomatic phase. Of equal importance in these criteria are the features of the screening test itself: it should be reliable, available, cost-effective relative to other strategies, and applicable in an ongoing fashion. These widely accepted criteria provide a useful framework for evaluation of new (and old) screening tests. Clearly, it is inadequate merely to use a test with face validity for detection of disease; rather, careful consideration of the potential benefits, risks, harms, and potential costs associated with screening must be undertaken before widespread clinical adoption.

Types of Screening

Mass or universal screening involves assessment of all individuals in a population or group (e.g., all school-aged children or all pregnant women). Case finding, or high-risk screening, involves application of a screening test to subgroups identified as being at higher risk than average because of the presence of known risk factors (e.g., a strong family history of disease). As discussed later, each of these approaches has merit, depending on the nature of the disease or condition being screened and the knowledge of important predisposing factors.

Assessment of Screening Tests

A list of commonly applied metrics for evaluation of screening tests in CVD is provided in Table 26-1. Some discussion of these tests is warranted for a fuller understanding of their implications. Classical metrics of test characteristics (sensitivity, specificity, and related metrics) can be understood most easily in comparison with a "gold standard" test indicating the definitive presence or absence of disease. However, they are also applicable to prognostic tests, in which the gold standard is the development (incidence) of disease during the follow-up interval of observation after testing.

As recently detailed by the American Heart Association,[2] appropriate consideration of traditional and novel screening tests for CVD (which may include single tests or multivariable risk scores) should entail assessment of a number of different metrics beyond simple association, sensitivity, specificity, and predictive values. Demonstration that a screening test has a significant statistical association with the outcome of

interest is necessary but clearly not sufficient for evaluation of its utility. A number of metrics are available to assist in the evaluation of the performance and utility of risk estimation models. These metrics assess characteristics of the test (similar to a diagnostic test), its ability to discriminate cases from non-cases, the calibration of the model, model fit, and the informativeness of the model for the outcome of interest. Newer methods of assessment, such as analysis of risk reclassification, also allow comparison of different risk stratification algorithms by use of novel markers or risk scores. Knowledge of a few of these metrics and concepts will suffice for most clinicians to interpret the utility of risk prediction models. Consideration of all of these factors is important to understanding the utility of a risk score.

Sensitivity, Specificity, and Predictive Values

As shown in Figure 26-1 and Table 26-1, sensitivity and specificity reflect the true-positive and true-negative rates, respectively. In other words, a test with high sensitivity will detect a large proportion of individuals who have disease; a test with high specificity will correctly be negative in individuals without disease. These are useful test characteristics that in most cases do not change on the basis of the prevalence of disease in the groups being tested. However, they do not necessarily answer the question that is of interest to a clinician and patient: Is disease present? Positive and negative predictive values typically may be more useful as assessments of diagnostic and screening tests because they indicate the likelihood of having or developing disease given a positive (or higher) or negative (lower) test result, but their heavy reliance on the incidence and prevalence of disease in the population may make them difficult to translate from one clinical scenario to another.

Measures of Model Fit and Informativeness

Other measures, such as the Bayes information criterion, are now commonly used to assess the utility of statistical risk prediction models that include screening tests. These tests can indicate whether a risk model is predicting disease incidence better than chance alone. They can further indicate whether the addition of new screening tests to a base model provides better risk prediction than the base model alone, provided all of the same individuals are being assessed by both models.

Discrimination

One of the most widely reported measures of model discrimination for screening tests generally, and CVD risk prediction models specifically, is the area under the receiver operating characteristic curve (AUC), or C-statistic. The C-statistic is a function of both the true-positive and false-positive rates of the screening tool across all of its values, and it represents the ability of the score to discriminate (future) cases from non-cases. In other words, the C-statistic indicates the probability that a randomly selected patient who has or develops the disease (a "case") will have a higher test result or risk score than a randomly selected non-case. The AUC or C-statistic can vary from 1.0 (perfect discrimination) to 0.5 (random chance, equivalent to flipping a coin to determine case status). Thus, a C-statistic of 0.75 for a given model would indicate that a randomly selected case has a higher score than a randomly selected non-case 75% of the time (Fig. 26-2). C-statistics below 0.70 are generally considered to indicate inadequate discrimination by a test, whereas those between 0.70 and 0.80 are considered "acceptable," and between 0.80 and 0.90, "excellent."[3]

The C-statistic is imperfect as a stand-alone metric for assessment of screening tools or risk prediction models. In general, the C-statistic indicates whether a test or risk score is generating appropriate rank-ordering of risk for cases and

TABLE 26-1 | Commonly Applied Measures and Terms for Assessment of the Utility of Screening Tests*

Measure	Definition	Comment
Sensitivity	Proportion of those with disease who have a positive test result [P(T+|D+)]	Detection rate, true-positive rate; high sensitivity is useful for ruling out disease
Specificity	Proportion of those without disease who have a negative test result [P(T−|D−)]	True-negative rate; high specificity is useful for ruling in disease
False-negative rate	Proportion of those with disease who have a negative test result [P(T−|D+)]	Equal to 1 − sensitivity; when low, useful for ruling out disease
False-positive rate	Proportion of those without disease who have a positive test result [P(T+|D−)]	Equal to 1 − specificity; when low, useful for ruling in disease
Positive predictive value (PV+)	Proportion of those with a positive test result who have disease [P(D+|T+)]	Dependent on the prevalence (incidence) of disease
Negative predictive value (PV−)	Proportion of those with a negative test result who do not have disease [P(D−|T−)]	Dependent on the prevalence (incidence) of disease
Likelihood ratio	Ratio of true-positive rate to false-positive rate [P(T+|D+)] / [P(T+|D−)]	Can be used to calculate post-test odds (and therefore post-test probability of disease) by multiplying with pretest odds
Pretest probability	Probability of disease based on available information (prevalence, or risk-adjusted prevalence)	
Post-test probability	Adjusted probability of disease after application of additional (screening) test	
Area under the receiver operating characteristic curve (AUC, or C-statistic)	Function of true-positive rate and false-positive rate across all values of diagnostic (screening) test	Indicates discrimination ability of test; likelihood that a randomly selected case will have a positive (or more adverse) test result compared with a randomly selected non-case
Model fit	Assessment of whether statistical model including test improves case detection/prediction compared with chance or base model	Information criteria or likelihood ratio test often used to assess the utility of the model
Calibration	Degree to which screening (prediction) test or model accurately predicts absolute levels of observed event rates	Usually assessed with Hosmer-Lemeshow test
Net reclassification improvement	Degree to which new test increases predicted risk (across a decision threshold) for those who subsequently have events and decreases predicted risk (across a decision threshold) for those who do not subsequently have events	
Integrated discrimination index	Indicates how far individuals are moving, on average, along the continuum of predicted risk after application of test	Equivalent to the difference in R^2 between the two models being compared

*In the case of screening tests related to prognosis (rather than to diagnosis), the definitions would be relevant to those who do or do not develop disease during observation.
P, probability; D+, disease present; D−, disease absent; T+, test positive; T−, test negative.

	Disease present	Disease absent	
Test positive	a (True positive; TP)	b (False positive; FP)	a + b
Test negative	c (False negative; FN)	d (True negative; TN)	c + d
	a + c	b + d	a + b + c + d

Sensitivity = True-positive rate = P(T+ | D+) = TP/(TP+FN) = a / (a+c)
Specificity = True-negative rate = P(T− | D−) = TN/(TN+FP) = b / (b+d)
Positive predictive value = P(D+ | T+) = TP/(TP+FP) = a / (a+b)
Negative predictive value = P(D− | T−) = TN/(TN+FN) = d / (c+d)

FIGURE 26-1 Calculation of utility measures for diagnostic or screening tests.

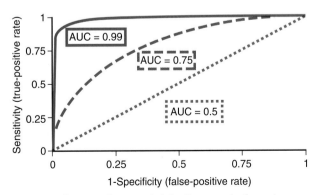

FIGURE 26-2 Representative curves depicting the area under the receiver operating characteristic curve (AUC or C-statistic).

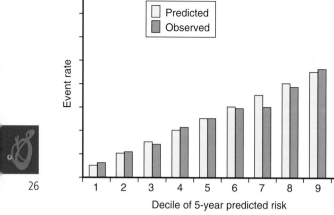

FIGURE 26-3 Assessment of calibration of a risk score or prediction test by comparing predicted 5-year risk with observed event rates, stratified by decile of predicted risk.

non-cases, not whether the predicted risk and observed outcome rates are similar (which is a function of calibration) or how much greater the estimated risk for disease is between selected cases and non-cases.[4,5]

Pepe and coworkers[6] have demonstrated that very large odds ratios (or relative risks) are required to reach meaningful levels in the C-statistic. For example, a univariate odds ratio of 9.0 or greater would be required to achieve a C-statistic that provides excellent discrimination of cases from non-cases for a continuous screening test (e.g., cholesterol or coronary calcium) in which the distribution of test scores differs by 2 or more standard deviations. These magnitudes of differences in distribution of test scores are rarely seen in clinical practice (where risk factor levels often overlap substantially), as are such high odds ratios. However, the combination of multiple, independent screening tests or risk markers, as in the Framingham risk score (FRS) and similar scores (see later), does provide these magnitudes of relative risk.

Calibration

Measures of calibration assess the ability of a screening test or risk prediction model to predict accurately the absolute level of risk that is subsequently observed. Demonstration that a risk prediction model is well calibrated would require that if the model estimates that the risk for a certain subgroup of individuals is 5% during 5 years, then the observed event rate should be close to 5%. Calibration is often assessed visually by dividing the population at risk into strata, such as deciles of predicted risk, and plotting the predicted risk versus the observed event rate for each decile (Fig. 26-3). The statistical metric used to test for the calibration of a risk model most often is the Hosmer-Lemeshow χ^2 test. A P value <0.05 for such a test would indicate poor calibration of the model for the population.

Assessment of Appropriate Risk Reclassification

A newer paradigm to assess the utility of screening tests and risk prediction models, which is recommended by the American Heart Association[2] for appropriate assessment of such tests, is risk reclassification analysis.[7] This approach requires measurement of the proportion of individuals who are reclassified from one risk stratum (e.g., intermediate risk) based on the estimated risk provided from a first model to a different risk stratum (e.g., high risk) based on estimated risk from a model that contains the additional test information. Some of these risk reclassifications end up being appropriate (based on subsequent observed events): some individuals who have

events are reclassified to higher predicted risk strata, and some who do not have events are reclassified to lower predicted risk strata. However, some reclassifications are inappropriate, moving future cases to lower predicted risk strata and future non-cases to higher predicted-risk strata.

Pencina and coworkers[7] have proposed two indices, the net reclassification improvement (NRI) and the integrative discrimination index (IDI), to attempt to quantify the appropriateness and the amount of overall reclassification. In general, the NRI indicates how much more appropriate reclassification occurs than inappropriate reclassification with use of the new model. The NRI can vary from −2, indicating that all individuals are reclassified inappropriately, to +2, indicating that all are reclassified appropriately. In other words, if the newer test reclassifies all of the people who have events upward, and all of the people who do not end up with events downward, the NRI would be +2. For this test, a P value <0.05 suggests that a significantly greater number are being reclassified appropriately than are being reclassified inappropriately. The IDI can be thought of as indicating how far individuals are reclassified, on average, along the continuum of predicted risk.[8] If the IDI is small (even if it is statistically significant), then a given individual's change in predicted risk with the new model will be small, on average. As an example, consider a new risk prediction model or test that is being compared with the FRS for stratifying a population into risk categories. The new model might have a significant NRI, reclassifying a net of 10% of people more appropriately; but if the IDI is small (e.g., less than 1%), then most of the net reclassification is occurring immediately adjacent to the decision thresholds that separate the risk categories, such as a change from a predicted risk of 19.8% with an old model to a predicted risk of 20.4% with a new model. This change might cross the decision threshold for treatment, but it would indicate no real impact in understanding or forecasting of the patient's risk, especially if the decision thresholds are relatively arbitrary. The significance of such small movements is also heavily dependent on the threshold selected. Indeed, this scenario is what is often observed in current studies comparing older and newer CVD risk prediction scores.[9]

Interpretation of Risk Information Provided by Screening Tests

Different types of information about risk for disease may be garnered from screening tests. The relative risk of disease is the ratio of disease or disease incidence among those with a positive test result compared with those who have a negative test result. As such, relative risk measures the strength of the association between the test and disease, but relative risks are poor indicators of clinical utility, and physicians and patients often have difficulty interpreting relative risk estimates[10-12] in the absence of an obvious comparison group. A relative risk for disease of 10 might seem very high, but if the incidence rate in the referent group is close to 0, it will also be close to 0 in the group with the relative risk of 10. Absolute risk of disease is often expressed as the estimated rate of development of new cases of disease per unit of time (or incidence) in individuals with a positive test result. Absolute risk estimates may be more easily understood than relative risks, and they allow clinical recommendations for interventions in individuals who exceed unacceptable risk thresholds.[10-12] This approach has been widely adopted for 5- and 10-year estimation of absolute risks for coronary heart disease (CHD) and CVD to guide clinical decision making for CVD prevention.[13] The attributable risk of a test result describes the proportion of the incidence of disease in a population associated with the test result, assuming a causal relationship exists. The population attributable risk takes into account the proportion of individuals in the population who test positive as well as the relative risk. Therefore, attributable risk is a useful concept in selecting screening tests that might be targeted for prevention programs.

In clinical trials, we often consider the concept of a number needed to treat (NNT) to prevent one event. The NNT is calculated as follows:

$$1 \bigg/ \left(\begin{array}{c} \text{rate of disease in the control group} - \text{rate of disease in} \\ \text{the intervention group} \end{array} \right)$$

Thus, an intervention that reduces mortality from 7% to 5% during 5 years would have an NNT of $1 / (0.07 - 0.05) = 1 / (0.02) = 50$. In other words, 50 people would need to be treated with the intervention for 5 years to prevent one event.

A similar concept, the number needed to screen (NNS), has been proposed.[14] Equivalently, the NNS represents the number of people who would have to be screened to detect one person with disease (as in mammography for breast cancer detection or fecal occult blood testing for colon cancer) or one person with a level of a risk marker that is deemed to be unacceptably high (e.g., detection of one individual with an Agatston coronary artery calcium score >300). The NNS is calculated as follows:

$$1 \bigg/ \left(\begin{array}{c} \text{rate of disease in the usual care group} - \text{rate of disease in} \\ \text{the screened group} \end{array} \right)$$

or

$$1 \bigg/ \left(\begin{array}{c} \text{prevalence of risk marker level greater than threshold in} \\ \text{a given group} \end{array} \right)$$

The NNS may be best calculated from clinical trial data that compare a screening strategy with usual care, but it can be derived from observational data as well. The concept has been expanded to adjust for willingness (or lack thereof) to undergo screening in certain groups, thus indicating a number needed to be invited for screening, which is generally a higher number among lower risk healthier populations, and a number actually needed to screen, a lower number among potentially motivated, higher risk screenees.[15,16]

Law[17] has pointed out several weaknesses of the NNS. First, there may be difficulty generalizing the NNS from one population to another that may have a different basal rate of disease. Similarly, it may be impossible to compare the NNS for two different screening modalities or two different diseases if they are performed in different populations. NNS estimates are also sensitive, meaning that small changes in factors that influence disease rates may have a large impact on NNS. In addition, events are not always prevented; some are postponed, which may also have significant value, but it is difficult to capture in shorter term studies.[17] Nonetheless, the NNS may represent a useful construct if appropriate comparisons are made.

Biases and Pitfalls of Screening Tests

Whereas it may seem intuitive that screening for disease would always be useful, a number of pitfalls related to screening are routinely encountered in clinical practice. It is thus important to determine objectively whether screening can ultimately improve outcomes.

Imperfection of Screening Tests: False-Positives, False-Negatives, and Implications

The discussion of metrics for assessment of screening tests introduced the concepts of false-positive and false-negative results of screening tests. False-negative results may be devastating, delaying diagnosis of a potentially deadly disease or

condition. If screening tests are selected for maximal sensitivity, this eventuality may be minimized. The implications of false-positive results are more subtle but potentially just as important because they will affect much larger numbers of individuals. If a disease is uncommon, with a prevalence of <50% in the population to be screened, it is virtually certain that there will be more false-positive than true-positive test results. For example, a seminal paper in the literature of screening mammography examined the 10-year risk of false-positive mammograms.[18] Based on data from 2400 women aged 40 to 69 years at entry, a group for whom mammography has consistently been shown to reduce risk for breast cancer deaths, there were an average of four mammograms performed during 10 years. Of the women who were screened, the false-negative rate was approximately 1%, but 24% had at least one false-positive mammogram, 13% had at least one false-positive breast examination, and a total of 32% had at least one false-positive result for either test, requiring further evaluation. Thus, a large proportion of women without breast cancer underwent further imaging or biopsy with associated anxiety, pain, potential harms of unnecessary procedures, and substantially increased costs due to false-positive results. The cumulative risk of a false-positive result after 10 mammograms was estimated to be 49%.[18] The issue of false-positives is further complicated when screening tests are used for prognosis because the gold standard is the occurrence of an event, which may not have happened (yet) within the observed follow-up but could happen soon thereafter, changing a false-positive into a true-positive.

Selection Bias, or Spectrum Bias

As discussed earlier, the utility of a screening test is dependent on the population being tested. For example, exercise treadmill testing is known to have higher sensitivity (i.e., higher detection rate) among people with three-vessel or left main coronary disease than among people with one-vessel coronary disease.[19] Thus, screening with treadmill testing will appear better among those selected to be at very high risk (or who may have unrecognized symptoms) than if it is applied to a more general healthy population. In addition, although one may invite entire groups or populations for screening, some individuals will be more likely than others to be screened. If people with a higher risk of disease are more likely to be screened, then the screening test could appear worse than it really is because adverse outcomes among the screened population will be higher than for the general population.[15] Conversely, if a test is selectively available to younger, healthier individuals, the screened group will have lower disease rates than the general population and will appear to have benefited from screening.

Adherence/Compliance Bias

Compared with the general population, people who are more likely to adhere to prescribed therapies may also be more willing to undergo screening, therefore improving the apparent impact of the screening strategy in preventing adverse outcomes.

Lead-Time Bias

The effectiveness of a screening test may be overestimated because it detects disease at a much earlier stage than would otherwise have been the case. Therefore, the time between "diagnosis" of disease and death will be prolonged, on average, compared with diagnosis at the time of symptom onset. However, if the outcome of early detection is similar to the outcome with symptomatic detection, this lead-time bias will give a false sense of effectiveness to the screening test: "survival with disease" is artifactually lengthened by earlier disease detection, even though age at death may be the same for both groups. In the meantime, the patient may have experienced anxiety or economic hardship related to the diagnosis. The amount of lead-time bias is a function of the sensitivity of the screening test as well as of the biologic rate of disease progression.

Length-Time Bias

Length-time bias has been best conceptualized in the framework of cancer detection, but it may have significant relevance to subclinical CVD detection as well. Many screening tests may perform better in detecting slower growing cancers that have a better prognosis than in detecting rapidly growing cancers because of a longer preclinical or latent phase in the slow-growing cancer. If true, then screening will tend to detect more cancers that would not have killed the patient or may not even have been symptomatic before death from other causes. In parallel, it is possible that some CVD screening tests could detect stable subclinical CVD better than they detect CVD that will become clinically manifested.

Prevalence Bias

A related concept is prevalence bias, in which early rounds of screening will tend to detect slower growing cancers, with good prognosis, whereas subsequent rounds of screening will detect newer, more rapidly growing cancers. This bias should be considered in the context of defining screening intervals.

Overdiagnosis Bias

Screening may also detect benign or harmless conditions that mimic the disease of interest. This may make the screening strategy appear to be more effective than it actually is because the harmless condition would not have resulted in an adverse outcome. However, it would likely have led to unnecessary treatment.

Combining Screening Tests

Use of multiple screening tests leads to several issues. First, they may be correlated; significant amounts of correlation and lack of independence may lead to false certainty when results are similar. For most screening situations, sequential testing will be preferred to use of concurrent multiple screening tests because the results from a first test may be sufficient, or they may revise the pretest probability to a point where a second test will be more useful.

Diagnostic Test Cutoffs

One final issue that merits consideration is the selection of appropriate thresholds (cutoffs) to define a positive test result for diagnostic or screening tests. The optimal cutoff point is a function of sensitivity and specificity, the prevalence of disease in the population to which it will be applied, and any benefits of correct diagnoses as well as risks and costs of incorrect diagnoses with regard to potential harm and downstream testing.

Presentation of Risks and Benefits of Screening

A substantial literature has addressed the issues related to presentation of data regarding the risks and benefits of screening. These issues include problems of framing risk estimates, with presentation of relative risk reductions, which may seem large, versus absolute risk reductions, which are usually very small for screening tests. Thus, a relative risk reduction of 15% in breast cancer mortality associated with mammographic screening may sound large, particularly for a scary disease like breast cancer, but this represents only 1 or 2 deaths prevented or postponed for 1000 women screened annually for 10 years. The "average" amount of life gained for a woman in her 40s is thus 3 days,[20] but it might be decades for the few women who are identified with breast

cancer. Other problems include physicians' and patients' perceptions of risk, their ability to assess the benefits and harms related to screening, and what value they might place on those outcomes, among many others.

However, if there exists a safe, inexpensive, and reasonable therapy that can provide substantial risk reduction, these problems may be surmountable by lowering the threshold for treatment substantially with little potential for harm. In such an environment, the implications of a false-positive result may be minimized. It is easy to suggest that we would rather overtreat than undertreat in such a situation. This paradigm may now be driving CVD screening, with the increasing availability of potent, generic statin medications.

Appropriate Evaluation and Application of Screening Tests

Given all of these potential pitfalls and biases in evaluating screening tests and strategies, it is imperative that new screening modalities be assessed rigorously before widespread application. This is particularly true for costly screening modalities. The best data come from randomized controlled clinical trials of screening strategies in appropriate populations across the spectrum of health and risk, with blinded evaluation of outcomes and appropriate gold standard or outcome definition. Subsequent analyses can then examine the relative and absolute reduction in disease, the number needed to screen (or harm), and the effectiveness and cost-effectiveness of the screening strategy in the general population or specific subgroups of interest.

SCREENING FOR CARDIOVASCULAR RISK FACTORS

Formal assessment of the risks, benefits, harms, and costs of screening for dyslipidemia, hypertension, and diabetes have been performed.[21-26] Although some data are lacking, the acknowledgment that these are causal risk factors for CVD, the available evidence on the ability of these risk factors to identify individuals at heightened risk for CHD, and the substantial data indicating efficacy, effectiveness, and cost-effectiveness of therapy (certainly for dyslipidemia and hypertension) have led to strong recommendations for universal screening among middle-aged and older adults and generally accepted practice of screening younger adults.[21-26] These are unlikely to be revised in the future.

SCREENING FOR GLOBAL CARDIOVASCULAR RISK

Current clinical practice guidelines from the U.S. National Cholesterol Education Program (ATP III),[13] international guidelines,[27,28] and American Heart Association guidelines[29] have adopted and thoroughly incorporated the strategy of "global" risk estimation using multivariable equations containing traditional risk factors as a means to identify those who should receive more intensive therapy. The U.S. Preventive Services Task Force (USPSTF) has supported the use of global risk estimation as a screening strategy for selection of patients warranting lipid-lowering therapy.[23]

Assessments of the Framingham Risk Score

In most cohorts studied to date, the FRS provides very good discrimination, as indicated by C-statistics that typically range from 0.75 to 0.80.[30-34] The FRS and similar risk scores discriminate risk better for women than they do for men, often having C-statistics in excess of 0.80 for women. In addition, the FRS has good discrimination in most populations (including those from outside the United States) in which it has been studied because it contains age as a covariate and because of the fairly universal associations between CVD and the major traditional risk factors the FRS also incorporates.

Calibration of the FRS in diverse populations may differ substantially, however, because of diverse CVD incidence rates in different settings. Studies to date indicate that the FRS discriminates CHD risk very well and is well calibrated for a wide range of white and African American populations in the United States. For other populations, such as Asian Americans, American Indians, Hispanic Americans, and native Chinese, discrimination remains acceptable, but the FRS tends to overestimate risk.[35,36] However, with simple steps to recalibrate the FRS model, it performs well in both discrimination and calibration.[35]

Given the overall acceptable to excellent risk discrimination provided by existing multivariable risk prediction models, they remain the logical standard to which new risk markers or subclinical disease measures from screening tests must be added to demonstrate improvement or against which newer models must be compared. The methods that should be used to evaluate novel markers of cardiovascular risk were recently summarized and recommended by a special panel of the American Heart Association.[2] All of the metrics discussed before should be examined and assessed for statistically significant improvement, and then clinical judgment applied to determine whether there is also clinically meaningful improvement that would affect decision making in a reasonable number of patients. That said, if the change in the C-statistic is small for a new compared with an existing risk score, or when a novel risk marker is added to an existing risk score, it is extremely unlikely that the novel risk score or marker will provide a clinically meaningful improvement as a screening tool across the population. However, the novel risk marker may still add value within certain subgroups. To demonstrate these concepts, it will be useful to consider some published examples.

Attempts to Improve Risk Prediction Through Addition of Novel Markers to Existing Risk Scores

A substantial body of literature during the last 5 years has been devoted to examining the addition of newer risk markers to traditional risk scores. Essentially all of the single additional markers studied to date have yielded little additional clinical benefit when considered as screening tests across the entire spectrum of risk. For example, Folsom and colleagues[37] observed minimal changes in the C-statistic (0.000 to 0.011) for prediction of CHD events using 19 different novel biomarkers added individually to the FRS. However, within subgroups predicted to be at intermediate risk by traditional models, addition of new risk markers can help reclassify some individuals, and this is often the group for which the addition of information from a new test is most clinically useful. In the Women's Health Study,[31] when C-reactive protein (CRP) was added to a model with traditional risk factors, the C-statistic did not improve measurably for the whole population (the reported C statistic was 0.81 for both models). However, women in the middle of the predicted risk spectrum in this cohort (FRS predicted risk of 5% to 9%) with a CRP level >3.0 had an observed event rate that was equal to or greater than that of some women with a FRS-predicted risk of ≥10%. However, the traditional risk model (FRS) determines a far greater magnitude of risk than does the level of CRP, indicating the important context provided by the traditional risk model.[38] Similar results have been observed with

addition of parental history information to traditional risk scores,[39] with minimal change in overall discrimination but potential benefit in intermediate-risk groups. More recent data suggest a larger change in the C-statistic associated with the addition of coronary artery calcium scores to the FRS, with increments in the C-statistic from 0.02 to 0.11 in different racial and ethnic groups.[30]

Because single risk markers have not added substantially to risk prediction, a number of investigators have examined the addition of multiple markers simultaneously to traditional risk equations. In the Cardiovascular Health Study, Shlipak and associates[40] reported that addition of six novel biomarkers (including interleukin-6, CRP, fibrinogen, lipoprotein(a), and factor VIII levels plus presence of anemia) to a traditional risk model improved the C-statistic from 0.73 to 0.74 in older individuals with chronic kidney disease but decreased the C-statistic from 0.73 to 0.72 in those with normal renal function. In the Framingham study, the addition of brain natriuretic peptide levels plus microalbuminuria to a traditional risk model for CVD events yielded an increase in the C-statistic from 0.76 to 0.77.[41]

More recent studies have extended these types of analyses to assess reclassification as well. In a cohort of 5067 Swedish individuals free of CVD at baseline, observed for a median of 12.8 years, models with traditional risk factors had C-statistics of 0.758 and 0.760 for CVD and CHD events, respectively. When two independently significant novel biomarkers were added to the traditional models, the C-statistics improved by 0.007 and 0.009, respectively, for CVD and CHD events, indicating minimal clinical utility. Likewise, the proportion of participants reclassified was modest (8% overall for CVD risk and 5% for CHD risk). The NRI was 0 for CVD events and 0.047% for CHD events, indicating no or only minimal net improvement in risk reclassification. Greater improvements in reclassification were observed in analyses restricted to intermediate-risk individuals, but any correct reclassification was almost entirely due to downward reclassification of individuals who did not experience events (yet).

The USPSTF recently evaluated nontraditional risk markers for CVD (including CRP, leukocyte count, fasting blood glucose, lipoprotein(a), and homocysteine) and made no recommendation for use of these markers because of insufficient evidence for potential benefits and harms.[42] The American Heart Association and the Centers for Disease Control and Prevention have recommended against routine screening with CRP or other inflammatory markers but concluded that it might be reasonable to aid in decision making for patients at intermediate predicted risk for CHD.[43]

Examples of Newer Risk Prediction Models

There now exists a large number of published risk prediction scores for various CVD or CHD endpoints that have been derived from a variety of different populations. One recent example, the Reynolds risk score for women,[9] included the traditional risk factors plus CRP levels and parental history as selected for inclusion in the model based on improvement in the Bayes information criterion. Compared with a Framingham-like model recalibrated for this study's endpoint, overall discrimination and calibration of the two models were similar. Internal validation of the Reynolds risk score revealed that 5.8% of 8149 women were reclassified when the Reynolds risk score was applied (compared with the FRS), with about half of those being reclassified upward and half downward. The clinical implications of downward reclassification are unclear because withholding of therapy from those potentially at higher risk on the basis of traditional risk factors does not seem warranted given available clinical trial data. The generalizability and utility of this score and many others are still being assessed.

Limitations of 10-Year Risk Prediction Models

Ten-year risk estimation represents a substantial improvement over clinician judgment alone for appropriate risk stratification.[44,45] However, it has some acknowledged limitations. For example, because age is the most heavily weighted variable in 10-year risk models derived from populations that span the adult age spectrum, in younger adults (<45 years old in men and <65 years old in women), modest elevations in risk factors have little effect on 10-year risk.[46,47] Even younger adults with substantial risk factor burden may still have 10-year risk estimates well below 10%, although their remaining lifetime risks may exceed 50% on the basis of these risk factors.[48] This is not a problem of the 10-year risk score per se, nor incorrect risk prediction, but rather a function of the decision thresholds that are imposed on the risk estimates and the short time horizon imposed by 10-year risk estimation.

The magnitude of risk factor levels that are needed to reach moderately high (10% to 20% 10-year predicted risk) and high-risk (>20%) thresholds in the ATP III risk assessment algorithm has recently been investigated. Cavanaugh-Hussey and colleagues[46] entered ranges of risk factor levels into the ATP III risk assessment tool for men and women from the age of 30 to 75 years. For almost all combinations of risk factors, even with extreme values, nonsmoking men <45 years old and essentially all women <65 years old have 10-year predicted risks below 10%. Thus, many younger patients with significant risk factor burden do not reach treatment thresholds based on current ATP III recommendations. A similar study[47] has recently evaluated the updated Framingham risk profile[49] for global CVD (not just CHD) risk, with somewhat similar findings, although the use of an expanded CVD endpoint does allow more men and particularly more women in their 50s to exceed 10% and 20% predicted 10-year risk.[47]

Several alternatives exist to address some of the limitations of 10-year risk estimates, particularly for younger adults. One alternative is to change the horizon for risk estimation, to provide long-term or lifetime risk estimates for CVD endpoints. Another possible solution would be to perform subclinical disease imaging in essentially all middle-aged adults to identify those with premature atherosclerosis.

SCREENING FOR SUBCLINICAL CARDIOVASCULAR DISEASE

Screening for presence of atherosclerotic coronary artery disease (CAD), or CVD in general, is potentially attractive on its face. However, it is fair to say that substantial further investigation of these screening strategies is warranted before widespread adoption of these technologies is implemented. Re-examination of Box 26-1 suggests that several of the World Health Organization criteria for screening have not been adequately investigated as yet.

Despite the immediate appeal of cardiovascular screening with such common tests as coronary calcium measurement,[50] B-mode ultrasound examination for intima-media thickness,[51] or other tests,[52] routine population-wide screening for subclinical CAD or CVD has met with nearly universal negative recommendations by expert panels to date.[29,53,54] A critical assessment of one of the most promising of the methods for early detection of CAD, coronary artery calcium (CAC) measured by rapid computed tomography, provides enlightening insights into the negatives of such screenings. On the

one hand, recent reports from the Multi-Ethnic Study of Atherosclerosis (MESA)[30] demonstrate convincingly that CAC testing is predictive of coronary events in whites, blacks, Hispanics, and Chinese Americans. Indeed, MESA investigators found that increased CAC scores are predictive over and above traditional risk factors in both men and women.[30,55] Despite showing unusually strong hazard ratios for major coronary events ranging as high as approximately 7 for those with elevated CAC scores compared with a reference group with CAC = 0, MESA results also showed that CAC has a low positive predictive value for near-term events regardless of the cutoff chosen for a positive test result.[30] Depending on the cutoff chosen for a positive test result, sensitivity is also relatively poor. In MESA, for a cutoff value of CAC >0 as the definition of a positive test result, sensitivity for near-term events was 91% but specificity was only 51% in this population of relatively low risk people (major coronary event rate during 3.9 years of median follow-up was slightly above 1%, with estimated 10-year risk extrapolated to approximately 5%).[42] With a cutoff of CAC >0 for a positive test result, positive predictive value is only 2%.[56] Furthermore, the positive predictive value would be substantially lower in younger populations than in the MESA cohort, which had a mean age of 62 years.

When a more stringent cutoff of CAC >100 is used, sensitivity for near-term major coronary events drops markedly to only 63%, and positive predictive value remains low at 3.5%.[56] Thus, although hazard ratios are impressive for CAC and far exceed those for carotid intima-media thickness,[37,51] CRP,[38] or any of the traditional risk factors for CHD,[30] positive predictive values for CAC measurement are poor. Indeed, even with these impressive hazard ratios, the C-statistic improves only from 0.79 for risk factors alone as a predictor of CHD events to 0.83 for risk factors plus CAC score. Thus, CAC scoring as a strategy to identify individuals at high risk of near-term events across essentially the entire population, as has been proposed by some,[57] will likely not be feasible. It may, however, still be very useful to reclassify risk among groups deemed to be at intermediate risk by traditional risk models, as current guidelines recommend.[50]

An important distinction between cancer screening tests and those available for cardiovascular risk assessment is availability (or the lack thereof for CVD tests) of robust cost-effectiveness or outcomes data from clinical trials of screening strategies incorporating these modalities. We do not have a full understanding of the risks of CVD screening; nor do we have a full accounting of benefits and costs. These issues have been the major cause for lack of endorsement of such tests as coronary calcium scoring for the general population by groups that include the USPSTF[54] and the U.K. National Health Service Research and Development Health Technology Assessment Program.[58] Not only do we lack evidence that these sorts of screening confer a substantial benefit, we know that there is also risk of harm. Harms of screening include false reassurance due to a test with low sensitivity, anxiety due to a false-positive test result, and in the case of certain tests such as mammography and coronary computed tomography, radiation exposures[59-61] as well as the additional anxiety and possible risks due to discovery and evaluation of incidental findings that result in considerable added medical expense and invasive procedures.[62] The added burden of follow-up invasive angiography (that might or might not be necessary) observed after coronary calcium scoring is a lesson that screening for vascular disease is not without hazards.

Radiographic mammography is recommended by the USPSTF,[63] with a quality rating of B (i.e., this level recommends that clinicians provide this service to eligible patients on the basis of at least fair evidence from clinical trials that the service improves important health outcomes and concludes that benefits outweigh harms). Evidence is strongest for women aged 50 to 69 years, the age group generally included in screening trials.[63] With the identical review standards, the USPSTF recommends against routine screening with resting electrocardiography, exercise treadmill testing, or rapid computed tomography scanning for coronary calcium for either the presence of severe coronary artery stenosis or the prediction of CHD events in adults at low risk for CHD events (i.e., screening of the general asymptomatic population). The USPSTF has concluded that there is at least fair evidence that these tests are ineffective or that harms outweigh benefits.[54]

The preceding discussion points regarding coronary calcium measurement pertain to what is arguably the best and best-studied screening test currently available for detection of subclinical CAD. Potential concerns are magnified when applied to measures with large potential sources of error (relative to signal), such as carotid intima-media thickness and arterial stiffness measures. There are substantial difficulties associated with broad application of these newer technologies in clinical practice, including technical issues (especially technician dependence of scanning), reader error and bias, and lack of agreement on the most appropriate parameters to be measured and the best instruments to use. It is also largely unclear how often any of the screening tests should be repeated or what a meaningful change in the results may be.

CONCLUSION

Additional studies of screening strategies, including their impact on patient outcomes, are urgently needed to define the role of novel risk markers and subclinical disease imaging in screening for risk and subclinical CVD. These studies should be designed to answer the full range of issues and criteria needed before routine screening for the asymptomatic patient is recommended. The literature on screening tests is full of lessons indicating that we cannot assume clinical benefit, effectiveness, or cost-effectiveness simply because the tests we employ are feasible, have anatomic or physiologic face validity, or are strongly predictive of outcomes.

The best approach at this time for CVD assessment and prevention appears to lie in routine testing for traditional, causal coronary risk factors and better implementation of existing preventive paradigms and clinical practice guidelines. As the USPSTF has noted, this is a proven approach to identify a group of patients who can benefit from preventive treatments shown in clinical trials of blood pressure lowering and cholesterol lowering. Indeed, the USPSTF has given blood pressure and cholesterol testing and screening its highest grade of quality, an A grade. Accordingly, the USPSTF strongly recommends that clinicians routinely provide these risk factor measurements to eligible patients on the basis of solid evidence that these services improve important health outcomes and the benefits of such tests substantially outweigh the harms.[21,22] The coming years present an exciting opportunity for researchers, policy makers, and clinicians to explore and to demonstrate the utility of novel risk markers and imaging modalities in appropriate subgroups of patients where benefits can be maximized, risks and costs can be justifiable and minimized, and therapies can be targeted to maximize the substantial promise of CVD prevention.

REFERENCES

1. Wilson JMG, Jungner G: Principles and practice of screening for disease. *WHO Chronicle* 22:473, 1968.
2. Hlatky MA, Greenland P, Arnett DK, et al: Criteria for evaluation of novel markers of cardiovascular risk: a scientific statement from the American Heart Association. *Circulation* 119:2408, 2009.
3. Hosmer DW, Lemeshow S: *Applied logistic regression*, ed 2, New York, 2000, Wiley.
4. Cook NR: Use and misuse of the receiver operating characteristic curve in risk prediction. *Circulation* 115:928, 2007.
5. Hilden J: The area under the ROC curve and its competitors. *Med Decis Making* 11:95, 1991.
6. Pepe MS, Janes H, Longton G, et al: Limitations of the odds ratio in gauging the performance of a diagnostic, prognostic, or screening marker. *Am J Epidemiol* 159:882, 2004.
7. Pencina MJ, D' Agostino RB, Sr, D'Agostino RB, Jr, Vasan RS: Evaluating the added predictive ability of a new marker: from area under the ROC curve to reclassification and beyond. *Stat Med* 27:157, 2008.
8. Pepe MS, Feng Z, Gu JW: Comments on "Evaluating the added predictive ability of a new marker: From area under the ROC curve to reclassification and beyond" by M. J. Pencina et al.. *Stat Med* 27:207, 2008.
9. Ridker PM, Buring JE, Rifai N, et al: Development and validation of improved algorithms for the assessment of global cardiovascular risk in women: the Reynolds Risk Score. *JAMA* 297:611, 2007.
10. Jackson R: Guidelines on preventing cardiovascular disease in clinical practice. Absolute risk rules—but raises the question of population screening. *BMJ* 320:659, 2000.
11. Rose G: Environmental health: problems and prospects. *J R Coll Physicians Lond* 25:48, 1991.
12. Vine DL, Hastings GE: Ischaemic heart disease and cholesterol. Absolute risk more informative than relative risk. *BMJ* 308:1040, 1994.
13. Third Report of the National Cholesterol Education Program (NCEP) Expert Panel on Detection, Evaluation, and Treatment of High Blood Cholesterol in Adults (Adult Treatment Panel III) Final Report. *Circulation* 106:3143, 2002.
14. Rembold CM: Number needed to screen: development of a statistic for disease screening. *BMJ* 317:307, 1998.
15. Richardson A: Screening and the number needed to treat. *J Med Screen* 8:125, 2001.
16. Tabar L, Vitak B, Yen M, et al: Number needed to screen: lives saved over 20 years of follow-up in mammographic screening. *J Med Screen* 11:126, 2004.
17. Law MR: The number needed to screen—an adaptation of the number needed to treat. *J Med Screen* 8:114, 2001.
18. Elmore JG, Barton MB, Moceri VM, et al: Ten year risk of false positive screening mammograms and clinical breast examinations. *N Engl J Med* 338:1089, 1998.
19. Pauker SG, Kassirer JP: Decision analysis. *N Engl J Med* 316:250, 1987.
20. Ransohoff DF, Harris RP: Lessons from the mammography screening controversy: can we improve the debate? *Ann Intern Med* 127:1029, 1997.
21. Screening for high blood pressure: U.S. Preventive Services Task Force reaffirmation recommendation statement. *Ann Intern Med* 147:783, 2007.
22. Screening for type 2 diabetes mellitus in adults: U.S. Preventive Services Task Force recommendation statement. *Ann Intern Med* 148:846, 2008.
23. Helfand M, Carson S: *Screening for lipid disorders in adults: selective update of 2001 U.S. Preventive Services Task Force Review*, Rockville, Md, 2008, Agency for Healthcare Research and Quality. AHRQ publication 08-05114-EF-1.
24. Norris SL, Kansagara D, Bougatsos C, et al: Screening adults for type 2 diabetes: a review of the evidence for the U.S. Preventive Services Task Force. *Ann Intern Med* 148:855, 2008.
25. Pignone MP, Phillips CJ, Lannon CM: *Screening for lipid disorders, systematic evidence review no. 4*, Rockville, Md, 2001, Agency for Healthcare Research and Quality. AHRQ publication AHRQ 01-S004.
26. Wolff T, Miller T: Evidence for the reaffirmation of the U.S. Preventive Services Task Force recommendation on screening for high blood pressure. *Ann Intern Med* 147:787, 2007.
27. Genest J, McPherson R, Frohlich J, et al: 2009 Canadian Cardiovascular Society/Canadian guidelines for the diagnosis and treatment of dyslipidemia and prevention of cardiovascular disease in the adult—2009 recommendations. *Can J Cardiol* 25:567, 2009.
28. Graham I, Atar D, Borch-Johnsen K, et al: European guidelines on cardiovascular disease prevention in clinical practice: full text. Fourth Joint Task Force of the European Society of Cardiology and other societies on cardiovascular disease prevention in clinical practice (constituted by representatives of nine societies and by invited experts). *Eur J Cardiovasc Prev Rehabil* 14:S1, 2007.
29. Mosca L, Banka CL, Benjamin EJ, et al: Evidence-based guidelines for cardiovascular disease prevention in women: 2007 update. *Circulation* 115:1481, 2007.
30. Detrano R, Guerci AD, Carr JJ, et al: Coronary calcium as a predictor of coronary events in four racial or ethnic groups. *N Engl J Med* 358:1336, 2008.
31. Ridker PM, Rifai N, Rose L, et al: Comparison of C-reactive protein and low-density lipoprotein cholesterol levels in the prediction of first cardiovascular events. *N Engl J Med* 347:1557, 2002.
32. Rutter MK, Meigs JB, Sullivan LM, et al: C-reactive protein, the metabolic syndrome, and prediction of cardiovascular events in the Framingham Offspring Study. *Circulation* 110:380, 2004.
33. van der Meer IM, de Maat MPM, Kiliaan AJ, et al: The value of C-reactive protein in cardiovascular risk prediction. *Arch Intern Med* 163:1323, 2003.
34. Wilson PWF, Nam BH, Pencina M, et al: C-reactive protein and risk of cardiovascular disease in men and women from the Framingham Heart Study. *Arch Intern Med* 165:2473, 2005.
35. D'Agostino RB, Grundy SM, Sullivan LM, et al: Validation of the Framingham coronary heart disease prediction scores: results of a multiple ethnic groups investigation. *JAMA* 286:180, 2001.
36. Liu J, Hong Y, D'Agostino RB, Sr, et al: Predictive value for the Chinese population of the Framingham CHD risk assessment tool compared with the Chinese Multi-Provincial Cohort Study. *JAMA* 291:2591, 2004.
37. Folsom AR, Chambless LE, Ballantyne CM, et al: An assessment of incremental coronary risk prediction using C-reactive protein and other novel risk markers: the Atherosclerosis Risk in Communities Study. *Arch Intern Med* 166:1368, 2006.
38. Lloyd-Jones DM, Liu K, Tian L, et al: Narrative review: assessment of C-reactive protein in risk prediction for cardiovascular disease. *Ann Intern Med* 145:35, 2006.

39. Lloyd-Jones DM, Nam B-H, D'Agostino RB, Sr, et al: Parental cardiovascular disease as a risk factor for cardiovascular disease in middle-aged adults: a prospective study of parents and offspring. *JAMA* 291:2204, 2004.

40. Shlipak MG, Fried LF, Cushman M, et al: Cardiovascular mortality risk in chronic kidney disease: comparison of traditional and novel risk factors. *JAMA* 293:1737, 2005.

41. Wang TJ, Gona P, Larson MG, et al: Multiple biomarkers for the prediction of first major cardiovascular events and death. *N Engl J Med* 355:2631, 2006.

42. Using nontraditional risk factors in coronary heart disease risk assessment: recommendation statement, topic page. U.S. Preventive Services Task Force. October 2009. Available at: http://www.uspreventiveservicestaskforce.org/uspstf/uspscoronaryhd.htm. Accessed March 31, 2010.

43. Markers of inflammation and cardiovascular disease: application to clinical and public health practice: a statement for healthcare professionals from the Centers for Disease Control and Prevention and the American Heart Association. *Circulation* 107:499, 2003.

44. Grover SA, Lowensteyn I, Esrey KL, et al: Do doctors accurately assess coronary risk in their patients? Preliminary results of the coronary health assessment study. *BMJ* 310:975, 1995.

45. Montgomery AA, Fahey T, MacKintosh C, et al: Estimation of cardiovascular risk in hypertensive patients in primary care. *Br J Gen Pract* 50:127, 2000.

46. Cavanaugh-Hussey MW, Berry JD, Lloyd-Jones DM: Who exceeds ATP-III risk thresholds? Systematic examination of the effect of varying age and risk factor levels in the ATP-III risk assessment tool. *Prev Med* 47:619, 2008.

47. Marma AK, Lloyd-Jones DM: Systematic examination of the updated Framingham Heart Study general cardiovascular risk profile. *Circulation* 120:384, 2009.

48. Lloyd-Jones DM, Leip EP, Larson MG, et al: Prediction of lifetime risk for cardiovascular disease by risk factor burden at 50 years of age. *Circulation* 113:791, 2006.

49. D'Agostino RB, Sr, Vasan RS, Pencina MJ, et al: General cardiovascular risk profile for use in primary care: the Framingham Heart Study. *Circulation* 117:743, 2008.

50. ACCF/AHA 2007 clinical expert consensus document on coronary artery calcium scoring by computed tomography in global cardiovascular risk assessment and in evaluation of patients with chest pain. *Circulation* 115:402, 2007.

51. O'Leary DH, Polak JF, Kronmal RA, et al: Carotid-artery intima and media thickness as a risk factor for myocardial infarction and stroke in older adults. *N Engl J Med* 340:14, 1999.

52. Cohn JN, Duprez DA: Time to foster a rational approach to preventing cardiovascular morbid events. *J Am Coll Cardiol* 52:327, 2008.

53. Screening for coronary heart disease, topic page. February 2004. U.S. Preventive Services Task Force. Available at: http://www.uspreventiveservicestaskforce.org/uspstf/uspsacad.htm. Accessed March 31, 2010.

54. Screening for coronary heart disease: recommendation statement. *Ann Intern Med* 140:569, 2004.

55. Lakoski SG, Greenland P, Wong ND, et al: Coronary artery calcium scores and risk for cardiovascular events in women classified as "low risk" based on Framingham risk score: the Multi-Ethnic Study of Atherosclerosis (MESA). *Arch Intern Med* 167:2437, 2007.

56. Greenland P, Lloyd-Jones D: Defining a rational approach to screening for cardiovascular risk in asymptomatic patients. *J Am Coll Cardiol* 52:330, 2008.

57. Naghavi M, Falk E, Hecht HS, et al: From vulnerable plaque to vulnerable patient—Part III: executive summary of the Screening for Heart Attack Prevention and Education (SHAPE) Task Force report. *Am J Cardiol* 98:2, 2006.

58. Waugh N, Black C, Walker S, et al: The effectiveness and cost-effectiveness of computed tomography screening for coronary artery disease: systematic review. *Health Technol Assess* 10:1, 2006.

59. Berrington de Gonzalez A, Mahesh M, Kim K-P, et al: Projected cancer risks from computed tomographic scans performed in the United States in 2007. *Arch Intern Med* 169:2071, 2009.

60. Kim KP, Einstein AJ, Berrington de Gonzalez A: Coronary artery calcification screening: estimated radiation dose and cancer risk. *Arch Intern Med* 169:1188, 2009.

61. Smith-Bindman R, Lipson J, Marcus R, et al: Radiation dose associated with common computed tomography examinations and the associated lifetime attributable risk of cancer. *Arch Intern Med* 169:2078, 2009.

62. Wald NJ: Screening: a step too far. A matter of concern. *J Med Screen* 14:163, 2007.

63. Screening for breast cancer: U.S. Preventive Services Task Force recommendation statement. *Ann Intern Med* 151:716, W-236, 2009.

CHAPTER 27

Role of Vascular Computed Tomography in Evaluation and Prevention of Cardiovascular Disease

Khurram Nasir, Roger S. Blumenthal, Nathan D. Wong, and Matthew J. Budoff

KEY POINTS

- Global risk assessment approaches for coronary heart disease, such as Framingham risk scores, underestimate long-term risks, especially in young men and postmenopausal women with multiple risk factors.

- Screening modalities, such as non–contrast-enhanced CT detection of coronary artery calcium, improve the ability to "accurately" predict risk in vulnerable groups and add information above and beyond global risk assessment.

- Absence of coronary artery calcification is associated with a very low risk of future CAD, significant stenosis, myocardial ischemia, and acute coronary syndrome during the next 5 years in nonsmokers.

- Guidelines reiterate that intermediate-risk individuals are the best patients for coronary artery calcium testing.

- Serial coronary artery calcium testing is currently not recommended because data for its prognostic significance are limited.

- Coronary artery calcium testing also appears to improve lifestyle changes and medication adherence.

- Coronary CTA has the potential to provide comprehensive information about the location, severity, and characteristics of atherosclerotic plaque, especially noncalcified plaque; however, there are currently no recommendations for its use as a screening tool in asymptomatic persons.

- The prognostic value of CTA-based plaque subtypes and burden above and beyond coronary artery calcium scores is not yet established.

Cardiovascular disease (CVD) is the leading cause of mortality worldwide, with coronary artery disease (CAD) accounting for nearly half of all CVD deaths.[1-3] Although it is highly prevalent in the Western world, in the next 15 years, an estimated 25 million people will die of stroke or heart disease, with 80% of this burden in developing countries.[2] Emerging data suggest that although the mortality rate after the occurrence of clinical heart disease (e.g., myocardial infarction [MI]) has significantly decreased during the last two decades, the incidence of new onset of CAD has remained relatively stable during this period.[4-6] This finding points to the fact that although we have made great strides in secondary prevention, we have failed in our primary efforts of decreasing the rate of new-onset CAD.

In approximately half of the individuals, the initial presentation of CAD is either MI or sudden death.[1] Unfortunately, conventional risk factor assessment predicts only 65% to 80% of future cardiovascular events,[1] leaving many middle-aged and older individuals to manifest a major cardiovascular event despite being classified as low risk by the Framingham risk estimate. Because half of first major coronary events occur in asymptomatic individuals, clinicians who want to implement appropriate primary prevention therapy must be able to accurately identify at-risk individuals.

Clinical decision making for primary prevention of CAD in asymptomatic individuals is traditionally guided by an initial estimate of the impact of single or clustered laboratory and physical factors as they relate to the risk of a coronary event. Preventive strategies are then modified and implemented after economic (personal, insurance provider, national impact) and individual (compliance, side effects) consequences of treatment versus no treatment are taken into account. Recommendations for diet, weight loss, and exercise offer little or no risk to the patient and yield significant long-term benefits.[7] Most decisions for clinical (i.e., pharmacologic) intervention, specifically those related to lipid lowering, are driven by perception of risk and attainment of goals for a given individual that are derived from large studies applied to both heterogeneous and homogeneous populations.

Screening for subclinical atherosclerosis in an effort to better identify persons at risk for CAD has been of increasing interest during the past decade. Cardiac computed tomography (CT) has shown promise in this regard, with a significant base of research and recent guidelines that have been established to support its use in selected groups of patients. Its use to better identify patients who might benefit from initiation or intensification of risk factor modification efforts is paramount to prevention efforts. This chapter details the current and future role of cardiac CT. The following discussion examines the methods, value, and future of cardiac CT in overall CAD in primary risk stratification and preventive strategies.

CURRENT CORONARY ARTERY DISEASE RISK STRATIFICATION GUIDELINES

A primary recommendation of the major advisory bodies is that all adults should undergo an office-based assessment as the initial step to identify those at higher risk for CAD events. One approach endorsed by both the American Heart Association (AHA) and the American College of Cardiology (ACC) and adopted by the National Cholesterol Education Program (NCEP) Adult Treatment Panel III (ATP III) is to apply a modification of the risk prediction algorithm derived from the Framingham Heart Study that incorporates a patient's age, total cholesterol concentration, high-density lipoprotein cholesterol (HDL-C) concentration, smoking status, and systolic blood pressure to estimate a person's 10-year risk for development of a "hard" coronary heart disease (CHD) event (MI or CHD death).[8]

Three levels of risk are defined on the basis of the probability of the occurrence of CHD in the next 10 years: <10% (low), 10% to 20% (intermediate), and >20% (high).[4] Individuals with CAD risk <10% are at presumed low risk of coronary events and can be reassured about their risk status without further risk assessment testing. Those with low risk are to be offered general public health recommendations in the short term, and they can usually avoid further risk assessments for approximately 5 years. At the other end of the risk spectrum, high-risk patients are those with established CAD or other clinical forms of atherosclerotic disease, suffer from diabetes mellitus, or frequently are older patients with multiple other CAD risk factors in accordance with NCEP ATP III guidelines; high-risk asymptomatic people should have all CAD risk factors treated to reduce CAD-specific and total CVD risk. Finally, a sizable group of individuals fall into the intermediate-risk category. Patients in this group do not currently qualify for the most intensive risk factor interventions, yet they have one or more risk factors that exceed desirable levels or multiple borderline risk factors. Often, there is not a definitive need to begin or to intensify therapy; however, many such persons do have underlying subclinical atherosclerosis that would place them at higher future risk of CAD than global risk assessment would predict. Intermediate-risk patients are the most likely to benefit from further risk stratification testing, if it is feasible, practical, targeted, and effective at further defining risk or in motivating effective behavioral changes.[8]

Determination of the intensity of treatment for primary prevention by use of global risk assessment algorithms such as the Framingham risk score (FRS) system employs data from population-based studies and does not take into account an individual's actual burden of atherosclerotic disease, which is believed to be the main culprit in development of clinical CAD. Indeed, such assessments may fall short if they are solely relied on for management decisions for the individual patient as these risk estimates are significantly age dependent; as a result, there is a great tendency to underestimate risk in younger individuals, who may be more appropriate candidates for early initiation of aggressive preventive strategies to reduce risk for development of clinical CAD.[9] In addition, the risk of a future CVD event in women is likely to be underestimated by these approaches, and nearly 90% of women younger than 70 years are considered low risk.[10]

This point can be illustrated in a study by Akosah and colleagues,[11] in which the authors assessed a simple question: How do NCEP guidelines classify young men and women presenting with an acute MI as their first manifestation of CAD? The study findings demonstrated that among adults aged <65 years with an acute MI, only 25% of patients would have met ATP III criteria, which are based on the FRS, for pharmacotherapy at the time of admission. The tendency of NCEP guidelines to underappreciate the risk for CAD was even more pronounced in women, with only 18% of women qualifying for pharmacotherapy for primary prevention; 58% of these patients had low-density lipoprotein cholesterol (LDL-C) concentration <130 mg/dL, and 40% had LDL-C <100 mg/dL.[11]

ATHEROSCLEROSIS AND CORONARY ARTERY DISEASE

Considering that atherosclerosis is the major underlying culprit for the development of clinical CAD, detection of individuals with subclinical atherosclerosis may aid in supplementing current global risk assessment approaches by more clearly identifying high-risk individuals who harbor advanced preclinical atherosclerosis. Screening studies to detect occult cancers, such as breast and colon cancer, are recommended in appropriate-risk adults to help prevent life-threatening conditions. Although atherosclerotic vascular disease accounts for more death and disability than all types of cancer, a screening tool to detect significant subclinical atherosclerosis and to target prevention of future cardiovascular events has not yet been adopted.[12]

A minority of patients with CAD do not exhibit traditional risk factors, such as hypertension, elevated cholesterol, obesity, and smoking. In addition, many patients with such risk factors do not develop CVD. Furthermore, there is substantial variation in the severity of CAD at every level of risk factor exposure. This variation in disease is probably due to a number of factors, including genetic susceptibility, presence of intrinsic biochemical and extrinsic environmental risk factors that are yet to be identified, and duration of exposure to the specific level of risk factors.[13]

Established noninvasive methods of evaluating CAD, such as stress testing, generally identify only patients with advanced atherosclerotic disease leading to a flow-limiting coronary stenosis and myocardial ischemia. The long-term risk of CAD, however, is more closely related to atherosclerosis plaque burden and stability than to the extent of a particular stenosis.[14] There is growing interest in quantifying and characterizing atherosclerosis in its preclinical, pre–flow-limiting phase so that appropriate preventive strategies can be instituted before an adverse event occurs.

With understanding of the need for noninvasive tests to assess atherosclerotic plaque, cardiac CT has evolved rapidly, with increasing ability to visualize the amount of coronary artery calcium.[15] Cardiac CT has been challenging, given rapid cardiac motion, small vessel diameters, tortuous anatomic patterns, and overlapping cardiac structures. Current 64-slice multirow detector computed tomography (MDCT) systems have faster gantry rotation speed, resulting in better temporal resolution and the better z-axis spatial resolution made possible by thin collimations with extensive volumetric acquisitions.

NON–CONTRAST-ENHANCED CORONARY COMPUTED TOMOGRAPHY: ASSESSMENT OF CORONARY ARTERY CALCIFICATION

During the past decade, there has been marked increased interest in the clinical use of cardiac CT scanning to identify and to quantify the amount of coronary artery calcified plaque (CAC). Calcification of the atherosclerotic plaque occurs by an active process of mineralization with deposition of hydroxyapatite crystals and not simple mineral precipitation. It begins in the very early stages of atherosclerosis. Studies have demonstrated that electron beam tomography (EBT) is a highly reliable method for identification of arterial calcification with a high sensitivity for detection of significant atherosclerosis. Rumberger and colleagues[16] have demonstrated a strong relationship ($r = 0.90$) between CAC measured by EBT and direct histologic plaque areas in autopsy hearts.

Although the total atherosclerotic plaque burden was associated strongly with the total calcium burden, not all plaques were found to be calcified. Moreover, within a given coronary artery, there is a poor correlation and wide variation between the degree of plaque calcification and extent of luminal stenosis on coronary angiography.[17,18] This may be due, at least in part, to individual variations in coronary artery remodeling, whereby the luminal cross-sectional area or external vessel dimensions enlarge in compensation for increasing area of mural plaque.

Despite the lack of a site-by-site correlation between calcification and luminal stenosis, coronary calcium scores calculated by EBT give a close approximation of the total atherosclerotic burden.[18] Because research has shown that burden of disease and cardiovascular risk are accounted for by more than focal luminal stenosis, non–contrast-enhanced cardiac CT is a potentially powerful tool for the identification of patients at risk.

METHODS OF ASSESSING CORONARY ARTERY CALCIUM

Modalities for Coronary Artery Calcium Determination

In the near past, CAC had generally been assessed by EBT; however, with a rapid explosion of use of MDCT in recent years. This has been a widely used modality to assess the extent and severity of underlying coronary calcification.[19] Neither modality requires intravenous administration of contrast material to determine CAC. In general, EBT uses a unique technology enabling ultrafast scan acquisition times in the high-resolution, single-slice mode with continuous, nonoverlapping slices of 3-mm thickness and an acquisition time of 100 msec/tomogram in a prospective manner. Electrocardiographic (ECG) triggering is done during end systole or early diastole at a time determined from the continuous ECG tracing recorded during scanning. Historically, the most common trigger time used is 80% of the R-R interval. However, this trigger occurs on or near the P wave during atrial systole, and the least cardiac motion among all heart rates occurs at 40% to 60% of the R-R interval.[19,20]

The current generation of MDCT systems is capable of acquiring up to 320 sections of the heart simultaneously with ECG gating in either a prospective or retrospective mode. These MDCT systems have two principal modes of scanning, which depend on whether the patient on the CT couch is advanced in a stepwise fashion (axial, sequential, or conventional mode) or continuously moved at a fixed speed relative to the gantry rotation (helical or spiral mode). Coronary calcification is determined in axial mode with use of prospective ECG triggering at predetermined offset from the ECG-detected R wave. With prospective gating, the temporal resolution of the MDCT system is proportional to the gantry speed, which determines the time to complete one 360-degree rotation.

For reconstruction of each slice, data from a minimum of 180 degrees plus the angle of the fan beam are required (approximately 220 degrees of the total 360-degree rotation). The most commonly used 64-slice scanners have rotation gantry speeds up to 330 msec.[19] MDCT imaging protocols vary among different camera systems and manufacturers. In general, 40 consecutive 2.5- to 3-mm-thick images are acquired per cardiac study. Calcified lesions are defined as two or three adjacent pixels with a tomographic density of >130 HU. Effective pixel size for a reconstruction matrix of 512×512 pixels with a common field of view of 26 cm is 0.26 mm^2.

Measurement of Coronary Artery Calcium Burden

On non–contrast-enhanced cardiac CT, CAC is in general defined as a hyperattenuated lesion above a threshold of 130 HU with an area of three adjacent pixels (at least 1 mm^2). There are currently two CT calcium scoring systems widely used, the original Agatston method[19] and the "volume" score method.[20] The Agatston method involves multiplication of the calcium area by a number related to CT density and, in the presence of partial volume artifacts, can be variable. With this method, area for all pixels above a threshold of 130 HU is calculated at every 3-mm slice and multiplied by a density factor.[19] Partial volume effects lead to higher peak values for small lesions (but not for large ones). On the other hand, the volume method developed by Callister and associates[20] appears to somewhat resolve the issue of slice thickness and spacing by computing a volume above threshold. As a result, it appears to be less dependent on minor changes in slice thickness. However, our group has previously demonstrated in nearly 10,000 patients that there appeared to be an excellent correlation between the scoring methods, and they show similar characterization when applied properly.[21] Both methods calculate lesion-specific scores within the left main, left circumflex, left anterior descending, and right coronary arteries and provide total scores for each artery and a sum total across all four arteries. An example of significant coronary calcium is shown in Figure 27-1.

MULTIDETECTOR COMPUTED TOMOGRAPHY COMPARED WITH ELECTRON BEAM TOMOGRAPHY FOR DETECTION OF CORONARY ARTERY CALCIUM

The comparability of MDCT- and EBT-derived CAC scores has been extensively explored.[22-24] The MDCT protocols vary considerably in these studies, ranging from conventional CT to single-slice CT (with either retrospective or prospective gating) to MDCT. EBT imaging was performed with the standard protocol conventionally used in routine clinical practice. Coronary calcification was defined as >130 HU for EBT but varied from 90 to 130 HU for MDCT. Although high correlation coefficients were reported between EBT and MDCT CAC scores, there was significant variability in individual CAC scores (range, 17% to 84%). In general, the interscan agreement for the presence of CAC between EBT and 64-slice

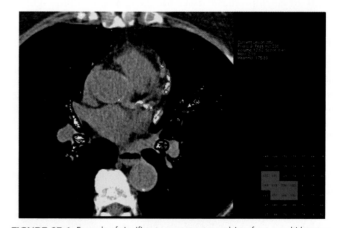

FIGURE 27-1 Example of significant coronary artery calcium from a multidetector CT scanner.

MDCT is excellent (99%). There was a significant linear relationship between the scores from the two scanners, and the interscanner variability between EBT and 64-slice MDCT was not significantly different. Bland-Altman analysis demonstrated a mean difference in scores of 8.3% by Agatston and 7.8% by volumetric calcium scoring. Compared with EBT, there were larger and more prevalent motion artifacts and larger mean Hounsfield units with 64-slice MDCT ($P < 0.001$). At CAC scanning, 64-slice MDCT and EBT were comparable in Agatston and volumetric scoring. The interscan variability between scanners is similar to interscan variability of two calcium scores done on the same equipment. However, heart rate control was achieved for this study for calcium scores. Whether these results are repeatable without heart rate control needs to be further assessed.

27

CLINICAL VALUE OF CORONARY ARTERY CALCIFICATION IN ASYMPTOMATIC INDIVIDUALS

Efforts have been made to develop noninvasive diagnostic tools to help determine the extent of atherosclerosis in asymptomatic patients and to improve detection of those who would benefit from more intensive preventive therapies, such as lipid-lowering medication and aspirin. This potential of coronary CT in the risk assessment protocol and management strategy is in accordance with the current philosophy of the NCEP and other organizations that stress the importance of matching therapy to level of assessed risks. However, to establish the role of CAC testing in primary preventive strategies, important questions need to be answered. Is the information gained from coronary CT additive to assessments made by cheaper office-based estimations of risk? If so, which populations of patients are expected to benefit from testing?

Does Coronary Artery Calcium Independently Predict Coronary Artery Disease Events?

The likelihood of plaque rupture and the development of acute cardiovascular events is related to the total atherosclerotic plaque burden.[13,18] Although controversy exists as to whether calcified or noncalcified plaques are more prone to rupture,[14] extensive calcification indicates the presence of both plaque morphologies.[16-18] There is a direct relationship between the CAC severity and the extent of atherosclerotic plaque; thus, the CAC score could be useful for risk assessment of asymptomatic individuals and potentially guide therapeutics.

Table 27-1 summarizes the findings of all major studies assessing the prognostic value of CAC burden among asymptomatic individuals.[25-38] In general, there appears to be a consensus among all studies that CAC is an independent predictor of CAD adverse outcome as well as of all-cause mortality after traditional risk factors are taken into account. Among 1172 asymptomatic patients observed for 3.6 years after an initial EBT screening, no events occurred in patients with a normal study, and the negative predictive value was 99.8% in patients with a CAC score <100. These results showed a 5%, 7%, and 13% hard cardiac event rate in individuals with a CAC score ≥80, ≥160, and ≥600, respectively.[25] The CAC score remained the best single predictor of risk after adjustment. Wong and colleagues[26] also showed that the CAC score severity predicted subsequent cardiovascular events independent of age, gender, and patient risk factor profile. Raggi and coworkers[27] studied more than 600 asymptomatic patients who were

referred for screening EBT and then observed for 32 ± 7 months. Both the absolute CAC score and the relative CAC score percentiles adjusted for age and gender predicted subsequent death and nonfatal MI. Hard cardiac events occurred in only 0.3% of subjects with a normal EBT study, but this increased to 13% in those with a CAC score >400. A very high CAC score ≥1000 may portend a particularly high risk of death or MI (25% per year) in individuals who are not treated with standard secondary prevention measures.

Larger studies have reported an approximately 10-fold increased risk with the presence of CAC. In one of the largest observational trials to date, Shaw and colleagues[29] reported all-cause mortality among 10,377 asymptomatic patients (4191 women and 6186 men) who had a baseline EBT study and were then observed for 5.0 ± 3.5 years (Fig. 27-2). Most subjects had cardiac risk factors including a family history of CAD (69%), hyperlipidemia (62%), hypertension (44%), and current cigarette smoking (40%). The CAC score was a strong independent predictor of mortality, with 43% additional predictive value contained within the CAC score beyond risk factors alone. Mortality significantly increased with increasing CAC score, within men and women separately as well as within each Framingham risk group (low-, intermediate-, and high-risk persons).[29] In addition, in the South Bay Heart Watch study, 1196 asymptomatic patients were observed (median = 7.0 years), and it was demonstrated that the CAC score added predictive power beyond that of standard coronary risk factors and C-reactive protein[30] (see Table 27-1). The results of the St. Francis Heart Study, which is a prospective registry of 5585 asymptomatic individuals, mirrored previous retrospective studies and confirmed the higher event rates associated with increasing CAC scores.[31] CAC scores >100 were associated with relative risks of 12 to 32, thus achieving secondary prevention equivalent event rates >2%/year.[31] The Rotterdam Heart Study[32] investigated 1795 asymptomatic participants (mean age, 71 years) who had CAC and measured risk factors. During a mean follow-up of 3.3 years, the multivariate-adjusted relative risk of coronary events was 3.1 for calcium scores of 101 to 400, 4.6 for calcium scores of 401 to 1000, and 8.3 for calcium scores >1000. Similarly, in a younger cohort of asymptomatic persons, the 3-year mean follow-up in 2000 participants (mean age, 43 years) showed that coronary calcium was associated with an 11.8-fold increased risk for incident CHD (CAD) ($P < 0.002$) in a Cox model controlling for the FRS.[33]

The Cooper Clinic Study[34] included more than 10,000 adults who were 22 to 96 years of age and free of known CAD. During a mean follow-up of 3.5 years, 81 hard events (CAD death, nonfatal MI) occurred. Age-adjusted rates (per 1000 person-years) of hard events were computed according to four CAC categories: no detectable CAC and incremental sex-specific thirds of detectable CAC; these rates were, respectively, 0.4, 1.5, 4.8, and 8.7 (trend $P < 0.0001$) for men and 0.7, 2.3, 3.1, and 6.3 (trend $P < 0.02$) for women. The association between CAC and CAD events remained significant after adjustment for CAD risk factors. Of note, in the largest single cohort study, Budoff and colleagues[35] showed risk-adjusted hazard ratios for total mortality ranging from 2.2 to 12.5 for CAC score categories of 11-100 to >1000 relative to 0, with CAC scores providing significant incremental information over risk factors. Finally, in a German study by Becker and coworkers,[36] the extent of CAC was determined by MDCT in 924 patients (443 men, 481 women, aged 59.4 ± 18.7 years). During the 3-year follow-up period, the event rates for coronary revascularization, MI, and cardiac death in patients with volume scores above the 75th percentile were significantly higher compared with the total study group, and no cardiovascular events occurred in patients with scores of zero. Receiver operating characteristic (ROC) analysis demonstrated that it outperformed both PROCAM and Framingham

TABLE 27–1	Summary of Outcomes Studies with Coronary Artery Calcification in Asymptomatic Individuals			
Author (Year)	**Type of Study and Population**	**Follow-up (years)**	**Number of Events**	**Results**
Arad et al[25] (2000)	Observational study, referral based N = 1172; age, 53 ± 11 yr	3.6	15 nonfatal MI, 21 revascularizations, 3 deaths	OR of 20 for CAC scores ≥160 compared with those with CAC scores <160
Wong et al[26] (2000)	Observational study, referral based N = 926; mean age, 54 yr	3.3	6 nonfatal MI, 20 revascularizations, 2 CVA	Overall, patients with CAC score ≥271 had a risk ratio of 9 for a CHD event.
Raggi et al[27] (2001)	Observational referral-based study N = 676; mean age, 52 yr	2.7	21 nonfatal MI, 9 deaths	CAC score was predictive of hard CAD events, with an OR of 22 for the CAC score 90% percentile.
Kondos et al[28] (2003)	Observational study, referral based N = 5635; age, 30-76 yr; 26% women	3.1	37 nonfatal MI, 166 revascularizations, 21 deaths	RR of 124 in men with soft events in the highest quartile (CAC 170-7000) Higher CAC scores added incremental prognostic information to conventional CAD risk assessment in men for hard CHD events.
Shaw et al[29] (2003)	Observation data series, referral based N = 10,377; age, 30-85 yr	5	249 all-cause mortality	CAC score an independent predictor of mortality with RR 4.0 for score of 401-1000
Greenland et al[30] (2004)	Prospective population-based study N = 1312; age, >45 yr	7	68 nonfatal MI, 16 deaths	HR of 3.9 for CAC score >301 CAC score able to modify predicted risk obtained from FRS alone (0.73 for FRS alone and 0.78 for FRS and CAC combined)
Arad et al[31] (2005)	Prospective population-based study N = 4613; age, 50 to 70 yr	4.3	40 nonfatal MI, 59 revascularizations, 7 CVA	RR for CAD events with CAC >100 was 11. Overall, it was superior to FRS in prediction of events (ROC curve of 0.79 versus 0.69; $P = 0.006$).
Vliegenthart et al[32] (2005)	Prospective population-based study N = 1795; age, 62 to 85 yr	3.3	40 nonfatal MI, 11 revascularizations, 38 CVA	Compared with those with CAC <100, the RR for events was 3.1, 4.6, and 8.3 for CAC 101-400, 401-1000, and >1000, respectively. There was a statistically significant high relative risk, >8, for those with CAC scores >1000 regardless of Framingham 10-year risk score ≤20% versus >20%.
Taylor et al[33] (2005)	Prospective cohort study 1627 men, 356 women; age, 40 to 50 yr (Army based)	3	9 ACS events	2% of men with CAC had events versus 0.2% without CAC ($P <0.0001$). Controlling for FRS, presence of CAC was associated with an independent 12-fold increase in relative risk. No events in women
LaMonte et al[34] (2005)	Retrospective study 6835 men, 3911 women; age, 22-96 yr	3.5	81 MI/CAD death, 206 revascularizations	Age-adjusted rates per 1000 person-years were computed according to 4 CAC categories: 0 CAC and incremental sex-specific thirds of detectable CAC. The rates were 0.4, 1.5, 4.8, and 8.7 for men and 0.7, 2.3, 3.1, and 6.3 for women.
Anand et al[37] (2006)	Prospective study 510 asymptomatic type 2 diabetic subjects; age, 53 ± 8 yr	2.2	22 (2 coronary deaths, 9 nonfatal MI, 3 ACS, 3 CVA, and 3 late revascularizations)	The overall rate of death or MI by CAC categories (<100, 101-400, 401-1000, and >1000) was 0 (n = 0), 2.6 (n = 2), 13.3 (n = 4), and 17.9% (n = 5), respectively ($P <0.0001$).
Budoff et al[35] (2007)	Observation data series, referral-based N = 25,253; mean age, 65 ± 11 yr	6.8	510 all-cause deaths	Compared with those without CAC, the risk-adjusted relative risk ratios for CAC were 2.2-, 4.5-, 6.4-, 9.2-, 10.4-, and 12.5-fold for scores of 11 to 100, 101 to 299, 300 to 399, 400 to 699, 700 to 999, and >1000, respectively ($P <0.0001$).
Detrano et al[39] (2008)	Prospective population-based study	3.4	162 CHD events (72 myocardial infarctions, 17 CHD deaths, 73 revascularizations)	Overall, the FRS-adjusted risk was 28% higher with doubling of CAC scores. CAC was equally predictive in all ethnic groups.
Becker et al[36] (2008)	Prospective population-based study	3.3	179 (65 cardiac death, 114 MI)	CAC score ≥75th percentile was associated with a significantly higher annualized event rate for MI (3.6% versus 1.6%; $P <0.05$). No cardiac events were observed in patients with CAC = 0.

27

Role of Vascular Computed Tomography in Evaluation and Prevention of Cardiovascular Disease

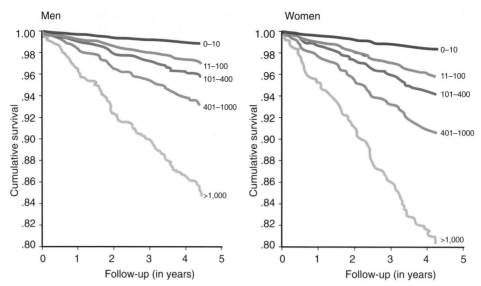

FIGURE 27-2 Risk of total mortality by calcium category in 10,377 asymptomatic individuals. *(From Shaw LJ, Raggi P, Schisterman E, et al: Prognostic value of cardiac risk factors and coronary artery calcium screening for all-cause mortality.* Radiology *228:826, 2003.)*

Summary RR Ratio	CACS	RR	(95% CI)	Events / N Higher Risk	Events / N Low Risk*	P
Average risk	1-112	1.9	(1.3-2.8)	67/9,514	45/12,163	0.001
Moderate risk	100-400	4.3	(3.1-6.1)	110/5,209	49/11,817	<0.0001
High risk	400-999	7.2	(5.2-9.9)	182/3,940	49/8,649	<0.0001
Very high risk	1,000	10.8	(4.2-27.7)	14/196	6/905	<0.0001

Lower risk ⟵ ⟶ Higher risk

FIGURE 27-3 Meta-analysis of relationship of CAC scores (CACS) with CHD outcomes. *(From Greenland P, Bonow RO, Brundage BH, et al: ACCF/AHA 2007 clinical expert consensus document on coronary artery calcium scoring by computed tomography in global cardiovascular risk assessment and in evaluation of patients with chest pain: a report of the American College of Cardiology Foundation Clinical Expert Consensus Task Force [ACCF/AHA Writing Committee to Update the 2000 Expert Consensus Document on Electron Beam Computed Tomography] developed in collaboration with the Society of Atherosclerosis Imaging and Prevention and the Society of Cardiovascular Computed Tomography.* J Am Coll Cardiol *49:378, 2007. Reproduced with permission.)*

models (*P* <0.0001), in which 36% and 34% of MIs occurred in the high-risk cohorts, respectively.

The utility of CAC testing was also recently described in CAD-equivalent individuals, that is, those with diabetes mellitus. Risk factors and CAC scores were prospectively measured in 510 asymptomatic type 2 diabetic subjects (mean age, 53 ± 8 years; 61% men) without prior CVD, with a median follow-up of 2.2 years.[37] In the multivariable model, the CAC score and extent of myocardial ischemia were the only independent predictors of outcome. ROC analysis demonstrated that CAC predicted cardiovascular events with the best area under the curve (0.92), significantly better than the United Kingdom Prospective Diabetes Study risk score (0.74) and Framingham score (0.60). The relative risk to predict a cardiovascular event for a CAC score of 101 to 400 was 10.13, and it increased to 58.05 for scores >1000 (*P* <0.0001). No cardiac events or perfusion abnormalities occurred in subjects with CAC ≤10 Agatston units up until 2 years of follow-up.

These findings were nicely summarized by the AHA/ACC expert consensus document on coronary artery calcium scoring, which took into account many of these studies. Compared with patients with no detectable coronary calcium, the relative risk ratio for CAC 100-400, 401-1000, and >1000 was 4.3 (95% CI, 3.5-5.2; *P* <0.0001), 7.2 (95% CI, 5.2-9.9;

P <0.0001), and 10.8 (95% CI, 4.2-27.7; *P* <0.0001), respectively. Importantly, patients with CAC score of zero have a very low rate of CAD death or MI (0.4%) during 3 to 5 years of observation[38] (Fig. 27-3).

At the same time, critics tend to point to limitations such as potential study generalizability of self-referral cohorts, validity of the risk factor measures and resultant multivariable models used in the studies, and risk of test-induced bias. However, these concerns have been addressed by a report from the Multi-Ethnic Study of Atherosclerosis (MESA), a population-based cohort, which reported the utility of CAC scores in predicting future events. According to Detrano and coworkers,[39] among nearly 6800 asymptomatic individuals observed for a median of 41 months, the hazard ratio for future hard CAD events (MI or MI-related death) with CAC 1-100 versus CAC = 0 was 5.3 (95% CI = 2.4-11.7; *P* <0.0001). The respective hazard ratios with CAC 101-300 and >300 were 10.8 (4.8-24.2; *P* <0.0001) and 12.0 (5.4-26.5; *P* <0.0001), with a 5-year cumulative incidence of CAD events directly associated with higher CAC scores, exceeding 10% in those with scores >300 (Fig. 27-4). These risk ratios are very much similar to those of published studies and confirm the pooled summary findings previously reported and lay to rest any concern about the prognostic value of CAC testing.[38]

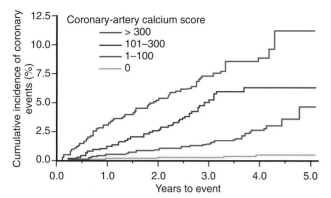

FIGURE 27-4 Cumulative incidence of CAD events according to increasing CAC score categories in the Multi-Ethnic Study of Atherosclerosis. *(From Detrano R, Guerci AD, Carr JJ, et al: Coronary calcium as a predictor of coronary events in four racial or ethnic groups.* N Engl J Med *358:1336, 2008.)*

TABLE 27–2	Prognostic Studies Demonstrating Improved Predicted Outcomes with Use of Coronary Artery Calcium Compared with Traditional Risk Factors		
Study	C-Statistic with Risk Factors, FRS	C-Statistic with Risk Factors, FRS plus CAC	P Value
Arad et al[31] (St. Francis Heart Study)	0.69	0.79	0.0006
Budoff et al[35]	0.611	0.813	<0.0001
Anand et al[37]	0.60	0.92	<0.0001
Becker et al[36]	0.68	0.77	<0.01
Detrano et al[39] (MESA)	0.77	0.82	<0.001

What Is the Value of Testing for Coronary Artery Calcium Across Ethnic and Racial Groups?

Most of the published data to date have related to white populations; however, two studies have addressed the value of CAC in other ethnic groups. First, Nasir and coworkers,[40] in nearly 15,000 ethnically diverse self-referred patients, assessed the role of CAC for the prediction of all-cause mortality. In comparison of prognosis by CAC scores in ethnic minorities and non-Hispanic whites, relative risk ratios were highest for African Americans, with scores ≥400 exceeding 16.1 ($P < 0.0001$). Hispanics with CAC scores ≥400 had relative risk ratios from 7.9 to 9.0; Asians with CAC scores ≥1000 had relative risk ratios 6.6-fold higher than those of non-Hispanic whites ($P <0.0001$). Second, the utility of CAC testing has also been reported in the prospective MESA study.[39] According to Detrano and coworkers, the risk associated with a doubling of the CAC score (a 1-unit increase in $\log_2$ [CAC + 1]) for a hard CAD event was 1.3 (1.2-1.4) in whites, 1.5 (1.3-1.7) in African Americans, 1.3 (1.1-1.5) in Hispanics, and 1.4 (1.1-1.8) in Chinese. These findings firmly establish that CAC scores provide significant information in all four major ethnic groups in the United States.

Does Coronary Artery Calcium Add Incremental Value to Global Risk Estimates?

The extent of CAC has been shown in several studies to predict cardiac events in symptomatic and asymptomatic individuals. However, decisions about the predictive utility of new tests should be based on the *additional* utility of a new test for risk prediction. The most important question about use for primary CAD risk stratification is whether it is predictive above and beyond the current standard risk assessment method of choice, the FRS, which is an inexpensive, easily available, and office-based tool. One way to determine additive utility of a new test is through the use of ROC curve analyses. The ROC curve is a plot of true-positive rate versus false-positive rate over the entire range of possible cutoff values. The area under the ROC curve (AUC) ranges between 1.0 for the perfect test and 0.5 for the useless test.

Studies comparing predictive capacity of conventional and newer biomarkers for prediction of cardiovascular events consistently demonstrate that adding a number of newer biomarkers (such as C-reactive protein, interleukins, and other proposed risk stratifiers) changes the C-statistic by only 0.009

($P = 0.08$). Small changes such as these in the C-statistic suggest limited or modest improvement in risk discrimination with additional risk markers. However, CAC scanning has been shown to markedly improve the C-statistic, suggesting robust improvement in risk discrimination (Table 27-2).

Raggi and colleagues[27] were among the first to assess the added contribution of CAC over and above the FRS. In a study of more than 10,000 asymptomatic individuals observed nearly 5 years, the C-statistic (from ROC curve analyses) for FRS in estimating risk of all-cause death was 0.67 (95% CI, 0.62-0.72; $P <0.0001$) for women and 0.68 (95% CI, 0.64-0.73; $P <0.0001$) for men. When CAC was added to this analysis, the C-statistic increased to 0.75 (95% CI, 0.70-0.80) for women ($P <0.0001$) and 0.72 (95% CI, 0.68-0.77) for men ($P <0.0001$), indicating a significant improvement in mortality prediction.[27]

In a similar fashion, Greenland and coworkers[30] found that the ROC curve for prediction of CAD death or nonfatal MI was 0.68 for FRS plus CAC, which was significantly greater than that of the FRS alone (0.63; $P <0.001$), with increasing levels of CAC associated with greater risk within each FRS group. Importantly, those in the intermediate-risk FRS group with high CAC scores had event rates as high as or higher than those of persons within the high-risk FRS group with lower CAC scores (Fig. 27-5). The recent population-based St. Francis Heart Study of 5585 asymptomatic individuals confirmed the findings of previous reports. The CAC score predicted CAD events independently of standard risk factors and C-reactive protein ($P = 0.004$), was superior to the FRS in the prediction of events (area under ROC curve of 0.79 ± 0.03 versus 0.69 ± 0.03; $P = 0.0006$), and enhanced stratification of those falling into the Framingham categories of low, intermediate, and high risk ($P <0.0001$).[31] Similarly, an improvement in AUC from 0.77 to 0.82 was noted in the landmark MESA study.[39]

More recently, Becker and coworkers[36] demonstrated that among 1726 asymptomatic individuals observed for a median of 40 months, the area under the ROC curve for CAC scores (0.81; 95% CI, 0.78-0.84) was significantly larger than that for the FRS risk (0.63; 95% CI, 0.59-0.65), PROCAM (0.65; 95% CI, 0.6-0.68), and European Society of Cardiology scores (0.66; 95% CI, 0.62-0.6) ($P = 0.03$). Most recently, Polonsky and colleagues reported in the Multiethnic Study of Atherosclerosis that the addition of CAC to models with age, gender, and risk factors resulted in a net reclassification of 0.25 ($P <0.001$), where 23% of subjects with events were reclassified as high risk and 13% of those without events were reclassified as low risk.[40a] In addition, in the Heinz Nixdorf Recall Study of 4129 subjects aged 45-75 without CHD at baseline, the addition of CAC to FRS not only improved the area under the curve from 0.68 to 0.75 ($P <0.003$) but also resulted in a

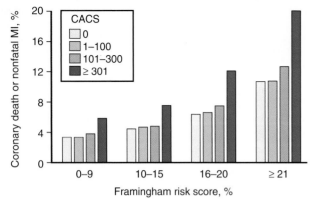

FIGURE 27-5 Predicted 7-year CHD event rates by CAC scores (CACS) within Framingham risk score groups. *(From Greenland P, LaBree L, Azen SP, et al: Coronary artery calcium score combined with Framingham score for risk prediction in asymptomatic individuals.* JAMA 291:210, 2004. *Reproduced with permission.)*

significant net reclassification of 21.7% of patients.[40b] Importantly, these findings not only support the contention that established cardiac risk factors possess a limited ability to quantitate CAD risk but also provide evidence that CAC may add unique information to risk assessment. As we go forward, it will be important to document the degree to which biomarkers or imaging tests, including CAC screening, can appropriately reclassify individuals from standard risk factor assessment for the purposes of more accurately targeting the intensity of treatment.

ABSENCE OF CORONARY ARTERY CALCIFICATION

There is increasing interest in the absence of CAC (a calcium score of zero) as a "negative" cardiovascular risk factor. Absence of CAC may reliably exclude obstructive coronary disease in asymptomatic and selected symptomatic individuals and appears to be associated with a low cardiovascular event rate, suggesting that less aggressive pharmacotherapy may be indicated in this population. However, published event rates for individuals with zero CAC vary, probably because of differences in baseline risk, follow-up period, and outcome ascertainment and verification. Our group has examined the literature for the relevance of the absence of CAC in the context of three major categories: (1) its prognostic utility in categorizing both asymptomatic and symptomatic patients according to their risk for adverse events, (2) its relationship with the presence or absence of significant coronary artery stenosis by invasive coronary angiography, and (3) the degree of myocardial ischemia detected in those with the absence of CAC.

Prognostic Value of Absence of Coronary Artery Calcification in Asymptomatic and Symptomatic Individuals

In our meta-analysis,[41] outcomes consisting of 71,595 *asymptomatic* individuals, 29,312 patients (41%) did not have any evidence of CAC. In a pooled follow-up of 50 months, only 0.47% of asymptomatic individuals without CAC (154 of 29,312) suffered a cardiovascular event during follow-up compared with 4.14% with CAC (1749 of 42,283). In a similar fashion, the meta-analysis revealed that among 3924 symptomatic patients (60% male), 921 patients (23%) did not have any evidence of CAC. In these symptomatic individuals, only 17 of 921 patients (1.8%) without CAC suffered a

cardiovascular event during follow-up of 42 months compared with 270 of 3003 patients (9.0%) with CAC.

Our group has further explored the prognostic value of absence of CAC in two different cohorts. Blaha and associates[42] showed that in a cohort of 44,052 asymptomatic middle-aged patients free of known CAD observed for up to 13 years, a CAC score of zero was associated with excellent survival, with all-cause mortality rates of 0.87 per 1000 person-years (<1% 10-year risk, or <0.1% per year). In a similar fashion, Budoff and colleagues,[43] in a multiethnic prospective cohort, demonstrated that those individuals with calcium scores of zero had a remarkably low rate of cardiovascular events. In a median of 4.1 years of follow-up, the event rate for hard CAD with CAC = 0 was 0.74 per 1000 participants (95% CI, 0.40-1.37); whereas for all CAD, those with CAC = 0 had 1.25 (95% CI, 0.78-2.02) events per 1000 person-years at risk.

However, even in the absence of CAC, relatively more events occur among those with higher risk, especially in diabetics and smokers.[42,43] The potential mechanisms may include presence of underlying noncalcified components, rapid development of atherosclerosis, and plaque destabilization. Whereas the relative risk of events is higher in the presence of low CAC, the absolute event rate remains low. In an appropriately selected non–high-risk patient, the absence of CAC could potentially be used as a rationale to emphasize lifestyle therapy, to scale back on costly preventive pharmacotherapy, and to refrain from frequent cardiac imaging and testing.

Given the low 1% 10-year risk in this population, a drug that produces a 30% relative risk reduction would have to be given to more than 300 patients for 10 years to prevent one death (number needed to treat, ~333 for 10 years).[42] Although current guidelines[38] do not recommend that preventive therapies such as lipid-lowering medications be downregulated in the absence of CAC, emerging data[41-43] suggest that aggressive management in this cohort is not warranted if one does not qualify according to NCEP guidelines. As such, physicians may consider emphasizing appropriate lifestyle therapy, using less pharmacotherapy, and not ordering costly cardiac imaging studies if there is no concerning history of exertional symptoms. This would allow those with the absence of CAC to follow healthy lifestyle modifications with little or no medical therapy, whereas intense therapy is focused on a smaller population of patients with an actual higher risk of events as demonstrated by increasing atherosclerotic burden. However, we do stress that individuals who smoke and have diabetes, even in the absence of CAC, should be treated according to existing guidelines.

Significant Coronary Artery Disease and Myocardial Ischemia in the Absence of Coronary Artery Calcification

Significant coronary artery stenosis (>50%) by angiography is frequently associated with the presence of CAC as assessed by EBT. The severity of angiographic coronary artery stenosis is not directly related to the total CAC. However, the absence of CAC can be extremely useful to rule out significant CAD among individuals presenting with chest pain. Our meta-analysis has shown that individuals with zero CAC are extremely unlikely to have obstructive coronary disease.[41] In our pooled analysis of 10,355 symptomatic patients who underwent coronary angiography (1941 with no CAC), the presence of CAC was highly sensitive (98%) in predicting a luminal stenosis >50% in any coronary artery, although the specificity was low (40%). Conversely, the absence of CAC had a high negative predictive value (93%) for ruling out any clinically significant coronary stenosis.[41] These data are consistent with direct pathologic comparisons.[16]

In fact, recent ACC/AHA guidelines also consider that "for the symptomatic patient, exclusion of measurable coronary calcium may be an effective filter before undertaking invasive diagnostic procedures or hospital admission."[38] Although absence of CAC is associated with a very low likelihood of significant CAD, approximately 2% of symptomatic individuals with significant CAD do not have evidence of CAC. These individuals (i.e., significant CAD without CAC) tend to be younger than 50 years.[44,45] As a result, one must exercise caution when evaluating younger patients for significant CAD in the absence of CAC.

Whereas the absence of calcification shows exceptional ability to predict the absence of a significant stenosis, the ability of CAC to predict myocardial ischemia by myocardial perfusion imaging is also encouraging although somewhat more modest. CAC scores below 100 are associated with a very low risk of cardiac ischemia,[46] which increases dramatically, especially when CAC scores are 400 or higher; however, the prevalence of other clinical conditions, such as metabolic syndrome or diabetes, may lower the threshold for identification by CAC of an increased likelihood of myocardial ischemia.[47] In nine studies examining 4870 patients referred for perfusion stress testing (1225 with no CAC), just 6% had evidence of ischemia.[41] The recent ACC/ASNC appropriateness criteria state that a low calcium score (especially in the absence of CAC) generally precludes the need for assessment by myocardial perfusion imaging.[48]

Ruling Out Acute Coronary Syndrome in the Absence of Coronary Artery Calcification

A pooled meta-analysis was composed of 431 patients complaining of acute chest pain with negative troponins and equivocal ECG findings based on three published studies.[41] The cohort consisted of 48% men (mean age, 51.4 years). There were only 2 of 183 patients (1.1%) without any CAC who were diagnosed with an acute coronary syndrome (ACS). Of the 248 patients with a positive CAC score, 77 (31%) were found to have an ACS. Overall, a positive CAC score had 99% sensitivity, 57% specificity, 24% positive predictive value, and 99% negative predictive value for the evaluation of ACS. The high sensitivity and negative predictive value may allow early discharge of those patients with nondiagnostic ECG findings and negative CAC score (score = 0). Long-term follow-up of this cohort demonstrates that patients without CAC at the time of the emergency visit are at very low risk of subsequent events.[49]

However, the current state of the literature is certainly small and inconclusive with respect to this important clinical entity. Whereas CAC can serve as a useful marker for exclusion of ACS in patients presenting to the emergency department, further studies in larger cohorts need to be done to establish its role in a clinical paradigm, especially with the excellent depiction not only of coronary anatomy but also of left ventricular function by contrast-enhanced coronary CT angiography.[41]

WHO ARE CANDIDATES FOR CORONARY ARTERY CALCIUM TESTING?

In 2007, the expert consensus document by the American College of Cardiology Foundation and the American Heart Association made recommendations to provide a perspective on the current state of the role of CAC testing in clinical practice. The consensus was that it may be reasonable to

consider use of CAC measurement in asymptomatic individuals who are at intermediate risk by the FRS.[38] This conclusion was based on the possibility that such individuals might be reclassified to a higher risk status on the basis of high CAC score and that subsequent patient management may be modified. However, at the same time, the committee did not find enough evidence for the utility of CAC testing in further risk stratification of those considered at low risk as well as of those considered at high risk for CAD in the next 10 years.

As far as those with 10-year risk >20%, they already meet eligibility criteria for aggressive lipid-lowering management with optional LDL-C goals of <70 mg/dL, and further CAC testing may not lead to changes in treatment goals. However, although recent guidelines have not recommended CAC testing for those with a 10-year estimated risk of <10% (low risk),[38] evidence is accumulating that such an approach may be problematic for the following reasons. If these guidelines are followed, most nondiabetic women who are younger than 70 years would not be candidates for further risk stratification with CAC testing, whereas the majority of men above 60 years will be candidates for further risk stratification.[50] Thus, a large number of women at higher risk for CAD risk may never become candidates for CAC testing. At the same time, the practicality of conducting additional screening for all such women becomes an important question. The important point is that those at <10% 10-year risk of CHD are frequently at significant longer term risk of CHD, warranting that this issue be revisited.

One approach would be to identify a subgroup of women in a low-risk group who are more likely to harbor significant CAC. Testing them may potentially be a cost-effective approach. Emerging evidence has strongly implicated the family history of premature CAD to be an independent risk factor associated strongly with higher burden of subclinical atherosclerosis[51-53]; however, a positive family history of CAD does not factor into most global risk algorithms, such as the FRS. Nasir and coworkers[51] demonstrated that among those with premature family history of CAD (especially with sibling history), nearly one third to one quarter of self-referred patients with no or one CAD risk factor had CAC ≥100. In a similar fashion, in the MESA cohort, at least 25% of individuals with family history of premature CAD had significant CAC.[52] In addition, it has been shown that among women with a family history of premature CAD along with multiple metabolic risk factors, a subgroup of women with FRS <10% will have significant atherosclerosis.[53]

Alternatively, based on the 2003 American College of Cardiology Bethesda Conference on atherosclerosis imaging, intermediate-risk groups could be reclassified as those at 6% to 20% risk, at least for women.[54] This strategy will identify more higher risk women who would not be placed in the intermediate-risk group, thus with lower thresholds for risk factor modification, especially regarding LDL-C control. Such persons may benefit from aggressive preventive strategies, such as statin, aspirin, and possibly blood pressure–lowering therapies, especially subsets in which the absolute risk of CAD events is increased, such as those who additionally have increased levels of CAC. Figure 27-6 provides a schematic algorithm to identify ideal candidates for CAC testing.

TRACKING PROGRESSION OF CORONARY ARTERY CALCIUM SCORES

A proposed use of CAC screening is to track atherosclerotic changes over time by serial measurements. There are several published studies of outcomes related to CAC progression. The first retrospective study demonstrated in 817 persons that CAC progression was greatest in those who experienced

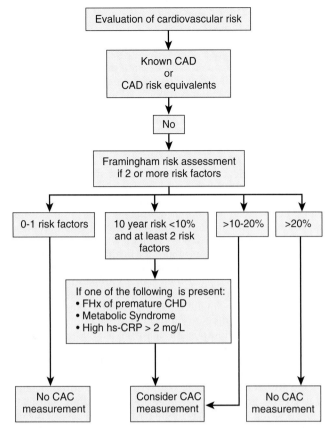

FIGURE 27-6 Schematic algorithm for identification of ideal candidates for CAC screening.

statins, representing a 61% decrease in the rate of progression with statin treatment. Similarly, Achenbach and colleagues[58] showed that with a standard dose of 0.3 mg/day of open-label cerivastatin in 66 dyslipidemic patients, the median annual relative increase in CAC scores was 25% during the untreated period before study entry versus 9% during the treatment period (P <0.0001). Reduction of CAC score was most prominent in those patients who achieved an LDL level <100 mg/dL.

However, to date, these results have not been replicated in randomized controlled trials. The SALTIRE trial (Scottish Aortic Stenosis and Lipid Lowering Trial, Impact on Regression) randomized 102 patients to atorvastatin or placebo and assessed CAC progression during an average follow-up of 2 years. Despite a significant reduction in LDL and C-reactive protein levels, there was a nonsignificant increase in percentage CAC progression (26%/year with atorvastatin versus 18%/year with placebo).[59] Schmermund and coworkers[60] also failed to show reduced progression of CAC in 366 asymptomatic patients randomized to either 10 mg or 80 mg of atorvastatin during 12 months. This was despite a 20% additional reduction in LDL level in the 80-mg atorvastatin treatment group. Similarly, the BELLES (Beyond Endorsed Lipid Lowering with EBCT Scanning) study, which randomized hyperlipidemic postmenopausal women to atorvastatin 80 mg or pravastatin 40 mg, found no effect on CAC progression in both arms. Although atorvastatin reduced LDL concentration by 47% ± 20% and pravastatin reduced LDL by 25% ± 19%, there was no significant difference in CAC progression after 12 months, with an increase of 15% and 14% in CAC scores noted in the atorvastatin and pravastatin arms, respectively.[61]

The St. Francis Heart Study is the only trial relating statin therapy and CAC progression to cardiac events.[62] This was a double-blind, randomized, controlled trial of atorvastatin 20 mg daily, vitamin C 1 g daily, and vitamin E (alpha-tocopherol) 1000 units daily versus matching placebos in 1005 patients with coronary calcium scores at or above the 80th percentile for age and gender. Despite significant reductions in LDL and triglyceride levels during a mean treatment course of 4.3 years, there was no effect on CAC progression. However, there was a significant 42% reduction in events in treated patients who had CAC scores ≥400 (8.7% versus 15.0%; P = 0.046).[62]

We believe more data are needed to justify the incremental population exposure to radiation and the cost associated with a repeated CT test to assess "change" until it is better understood what therapies may be of benefit and how clinicians should use these data in clinical practice. MESA and other population-based studies are evaluating the prognostic value of change of CAC. Until then, consensus guidelines do not support serial measurement of CAC for the purposes of tracking the effects of therapeutic interventions.[38]

a future MI.[55] A second study measured the change in CAC in 495 asymptomatic subjects submitted to sequential CT scanning. The associated relative risk for acute MI for patients exhibiting ≥15% CAC progression was elevated 17.2-fold (95% CI, 4.1 to 71.2) compared with those without CAC progression (P <0.0001).

A large prospective study using CT to measure progression of CAC has also been reported. This study was designed as a clinical trial to evaluate the impact of aggressive lipid-lowering and antioxidant therapy on the progression of CAC in 4613 asymptomatic persons aged 50 to 70 years, with EBT scanning of the coronary arteries at baseline and again at 2 years and follow-up for 4.3 years.[31] Whereas the intervention failed to significantly affect progression of CAC, those who sustained a coronary event had a median increase in CAC score of 247 compared with only 4 in those who did not sustain a coronary event at any time during the study. Multiple logistic regression demonstrated that only age (P = 0.03), male gender (P = 0.04), LDL-C (P = 0.01), HDL-C (P = 0.04), and 2-year change in calcium score (P = 0.0001) were significantly associated with subsequent CAD events. Increasing calcium scores were most strongly related to coronary events in this clinical study, similar to prior observational studies.

The effect of therapeutic intervention, especially statins, on rate of progression of CAC is controversial. The earlier published retrospective and prospective cohort studies suggested a reduction in the rate of CAC progression. Callister and associates,[56] who retrospectively studied 149 asymptomatic patients referred for sequential EBT scans at least 1 year apart, demonstrated a 45% slowing in the rate of CAC progression in those receiving statins. Budoff and coworkers,[57] in one of the first prospective studies in this regard, demonstrated that rate of CAC progression was 39% in those patients with dyslipidemia versus 15% in those receiving

CORONARY ARTERY CALCIUM TESTING AND DOWNSTREAM MEDICATION INITIATION AND ADHERENCE

Adequate control of risk factors with behavioral modification and medications to control lipids, blood pressure, and other risk factors in asymptomatic patients has been the cornerstone of preventive efforts to reduce the occurrence of cardiovascular events. Among individuals with higher CAD risk, such as those with elevated CAC, these established preventive therapies are appropriate interventions. Emerging evidence also indicates that CAC may be associated with initiation of and improved adherence with cardioprotective medications. For example, Wong and coworkers,[63] in a retrospective study of 703 self-referred adults, reported that the extent of CAC is independently associated with beginning of lipid-lowering medications and aspirin as well as with initiation of healthful lifestyle changes, including losing weight and decreasing dietary fat. Taylor and colleagues,[64] who compared statin and aspirin use in 1640 young men, reported that at 6-year follow-up after a CAC test, statin use was threefold more likely among those with any CAC compared with CAC = 0 (48% versus 15%; P <0.001) and aspirin use was nearly twice as likely (53% versus 32%; P <0.01). Our group has also previously shown that those with elevated CAC scores are almost three times more likely to initiate aspirin therapy compared with subjects with absent CAC scores.[65] Overall, aspirin initiation was lowest (29%) among those with CAC = 0 and gradually increased with higher CAC scores (1 to 99, 55%; 100 to 399, 61%; ≥400, 63%; P <0.001 for trend). In a multiethnic cohort, Nasir and colleagues[66] demonstrated that after demographics, CAD risk factors, and socioeconomic factors are taken into account, a high CAC score (>400) is associated with a 32% to 55% higher likelihood of initiation of these cardioprotective medications in a mean follow-up of 1.6 years.

Although there appears to be a consistent relationship of elevated CAC scores with initiation of preventive therapies, data on whether atherosclerosis imaging improves medication adherence are conflicting. Our group reported in a study of 505 asymptomatic individuals that continuation of lipid-lowering medication was lowest (44%) among those with a CAC score in the first quartile (0-30), whereas 91% of individuals with a baseline CAC score in the fourth quartile (>526) adhered to lipid-lowering medication.[67] In multivariable analysis, after adjustment for cardiovascular risk factors, age, and gender, higher baseline CAC scores were strongly associated with adherence to statin therapy. However, no significant differences were noted in continuation of either lipid-lowering medication (87% versus 79%; P = 0.06) or aspirin (79% versus 83%; P = 0.36) according to presence or absence of CAC. Nasir and colleagues[66] showed that the risk ratios for medication continuation with elevated CAC scores were 1.10 (95% CI, 1.01-1.20) for lipid-lowering medication, 1.05 (1.02-1.08) for blood pressure–lowering medication, and 1.14 (1.04-1.25) for aspirin initiation. Moreover, in the only published randomized clinical trial assessing the effects of CAC scanning on estimated risk of CAD after 1 year determined by changes in FRS,[68] there was no difference in mean absolute risk change in 10-year FRS (+0.30 versus +0.36; P = 0.81) comparing overall groups who received CAC score results with those who did not; however, those who received intensive case management of risk factors versus usual care had a significantly better outcome (change in FRS of −0.06 versus +0.74; P = 0.003). In this study, the prevalence of CAC was fairly low (15%), with generally low CAC scores in those with CAC; thus, it is possible that power was limited to impact on change in risk among most of the participants who did not have CAC.

In general, we think that CAC assessment not only may have a role in diagnosis of coronary atherosclerosis but also may improve the likelihood of individuals at highest risk of coronary events to be on appropriate preventive medication. Emerging evidence indicates that the rate of use of these medications in the group that would most likely benefit from lipid-lowering therapy (those patients with increased levels of subclinical atherosclerosis) is substantially higher. The results of these studies in general suggest that CAC found on cardiac CT may add much needed motivation to asymptomatic patients recommended for lifestyle modification and drug therapy; however, properly designed randomized trials remain necessary to evaluate the true role of CAC testing in improving clinical outcomes that may be a result of any such risk factor modification efforts.

CORONARY ARTERY CALCIUM TESTING AND DOWNSTREAM TESTING AND COSTS

From a societal standpoint, apart from the ability of CAC testing to predict future CAD outcomes, a key point to be demonstrated is that atherosclerosis imaging for adults will not lead to a cascade of costly downstream testing. This issue becomes even more relevant in the current economic climate, and there are active governmental efforts to curtail health care expenditures.[69] Shaw and coworkers[70] showed that the majority of individuals who had either no CAC or minimal CAC scores of 1 to 10 had very few downstream additional cardiac tests, whereas the majority of testing was performed in those with advanced CAC. Noninvasive testing was infrequent and medical costs were low among subjects with low CAC scores, both rising progressively with increasing CAC scores (P < 0.001), particularly in the 31 (2.2% of subjects) who had CAC scores ≥1000. Similarly, invasive coronary angiography rose progressively with increasing scores (P <0.001) but occurred exclusively among subjects first undergoing noninvasive testing and overall was performed in only 19.4% of subjects with CAC scores ≥1000. It was clearly shown that invasive procedures were not performed immediately after CAC testing, and they were performed in a stepwise manner preceded by functional imaging with either exercise stress testing or stress myocardial perfusion imaging.[70]

On the basis of our assumptions derived from the MESA study, among every 100 individuals screened for CAC, only 8 would have CAC scores ≥400, with the majority of these eventually undergoing stress echocardiography or myocardial perfusion testing (5 to 7 individuals) and nearly half undergoing invasive coronary angiography (approximately 4 individuals). In comparison, only 14 individuals of the 78 of 100 screened with CAC scores of 0 to 10 would undergo some sort of stress imaging, and only 1 will proceed with invasive coronary angiography in 6 years of follow-up. For the majority of individuals with no or low CAC (78% of those screened with CAC), the median costs were minimal ($25 to $35), mostly incurred by ECG testing, which is often part of the initial assessment of individuals with hypertension (a feature observed in nearly 60% of this low-risk group).[69]

Although the emerging data are encouraging, we hope that the various stakeholders in determining health care resource allocation will quickly move in the direction of addressing whether selective use of atherosclerosis imaging should play any role in halting the epidemic of atherosclerotic vascular disease by better refining which middle-aged and older adults are truly at relatively high risk versus very low risk for a CVD event during the next 5 to 10 years. There is an urgent need of a randomized trial that compares the current traditional risk factors–based approach with one supplemented by subclinical atherosclerotic screening to determine whether this approach can save lives in a manner that is at least moderately cost-effective.

USING INFORMATION FROM CORONARY ARTERY CALCIUM TESTING TO MODIFY TREATMENT

Incorporation of CAC into preventive strategies applied in the context of conventional clinical profiles can potentially refine risk definition or understanding of the consequences of risk factors into a more complete or comprehensive assessment in any given person. At the moment, we have proposed that the CAC scoring can be used to modify the number of points assigned to chronologic age in determining global risk

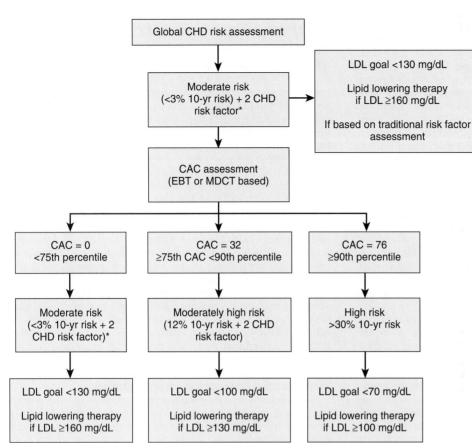

* If only one risk factor, then LDL goals <160 mg/dL in presence of 10-year risk <10%

FIGURE 27-7 Incorporation of the CAC score with global risk assessment for a 40-year-old asymptomatic man, past but not current smoker, no diabetes, with total cholesterol of 205 mg/dL and HDL of 41 mg/dL, and mild untreated hypertension [systolic blood pressure of 150 mm Hg].

assessment, such as in the Framingham risk or European risk score estimates, for more accurate prediction of 10-year cardiovascular risk.[71] The use of CAC scoring in combination with conventional risk factor assessment to define a "modified" FRS allows the inclusion of subclinical disease definition into the context of modifiable risk factors.

Merely finding subclinical disease does not imply which treatable factors require modification. Merely establishing an elevated blood cholesterol level or smoking status does not imply that these factors have contributed to the actual development of disease because genetics and other unidentified factors will also influence the presence of disease in any given individual. In the FRS, age can be largely considered a proxy for the atherosclerotic burden, which increases progressively with age but may vary greatly between individuals. The employment of CAC scores to identify the "heart age" allows accounting for the variability in atherosclerotic burden at a given age and can be easily incorporated into FRS as well as the NCEP guidelines.

An example of the incorporation of the CAC score with estimation of global risk score is shown in Figure 27-7. For example, in a person determined to be at low risk by global risk assessment, consistent with high event rates associated with higher CAC burden, it seems appropriate to initiate drug therapy at lower thresholds of LDL-C (e.g., 130 mg/dL instead of 160 mg/dL) in those with CAC scores in the ≥75th percentile group and at even lower cut points (e.g., 100 mg/dL) when CAC is ≥90th percentile for age or gender in the presence of multiple risk factors. This is especially true among individuals with a strong family history of premature CAD as

they tend to have higher CAD event rates even at lower levels of predicted risk. In these persons, especially with CAC scores >400, further evaluation by functional testing, such as myocardial perfusion imaging, may be considered.

Use of cardiac CT screening, even at as high a cost as $500 per study, will still be about half the cost of a brand name statin therapy for a year. In recent years, many cities and academic centers charge $100 or less for a coronary calcium scan. Identification of those with no or very mild CAC as those in whom a more conservative LDL goal may be acceptable has been previously suggested to provide a cost-effective use of EBT/CT technology in clinical practice.[72]

CONTRAST-ENHANCED CORONARY COMPUTED TOMOGRAPHY: ASSESSMENT OF NATIVE CORONARY ARTERIES

The explosive growth of cardiovascular imaging during the past few decades has facilitated the noninvasive detection of CAD. Although the CAC score correlates well with disease burden, calcified plaques represent only a portion of the total atherosclerosis plaque burden.[15] With the advent of multislice CT technology, coronary computed tomographic angiography (CTA) has the potential to provide comprehensive information about the location, severity, and characteristics of atherosclerotic plaque. It is able to differentiate plaques that are calcified, noncalcified, and mixed (containing both components).[73] As the reliability of MDCT in the detection and grading of coronary artery stenosis has been established, the challenge now is to define the ability of this diagnostic tool to distinguish the coronary artery plaque prone to rupture with findings suggestive of instability. In the following section, we describe briefly the image acquisition and analyses and mainly elucidate our current understanding, explore the relationship of plaque subtypes with current and future cardiovascular risk, and assess the potential role of CTA in primary preventive strategies.

Image Acquisition

MDCT scanners produce images by rotating an x-ray tube around a circular gantry through which the patient advances on a moving table. Pitch is the speed of the table relative to the speed of the gantry rotation, which allows each cross-sectional level of the heart to be imaged during more than one cardiac cycle. The number of image slices acquired during each gantry rotation (4 to 320) determines the overall duration of the MDCT scan. Developments in MDCT technology have led to the rapid advancement from 4-slice MDCT machines in 1998 to 64-multislice scanners available for clinical use in 2004.[24] The current 64-slice MDCT systems are capable of simultaneously acquiring 64 sections of the heart with the fastest gantry speeds of 330 msec per rotation. The increased numbers of detectors have greater craniocaudal coverage per rotation, which results in faster scan times and allows the entire cardiac anatomy to be imaged in less than 10 seconds.

Cardiac CT is performed with ECG gating in a prospective or retrospective mode. ECG gating synchronizes image acquisition with the cardiac cycle. The optimal phase or interval for image analysis is the period during which the heart is the least mobile (usually end diastole) and the least degraded by motion artifact. Prospective ECG gating entails scan initiation at a defined interval after the R wave, continues for a pre-specified duration, and then stops until the same optimal period is reached in the subsequent cardiac cycle, at which time scanning resumes.

Retrospective ECG gating employs continuous acquisition of images throughout the cardiac cycle. The images from multiple consecutive heartbeats are then reconstructed at various percentages of the R-R interval (e.g., from 0% to 90% of the R-R cycle at 10% intervals). With retrospective gating, several thousand images can be acquired during a single cardiac study, allowing the interpreting physician to select the images with the least amount of motion-related distortion before final image reconstruction. Gating is the most advantageous at slow heart rates (less than 60 beats/min), when the R-R interval is >1000 msec and the fastest imaging protocols are used.

Cardiac motion is minimized with the oral or intravenous administration of beta blockers before scanning, thereby reducing the heart rate and prolonging the time during the cardiac cycle at which coronary artery velocity is low. For those individuals without contraindication to beta blockade, these drugs are the medication of choice because they not only decrease the heart rate through the reduction of sympathetic tone but also may reduce the number of premature atrial or ventricular beats, which adversely affect the overall quality of the images. Another crucial element for high-quality coronary images to be obtained is maximal dilation of the coronary vessels with nitroglycerin through the use of sublingual tablets or spray. Respiratory motion is excluded by performance of the scan during a breath-hold.

Coronary CTA requires the intravenous administration of an iodinated contrast medium (which is contraindicated in persons with renal impairment). Approximately 50 to 100 mL of contrast medium is necessary for adequate coronary artery enhancement. The accurate timing of image acquisition relative to the injection of contrast material is a major determinant of overall image quality. A test bolus or bolus tracking technique is used to optimize this timing by determining the amount of time necessary to peak enhancement in the aorta.

Advancements in MDCT technology have led to shorter scan times, reduced breath-hold duration, smaller injections of intravenous contrast material, and decreased motion-related artifacts, resulting in lower radiation exposure and improved diagnostic accuracy.

Image Interpretation

The coronary vasculature on cardiac CTA is evaluated through axial images, multiplanar (coronal, sagittal, or oblique) reformations, and three-dimensional data sets constructed from specific phases during the cardiac cycle. Maximum intensity projection images allow the evaluation of longer segments of the coronary vessels but can be limited by overlapping structures adjacent to the artery of interest. Curved multiplanar reformations are reconstructed on a plane to fit a curve and allow display of the entire vessel in a single image. Three-dimensional volume-rendered images are useful for selection of images with the least motion artifact and for assessment of the relationships among different anatomic structures. Most assessments of plaque, however, have been qualitative in nature, and there is yet to be any reliable software that can reproducibly quantitate the amounts of soft or mixed plaque burden and that is not cumbersome to use.

Association of CTA-Detected Plaque Subtypes with Traditional Risk Factors

There has been increasing interest in the detection and quantitation of plaque subtypes by CTA, including calcified, mixed, and noncalcified plaque. Figure 27-8 shows examples of CTA-assessed calcified and noncalcified plaque, including correlation with intravascular ultrasound (Fig. 27-8A). Figure 27-9 shows a volume-rendered image demonstrating severe coronary atherosclerosis affecting the distal left main, proximal left anterior descending, and first diagonal and the proximal right coronary artery. Few studies have assessed the relationship of traditional risk factors with coronary plaque subtypes determined on CTA.[74-80] Rivera and associates[74] reported on the relationship of traditional cardiovascular risk factors with the presence and burden of plaque subtypes in more than 1000 asymptomatic Korean individuals who underwent CTA. In agreement with what has been previously shown with CAC, age and male gender were overall the strongest predictors for the presence of any plaque as well as for an increased burden of calcified, mixed, or noncalcified plaque. The study found that specific plaque types are more strongly associated with certain risk factors. For example, age and hypertension were the strongest predictors of mixed plaque burden, whereas smoking was strongly associated with the burden of noncalcified plaque; LDL-C related only to the presence and burden of mixed plaque.

It is also well known that individuals with diabetes have a significantly higher risk for the development of coronary events. For this reason, there is increased interest in the noninvasive assessment of coronary plaque in this population of patients. It is postulated that underlying coronary plaque differences may in part explain the increased risk of CVD in this vulnerable group. Our group assessed 416 symptomatic patients (64% men; mean age, 61 ± 13 years), with 61 (15%) reporting type 2 diabetes, who underwent CTA. Enrolled patients had an intermediate pretest probability of obstructive CAD.[77] Patients with diabetes had a higher number of coronary segments with mixed plaques compared with

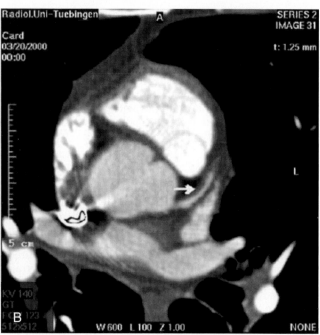

FIGURE 27-8 A, Correlation of CTA of the coronary arteries with intravascular ultrasound illustrates the ability of MDCT to demonstrate calcified and noncalcified coronary plaques. **B,** Noncalcified, soft, lipid-rich plaque in left anterior descending artery (arrow) (Somatom Sensation 4, 120 mL Imeron 400). The plaque was confirmed by intravascular ultrasound. (**A** from Becker CR, Ohnesorge BM, Schoepf UJ, Reiser MF: Current development of cardiac imaging with multidetector-row CT. Eur J Radiol 36:97, 2000. **B** from Kopp AF, Küttner A, Trabold T, et al: Multislice CT in cardiac and coronary angiography. Br J Radiol 77:S87, 2004. Reproduced with permission.)

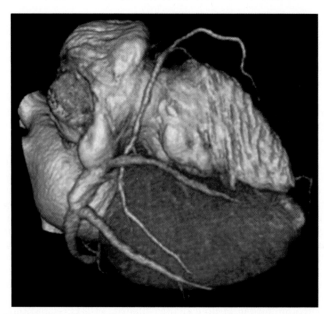

FIGURE 27-9 Volume-rendered image from 16-slice Toshiba Aquilion multidetector scanner showing distal right coronary artery and veins. Severe coronary atherosclerosis, with significant obstructions affecting the distal left main, proximal left anterior descending, and first diagonal and the proximal right coronary artery. (Courtesy of Toshiba, Inc.)

nondiabetic patients (1.67 ± 2.01 versus 1.23 ± 1.61; $P = 0.05$), whereas no such differences were observed for noncalcified and calcified components. Even after traditional risk factors were taken into account, patients with diabetes were more likely to have an elevated burden (three or more segments) of mixed coronary plaque (odds ratio, 2.34; 95% CI, 1.14-4.83). On the other hand, no significant burden association

was observed with noncalcified (0.38; 95% CI, 0.08-1.71) or calcified (0.98; 95% CI, 0.50-1.95) plaques.

Similar findings have also been reported by Rivera and associates,[78] who studied 217 asymptomatic Korean outpatients with type 2 diabetes who had no prior history of CAD. A total of 138 individuals (64%) had occult CAD (any plaque) on CTA. Similar to prior reports, most subjects (62 of 138; 45%) had a combination of noncalcified, calcified, and mixed coronary plaques, whereas exclusively noncalcified, calcified, and mixed plaques were seen in 9% (13 of 138), 20% (27 of 138), and 26% (36 of 138), respectively.[78] Rivera and associates[79] also investigated the association of coronary plaque subtypes with the level of glycosylated hemoglobin in a group of 906 asymptomatic individuals without diabetes. Unadjusted analyses demonstrated a positive association between increasing levels of hemoglobin A1c and the number of coronary segments with mixed plaques ($P < 0.0001$). After traditional risk factors were taken into account, those with hemoglobin A1c in the highest tertile (5.9% to 7.0%) versus the lowest tertile (<5.4%) had a relative risk of 4.6 (95% CI, 1.3-16.5) of having two or more segments with mixed plaque. No relationship was seen with calcified or noncalcified plaques.

Another key area of interest that relates to coronary plaque morphology is the difference in plaque composition between men and women. This could potentially help determine the natural history of atherosclerosis in the two genders as well as pinpoint the possible difference in prevalence of plaque subtypes. These findings could be relevant, taking into consideration that women at almost all age strata are at a lower risk of experiencing cardiovascular events. Few reports based on intravascular ultrasound studies have identified sex differences in morphology of coronary artery plaques, suggesting that coronary plaques in women contain relatively large amounts of cellular tissue and relatively little dense fibrous tissue and calcium. However, these evaluations are limited by the invasive nature of the procedure as well as by limited assessment of few coronary segments and thus may not reflect differences in the overall plaque burden. Nasir and coworkers[80] demonstrated that among symptomatic individuals undergoing CTA, women presented with a significantly lower mean number of segments containing calcified plaques (1.43 ± 2.04 versus 2.25 ± 2.30; $P = 0.004$) as well as mixed plaques (1.67 ± 1.23 versus 2.25 ± 2.30; $P = 0.05$), whereas no such relationship was seen with noncalcified plaques (0.72 ± 1.01 versus 0.86 ± 1.06; $P = 0.21$). On the other hand, the relative proportion of overall plaque burden was more likely to be noncalcified (40% versus 28%) and less likely to be mixed (22% versus 28%) as well as calcified (38% versus 43%). In other words, despite similar overall noncalcified plaque burden, women were found to have a higher proportion of noncalcified to total plaque (i.e., larger relative burden of noncalcified plaque). The potential mechanisms of the higher proportion of noncalcified plaque in women are not entirely clear, and further research is needed into whether endogenous hormonal factors, such as estrogen, may play a role.

Association of CTA-Detected Plaque Subtypes with Myocardial Perfusion Defects

Detection of myocardial perfusion abnormalities in a noninvasive manner by modalities such as single-photon emission computed tomography (SPECT) is a method for identification of high-risk patients and stratification according to cardiovascular prognosis. In one study, Lin and colleagues[81] evaluated 163 consecutive low- to intermediate-risk symptomatic patients without known CAD who underwent both stress SPECT and MDCT. Overall, 33 (17%) had a summed stress score of >8 (abnormal myocardial perfusion). Among individuals with a summed stress score >8 versus ≤8, a significant difference only in the number of mixed plaques was reported (2.10 ± 2.50 versus 1.16 ± 1.69; $P = 0.01$), whereas no differences were seen in noncalcified (1.03 ± 1.67 versus 0.97 ± 1.44; $P = 0.83$) and calcified (2.10 ± 2.50 versus 1.56 ± 1.59; $P = 0.54$) plaque. In multivariate analyses, adjusting for traditional risk factors, mixed plaque burden remained associated with summed stress score >8 (odds ratio, 1.28; 95% CI, 1.05-1.56). Although the study findings implicate a potential role of assessment of mixed plaque burden, studies are needed to confirm these findings in large heterogeneous populations.

Association of CTA-Detected Plaque Subtypes with Features of Plaque Vulnerability on Intravascular Ultrasound Examination

Autopsy studies have demonstrated that individuals suffering sudden cardiac death have multiple plaques containing a large amount of necrotic core with an overlying thin-cap fibroatheroma, which are traits believed to be linked to plaque rupture.[14] Although intravascular ultrasound is well equipped to assess plaque subtypes as well as thin-cap fibroatheroma, whether certain plaque types now detected on coronary MDCT provide clues to these vulnerability features is not well studied. In a landmark study, Pundziute and coworkers[82] assessed the prevalence of plaque subtypes on MDCT and the relationship with thin-cap fibroatheroma based on intravascular ultrasound in 25 patients with ACS. In these vulnerable patients, 32% of plaques were noncalcified on MDCT and 59% were mixed. More interestingly, intravascular ultrasound–derived thin-cap fibroatheromas were most frequently

observed in lesions classified as mixed (68%) compared with noncalcified (19%) and calcified (13%; $P = 0.001$) on contrast-enhanced MDCT. These findings are consistent with prior invasive report that more plaques with tiny calcific deposits are noted with culprit lesions in ACS patients.[33]

Association of CTA-Detected Plaque Subtypes with Cardiovascular Disease Outcomes

On non–contrast-enhanced cardiac CT, the identification and quantification of CAC provide prognostic information incremental to conventional risk factors in predicting adverse cardiac events. There is significant lack of knowledge about the "prognostic" significance of noncalcified versus calcified plaque detectable with CTA on top of overall plaque burden assessment, for which the CAC score is an excellent surrogate. To date, to the best of our knowledge, only one study has attempted to assess the relationship of coronary plaque subtypes detected by MDCT and future events. Pundziute and coworkers[83] observed a total of 100 symptomatic patients who underwent coronary MDCT for the occurrence of cardiac death, nonfatal MI, unstable angina requiring hospitalization, and revascularization. During a mean follow-up of 16 months, 33 events occurred in 26 patients. Among all plaque subtypes, only mixed plaque burden was associated with adverse events (hazard ratio, 1.6; 95% CI, 1.6-2.0).

In recent years, the development of contrast-enhanced coronary CTA has enabled the identification of different plaque subtypes (exclusively calcified or mixed plaques) and has generated great enthusiasm, given the potential of identifying "vulnerable plaques." The emerging literature provides insights into the relationship between plaque characterization with MDCT and varying clinical scenarios, suggesting that plaque composition could have incremental value and potentially be included in overall risk stratification strategies. Currently, it is not entirely clear whether exclusively calcified or noncalcified plaque subtypes predispose to higher cardiovascular risk; however, data from the limited studies in this regard suggest that mixed plaque burden is more likely to be associated with high-risk groups, such as patients with diabetes mellitus and those with elevated inflammatory biomarkers. In addition, mixed plaque has been shown to be strongly associated with myocardial perfusion defects and features of plaque instability such as thin-cap fibroatheroma. Recently, CT-assessed characteristics such as positive vessel remodeling and low-attenuation plaques have also been shown to be associated with subsequent development of ACS.[84]

Although one small study has suggested mixed plaque burden to predict future outcomes, it is not entirely clear if there is additional prognostic value above and beyond the CAC score, an established marker of future CAD events, especially in the absence of detectable CAC.[85] We believe that large long-term studies are needed to clearly elucidate the role of these plaque subtypes in the overall risk assessment strategies. Until then, we believe the value of plaque assessment by CTA appears to be less on the extremes (noncalcified and calcified), but the eventual prognostic importance of mixed plaque may eventually be seen in future long-term studies.

RADIATION DOSE

Increased awareness of radiation in the medical community and general population has raised warnings about unnecessary testing, especially in the context of CTA, for which the mean doses are rather high compared with some other forms of cardiac testing. Radiation doses with coronary calcium scores are sufficiently low (approximately 1 mSv) with either EBT or MDCT, which is far below background annual radiation exposures.[24] CTA doses for retrospective triggering are in the range of 10 to 18 mSv (which is similar to cardiac nuclear doses). Since the increased awareness and concern about radiation, several radiation dose reduction techniques have been introduced. These include dose modulation (lowers radiation dose 30% to 48%), reduction of kilovoltage to 100 kVp for thinner patients (lowers radiation dose by 40%), limitation of the top and bottom of the scan field (lowers radiation dose by 20%),[86] and prospective triggering (lowers radiation dose by 70%).[87] Collectively, the dose reduction will be approximately 80% to 90%.

One study, without use of any other dose reduction technique except for prospective imaging, reported that the mean radiation dose to the patient was 77% lower for prospective gating (4.2 mSv) than for retrospective gating (18.1 mSv) ($P < 0.01$), without compromising image quality or diagnostic accuracy.[88] Another study similarly reported that use of prospective triggering reduced radiation exposure by 80% without compromising image quality compared with traditional retrospective acquisition.[89]

GUIDELINES FOR CORONARY ARTERY CALCIUM TESTING AND COMPUTED TOMOGRAPHIC ANGIOGRAPHY IN ASYMPTOMATIC INDIVIDUALS

The American Heart Association recommendations for calcium scanning from the 2006 Scientific Statement are summarized as follows: (1) CAC scanning may be suitable in patients at intermediate CAD risk to refine risk prediction and to select patients for altered targets of lipid-lowering therapies; (2) CAC assessment may be reasonable for the assessment of symptomatic patients, especially in the setting of equivocal treadmill or functional testing; and (3) CAC scanning may be considered for triage of patients with chest pain with equivocal or normal electrocardiograms and negative cardiac enzyme studies.[24]

Other scientific statements also have endorsed the conceptual approach to refining the cardiovascular risk assessment through CAC detection. For example, the NCEP ATP III stated that "in persons with multiple risk factors, high coronary calcium scores (e.g., >75th percentile for age and sex) denote advanced coronary atherosclerosis and provide a rationale for intensified LDL-lowering therapy."[8]

A clinical expert consensus document of the American College of Cardiology published in 2007 specified that coronary calcium measurement in clinically selected patients at intermediate CAD risk (e.g., those with a 10% to 20% Framingham 10-year risk score) is a reasonable option to refine clinical risk prediction and to select patients for altered targets for lipid-lowering therapies.[38] The recommendations from the American Heart Association and the American College of Cardiology are similar to those of the European guidelines.[89] The European guidelines state, "The resulting calcium score is an important parameter to detect asymptomatic individuals at high risk for future CVD events, independent of the traditional risk factors." The guidelines state that calcium scanning should be used as a tool to improve risk assessment in individual patients. This organization further acknowledged that the prognostic relevance of CAC has been demonstrated in several prospective studies, not only in asymptomatic individuals but also in patients undergoing coronary angiography. However, screening for CAC should be reserved for individuals at intermediate risk and in men older than 45 years and women older than 55 years.

At the same time, the current guidelines do not recommend the use of CAC scanning in subjects at high risk (e..g, >20% risk of a CAD event in 10 years) or with preexisting CAD or diabetes, for which aggressive guidelines already exist, so results of CAC scanning should not influence therapeutic decisions, or in those at low risk (e.g., population screening in those with <10% risk of a CAD event in 10 years). Moreover, serial imaging for assessment of progression of coronary calcification is not recommended, nor are there any indications for performing CTA for risk assessment in asymptomatic individuals or for monitoring disease progression in any group of patients.[24,38]

CONCLUSION

Global risk assessment seems to underestimate the CAC burden as well as the CVD risk, especially in selected young men and postmenopausal women with multiple risk factors. CAC is an independent predictor of CAD events and provides prognostic information above and beyond the FRS. Assessment of coronary artery calcification with non–contrast-enhanced CT appears to be most predictive among individuals with intermediate risk. Although current recommendations do not support its use as a screening tool in low-risk patients, emerging data suggest that many of these individuals with a family history of premature CAD may potentially benefit from this testing.

At the other end of the spectrum, those with high pretest probability are essentially at CAD-equivalent risk regardless of calcium score, and treatment of risk factors rather than screening would be more appropriate. Integration of the information generated from the FRS with CAC, especially by incorporation of age as another criterion in risk assessment, appears to be an effective system for assessment of actual cardiac risk to optimally target and follow the effect of preventive measures. In addition to providing information on risk stratification, CAC testing may improve adherence to preventive medication use in appropriate high-risk individuals. To date, there does not seem to be evidence for a substantial increase in downstream testing with CAC testing in asymptomatic individuals. There is an important need, however, for randomized clinical trials to better document the clinical utility of both CAC scanning and CTA with respect to clinical outcomes.

REFERENCES

1. Rosamond W, Flegal K, Furie K, et al: Heart disease and stroke statistics—2008 update: a report from the American Heart Association Statistics Committee and Stroke Statistics Subcommittee. *Circulation* 117:e25, 2008.
2. Yusuf S, Reddy S, Ounpuu S, Anand S: Global burden of cardiovascular diseases: part I: general considerations, the epidemiologic transition, risk factors, and impact of urbanization. *Circulation* 104:2746, 2001.
3. Fuster V, Voute J, Hunn M, Smith SC, Jr: Low priority of cardiovascular and chronic diseases on the global health agenda: a cause for concern. *Circulation* 116:1966, 2007.
4. Rosamond WD, Chambless LE, Folsom AR, et al: Trends in the incidence of myocardial infarction and in mortality due to coronary heart disease, 1987 to 1994. *N Engl J Med* 339:861, 1998.
5. Ergin A, Muntner P, Sherwin R, He J: Secular trends in cardiovascular disease mortality, incidence, and case fatality rates in adults in the United States. *Am J Med* 117:219, 2004.
6. Davies AR, Smeeth L, Grundy EM: Contribution of changes in incidence and mortality to trends in the prevalence of coronary heart disease in the UK: 1996-2005. *Eur Heart J* 28:2142, 2007.
7. Ornish D, Scherwitz LW, Billings JH, et al: Intensive lifestyle changes for reversal of coronary heart disease. *JAMA* 280:2001, 1998.
8. Expert Panel on Detection, Evaluation, and Treatment of High Blood Cholesterol in Adults. Executive Summary of the Third Report of the National Cholesterol Program (NCEP) Expert Panel on detection, evaluation and treatment of high blood cholesterol in adults (Adult Treatment Panel III). *JAMA* 285:2486, 2001.
9. Nasir K, Michos ED, Blumenthal RS, Raggi P: Detection of high-risk young adults and women by coronary calcium and National Cholesterol Education Program Panel III guidelines. *J Am Coll Cardiol* 46:1931, 2005.
10. Ford ES, Giles WH, Mokdad AH: The distribution of 10-year risk for coronary heart disease among US adults: findings from the National Health and Nutrition Examination Survey III. *J Am Coll Cardiol* 43:1791, 2004.

27

11. Akosah KO, Schaper A, Cogbill C, Schoenfeld P: Preventing myocardial infarction in the young adult in the first place: how do the National Cholesterol Education Panel III guidelines perform? *J Am Coll Cardiol* 41:1475, 2003.
12. Shaw LJ, Blumenthal RS, Raggi P: Screening asymptomatic low-risk individuals for coronary heart disease: issues and controversies. *J Nucl Cardiol* 11:382, 2004.
13. Kullo IJ, Ballantyne CM: Conditional risk factors for atherosclerosis. *Mayo Clin Proc* 80:219, 2005.
14. Stary HC, Chandler RE, Dinsmore RE, et al: A definition of advanced types of atherosclerotic lesions and a histological classification of atherosclerosis. A report from the Committee on Vascular Lesions of the Council on Arteriosclerosis. American Heart Association. *Circulation* 92:1355, 2005.
15. Budoff MJ, Achenbach S, Duerinckx A: Clinical utility of computed tomography and magnetic resonance techniques for noninvasive coronary angiography. *J Am Coll Cardiol* 42:1867, 2003.
16. Rumberger JA, Simons DB, Fitzpatrick LA, et al: Coronary artery calcium area by electron-beam computed tomography and coronary atherosclerotic plaque area. A histopathologic correlative study. *Circulation* 92:2157, 1995.
17. Rumberger JA, Sheedy PF, Breen JF, Schwartz RS: Electron beam computed tomographic coronary calcium score cutpoints and severity of associated angiographic lumen stenosis. *J Am Coll Cardiol* 29:1542, 1997.
18. Sangiorgi G, Rumberger JA, Severson A, et al: Arterial calcification and not lumen stenosis is highly correlated with atherosclerotic plaque burden in humans: a histologic study of 723 coronary artery segments using nondecalcifying methodology. *J Am Coll Cardiol* 31:126, 1998.
19. Agatston AS, Janowitz WR, Hildner FJ, et al: Quantification of coronary artery calcium using ultrafast computed tomography. *J Am Coll Cardiol* 15:827, 1990.
20. Callister TQ, Cooil B, Raya SP, et al: Coronary artery disease: improved reproducibility of calcium scoring with an electron-beam CT volumetric method. *Radiology* 208:807, 1998.
21. Nasir K, Raggi P, Rumberger JA, et al: Coronary artery calcium volume scores on electron beam tomography in 12,936 asymptomatic adults. *Am J Cardiol* 93:1146, 2004.
22. Mao SS, Pal RS, McKay CR, et al: Comparison of coronary artery calcium scores between electron beam computed tomography and 64-multidetector computed tomographic scanner. *J Comput Assist Tomogr* 33:175, 2009.
23. Daniell AL, Wong ND, Friedman JD, et al: Concordance of coronary calcium estimation between multidetector computed tomography and electron beam tomography. *Am J Roetonogy* 185:1542, 2005.
24. Budoff MJ, Achenbach S, Blumenthal RS, et al: Assessment of coronary artery disease by cardiac computed tomography: a scientific statement from the American Heart Association Committee on Cardiovascular Imaging and Intervention, Council on Cardiovascular Radiology and Intervention, and Committee on Cardiac Imaging, Council on Clinical Cardiology. *Circulation* 114:1761, 2006.
25. Arad Y, Spadaro LA, Goodman K, et al: Prediction of coronary events with electron beam computed tomography. *J Am Coll Cardiol* 36:1253, 2000.
26. Wong ND, Hsu JC, Detrano RC, et al: Coronary artery calcium evaluation by electron beam computed tomography and its relation to new cardiovascular events. *Am J Cardiol* 86:495, 2000.
27. Raggi P, Cooil B, Callister TQ: Use of electron beam tomography data to develop models for prediction of hard coronary events. *Am Heart J* 141:375, 2001.
28. Kondos GT, Hoff JA, Sevrukov A, et al: Electron-beam tomography coronary artery calcium and cardiac events: a 37-month follow-up of 5635 initially asymptomatic low- to intermediate-risk adults. *Circulation* 107:2571, 2003.
29. Shaw LJ, Raggi P, Schisterman E, et al: Prognostic value of cardiac risk factors and coronary artery calcium screening for all-cause mortality. *Radiology* 228:826, 2003.
30. Greenland P, LaBree L, Azen SP, et al: Coronary artery calcium score combined with Framingham score for risk prediction in asymptomatic individuals. *JAMA* 291:210, 2004.
31. Arad Y, Goodman KJ, Roth M, et al: Coronary calcification, coronary disease risk factors, C-reactive protein, and atherosclerotic cardiovascular disease events: the St. Francis Heart Study. *J Am Coll Cardiol* 46:158, 2005.
32. Vliegenthart R, Oudkerk M, Hofman A, et al: Coronary calcification improves cardiovascular risk prediction in the elderly. *Circulation* 112:572, 2005.
33. Taylor AJ, Bindeman J, Feuerstein I, et al: Coronary calcium independently predicts incident premature coronary heart disease over measured cardiovascular risk factors: mean three-year outcomes in the Prospective Army Coronary Calcium (PACC) project. *J Am Coll Cardiol* 46:807, 2005.
34. LaMonte MJ, FitzGerald SJ, Church TS, et al: Coronary artery calcium score and coronary heart disease events in a large cohort of asymptomatic men and women. *Am J Epidemiol* 162:421, 2005.
35. Budoff MJ, Shaw LJ, Liu ST, et al: Long-term prognosis associated with coronary calcification: observations from a registry of 25,253 patients. *J Am Coll Cardiol* 49:1860, 2007.
36. Becker A, Leber A, Becker C, Knez A: Predictive value of coronary calcifications for future cardiac events in asymptomatic individuals. *Am Heart J* 155:154, 2008.
37. Anand DV, Lim E, Hopkins D, et al: Risk stratification in uncomplicated type 2 diabetes: prospective evaluation of the combined use of coronary artery calcium imaging and selective myocardial perfusion scintigraphy. *Eur Heart J* 27:713, 2006.
38. Greenland P, Bonow RO, Brundage BH, et al: ACCF/AHA 2007 clinical expert consensus document on coronary artery calcium scoring by computed tomography in global cardiovascular risk assessment and in evaluation of patients with chest pain: a report of the American College of Cardiology Foundation Clinical Expert Consensus Task Force (ACCF/AHA Writing Committee to Update the 2000 Expert Consensus Document on Electron Beam Computed Tomography) developed in collaboration with the Society of Atherosclerosis Imaging and Prevention and the Society of Cardiovascular Computed Tomography. *J Am Coll Cardiol* 49:378, 2007.
39. Detrano R, Guerci AD, Carr JJ, et al: Coronary calcium as a predictor of coronary events in four racial or ethnic groups. *N Engl J Med* 358:1336, 2008.
40. Nasir K, Shaw LJ, Liu ST, et al: Ethnic differences in the prognostic value of coronary artery calcification for all-cause mortality. *J Am Coll Cardiol* 50:953, 2007.
40a. Polonsky TS, McClelland RL, Jorgensen NW, et al: Coronary artery calcium score and risk classification for coronary heart disease prediction. *JAMA* 303:1610, 2010.
40b. Erbel R, Möhlenkamp S, Moebus S, et al; Heinz Nixdorf Recall Study Investigative Group: Coronary risk stratification, discrimination, and reclassification improvement based on quantification of subclinical coronary atherosclerosis: the Heinz Nixdorf Recall study. *J Am Coll Cardiol* 56:1397, 2010.
41. Sarwar A, Shaw LJ, Shapiro MD, et al: Diagnostic and prognostic value of absence of coronary artery calcification. *JACC Cardiovasc Imaging* 2:675, 2009.
42. Blaha MJ, Budoff MJ, Shaw LJ, et al: Absence of coronary artery calcification and all-cause mortality. *JACC Cardiovasc Imaging* 2:692, 2009.
43. Budoff MJ, McClelland RL, Nasir K, et al: Cardiovascular events with absent or minimal coronary calcification: the Multi-Ethnic Study of Atherosclerosis (MESA). *Am Heart J* 158:554, 2009.
44. Rumberger JA, Sheedy PF 3rd, Breen JF, Schwartz RS: Coronary calcium, as determined by electron beam computed tomography, and coronary disease on arteriogram. Effect of patient's sex on diagnosis. *Circulation* 91:1363, 1995.
45. Budoff MJ, Georgiou D, Brody A, et al: Ultrafast computed tomography as a diagnostic modality in the detection of coronary artery disease: a multicenter study. *Circulation* 93:898, 1996.
46. Berman DS, Wong ND, Gransar H, et al: Relationship between abnormality on stress myocardial perfusion SPECT and extent of atherosclerosis by coronary calcium tomography in patients without known coronary artery disease. *J Am Coll Cardiol* 44:923, 2004.
47. Wong ND, Rozanski AR, Gransar H, et al: Metabolic syndrome increases the likelihood of inducible myocardial ischemia among patients with subclinical atherosclerosis. *Diabetes Care* 28:1445, 2005.
48. Brindis RG, Douglas PS, Hendel RC, et al: ACCF/ASNC appropriateness criteria for single-photon emission computed tomography myocardial perfusion imaging (SPECT MPI): a report of the American College of Cardiology Foundation Quality Strategic Directions Committee Appropriateness Criteria Working Group and the American Society of Nuclear Cardiology endorsed by the American Heart Association. *J Am Coll Cardiol* 46:1587, 2005.
49. Georgiou D, Budoff MJ, Kaufer E, et al: Screening patients with chest pain in the emergency department using electron beam tomography: a follow-up study. *J Am Coll Cardiol* 38:105, 2001.
50. Ford ES, Giles WH, Mokdad AH: The distribution of 10-year risk for coronary heart disease among US adults: findings from the National Health and Nutrition Examination Survey III. *J Am Coll Cardiol* 43:1791, 2004.
51. Nasir K, Michos ED, Rumberger JA, et al: Coronary artery calcification and family history of premature coronary heart disease: sibling history is more strongly associated than parental history. *Circulation* 110:2150, 2004.
52. Nasir K, Budoff MJ, Wong ND, et al: Family history of premature coronary heart disease and coronary artery calcification: Multi-Ethnic Study of Atherosclerosis (MESA). *Circulation* 116:619, 2007.
53. Michos ED, Nasir K, Braunstein JB, et al: Framingham risk equation underestimates subclinical atherosclerosis risk in asymptomatic women. *Atherosclerosis* 184:201, 2006.
54. Wilson PW, Smith SC, Jr, Blumenthal RS, et al: 34th Bethesda Conference: Task force #4—How do we select patients for atherosclerosis imaging? *J Am Coll Cardiol* 41:1898, 2003.
55. Raggi P, Callister TQ, Shaw LJ: Progression of coronary artery calcium and risk of first myocardial infarction in patients receiving cholesterol-lowering therapy. *Arterioscler Thromb Vasc Biol* 24:1272, 2004.
56. Callister TQ, Raggi P, Cooil B, et al: Effect of HMG-CoA reductase inhibitors on coronary artery disease as assessed by electron-beam computed tomography. *N Engl J Med* 339:1972, 1998.
57. Budoff MJ, Lane KL, Bakhsheshi H, et al: Rates of progression of coronary calcium by electron beam tomography. *Am J Cardiol* 86:8, 2000.
58. Achenbach S, Ropers D, Pohle K, et al: Influence of lipid-lowering therapy on the progression of coronary artery calcification: a prospective evaluation. *Circulation* 106:1077, 2002.
59. Houslay ES, Cowell SJ, Prescott RJ, et al: Progressive coronary calcification despite intensive lipid-lowering treatment: a randomised controlled trial. *Heart* 92:1207, 2006.
60. Schmermund A, Achenbach S, Budde T, et al: Effect of intensive versus standard lipid-lowering treatment with atorvastatin on the progression of calcified coronary atherosclerosis over 12 months: a multicenter, randomized, double-blind trial. *Circulation* 113:427, 2006.
61. Raggi P, Davidson M, Callister TQ, et al: Aggressive versus moderate lipid-lowering therapy in hypercholesterolemic postmenopausal women: Beyond Endorsed Lipid Lowering with EBT Scanning (BELLES). *Circulation* 112:563, 2005.
62. Arad Y, Spadaro LA, Roth M, et al: Treatment of asymptomatic adults with elevated coronary calcium scores with atorvastatin, vitamin C, and vitamin E: the St. Francis Heart Study randomized clinical trial. *J Am Coll Cardiol* 46:166, 2005.
63. Wong ND, Detrano RC, Diamond G, et al: Does coronary artery screening by electron beam computed tomography motivate potentially beneficial lifestyle behaviors? *Am J Cardiol* 78:1220, 1996.
64. Taylor A, Bindeman J, Feuerstein I, et al: Community-based provision of statin and aspirin after the detection of coronary artery calcium within a community-based screening cohort. *J Am Coll Cardiol* 51:1337, 2008.
65. Orakzai R, Nasir K, Orakzai S, et al: Effect of patient visualization of coronary calcium by electron beam computed tomography on changes in beneficial lifestyle behaviors. *Am J Cardiol* 101:999, 2008.
66. Nasir K, McClelland R, Blumenthal RS, et al: Coronary artery calcium in relation to initiation and continuation of cardiovascular medications: the Multi-Ethnic Study of Atherosclerosis (MESA). *Circ Cardiovasc Qual Outcomes* 3:228, 2010.

67. Kalia NK, Miller LG, Nasir K, et al: Visualizing coronary calcium is associated with improvements in adherence to statin therapy. *Atherosclerosis* 185:394, 2006.

68. O'Malley PG, Feuerstein IM, Taylor AJ: Impact of electron beam tomography with or without case management on motivation, behavioral change, and cardiovascular risk profile. A randomized controlled trial. *JAMA* 289:2215, 2003.

69. Blumenthal RS, Huang C, Nasir K: Selective use of coronary artery calcium screening: worth the cost? *J Am Coll Cardiol* 54:1268, 2009.

70. Shaw LJ, Min JK, Budoff MJ, et al: Induced cardiovascular procedural costs and resource consumption patterns after coronary artery calcium screening: results from the EISNER (Early Identification of Subclinical Atherosclerosis by Noninvasive Imaging Research) study. *J Am Coll Cardiol* 54:1258, 2009.

71. Nasir K, Vasamreddy C, Blumenthal RS, Rumberger JA: Comprehensive coronary risk determination in prevention: an imaging and clinical based definition combining computed tomographic coronary artery calcium score and Framingham/NCEP risk score. *Int J Cardiol* 110:129, 2006.

72. Rumberger JA: Cost effectiveness of coronary calcification scanning using electron beam tomography in intermediate and high-risk asymptomatic individuals. *J Cardiovasc Risk* 7:113, 2000.

73. Leber AW, Knez A, Becker A, et al: Accuracy of multidetector spiral computed tomography in identifying and differentiating the composition of coronary atherosclerotic plaque: a comparative study with intracoronary ultrasound. *J Am Coll Cardiol* 43:1241, 2004.

74. Rivera JJ, Nasir K, Cox PR, et al: Association of traditional cardiovascular risk factors with coronary plaque sub-types assessed by 64-slice computed tomography angiography in a large cohort of asymptomatic subjects. *Atherosclerosis* 206:451, 2009.

75. Bamberg F, Dannemann N, Shapiro MD, et al: Association between cardiovascular risk profiles and the presence and extent of different types of coronary atherosclerotic plaque as detected by multidetector computed tomography. *Arterioscler Thromb Vasc Biol* 28:568, 2008.

76. Cheng VY, Wolak A, Gutstein A, et al: Low-density lipoprotein and noncalcified coronary plaque composition in patients with newly diagnosed coronary artery disease on computed tomographic angiography. *Am J Cardiol* 105:761, 2010.

77. Ibebuogu UN, Nasir K, Gopal A, et al: Comparison of atherosclerotic plaque burden and composition between diabetic and nondiabetic patients by non invasive CT angiography. *Int J Cardiovasc Imaging* 25:717, 2009.

78. Rivera JJ, Nasir K, Choi EK, et al: Detection of occult coronary artery disease in asymptomatic individuals with diabetes mellitus using non-invasive cardiac angiography. *Atherosclerosis* 203:442, 2009.

79. Rivera JJ, Nasir K, Choi EK, et al: Association between increasing levels of hemoglobin A1c and coronary atherosclerosis in asymptomatic individuals without diabetes mellitus. *Coron Artery Dis* 21:157, 2010.

80. Nasir K, Gopal A, Blankstein R, et al: Noninvasive assessment of gender differences in coronary plaque composition with multidetector computed tomographic angiography. *Am J Cardiol* 105:453, 2010.

81. Lin F, Shaw LJ, Berman DS, et al: Multidetector computed tomography coronary artery plaque predictors of stress-induced myocardial ischemia by SPECT. *Atherosclerosis* 197:700, 2008.

82. Pundziute G, Schuijf JD, Jukema JW, et al: Evaluation of plaque characteristics in acute coronary syndromes: non-invasive assessment with multi-slice computed tomography and invasive evaluation with intravascular ultrasound radiofrequency data analysis. *Eur Heart J* 29:2373, 2008.

83. Pundziute G, Schuijf JD, Jukema JW, et al: Prognostic value of multislice computed tomography coronary angiography in patients with known or suspected coronary artery disease. *J Am Coll Cardiol* 49:62, 2007.

84. Motoyama S, Sarai M, Harigaya H, et al: Computed tomographic angiography characteristics of atherosclerotic plaques subsequently resulting in acute coronary syndrome. *J Am Coll Cardiol* 54:49, 2009.

85. Nasir K, Budoff MJ, Shaw LJ, Blumenthal RS: Value of multislice computed tomography coronary angiography in suspected coronary artery disease. *J Am Coll Cardiol* 49:2070, 2004.

86. Gopal A, Budoff MJ: A new method to reduce radiation exposure during multi-row detector cardiac computed tomographic angiography. *Int J Cardiol* 132:435, 2009.

87. Earls JP, Berman EL, Urban BA, et al: Prospectively gated transverse coronary CT angiography versus retrospectively gated helical technique: improved image quality and reduced radiation dose. *Radiology* 246:742, 2008.

88. Hirai N, Horiguchi J, Fujioka C, et al: Prospective versus retrospective ECG-gated 64-detector coronary CTA: assessment of image quality, stenosis, and radiation dose. *Radiology* 248:424, 2008.

89. De Backer G, Ambrosioni E, Borch-Johnsen K, et al: Third Joint Task Force of European and Other Societies on Cardiovascular Disease Prevention in Clinical Practice: European guidelines on cardiovascular disease prevention in clinical practice. *Eur Heart J* 24:1601, 2003.

27

Use of Cardiac Magnetic Resonance Imaging and Positron Emission Tomography in Assessment of Cardiovascular Disease Risk and Atherosclerosis Progression

Prabhakar Rajiah and Milind Y. Desai

KEY POINTS

- Atherosclerosis is a chronic immunoinflammatory disorder of the vascular, metabolic, and immune systems.

- Detection of subclinical atherosclerotic disease will enable initiation of earlier treatment and prevent the progression of atherosclerotic vascular disease and plaque disruption.

- MRI can evaluate various aspects of cardiovascular disease, including plaque morphology, vascular physiology, and myocardial function.

- High-resolution multicontrast MRI is used to characterize the specific tissue components of complex plaques, which aids in the detection of vulnerable plaque.

- Because of high reproducibility, MRI is valuable in assessment of plaque progression and regression.

- Molecular imaging elucidates the biology of various cellular and molecular targets in atherosclerosis before the development of gross phenotypic changes.

- MRI is an ideal molecular imaging modality because of its high spatial and temporal resolutions, noninvasive nature, lack of ionizing radiation, and excellent reproducibility.

- PET can assess inflammatory activity within atherosclerotic plaque because of avid FDG uptake and accumulation within the macrophages in inflamed plaque.

- PET can simultaneously evaluate cardiac perfusion and metabolism and hence plays a vital role in evaluation of selected patients with cardiovascular risk factors or disease.

Atherosclerosis is a diffuse, chronic immunoinflammatory disease of the vascular, metabolic, and immune systems characterized by deposition of lipid and fibrous products in the arterial wall. It is the result of complex biologic processes, resulting in various local and systemic manifestations after a long asymptomatic period. Genetic predisposition is part of the variability in development of atherosclerotic disease, plaque destabilization, and subsequent thrombosis.

Atherosclerosis is the single most important contributor to the burden of cardiovascular disease.[1] In spite of advances in prevention, risk assessment, and treatment, cardiovascular disease is the major global cause of morbidity and mortality. An estimated 80 million American adults have cardiovascular disease, which accounted for 35% of deaths and an estimated cost of $475.3 billion dollars in 2009.[2] The large population at risk for coronary events and frequent first presentation with a significant cardiovascular event or sudden death makes it seem reasonable to detect subclinical disease for initiation of earlier treatment to prevent the progression of atherosclerotic vascular disease and plaque disruption.

Conventionally, imaging has focused on detection and grading of stenotic lesions and perfusion abnormalities in organs distal to the stenosis. However, major acute events, such as myocardial infarction (MI) and stroke, are generally produced not by plaques with high-grade stenosis but by disruption of plaques that did not produce significant stenosis or perfusion abnormalities

in stress tests, the so-called vulnerable plaque. In addition, recent evidence suggests that interventional treatment of coronary stenosis does not significantly improve MI and death rates in many persons with stable angina compared with a strategy of aggressive medical and lifestyle changes.[3]

Hence, there is a need for new diagnostic tests that will be able to detect, quantify, and characterize the plaque, including its biologic activity and stability, ideally at an earlier subclinical stage in the disease process so that high-risk patients can be identified and treatment initiated earlier in the long asymptomatic phase to modify the disease progression and to reduce the risk of a major event. Because atherosclerosis is a diffuse disease, detection in one vascular territory implies involvement of other vascular territories, and treatment has to be both local and global.[4] Novel therapeutic strategies include targeted transport vehicles allowing drug delivery to specific cells or cell structures.

IMAGING OF ATHEROSCLEROSIS

The purposes of imaging in atherosclerosis are understanding of the natural history and pathobiology of atherosclerosis, diagnosis of subclinical disease and risk stratification, evaluation of plaque burden (location, size, chemical composition, biologic activity), and identification of vulnerable plaque. Serial imaging is performed to assess plaque progression or regression. Assessment of the impact of drug therapy on atherosclerosis directly is a surrogate endpoint for trials, reducing the need for expensive multicenter clinical trials or triaging which drugs go into expensive phase III clinical trials.

The ideal imaging technique should be sufficiently sensitive and specific for detection of atherosclerosis, inexpensive, reproducible, easy to perform, widely available, tolerated by patients, and noninvasive or minimally invasive. It should have no or minimal radiation, provide immediate results, quantify plaque components, be feasible in all vascular beds, add predictive value over measurement of established risk factors, and correlate highly with risks of subsequent major events.[5]

28

The various available imaging options include invasive techniques, such as coronary angiography, intravascular ultrasound, palpography, and optical coherence tomography, and noninvasive techniques, such as high-resolution ultrasound, computed tomography (CT), single-photon emission computed tomography (SPECT), positron emission tomography (PET), and magnetic resonance imaging (MRI). Each has its advantages and disadvantages.

MAGNETIC RESONANCE IMAGING

MRI uses the magnetic characteristics of the most abundant proton in the human body, hydrogen, to generate images. When they are placed in a powerful magnet, these protons align with the magnetic field; but on application of radiofrequency pulses, this alignment can be altered, causing the hydrogen protons to produce a varying magnetic field that can be detected by the scanner. The signal can be manipulated by multiple, additional magnetic fields for reconstruction of an image of the tissues of interest. The combination of radiofrequency and gradient waveforms used to obtain an image is called a pulse sequence. The appearance and signal intensity of any tissue on MRI depend on the type of pulse sequence and imaging parameters.

Rapid advances in the last 10 years have resulted in the emergence of MRI as an important tool in evaluation of cardiovascular disease. This is attributed to improved hardware, particularly the high–field strength magnets and high-sensitivity coils, and novel contrast agents, including those labeled with molecular targets. MRI is noninvasive and has no ionizing radiation; it has high inherent soft tissue contrast, spatiotemporal resolution, large field of view, and multiplanar imaging capabilities. Intravenous chelated gadolinium contrast material is useful for further characterization, but it is best avoided in patients with severe renal dysfunction because of the association with nephrogenic systemic fibrosis, a debilitating fibrosing condition believed to be secondary to an immune reaction to gadolinium particles deposited in the layers of skin, most probably due to high serum concentrations in patients with impaired renal function.

MRI Techniques in Cardiovascular Diseases

MRI plays an important role in the evaluation of various aspects of cardiovascular disease (Table 28-1).

High-Resolution Multicontrast Imaging

High-resolution MRI is used to characterize the atherosclerotic plaque. The normal arterial wall has three layers, namely, the tunica intima, media, and adventitia, which cannot be separately distinguished on MRI. However, plaques are composed of variable quantities of cells, connective tissue, lipids, calcification, and debris, which can be evaluated by MRI (Table 28-2, Fig. 28-1).[6,7]

TABLE 28–1	Role of MRI in Evaluation of Various Aspects of Cardiovascular Disease
Technique	**Assessment**
MR angiography	Stenosis, dilation
Whole-body MRA	Screening
High-resolution MRI	Plaque detection, quantification, characterization
Vascular physiology	Compliance, aortic stiffness with pulse wave velocity, flow-mediated vasodilation
Functional data	Wall shear stress, neovascularization density
Molecular imaging	Detection of cellular and molecular targets
	Assessment of vulnerable plaque
Myocardial function	Volumes, mass, function
	Regional function
Stress perfusion study	Ischemia
Delayed enhancement	Viability
Coronary MRA	Coronary luminal assessment
Peripheral arterial MRI	MRA luminal assessment
	High-resolution MRI for plaque characterization
	Phosphocreatine kinetics
Intravascular MRI	Plaque assessment and characterization
	Guidance for coronary intervention

Signals on MRI depend on proton density and T1 (longitudinal) and T2 (transverse) relaxation times of protons in water and fat. Differences in relaxation times of different tissues produce the contrast in MRI images, which can be manipulated by changing scan parameters or with contrast agents that modify relaxation times. MRI has high inherent soft tissue contrast that is ideal for characterization and differentiation of plaque components on the basis of biophysical and biochemical parameters, such as chemical composition, concentration, water content, physical state, molecular motion, and diffusion.

High-resolution MRI with multicontrast black blood techniques and dynamic contrast-enhanced angiography is used to characterize the specific tissue components of complex plaques, which aids in the detection of vulnerable plaque. High field magnets (1.5T or above) and phased array surface coils are used. Electrocardiography-gated axial images of the thoracic aorta are acquired in expiratory breath-hold. Multicontrast techniques use a combination of black and bright blood techniques that usually include T1 weighting, T2 weighting, proton density weighting, and three-dimensional time of flight, followed by postcontrast T1 weighting and time of flight.

Black blood images are acquired by the double inversion recovery fast spin-echo technique,[8] which eliminates signal from flowing blood, resulting in high contrast between the dark blood and arterial wall with signal, enabling precise identification of the lumen-wall interface that is critical for assessment of plaque composition. T1, T2, and proton density weighting are achieved by use of different relaxation time (TR) and echo time (TE). Magnetization transfer and diffusion imaging are used in some protocols.[9] Combinations of these different weightings help distinguish all the major plaque components, such as the lipid-rich necrotic core, fibrous cap, loose matrix, calcification, and intraplaque hemorrhage, all of which have different signal characteristics (Table 28-3).[6,10] The MRI findings have been validated in histologic studies and are highly reproducible both qualitatively and quantitatively, thus making MRI useful for serial evaluation of plaque progression or regression.

TABLE 28–2 | Conventional and Modified American Heart Association Classification of Atherosclerotic Plaques for Histologic Diagnosis and MRI

Stage	Histologic Appearance	MRI Stage	MRI Appearance
I	Not grossly apparent; isolated macrophages with oxidized lipid droplets (foam cells)	I-II	Normal wall thickness; thin plaque, no calcification, <10% stenosis
II	Fatty streak with multiple foam layers		
III	Preatheroma: raised fatty streak; multiple, small extracellular lipid cores; foam cells with lipid droplets; increasing smooth muscle cells	III	Diffuse intimal thickening; small eccentric plaque, no calcification
IV	Atheroma: single, massive extracellular lipid pool, covered by proteoglycan-rich layer infiltrated with foam cells and smooth muscle cells with and without lipid droplet inclusion	IV-V	Plaque with lipid or necrotic core, covered by fibrous cap, possible small calcifications
V	Fibroatheroma: type IV, but with a surrounding cap rich in fibrosis, possible small calcifications		
VI	Complex plaque with possible surface defect, hemorrhage, or thrombus	VI	Complex plaque with possible surface defect, hemorrhage, or thrombus
VII	Calcified plaque	VII	Calcified plaque
VIII	Fibrotic plaque without lipid core; fibrous tissue, no lipid core	VIII	Fibrous tissue, no lipid core, possible small calcifications

Modified from Cai JM, Hatsukami T, Ferguson MS, et al: Classification of human atherosclerotic lesions with in vivo multicontrast magnetic resonance imaging. *Circulation* 106:1368, 2002.

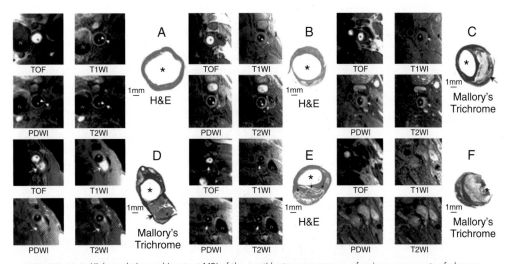

FIGURE 28-1 High-resolution multicontrast MRI of the carotid artery: appearances of various components of plaques. **A,** Type I-II lesion in common carotid artery (layered foam cells were detected by histology). On multicontrast-weighted MR images, carotid wall appears normal (arrow). The asterisk indicates the lumen; H&E, hematoxylin and eosin. **B,** Type III lesion in common carotid artery (extracellular lipid pool was detected by histology). On MR images, carotid wall shows slight eccentric thickening (arrow). **C,** Type IV-V lesion in internal carotid artery (lipid-rich necrotic core was detected by histology). On MR images, lipid-rich necrotic core (arrow) had iso-signal intensity on both T1WI and TOF but iso-signal intensity to slightly high signal intensity on PDWI and T2WI. Lumen is moderately stenosed. **D,** Type VI lesion just distal to carotid bifurcation (acute to subacute mixed hemorrhages were detected by histology). On MR images, acute and subacute mixed hemorrhage had high signal intensity on both TOF and T1WI, iso-signal intensity to slightly high signal intensity on PDWI and T2WI (arrow). **E,** Type VII lesion in common carotid artery. Extensive calcification was present in plaque by histology (boundary of calcified region is outlined for clarification). Calcified region (arrow) had low signal intensity on all images. **F,** Type VIII lesion in internal carotid artery. Connective tissue was characterized by immunocytochemistry as proteoglycan-rich early matrix. MR images show varied signal intensity. PDWI, proton density–weighted imaging; T1WI, T1-weighted imaging; T2WI, T2-weighted imaging; TOF, time of flight. *(Modified from Cai JM, Hatsukami T, Ferguson MS, et al: Classification of human atherosclerotic lesions with in vivo multicontrast magnetic resonance imaging.* Circulation *106:1368, 2002.)*

28

Use of Cardiac Magnetic Resonance Imaging and Positron Emission Tomography in Assessment

Vulnerable plaque refers to thrombosis-prone plaques and plaques with high probability of undergoing rapid progression and thus becoming culprit plaques.[11] The salient characteristics of vulnerable and stable plaques are listed in Table 28-4.[12]

Large Lipid-Rich Necrotic Core. The large lipid-rich necrotic core is composed of extracellular lipids (cholesteryl

TABLE 28–3	MRI Characteristics of Various Tissue Components in Different MRI Sequences			
	T1	T2	Proton Density	Enhancement
Lipid	Hyper	Hypo	Hyper	None
Fibrocellular	Hyper	Hyper	Hyper	None
Calcium	Hypo	Hypo	Hypo	None
Necrotic core	Low	High	High	None
Fibrous cap	Low	Low	Low	Enhancement
Hemorrhage	High	Low	Intermediate	None

TABLE 28–4	Characteristic Features of Vulnerable and Stable Plaques
Vulnerable Plaque	**Stable Plaque**
Large lipid-rich core (>40% plaque volume) Thin fibrous cap (<65-100 μm) Active inflammation Endothelial denudation with superficial platelet aggregation Fissured plaque Stenosis >90%	Small lipid core Thick fibrous cap Abundant smooth muscle cells No inflammation
Minor	
Superficial calcified nodule Glistening yellow (large lipid-rich core, thin cap) Intraplaque hemorrhage Endothelial dysfunction Outward remodeling	

monohydrate or unesterified cholesterol) and cellular debris. Necrotic core has low intensity on T2-weighted images because of short T2 and no contrast enhancement.

Thin Fibrous Cap. The fibrous cap is made up of intimal smooth muscle cells and connective tissue. Fibrous tissue has short T1, which results in bright signal on T1-weighted images and contrast enhancement. Rupture-prone plaques are very thin (65 to 150 μm), which is below the spatial resolution of MRI. In three-dimensional time of flight, the fibrous cap is seen at the interface of the bright lumen and dark wall,[13] making it possible to assess its integrity (Fig. 28-2).[14] Higher strength magnets and multiple-channel coils may be necessary for further characterization. Easy visualization of a cap on MRI generally indicates that it is relatively thick. Nonvisualization (implying a thin cap) or disruption of the fibrous cap indicates potentially high risk plaques (Fig. 28-3).

Active Inflammation. Inflamed plaques are characterized by rich and active macrophages, mast cells, T cells, proinflammatory cytokines, procoagulant mediators, increased matrix metalloproteinase expression, and reduced smooth muscle cells. Inflammation can be detected by contrast enhancement because of increased vascular permeability and edema[9] or by molecular MRI techniques (see later).

Erosion or Fissure of Plaque Surface. Ulcerations are more common in symptomatic patients, regardless of the intensity of symptoms. In addition to the multicontrast black blood MRI, longitudinal black blood magnetic resonance angiography (MRA) increases the ability to identify ulcerations.

Superimposed Thrombus. Thrombus is more prevalent in symptomatic patients, especially with ipsilateral symptoms and plaque ulceration. Thrombotically active plaque associated with high inflammatory infiltrate is seen in 74% of patients presenting with major stroke. Thrombus is the plaque component that is more heterogeneous and difficult to detect.

Luminal Stenosis >90%. Shear stress imposes significant risk of thrombosis and sudden occlusion. It also indicates the presence of many nonstenotic or less stenotic plaques that are vulnerable for rupture and thrombosis.

Superficial Calcified Nodules. Calcified nodules within or close to the cap can protrude through and rupture the cap. Surface calcified nodules can have an exposed thrombogenic surface or can be encapsulated. Calcification (mainly calcium hydroxyapatite) has a low signal because of low proton density and diffusion-mediated susceptibility effects, making

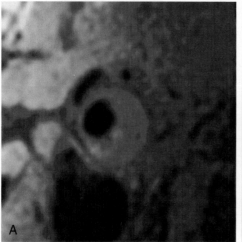
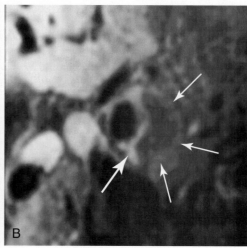

FIGURE 28-2 Axial precontrast **(A)** and postcontrast **(B)** double inversion recovery fast spin-echo black blood images of the carotid artery with fat saturation show heterogeneous enhancement along the outer wall of the atheroma (arrows) and along the margin of the lumen, indicating a fibrous cap. *(Modified from Wasserman BA, Smith WI, Trout HH, et al: Carotid atherosclerosis: in vivo morphologic characterization with gadolinium enhanced double oblique MR imaging. Initial results. Radiology 223:566, 2002.)*

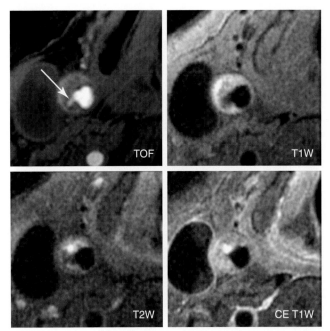

measured manually or by automated techniques, such as MEPPS (morphology-enhanced probabilistic plaque segmentation algorithm) and CASCADE (computer-aided system for cardiovascular disease evaluation), which are based on probabilistic assumptions. The system determines the probability that each MRI pixel belongs to each of the four tissue types, namely, lipid, calcification, fibrous tissue, and loose matrix, and uses computing active contours to identify the boundaries of high probability regions of each tissue, which are then segmented and displayed in three dimensions.[13] This reduces analysis time and reader bias and improves reproducibility. Quantitative measurements have been correlated with histology and are highly reproducible.[13]

MRI of Individual Vascular Territories

The majority of the work on morphologic MRI of the atherosclerotic plaque has been performed in the carotid arteries and aorta because of their superficial location and large size, respectively. New studies are reporting assessment of plaques in coronary and other arterial territories, which are limited by small size and deep location. In all these territories, MRI acquisition takes a long time because of the need for high-resolution images.

Carotid Plaques. Black blood multicontrast MRI with surface coils has been well established and validated with histology in the demonstration of carotid plaque morphology (volume, area, and thickness), structure, and composition.[19] There is a correlation between thinning or rupture of the fibrous cap and recent history of transient ischemic attack or stroke.[20] Ipsilateral arteries in symptomatic patients have a higher prevalence of intraplaque hemorrhage and fibrous cap rupture. Intraplaque hemorrhage indicates an increase in plaque burden (increased necrotic core size), decreased lumen size, repeated intraplaque hemorrhage, and subsequent plaque rupture, making it a superior prognostic indicator (Fig. 28-4).

A greater plaque burden and plaque eccentricity are prevalent among patients with prior major cardiovascular or cerebrovascular events.[21] A prospective study of asymptomatic patients with a 50% to 79% stenosis showed that intraplaque hemorrhage, larger necrotic core area, and thinned or ruptured fibrous cap are associated with a high hazard ratio for subsequent clinical events (Fig. 28-5). Increases in thickness of arterial wall, average area of intraplaque hemorrhage, and necrotic core area were associated with increased hazard ratio for subsequent clinical areas.[22] MRI was also useful for evaluation of plaque regression in carotids (e.g., ORION [Outcome of Rosuvastatin treatment on carotid artery atheroma: a magnetic resonance Imaging ObservatioN] trial).

Aortic Plaque. Multiple studies have established a correlation between aortic plaques and coronary artery lesions. Thoracic aortic plaques are associated with hypercholesterolemia, and a correlation with low-density lipoprotein cholesterol (LDL-C) level has been shown.[5] Abdominal aortic plaques are not associated with LDL-C levels, but they are associated with smoking. Although the exact reason for this variable susceptibility to different risk factors is not known, there are slight differences in the vascular beds. The abdominal aorta has less prominent vasa vasorum, resulting in nutrition only by diffusion, and it has higher blood pressures and higher stiffness with more collagen and less elastin and geometric tapering. Plaques in both the thoracic and abdominal aorta are associated with age and high blood pressure.[18]

There is a high association between thoracic aortic plaques and coronary artery disease (CAD), more than with carotid or femoral artery plaques. Complex plaques are associated with cardiovascular events. Autopsy studies have shown a relationship between severe abdominal aortic plaques and cardiac events, but no association has been shown between CAD and abdominal plaques. An MRI study[18] showed a higher

FIGURE 28-3 Multicontrast MR images demonstrating rupture of fibrous cap in a carotid artery plaque (arrow). High signal intensity in T2-weighted and postcontrast T1-weighted images indicates plaque inflammation and neovasculature. *(Modified from Chu B, Ferguson MS, Chen H, et al: Cardiac magnetic resonance features of the disruption-prone and the disrupted carotid plaque.* JACC Cardiovasc Imaging *2:883, 2009.)*

it difficult to be detected in black blood imaging, but it can be seen clearly in time-of-flight images.

Intraplaque Hemorrhage. Intraplaque hemorrhage is due to rupture of fragile microvessels. It has a variable signal, depending on the blood breakdown products. Methemoglobin, which is seen in the subacute stage, shows T1 shortening and high signal on T1 imaging. The window for observation of these changes is small, and it is essential to localize the hemorrhage within the plaque. Hemorrhages close to the lumen and intraluminal thrombosis are more often associated with embolism and symptoms than deep plaque hemorrhages are.

Outward Positive Remodeling. Vulnerable plaques are often associated with positive remodeling, which prevents luminal narrowing; as a result, the patient may be asymptomatic, and stress perfusion imaging is often normal.[15] This is a surrogate marker of plaque vulnerability.

Adventitial Inflammation and Neovascularity. Adventitial inflammation and neovascularity are associated with high risk of plaque rupture. Gadolinium enhancement in T1-weighted MRI has high sensitivity for neovascularity (80%). Dynamic enhancement indicates vascular density, which is a marker of neovascularity, and delayed enhancement reflects increased permeability of inflamed vessels.[16]

Post–Gadolinium Contrast Enhancement

Intense contrast enhancement indicates neovascularity and increased endothelial permeability, which results in entry of the contrast agent from blood plasma into the plaque. Strong enhancement is an indicator of plaque inflammation, which is a sign of vulnerability. The amount of enhancement is a marker of extent of acute inflammation. Late gadolinium enhancement is used to identify fibrous plaque.[13,17]

Plaque Quantification

Plaque seen on black blood MRI has been validated with transesophageal echocardiography[18] and with histopathology in animal models in multiple studies. Plaque can be

28

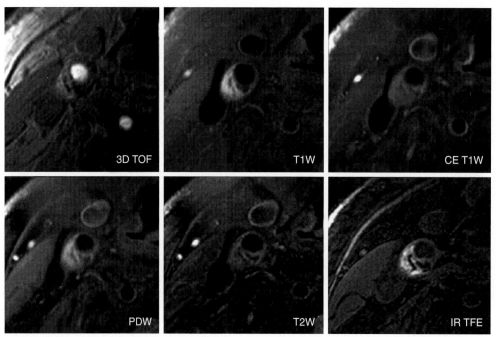

FIGURE 28-4 Hyperintense signal in the plaque is due to intraplaque hemorrhage on the three-dimensional time-of-flight (3D TOF), T1-weighted (T1W), and inversion recovery turbo field-echo (IR TFE) sequences. Hypointense signals in both TOF and IR TFE techniques are the densely calcified areas. *(Modified from Chu B, Ferguson MS, Chen H, et al: Cardiac magnetic resonance features of the disruption-prone and the disrupted carotid plaque. JACC Cardiovasc Imaging 2:883, 2009.)*

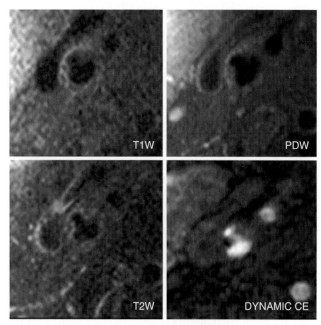

FIGURE 28-5 Multicontrast MR images show a large surface ulceration in a carotid artery plaque. *(Modified from Chu B, Ferguson MS, Chen H, et al: Cardiac magnetic resonance features of the disruption-prone and the disrupted carotid plaque. JACC Cardiovasc Imaging 2:883, 2009.)*

prevalence of plaques in the thoracic (73%) and abdominal aorta (94%) in patients with CAD than in those without it. The extent of plaques correlated with the extent of coronary artery stenosis. Whereas the thoracic plaques were independently associated with CAD, the abdominal aortic plaques were not associated independently with CAD. There was no difference in prevalence between CAD with and without MI.

Complex plaques in the abdominal aorta were more prevalent in CAD patients with MI than without MI. Among patients without MI, complex aortic plaques were more prevalent in patients with complex coronary lesions than without complex coronary lesions. All these suggest that complex aortic plaques are linked to coronary plaque instability, which leads to development of MI and complex coronary lesions. Complex aortic plaque, especially in the abdominal aorta, is a good marker of coronary plaque instability. CT studies have also shown a better association between thoracic aortic plaques and CAD. Hence, thoracic aortic plaque is a better marker of coexisting CAD.[5]

Coronary Artery Plaque. Plaque imaging in coronary arteries is hampered by the small diameter, tortuosity, deep location, and high mobility of the coronary arteries and the small volume of plaque. In addition, not all ruptured plaques cause acute coronary syndromes, and vulnerability is not static. A vulnerable plaque one day may look stable another day.[23] There has been a good correlation between black blood MRI–measured coronary wall thickness and matched pathology sections, with good reproducibility. Increased wall thickness is seen in patients with more than 40% stenosis on angiography.[24] Because of low resolution, MRI may overestimate coronary wall thickness in normal patients.

In asymptomatic type 1 diabetes mellitus, coronary wall MRI reveals higher plaque burden in subjects with nephropathy than with normoalbuminuria.[25] Hyperintense plaque in T1-weighted sequences indicates an unstable plaque due to intraplaque hemorrhage, and it correlates with positive remodeling, ultrasound attenuation, lower Hounsfield units in CT, and transient flow after percutaneous coronary intervention. These findings are similar to those in carotid plaque characterization, which has been validated with histology.[26] T1-weighted coronary plaque imaging has the potential for identification of complex coronary lesions in patients with unstable CAD.

High-resolution coronary plaque imaging has been performed in humans by 3T scanners with a 32-channel cardiac coil (0.5 × 0.5 × 3-mm resolution) and in animals by a 9T scanner (97-μm resolution) and intravascular MRI (117 ×

areas at 18 months was lower in those who took statins compared with the non-statin group.[33] In a similar study of CAD patients, MRI showed significantly less lipid core area and lipid composition in patients who were receiving intensive lipid-lowering therapy compared with a nontreated group.[34] MRI of the thoracic aorta demonstrated changes in plaque volume and lumen after simvastatin (20 to 80 mg) therapy for 6 months that correlated with LDL reduction.[35] Other studies have shown continued decrease in plaques in the aorta and carotid arteries at 12 months and after 18 to 24 months of statin treatment,[36] with minimal changes in luminal dimension.

A study comparing 5 mg versus 20 mg of atorvastatin for 12 months in hypercholesterolemic patients showed greater reduction of thoracic aortic plaque in the 20-mg than in the 5-mg group that correlated with reduced LDL-C levels. Abdominal aortic plaque did not change with the 20-mg dose but became worse with just 5 mg[37] (Fig. 28-7). Similar results were shown in a Japanese study that used 20 mg of atorvastatin. Another study that compared 20 mg versus 80 mg of simvastatin showed greater reduction of carotid and aortic plaque at 12 months in the higher dose group.[38] All these studies prove that intensive atorvastatin therapy reduces LDL-C and causes plaque regression in thoracic aorta and carotid and coronary arteries.[38]

Fibrates reduce triglyceride and increase high-density lipoprotein cholesterol (HDL-C) levels. An MRI study of hypertriglyceridemic patients after 400 mg of bezafibrate showed regression of thoracic aortic wall plaques without change in cross-sectional area, regression of abdominal aortic plaques with increase in cross-sectional area, and correlation between wall area change and triglyceride reduction and HDL-C increase.[39] The change in abdominal plaques alone correlated with HDL particle size reduction and LDL size increase by nuclear magnetic resonance, implying that there might be different mechanisms in the thoracic and abdominal aorta for plaque regression and that triglyceride plays an important role in atherosclerosis in the abdominal aorta.

Because the abdominal aorta has no vasa vasorum and reverse lipid transport happens through diffusion into the lumen, there might be an increase in area after therapy, compared with the thoracic aorta, in which reverse transport occurs because of the presence of vasa vasorum and there is no significant reduction.[18] MRI has also been used to compare the effects of statins versus statins plus the peroxisome proliferator activated receptor γ agonist on plaque.[40]

Advances in Morphologic MRI

Higher field strength of magnets, dedicated multichannel phase array coils to increase signal-to-noise ratio, multislice motion-sensitized driven-equilibrium turbo spin-echo sequences to suppress plaque-mimicking artifacts, and three-dimensional isotropic sequences for evaluation of luminal surface and plaque definition are some of the latest advances in morphologic MRI. T2* imaging of iron forms within the plaque has demonstrated lower T2* values in symptomatic plaques.[41]

High-Field MRI

3T MRI has the advantages of having twice the signal of 1.5T MRI and higher contrast-to-noise ratio, although it has higher chemical shift and susceptibility artifacts. Double inversion delay time is increased to accommodate increased blood T1. High spatial resolution images are acquired by parallel imaging and multiple averages, and these are useful for detection, characterization, and quantification of early and moderate plaques, with a high correlation between plaque quantity and components and histopathology. An 18-month follow-up study using 3T MRI showed 50% reduction in lipid content with minimal change in plaque size in a subject receiving

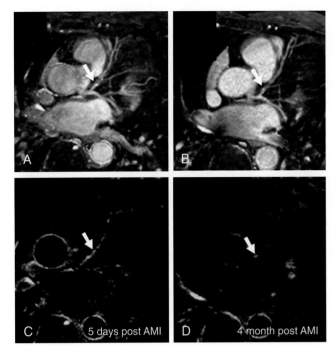

FIGURE 28-6 Coronary MRA of a 62-year-old patient with inferolateral infarction shows a luminal stenosis in the proximal left anterior descending (LAD) coronary artery (arrow) that corresponds to 50% stenosis in x-ray angiography **(A)**. MRA 5 days after infarction **(C)** shows contrast uptake within proximal LAD. MRA 4 months after MI **(B, D)** shows marked reduction of coronary enhancement in proximal LAD; the stenotic region shows mild uptake (arrow). **A** and **B** are fused images, which fused the enhancement in **C** and **D** with MRA. *(Modified from Ibrahim T, Makowski M, Jankauskas A, et al: Serial contrast-enhanced cardiac MRI demonstrates regression of hyperenhancement within the coronary artery wall in patients after acute myocardial infarction.* JACC Cardiovasc Imaging *2:580, 2009.)*

156-μm resolution).[27] A study demonstrated coronary arterial wall enhancement during acute MI due to edema and inflammation and resolution during delayed phase (6 months later), which offers the potential for visualization of inflammation in coronary atherosclerosis (Fig. 28-6).[28,29] However, enhancement was diffuse and not localized to the occlusive site.

MRI in Plaque Progression and Regression

Because of its high reproducibility, MRI is useful in the evaluation of plaque progression and regression and has been well established in numerous animal and human studies. The use of MRI has significantly reduced the sample size required for evaluation of pharmacologic regression of atherosclerosis in clinical trials. In an early study,[30] with balloon-injured rabbits fed a high- versus low-cholesterol diet, MRI at 4 and 20 months showed higher wall thickness and stenosis in the high-cholesterol group. A similar MRI study with hypercholesterolemic rabbits fed a high-cholesterol diet for 12 weeks followed by a normal diet for 12 weeks showed increased wall volume during a high-cholesterol diet phase and decreased wall volume during the normal diet phase.[31]

Numerous MRI studies have evaluated the response of carotid and aortic atherosclerotic lesions to various doses and regimens of medical therapy.[5] MRI can measure plaque reduction and map changes in plaque composition in response to intensive lipid-lowering treatment and has been validated with histology. MRI has good reproducibility and low interscan variability and is able to detect a 10% change in wall volume and a 20% change in percentage of lipid-rich or necrotic core components.[32]

In a study of asymptomatic subjects with 50% carotid stenosis, MRI showed that the rate of increase in carotid wall

28

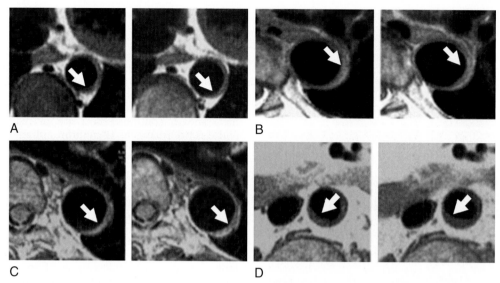

A   B

C   D

FIGURE 28-7 MRI at baseline and after 1 year of atorvastatin treatment. In **A,** a thoracic aortic plaque showed 28% vessel wall area reduction with a 20-mg dose of atorvastatin. In **B,** a thoracic aortic plaque showed 10% regression with a 5-mg dose. In **C,** a thoracic aortic plaque showed 15% progression with a 5-mg dose. In **D,** an abdominal plaque showed 9% progression despite a 20-mg dose. *(Modified from Yonemura A, Momiyama Y, Fayad ZA, et al: Effect of lipid lowering therapy with atorvastatin on atherosclerotic aortic plaques detected by noninvasive MRI. J Am Coll Cardiol 45:733, 2005.)*

aggressive statin therapy. Similar studies have been performed in coronary arteries, thoracic aorta, and femoral arteries. Higher field strengths, such as 7T and 9.4T, increase spatial resolution further and suggest potential for spectroscopic methods.[42]

Coronary Magnetic Resonance Angiography

Coronary MRA provides information on the coronary artery lumen and vessel wall including plaque, which can be three-dimensionally reconstructed in multiple planes, without radiation or intravenous administration of contrast material. However, valuation of coronary arteries requires high spatial resolution (3 to 4 mm) and temporal resolution (<75 msec). A three-dimensional steady-state free precession whole-heart sequence with T2 preparation to decrease myocardial signal and fat saturation to decrease epicardial fat signal is used to image coronary arteries. Blood vessels appear bright because of intrinsic contrast. Images are acquired in diastole and expiration with free breathing technique using navigator gating of the diaphragm (Fig. 28-8). To obtain high-resolution images (0.7 to 0.8 mm), acquisition time can be very long, up to 12 to 15 minutes. MRI has a sensitivity of 80% to 90%, specificity of >90%, and negative predictive value of 81% for identification of coronary artery stenosis.[43] However, coronary MRA is not as widely used as CT angiography because of low sensitivity, long acquisition time, and lack of expertise in many hospitals.

Magnetic Resonance Angiography

Whole-body MRA can examine the entire arterial tree excluding the intracranial and coronary vessels in one sitting by use of bolus chase technique, multichannel receiver surface coils, and parallel imaging techniques, without radiation or arterial cannulation, and it is less nephrotoxic. Multistation techniques are used, typically a four-station technique; the first station covers supra-aortic arteries and the thoracic aorta, the second station covers the abdominal aorta, the third station

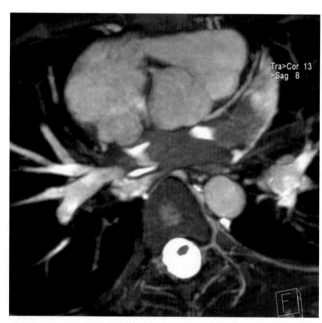

FIGURE 28-8 Three-dimensional whole-heart steady-state free precession MRI sequence demonstrates the origins and proximal segments of all the left and right coronary arteries.

covers the external iliac to popliteal areas, and the fourth station covers up to the ankle. Subsystolic venous compression in the calf can reduce venous contamination and increase signal-to-noise and contrast-to-noise ratios. Higher resolution scans can be performed at sites of plaques to characterize them and to quantify luminal stenosis. 3T magnet (higher signal), surface multichannel coils, parallel imaging, and blood pool agent (MS-325) will potentially improve the quality of MRA. MRA has been validated for pelvic and lower limb arteries. However, reproducibility has not been completely assessed yet, and it can overestimate stenosis.

The ability to image multiple vascular beds makes it useful in evaluation of atherosclerosis. MRA can be combined with volume, assess disease severity, and monitor plaque progression or regression in response to therapy.

The superficial femoral artery is the ideal vessel because it is superficial and nonmobile. Popliteal arteries have also been evaluated to demonstrate the changes that occur with remodeling and restenosis after angioplasty.[46] First-pass contrast-enhanced dual contrast perfusion imaging of calf muscle at peak exercise with an MR-compatible pedal ergometer and ^{31}P MR spectroscopy at peak exercise measure phosphocreatine recovery kinetics, which varies greatly between normals and patients with peripheral arterial disease, particularly at maximal workload.[47]

Myocardial Function

Global Myocardial Function

Left ventricular volumes, mass, and ejection fraction are important markers of cardiovascular disease and independent predictors of cardiovascular events, with changes seen before onset of symptoms. Left ventricular hypertrophy is considered an abnormal response to conditions such as hypertension, not physiologic or compensatory, and it is an independent predictor of cardiovascular events.[23] Left ventricular mass is an important marker of subclinical disease and decreases after therapy reduces adverse events.[23] The MESA study has demonstrated an 18-fold higher rate of congestive heart failure during a short period of observation in those with left ventricular hypertrophy, after accounting for traditional risk factors and coronary calcium score.[43]

MRI is the most accurate technique in the evaluation of cardiac volumes and mass, with only 5% standard errors compared with 20% for echocardiography.[48] Volumes are measured manually or semiautomatically by steady-state free precession sequences obtained in the short-axis plane, by drawing manual or automatic endocardial and epicardial contours. Mass is obtained by multiplying the wall volume with myocardial density (1.05 g/cm^3) (Fig. 28-10). With increasing age, particularly in men, the mass-to-volume ratio increases, although left ventricular mass is maintained because of decrease of end-diastolic volume due to concentric remodeling.

Regional Myocardial Function

Regional changes often precede global abnormalities in cardiac function. Strain is fractional change in length from the resting state in diastole to contraction in systole. Radial, circumferential, and longitudinal strains can be measured on MRI by myocardial tagging techniques, such as SPAMM (spatial modulation of magnetization) or CSPAMM (complementary spatial modulation of magnetization), which produces dark saturation bands perpendicular to the scanning plane[43] (Fig. 28-11). Strain is quantified by harmonic phase analysis, which is more accurate than visual estimation of regional function. Strains can be measured separately in the subendocardial, mid-wall, and subepicardial layers. Other techniques for tagging are strain-encoded imaging (tags are parallel to imaging plane), displacement encoding with stimulated echoes (DENSE), and velocity encoding phase shifts with phase contrast imaging.

With age, although the ejection fraction is maintained in normal range, peak strain decreases, particularly in the left anterior descending territory of men. In women, strain increases with concentric remodeling in all but the highest quartile of mass-to-volume ratio. A direct relationship between regional diastolic dysfunction (decreased diastolic strain) and increasing left ventricular mass is demonstrated in asymptomatic individuals. After control for established risk factors, increased diastolic blood pressure was associated

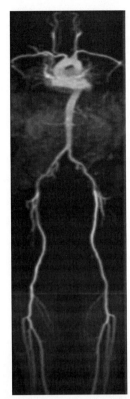

FIGURE 28-9 Maximum intensity projection of whole-body MRA shows all the arteries from the head to the leg, which are used to calculate the atherosclerotic score index. *(Modified from Lehrke S, Egenlauf B, Steen H, et al: Prediction of coronary artery disease by a systemic atherosclerosis score index derived from whole-body MRI angiography.* J Cardiovasc Magn Reson *11:36, 2009.)*

whole-body MR screening.[44] MRA has detected unknown arterial disease in different populations, such as those characterized by advanced age, diabetes, and post-MI.[45] MRA is useful for repeated clinical examinations but has not yet been studied or validated to predict future cardiovascular events. An atherosclerotic score index (ASI) has been measured by scoring luminal narrowing (1, normal; 2, <25%; 3, 26% to 50%; 4, 51% to 75%; 5, 76% to 99%; 6, occlusion) in 40 extracardiac segments and dividing the sum by the number of analyzable segments (Fig. 28-9). ASI was higher in patients with CAD than in those without and correlated with Framingham and PROCAM risk scores. An ASI >1.54 has 59% sensitivity, 86% specificity, and 84% positive predictive value for predicting CAD and confirming increased risk of CAD in those with extracardiac atherosclerosis, in addition to giving an estimate of total atherosclerotic burden in the body.[45]

Peripheral MRI

Peripheral arterial atherosclerosis is the most common cause of peripheral arterial disease, often leading to vascular obstruction. MRA, high-resolution black blood imaging, and first-pass contrast-enhanced dual contrast perfusion imaging of the calf are the MRI techniques used in assessment of peripheral arterial disease. MRA can detect and quantify luminal stenosis, although it is technically challenging because of artifacts such as signal loss from in-plane saturation, turbulent flow, metallic clips and stents, and end-organ effects of peripheral arterial disease. High-resolution black blood imaging using surface coil and flow saturation can diagnose preclinical vascular disease, measure plaque

LV analysis: pr2 (not validated).

ANALYSIS SETTINGS INFORMATION:

Blood volume results are not filtered
and not corrected.

RESULTS SUMMARY:

Ejection fraction : 37.7%
Stroke volume   : 56.4 mL
Stroke index   : n/a
Cardiac output : 3.4 1/min
Cardiac index   : n/a

ED time   :   0.00 ms (phase 1)
ED volume   :   149.39 mL
ES time   :   376.00 ms (phase 12)
ES volume   :   93.00 mL
ED wall mass   :   81.47 9
ED wall + papillary mass   :   n/a
ED wall − correct. mass   :   n/a
ED wall + papillary   :   n/a
  − correct. mass
Heart rate   :   60.00 bpm
Patient height   :   n/a
Patient weight   :   80.00 kg

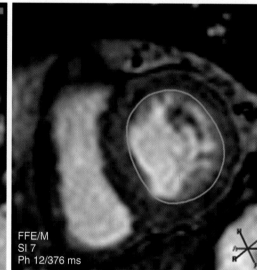

FIGURE 28-10 MRI measurement of left ventricular volumes, function, and mass. Endocardial (green) and epicardial (yellow) contours are shown.

with decreased circumferential strain in asymptomatic individuals,[43] particularly in smokers.

Stress Perfusion MRI

First-pass myocardial perfusion imaging with MRI is a sensitive technique to detect myocardial ischemia, with high detection of CAD compared with coronary angiography,[49] and it has a 100% negative predictive value for subsequent CAD.[50] Perfusion MRI is performed both at rest and after pharmacologic stress (adenosine or dipyridamole). Intravenous contrast produces T1 shortening of normal myocardium, resulting in bright signal on T1-weighted sequences. Hypoperfused areas (ischemic or revascularized infarct) appear dark (Fig. 28-12). Microvascular dysfunction is seen as a subendocardial perfusion defect in a nonvascular distribution. Sequences used for perfusion are typically multislice T1-weighted two-dimensional sequences, which could be steady-state free precession (SSFP), fast low-angle shot (FLASH), or gradient-recalled echo planar imaging (GRE EPI), either inversion or saturation

recovery based or hybrid, each with its advantages and disadvantages.[51] Typically, perfusion studies are followed by delayed enhancement images to evaluate myocardial viability,[52] and this enhances the performance of adenosine stress cardiovascular magnetic resonance. Detection of even small amounts of myocardial delayed enhancement in patients without known MI is an adverse prognostic indicator. Direct assessment of myocardial perfusion after adenosine stress is sensitive, whereas adenosine-induced wall motion abnormalities are highly specific.[53]

Semiquantitative analysis of the blood flow could be obtained by analysis of the postcontrast myocardial signal intensity as a function of time. Myocardial perfusion reserve index is the ratio of the maximal upslope of the time-intensity profiles at stress and at rest, which is a good indicator of perfusion. After vasodilation in a normal vessel, there is a peak followed by washout before plateau. If there is no overshoot, it indicates no vasodilator response. Absolute quantification is possible if there is an accurate estimate of arterial input function, which is measured from the left ventricular

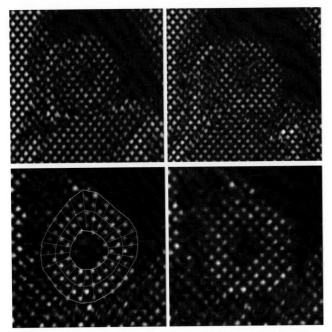

FIGURE 28-11 Regional myocardial function evaluated by grid tags with SPAMM technique. Endocardial and epicardial contours are drawn to estimate strain at multiple levels (bottom left). Strain map is illustrated in the bottom right image.

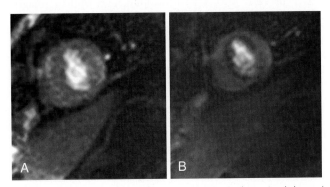

FIGURE 28-12 MRI in a 46-year-old woman presenting with exertional chest pain shows normal rest perfusion scan (A), but there is a dark band of hypoperfusion in the apical septal, anterior, and inferior walls in the stress image (B) consistent with ischemia in the distal left anterior descending territory.

blood pool signal. Dual bolus or dual sequence methods improve accuracy. Quantification of myocardial blood flow and myocardial perfusion reserve can be performed through deconvolution models or model-independent analysis. MRI has a higher accuracy for subendocardial than for transmural perfusion analysis.[54]

Perfusion imaging can also be performed without intravenous contrast material by endogenous contrast mechanisms. In the BOLD (blood oxygen level dependent) technique, normally perfused areas have oxyhemoglobin, which is slightly diamagnetic, producing normal MRI signal, but hypoperfused areas have deoxyhemoglobin, which is paramagnetic and causes signal loss in T2*/T2-weighted images.[55] ASL (arterial spin labeling) works by magnetically labeling blood flowing into slices of interest, which then exchanges with tissue water, altering the tissue magnetization. Subtraction of the image with labeled inflowing spins from an image without spin labeling gives a perfusion-weighted image.

Dobutamine MRI

Dobutamine infusion makes ischemic segments dysfunctional, which could be assessed by cardiac MRI as an alternative test for the diagnosis of CAD and quantifying myocardium at risk, particularly useful in patients in whom echocardiography cannot be performed. The sensitivity of dobutamine MRI is higher than that of echocardiography,[56] and it can be further enhanced by myocardial tagging.[57] It is also useful in predicting left ventricular functional recovery after coronary revascularization.[58] Combined adenosine and dobutamine stress imaging showed 99% survival in patients with normal images and 84% with abnormal images in a series of 513 patients with known or suspected coronary disease during a mean follow-up of 2.3 years.[59] In a multicenter, multivendor trial, perfusion cardiovascular magnetic resonance was proven to be a valuable alternative to SPECT for CAD detection, showing equal performance in the head-to-head comparison.[49] It is also useful in assessing the results of a percutaneous coronary intervention.

Intravascular MRI

Intravascular MRI (IVMR) can be used to image small vessels, such as coronary arteries and iliac or renal arteries, with high signal-to noise-ratio, spatial resolution, and temporal resolution.[60] Intravascular coils have been used for lesion assessment and characterization in carotid and iliac arteries, although there was not enough spatial resolution to visualize thin fibrous cap or atheroma thickness. IVMR can also evaluate increased lipid levels associated with potentially vulnerable plaques, with the help of an integrated, self-contained MRI probe, with magnets and transmit-receive radiofrequency coils on the tip of the catheter that measure lipid concentration in the arterial wall based on apparent diffusion coefficient (ADC). Fibrous tissue has high ADC (unrestricted diffusion), but lipid-rich tissue has low ADC (restricted because of large cholesterol esters).

Intravascular coils within the venous system can evaluate the adjacent arterial system. IVMR is potentially useful for guiding coronary interventions such as angioplasty and stent placement, with good real-time visualization of the catheter and three-dimensional multiplanar reconstruction capabilities and without need for fluoroscopy, radiation, or nephrotoxic contrast agents. IVMR is also used to confirm delivery of local gene therapy or nanoparticles to plaques or vascular wall by a special balloon catheter system. Limitations of intravascular systems are their invasiveness, catheter size, length of imaging protocols, and local heating.

Shear Stress

Plaque rupture is frequently seen at areas exposed to high wall shear stress, typically upstream to maximal stenosis. High wall shear stress also induces antiproliferative activity by endothelial cells on the upstream side, which enhances plaque vulnerability. Information on vascular geometry, inflow conditions, and plaque is acquired from MRI including angiography, and a computational fluid dynamic model is created from which shear stress acting on the luminal surface can be computed from the velocity field. It is unclear how variable geometric reconstruction and restricting assumptions on blood rheology or vessel wall compliance affect the accuracy of results.[13] Wall shear stress can also be calculated semiautomatically and with good reproducibility with model-based segmentation of phase contrast MRI by determination of flow volume and maximal flow velocity in cross sections of these vessels (Fig. 28-13). There is site-specific variation of wall shear stress based on this method.

Vascular Function

Vascular function is an early marker of cardiovascular disease. Arterial compliance is both a cause and a consequence of

Baseline

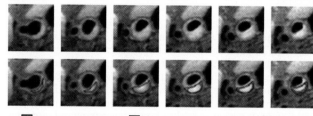

■ Lipid/necrotic core   □ Intraplaque hemorrhage   ■ Ulcer

Follow-up

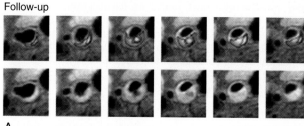

A

Baseline   Follow-up

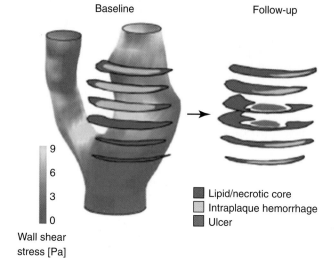

Wall shear stress [Pa]

9
6
3
0

■ Lipid/necrotic core
□ Intraplaque hemorrhage
■ Ulcer

B

FIGURE 28-13 Morphologic MR images and vessel wall segmentation at baseline and 10-month follow-up. Initial scan shows lipid-rich necrotic core (blue) and intraplaque hemorrhage (teal) in internal carotid artery. Follow-up MRI shows large ulcer in proximal internal carotid artery. Ulceration developed in the region that had the highest wall shear stress at baseline. (Modified from Chu B, Ferguson MS, Chen H, et al: Cardiac magnetic resonance features of the disruption-prone and the disrupted carotid plaque. JACC Cardiovasc Imaging 2:883, 2009.)

vascular disease. Aortic stiffness is associated with cardiovascular risk factors, morbidity, and mortality. It has been shown to be independently associated with CAD. In addition, decreased central aortic compliance causes systolic hypertension, left ventricular hypertrophy, and diastolic dysfunction. Velocity-encoded phase contrast MRI is a useful noninvasive technique in the assessment of various vascular parameters compared with invasive techniques, which often make assumptions on central arterial pressure and the path length.[61] Various vascular parameters could be assessed by MRI (Table 28-5).

Molecular Imaging

Molecular imaging elucidates the biology of physiologically relevant cellular and molecular targets in atherosclerosis by use of specific contrast agents, which enables detection before

TABLE 28–5	Vascular Functional Parameters That Could Be Assessed by MRI
Parameter	**Measurement**
Aortic strain	(systolic diameter − diastolic diameter)/ diastolic diameter
Aortic stiffness index (β)	ln(systolic blood pressure/diastolic blood pressure)/[(systolic diameter − diastolic diameter)/diastolic diameter]
Aortic distensibility	2 × (systolic diameter − diastolic diameter)/[systolic blood pressure − diastolic blood pressure) × diastolic diameter]
Aortic elastic modulus E_p	(systolic blood pressure − diastolic blood pressure)/[(systolic diameter − diastolic diameter)/diastolic diameter]
Young's circumferential static elastic modulus E_s	E_p × diastolic diameter/2h, where h is the diastolic intima-media thickness
Pulse wave velocity (m/sec)	Distance between two points/transit time of pulse wave between points

the development of gross phenotypic changes. Molecular imaging complements anatomic and physiologic imaging and can be performed with nuclear medical techniques such as SPECT or PET, MRI, CT, ultrasound, and optical imaging, either as stand-alone or hybrid modalities.[62] Although many of these techniques are still in basic and translational research stages, recent advances in understanding of pathophysiology, imaging agent chemistry, and imaging platforms have led to progression of many agents to clinical evaluation and application, which includes therapy.[63]

Molecular imaging provides insights into pathophysiology that reveal disease diversity. Its advantages include early and refined diagnosis, identification of vulnerable plaque and high-risk patients, and multimodality imaging options. Initiation and titration of therapy targets the biology and molecular profile of vulnerable plaque rather than the lipid profile. It provides opportunities for image-guided therapy and local drug release, and systemic toxicity is decreased. Immediate and accurate follow-up is possible because the molecular response to therapy is quantified. Surrogate imaging endpoints for clinical trials enable assessment of the efficacy of novel drugs that are faster and cheaper.

Components of Molecular Imaging

Molecular imaging involves target molecules, ligands, carrier vehicles, and signal elements (Fig. 28-14). Although there are various possible target molecules for atherosclerosis, imaging of them is challenging because of their location in vessels deep inside the body, small quantities, motion, and high shear stress in large arteries.[64] Ligands are molecules such as monoclonal antibodies, fragments, small molecules, small peptides, or carbohydrates that have high affinity and specificity for the target molecule. Probes can also be modified to be taken by specific cells.[64] Carrier vehicles such as cells, liposomes, microbubbles, perfluorocarbon emulsions, and cross-linked iron oxide transport the ligands to the target molecules. In addition, carriers are also attached to signal elements that generate the signal to be detected by imaging. These include microbubbles (ultrasound), radioactive isotopes (SPECT and PET), paramagnetic and superparamagnetic compounds (MRI), iodinated compounds (CT), and fluorochromes (optical imaging).

Signal elements can be delivered in quenched form to be liberated only after specific enzymatic cleavage or emit signal when the ligand binds to the target.[65] The ligand can be

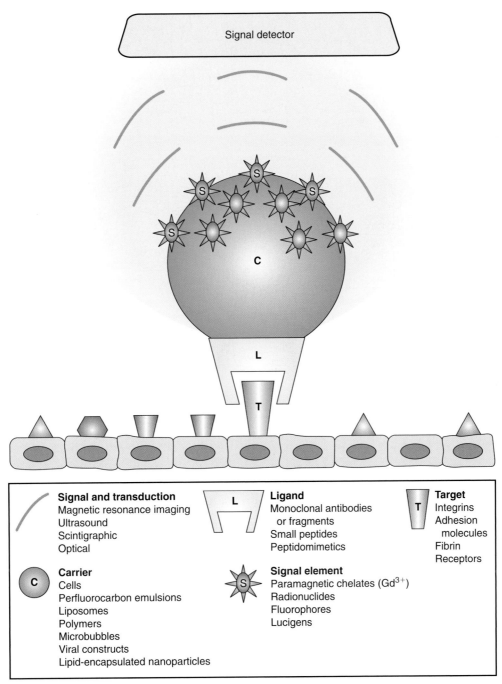

Signal and transduction
Magnetic resonance imaging
Ultrasound
Scintigraphic
Optical

Ligand
Monoclonal antibodies
 or fragments
Small peptides
Peptidomimetics

Target
Integrins
Adhesion
 molecules
Fibrin
Receptors

Carrier
Cells
Perfluorocarbon emulsions
Liposomes
Polymers
Microbubbles
Viral constructs
Lipid-encapsulated nanoparticles

Signal element
Paramagnetic chelates (Gd^{3+})
Radionuclides
Fluorophores
Lucigens

FIGURE 28-14 Schematic diagram illustrating a model of targeted contrast agents. The molecule of interest (T) is targeted by the specific ligand (L), which is conjugated to a carrier particle (C), which concentrates the signal molecules (S) at the binding site. *(Modified from Choudhury RP, Fuster V, Fayad ZA: Molecular, cellular and functional imaging of atherosclerosis.* Nat Rev Drug Discov *3:913, 2004.)*

conveyed to the target by diffusion, mass flow, receptor-mediated internalization, pinocytosis, or intracellular carriage. The sensitivity of agents can be increased by use of multivalent compounds, by conjugation of multiple ligands to a signal moiety, or by conjugation of multiple signal compounds to the target.[66,67]

MRI has the advantages of being noninvasive and requiring no radiation, making it ideal for serial tracking. It has good spatial and temporal resolution, which is ideal for dynamic studies, and it has excellent reproducibility and is good for evaluation of multiple beds. However, it has lower sensitivity than PET or SPECT for detection of sparse targets and has prolonged imaging times.

Molecular imaging can be used at many targets (Fig. 28-15) for the diagnosis of atherosclerotic plaque, including its activity (Table 28-6).

Molecular MRI Contrast Agents

Molecular MRI contrast agents can be broadly divided into nonspecific, targeted, and activatable types. Nonspecific agents operate by passive targeting and are used to detect physiologic changes. Targeted contrast agents are used to determine structure and work by localizing proteins. Low-molecular-weight target-specific contrast agents are suitable for imaging of dense or common epitopes. Activatable contrast agents are used to localize enzymes and to determine

Modality	Flow-mediated vasodilation	Adhesion molecules	Macrophages	MMPs Cathepsin	Lipid core Fibrous cap	$\alpha_v\beta_3$ integrin	Florin Platelets $\alpha_{IIb}\beta_3$ integrin Tissue factor
MRI	+	+	+	+	+	+	+
Ultrasound	+	+	+	–	±	+	+
Fluorescence	–	+	+	+	–	+	+
PET	–	+	+	+	–	+	+
Process	Endothelial dysfunction	Endothelial activation	Inflammation	Proteolysis Apoptosis		Angiogenesis	Thrombosis

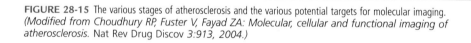

FIGURE 28-15 The various stages of atherosclerosis and the various potential targets for molecular imaging. *(Modified from Choudhury RP, Fuster V, Fayad ZA: Molecular, cellular and functional imaging of atherosclerosis. Nat Rev Drug Discov 3:913, 2004.)*

function. Signal can be amplified and background signal minimized by use of smart agents (protease activatable, oligomerization of signal-producing substrates), cellular trapping of phosphorylated substrates, or covalent binding.[68]

T1 Contrast Agents (Positive Agents). T1 agents, such as gadolinium, iron, and manganese, have unpaired electrons in their outer shells, which because of their paramagnetic effect produce T1 shortening of adjacent tissue protons, resulting in high signal. These agents are usually chelated to avoid the toxicity of free ions. The commonly used gadolinium agents include micelles (10 to 20 nm), lipoproteins (10 to 20 nm), and perfluorocarbon nanoparticles (200 nm). Signal from the contrast agent can be further augmented by increasing either the relaxivity or the concentration of the contrast agent.

T2/T2* Contrast Agents (Negative Agents). T2 agents produce a large dipolar magnetic field gradient because of their strong magnetic moment that accelerates dephasing of adjacent protons. The most commonly used iron-based agents have microcrystalline magnetite or maghemite cores with dextran or siloxane coating that binds to scavenger receptors in macrophages and is phagocytosed, depending on macrophage activation status. Iron-based contrast agents have both T1 and T2 shortening effects, with the predominant effect determined by the relaxivity ratio (r2/r1). If the ratio is low (i.e., in dispersed agents, low concentration, or short TE/TR sequences), they produce more T1 shortening with positive

contrast; but if the ratio is high (clustered together, long TE/TR sequences), they produce more T2 and T2* shortening with negative contrast. In addition, the extent of darkening does not directly correlate with the concentration of contrast agent because it is associated with blooming and technical parameters. No toxicity has been demonstrated so far with iron agents, and iron uptake is not inhibited by statins.[69] T2 agents are classified on the basis of their size.

1. Nanoparticles (10 nm-1 μm) have high relaxivity, with predominantly intravascular distribution, slow extracellular distribution, and hepatic clearance (see section later).
2. MPIO (microparticles of iron oxide) are the largest iron particles (0.9-4.5 μm), with high iron payload and high specificity due to less extravasation and nonspecific endothelial uptake. They distribute only in the intravascular space without any plaque uptake, making them useful for imaging of adhesion molecules[70] and activated platelets.
3. SPIO (superparamagnetic iron oxide, 50-300 nm) is made up of an iron oxide core surrounded by a thin and incomplete dextran coating (e.g., ferrum oxide, ferucarbotran [Resovist]). These particles usually aggregate in solution into large clusters and are rapidly cleared by reticuloendothelial cells ($t_{1/2}$, 5 minutes), which limits passive diffusion, with rapid extracellular space distribution, fast renal clearance, and moderate relaxivity. Uptake in macrophages of atherosclerotic plaque has been demonstrated in mice

Process	Target	Contrast Agent	Mechanism of Action
Endothelial dysfunction	HDL Oxidized LDL MPO	HDL-like nanoparticle (37pA,18aA) Micelles with IK17 Fab Oligomerized MPO substrates	Reverse cholesterol transport Binds to oxidized LDL Binds to MPO
Endothelial activation	VCAM-1 VCAM-1, P-selectin	VINP-28 VNP Trimodality nanoparticle Dual ligand	Ligand homologous to VLA-4 VLA-4 homologue for MRI and NIRF MRI, NIRF, PET Binds to VCAM-1 and P-selectin
Inflammation	Macrophages Scavenger receptors SRA, CD36	USPIO Trimodality nanoparticle Gadolinium immunomicelles with antibodies to MSR	Phagocytosed by macrophages, T2* shortening Positive markers available Macrophage phagocytosis MRI, PET, NIRF Binds to MSR
Proteolysis	Matrix metalloproteinases (1, 2, 3, 8, 9, 13)	P947	Contains matrix metalloproteinase inhibitory peptide
Apoptosis	Cell membrane phosphatidylserine Enzymes, cathepsins (K, B), caspases, scramblases	Annexin V–cross-linked iron oxide–Cy5.5	High affinity for phosphatidylserine
Proliferation	Smooth muscle cells		
Extracellular matrix formation	Collagen, elastin, tenascin-C	Gadofluorine Elastin-binding Gd-DTPA	Binds to extracellular matrix components, elastin
Lipid core, fibrous core formation	Lipid core, fibrous cap		LDL pathway
Angiogenesis	$\alpha_v\beta_3$ integrin Increased vascularity and leakage	Paramagnetic nanoparticles Fumagillin nanoparticle Perfusion markers Gadofluorine micelles Gadofosveset	Target $\alpha_v\beta_3$ integrin Theranostic agent against angiogenesis Dynamic contrast-enhanced MRI; increased enhancement
Thrombus	Fibrin Thrombus Platelets Tissue factor	Fibrin-binding nanoparticles EP-2104R Peptides Antibodies to glycoprotein IIb/IIIa	Peptide with high affinity for fibrin Peptide with high affinity for $\alpha_v\beta_3$ integrin; integrated into thrombi
Cell trafficking	Monocytes Lymphocytes Stem cells Oxidized LDL	Labeled antibodies	

TABLE 28-6 | Molecular Imaging Targets and Agents in Atherosclerosis

and humans,[71,72] further accelerated by injection of proinflammatory cytokines.[71]

4. USPIO (ultrasmall paramagnetic iron oxide, 20-40 nm) particles have a thick and complete dextran coating surrounding a small nucleus of iron oxide to minimize aggregation (e.g., ferumoxtran). They have a long half-life in blood (24 to 36 hours) because of small size, dextran coating, and slow reticuloendothelial system clearance, which results in passive extravasation, nonspecific uptake, and high background contrast. Uptake in atherosclerotic plaque[73] could be by passive diffusion across a leaky inflamed endothelium or endocytosis by activated blood monocytes followed by transcytosis through endothelium or transport through neovasculature. Uptake in macrophages is by pinocytosis for small particles and receptor-mediated endocytosis and phagocytosis for large particles, both of which are dependent on scavenger receptor SR-A and cytokine activation including interferon-γ and interleukin-4. The intensity of ferumoxtran phagocytosis, rather than macrophage density, is decreased after treatment with p38 MAPK inhibitor.[74]

5. CLIO (cross-linked iron oxides, 30-50 nm) have functionalized exteriors that permit covalent conjugation of surface ligands, such as antibodies and peptides (e.g.,VINP-29 for VCAM-1).

6. VSOP (very small iron oxide particles, 4-8 nm) have a citrate coating, with electrostatic stabilization (e.g., VSOP-C184).

Chemical Exchange Saturation Agents. Chemical exchange saturation agents are based on the principle of magnetization transfer. One or more pools of exchangeable protons with sharply defined resonance frequency and large chemical shifts are well separated from free water peak. Selective radiofrequency radiation of exchangeable protons results in transfer of saturated magnetization to water resonance peak and causes drop in signal intensity. These agents include small diamagnetic compounds, such as sugars and amino acids; paramagnetic lanthanides, such as europium, dysprosium, holmium, erbium, thulium, and ytterbium chelates; and macromolecular systems, such as dendrimers, polymers, single-stranded RNA, and LIPOCEST (liposomes with 0.1 mm concentration of Tm-DOTMA).[68]

Fluorine 19–Based Agents. The nucleus of fluorine 19 has a high magnetogyric ratio; it is abundant in nature although minimally seen in the human body, which results in minimal background noise during imaging. Fluorinated compounds such as perfluorocarbon and perfluoropolyether oils stabilized with surfactants such as water form emulsions and can be used to label cells or function as target-specific contrast agents.[68] [19]F MRI data can be superimposed on ^{1}H MRI that depicts anatomic information.

Selective Gadolinium Agents. MRI contrast agents can be engineered to conceal gadolinium from tissue water, revealed only when a specific enzyme-mediated cleavage occurs. This has been used in imaging of β-galactosidase activity as a marker of transgene expression. Similarly, a conditionally activated probe that on exposure to myeloperoxidase causes oligomerization of gadolinium-rich generating particles with higher T1 relaxivity than a monomeric source compound has also been used.[65]

Nanoparticles. Nanotechnology combines materials by precisely engineering atoms and molecules to yield new molecular assemblies on the scale of individual cells, organelles, or even smaller (5 to 500 nm), with unique chemical and biologic properties that can easily integrate multiple properties (multiple contrast, diagnostic and therapeutic, multiple targeting groups), resulting in higher payloads, higher contrast, and lengthy circulation times. Nanoparticles have a core surrounded by a coating on which are attached ligands and biocompatible polymers. Sources of contrast and therapeutics are included in the core or in the coating.[75] The various types of nanoparticles are liposomes with lipid bilayer (50 to 700 nm); emulsions—oil in water type mixtures, stabilized with surfactants (e.g., perfluorocarbons, 200 to 400 nm); polymers—flexible designer approach with controlled size (40 to 200 nm) and shape (e.g., polyhydroxy acids, dendrimers); and metallic (15 to 60 nm; e.g., iron oxide, gold nanoparticles, carbon nanotubes, fullerenes). However, toxicity information on nanoparticles is limited. Oxidative damage, dermal toxicity, and granulomas have been reported.[76]

Theranostic Agents. Theranostic agents are integrated therapeutic and diagnostic molecules. Addition of a diagnostic moiety enables temporal and spatial monitoring of the therapeutic agent, confirms delivery at the desired target, identifies the need for dose modification, and quantifies the molecular efficiency. Nanoparticles can deliver drugs by liposomes through endocytosis or contact-facilitated drug delivery that requires close apposition between the carrier and the targeted cell membrane. Examples include fumagillin nanoparticle against angiogenesis and CLIO-THPC and CLIO-Cy5.5 against inflammation.[66] Iron oxide nanoparticles with attached Cy5.5 (near-infrared fluorescence [NIRF]), MPAP (membrane translocation myristoylated polyarginine peptide), and siRNA can be detected by both MRI and fluorescence and are efficiently taken up by cells and silence specific genes such as green fluorescence protein. siRNA attached to antisense to survivin, an inhibitor of apoptosis proteins, is used in mice for the treatment for cancer.[68]

Targets and Agents in Atherosclerosis

The various techniques of molecular MRI are described in Table 28-7.

Endothelial Adhesion Molecules. Endothelial adhesion molecules are involved in early stages of atherogenesis with increased expression. Vascular cell adhesion molecule 1 (VCAM-1) is a ligand for very late antigen 4 (VLA-4) and $\alpha_4\beta_1$ integrin. VINP-28 (VCAM-1 internalizing nanoparticle 28), a magnetofluorescent nanoparticle with iron oxide and the ligand VHPKQHR that is homologous to VLA-4, is trapped in VCAM-1–expressing cells. Uptake in atherosclerotic plaques has been shown in mice and human carotid artery plaques.[77]

TABLE 28–7	Molecular MRI Techniques in Atherosclerosis
Technique	**Mechanism**
Dynamic contrast-enhanced MRI	Assessment of permeability of neovasculature due to angiogenesis
Enhanced permeability and retention	Long-circulating macromolecular agent that accumulates in inflamed plaque over time because of enhanced permeability
Ex vivo labeled cells	Cells are labeled ex vivo (e.g., monocytes) and injected into body and tracked in vivo
In vivo labeled cells	Intravenous injection of probe or contrast agent that is taken up by cells of interest (e.g., monocyte tracking)
Conjugate imaging probe with one or several targeting ligands that will recognize and bind receptors	Targeting of cell surface receptors expressed in endothelium or inside plaque with increased permeability
Modified lipoproteins	Enriched lipoproteins follow the HDL pathway and localize to the lipid core

Another ligand, VHHSPNKK, with homology to a chain of VLA-4, also showed similar results.[78] VINP-28 can also be conjugated to fluorescence, infrared, or radioactive probes. The trimodality nanoparticle for detection by MRI, PET, and NIRF is made up of dextrinated and DTPA-modified nanoparticle (20 nm), labeled [64]Cu (PET tracer), and a fluorophore.[79] Dual ligand technique (binding to VCAM-1 and P-selectin) has also been demonstrated.[80]

Inflammation. Inflammation plays an important role in pathogenesis of atherosclerosis, resulting in plaque rupture, thrombotic vessel occlusion, and major vascular events. Macrophages are involved in atheroma initiation, propagation, and rupture.

USPIO or magnetic nanoparticles coated with dextran, such as ferumoxtran-10 and ferumoxytol, are taken up by macrophages in atherosclerotic plaques and produce dark signal in MRI due to T2* shortening,[69] with good histopathologic correlation to plaque macrophage activity and iron deposition in carotid endarterectomy specimens[81] but no correlation with luminal stenosis, indicating that they are independent risk factors. In stroke patients, USPIO uptake was seen even on the asymptomatic side; and in patients undergoing coronary artery bypass grafting, uptake was seen in asymptomatic atheromas, indicating the systemic nature of disease.[69,81] Vessel inflammation may be quantified to identify high-risk plaques. Imaging of coronary plaques by this technique would require high resolution and signal-to-noise ratio, probably achievable with intravascular coils or novel pulse sequences.[70] Bimodality nanoparticles (CLIO-Cy5.5, CLIO-VT680, CLIO-Cy7, CLIO-VT570) for NIRF and MRI and trimodality nanoparticles (^{64}Cu, CLIO-VT680) for NIRF, PET, and MRI are available and have higher signal and sensitivity.[79]

USPIOs have been used in plaque progression and regression trials, both in animals and in humans. Anti-inflammatory treatment reduced USPIO uptake by 70% in a mouse model. In the ATHEROMA study, in which subjects received either 10 mg or 80 mg of atorvastatin, imaging at 12 weeks with ferumoxtran showed significant reduction of inflammation in the higher dose group (Fig. 28-16).[82] However, these studies are based on visual estimation, and quantitative techniques are required. In another study,[74] an anti-inflammatory agent, p38 MAPK (mitogen-activated protein kinase) inhibitor SB-239063, was given to knockout mice, which resulted

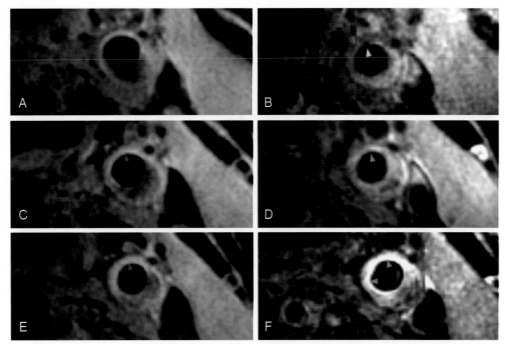

FIGURE 28-16 T2*-weighted imaging of a left common carotid artery before and after ultrasmall superparamagnetic iron oxide (USPIO) infusion at the three time points of 0 (**A** and **B**), 6 (**C** and **D**), and 12 weeks (**E** and **F**). **B,** USPIO uptake can clearly be seen in the plaque at baseline (arrowhead). **C** and **E,** Pre-USPIO imaging remains similar at all three time points with Sinerem having been cycled out of the plaque before reimaging (arrowhead). **D,** The plaque begins to enhance at 6 weeks (arrowhead). This signifies that there is a predominant T1 effect, indicating minimal USPIO uptake and a lack of activated macrophages (minimal inflammation). **E,** No residual USPIO signal is also seen in the pre-USPIO imaging at 12 weeks. **F,** Signal enhancement post-USPIO can be seen with no evidence of signal voids (arrowheads). *(Modified from Tang TY, Howarth SPS, Miller SR, et al: The ATHEROMA [Atorvastatin Therapy: Effects on Reduction of Macrophage Activity] Study. Evaluation using ultrasmall superparamagnetic iron oxide-enhanced magnetic resonance imaging in carotid disease. J Am Coll Cardiol 53:2039, 2009.)*

in no change in plaque macrophage content between SB-239063 animals and normal controls, but diminished iron oxide uptake on MRI was seen in SB-239063–treated mice, suggesting decrease in macrophage phagocytic activity.[69,81]

Signal produced by iron agents is highly dependent on technical parameters. In addition, signal is limited by long delay for imaging and background imaging artifacts. Bright signal can be obtained with use of iron agents, in appropriate sequences and concentration. Serial inversion recovery MRI with monocrystalline iron oxide nanoparticle-47 produced high signal in rabbits.[83] Other techniques include gradient echo acquisition for SPIO, inversion recovery on resonance water suppression, and ultrashort echo time, all of which enhance the signal.[84] Postcontrast T1-weighted MRA done 5 days after introduction of USPIO will generate high signal in the lumen because of low concentration of luminal USPIO (T1 shortening) at 5 days and signal drop in the plaques because of high concentration in plaque (T2/T2* shortening),[73] which is ideal for visualization of both the lumen and the plaques. Another interesting study found that in carotid stenosis, dark signal is seen in symptomatic patients because of high macrophage content, high uptake, and high concentration, but mild high signal is seen in asymptomatic patients because of large fibrous caps, fewer macrophages, and low concentration of USPIO.[85]

Nanoparticles containing immunomicelles with monoclonal antibodies targeting scavenger receptors (MSR) and high payload of gadolinium (5900 molecules) have been used in mice (Fig. 28-17)[86] to demonstrate high signal at 1 and 24 hours in actively inflamed plaques, with good histopathologic correlation. USPIOs can potentially be used in the future to target macrophage markers such as MAC387 and CD68.[69]

Angiogenesis. Angiogenesis results in enhanced permeability of neovasculature, which can be detected by dynamic contrast-enhanced MRI (DCE-MRI) or by use of long-circulating contrast agents that progressively accumulate in the plaque.

Dynamic Contrast-Enhanced MRI. Post–gadolinium contrast enhancement kinetics measured by DCE-MRI has been shown to correlate with plaque neovascularity and vulnerability. Kinetic modeling and integrated area under the enhancement versus time curve are useful in characterizing enhancement dynamics in plaque. Fractional plasma volume (V_p) correlates strongly with histologically validated neovasculature content, which is the main source of entry of inflammatory cells into atherosclerotic plaques. Transfer constant (K^{trans}) is also a potential marker of plaque inflammation because it correlates with macrophage density,[87] neovasculature,[88] loose matrix content, serum markers of inflammation, and proinflammatory risk factors (C-reactive protein, LDL, smoking). There is mild overestimation of neovasculature as measured by dynamic MRI because of rapid exchange of contrast agent between the plasma and interstitial volumes. Any region that comes to equilibrium within one time frame of dynamic sequence will be indistinguishable from blood[13] (Fig. 28-18).

Macromolecular Agents. Macromolecular agents such as gadofluorine and paramagnetic micellar agents accumulate over time in atherosclerotic plaques because of increased vascular permeability and retention. In addition, because of its lipophilic nature, gadofluorine forms 5-nm micelles in aqueous solution and preferentially labels the fatty cores of plaques in cholesterol-fed rabbits.[89]

Gadofosveset (Vasovist, MS-325) is a new gadolinium-based contrast agent that heavily (>75%) binds to serum

28

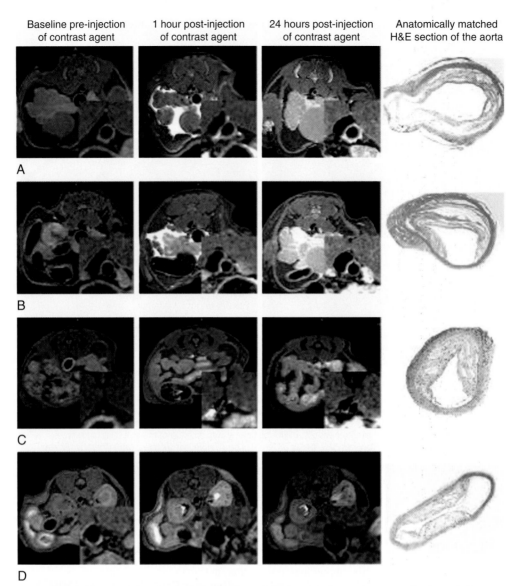

Baseline pre-injection of contrast agent | 1 hour post-injection of contrast agent | 24 hours post-injection of contrast agent | Anatomically matched H&E section of the aorta

FIGURE 28-17 In vivo MR images obtained at baseline and after injection of macrophage-targeted immunomicelles **(A, B)**, untargeted micelles **(C)**, and Gd-DTPA **(D)** in ApoE⁻/⁻ mice. The MRI insets are enlargements of the aortas. **A-D, right,** Hematoxylin and eosin sections of the aorta at the identical anatomic level as the MRI images from the same animal. Very significant heterogeneous enhancement of the aortic wall was seen, at least twofold higher than untargeted micelles. *(Modified from Amirbekian V, Lipinski MJ, Briley-Saebo KC, et al: Detecting and assessing macrophages in vivo to evaluate atherosclerosis noninvasively using molecular MRI. Proc Natl Acad Sci U S A 104:961, 2007.)*

albumin (>75%), resulting in a long elimination half-life and high relaxivity. It produces higher enhancement than gadopentetate dimeglumine (Gd- DTPA) in atherosclerotic plaques of rabbits, either because of increased entry into a leaky microvasculature due to its small size or through normal microvasculature due to albumin binding (Fig. 28-19). Once inside the plaque, it binds to albumin, which is present in higher quantities in plaques, resulting in increased relaxivity, which causes increased signal.[90]

Gadofluorine M (GdF) enhancement correlates directly with plaque instability because it preferentially binds to collagenous material within plaques, and it accumulates more and penetrates deeper into plaques with large numbers of foam cells.[91] It also has a long plaque half-life (24 hours), which improves the conspicuity of atherosclerotic vessel wall both at 1 and 24 hours. Multiple plaques and multiple vascular territories can be imaged with a single injection.

Angiogenesis Marker Imaging. $\alpha_V\beta_3$ integrin (glycoprotein)–specific antibodies and $\alpha_V\beta_3$-specific RGD peptides or peptidomimetics are molecules that target markers expressed on angiogenically activated endothelial cells. Nanoparticle targeted to $\alpha_V\beta_3$ integrin is a perfluorocarbon type, with a high payload of gadolinium (Gd-DTPA bis-oleate, 90,000 atoms per particle) that can be imaged by both ultrasound and MRI.[68]

Theranostic Agent. Fumagillin, an antiangiogenic drug, has been delivered along with integrin-targeted nanoparticles in rabbits, which showed decreased MRI enhancement 1 week after treatment. Baseline enhancement predicted therapeutic response, with low response in those with higher baseline enhancement. Dual angiogenesis-targeted fumagillin nanoparticle (integrin $\alpha_V\beta_3$, $\alpha_5\beta_1$) is more effective than single. Fumagillin has also been shown to have a synergistic antiangiogenic effect with statins.[92]

Proteases. Inflammatory proteases promote extracellular matrix digestion, plaque remodeling, and fibrous cap rupture.

Matrix Metalloproteinase. Matrix metalloproteinase is a surrogate marker for the presence of macrophages. P947 is a gadolinium chelate (Gd-DOTA) covalently bound to a peptide that specifically binds to matrix metalloproteinases at the enzymatic active site; it has been shown to localize to the fibrous cap of atherosclerotic plaque in mice and human carotid arteries, producing greater and longer contrast effects than Gd-DTPA.[87,93]

Myeloperoxidase. Myeloperoxidase is a heme peroxidase enzyme that generates oxidant species hypochlorous acid. It is produced by macrophages within the plaque and promotes atherogenesis by modifying LDL, inactivating HDL and nitric oxide, activating matrix metalloproteinases, releasing tissue factor, and causing apoptosis. Myeloperoxidase substrates are available that, when oligomerized, produce high signal with MRI.[66]

Cathepsins. Cathepsins include cysteine proteases that are produced by macrophages, endothelial cells, and smooth muscle cells. Cathepsins S and K degrade extracellular matrix through their elastase and collagenase properties and destabilize plaque. Cathepsin K localizes to the shoulder of ruptured atherosclerotic plaques, which can be imaged by NIRF or MRI with an activatable imaging agent that becomes fluorescent after enzymatic cleavage by cathepsin B and is detected by fluorescence-mediated tomography co-registered with MRI.[94]

Apoptosis. Apoptotic cells express on their surface phosphatidylserine, a phospholipid that is normally seen in the inner cell membrane of viable cells. Annexin A binds to phosphatidylserine, which, when it is cross-linked to iron oxide, can be used for MRI in humans and animals. Dual modality particles (CLIO-annexin-Cy5.5) use iron oxide and Cy5.5 for MRI and optical imaging.[68] Annexin V has been shown to localize with nonapoptotic macrophages and intraplaque hemorrhages.[64]

Extracellular Matrix Production. Elastin-binding Gd-DTPA, a novel low-molecular-weight gadolinium chelate ([153]Gd-labeled BMS753951) with high affinity to elastin and a high relaxivity, localizes preferentially in the arterial wall of hypercholesterolemic rabbits, facilitating MRI imaging of plaque location, lesion burden, and remodeling. Uptake was seen in ApoE mice at the sites of extracellular matrix

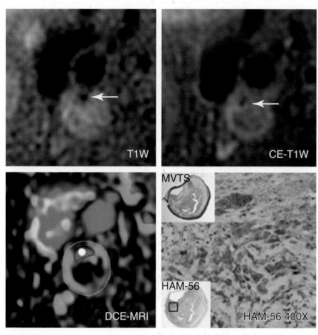

FIGURE 28-18 Dynamic contrast-enhanced MRI of an inflamed fibrous cap of plaque (in T1W and CE-T1W) shows high transfer constant (green) in the adventitial vasa vasorum (near the outer vessel wall boundary) and along the lumen boundary (inner boundary demarcating red lumen region). *(Modified from Chu B, Ferguson MS, Chen H, et al: Cardiac magnetic resonance features of the disruption-prone and the disrupted carotid plaque. JACC Cardiovasc Imaging 2:883, 2009.)*

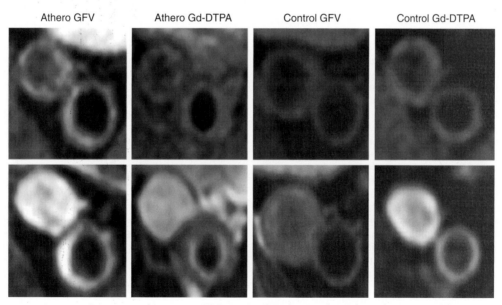

FIGURE 28-19 Precontrast and postcontrast MR images in atherosclerotic and control animals receiving gadofosveset (GFV) and Gd-DTPA. **Top row,** Precontrast images. **Bottom row,** Postcontrast images. Athero, atherosclerotic rabbit; Gd-DTPA, gadopentetate dimeglumine. Signal enhancement after contrast agent administration is seen in all groups except control animals receiving gadofosveset. The signal enhancement is higher for atherosclerotic than for control animals imaged with gadofosveset. Gd-DTPA could not enable discrimination between normal and atherosclerotic vessel walls. *(Modified from Lobbes MBI, Miserus RJ, Heeneman S, et al: Atherosclerosis: contrast-enhanced MR imaging of vessel wall in rabbit model—comparison of gadofosveset and gadopentetate dimeglumine. Radiology 250:682, 2009.)*

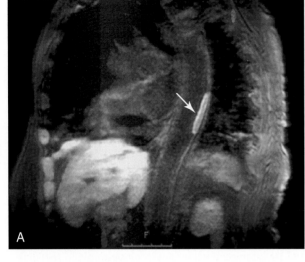

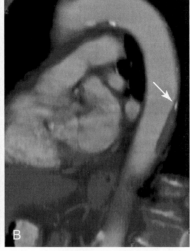

FIGURE 28-20 Sagittal black blood MRI **(A)** after injection of EP-2104R shows high uptake within thrombus (arrow) in descending thoracic aorta. In the CT scan **(B),** plaque is seen as a dark structure (arrow). *(Modified from Spuentrup E, Botnar RM, Wiethoff AJ, et al: MR imaging of thrombi using EP-2104R, a fibrin specific contrast agent: initial results in patients,* Eur Radiol *18:1995, 2008.)*

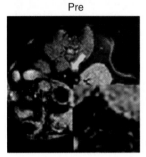

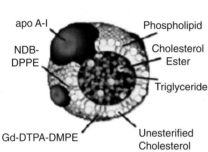

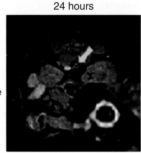

Pre

24 hours

apo A-I

NDB-DPPE

Phospholipid

Cholesterol Ester

Triglyceride

Gd-DTPA-DMPE

Unesterified Cholesterol

FIGURE 28-21 In vivo MR images of abdominal aorta in 8-week-old mouse, before **(left image)** and after **(right image)** injection of recombinant HDL-like nanoparticles **(middle image),** show uptake within the abdominal aortic plaque (arrow). *(Modified from Frias JC, Williams KJ, Fisher EA, et al: Recombinant HDL-like nanoparticles: a specific agent for MRI of atherosclerotic plaques.* J Am Chem Soc *126:16316, 2004.)*

formation (intimal hyperplasia), aneurysm (elastin degradation), and hypertension (excess elastin formation), including coronary artery plaques and poststent injuries.[95]

Thrombus. Thrombus can be imaged with use of ligands against targets such as fibrin, platelet integrins, tissue factor, and factor XIIIa.

Fibrin-specific probes using paramagnetic perfluorocarbon nanoparticles with a high payload of gadolinium chelates (50,000 to 90,000 gadolinium atoms) conjugated with fibrin-specific antibodies localize to disrupted carotid plaques.[96] Fibrin-binding gadolinium-labeled peptide with only four gadolinium chelates per targeting moiety can also be used if there is abundant fibrin. Iron particles with antifibrin antibodies have also been used in animal studies.[97]

EP-2104R is a novel fibrin-specific gadolinium-based agent that localizes to and enhances in the intraluminal thrombus layer. With use of this agent, a vulnerable plaque with plaque erosion and thrombus can be localized with single delayed postcontrast heavily T1-weighted electrocardiography-gated black blood sequence[97] (Fig. 28-20). Thrombi of various ages can be localized in various vascular territories and the heart. In humans, its use has been demonstrated in patients with transient ischemic attack, but coronary arterial imaging would be challenging.

Platelets could be targeted by arginine–glycine–aspartic acid peptides or single-chain antibody that is specific for activated conformation of glycoprotein IIb/IIIa. Tissue factor and factor XIIIa have also been imaged in vitro with MRI.[76]

Lipoproteins. Enriched lipoproteins with contrast-inducing species can be used to localize to the lipid core because they will follow the HDL pathways into plaque macrophages. HDL for molecular imaging can be reconstituted from humans

or can be recombinant. Reconstituted HDL particle (9 nm) contains phospholipids with human apolipoprotein A-I, with or without unesterified cholesterol and Gd-DTPA-DMPE. Recombinant HDL is made up of apolipoprotein A-I–mimicking peptide 37pA (7.6 nm) or 18aA (8.0 nm), phospholipid, Gd-DTPA-DMPE (15 to 20 molecules per particle), and fluorescent phopholipid[98] (Fig. 28-21). Both these molecules are localized to the intima of atherosclerotic plaques in mice and enhanced in 24 hours.[99]

Oxidized LDL is a key factor in initiation and progression of atherosclerosis that indicates an unstable plaque because it upregulates matrix metalloproteinases and apoptosis. Micelles containing gadolinium and IK17 Fab (antibodies to oxidation-specific isotopes) localize to atherosclerotic plaques in apolipoprotein E–deficient mice at 72 hours.[100]

Osteogenesis and Calcification. The superficial calcified nodule is a marker of vulnerable plaque, and this can be detected by macrophage-avid MRI magnetofluorescent nanoparticles coupled with intravital confocal fluorescence microscopy. Bisphosphonate probes have been used to detect osteogenesis in early-stage carotid plaques.[101]

POSITRON EMISSION TOMOGRAPHY

PET is based on beta decay of radioisotopes that results in the emission of a positron, a positively charged beta particle. After emission, the positron travels a few millimeters in tissue and collides with an electron, which results in complete annihilation of both the positron and electron and conversion to energy in the form of two high-energy (511 keV) gamma rays that are released at 180 degrees from each other.

PET detectors register only events with temporal coincidence of photons striking at directly opposite detectors, which enhances the spatial and temporal resolution of PET compared with SPECT. Easy labeling of primary substrates for energy metabolism and membrane receptor subtypes in the heart allows highly sensitive investigation of physiologic pathways and quantization of tissue metabolism.

PET uses positron-emitting isotopes (oxygen 15, carbon 11, nitrogen 13, and fluorine 18) that are incorporated into physiologically active molecules. Rubidium Rb 82 chloride, [13N]ammonia, and [15O]water are tracers that evaluate perfusion; [18F]fluorodeoxyglucose (FDG), [11C]acetate, and [11C] palmitate evaluate metabolism. Dynamic-mode PET allows evaluation of rate of change of physiologic processes. However, PET scanning is associated with significant ionizing radiation and has limited spatial resolution to evaluate coronary arteries.

PET/CT is a type of hybrid imaging that combines the images from PET and CT scans performed at the same time on the same machine, which helps in correlation of anatomic and functional information, thereby improving accuracy; at the same time, it reduces scanning time (faster CT acquisition for co-registration and attenuation correction of PET data) and radiation dose. Multiple targets can also be evaluated in the same examination.[39] PET/MRI co-registers low spatial resolution PET with high spatial resolution MRI images, with significantly lower radiation dose than in PET/CT.

In the cardiovascular system, PET can be used in direct evaluation of the atherosclerotic plaque and also in the assessment of myocardial ischemia.

PET Imaging of Atherosclerotic Plaque

Imaging of Macrophages

FDG is taken up into cells similar to glucose, but it does not have the metabolic pathway for further metabolism and excretion. Linked to ^{18}F, a positron emitter, FDG can be used to detect and to quantify FDG within the tissue of interest. FDG-PET is useful in assessment of inflammatory activity within atherosclerotic plaque because the macrophages in inflamed plaque show avid FDG uptake and accumulation. The efficacy of PET in detecting atherosclerotic inflammation in various vascular beds has been extensively demonstrated in various human and animal[5] studies that used PET/CT or co-registered information with CT or MRI.

Higher FDG uptake has been demonstrated in symptomatic than in asymptomatic carotid plaques.[102] Autoradiography confirmed that the uptake was within macrophages, and there was a direct correlation between FDG uptake and macrophage burden in the plaque (Fig. 28-22).[103] The carotid FDG uptake was higher in men, older age, and those with higher inflammatory biomarkers, metabolic syndrome, hypertension, hyperlipidemia, low HDL concentration, high levels of high-sensitivity C-reactive protein, and CAD.[104,105] In symptomatic patients with transient ischemic attack, uptake was also seen in asymptomatic nonstenotic areas on the opposite and same side, indicating that angiography may not always identify the culprit lesion.[106] There was no overlap between inflammation and calcification, indicating that calcification represents a much later stage of the disease process.

Combined MRI and PET can identify lesions responsible for embolic events, with MRI delineating the vascular lumen and PET identifying inflammation.[107] In addition, FDG uptake may predict plaque rupture and clinical events. In a rabbit atherosclerotic model, plaque thrombosis was promoted by Russell viper venom injection, and FDG-PET was done before and after triggering of thrombus. Segments that developed thrombus had the highest FDG uptake and highest macrophage activity. FDG uptake and hence plaque inflammation

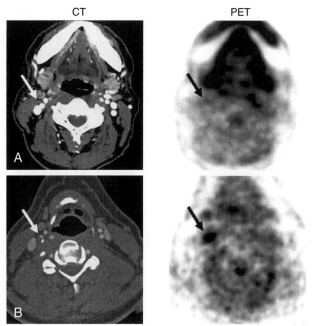

CT   PET

FIGURE 28-22 Axial PET images and the co-registered CT images from two patients, one (patient A) who manifested low ^{18}F-fluorodeoxyglucose (FDG) uptake in the region of the carotid plaque and one (patient B) with high FDG uptake in the region of the carotid plaque. The region of the excised carotid plaque is noted with arrows. **A,** Trichrome-stained histologic specimen from patient A demonstrated a collagen-rich plaque with low lipid content, and CD68 staining on the high-powered images demonstrated limited macrophage infiltration. These histologic features are consistent with a metabolically stable and potentially clinically stable plaque. **B,** Trichrome-stained histologic specimen from patient B demonstrated a complex plaque with a necrotic core, and the CD68 staining demonstrated intense macrophage infiltration. These histologic features are consistent with a metabolically unstable plaque that is vulnerable to rupture. *(Modified from Tawakol A, Migrino RQ, Bashian GG, et al: In vivo 18F-fluorodeoxyglucose positron emission tomography imaging provides a noninvasive measure of carotid plaque inflammation in patients.* J Am Coll Cardiol 48:1818, 2006.)

increased proportionally with duration of cholesterol feeding.[108] In a study of 2000 cancer patients, patients with the highest arterial FDG uptake were more likely to have previously suffered a vascular event.[109]

FDG-PET is a proven, reproducible technique in the detection of inflammation in different arterial beds, such as the aorta[110] and the vertebral,[107] brachial, subclavian, and peripheral arteries, including femoral and iliac arteries.[111] However, PET imaging of coronary arteries is limited by significant background FDG uptake by metabolically active myocardium, small size of the coronary arteries and plaque,[112] and deep location, tortuosity, and mobility of coronary arteries. Myocardial FDG uptake could be bypassed by use of high-fat/low-glucose protein preferred diet or beta blockers before imaging. Spatial resolution can be improved by co-registering with CT or MRI or by use of intravascular radiation detectors. Electrocardiographic or respiratory gating is used to reduce motion.[110]

PET has also been well established as a useful technique in serial follow-up for evaluation of plaque for progression or regression, with high interobserver and intraobserver reproducibility,[5] although there might be a change in pattern of uptake due to waxing and waning of atherosclerosis.[113] Decreased FDG uptake has been demonstrated in aortic wall of atherosclerotic rabbits after the use of statins[114] and after 3-month treatment with probucol.[115] In humans, reduction of carotid plaque inflammation that correlated with HDL elevation was demonstrated after just 3 months of simvastatin therapy in 43 oncology patients (Fig. 28-23). MRI typically takes up to a year for changes to be visualized.[116]

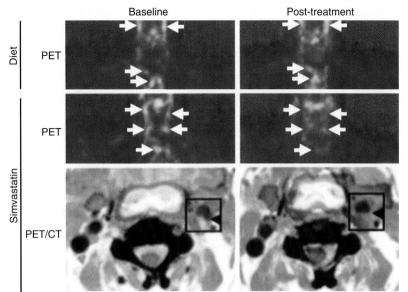

Baseline Post-treatment

Diet — PET

Simvastatin — PET

PET/CT

FIGURE 28-23 Effects of simvastatin on [18]FDG uptake in atherosclerotic plaque inflammation. Representative [18]FDG-PET images at baseline and after 3 months of treatment (post-treatment) with dietary management alone (diet) or simvastatin. **Top,** Dietary management alone had no effect on [18]FDG uptakes (arrows) in the aortic arch and the carotid arteries. **Middle,** ^{18}F-FDG uptakes were attenuated by simvastatin treatment. **Bottom,** The co-registered images of [18]FDG-PET and CT clearly show that the plaque [18]FDG uptakes (arrowheads) disappeared after 3-month treatment with simvastatin. *(Modified from Tahara N, Kai H, Ishibashi M, et al: Simvastatin attenuates plaque inflammation.* J Am Coll Cardiol *48:1825, 2006.)*

The limitations of FDG-PET for macrophages are nonspecific uptake in endothelial cells and lymphocytes and partial volume artifact. This could be overcome by concomitant use of high-resolution MRI/CT.

Other Macrophage Targets

Other targets for imaging of macrophages include benzodiazepine receptors in mitochondrial membranes, particularly in macrophages, using targeted agents such as [^{11}C](R)-PK11195[117] or PBR28.[70]

Other PET Targets

Proliferating smooth muscle cells in the plaque can be imaged by indium In 111–labeled Z2D3. LDL labeled with indium In 125 and technetium Tc 99m accumulates in the lipid core of atherosclerosis and can be imaged. Annexin V and other markers also can be used, labeled with PET-compatible tracers such as [124]I and [18]F.

VCAM

With use of ^{18}F-labeled 4V (linear, multivalent tetrameric synthetic peptide VHPKQHR, which has sequence homology to VLA-4 and increased affinity to VCAM-1), PET/CT showed high uptake in endothelium of atherosclerotic lesions in hypercholesterolemic mice and low uptake in mice receiving an atorvastatin-enriched diet.[118] This tracer has good potential for human use because of its short circulating half-life and high ratio of atherosclerotic/nonatherosclerotic lesion uptake.

RAGE

RAGE (receptor of advanced glycation end products) is an important target in the vessel wall that has been implicated in atherosclerotic progression. It belongs to the immunoglobulin superfamily of cell surface receptors that is expressed in endothelial cells, smooth muscle cells, monocytes-macrophages, and lymphocytes. The three important RAGE ligands are advanced glycation end products, S100/calgranulins, and high-mobility group box 1/amphoterin. The interaction of RAGE ligands with RAGE in inflammatory cells leads to activation of transcription factors, which leads to upregulation of cytokines, adhesion molecules, matrix metalloproteinases, and tissue factor, resulting in chronic cellular activation, vascular inflammation, and endothelial dysfunction. ^{99m}Tc-labeled anti-RAGE F(ab')$_2$ antibodies have been used in atherosclerotic mice.[119] PET studies have been done in rats with use of recombinant human S100A1, S100B, and S100A12 proteins labeled with the positron emitter fluorine 18 (^{18}F) by conjugation with *N*-succinimidyl-[^{18}F]fluorobenzoate ([^{18}F]SFB).[120]

Assessment of Myocardial Ischemia and Adequacy of Risk Factor Reduction

The majority of the burden of CAD is accounted for by traditional risk factors.[121] Asymptomatic silent ischemia is the most common manifestation of CAD and a predictor of adverse clinical outcomes, such as coronary events and cardiac death.[122] Silent ischemia carries similar adverse prognosis in patients after an episode of unstable angina,[123] MI,[124] or chronic stable angina.[125] Decisions for invasive workup and intervention cannot be based solely on symptoms and morphologic detection of stenosis.

Hyperlipidemia-induced endothelial dysfunction can also cause vasoconstriction of established coronary stenosis and result in silent or overt ischemia,[126] which could be partially reversed by use of a statin.[127] Low–saturated fat, vegetarian diets with mild to moderate exercise and stress management reduced size and severity of perfusion abnormalities on PET scan with only modest regression on angiographic score.[128] Stress reduction has also been shown to treat ischemic episodes.[129]

Repeated episodes of silent ischemia caused by obstruction of epicardial coronary arteries decrease downstream blood flow and perfusion, resulting in small areas of subendocardial necrosis, which eventually leads to fibrosis and left ventricular dysfunction. Cardiac risk increases with severity of ischemia.[130] Functional tests are necessary to identify the presence, extent, and severity of myocardial ischemia, which is associated with outcome. A normal perfusion scan excludes myocardial ischemia, with an event rate of less than 1% per year.[131] These tests can act as a gatekeeper for coronary angiography and help in choosing the optimal therapeutic pathway.

Ischemia can be managed by either anti-ischemic drugs (beta blockers, calcium channel blockers, nitrates, or combination) or revascularization procedures. There is no strong evidence to suggest that complete suppression of ischemia with aggressive drug therapy improves the adverse clinical outcomes. Several studies have shown improved outcomes in silent ischemia after revascularization. The Asymptomatic Cardiac Ischemia Pilot (ACIP) study[132] found that coronary artery bypass grafting suppressed ischemia more than percutaneous transluminal coronary angioplasty at 12 weeks, and 1- or 2-year mortality was lower for revascularized patients than for those receiving medical therapy. The DANAMI[133] and SWISSI II[134] trials showed better outcomes for percutaneous coronary intervention compared with medical therapy for post-MI ischemia, although both trials did not use optimal medical therapy or optimized interventional therapy. The COURAGE trial compared optimal medical therapy with optimal medical therapy and percutaneous coronary intervention with bare metal stents and found no difference between both groups in the primary endpoint of death from any cause and nonfatal MI in 4.6 years.[129]

Investigative procedures are necessary for objective assessment of therapeutic response to ischemia. Although Holter monitoring and elimination of ST-segment depression on electrocardiography can be used to evaluate the efficacy of these therapies, they are not accurate or reliable because of marked variability in the number and duration of ischemic episodes as detected by this technique.[135] PET is an ideal technique for evaluation of silent or overt ischemia and assessment of response to various therapies because of its high accuracy and reliability in quantitative estimation of myocardial blood flow and perfusion reserve.

Detection of myocardium previously exposed to ischemia can be useful in identification of myocardium at risk for acute coronary syndromes. Annexin V and ^{123}I-labeled β-methyl-p-iodophenyl-pentadecanoic acid are potential ischemic molecular markers.[130]

Evaluation of Ischemia by PET

Coronary Blood Reserve

Coronary or myocardial blood reserve (MBR) is the increase of myocardial blood flow (MBF) from rest to stress (MBR = MBF during stress – MBF during rest). Coronary blood flow normally adapts rapidly to meet the changing myocardial oxygen demands to maintain normal contraction. Because oxygen extraction at rest is already at maximum, oxygen supply can be maintained at stress only by increasing coronary blood flow. Coronary blood flow depends on aortic diastolic pressure and downstream resistance. Aortic diastolic pressure does not vary much from rest, and hence blood flow can be maintained only by decreased resistance.

In animals, resistance to coronary flow is provided by large epicardial vessels (R1), coronary arterioles (R2), and wall tension from ventricular chambers (R3). R2 predominates at rest, but with stress, blood flow increases up to four times because of reduction of R2 resistance and mild dilation of epicardial vessels with normal endothelial cell function. R3 may be increased or unchanged, depending on increase in chamber radius and wall tension. In mild coronary stenosis, flow is maintained at rest and stress by autoregulatory dilation of downstream arteriolar resistance vessels. With moderate stenosis, rest flow is maintained by use of coronary reserve, but inadequate vasodilatory reserve is available during stress to decrease resistance and to increase flow. With severe stenosis, there is no vasodilatory reserve to maintain even resting circulation.

In humans, CAD is more complex, with the coronary blood reserve affected by length and complexity of stenosis. The presence and extent of CAD are not always related to clinical manifestations of ischemic heart disease, and it is not always possible to predict its progression and response to treatment. In humans with normal endothelial function, during stress, coronary flow increases because of coronary arterial and arteriolar vasodilation, resulting in maximal coronary flow reserve.

Subjects with traditional coronary risk factors demonstrate abnormal coronary vasoreactivity in both epicardial and resistance vessels (through passive elastic behavior of microvascular walls at vasodilation). Coronary functional and microvascular alterations may coexist with epicardial coronary artery lesions and contribute to ischemia. In addition, endothelial dysfunction without significant coronary artery stenosis can also cause ischemia by coronary vascular and blood flow abnormalities that reduce coronary vasodilating properties at macrovascular and microvascular levels. In addition, a stenosis may not be discrete. Development of collaterals also changes the blood flow patterns.

Role of PET in the Evaluation of Myocardial Ischemia

PET plays a vital role in evaluation of patients with cardiovascular risk factors or cardiovascular disease and is a well-established modality for evaluation of myocardial perfusion, viability, and metabolism.[136] SPECT measures only regional differences in flow. Balanced ischemia due to multivessel CAD will not be detected on SPECT because of uniform decrease in flow reserve in all vascular territories. PET can quantify absolute regional coronary blood flow at rest and stress and calculate the coronary blood flow reserve.

Detection of mild abnormalities in myocardial blood flow reserve with PET potentially allows early identification of CAD that is characterized by endothelial dysfunction in asymptomatic patients with elevated cholesterol, smoking, hypertension, and insulin resistance. Abnormal blood flow reserve may be a predictor of future cardiovascular outcomes among patients with cardiomyopathies in the absence of CAD.[137]

Compared with SPECT, PET has higher spatial resolution, improved attenuation and scatter correction, and higher sensitivity and specificity in detection of CAD. PET also provides information on cardiac metabolism in absolute terms. The main limitation of PET is the short half-life of the tracers, [13N]ammonia and [82]Rb, which necessitates an on-site cyclotron for [13N]ammonia and expensive monthly replacement of the generator for [82]Rb. Use of drugs instead of exercise is another limitation of PET because exercise is an important component of myocardial perfusion imaging studies with independent prognostic and diagnostic value (Fig. 28-24).

Cardiac Metabolism

Fasting Metabolism

ATP is generated by oxidative phosphorylation and glycolysis. The major energy sources of the heart are fatty acids, glucose, and lactate, depending on the physiologic condition and arterial concentrations. During fasting, energy is mainly derived from long-chain free fatty acids and to a lesser extent (15% to 20%) from glucose. With normal oxygen supply, ATP and tissue citrate formed by breakdown of fatty acids suppress glucose oxidation. With decreased oxygen supply, ATP and citrate levels fall, and glycolysis is accelerated. Anaerobic glycolysis is maintained only if lactate and hydrogen ions are removed without accumulation. In severe hypoperfusion, lactate and hydrogen accumulate, which inhibits glycolytic enzymes, thus depleting high-energy phosphates, resulting in cell membrane disruption and death.

[18F]FDG

FDG is used for imaging of myocardial glucose use. FDG exchanges across capillaries and cell membranes and is

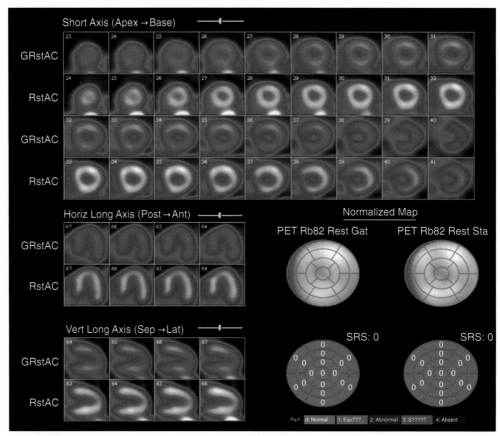

FIGURE 28-24 Normal appearances of PET perfusion scan using ^{82}Rb in a 52-year-old man. No defect is seen in either the rest scan or the post-dipyridamole ^{82}Rb stress scan, indicating absence of ischemia.

phosphorylated by hexokinase to FDG 6-phosphate, but it is not metabolized further or used in glycogen synthesis and is trapped in myocardium because of slow dephosphorylation, thus permitting imaging. PET scan is performed after loading of 50 to 75 g of glucose 1 to 2 hours before injection of 5 to 10 mCi of FDG. In diabetics, image quality may not be good because of low plasma insulin, noninhibition of tissue lipolysis, and high free fatty acid levels. Intravenous insulin after glucose loading, hyperinsulinemic euglycemic clamping, and nicotinic acid derivative are used in diabetics.

PET in Early-Stage Coronary Artery Disease

Abnormal impairment of myocardial perfusion reserve (MPR) without angiographically demonstrated coronary stenosis indicates either undetected atherosclerosis or coronary microvascular or endothelial dysfunction after hemodynamic and extravascular factors are excluded (Fig. 28-25). Myocardial blood flow and MPR can be globally reduced in remote myocardium supplied by angiographically normal coronary arteries in patients with CAD elsewhere. Few studies[137] have shown preserved MPR in regions supplied by angiographically normal coronary arteries in patients with one-vessel CAD. This information is useful to stratify prognosis, to determine treatment, and to monitor treatment.

MPR measured by PET is inversely related to 10-year CHD risk in a population with no known CAD but with low to intermediate CAD risk based on Framingham score.[138] This reflects preclinical disease, which could be a combination of subclinical atherosclerosis and endothelial dysfunction, either of which is not severe enough to be manifested as an overt perfusion defect (in SPECT scan) but is detected by

more sensitive measure of myocardial blood flow with PET; 50% of patients with normal myocardial perfusion PET images show evidence of non–flow-limiting coronary atherosclerosis on CT scan.

Progression of subclinical disease over time contributes to higher future CHD risk, facilitated by underlying endothelial dysfunction that promotes coronary vasoconstriction and thrombosis. Clinically overt abnormalities in flow reserve signify advanced coronary atherosclerosis and merit aggressive risk factor modification and possible revascularization. However, preclinical abnormalities in vasodilator reserve on quantitative PET (but with low to intermediate risk based on Framingham score) also relate to higher estimated CHD risk and might necessitate more aggressive risk factor modification for these subjects. MPR provides a way to document how risk factors translate into measurable damage to coronary circulation, predicting future cardiovascular events, independent of significant coronary stenosis.

In patients with known CAD, there was a significantly worse prognosis in patients with higher reduction of global MPR, making it a more sensitive predictor of sudden death and other adverse outcomes than left ventricular ejection fraction. The prognosis was dependent on global impairment of myocardial perfusion and independent of extent of regional ischemia. This global impairment is common in left ventricular dysfunction due to either primitive myocardial disease or CAD. Coronary vasodilating capability is an independent prognostic determinant.

PET in Advanced Cardiovascular Disease

In patients with established CAD, PET identifies patients with moderate to severe ischemia but with viable

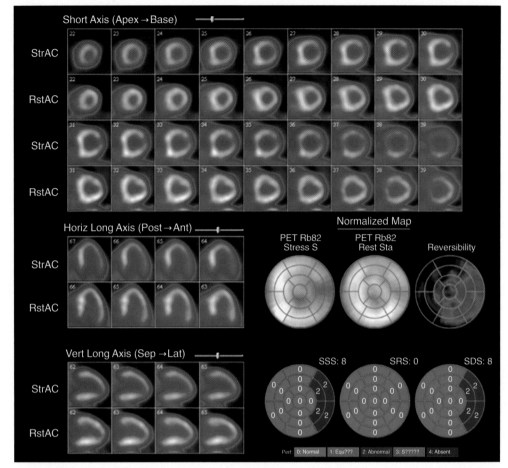

FIGURE 28-25 ⁸²Rb PET perfusion scan in a 62-year-old man with chest pain. The rest scans are normal, but there is a mild perfusion defect in the stress scan in the basal and mid anterolateral and inferolateral segments, consistent with reversible ischemia in the distribution of the left circumflex artery.

TABLE 28–8	Stages of Cardiovascular Ischemia Detected by PET Scan				
	Rest Perfusion	**Stress Perfusion**	**Contraction**	**Coronary Arteries**	**Metabolism**	**Diagnosis**
1	Normal	Normal	Normal	Normal	Normal	Normal
2	Normal	Decreased	Normal	Normal	Normal	Endothelial or microvascular dysfunction Undetected atherosclerosis
3	Normal	Decreased	Normal	Stenosis	Normal	Ischemia by coronary artery stenosis
4	Decreased	Decreased	Decreased	Stenosis	Absent	Infarcted myocardium
5	Present	Decreased	Decreased	Stenosis	Present	Stunned myocardium
6	Decreased	Decreased	Decreased	Stenosis	Present	Hibernating myocardium

myocardium, the subset of patients who will benefit from revascularization. With prolonged imbalance between myocardial supply and demand, high-energy phosphates are depleted, resulting in impaired contraction, which is persistent and results in cell death or infarct. In stunned and hibernating myocardium, myocardial function is depressed at rest, but the myocytes are viable. Stunned myocardium is seen after single or multiple, brief or prolonged transient ischemic episodes followed by reperfusion, resulting in depressed resting function with normal perfusion. Hibernating myocardium is seen after repetitive ischemic episodes resulting in hypoperfusion at rest with depressed myocardial function. Both stunned and hibernating myocardium can recover function after revascularization.

In ischemia, the myocyte metabolism shifts from fatty acids to glucose. Therefore, uptake of an ¹⁸F-labeled glucose analogue (FDG) in a region of myocardium indicates metabolic activity and thus viability. This enables PET to differentiate hibernating and stunned myocardium from infarct. The presence of enhanced FDG uptake in a region of decreased flow (known as a PET perfusion-metabolism mismatch) indicates hibernating myocardium, whereas a reduction in both the metabolism and flow (perfusion-metabolism match) reflects nonviable infarcted myocardium. Dysfunction with normal perfusion and metabolism suggests stunned myocardium (Table 28-8, Fig. 28-26).

PET has mean sensitivity, specificity, and positive and negative predictive values of 93%, 58%, 71%, and 86%,

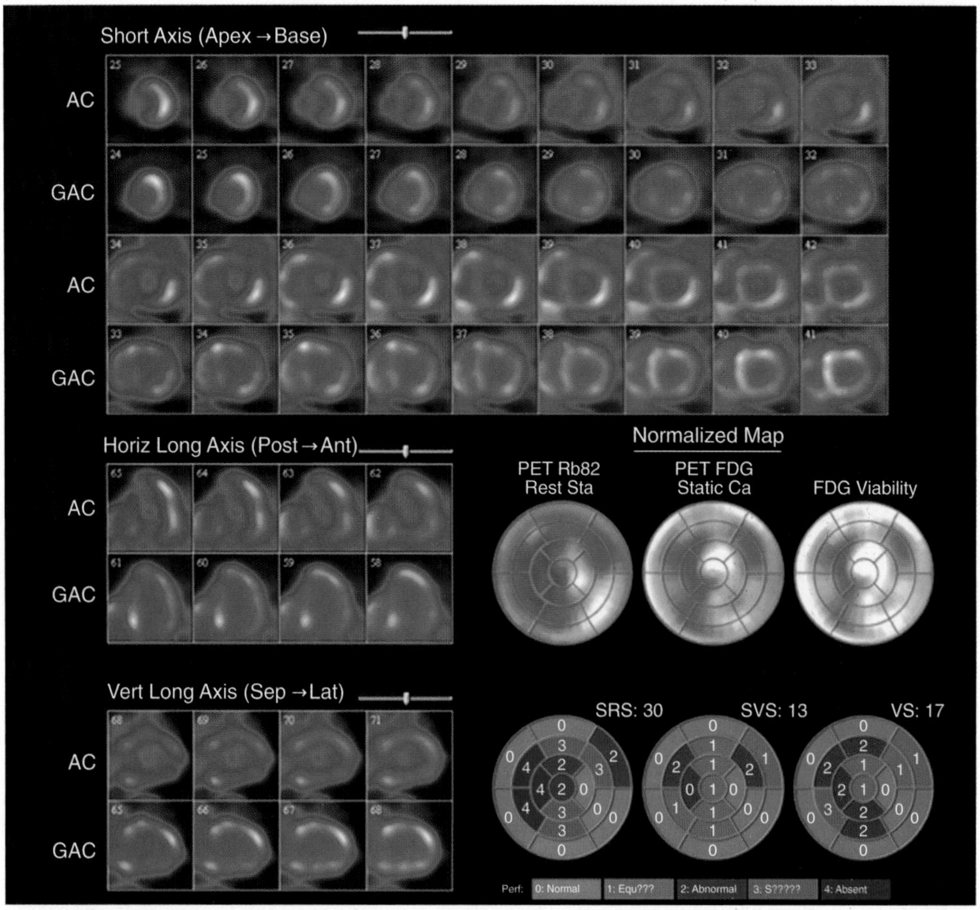

FIGURE 28-26 PET scan in advanced disease. In the rest perfusion images, reduced tracer uptake is seen in the basal and mid anterolateral, mid and apical anterior, inferior, and septal segments and the apex. In the FDG metabolic scan, there is unmatched FDG uptake in the basal anterolateral wall, mid and apical anterior and inferior segments, apex, mid inferior septum, and basal anterolateral wall, indicating hibernating segments in left anterior descending and right coronary artery territories (40% of myocardium). There is no FDG uptake in the mid anterior septum, anterolateral segments, and apical septum, indicating scar (18% of myocardium).

respectively, to detect myocardial viability.[139] Infarcted myocardium has only a 20% chance of functional improvement after revascularization, compared with an 80% to 85% chance for hibernating or stunned myocardium.[140] The scar size on FDG-PET is an independent predictor of improvement in ejection fraction after revascularization.[141] PET may be superior to SPECT in the setting of very severe left ventricular dysfunction.[142]

Thus, PET is a useful noninvasive imaging modality to detect abnormal myocardial blood flow and MPR, which are reliable markers for disease progression and new endpoints of treatment aimed at improving global vascular function. Myocardial perfusion abnormalities in PET have been shown to improve after long-term intense risk factor modification.

CONCLUSION

MRI and PET are useful imaging techniques in the evaluation of different stages of atherosclerosis and assessment of cardiovascular risk factors. High-resolution multicontrast MRI is a valuable noninvasive technique in plaque characterization and quantification. Molecular MRI can detect subclinical stages of atherosclerosis. MRI is also useful in the evaluation of global and regional myocardial function, myocardial ischemia, and various vascular factors. Whole-body MRA can be used to evaluate multiple vascular beds in a single examination, particularly in the asymptomatic intermediate-risk

group. PET scanning can be used in targeted imaging of atherosclerosis with molecular probes and also in the evaluation of myocardial ischemia. Both MRI and PET are useful in the assessment of plaque progression or regression, particularly as a surrogate endpoint of treatment in response to novel drugs.

REFERENCES

1. Libby P: Inflammation in atherosclerosis. *Nature* 420:868, 2002.
2. Lloyd-Jones D, Adams R, Carnethon M, et al: Heart disease and stroke statistics—2009 update: a report from the American Heart Association Statistics Committee and Stroke Statistics Subcommittee. *Circulation* 119:e21, 2009.
3. Boden WE, O'Rourke RA, Teo KK, et al: Optimal medical therapy with or without PCI for stable coronary disease. *N Engl J Med* 356:1503, 2007.
4. Libby P: Act local, act global: inflammation and the multiplicity of vulnerable coronary plaques. *J Am Coll Cardiol* 41:1600, 2005.
5. Rudd JH, Myers KS, Sanz J, et al: Multimodality imaging of atherosclerosis. *Top Magn Reson Imaging* 18:379, 2007.
6. Cai JM, Hatsukami T, Ferguson MS, et al: Classification of human atherosclerotic lesions with in vivo multicontrast magnetic resonance imaging. *Circulation* 106:1368, 2002.
7. Serfaty JM, Chaabane L, Tabib A, et al: Atherosclerotic plaques: classification and characterization with T2 weighted high spatial resolution MR imaging. *Radiology* 219:403, 2001.
8. Fayad ZA, Fallon JT, Shinnar M, et al: Noninvasive in vivo high resolution MRI of atherosclerotic lesions in genetically engineered mice. *Circulation* 98:1541, 1998.
9. Yuan C, Beach KW, Smith LH, et al: Measurement of atherosclerotic carotid plaque size in vivo using high resolution magnetic resonance imaging. *Circulation* 98:2666, 1998.
10. Toussaint JF, LaMuraglia GM, Southern JF, et al: Magnetic resonance images lipid, fibrous, calcified, hemorrhagic and thrombotic components of human atherosclerosis in vivo. *Circulation* 94:932, 1996.

11. Naghavi M, Libby P, Falk E, et al: From vulnerable plaque to vulnerable patient: a call for new definitions and risk assessment strategies: part I. *Circulation* 108:1664, 2003.

12. Libby P, Aikawa M: Stabilization of atherosclerotic plaques: new mechanisms and clinical targets. *Nat Med* 8:1257, 2003.

13. Chu B, Ferguson MS, Chen H, et al: Cardiac magnetic resonance features of the disruption-prone and the disrupted carotid plaque. *JACC Cardiovasc Imaging* 2:883, 2009.

14. Wasserman BA, Smith WI, Trout HH, et al: Carotid atherosclerosis: in vivo morphologic characterization with gadolinium enhanced double oblique MR imaging. Initial results. *Radiology* 223:566, 2002.

15. Glagov S, Weisenberd E, Zarins C, et al: Compensatory enlargement of human atherosclerotic coronary arteries. *N Engl J Med* 316:1371, 1987.

16. Sanz J, Fayad ZA: Imaging of atherosclerotic cardiovascular disease. *Nature* 451:953, 2008.

17. Yuan C, Kerwin WS, Ferguson MS, et al: Contrast enhanced high resolution MRI for atherosclerotic carotid artery tissue characterization. *J Magn Reson Imaging* 15:62, 2002.

18. Momiyama Y, Fayad ZA: Aortic plaque imaging and monitoring atherosclerotic plaque interventions. *Top Magn Reson Imaging* 18:349, 2007.

19. Kerwin W, Xu D, Liu F, et al: Magnetic resonance imaging of carotid atherosclerosis. Plaque analysis. *Top Magn Reson Imaging* 18:371, 2007.

20. Gao T, Zhang Z, Yu W, et al: Atherosclerotic carotid vulnerable plaque and subsequent stroke: a high resolution MRI study. *Cerebrovasc Dis* 27:345, 2009.

21. Mani V, Muntner P, Gidding SS, et al: Cardiovascular magnetic resonance parameters of atherosclerotic plaque burden improve discrimination of prior major adverse cardiovascular events. *J Cardiovasc Magn Reson* 11:10, 2009.

22. Takaya N, Yuan C, Chu B, et al: Presence of intraplaque hemorrhage stimulates progression of carotid atherosclerotic plaques: a high-resolution MRI study. *Circulation* 111:2768, 2005.

23. Flice R, Lima JAC, Bluemke DA: Subclinical disease detection—advanced imaging applications. *Top Magn Reson Imaging* 18:339, 2007.

24. Fayad ZA, Fuster V, Fallon JT, et al: Noninvasive in vivo human coronary artery lumen and wall imaging using black blood magnetic resonance imaging. *Circulation* 102:506, 2000.

25. Botnar RM: Coronary plaque characterization by T1 weighted cardiac magnetic resonance. *JACC Cardiovasc Imaging* 2:729, 2009.

26. Kawasaki T, Koga S, Koga N, et al: Characterization of hyperintense plaque with non-contrast T1-weighted cardiac magnetic resonance coronary plaque imaging: comparison with multislice CT and intravascular ultrasound. *JACC Cardiovasc Imaging* 2:720, 2009.

27. Pasterkamp G, Falk E, Woutman H, et al: Techniques characterizing the coronary atherosclerotic plaque: influence on clinical decision making? *J Am Coll Cardiol* 36:13, 2000.

28. Ibrahim T, Makowski M, Jankauskas A, et al: Serial contrast-enhanced cardiac MRI demonstrates regression of hyperenhancement within the coronary artery wall in patients after acute myocardial infarction. *JACC Cardiovasc Imaging* 2:580, 2009.

29. Virmani R, Burke AP, Farb A, et al: Pathology of the vulnerable plaque. *J Am Coll Cardiol* 47:C13, 2006.

30. McConnell MV, Aikawa M, Maier SE, et al: MRI of rabbit atherosclerosis in response to dietary cholesterol lowering. *Arterioscler Thromb Vasc Biol* 19:1956, 1999.

31. Hegyi L, Hockings P, Benson M, et al: Short term arterial remodelling in the aortae of cholesterol fed New Zealand white rabbits shown in vivo by high resolution magnetic resonance imaging—implications for human pathology. *Pathol Oncol Res* 10:159, 2004.

32. Saam T, Kierwin WS, Chu B, et al: Sample size calculation for clinical trials using MRI for the quantitative assessment of carotid atherosclerosis. *J Cardiovasc Magn Reson* 7:799, 2005.

33. Saam T, Yuan C, Chu B, et al: Predictors of carotid atherosclerotic plaque progression as measured by noninvasive MRI. *Atherosclerosis* 194:e34, 2007.

34. Zhao XQ, Yuan C, Hatsukami TS, et al: Effects of prolonged intensive lipid lowering therapy on the characteristics of carotid atherosclerotic plaques in vivo by MRI: a case-control study. *Arterioscler Thromb Vasc Biol* 21:1623, 2001.

35. Lima JA, Desai MY, Steen H, et al: Statin induced cholesterol lowering and plaque regression after 6 months of magnetic resonance imaging monitored therapy. *Circulation* 110:2336, 2004

36. Corti R, Fuster V, Fayad ZA, et al: Lipid lowering by simvastatin induces regression of human atherosclerotic lesions. *Circulation* 106:2884, 2002.

37. Yonemura A, Momiyama Y, Fayad ZA, et al: Effect of lipid lowering therapy with atorvastatin on atherosclerotic aortic plaques detected by noninvasive MRI. *J Am Coll Cardiol* 45:733, 2005.

38. Corti R, Fuster V, Fayad ZA, et al: Effects of aggressive versus conventional lipid lowering therapy by simvastatin on human atherosclerotic lesions: a prospective, randomized, double-blind trial with high-resolution MRI. *J Am Coll Cardiol* 46:106, 2005.

39. Ayaori M, Momiyama Y, Fayad ZA, et al: Effect of bezafibrate therapy on atherosclerotic aortic plaques detected by MRI in dyslipidemic patients with hypertriglyceridemia. *Atherosclerosis* 196:425, 2008.

40. Corti R, Osende JI, Fallon JT, et al: The selective peroxisomal proliferator activated receptor gamma agonist has an additive effect on plaque regression in combination with simvastatin in experimental atherosclerosis: in vivo study by high resolution magnetic resonance imaging. *J Am Coll Cardiol* 43:464, 2004.

41. Raman SV, Winner MW, III, Tran T, et al: In vivo atherosclerotic plaque characterization using magnetic susceptibility distinguishes symptom producing plaques. *J Am Coll Cardiol* 1:49, 2008.

42. Hinton-Yates DP, Cury RC, Wald LL, et al: 3.0 T plaque imaging. *Top Magn Reson Imaging* 18:389, 2007.

43. Bild DE, Bluemke DA, Burke GL, et al: Multi-ethnic study of atherosclerosis: objectives and design. *Am J Epidemiol* 156:871, 2002.

44. Hansen T, Ahlstrom H, Johansson L: Whole-body screening of atherosclerosis with magnetic resonance angiography. *Top Magn Reson Imaging* 18:329, 2007.

45. Lehrke S, Egenlauf B, Steen H, et al: Prediction of coronary artery disease by a systemic atherosclerosis score index derived from whole-body MRI angiography. *J Cardiovasc Magn Reson* 11:36, 2009.

46. Coulden RA, Moss H, Graves MJ, et al: High resolution magnetic resonance imaging of atherosclerosis and the response to balloon angioplasty. *Heart* 83:188, 2000.

47. Kramer CM: Peripheral arterial disease assessment—wall, perfusion and spectroscopy. *Top Magn Reson Imaging* 18:357, 2007.

48. Myerson SG, Bellenger NG, Pennell DJ: Assessment of LV mass by cardiovascular magnetic resonance. *Hypertension* 39:750, 2002.

49. Schwitter J, Wacker CM, Van Rossum AC, et al: MR-IMPACT: comparison of perfusion CMR with SPECT for the detection of coronary artery disease in a multicentre, multivendor, randomized trial. *Eur Heart J* 29:480, 2008.

50. Ingkanisorn W, Kwong R, Bohme N, et al: Prognosis of negative adenosine stress magnetic resonance in patients presenting to an emergency department with chest pain. *J Am Coll Cardiol* 47:1427, 2006.

51. Kellman P, Arai AE: Imaging sequences for first pass perfusion—a review. *J Cardiovasc Magn Reson* 9:525, 2007.

52. Klem I, Heitner JF, Shah DJ, et al: Improved detection of coronary artery disease by stress perfusion cardiovascular magnetic resonance with the use of delayed enhancement infarction imaging. *J Am Coll Cardiol* 47:1630, 2006.

53. Paetsch I, Jahnke C, Wahl A, et al: Comparison of dobutamine stress magnetic resonance, adenosine stress magnetic resonance, and adenosine stress magnetic resonance perfusion. *Circulation* 110:835, 2004.

54. Barmeyer AA, Stork A, Muellerleile K, et al: Contrast enhancing cardiac MR imaging in the detection of reduced coronary flow reserve. *Radiology* 243:377, 2007.

55. Fieno DS, Shea SM, Li Y, et al: Myocardial perfusion imaging based on blood oxygen level dependent effect using T2 prepared SSFP MRI. *Circulation* 110:1284, 2004.

56. Nagel E, Lehmkuhl HB, Bocksch W, et al: Noninvasive diagnosis of ischemia-induced wall motion abnormalities with the use of high-dose dobutamine stress MRI: comparison with dobutamine stress echocardiography. *Circulation* 99:763, 1999.

57. Kuijpers D, Ho KY, Van Dijkman PR, et al: Dobutamine cardiovascular magnetic resonance for the detection of myocardial ischemia with the use of myocardial tagging. *Circulation* 107:1592, 2003.

58. Wellnhofer E, Olariu A, Klein C, et al: Magnetic resonance low-dose dobutamine test is superior to scar quantification for the prediction of functional recovery. *Circulation* 109:2172, 2004.

59. Jahnke C, Nagel, E, Gebker R, et al: Prognostic value of cardiac magnetic resonance stress tests: adenosine stress perfusion and dobutamine stress wall motion imaging. *Circulation* 115:1769, 2007.

60. Ferrari VA, Wilensky RL: Intravascular magnetic resonance imaging. *Top Magn Reson Imaging* 18:401, 2007.

61. Herrington DM, Kesler K, Reiber JHC, et al: Arterial compliance adds to conventional risk factors for prediction of angiographic coronary artery disease. *Am Heart J* 146:662, 2003.

62. Osborn EA, Jaffer FA: Advances in molecular imaging of atherosclerotic vascular disease. *Curr Opin Cardiol* 23:620, 2008.

63. Jaffer FA, Libby P, Weissleder R, et al: Molecular and cellular imaging of atherosclerosis: emerging applications. *J Am Coll Cardiol* 47:1328, 2006.

64. Jaffer FA, Libby P, Weissleder R: Molecular imaging of cardiovascular disease. *Circulation* 116:1052, 2007.

65. Choudhry RP, Fisher EA: Molecular imaging in atherosclerosis, thrombosis, and vascular inflammation. *Arterioscler Thromb Vasc Biol* 29:983, 2009.

66. Jaffer FA, Libby P, Weissleder R: Optical and multimodality molecular imaging: insights into atherosclerosis. *Arterioscler Thromb Vasc Biol* 29:1017, 2009.

67. Choudhury RP, Fuster V, Fayad ZA: Molecular, cellular and functional imaging of atherosclerosis. *Nat Rev Drug Discov* 3:913, 2004.

68. Mulder WJM, Strijkers GJ, Vucic E, et al: Magnetic resonance molecular imaging contrast agents and their application in atherosclerosis. *Top Magn Reson Imaging* 18:409, 2007.

69. Tang TY, Muller KH, Graves MJ, et al: Iron oxide particles for atheroma imaging. *Arterioscler Thromb Vasc Biol* 29:1, 2009.

70. Rudd JHF, Hyafil F, Fayad ZA: Inflammation imaging in atherosclerosis. *Arterioscler Thromb Vasc Biol* 29:1009, 2009.

71. Litovsky S, Madjid M, Zarrabi A, et al: Superparamagnetic iron oxide–based method for quantifying recruitment of monocytes to mouse atherosclerotic lesions in vivo: enhancement by tissue necrosis factor-α, interleukin-1β, and interferon-γ. *Circulation* 107:1545, 2003.

72. Kawahara I, Nakamoto M, Kitagawa N, et al: Potential of magnetic resonance plaque imaging using superparamagnetic particles of iron oxide for the detection of carotid plaque. *Neurol Med Chir* 48:157, 2009.

73. Ruehm SG, Corot C, Vogt P, et al: MRI of atherosclerotic plaque with USPIO in hyperlipidemic rabbits. *Circulation* 103:413, 2001.

74. Morris JB, Olzinski AR, Bernard RE, et al: p38 MAPK inhibition reduces aortic USPIO uptake in a mouse model of atherosclerosis: MRI assessment. *Arterioscler Thromb Vasc Biol* 28:265, 2008.

75. Cormode DP, Skaja T, Fayad ZA, et al: Nanotechnology in medical imaging; probe design and applications. *Arterioscler Thromb Vasc Biol* 22:992, 2009.

76. Wickline SA, Neubauer AM, Winter P, et al: Applications of nanotechnology to atherosclerosis, thrombosis, and vascular biology. *Arterioscler Thromb Vasc Biol* 26:435, 2006.

77. Nahrendorf M, Jaffer FA, Kelly KA, et al: Noninvasive VCAM-1 imaging identifies inflammatory activation of cells in atherosclerosis. *Circulation* 114:1504, 2006.

78. Kelly KA, Allport JR, Tsourkas A, et al: Detection of vascular adhesion molecule-1 expression using a novel multimodal nanoparticle. *Circ Res* 96:327, 2005.

79. Nahrendorf M, Zhang H, Hembrador S, et al: Nanoparticle PET-CT imaging of macrophages in inflammatory atherosclerosis. *Circulation* 117:379, 2008.

488

80. McAteer MA, Schneider JE, Ali ZA, et al: Magnetic resonance imaging of endothelial adhesion molecules in mouse atherosclerosis using dual targeted microparticles of iron oxide. *Arterioscler Thromb Vasc Biol* 28:77, 2008.

81. Tang TY, Howarth SPS, Miller SR, et al: Correlation of carotid atheromatous plaque inflammation using USPIO-enhanced MR imaging with degree of luminal stenosis. *Stroke* 39:2144, 2008.

82. Tang TY, Howarth SPS, Miller SR, et al: The ATHEROMA (Atorvastatin Therapy: Effects on Reduction of Macrophage Activity) Study. Evaluation using ultrasmall superparamagnetic iron oxide-enhanced magnetic resonance imaging in carotid disease. *J Am Coll Cardiol* 53:2039, 2009.

83. Briley-Saebo KC, Mani V, Hyafil F, et al. Fractionated Feridex and positive contrast: in vivo MR imaging of atherosclerosis. *Magn Reson Med* 59:721, 2008.

84. Fayad ZA, Razzouk L, Briley-Saebo KC, et al: Iron oxide magnetic resonance imaging for atherosclerosis therapeutic evaluation: still "rusty"? *J Am Coll Cardiol* 22:2051, 2009.

85. Howarth SP, Tang TY, Trivedi R, et al: Utility of USPIO enhanced MR imaging to identify inflammation and fibrous cap: a comparison of symptomatic and asymptomatic individuals. *Eur J Radiol* 70:555, 2009.

86. Amirbekian V, Lipinski MJ, Briley-Saebo KC, et al: Detecting and assessing macrophages in vivo to evaluate atherosclerosis noninvasively using molecular MRI. *Proc Natl Acad Sci U S A* 104:961, 2007.

87. Lancelot E, Amirbekian V, Brigger I, et al: Evaluation of matrix MMPs in atherosclerosis using a novel noninvasive imaging approach. *Arterioscler Thromb Vasc Biol* 28:425, 2008.

88. Kerwin W, Hooker A, Spilker M, et al: Quantitative magnetic resonance imaging analysis of neovasculature volume in carotid atherosclerotic plaque. *Circulation* 107:851, 2003.

89. Sirol M, Itskovich VV, Mani V, et al: Lipid-rich atherosclerotic plaques detected by gadofluorine-enhanced in vivo magnetic resonance imaging. *Circulation* 109:2890, 2004.

90. Lobbes MBI, Miserus RJ, Heeneman S, et al: Atherosclerosis: contrast-enhanced MR imaging of vessel wall in rabbit model—comparison of gadofosveset and gadopentetate dimeglumine. *Radiology* 250:682, 2009.

91. Ronald JA, Chen Y, Belisle AJL, et al: Comparison of gadofluorine-M and Gd-DTPA for noninvasive staging of atherosclerotic plaque stability using MRI. *Circ Cardiovasc Imaging* 2:225, 2009.

92. Winter PM, Neubauer AM, Caruthers SD, et al: Endothelial $\alpha_v\beta_3$ integrin–targeted fumagillin nanoparticles inhibit angiogenesis in atherosclerosis. *Arterioscler Thromb Vasc Biol* 26:2103, 2006.

93. Amirbekian V, Aguinaldo JGS, Amirbekian BS, et al: Atherosclerosis and matrix metalloproteinases: experimental molecular MR imaging in vivo. *Radiology* 251:429, 2009.

94. Ntziachristoas V, Tung CH, Bremer C, et al: Fluorescence molecular tomography resolves protease activity in vivo. *Nat Med* 8:757, 2002.

95. Saraste A, Knoedler, Weidl E, et al: MR vessel wall imaging of the descending aorta using an elastin binding contrast agent in ApoE$^{-/-}$ TFDeltact double knockout mouse model of advanced atherosclerosis. *J Cardiovasc Magn Reson* 10(Suppl 1):A54, 2008.

96. Flacke S, Fischer S, Scott MJ, et al: Novel MRI contrast agent for molecular imaging of fibrin: implications for detecting vulnerable plaques. *Circulation* 104:1280, 2001.

97. Spuentrup E, Botnar RM, Wiethoff AJ, et al: MR imaging of thrombi using EP-2104R, a fibrin specific contrast agent: initial results in patients. *Eur Radiol* 18:1995, 2008.

98. Frias JC, Williams KJ, Fisher EA, Fayad ZA: Recombinant HDL-like nanoparticles: a specific agent for MRI of atherosclerotic plaques. *J Am Chem Soc* 126:16316, 2004.

99. Briley-Saebo KC, Geninatti-Crich S, Cormode DP, et al: High relaxivity gadolinium-modified HDL as MRI contrast agents. *J Phys Chem B* 113:6283, 2009.

100. Briley-Saebo KC, Shaw PX, Mulder WJM, et al: Targeted molecular probes for imaging atherosclerotic lesions with magnetic resonance using antibodies that recognize oxidation specific epitopes. *Circulation* 117:3206, 2008.

101. Aikawa E, Nahrendorf M, Figueiredo JL, et al: Osteogenesis associates with inflammation in early-stage atherosclerosis evaluated by molecular imaging in vivo. *Circulation* 116:2841, 2007.

102. Rudd JH, Warburton EA, Fryer TD, et al: Imaging atherosclerotic plaque inflammation with [^{18}F]-fluorodeoxyglucose positron emission tomography. *Circulation* 105:2708, 2002.

103. Tawakol A, Migrino RQ, Bashian GG, et al: In vivo ^{18}F-fluorodeoxyglucose positron emission tomography imaging provides a noninvasive measure of carotid plaque inflammation in patients. *J Am Coll Cardiol* 48:1818, 2006.

104. Rudd JH, Myers KS, Bansilal S, et al: ^{18}Fluorodeoxyglucose positron emission tomography imaging of atherosclerotic plaque inflammation is highly reproducible: implications for atherosclerosis therapy trials. *J Am Coll Cardiol* 50:892, 2007.

105. Tahara N, Imaizumi T, Virmani R, et al: Clinical feasibility of molecular imaging of plaque inflammation in atherosclerosis. *J Nucl Med* 50:331, 2009.

106. Davies JR, Rudd JH, Weissberg PL: Molecular and metabolic imaging of atherosclerosis. *J Nucl Med* 45:1898, 2004.

107. Davies JR, Rudd JH, Fryer RD, et al: Identification of culprit lesions after transient ischemic attack by combined ^{18}F fluorodeoxyglucose positron-emission tomography and high-resolution MRI. *Stroke* 36:2642, 2005.

108. Aziz K, Berger K, Claycombe K, et al: Noninvasive detection and localization of vulnerable plaque and arterial thrombosis with computed tomography angiography/positron emission tomography. *Circulation* 117:2061, 2008.

109. Paulmier B, Duet M, Khayat R, et al: Arterial wall uptake of fluorodeoxyglucose on PET imaging in stable cancer patients indicates higher risk of cardiovascular events. *J Nucl Cardiol* 15:209, 2009.

110. Dunphy MP, Freiman A, Larson SM, et al: Association of vascular ^{18}F-FDG uptake with vascular calcification. *J Nucl Med* 46:1278, 2005.

111. Rudd JH, Myers KS, Bansilal S, et al: Atherosclerosis inflammation imaging with ^{18}F-FDG PET: carotid, iliac and femoral uptake reproducibility, quantification methods, and recommendations. *J Nucl Med* 49:871, 2008.

112. Virmani R, Burke AP, Kolodgie FD, Farb A: Vulnerable plaque: the pathology of unstable coronary lesions. *J Interv Cardiol* 15:439, 2002.

113. Ben-Haim S, Kupzov E, Tamir A, et al: Changing patterns of abnormal vascular wall F-18 FDG uptake on follow-up PET/CT studies. *J Nucl Cardiol* 13:791, 2006.

114. Ibanez B, Badimon JJ, Garcia MJ: Diagnosis of atherosclerosis by imaging. *Am J Med* 122:S15, 2009.

115. Ogawa M, Magata Y, Kato T, et al: Application of ^{18}F-FDG PET for monitoring the therapeutic effect of anti-inflammatory drugs on stabilization of vulnerable atherosclerotic plaques. *J Nucl Med* 47:1845, 2006.

116. Tahara N, Kai H, Ishibashi M, et al: Simvastatin attenuates plaque inflammation. *J Am Coll Cardiol* 48:1825, 2006.

117. Venneti S, Lopresti BJ, Wang G, et al: PET imaging of brain macrophages using the peripheral benzodiazepine receptor in a macaque model of neuro AIDS. *J Clin Invest* 113:981, 2004.

118. Nahrendorf M, Keliher E, Panizzi P, et al: ^{18}F-4V for PET-CT imaging of VCAM-1 expression in atherosclerosis. *JACC Cardiovasc Imaging* 2:1213, 2009.

119. Fayad ZA, Vucic E: "Feeling the RAGE" in the atherosclerotic vessel wall. *Circ Cardiovasc Imaging* 1:178, 2008.

120. Hoppmann S, Haase C, Richter S, Pietzsch J: Expression, purification and fluorine-18 radiolabeling of recombinant S100 proteins—potential probes for molecular imaging or receptor for advanced glycation end products (RAGE) in vivo. *Protein Expr Purif* 57:143, 2008.

121. Weintrab HS: Identifying the vulnerable patient with rupture prone plaque. *Am J Cardiol* 101:3F, 2008.

122. Exercise electrocardiogram and coronary heart disease mortality in the Multiple Risk Factor Intervention Trial. Multiple Risk Factor Intervention Trial Research Group. *Am J Cardiol* 55:16, 1985.

123. Norgaard BL, Andersen K, Dellborg M, et al; TRIM Study Group: Admission risk assessment by cardiac troponin T in unstable coronary artery disease: additional prognostic information from continuous ST segment monitoring. *J Am Coll Cardiol* 33:1519, 1999.

124. Deedwania PC: Asymptomatic ischemia during predischarge Holter monitoring predicts poor prognosis in the postinfarction period. *Am J Cardiol* 71:859, 1993.

125. Forslund L, Hjemdahl P, Held C, et al: Prognostic implications of ambulatory myocardial ischemia and arrhythmias and relations to ischemia on exercise in chronic stable angina pectoris (the Angina Prognosis Study in Stockholm [APSIS]). *Am J Cardiol* 84:1151, 1999.

126. Vita JA, Treasure CB, Nabel EG, et al: Coronary vasomotor response to acetylcholine relates to risk factors for coronary artery disease. *Circulation* 81:491, 1990.

127. Andrews TC, Raby K, Barry J, et al: Effect of cholesterol reduction on myocardial ischemia in patients with coronary disease. *Circulation* 95:324, 1997.

128. Gould KL, Ornish D, Scherwitz L, et al: Changes in myocardial perfusion abnormalities by PET after long-term, intense risk factor modification. *JAMA* 274:894, 1995.

129. Blumenthal JA, Jiang W, Babyak MA, et al: Stress management and exercise training in cardiac patients with myocardial ischemia. Effects on prognosis and evaluation of mechanisms. *Arch Intern Med* 157:2213, 1997.

130. Wu JC, Bengel FM, Gambhir SS: Cardiovascular molecular imaging. *Radiology* 244:337, 2007.

131. Iskander S, Iskandrian AE: Risk assessment using single-photon emission computed tomographic technetium-99m sestamibi imaging. *J Am Coll Cardiol* 32:57, 1998.

132. Davies RF, Goldberg AD, Forman S, et al; ACIP Investigators: Asymptomatic Cardiac Ischemia Pilot (ACIP) study two-year follow up. *Circulation* 95:2037, 1997.

133. Madsen JK, Grande P, Saunamaki K, et al: Danish multicenter randomized study of invasive versus conservative treatment in patients with inducible ischemia after thrombolysis in acute myocardial infarction (DANAMI). *Circulation* 96:748, 1997.

134. Erne P, Schoenenberger AW, Burckhardt D, et al: Effects of percutaneous coronary interventions in silent ischemia after myocardial infarction: the SWISSI II randomized controlled trial. *JAMA* 297:1985, 2007.

135. Patel DJ, Mulcahy D, Norrie J, et al: Natural variability of transient myocardial ischemia during daily life: an obstacle when assessing efficacy of anti-ischemic agents? *Heart* 76:477, 1996.

136. Schelbert HR: Metabolic imaging to assess myocardial viability. *J Nucl Med* 35:85, 1994.

137. Neglia D, L'Abbate A: Myocardial perfusion reserve in ischemic heart disease. *J Nucl Med* 50:175, 2009.

138. Dorbala S, Hassan A, Heinonen T, et al: Coronary vasodilator reserve and Framingham risk scores in subjects at risk for coronary artery disease. *J Nucl Cardiol* 13:761, 2006.

139. Bax JJ, Poldermans D, Elhendy A, et al: Sensitivity, specificity, and predictive accuracies of various noninvasive techniques for detecting hibernating myocardium. *Curr Probl Cardiol* 26:147, 2001.

140. Tamaki N, Yonekura Y, Yamashita K, et al: Positron emission tomography using fluorine-18 deoxyglucose in evaluation of coronary artery bypass grafting. *Am J Cardiol* 64:860, 1989.

141. Beanlands RS, Ruddy TD, deKemp RA, et al: PET and recovery following revascularization (PARR-1); the importance of scar and development of a prediction rule for the degree of recovery of left ventricular function. *J Am Coll Cardiol* 40:1735, 2002.

142. Marin-Neto JA, Dilsizian V, Arrighi JA, et al: Thallium scintigraphy compared with ^{18}F-fluorodeoxyglucose positron emission tomography for assessing myocardial viability in patients with moderate versus severe LV dysfunction. *Am J Cardiol* 82:1001, 1998.

28

CHAPTER 29

Exercise Treadmill Stress Testing With and Without Imaging

Amil M. Shah and Samia Mora

Data from 2006 indicate that 16,800,000 U.S. adults aged 20 years or older have coronary heart disease (CHD), with an annual incidence of myocardial infarction (MI) of 1,450,000.[1] Among patients experiencing sudden death, it is the first presentation of CHD in about 25%.[2] For these reasons, there has been considerable interest in risk stratification of asymptomatic individuals without a diagnosis of CHD to prevent future events.[3] Given its noninvasive nature and the prognostic information it provides in established CHD, exercise testing has generated considerable interest.

A promising avenue for improving cardiac risk stratification has come from studies evaluating the prognostic value of exercise testing in asymptomatic populations with test variables that are not related to exercise-induced ST-segment depression. In particular, functional measures such as exercise capacity, blood pressure, and heart rate recovery have been linked to increased CHD and all-cause death in both women and men.

Additional imaging with myocardial perfusion or echocardiography may further identify another subgroup of asymptomatic individuals at higher risk for future events. However, despite the increased risk associated with certain aspects of the exercise test, the low cardiac event rate and low positive predictive value of abnormal test results in asymptomatic populations do not support a strategy of routine screening of adult asymptomatic populations. Clinical trial data are scarce and are eagerly awaited to answer the important question facing clinicians and patients alike: to screen or not to screen asymptomatic adults for CHD?

CURRENT GUIDELINES AND LIMITATIONS

Current guidelines do not recommend exercise testing for routine screening in asymptomatic subjects. Recent guidelines from the U.S. Preventive Services Task Force found insufficient evidence to recommend routine screening because of the low positive predictive value (estimates ranging from 6% to 48%) among asymptomatic men.[4] Similarly, there are no Class I indications for exercise testing in asymptomatic adults in the 2002 American College of Cardiology/American Heart Association (ACC/AHA) guidelines (Table 29-1). However, these guidelines have been based largely on data regarding the performance of stress electrocardiography for diagnosis of coronary disease in a low-risk population.[5]

There is a growing body of literature suggesting the utility of nonelectrocardiographic exercise testing parameters in determining prognosis in asymptomatic subjects, beyond current risk stratification with commonly used global risk scores.[5] As reviewed in more detail later, these parameters include exercise capacity, chronotropic response, exercise blood pressure, heart rate recovery, and ventricular arrhythmias. All have demonstrated prognostic utility even after accounting for traditional risk factors or global risk scores (e.g., the Framingham risk score).

USE AS A SCREENING TEST

Broadly conceived, the purpose of a screening test is either earlier diagnosis of disease or risk stratification to allow effective interventions to prevent adverse outcomes. Current guidelines recommend office-based risk stratification of all individuals with multiple risk factor scores to determine global risk.[6] This is most commonly accomplished by the Framingham risk score as modified by the National Cholesterol Education Program Adult Treatment Panel III. In this framework, patients can be stratified into low-risk (predicted 10-year absolute risk of MI or CHD death <10%), intermediate-risk (6% to 20%), and high-risk (>20%) groups.[6] Whereas aggressive medical interventions are clearly indicated in high-risk patients, population-based studies suggest that less than 3% of asymptomatic subjects fall into the high-risk group, particularly among women.[7] Although all patients should control known risk factors, some have argued that given the substantial variation in risk among intermediate-risk patients and the sizable proportion of patients falling in this category, these patients would benefit from further risk stratification (Fig. 29-1).[3]

As presented in the following sections, multiple stress testing parameters have been demonstrated to add prognostic information beyond risk factor scores. However, data are still lacking that such refinements in prognostic assessment actually influence patient management and outcomes.[5] As discussed more fully in a later section, this critical information still awaits large-scale randomized clinical trials to assess the impact of risk stratification by exercise testing on outcomes.[5]

TABLE 29–1	2002 ACC/AHA Guidelines for the Use of Exercise Testing in Asymptomatic Individuals Without Known Coronary Heart Disease
Class I	None
Class IIa	Evaluation of asymptomatic persons with diabetes mellitus who plan to start vigorous exercise (*Level of Evidence: C*)

Class IIb	Evaluation of persons with multiple risk factors as a guide to risk reduction therapy
	Evaluation of asymptomatic men older than 45 years and women older than 55 years:
	  Who plan to start vigorous exercise (especially if sedentary), or
	  Who are involved in occupations in which impairment might impact public safety, or
	  Who are at high risk for CAD due to other diseases (e.g., peripheral vascular disease and chronic renal failure)

Class III	Routine screening of asymptomatic men or women

From Gibbons RJ, Balady GJ, Bricker JT, et al: ACC/AHA 2002 guideline update for exercise testing: summary article: a report of the American College of Cardiology/American Heart Association Task Force on Practice Guidelines (Committee to Update the 1997 Exercise Testing Guidelines), *Circulation* 106:1883, 2002. © 2002 American Heart Association, Inc.

EXERCISE STRESS TEST PERFORMANCE

Safety, Contraindications, and Indications for Test Termination

Exercise stress testing is a generally safe procedure. Recognized serious complications of exercise testing include MI, malignant ventricular arrhythmias, and sudden death (Table 29-2). Large survey studies have reported acute MI in 0.9 to 3.6 per 10,000 tests, serious arrhythmias in 0.3 to 4.8 per 10,000 tests, and death in 0 to 0.5 per 10,000 tests.[8-10] The risk of adverse events is higher in post-MI patients and patients undergoing evaluation for malignant ventricular arrhythmias.[11] Given the potential for serious risks (although rare), clinical judgment is essential in selecting patients appropriate for stress testing, as is careful monitoring by appropriately trained staff before, during, and after testing.[12]

Absolute and relative contraindications to exercise testing are listed in Table 29-3.[13] In general, any patient with evidence of clinical or hemodynamic instability should not undergo exercise testing until the condition is stabilized. Absolute and relative indications for termination of exercise testing are listed in Table 29-4.[11]

Commonly Used Exercise Protocols

In general, exercise protocols are designed to assess exercise capacity. Maximum oxygen consumption ($\dot{V}O_2$ max), defined

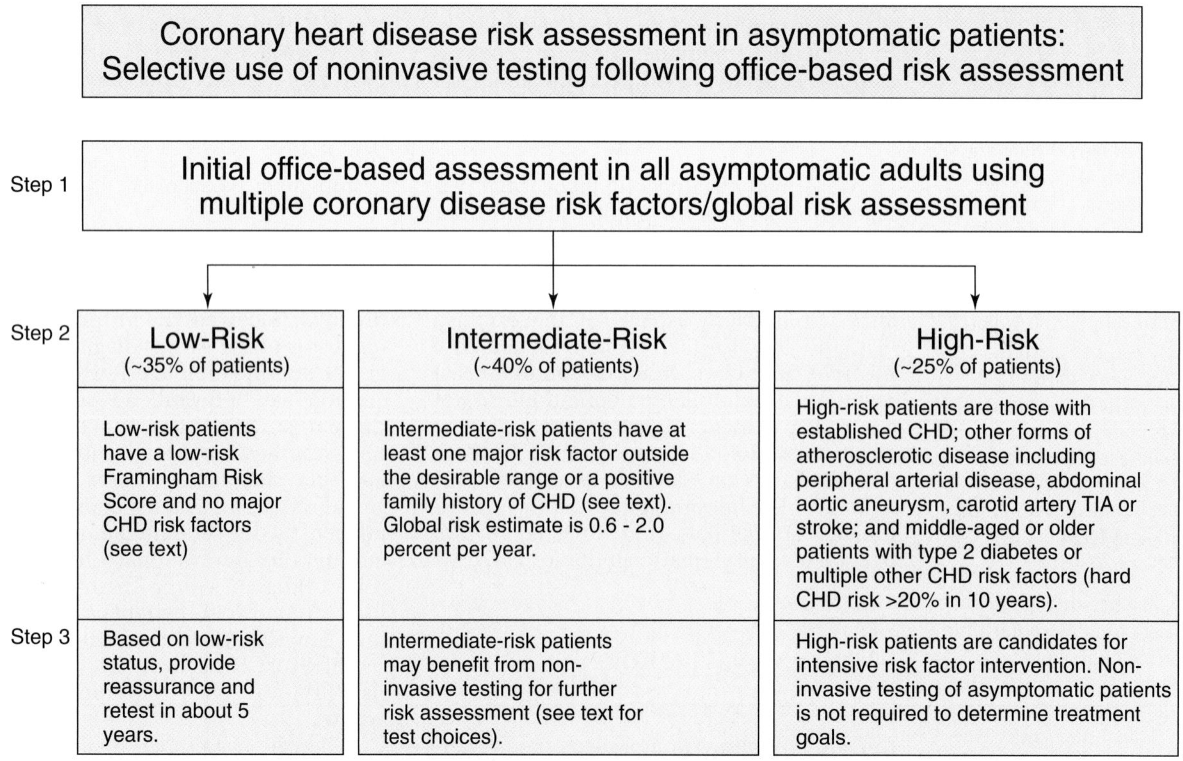

Coronary heart disease risk assessment in asymptomatic patients: Selective use of noninvasive testing following office-based risk assessment

Step 1 — Initial office-based assessment in all asymptomatic adults using multiple coronary disease risk factors/global risk assessment

Step 2

Low-Risk (~35% of patients)	Intermediate-Risk (~40% of patients)	High-Risk (~25% of patients)
Low-risk patients have a low-risk Framingham Risk Score and no major CHD risk factors (see text)	Intermediate-risk patients have at least one major risk factor outside the desirable range or a positive family history of CHD (see text). Global risk estimate is 0.6 - 2.0 percent per year.	High-risk patients are those with established CHD; other forms of atherosclerotic disease including peripheral arterial disease, abdominal aortic aneurysm, carotid artery TIA or stroke; and middle-aged or older patients with type 2 diabetes or multiple other CHD risk factors (hard CHD risk >20% in 10 years).
Step 3 — Based on low-risk status, provide reassurance and retest in about 5 years.	Intermediate-risk patients may benefit from non-invasive testing for further risk assessment (see text for test choices).	High-risk patients are candidates for intensive risk factor intervention. Non-invasive testing of asymptomatic patients is not required to determine treatment goals.

FIGURE 29-1 Potential role of exercise stress testing for further risk stratification of patients with intermediate risk of CHD based on global risk assessment. See text for further discussion. (*From Greenland P, Smith SC, Grundy SM: Improving coronary heart disease risk assessment in asymptomatic people: role of traditional risk factors and noninvasive cardiovascular tests.* Circulation 104:1863, 2001.)

TABLE 29-2	Recognized Serious Complications of Exercise Testing

Cardiac
Bradyarrhythmias
Tachyarrhythmias
Acute coronary syndromes
Heart failure
Hypotension, syncope, and shock
Death

Noncardiac
Musculoskeletal trauma
Soft tissue injury

Miscellaneous
Severe fatigue (malaise), sometimes persisting for days; dizziness; fainting; body aches; delayed feelings of illness

From Fletcher GF, Balady GJ, Amsterdam EA, et al: Exercise standards for testing and training: a statement for healthcare professionals from the American Heart Association. *Circulation* 104:1694, 2001. © 2001 American Heart Association, Inc.

TABLE 29-3	Absolute and Relative Contraindications to Exercise Stress Testing

Absolute
Acute myocardial infarction (within 2 days)
High-risk unstable angina (as defined in the ACC/AHA Guidelines for the Management of Patients with Unstable Angina/Non–ST-Segment Elevation Myocardial Infarction)
Uncontrolled cardiac arrhythmias causing symptoms or hemodynamic compromise
Symptomatic severe aortic stenosis
Uncontrolled symptomatic heart failure
Acute pulmonary embolus or pulmonary infarction
Acute myocarditis or pericarditis
Acute aortic dissection

Relative
Left main coronary stenosis
Moderate stenotic valvular heart disease
Electrolyte abnormalities
Severe arterial hypertension (systolic blood pressure >200 mm Hg and/or diastolic blood pressure >110 mm Hg)
Tachyarrhythmias or bradyarrhythmias
Hypertrophic cardiomyopathy and other forms of outflow tract obstruction
Mental or physical impairment leading to inability to exercise adequately
High-degree atrioventricular block

From Gibbons RJ, Balady GJ, Bricker JT, et al: ACC/AHA 2002 guideline update for exercise testing: summary article: a report of the American College of Cardiology/American Heart Association Task Force on Practice Guidelines (Committee to Update the 1997 Exercise Testing Guidelines). *Circulation* 106:1883, 2002. © 2002 American Heart Association, Inc.

TABLE 29-4	Absolute and Relative Indications for Termination of an Exercise Stress Test

Absolute
Drop in systolic blood pressure of >10 mm Hg from baseline blood pressure despite an increase in workload, when accompanied by other evidence of ischemia
Moderate to severe angina
Increasing nervous system symptoms (e.g., ataxia, dizziness, or near-syncope)
Signs of poor perfusion (cyanosis or pallor)
Technical difficulties in monitoring ECG or systolic blood pressure
Subject's desire to stop
Sustained ventricular tachycardia
ST elevation (≥1.0 mm) in leads without diagnostic Q waves (other than V_1 or aVR)

Relative
Drop in systolic blood pressure of >10 mm Hg from baseline blood pressure despite an increase in workload, in the absence of other evidence of ischemia
ST or QRS changes such as excessive ST depression (>2 mm of horizontal or downsloping ST-segment depression) or marked axis shift
Arrhythmias other than sustained ventricular tachycardia, including multifocal PVCs, triplets of PVCs, supraventricular tachycardia, heart block, or bradyarrhythmias
Fatigue, shortness of breath, wheezing, leg cramps, or claudication
Development of bundle branch block or IVCD that cannot be distinguished from ventricular tachycardia
Increasing chest pain
Hypertensive response (systolic blood pressure >250 mm Hg and/or diastolic blood pressure >115 mm Hg)

ECG, electrocardiogram; IVCD, intraventricular conduction delay; PVCs, premature ventricular contractions.
From Gibbons RJ, Balady GJ, Bricker JT, et al: ACC/AHA 2002 guideline update for exercise testing: summary article: a report of the American College of Cardiology/American Heart Association Task Force on Practice Guidelines (Committee to Update the 1997 Exercise Testing Guidelines). *Circulation* 106:1883, 2002. © 2002 American Heart Association, Inc.

as the maximal amount of oxygen a subject can take in from inspired air during dynamic exercise, is considered the best measure of cardiovascular fitness and exercise capacity.[11] When peak consumption is achieved, $\dot{V}_{O_2}$ max can estimate cardiac output. Oxygen uptake can be expressed in units of sitting/resting requirements or metabolic equivalents (METs); a MET is defined as a unit of sitting/resting oxygen uptake (approximately 3.5 mL O_2/kg/min). $\dot{V}_{O_2}$ max varies significantly with age (declining by 8% to 10% per decade[14]), gender (generally lower in women), physical activity (nearly 25% reduction noted with 3 weeks of bed rest[11]), heredity,[15] and degree of myocardial impairment.

Exercise protocols with progressive incremental increases in workload tend to estimate $\dot{V}_{O_2}$ max more accurately.[16] The optimal protocol will vary by patient and should last for 6 to 12 minutes to reliably reflect the upper limit of the patient's cardiorespiratory function.[11,16] Exercise is most commonly performed with bicycle ergometry or treadmill. Commonly used protocols are illustrated in Figure 29-2. Compared with the cycle ergometer, treadmill tests tend to demonstrate 10% to 15% higher $\dot{V}_{O_2}$ max, 5% to 20% higher peak heart rate, and more frequent ST-segment changes.[16]

The most commonly used treadmill protocol in the United States is the Bruce protocol.[8,9] Whereas a large amount of published data exist with use of the Bruce protocol, the relatively large increments in work between stages can make $\dot{V}_{O_2}$ max estimation less accurate and cause some patients to terminate exercise before $\dot{V}_{O_2}$ max is achieved.[11,16] Estimation of $\dot{V}_{O_2}$ max appears more accurate with use of exercise duration–targeted ramp protocols, which constantly increase work by increasing incline at set brief intervals and increasing ramp speed on the basis of estimated functional capacity.[17] The major limitation is the need to accurately predict a patient's functional capacity.

EXERCISE STRESS TEST INTERPRETATION

Exercise testing produces both electrocardiographic and non-electrocardiographic data that can be used both for diagnosis of CHD and for prognosis. Interpretation of exercise testing data must incorporate the clinical context of the test and, most important, the pretest probability of disease.

29

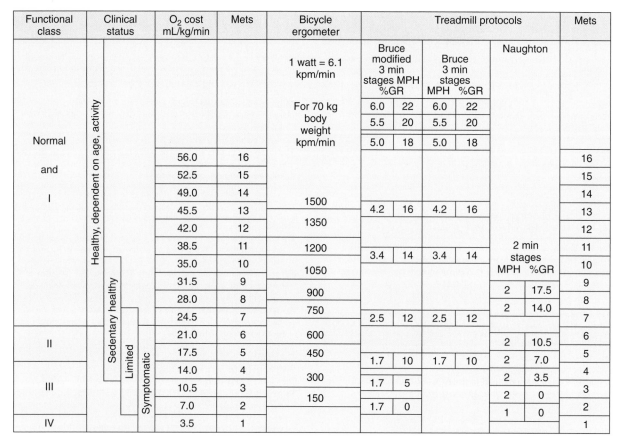

FIGURE 29-2 Commonly used treadmill and bike exercise protocols with the relationship between METs achieved and protocol stage. kpm, kilopond-meters; MPH, miles per hour; %GR, percent grade. *(From Fletcher GF, Balady GJ, Amsterdam EA, et al: Exercise standards for testing and training: a statement for healthcare professionals from the American Heart Association.* Circulation *104:1694, 2001. © 2001 American Heart Association, Inc.)*

Performance Characteristics of Exercise Testing and Bayes' Theorem

Definitions of parameters used to quantify the diagnostic accuracy of a test are listed in Table 29-5.[13] Sensitivity defines the probability that a patient with disease will have a positive test result, and specificity defines the probability that a patient without disease will have a negative test result. However, the clinically relevant information in interpreting the results of any given test is the likelihood that a positive result is truly indicative of disease (positive predictive value) and that a negative result truly excludes disease (negative predictive value). As Table 29-5 illustrates, these parameters are dependent not only on the test but also on the prevalence of disease in the population (i.e., the pretest probability).

Bayes' theorem states that the probability of disease after a diagnostic test is equal to the pretest probability of disease multiplied by the probability of a true positive result from the test.[13] A corollary is that the chances of a positive result truly reflecting disease (i.e., positive predictive value) will be higher in high-prevalence populations and lower in low-prevalence populations. This point is illustrated in Figure 29-3. Bayesian analysis is critical in the appropriate interpretation of stress testing.

Test Interpretation: Diagnosis

Estimates of the diagnostic accuracy of electrocardiographic exercise stress testing for the diagnosis of hemodynamically significant coronary disease vary widely and are confounded

TABLE 29–5	Definitions of Sensitivity, Specificity, Positive Predictive Value, and Predictive Accuracy
Sensitivity	$[TP/(TP + FN)] \times 100$
Specificity	$[TN/(FP + TN)] \times 100$
Positive predicted value	$\dfrac{\text{Sensitivity} \times P(CAD)}{[\text{Sensitivity} \times P(CAD)] + [(1 - \text{specificity})(1 - P(CAD))]}$
Predictive accuracy	$[\text{Sensitivity} \times P(CAD)] + [(1 - \text{specificity})[1 - P(CAD)]]$

Note that the calculated positive predictive value (PPV) and negative predictive value (NPV) are dependent on the population prevalence of disease. FN, false negative; FP, false positive; P(CAD), pretest probability; TN, true negative; TP, true positive.

From Gibbons RJ, Balady GJ, Bricker JT, et al: ACC/AHA 2002 guideline update for exercise testing: summary article: a report of the American College of Cardiology/American Heart Association Task Force on Practice Guidelines (Committee to Update the 1997 Exercise Testing Guidelines). *Circulation* 106:1883, 2002. © 2002 American Heart Association, Inc.

by the fact that the majority of studies suffer from workup bias, discussed in further detail later.

Determining the Pretest Probability of CHD

Multiple predictive models have been developed to assist the clinician in assessing the pretest probability of CHD in a given patient.[13,18-20] These models consistently show age, gender, and chest pain history to be the most powerful predictors of CHD, although additional factors such as smoking and history of diabetes are also predictors.[18,19] The most commonly used assessment tool is demonstrated in Table 29-6.[13,20] Pretest probability of CHD is determined as high (>90%), intermediate (10% to 90%), low (5% to 10%), and very low (<5%). On the basis of the previous discussion of bayesian conditional probabilities, the results of exercise testing will have the greatest effect on post-test probability of CHD in subjects with intermediate pretest probabilities.

Interpretation of Electrocardiographic Response

Normally encountered electrocardiographic changes with exercise include increased P wave magnitude in the inferior leads with shortening of the PR interval, decreased R wave amplitude in the lateral leads, and depression of the J-point in the lateral leads.[11] Assessment of electrocardiographic manifestations of exercise-induced myocardial ischemia focuses on the ST segment.

In exercise electrocardiography, the ST-segment deviation is measured relative to the P-Q junction.[11] Generally accepted criteria for abnormal ST-segment depression are horizontal and downsloping ST-segment depression of ≥0.10 mV (1 mm) for 80 msec, with downsloping ST-segment depression being more specific than horizontal or upsloping ST-segment depression (Fig. 29-4).[11]

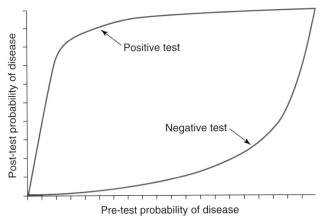

FIGURE 29-3 Graphic illustration of the post-test probability of disease (*y*-axis) for a positive versus negative test as a function of the pretest probability of disease (*x*-axis). (*Modified from Schwartz JS: Clinical decision-making in cardiology.* In *Zipes DP, Libby P, Bonow RO, Braunwald E, editors:* Braunwald's heart disease: a textbook of cardiovascular medicine, *ed 7, Philadelphia, Elsevier Saunders, 2005, pp 27-34.*)

ST-Segment Depression. Resting ST-segment depression is a risk marker of adverse cardiac prognosis in itself.[21] Resting ST-segment depression of <1 mm has been shown to increase the sensitivity but to decrease the specificity of exercise testing,[22,23] and exercise testing is still considered a reasonable first test in these patients.[13] Importantly, ischemic ST-segment depression occurring only during the recovery phase of an exercise test appears to have comparable diagnostic significance to ST-segment depression occurring during exercise.[24]

Exercise-induced ST-segment depression has diagnostic properties that vary widely. Important methodologic limitations that may inflate estimates of ST-segment depression sensitivity are inclusion of subjects with high probability of having disease (e.g., prior MI) and workup bias.[13] Workup bias refers to inclusion of subjects based on the results of the test being evaluated, that is, only subjects undergoing both stress testing and coronary angiography are included, although the decision to pursue angiography is influenced by the results of the exercise test.[13]

A meta-analysis of 147 studies involving 24,074 patients and comparing exercise-induced ST depression with coronary angiography reported a mean sensitivity and specificity of 68% and 77%, respectively.[25] However, both the sensitivity and specificity calculations varied widely; the range of reported sensitivity was 23% to 100%, and the range of reported specificity was 17% to 100%.[25] Studies that avoided workup bias and did not include many patients with high pretest probability of disease suggest a sensitivity of 50% and a specificity of 90% associated with exercise-induced 1-mm ST-segment depression.[13]

ST-Segment Elevation. The development of ST-segment elevation, measured from the baseline ST level, is not infrequent in leads with preexisting Q waves and is of unclear significance among patients with prior MI.[13] Exercise-induced ST-segment elevation in subjects without preexisting Q waves is rare, occurring in an estimated 0.1% of patients in a clinical laboratory. It is associated with transmural ischemia and reliably localizes the area of ischemia.[13]

Gender Differences in ST-Segment Changes. It is notable that exercise-induced ST-segment depression has not been found to be associated with higher risk in asymptomatic women,[26-28] in contrast to findings in asymptomatic men, in whom ischemic electrocardiographic changes have been associated with higher mortality.[29-32] This sex difference in the prognostic accuracy of the ST segment is consistent with previously reported sex differences regarding its diagnostic accuracy[33] and may be related to hormonal effects on the electrocardiogram[34] or sex differences in endothelial function.[35] Other measures obtained from exercise testing that add

TABLE 29-6	Commonly Used Table Incorporating Age, Gender, and Character of Chest Pain to Estimate Pretest Probability of Coronary Heart Disease				
Age (years)	Gender	Typical/Definite Angina Pectoris	Atypical/Probable Angina Pectoris	Nonanginal Chest Pain	Asymptomatic
30-39	Men	Intermediate	Intermediate	Low	Very low
	Women	Intermediate	Very low	Very low	Very low
40-49	Men	High	Intermediate	Intermediate	Low
	Women	Intermediate	Low	Very low	Very low
50-59	Men	High	Intermediate	Intermediate	Low
	Women	Intermediate	Intermediate	Low	Very low
60-69	Men	High	Intermediate	Intermediate	Low
	Women	High	Intermediate	Intermediate	Low

See text for further discussion.

From Gibbons RJ, Balady GJ, Bricker JT, et al: ACC/AHA 2002 guideline update for exercise testing: summary article: a report of the American College of Cardiology/American Heart Association Task Force on Practice Guidelines (Committee to Update the 1997 Exercise Testing Guidelines). *Circulation* 106:1883, 2002. © 2002 American Heart Association, Inc.

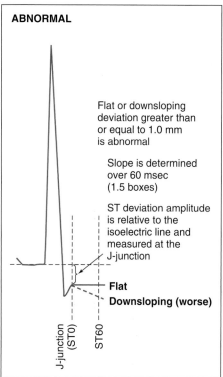

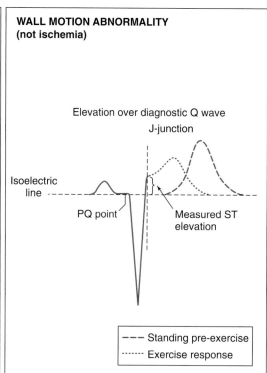

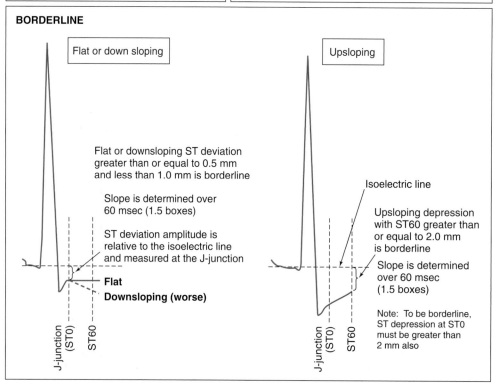

FIGURE 29-4 Standard interpretation of ST-segment deviation for exercise electrocardiography. *(From Fletcher GF, Balady GJ, Amsterdam EA, et al: Exercise standards for testing and training: a statement for healthcare professionals from the American Heart Association. Circulation 104:1694, 2001. © 2001 American Heart Association, Inc.)*

useful prognostic information in women are discussed later and include functional capacity and heart rate recovery.

Test Interpretation: Prognosis

Use of Common Prognostic Scores (Duke Treadmill Score)

Multiple parameters measured during the exercise stress test yield prognostic information. Many are discussed in greater detail later. Multiple studies have demonstrated the prognostic importance of exercise capacity, measured as treadmill stage, exercise duration, metabolic equivalents, watts, or double product.[13] In addition, studies evaluating the most predictive independent prognostic parameters from exercise tests consistently also identify the presence of exercise-induced myocardial ischemia, generally reflected in ST-segment deviation or anginal symptoms.[13] Whereas

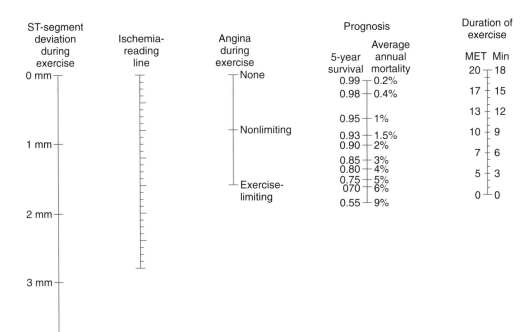

FIGURE 29-5 Nomogram to predict prognosis (annual mortality rate and 5-year survival) based on the Duke treadmill score. *(From Gibbons RJ, Balady GJ, Bricker JT, et al: ACC/AHA 2002 guideline update for exercise testing: summary article: a report of the American College of Cardiology/American Heart Association Task Force on Practice Guidelines [Committee to Update the 1997 Exercise Testing Guidelines]. Circulation 106:1883, 2002. © 2002 American Heart Association, Inc.)*

multiple risk scores integrating these various prognostic markers have been developed,[13] the most widely used is the Duke treadmill score (DTS).[36,37]

The DTS was initially developed in 2842 subjects referred for cardiac catheterization who had also undergone exercise testing for evaluation of symptoms of CHD.[36] The investigators identified three prognostic variables: ST-segment depression, exercise time on Bruce protocol, and Duke angina index. In the Duke angina index, angina index 0 = no angina, 1 = typical angina occurred, and 2 = angina was reason for test termination.

The resulting DTS is calculated as

$$DTS = \text{Exercise time (in minutes)} - (5 \times \text{ST deviation in mm})$$
$$- (4 \times \text{Duke angina index})$$

This score effectively stratified subjects in terms of 5-year risk of death or MI and provided incremental prognostic value beyond clinical and angiographic data. In subjects with low-risk treadmill scores (≥+5), 5-year event-free survival (death or MI) was 93%; in intermediate-risk subjects (score −10 to +4), it was 86%; and in high-risk subjects (score ≤ −11), it was 63%.[36] The investigators subsequently validated the score in unselected outpatients, demonstrating that in this population, the 4-year survival among low-risk patients was 99%, whereas among high-risk patients, it was 79% (Fig. 29-5).[37] An important limitation of the DTS is its limited discrimination in elderly subjects.[38]

Nonelectrocardiographic Prognostic Parameters

Exercise Capacity. Exercise (or functional) capacity refers to the maximal oxygen extraction obtainable during exercise and is commonly measured in METs. METs are multiples of basal metabolism; one MET is the basal oxygen uptake during quiet sitting and is equal to 3.5 mL/kg/min. Exercise capacity is influenced by factors outside of cardiovascular fitness,

most importantly age and gender.[39,40] Nomograms have been developed to estimate age-predicted exercise capacity among men [18.0 − (0.15 × age)][39] and women [14.7 − (0.13 × age)][40] (Fig. 29-6). For example, with use of this nomogram, women who did not achieve 85% of their age-predicted exercise capacity had a twofold higher risk of cardiovascular death.[40]

Exercise capacity is the most powerful prognostic parameter from an exercise test. Multiple large studies in both asymptomatic and symptomatic subjects have reported similar findings.[39,40-44] This relationship is present in both men[31,39] and women.[26,40] In one landmark study of more than 14,000 healthy men and women, physical fitness measured by maximal treadmill time was significantly associated with mortality during 8-year follow-up, independent of demographics and standard risk factors.[45]

A study of 2994 asymptomatic women observed for 20 years demonstrated that women who were below the median at baseline for exercise capacity (<7.5 METs) and heart rate recovery (<55 beats/min difference between peak exercise heart rate and heart rate at 2-minute recovery) had a 3.5-fold higher risk of cardiovascular death independent of traditional risk factors.[26] Importantly, functional capacity provides prognostic information beyond traditional risk stratification by the Framingham risk score in both men[27] and women,[46] as discussed later.

Chronotropic Incompetence. Chronotropic incompetence refers to an inability to achieve the expected increase in heart rate with exercise.[5] Multiple parameters have been used to assess chronotropic incompetence. It is most commonly evaluated by the proportion of age-predicted maximal heart rate (HR) achieved during the stress test (peak HR/220 − age).[5] However, in addition to age, the chronotropic response to exercise is also affected by resting heart rate and physical fitness.[47] The proportion of heart rate reserve used is defined as [(peak HR − rest HR)/(maximum age-predicted HR − rest HR)] × 100 and incorporates information about resting heart rate.[48] The chronotropic index incorporates data for both

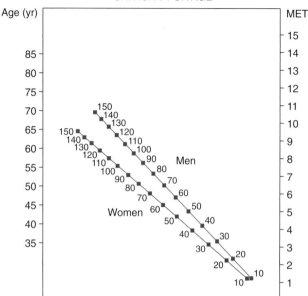

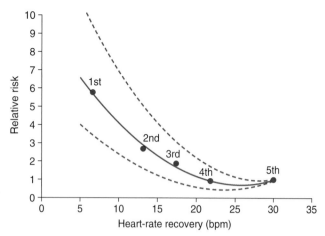

FIGURE 29-6 Nomograms for determination of age-predicted exercise capacity among men and women. *(From Gulati M, Black HR, Shaw LJ, et al: The prognostic value of a nomogram for exercise capacity in women.* N Engl J Med *353:468, 2005. © 2005 Massachusetts Medical Society. All rights reserved.)*

FIGURE 29-7 Relationship between heart rate recovery (beat per minute reduction during the first minute after exercise) and all-cause mortality at 6-year follow-up among a referral population of more than 2400 individuals. Relative risks for each quintile of heart rate recovery compared with the highest quintile (5th) are presented. *(From Cole CR, Blackstone EH, Pashkow FJ, et al: Heart-rate recovery immediately after exercise as a predictor of mortality.* N Engl J Med *341:1351, 1999. ©1999 Massachusetts Medical Society. All rights reserved.)*

resting heart rate and physical fitness and is defined as the ratio of the metabolic reserve to the heart rate reserve:[47]

Chronotropic index at any stage of the exercise test =

$$[(\text{METs}_{\text{stage}} - \text{METs}_{\text{rest}})/(\text{METs}_{\text{peak}} - \text{METs}_{\text{rest}})]/$$
$$(\text{HR}_{\text{peak}} - \text{HR}_{\text{rest}})/(\text{HR}_{\text{max predicted}} - \text{HR}_{\text{rest}})$$

Chronotropic incompetence measured by all three indices has been consistently associated with increased risk of all-cause and cardiovascular mortality, even after adjustment for demographics and standard risk factors.[47-50] This has been shown in both referral populations[48,49,50] and studies of healthy asymptomatic individuals.[47] In studies involving nuclear perfusion imaging, measures of chronotropic incompetence consistently provide additional prognostic information beyond the findings on perfusion imaging.[48,49] In asymptomatic individuals, measures of chronotropic incompetence appear to provide additional prognostic information beyond Framingham risk score.[27] Importantly, the majority of studies assessing the prognostic role of chronotropic incompetence excluded patients receiving beta blocker therapy at the time of the exercise test.

Mechanistically, the increase in heart rate with exercise is thought to reflect physiologic parasympathetic withdrawal and increased sympathetic activity with exercise.[5] An early study comparing chronotropic response among subjects with heart failure and normal controls suggested that in this population at least, chronotropic incompetence is at least partially mediated by postsynaptic beta-adrenergic desensitization with resulting decreased sensitivity of the sinus node to sympathetic activity.[5,51]

Heart Rate Recovery. Whereas chronotropic response to exercise is thought to reflect sympathetic sensitivity, the rate of decrease in heart rate after exercise, termed heart rate recovery, likely reflects parasympathetic reactivation.[5]

Heart rate recovery = heart rate$_{\text{peak exercise}}$ −

heart rate$_{\text{1 or 2 minutes post exercise}}$

Heart rate recovery is a measure of parasympathetic nervous system function and autonomic balance.[52] Impaired heart rate recovery is commonly defined as a decrease in heart rate of ≤12 beats/min within the first minute after exercise,[53-55] although some have proposed a decrease of <22 beats/min at 2 minutes after exercise as the optimal cut point for prediction of risk of mortality.[56]

Impaired heart rate recovery is associated with an increased risk of death, even after adjustment for patient demographics, standard risk factors, and perfusion abnormalities on nuclear imaging (Fig. 29-7).[53-55] The relationship between heart rate recovery and risk of death is also independent of exercise capacity and peak chronotropic response.[53,55] Importantly, impaired heart rate recovery, in combination with exercise capacity, provides incremental prognostic information beyond established global risk scores, including the Framingham risk score[46] and the European SCORE,[57] as discussed in the next section.

How concurrent use of beta blockers affects the predictive power of heart rate recovery is unclear. In multiple studies, subjects with abnormal heart rate recovery do appear more likely to be receiving beta blocker therapy.[54,55] However, sub-group analysis in more than 2400 subjects referred for exercise testing, 13% of whom were receiving beta blocker therapy, did not find any significant modification of the relationship between impaired heart rate recovery and risk of death by concurrent beta blocker use.[53]

Incremental Value of Exercise Capacity and Heart Rate Recovery Beyond Traditional Risk Scores. Recent data demonstrated that these two variables added important prognostic information to the Framingham risk score. Asymptomatic individuals with low- or intermediate-risk Framingham scores had 8- to 10-fold higher risk of cardiovascular death if they also had low values of these two exercise measures combined (Fig. 29-8).[46] Using annual cardiovascular mortality rates and receiver operating curves, the study found that half of women and just under half of men with Framingham risk scores of 10% to 19%, in addition to half of women with Framingham risk scores of 6% to 9%, would be reclassified as high risk on the basis of having low heart rate recovery/low METs, thus providing clinically important risk information.

By applying the simple measurements of heart rate recovery and exercise capacity, this study accurately reclassified

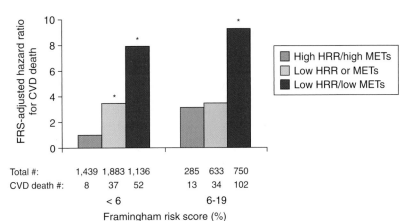

FIGURE 29-8 Framingham risk score (FRS)–adjusted hazard ratios for cardiovascular death from Cox proportional hazards models according to FRS categories and heart rate recovery/metabolic equivalents (HRR/METs) groups at 20-year follow-up. P_{trend} values are for tests of significance for trend across the three HRR/METs groups in each FRS category. An asterisk is shown for each of the hazard ratios that were statistically significant in a pairwise comparison to individuals with high HRR/high METs in the same FRS group (all <0.001). (*From Mora S, Redberg RF, Sharrett AR, Blumenthal RS: Enhanced risk assessment in asymptomatic individuals with exercise testing and Framingham risk scores.* Circulation *112:1566, 2005.*)

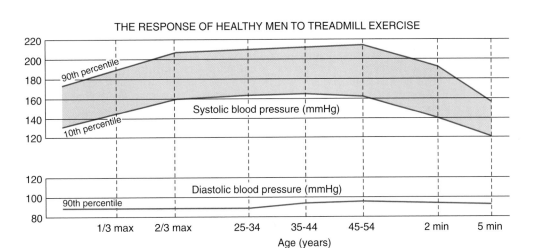

FIGURE 29-9 Illustration of the normal blood pressure response to exercise. (*From Fletcher GF, Balady GJ, Amsterdam EA, et al: Exercise standards for testing and training: a statement for healthcare professionals from the American Heart Association.* Circulation *104:1694, 2001. © 2001 American Heart Association, Inc.*)

as high risk approximately 50% of asymptomatic individuals who were deemed to be at intermediate risk by Framingham criteria. These findings have been substantiated in other populations.[27,57,58] Finally, both exercise capacity and heart rate recovery are at least partially modifiable and may be improved with moderate regular physical activity and exercise training by approximately 15% to 30% in a period of several months.[59]

Blood Pressure Responses. The normal blood pressure response to exercise (Fig. 29-9) is characterized by a steady rise in systolic blood pressure with little change in diastolic blood pressure, thereby resulting in an increase in pulse pressure (systolic minus diastolic blood pressure).[11] Exercise-induced hypotension is often defined as an initial increase in blood pressure followed by a decrease of 20 mm Hg during exercise or by a decrease in blood pressure during exercise >10 mm Hg below standing rest blood pressure.[11,60] It is associated with an increased prevalence of three-vessel disease or left main coronary artery disease and up to threefold increased risk of death at 2-year follow-up.[60]

Studies including normotensive men, women, whites, and African Americans have suggested that exaggerated systolic blood pressure response to exercise (commonly defined as peak systolic blood pressure >200 to 220 mm Hg) is associated with an increased risk of subsequent hypertension.[61,62] However, studies have been conflicting.

Fagard and colleagues[63] first reported on this association in their study of 143 hypertensive men, demonstrating that

blood pressure attained at submaximal or maximal workloads was not predictive of death from cardiovascular disease once baseline blood pressure was taken into account. Contrary to this, several studies showed that systolic exercise blood pressure could independently predict death from cardiovascular disease.[64-66] In particular, two landmark studies examining more that 7000 individuals found that submaximal exercise systolic blood pressure was, in fact, predictive of future cardiovascular death, even after controlling for rest blood pressure.[64,65] However, these findings were controversial because the relative contribution of rest blood pressure may have been underestimated in these studies, and the findings were attenuated once subjects were asked to exercise to maximum capacity. Given these conflicting data on the association of systolic blood pressure during exercise and cardiovascular endpoints, the ACC/AHA guidelines on exercise testing included exercise-induced hypertension as a marker for future clinical hypertension, but they did not link it with cardiovascular disease or mortality outcomes.[13]

The relative contribution of diastolic blood pressure to cardiovascular endpoints remained unclear until recently. In 2008, investigators for the Framingham Offspring Study noted an association between low-level exercise diastolic blood pressure and cardiovascular disease events in asymptomatic individuals independent of traditional risk factors and rest blood pressure.[67] Recently, a study was performed that found significant positive association for blood pressure (both systolic and diastolic) at rest, low-level (Bruce stage 2) exercise, and maximum exercise with death from cardiovascular disease in an asymptomatic population consisting of more than 6500 individuals.[68] The strongest association existed for rest blood pressure, followed by Bruce stage 2, and then maximal blood pressure during exercise. Among hypertensives, whether they had normal (<120/80) or prehypertension, Bruce stage 2 blood pressure >180/90 versus ≤180/90 mm Hg carried a 1.5- to 2.0-fold increased risk of cardiovascular death, independent of rest blood pressure risk factors.

In addition, exercise blood pressure added predictive value (net reclassification improvement, 10%-12%). These findings could potentially identify individuals who warrant more aggressive treatment than is currently recommended and deserve further investigation.

Ventricular Arrhythmias. The prognostic role of exercise-induced ventricular ectopy remains controversial,[11] with conflicting data.[69-71] Studies among population-based cohorts[72,73] and referral populations[74] suggest that exercise-induced frequent ventricular ectopy is associated with increased long-term all-cause and cardiac mortality. In these analyses, frequent ventricular ectopy is generally defined as increased frequency of premature ventricular contractions (e.g., >7 per minute or >10% of beats in a 30-second period), ventricular bigeminy or trigeminy, couplets or triplets, or ventricular tachycardia.

In a study of 6101 asymptomatic men who underwent exercise testing, exercise-induced frequent ventricular ectopy was associated with increased risk of cardiovascular death at 23-year follow-up.[72] This association was independent of and similar in magnitude to the relationship between exercise-induced ST-segment depression and risk of cardiovascular death (2.5-fold increased risk).[72] Similarly, an analysis of 2885 asymptomatic subjects from the Framingham Offspring Study found that subjects with exercise-induced premature ventricular contractions were at increased risk of all-cause mortality at 15-year follow-up, with a multivariable adjusted hazard ratio of nearly twofold.[73] A recent report from a referral population of 29,244 patients found that the presence of frequent ventricular ectopy during recovery phase was an even stronger predictor of mortality than frequent ectopy during exercise at 5 years of follow-up.[74]

Data exist that the occurrence of exercise-induced frequent ventricular ectopy is associated with increased risk of death, but more data are needed to clarify this association. The strength and magnitude of this relationship likely vary with the definition of frequent ventricular ectopy employed, the phase of exercise test when measured (exercise versus recovery), the population being assessed (asymptomatic screening versus referral versus known CHD), and the duration of follow-up.

Silent Ischemia

Silent ischemia is defined as the presence of demonstrable myocardial ischemia in the absence of angina symptoms. Most investigations of the clinical relevance of silent ischemia have been done in subjects with established coronary disease, either prior treated angina or prior acute coronary syndrome.[75-77] In the Asymptomatic Cardiac Ischemia Pilot (ACIP) study, 496 subjects with stable coronary disease, evidence of ischemia by exercise testing and ambulatory electrocardiographic monitoring, and coronary disease amenable to revascularization by angiography were randomized to medical therapy (angina guided or ischemia guided) or revascularization.[78]

Among the medically treated subjects, the burden of ischemia reflected in the number of ischemic episodes on ambulatory electrocardiographic monitoring was significantly associated with the incidence of ischemic events at 1-year follow-up.[78] The presence of myocardial ischemia was also associated with increased risk of cardiac events after revascularization[75] and MI.[77]

Fewer data exist for the prevalence and prognostic significance of silent ischemia in asymptomatic subjects without known coronary disease. Ischemic electrocardiographic response to stress has been associated with increased risk of subsequent cardiac events but has poor predictive value because of the high false-positive rate in low-risk populations.[79] Studies of asymptomatic ischemia on exercise testing confirmed by angiography suggest a prevalence among otherwise healthy men of roughly 2.5% to 2.7%.[80,81]

In a report of 407 subjects from the Baltimore Longitudinal Study of Aging, investigators noted an age-dependent increase in the prevalence of concordant abnormal electrocardiographic and nuclear perfusion responses to exercise stress testing, from 2% for subjects younger than 60 years to 15% for subjects older than 80 years.[79]

Even greater uncertainty exists about the prognostic implications of silent ischemia in asymptomatic populations. In the analysis from the Baltimore Longitudinal Study of Aging, during an average follow-up of 4.6 years, subjects with concordant electrocardiographic and perfusion abnormalities with stress testing were at a higher risk (48%) of subsequent angina, MI, or cardiac death than were those with normal results (7%) or with abnormal response of only one parameter (8%).[79] Importantly, the majority of events among those with concordant abnormalities consisted of development of angina (6 of 11), and the number of subjects with concordant abnormalities was small (n = 23).

Results of studies using ambulatory electrocardiographic recording to detect asymptomatic ischemia have been conflicting.[82,83] In a study of 394 men born in 1914 from Sweden, 79 of 341 subjects without a history of CHD had at least one episode of horizontal or downsloping ST depression of at least 0.1 mV. During an average follow-up of 43 months, these 79 subjects were at a higher risk of fatal or nonfatal MI (10.1% versus 2.3%).[83] However, not all studies have found this association with hard outcomes.

STRESS TESTING WITH IMAGING FOR SCREENING RISK ASSESSMENT OF ASYMPTOMATIC INDIVIDUALS

Current guidelines do not recommend routine screening with an exercise test for detection of CHD but do allow exercise testing in individuals with risk factors before starting of a vigorous exercise program other than walking (see Table 29-1). Whereas both exercise myocardial perfusion scintigraphy and exercise echocardiography have been shown to have prognostic value in symptomatic patients, their role for screening or prognostic purposes in asymptomatic individuals has not been well examined. Here, we summarize accepted indications for testing with imaging and examine the few prospective studies that have evaluated the use of stress imaging in asymptomatic or mildly symptomatic populations.

Although some studies, but not all, found additional prognostic value to stress-induced imaging abnormalities, absolute event rates were consistently low (even in subjects with abnormal test results), and the sensitivity was too low to justify cost-effective use of these tests. One randomized clinical trial, the Detection of Ischemia in Asymptomatic Diabetics (DIAD) study, was performed with pharmacologic stress but is discussed in detail because it is the only randomized clinical trial to test a strategy of screening stress myocardial perfusion imaging (MPI) versus no screening in asymptomatic individuals and found no benefit in outcomes for screening.

Indications for Testing with Imaging

In the diagnosis of CHD, exercise testing with imaging as an initial test is recommended only in a limited number of circumstances (Table 29-7).[84] These are situations in which baseline electrocardiographic abnormalities make interpretation of ischemic ST-segment deviation unreliable: preexcitation syndrome (Wolff-Parkinson-White), electrically paced ventricular rhythm, more than 1 mm of resting ST-segment depression, and complete left bundle branch block.[13] Subjects with ventricular paced rhythms and complete left bundle branch block should generally undergo vasodilator stress perfusion studies because of the increased false-positive rate associated with exercise stress and echocardiographic imaging.[84] Resting ST-segment depression <1 mm does not require imaging. Subjects unable to exercise should undergo a pharmacologic stress imaging study.

TABLE 29–7	2002 ACC/AHA Guidelines for the Use of Imaging as a First-Line Test for the Diagnosis of Coronary Heart Disease in Patients Who Are Able to Exercise

Class I

Exercise myocardial perfusion imaging or exercise echocardiography in patients with an intermediate pretest probability of CHD who have one of the following baseline ECG abnormalities:
  Preexcitation syndrome (Wolff-Parkinson-White) (Level of Evidence: B)
  More than 1-mm ST-segment depression at rest (Level of Evidence: B)
Exercise myocardial perfusion imaging or exercise echocardiography in patients with prior revascularization (PCI or CABG) (Level of Evidence: B)
Vasodilator (adenosine or dipyridamole) myocardial perfusion imaging in patients with an intermediate pretest probability of CAD and one of the following baseline ECG abnormalities:
  Paced ventricular rhythm (Level of Evidence: C)
  Left bundle branch block (Level of Evidence: B)

Class IIb

Exercise myocardial perfusion imaging or exercise echocardiography in patients with a low or high probability of CHD who have one of the following baseline ECG abnormalities:
  Preexcitation syndrome (Wolff-Parkinson-White) (Level of Evidence: B)
  More than 1-mm ST-segment depression at rest (Level of Evidence: B)
Vasodilator (adenosine or dipyridamole) myocardial perfusion imaging in patients with a low or high pretest probability of CAD and one of the following baseline ECG abnormalities:
  Paced ventricular rhythm (Level of Evidence: C)
  Left bundle branch block (Level of Evidence: B)
Exercise myocardial perfusion imaging or exercise echocardiography in patients with an intermediate probability of CHD who have one of the following:
  Digoxin use with less than 1-mm ST depression on the baseline ECG (Level of Evidence: B)
  LVH with less than 1-mm ST depression on the baseline ECG (Level of Evidence: B)
Exercise myocardial perfusion imaging, exercise echocardiography, adenosine or dipyridamole myocardial perfusion imaging, or dobutamine echocardiography as the initial stress test in a patient with a normal rest ECG who is not taking digoxin (Level of Evidence: B)
Exercise or dobutamine echocardiography in patients with left bundle branch block (Level of Evidence: C)

CABG, coronary artery bypass grafting; CAD, coronary artery disease; CHD, coronary heart disease; ECG, electrocardiogram; LVH, left ventricular hypertrophy; PCI, percutaneous coronary intervention.

From Gibbons RJ, Balady GJ, Bricker JT, et al: ACC/AHA 2002 guideline update for exercise testing: summary article: a report of the American College of Cardiology/American Heart Association Task Force on Practice Guidelines (Committee to Update the 1997 Exercise Testing Guidelines). *Circulation* 106:1883, 2002.
© 2002 American Heart Association, Inc.

Myocardial Perfusion Imaging

The Baltimore Longitudinal Study of Aging evaluated the predictive value of exercise testing with imaging in a community-based study.[79] Individuals with an abnormal exercise electrocardiogram and abnormal thallium scan had 3.6-fold increased risk of clinical CHD during a 5-year period. However, the prevalence of ischemia was low as expected for a general community-based population, and the authors concluded that it was not cost-effective to screen unselected individuals, especially those younger than 60 years.

For higher risk asymptomatic patients enriched with risk factors and having a family history of premature CHD, thallium imaging combined with exercise testing improved the predictive value of the test.[85] In the Johns Hopkins Sibling Study, 264 asymptomatic siblings (mean age, 46 years) of individuals with premature CHD underwent exercise thallium testing. The relative risk for development of clinical CHD (death, MI, or revascularization) during a follow-up period of 6 years was fourfold for an abnormal exercise electrocardiogram and fivefold for an abnormal scan, defined as a moderate reversible segmental perfusion defect. Siblings with an abnormal exercise electrocardiogram and abnormal thallium scan had a relative risk of 14.5 compared with siblings who had both normal. In a subsequent report from the same study but with a larger sample size of 734 siblings, abnormal thallium scan combined with abnormal exercise electrocardiogram correlated with generally mild obstructive coronary disease on angiography.[86]

The DIAD Study

The primary objective of the DIAD study was to determine whether screening of type 2 asymptomatic diabetic patients with pharmacologic (adenosine) MPI would reduce cardiac events, defined as fatal and nonfatal coronary events.[87] A total of 1123 type 2 diabetic patients with no history of CHD (mean age, 60 years; mean diabetes duration, 8 to 9 years; >60% with two or more additional cardiac risk factors at baseline) were randomized to screening with adenosine MPI versus no screening. Patients were then referred to their medical providers for appropriate care without mandating angiography in those with abnormal stress test results.

During a mean follow-up of 5 years, the primary endpoint was not significantly different (*P* = 0.73; Fig. 29-10A) among those screened with MPI (2.7%) versus those not screened (3.0%), despite a higher use of angiography in the MPI compared with the nonscreened group (4.4% versus 0.5%). Overall, the cardiac event rate during follow-up was low (0.6%/year), with most patients receiving statins and aspirin. This low cardiac event rate in this asymptomatic diabetic population is lower by up to fourfold compared with diabetic patients referred for stress testing (workup/referral bias).

Whereas moderate or large perfusion abnormalities on MPI had sixfold higher relative risk of cardiac events compared with normal studies or small perfusion abnormalities (Fig. 29-10B), the positive predictive value was low (12%), with more than half of the cardiac events occurring in patients with normal studies. Thus, the DIAD study found no clinical benefit during a 5-year period for routine screening of type 2 diabetic patients without history of CAD with adenosine MPI, despite the higher risk associated with moderate to large perfusion abnormalities, calling into question certain guideline recommendations for screening of asymptomatic individuals (see Table 29-1).[13]

Exercise Echocardiography

The predictive value of exercise echocardiography was evaluated in 1859 individuals (mean age, 51 years) with no anginal

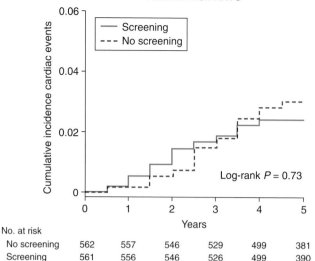

ALL PARTICIPANTS

A

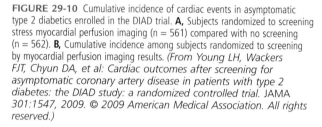

FIGURE 29-10 Cumulative incidence of cardiac events in asymptomatic type 2 diabetics enrolled in the DIAD trial. **A,** Subjects randomized to screening stress myocardial perfusion imaging (n = 561) compared with no screening (n = 562). **B,** Cumulative incidence among subjects randomized to screening by myocardial perfusion imaging results. *(From Young LH, Wackers FJT, Chyun DA, et al: Cardiac outcomes after screening for asymptomatic coronary artery disease in patients with type 2 diabetes: the DIAD study: a randomized controlled trial. JAMA 301:1547, 2009. © 2009 American Medical Association. All rights reserved.)*

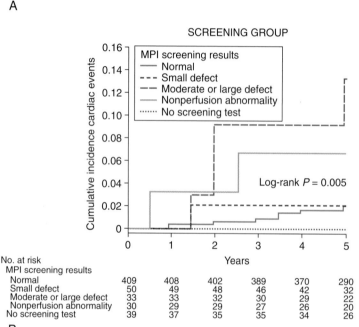

SCREENING GROUP

B

or heart failure symptoms and no history of CHD but who were referred for exercise testing by their health care providers.[88] No increased risk of death associated with exercise-induced ischemia was found on echocardiography during a 10-year follow-up, even in the subgroups of individuals with several risk factors or who were at intermediate risk. By contrast, the DTS as well as resting left ventricular dysfunction (most of which was mild dysfunction) imparted increased risk. Thus, this study found no additional prognostic value to exercise echocardiography for screening of these relatively asymptomatic individuals but confirmed the value of exercise capacity or DTS in predicting risk.

By contrast, in a prior study of patients who were mildly symptomatic but at low pretest probability of disease, exercise-induced ischemia on echocardiography was associated with increased risk of events during a 3-year period.[89] However, the event rate was low during follow-up, as was the sensitivity of the test (47%), and the authors concluded that exercise echocardiography is not cost-effective in this setting.

Need for Randomized Clinical Trial Data

There are several potential important implications of the DIAD study for clinical guidelines and future design of clinical trials in asymptomatic individuals. First, the DIAD study demonstrated that it is feasible to conduct well-designed screening trials in asymptomatic individuals to determine the utility of screening tests with respect to clinical outcomes. Second, the low rates of cardiac events in asymptomatic individuals in DIAD, even when stress test results were abnormal, and the low positive predictive value of these abnormalities are consistent with results from prior prospective nonrandomized studies. Thus, it is not surprising that there was no clinical benefit associated with screening of these asymptomatic individuals, even though they were diabetic and had several other risk factors. Finally, this underscores the importance of conducting randomized clinical trials in asymptomatic populations to evaluate the clinical utility of screening stress testing, as called for by the AHA expert group.[5]

CONCLUSION

Exercise stress testing is a safe procedure and provides both diagnostic and prognostic information in asymptomatic or minimally symptomatic individuals. A growing body of literature supports the utility of nonelectrocardiographic parameters—in particular, exercise capacity, chronotropic response, exercise blood pressure, and heart rate recovery—in determining prognosis in asymptomatic subjects beyond traditional risk factors or global risk scores. However, data are still lacking that the screening use of exercise testing results in improved patient outcomes. There are currently no Class I indications for exercise testing in asymptomatic adults in the ACC/AHA guidelines. Guidelines suggest that testing in asymptomatic individuals may be reasonable in the following situations: before vigorous exercise is started in the presence of diabetes, older age (men >45 years, women >55 years), or higher absolute risk for CHD due to comorbid conditions such as peripheral vascular disease and chronic kidney disease and for individuals involved in occupations potentially having an impact on public safety. Exercise testing with imaging should be used as an initial test in the following situations: preexcitation syndrome (Wolff-Parkinson-White), electrically paced ventricular rhythm, more than 1 mm of resting ST-segment depression, and complete left bundle branch block. Although some studies suggest additional prognostic value of imaging along with stress testing in asymptomatic subjects, stress testing with imaging is not cost-effective in this population because of consistently low event rates and low test specificity. Of note, the results of the DIAD trial further call into question the utility of screening stress testing in asymptomatic diabetic patients. More data from randomized clinical trials in asymptomatic populations are needed to evaluate the utility of screening exercise testing.

REFERENCES

1. Lloyd-Jones D, Adams R, Carnethon M, et al: Heart disease and stroke statistics—2009 update: a report from the American Heart Association Statistics Committee and Stroke Statistics Subcommittee. *Circulation* 119:e21, 2009.
2. Myerburg RJ, Kessler KM, Castellanos A: Sudden cardiac death: epidemiology, transient risk, and intervention assessment. *Ann Intern Med* 119:1187, 1993.
3. Greenland P, Smith SC, Grundy SM: Improving coronary heart disease risk assessment in asymptomatic people: role of traditional risk factors and noninvasive cardiovascular tests. *Circulation* 104:1863, 2001.
4. *Screening for coronary heart disease,* topic page. February 2004. U.S. Preventive Services Task Force. Available at: http://www.uspreventiveservicestaskforce.org/uspstf/uspsacad.htm.
5. Lauer M, Froelicher ES, Williams M, Kligfield P: Exercise testing in asymptomatic adults: a statement for professionals from the American Heart Association Council on Clinical Cardiology, Subcommittee on Exercise, Cardiac Rehabilitation, and Prevention. *Circulation* 112:771, 2005.
6. Grundy SM, Pasternak R, Greenland P, et al: AHA/ACC scientific statement: assessment of cardiovascular risk by use of multiple-risk-factor assessment equations: a statement for healthcare professionals from the American Heart Association and the American College of Cardiology. *J Am Coll Cardiol* 34:1348, 1999.
7. Ford ES, Giles WH, Mokdad AH: The distribution of 10-year risk for coronary heart disease among US adults: findings from the National Health and Nutrition Examination Survey III. *J Am Coll Cardiol* 43:1791, 2004.
8. Stuart RJ, Ellestad MH: National survey of exercise stress testing facilities. *Chest* 77:94, 1980.
9. Myers J, Voodi L, Umann T, Froelicher VF: A survey of exercise testing: methods, utilization, interpretation, and safety in the VAHCS. *J Cardiopulm Rehab* 20:251, 2000.
10. Senaratne MP, Smith G, Gulamhusein SS: Feasibility and safety of early exercise testing using the Bruce protocol after acute myocardial infarction. *J Am Coll Cardiol* 35:1212, 2000.
11. Fletcher GF, Balady GJ, Amsterdam EA, et al: Exercise standards for testing and training: a statement for healthcare professionals from the American Heart Association. *Circulation* 104:1694, 2001.
12. Schlant RC, Friesinger GC, Leonard JJ: Clinical competence in exercise testing. A statement for physicians from the ACP/ACC/AHA Task Force on Clinical Privileges in Cardiology. *J Am Coll Cardiol* 16:1061, 1990.
13. Gibbons RJ, Balady GJ, Bricker JT, et al: ACC/AHA 2002 guideline update for exercise testing: summary article: a report of the American College of Cardiology/American Heart Association Task Force on Practice Guidelines (Committee to Update the 1997 Exercise Testing Guidelines). *Circulation* 106:1883, 2002.
14. Cohn JN: Quantitative exercise testing for the cardiac patient: the value of monitoring gas exchange: introduction. *Circulation* 76(Suppl VI):VI-1, 1987.
15. Bouchard C, An P, Rice T, et al: Familial aggregation of VO_2max response to exercise training: results from the HERITAGE Family Study. *J Appl Physiol* 87:1003, 1999.
16. Myers J, Froelicher VF: Optimizing the exercise test for pharmacological investigations. *Circulation* 82:1839, 1990.
17. Whipp BJ, Davis JA, Torres F, Wasserman K: A test to determine parameters of aerobic function during exercise. *J Appl Physiol* 50:217, 1981.
18. Morise AP, Haddad WJ, Beckner D: Development and validation of a clinical score to estimate the probability of coronary artery disease in men and women presenting with suspected coronary disease. *Am J Med* 102:350-356, 1997.
19. Pryor DB, Harrell FE, Lee KL, Califf RM, Rosati RA: Estimating the likelihood of significant coronary artery disease. *Am J Med* 75:771, 1983.
20. Diamond GA, Forrester JS: Analysis of probability as an aid in the clinical diagnosis of coronary-artery disease. *N Engl J Med* 300:1350, 1979.
21. Miranda CP, Lehmann KG, Froelicher VF: Correlation between resting ST segment depression, exercise testing, coronary angiography, and long-term prognosis. *Am Heart J* 122:1617, 1991.
22. Fearon WF, Lee DP, Froelicher VF: The effect of resting ST segment depression on the diagnostic characteristics of the exercise treadmill test. *J Am Coll Cardiol* 35:1206, 2000.
23. Rywik TM, O'Connor FC, Gittings NS, et al: Role of nondiagnostic exercise-induced ST-segment abnormalities in predicting future coronary events in asymptomatic volunteers. *Circulation* 106:2787, 2002.
24. Rywik TM, Zink RC, Gittings NS, et al: Independent prognostic significance of ischemic ST-segment response limited to recovery from treadmill exercise in asymptomatic subjects. *Circulation* 97:2117, 1998.
25. Gianrossi R, Detrano R, Mulvihill D, et al: Exercise-induced ST depression in the diagnosis of coronary artery disease. A meta-analysis. *Circulation* 80:87, 1989.
26. Mora S, Redberg RF, Cui Y, et al: Ability of exercise testing to predict cardiovascular and all-cause death in asymptomatic women: a 20-year follow-up of the lipid research clinics prevalence study. *JAMA* 290:1600, 2003.
27. Balady GJ, Larson MG, Vasan RS: Usefulness of exercise testing in the prediction of coronary disease risk among asymptomatic persons as a function of the Framingham risk score. *Circulation* 110:1920, 2004.
28. Gulati M, Arnsdorf MF, Shaw LJ, et al: Prognostic value of the Duke treadmill score in asymptomatic women. *Am J Cardiol* 96:369, 2005.
29. Rautaharju PM, Prineas RJ, Eifler WJ, et al: Prognostic value of exercise electrocardiogram in men at high risk of future coronary heart disease: Multiple Risk Factor Intervention Trial experience. *J Am Coll Cardiol* 8:1, 1986.
30. Ekelund LG, Haskell WL, Johnson JL, et al: Physical fitness as a predictor of cardiovascular mortality in asymptomatic North American men. The Lipid Research Clinics Mortality Follow-up Study. *N Engl J Med* 319:1379, 1988.
31. Myers J, Prakash M, Froelicher V, et al: Exercise capacity and mortality among men referred for exercise testing. *N Engl J Med* 346:793, 2002.
32. Bruce RA, Hossak KF, DeRouen TA, Hofer V: Enhanced risk assessment for primary coronary heart disease events by maximal exercise testing: 10 years' experience of Seattle Heart Watch. *J Am Coll Cardiol* 2:565, 1983.
33. Kwok Y, Kim C, Grady D, et al: Meta-analysis of exercise testing to detect coronary artery disease in women. *Am J Cardiol* 83:660, 1999.
34. Bokhari S, Bergmann SR: The effect of estrogen compared to estrogen plus progesterone on the exercise electrocardiogram. *J Am Coll Cardiol* 40:1092, 2002.
35. Palinkas A, Toth E, Amyot R, et al: The value of ECG and echocardiography during stress testing for identifying systemic endothelial dysfunction and epicardial artery stenosis. *Eur Heart J* 23:1587, 2002.
36. Mark DB, Hlatky MA, Harrell FE, et al: Exercise treadmill score for predicting prognosis in coronary artery disease. *Ann Intern Med* 106:793, 1987.
37. Mark DB, Shaw L, Harrell EF, et al: Prognostic value of a treadmill exercise score in outpatients with suspected coronary artery disease. *N Engl J Med* 325:849, 1991.
38. Kwok JM, Miller TD, Hodge DO, Gibbons RJ: Prognostic value of the Duke treadmill score in the elderly. *J Am Coll Cardiol* 39:1475, 2002.
39. Morris CK, Myers J, Froelicher VF, et al: Nomogram based on metabolic equivalents and age for assessing aerobic exercise capacity in men. *J Am Coll Cardiol* 22:175, 1993.
40. Gulati M, Black HR, Shaw LJ, et al: The prognostic value of a nomogram for exercise capacity in women. *N Engl J Med* 353:468, 2005.
41. Ekelund LG, Haskell WL, Johnson JL, et al: Physical fitness as a predictor of cardiovascular mortality in asymptomatic North American men. The Lipid Research Clinics Mortality Follow-up Study. *N Engl J Med* 319:1379, 1988.
42. Blair SN, Kohl HW, Barlow CE, et al: Changes in physical fitness and all-cause mortality. A prospective study of healthy and unhealthy men. *JAMA* 273:1093, 1995.
43. Kannel WB, Wilson P, Blair SN: Epidemiological assessment of the role of physical activity and fitness in development of cardiovascular disease. *Am Heart J* 109:876, 1985.
44. Myers J, Prakash M, Froelicher V, et al: Exercise capacity and mortality among men referred for exercise testing. *N Engl J Med* 346:793, 2002.
45. Blair SN, Kohl HW, Paffenbarger RS, et al: Physical fitness and all-cause mortality. A prospective study of healthy men and women. *JAMA* 262:2395, 1989.
46. Mora S, Redberg RF, Sharrett AR, Blumenthal RS: Enhanced risk assessment in asymptomatic individuals with exercise testing and Framingham risk scores. *Circulation* 112:1566, 2005.
47. Lauer MS, Okin PM, Larson MG, et al: Impaired heart rate response to graded exercise. Prognostic implications of chronotropic incompetence in the Framingham Heart Study. *Circulation* 93:1520, 1996.
48. Azarbal B, Hayes SW, Lewin HC, et al: The incremental prognostic value of percentage of heart rate reserve achieved over myocardial perfusion single-photon emission computed tomography in the prediction of cardiac death and all-cause mortality: superiority over 85% of maximal age-predicted heart rate. *J Am Coll Cardiol* 44:423, 2004.
49. Lauer MS, Francis GS, Okin PM, et al: Impaired chronotropic response exercise stress testing as a predictor of mortality. *JAMA* 281:524, 1999.

502

50. Elhendy A, Mahoney DW, Khandheria BK, et al: Prognostic significance of impairment of heart rate response to exercise: impact of left ventricular function and myocardial ischemia. *J Am Coll Cardiol* 42:823, 2003.
51. Colucci WS, Ribeiro JP, Rocco MB, et al: Impaired chronotropic response to exercise in patients with congestive heart failure. Role of postsynaptic beta-adrenergic desensitization. *Circulation* 80:314, 1989.
52. Lauer MS: Exercise electrocardiogram testing and prognosis. Novel markers and predictive instruments. *Cardiol Clin* 19:401, 2001.
53. Cole CR, Blackstone EH, Pashkow FJ, et al: Heart-rate recovery immediately after exercise as a predictor of mortality. *N Engl J Med* 341:1351, 1999.
54. Nishime EO, Cole CR, Blackstone EH, et al: Heart rate recovery and treadmill exercise score as predictors of mortality in patients referred for exercise ECG. *JAMA* 284:1392, 2000.
55. Vivekananthan DP, Blackstone EH, Pothier CE, Lauer MS: Heart rate recovery after exercise is a predictor of mortality, independent of the angiographic severity of coronary disease. *J Am Coll Cardiol* 42:831, 2003.
56. Shetler K, Marcus R, Froelicher VF, et al: Heart rate recovery: validation and methodologic issues. *J Am Coll Cardiol* 38:1980, 2001.
57. Aktas MK, Ozduran V, Pothier CE, et al: Global risk scores and exercise testing for predicting all-cause mortality in a preventive medicine program. *JAMA* 292:1462, 2004.
58. Gulati M, Pandey DK, Arnsdorf MF, et al: Exercise capacity and the risk of death in women: the St. James Women Take Heart Project. *Circulation* 108:1554, 2003.
59. American College of Sports Medicine Position Stand: The recommended quantity and quality of exercise for developing and maintaining cardiorespiratory and muscular fitness, and flexibility in healthy adults. *Med Sci Sports Exerc* 30:975, 1998.
60. Dubach P, Froelicher VF, Klein J, et al: Exercise-induced hypertension in a male population. Criteria, causes, and prognosis. *Circulation* 78:1380, 1988.
61. Miyai N, Arita M, Miyashita K, et al: Blood pressure response to heart rate during exercise test and risk of future hypertension. *Hypertension* 39:761, 2002.
62. Manolio TA, Burke GL, Savage PJ, et al: Exercise blood pressure response and 5-year risk of elevated blood pressure in a cohort of young adults: the CARDIA study. *Am J Hypertens* 7:234, 1994.
63. Fagard R, Staessen J, Thijs L, Amery A: Prognostic significance of exercise versus resting blood pressure in hypertensive men. *Hypertension* 17:574, 1991.
64. Filipovsky J, Ducimetiere P, Safar ME: Prognostic significance of exercise blood pressure and heart rate in middle-aged men. *Hypertension* 20:333, 1992.
65. Mundal R, Kjeldsen SE, Sandvik L, et al: Exercise blood pressure predicts cardiovascular mortality in middle-aged men. *Hypertension* 24:56, 1994.
66. Allison TG, Coreiro MA, Miller TD, et al: Prognostic significance of exercise-induced systemic hypertension in healthy subjects. *Am J Cardiol* 83:371, 1999.
67. Lewis GD, Gona P, Larson MG, et al: Exercise blood pressure and the risk of incident cardiovascular disease (from the Framingham Heart Study). *Am J Cardiol* 101:1614, 2008.
68. Weiss SD, Blumenthal RS, Sharrett AR, et al: Exercise blood pressure and future cardiovascular death in asymptomatic individuals. *Circ* 121:2109, 2010.
69. Udall JA, Ellestad MH: Predictive implications of ventricular premature contractions associated with treadmill stress testing. *Circulation* 56:985, 1977.
70. Califf RM, McKinnis RA, McNeer JF, et al: Prognostic value of ventricular arrhythmias associated with treadmill exercise testing in patients studied with cardiac catheterization for suspected ischemic heart disease. *J Am Coll Cardiol* 2:1060, 1983.
71. Sami M, Chaitman B, Fisher L, et al: Significance of exercise-induced ventricular arrhythmia in stable coronary artery disease: a coronary artery surgery subject project. *Am J Cardiol* 54:1182, 1984.

72. Jouven X, Zureik M, Desnos M, et al: Long-term outcome in asymptomatic men with exercise-induced premature ventricular depolarizations. *N Engl J Med* 343:826, 2000.
73. Morshedi-Meibodi A, Evans JC, Levy D, et al: Clinical correlates and prognostic significance of exercise-induced ventricular premature beats in the community: the Framingham Heart Study. *Circulation* 109:2417, 2004.
74. Frolkis JP, Pothier CE, Blackstone EH, Lauer MS: Frequent ventricular ectopy after exercise as a predictor of death. *N Engl J Med* 348:781, 2003.
75. Weiner DA, Ryan TJ, McCabe CH, et al: Risk of developing an acute myocardial infarction or sudden coronary death in patients with exercise-induced silent myocardial ischemia. A report from the Coronary Artery Surgery Study (CASS) registry. *Am J Cardiol* 62:1155, 1988.
76. Cohn PF, Fox KM, Daly C: Silent myocardial ischemia. *Circulation* 108:1263, 2003.
77. Gutterman DD: Silent myocardial ischemia. *Circ J* 73:785, 2009.
78. Stone PH, Chaitman BR, Forman S, et al: Prognostic significance of myocardial ischemia detected by ambulatory electrocardiography, exercise treadmill testing, and electrocardiogram at rest to predict cardiac events by one year (the Asymptomatic Cardiac Ischemia Pilot [ACIP] study). *Am J Cardiol* 80:1395, 1997.
79. Fleg JL, Gerstenblith G, Zonderman AB, et al: Prevalence and prognostic significance of exercise-induced silent myocardial ischemia detected by thallium scintigraphy and electrocardiography in asymptomatic volunteers. *Circulation* 81:428, 1990.
80. Froehicker VF, Thompson AJ, Longo MR, et al: Value of exercise testing for screening asymptomatic men for latent coronary artery disease. *Prog Cardiovasc Dis* 18:265, 1976.
81. Thaulow E, Erikssen J, Sandik L, et al: Initial clinical presentation of cardiac disease in asymptomatic men with silent myocardial ischemia and angiographically documented coronary artery disease (the Oslo Ischemia Study). *Am J Cardiol* 72:629, 1993.
82. Fleg J, Kennedy H: Long term prognostic significance of ambulatory electrocardiographic findings in apparently healthy subjects greater than or equal to 60 years of age. *Am J Cardiol* 70:748, 1992.
83. Hedblad B, Juul-Moller S, Svensson K, et al: Increased mortality in men with ST segment depression during 24h ambulatory long-term ECG recording: results from prospective population study "Men born in 1914," from Malmö, Sweden. *Eur Heart J* 10:149, 1989.
84. Fraker TD, Jr, Fihn SD; 2002 Chronic Stable Angina Writing Committee; American College of Cardiology; American Heart Association: 2007 chronic angina focused update of the ACC/AHA 2002 guidelines for the management of patients with chronic stable angina: a report of the American College of Cardiology/American Heart Association Task Force of Practice Guidelines Writing Group to develop the focused update of the 2002 guidelines for the management of patients with chronic stable angina. *J Am Coll Cardiol* 50:2264, 2007.
85. Blumenthal RS, Becker DM, Moy TF, et al: Exercise thallium tomography predicts future clinically manifest coronary heart disease in a high-risk asymptomatic population. *Circulation* 93:915, 1996.
86. Blumenthal RS, Becker DM, Yanek LR, et al: Detecting occult coronary disease in a high-risk asymptomatic population. *Circulation* 107:702, 2003.
87. Young LH, Wackers FJT, Chyun DA, et al: Cardiac outcomes after screening for asymptomatic coronary artery disease in patients with type 2 diabetes: the DIAD study: a randomized controlled trial. *JAMA* 301:1547, 2009.
88. Marwick TH, Case C, Short L, Thomas JD: Prediction of mortality in patients without angina: use of an exercise score and exercise echocardiography. *Eur Heart J* 24:1223, 2003.
89. Elhendy A, Shub C, McCully RB, et al: Exercise echocardiography for the prognostic stratification of patients with low pretest probability of coronary artery disease. *Am J Med* 111:18, 2001.

29

Carotid Intima-Media Thickness Measurement and Plaque Detection for Cardiovascular Disease Risk Prediction

Heather M. Johnson and James H. Stein

KEY POINTS

- Measurement of carotid intima-media thickness (CIMT) with B-mode ultrasound is a noninvasive, sensitive, and highly reproducible technique for identifying and quantifying arterial injury and cardiovascular disease risk.

- The relationship between increasing CIMT and incident cardiovascular disease events has been established across a wide age range; however, the strongest data are for individuals between 42 and 74 years of age.

- Several prospective, population-based studies demonstrated that carotid plaque presence is associated with a significantly increased risk for myocardial infarction, stroke, and coronary heart disease death, independent of traditional risk factors.

- The relative risks associated with the presence of plaque are similar to or slightly higher than those observed with increased CIMT.

- The most recent, comprehensive recommendations on the use of carotid ultrasound for cardiovascular disease risk assessment are contained in a Consensus Statement published in 2008 by the American Society of Echocardiography.

- The ASE Consensus Statement recommended that carotid ultrasound with CIMT measurement and evaluation for plaque presence be considered in intermediate-risk patients, in patients with a family history of premature cardiovascular disease in a first-degree relative, in individuals younger than 60 years old with severe abnormalities of a single risk factor, and in women younger than 60 years old with two or more risk factors.

- Randomized outcome studies are needed to determine if improved risk prediction, behavior changes, and changes in physician practice that occur with CIMT or carotid plaque imaging lead to improved patient outcomes and cardiovascular disease risk reduction.

Cardiovascular disease (CVD) is the leading cause of death in the United States, accounting for approximately 864,480 (35.3%) deaths annually.[1] Each year, approximately 1.2 million individuals experience a myocardial infarction (MI), approximately one third of which are fatal.[1] Unfortunately, for a majority of individuals, the first symptom of heart disease is sudden cardiac death or MI.[1,2] Atherosclerosis, the anatomic substrate for MI, begins in childhood and progresses over decades.[3] To prevent death and morbidity from coronary heart disease, there is great interest in identifying high-risk, asymptomatic patients who would be candidates for more intensive, evidence-based medical interventions that prevent progression of atherosclerosis and reduce CVD risk.[4]

Arterial imaging to identify and to quantify subclinical vascular disease has been suggested to further refine coronary heart disease risk assessment.[4,5] As a screening test, imaging must be safe, sensitive, affordable, and lead to interventions that can favorably alter the natural history of CVD. Measurement of carotid intima-media thickness (CIMT) with B-mode ultrasound is a noninvasive, sensitive, and highly reproducible technique for identifying and quantifying arterial injury and CVD risk. It is a well-validated research tool that increasingly is being used as a clinical tool.[6-15] The United States Centers for Medicare and Medicaid has established a Current Procedural Terminology code (0126T) for "common carotid intima-media thickness (IMT) study for evaluation of atherosclerotic burden or coronary heart disease risk factor assessment."

CAROTID INTIMA-MEDIA THICKNESS AND PLAQUE IMAGING

The extent of carotid artery atherosclerosis is strongly related to the extent of coronary artery atherosclerosis.[16] Carotid duplex ultrasound is used to evaluate for the presence and extent of occlusive, advanced, flow-limiting carotid artery atherosclerosis.[17] Ultrasound imaging of carotid artery wall thickness is a distinctly different test that is used to assess CVD risk. The superficial location and easy accessibility of the common carotid artery permit accurate, reproducible ultrasound imaging. The walls of the carotid artery are composed of the lumen-intima interface and the media-adventitia interface that together produce two echogenic lines in the far wall of the carotid artery (Fig. 30-1).[9] Measurement of the combined thickness of these interfaces comprises the CIMT (Fig. 30-2). The presence of subclinical arterial injury is demonstrated by increased CIMT, and the presence of carotid plaque represents subclinical atherosclerotic disease.

RELATIONSHIP BETWEEN CAROTID INTIMA-MEDIA THICKNESS AND CARDIOVASCULAR DISEASE EVENTS

There are 11 published prospective, population-based studies of CIMT and CVD risk that included at least 1000 participants and

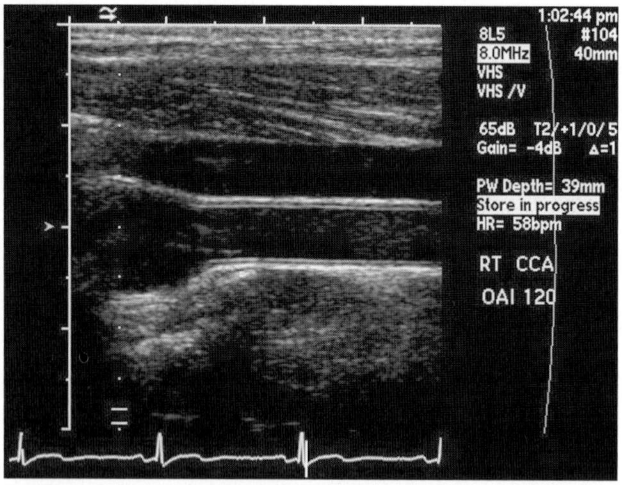

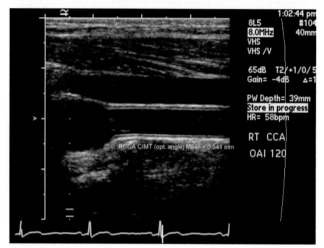

FIGURE 30-1 Longitudinal plane demonstrating "double-line sign" on near and far walls of the common carotid artery.

FIGURE 30-2 Leading edge–to–leading edge measurement of the far-wall common carotid artery CIMT.

presented odds ratios or relative risks adjusted for CVD risk factors (Table 30-1).[7,8,18-26] Many of these studies recently were reviewed in detail.[27] These studies demonstrated that increased CIMT is associated with significantly increased risk for MI, stroke, and/or coronary heart disease death.[7,8,18-26] Two additional large studies had similar findings.[28,29] In several studies, the adjusted relative risks associated with the greatest degrees of wall thickness (see cut points in Table 30-1) were high enough (>2.0) that they would be expected to improve coronary heart disease risk prediction in appropriately selected patients.[7,8,18,20,23,29] Furthermore, CIMT measurements improve on traditional risk factors for classification of patients in regard to the presence of significant angiographic coronary artery disease[30] and risk of recurrent CVD events.[31] In an analysis of unselected participants in the Atherosclerosis Risk in Communities (ARIC) study, CIMT values significantly (albeit modestly, ~0.02) increased the area under the receiver operator characteristic curve (AUC) for prediction of cardiovascular events in men.[32] In the Multi-Ethnic Study of Atherosclerosis (MESA), increased CIMT was positively associated with CVD events and stroke.[25] As in ARIC, CIMT values modestly increased the AUC (by ~0.01) for prediction of CVD compared with traditional risk factors alone.[25]

The relationship between increasing CIMT and incident cardiovascular events has been established across a wide age range. However, the strongest data are for individuals between 42 and 74 years of age; several studies of individuals in this age range show similar results (see Table 30-1). For younger adults (18 to 42 years old), consistent, strong relationships between increasing risk factor burden and CIMT, as well as between CIMT and emerging risk factors, have been demonstrated.[33-40] In the Carotid Atherosclerosis Progression Study (CAPS), CIMT predicted CVD events even among 2436 individuals <50 years old (mean, 38.7 years; standard deviation, 7.0 years).[19] In that study, the relative risk associated with increased CIMT appeared to be higher among younger than older adults.[19]

In the Tromsø Study of 6226 subjects, there were conflicting data regarding the predictive value of CIMT and CVD events. The CIMT in the common carotid artery did not demonstrate a statistically significant relationship between CIMT and first MI,[24] but there was a significant relationship, in both men and women, when CIMT was evaluated with use of both the common carotid artery and bulb segments.[24] However, this study measured CIMT only in the right carotid artery. The American Society of Echocardiography (ASE) Consensus Statement recommends that CIMT be evaluated with the far wall of both the right and left common carotid arteries, in conjunction with plaque imaging in the common carotid, bulb, and internal carotid artery segments, because atherosclerosis progresses more rapidly in the bulb and internal carotid artery segments, and the effects of risk factors on CIMT can vary by segment.[9,41-44] This approach has been validated, and its predictive value has been rigorously demonstrated in other studies (see Table 30-1).[9]

RELATIONSHIP BETWEEN CAROTID PLAQUES AND CARDIOVASCULAR DISEASE EVENTS

Carotid plaque presence is associated with the presence of coronary artery plaque and the occurrence of future cardiovascular and cerebrovascular disease events.[24,26,30] Most carotid plaques are found in the bulb and proximal internal carotid artery segments because of turbulent flow.[45] Atherosclerosis and CIMT progress more rapidly in the bulb and internal carotid segments compared with the common carotid artery.[41,42] Seven population-based studies that included at least 1000 participants and presented relative risks or hazard ratios adjusted for CVD risk factors have demonstrated the predictive power of carotid plaque (Table 30-2).[21-23,26,46-48] In these studies, the relative risks associated with the presence of plaque were similar to or slightly higher than those observed with increased CIMT. Two additional large studies of carotid plaque presence and two studies that evaluated plaque area had similar results.[24,29,49,50] The presence of carotid plaque predicted future CVD events among young, middle, and elderly subjects.[24,49] A prospective study of 367 elderly men (>70 years old) demonstrated that the presence of carotid plaque significantly improved the AUC for prediction of all-cause mortality and cardiovascular mortality, even after considering traditional cardiovascular risk factors and use of medications (by ~0.03 to 0.04).[49] In San Daniele Township, the presence of carotid plaque or CIMT >1 mm had greater predictive value than the Framingham risk score for ischemic cerebrovascular disease events and a small increase in AUC (by ~0.01).[26]

Unfortunately, the definition of carotid plaque in most reported studies was not uniform.[51] Most studies identified plaque as focal widening relative to adjacent segments with protrusion into the lumen and/or had a minimum wall thickness.[51] The Mannheim Carotid Intima-Media Thickness Consensus Report suggested that plaque should be defined as "a focal structure that encroaches into the arterial lumen of at least 0.5 mm or 50% of the surrounding IMT or demonstrates

| TABLE 30–1 | Prospective Studies of Carotid Intima-Media Thickness and Risk for Cardiovascular Disease Events in Individuals Without Known Cardiovascular Disease (N >1000 participants each) |

Study	N	Age, years (% W)	Follow-up, years	Measurement and Site(s)	Event	Δ CIMT (mm), Adjusted RR (95% CI)*	CIMT Cut Point, Adjusted RR (95% CI)*,†
ARIC[7]	12,841	45-64 (57%)	5.2	Mean of mean CCA, bulb, ICA	MI, CHD death	0.19 W: 1.38 (1.21-1.58) M: 1.17 (1.04-1.31)	Highest tertile W: 2.53 (1.02-6.26) M: 2.02 (1.32-3.09)
				Mean CCA	MI, CHD death	0.19 W: 1.46 (1.22-1.74) M: 1.08 (0.91-1.1.27)	—
ARIC[18]	14,214	45-64 (55%)	7.2	Mean of mean CCA, bulb, ICA	Stroke	0.19 W: 1.36 (1.16-1.59) M: 1.21 (1.05-1.39)	Highest tertile W: 2.32 (1.09-4.94) M: 2.24 (1.26-4.00)
				Mean CCA	Stroke	0.18 W: 1.32 (1.10-1.58) M: 1.38 (1.16-1.65)	Highest tertile W: 1.65 (0.85-3.19) M: 2.69 (1.49-4.87)
CAPS[19]	5056	19-90 (49.7%)	4.2	Mean Far-wall CCA	MI	0.16 1.16 (1.05-1.27)	Highest quartile 1.83 (0.97-3.45)
				Mean Far-wall CCA	Stroke	0.16 1.11 (0.97-1.28)	Highest quartile 1.82 (0.64-5.16)
				Mean Far-wall CCA	MI, stroke, death	0.16 1.17 (1.08-1.26)	Highest quartile 1.85 (1.09-3.15)
CHS[8]	4476	>65 (39%)	6.2	Mean of maximum Near + far CCA, ICA	MI	1 SD 1.36 (1.23-1.52)	Highest quintile 3.61 (2.13-6.11)
				Maximum Near + far CCA	MI	0.20 1.24 (1.12-1.38)	Highest quintile 2.46 (1.51-4.01)
				Mean of maximum Near + far CCA, ICA	Stroke	1 SD 1.33 (1.20-1.47)	Highest quintile 2.57 (1.64-4.02)
				Maximum Near + far CCA	Stroke	0.20 1.28 (1.16-1.42)	Highest quintile 2.13 (1.38-3.28)
KIHD[20]	1257	42-60 (0%)	3	Maximum Far-wall CCA	MI	0.11 1.11 (1.06-1.16)	>1.0 mm 2.1 (0.8-5.2)
MDCS[22]	5163	46-68 (60%)	7	Maximum Far-wall CCA	MI, CHD death	0.15 1.23 (1.07-1.41)	Highest tertile 1.50 (0.81-2.59)
MESA[25]	6698	48-84	5.3	Mean of maximum Near + far CCA, ICA	CHD, stroke, cardiovascular death	1 SD 1.2 (1.0-1.3)	Highest quartile 1.7 (1.2-2.5)
Rotterdam[23]	6389	>55 (62%)	7-10	Maximum Near + far CCA	MI	0.21 1.28 (1.14-1.44)	Highest quartile 1.95 (1.19-3.19)
San Daniele[26]	1348	18-99 (53%)	12.7	Mean of maximum Far-wall CCA	Ischemic stroke, TIA, vascular death	—	>1.0 mm 5.6 (3.2-10.1)
Tromsø[24]	6226	25-84 (52%)	5.4	Mean of mean Near + far CCA, bulb, ICA	MI	—	Highest quartile W: 2.86 (1.07-7.65) M: 1.73 (0.98-3.06)
Yao City[21]	1289	60-74 (0%)	4.5	Mean of maximum Near + far CCA, ICA	Stroke	—	Highest quartile 4.9 (1.9-12.0)

*Adjusted for age, sex, and traditional risk factors.

†Highest tertile or quartile compared with lowest tertile or quartile.

CCA, common carotid artery; CHD, coronary heart disease; CI, confidence interval; CIMT, carotid intima-media thickness; ICA, internal carotid artery; M, men; MI, myocardial infarction; RR, relative risk; SD, standard deviation; TIA, transient ischemic attack; W, women.

a thickness of ≥1.5 mm."[52,53] An ASE report defined nonobstructive plaque as "the presence of focal thickening at least 50% greater than that of the surrounding vessel wall."[54] These definitions are similar to those used in the ARIC study, the largest prospective cohort study that demonstrated the predictive value of plaque in cardiovascular risk assessment.[46]

The ASE Consensus Statement recommended that carotid plaque be defined as the presence of focal wall thickening that is at least 50% greater than that of the surrounding vessel wall or as a focal region with CIMT >1.5 mm that protrudes into the lumen and is distinct from the adjacent boundary.[9,46,52-54]

TABLE 30–2 | **Prospective Studies of Carotid Plaque Presence and Risk for Cardiovascular Disease Events in Individuals Without Known Cardiovascular Disease (N >1000 participants each)**

Study	N	Age, years (% W)	Follow-up, years	Event	Plaque Presence, Adjusted HR (95% CI)*	Plaque Presence, Adjusted RR (95% CI)*
ARIC[46]	12,375	45-64 (54%)	7	MI, CHD death	With AS: 2.96 (1.54-3.30) Without AS: 2.02 (1.42-2.41)	—
KIHD[47]	1288	42-60 (0%)	≤2	MI	4.15 (1.5-11.47)	—
MDCS[22]	5163	46-68 (60%)	7	MI, CHD death	1.81 (1.14-2.87)	—
Northern Manhattan[48]	1939	>40 (59%)	6.2	Stroke	3.1 (1.1-8.5)	—
Rotterdam[23]	6389	>55 (62%)	7-10	MI	Severe 1.83 (1.27-2.62)	—
San Daniele[26]	1348	18-99 (53.3%)	12.7 (mean)	Ischemic stroke, TIA, vascular death	—	10.4 (6.4-17.1)
Yao City[21]	1289	60-74 (0%)	4.5	Stroke	—	3.2 (1.4-7.1)

*Adjusted for age, sex, and traditional risk factors.

AS, acoustic shadowing; CHD, coronary heart disease; CV, cardiovascular; HR, hazard ratio; RR, relative risk; MI, myocardial infarction; TIA, transient ischemic attack; W, women.

Quantification of carotid plaque area also is a strong predictor of future CVD events.[24,50,55] In some studies, the two-dimensional total carotid plaque area was more predictive of MI than CIMT, after adjustment for traditional CVD risk factors.[24,56] In the Tromsø Study, baseline carotid plaque area was a stronger predictor of future MI than CIMT (see Tables 30-1 and 30-2), especially in women. In both men and women, there was a direct correlation between total plaque area and MI incidence.[24] In a report of 1686 individuals in an atherosclerosis prevention clinic, those in the highest quartile of carotid plaque had the greatest risk of future vascular events (see Table 30-2), and subjects with progression of carotid plaque area doubled their risk of future events compared with subjects with stable plaque area.[24]

The ASE does not currently recommend risk stratification based on carotid plaque measurements outside of the research setting because of their complex geometry and the absence of a published, widely applicable standard for imaging and measurement of carotid plaque area.[54,57] Carotid plaque area and even volume have been used in limited clinical settings to assist with risk stratification and to evaluate the efficacy of atherosclerosis disease management.[12,50,55,58] However, the incremental predictive value of the quantification of carotid plaque, beyond defining the presence of plaque, is unknown.

GUIDELINE AND CONSENSUS STATEMENT RECOMMENDATIONS FOR CAROTID INTIMA-MEDIA THICKNESS

The use of carotid ultrasound for evaluation of CIMT and carotid plaque as a clinical risk prediction tool has been addressed in several guidelines and consensus statements.[9] In 2000, the American Heart Association Prevention Conference V concluded that CIMT "can now be considered for further clarification of coronary heart disease risk assessment at the request of a physician," provided it is performed by an experienced laboratory.[4] In 2001, the National Cholesterol Education Program Adult Treatment Panel III stated that CIMT "could be used as an adjunct in coronary heart disease risk assessment … the finding of an elevated carotid IMT (e.g.,

≥75th percentile for age and sex) could elevate a person with multiple risk factors to a higher risk category."[59] This expert panel concluded that "if carried out under proper conditions, carotid IMT could be used to identify persons at higher risk than that revealed by the major risk factors alone."[59] In 2003, the 34th Bethesda Conference supported the use of CIMT as a screening test for subclinical vascular disease.[5] The clinical application of CIMT methodology was reviewed and supported in 2006 in a report from the American Society of Echocardiography and the Society of Vascular Medicine and Biology.[54] In 2007, the European Society of Cardiology described increased CIMT as a marker of hypertensive target organ damage.[60] The most recent, comprehensive recommendations on the use of carotid ultrasound, including CIMT and carotid plaque presence, for cardiovascular risk assessment are contained in a Consensus Statement published in 2008 by the American Society of Echocardiography and were endorsed by the Society of Vascular Medicine.[9]

APPLICATION OF CAROTID ULTRASOUND FOR CARDIOVASCULAR DISEASE RISK ASSESSMENT

Carotid ultrasound is a noninvasive tool to identify asymptomatic patients at increased CVD risk. In traditional CVD risk assessment, risk factors are used to estimate a 10-year CVD event risk; however, this estimate may not accurately reflect elevated long-term risks, especially in young and middle-aged adults, women, and ethnic minorities.[61-68] A longitudinal study that included subjects from the Coronary Artery Risk Development in Young Adults (CARDIA) and MESA studies demonstrated that subjects with a low 10-year but high lifetime CVD risk had higher common and internal CIMT compared with those at low lifetime risk and had greater progression of coronary artery calcification during 15 years.[69] Cross-sectional and longitudinal studies have integrated CIMT with CVD risk assessment algorithms and demonstrated significant reclassification[10-13] and improvement in CVD risk stratification by individualizing vascular risks with use of CIMT results, especially in intermediate-risk patients.[6,14,70]

The ASE Consensus Statement[9] recommended that carotid ultrasound with CIMT measurement and evaluation for plaque presence could be considered in the following types of patients if the level of aggressiveness of therapy (e.g., pharmacotherapy) or additional information about the burden of subclinical vascular disease or future CVD risk is needed:

- intermediate risk (Framingham risk score 6% to 20% without established coronary heart disease, peripheral arterial disease, cerebrovascular disease, diabetes mellitus, or abdominal aortic aneurysm);
- family history of premature CVD in a first-degree relative (men <55 years old, women <65 years old);
- individuals <60 years old with severe abnormalities in a single risk factor (such as genetic dyslipidemia) who are not being treated with medications; or
- women <60 years old with at least two CVD risk factors.

COMPARISON OF CAROTID INTIMA-MEDIA THICKNESS AND CORONARY ARTERY CALCIUM

Fast computed tomography for measurement of coronary artery calcium is another technique that evaluates for the presence and extent of subclinical vascular disease and predicts future CVD events.[71-73] A report from the MESA study compared the prognostic value of CIMT and coronary artery calcium in predicting fatal CVD events, development of coronary heart disease, and stroke in 6698 participants (45 to 84 years old) during 5.3 years of follow-up.[25,74] Both imaging modalities predicted the primary outcomes; however, coronary artery calcium was a stronger predictor of incident CVD than was CIMT. After adjustment for each other (coronary calcium and CIMT) and traditional risk factors, the hazard ratio for each standard deviation increase in coronary artery calcium increased by 2.1-fold compared with 1.3-fold for each standard deviation increase in maximum CIMT, and the change in the AUC for prediction of CVD events was greater with coronary artery calcification (~0.03) than with CIMT (~0.01).[25] CIMT, but not coronary artery calcification, predicted incident stroke.[25] In the Cardiovascular Health Study (CHS) of adults older than 65 years old, common carotid artery CIMT (hazard ratio, 11.25 [2.28-55.61]) was a stronger predictor of strokes compared with coronary artery calcium (hazard ratio, 3.73 [0.81-17.11]).[75] The hazard ratios for coronary heart disease and total CVD were not statistically different between CIMT and coronary artery calcium.

The clinical predictive value of coronary calcium in younger men, women, and African Americans is less clear because of a lower prevalence of coronary artery calcium in these subgroups. CIMT has the advantage of being a continuous measure that could be used, if clinically indicated, to stratify risk in individuals for whom coronary artery calcium scoring may have limited discriminatory power because of a high predicted prevalence of a zero calcium score.[76] In a report from MESA, increased CIMT predicted total CVD events (hazard ratio, 2.2; 95% confidence interval, 1.2-4.0) among individuals with low coronary artery calcium scores (<10), along with increasing age, family history of CVD, use of lipid-lowering medications, and smoking.[77] CIMT (hazard ratio, 3.2; 95% confidence interval, 1.5-6.6) and former and current smoking were independent predictors of hard CVD events.[77]

As a screening test, carotid ultrasound has additional advantages that should be considered. Although the amount of radiation exposure with modern calcium screening by non–contrast-enhanced fast computed tomography is relatively low, carotid ultrasound does not involve any exposure to ionizing radiation, an important consideration when

imaging healthy young and middle-aged adults.[78] Compared with computed tomography, CIMT is an inexpensive, portable predictive tool that can be used in the office setting.[79] Also, carotid ultrasound can be performed serially to monitor the clinical effectiveness of therapeutic intervention or changes in arterial injury over time without risk of recurrent radiation exposure[55]; however, serial monitoring is not recommended by the ASE Consensus Statement at this time.[9]

EFFECTS OF CAROTID INTIMA-MEDIA THICKNESS SCREENING PROGRAMS ON CLINICAL PRACTICE AND OUTCOMES

Several clinical CVD risk assessment programs have used carotid ultrasound to measure CIMT.[6,10-15,80] In clinical practice, CIMT has been shown to help reclassify patients at intermediate risk,[6,10-12] to discriminate between patients with and without prevalent CVD,[28] and to predict major adverse cardiovascular events.[6,14] Most of these studies considered the patient's age and sex by use of normative percentile values.[10,11,13-15] The METEOR (Measuring Effects on Intima-Media Thickness: An Evaluation of Rosuvastatin) study demonstrated that middle-aged adults at apparently low to intermediate CVD risk but with increased CIMT benefited from statin therapy that they otherwise would not have qualified for on the basis of current treatment guidelines.[59,81] In this prospective, randomized multicenter clinical trial, the magnitude of the difference in CIMT progression rates (−0.145 mm/year) was similar to that observed in secondary prevention trials that were associated with a reduction in CVD events.[81,82] Although not definitive, this study suggests that use of CIMT to modify preventive treatment strategies is feasible and associated with a delay in the progression of arterial wall thickening, which is associated with reduced CVD risk.

Some data suggest that increased CIMT or carotid plaque presence can influence the behavior of patients and physicians. A small study (N = 153) randomly assigned smokers to a smoking cessation intervention or smoking cessation plus carotid ultrasound, after which they were shown a picture of their carotid plaque. Smoking cessation rates were 22.2% in the 54 participants with at least one plaque compared with 5% and 6.3% among those without plaque or who did not have ultrasonography (P = 0.003).[83] In a small (N = 23), pilot study of visual feedback from carotid ultrasound imaging compared with verbal feedback, the intervention increased perception of smoking-related illness and smoking cessation behavior and intention; however, intention increased only in people with high levels of self-efficacy (P < 0.03).[84] In a study of 210 individuals reported in abstract form and described in a review paper, patients were more likely to adhere to recommendations for diet, exercise, and smoking cessation 12 months after seeing pictures of their CIMT examination.[85]

In another promising pilot study, carotid plaque screening was performed on asymptomatic patients with at least two CVD risk factors to assess the impact of carotid plaque screening on the physician's and patient's behavior in an office practice setting. Identification of carotid plaques increased the likelihood that physicians would prescribe aspirin (P = 0.031) and lipid-lowering therapy (P = 0.004), but did not change patients' motivation to make lifestyle changes.[86] In a subsequent multicenter trial of 253 patients, CIMT and carotid plaques were assessed in a clinical office setting by non-sonographer clinicians using a handheld ultrasound system. When increased CIMT or carotid plaque was detected, physicians significantly changed their behavior by ordering aspirin and lipid-lowering therapy (odds ratios, 2.9-7.4; P < 0.001), interventions that are proven to reduce CVD risk in patients at increased risk.[79] Furthermore, patients had a greater perceived likelihood of having or developing heart disease ($P = 0.004$) and reported greater intentions to take cholesterol-lowering medication ($P = 0.002$); however, even subjects without ultrasound abnormalities reported increased motivation to exercise ($P = 0.003$) and make dietary changes ($P = 0.051$), illustrating the complexity of affecting a patient's behavior with imaging.[79] The coronary artery calcium screening literature also suggests that the behavior of physicians is affected more than that of patients and is missing long-term data showing that a strategy for atherosclerosis screening is superior to current strategies or case management.[87-91] Large, randomized outcome studies are needed to determine if improved risk prediction, behavior changes, and changes in the practice of physicians that occur with CIMT and/or carotid plaque imaging translate into improved patient outcomes and reduced cardiovascular events.

CAROTID INTIMA-MEDIA THICKNESS AND CAROTID PLAQUE SCANNING TECHNIQUE

The following recommendations are from the recent ASE Consensus Statement.[9] Before the study is started, both the sonographer and patient must be positioned comfortably to facilitate accurate, high-quality, and reproducible images. The patient should lie supine with their head on the scan table. The ideal position of the neck is a slight hyperextension and rotation in the direction opposite the probe. Use of external landmarks and a 45-degree angle wedge pillow can help standardize the transducer's angle relative to the patient's head position (Fig. 30-3). Standard three-lead electrocardiographic monitoring should be performed with acquisition of easily discernible R-wave deflections. Scan time can vary according to protocol requirements and sonographer experience.[92]

Carotid arteries should be imaged with a state-of-the-art ultrasound system with a linear array transducer operating at a fundamental frequency of at least 7 MHz. Most subjects can

be scanned at a standard depth of 4 cm from anterior to posterior planes. With increased depth, there is decreased resolution (larger pixel size). A single focal zone, high dynamic range, and fundamental frequencies without harmonic or compound imaging should be used. Use of ultrasound contrast, although a promising research technique, is not recommended for clinical assessment of CIMT at this time. B-mode imaging, rather than M-mode imaging, is recommended. All reported observational studies relating CIMT values to cardiovascular events used B-mode measurements averaged over at least a 1-cm segment. Multiple measurements of multiple extended segment lengths permit expression of CIMT values at higher levels of precision instead of simple multiples of pixel size.

Carotid ultrasound imaging should follow a protocol from a large epidemiologic study that reported CIMT values in percentiles by age, sex, and race or ethnicity. ARIC, MESA, Bogalusa Heart Study, and CHS are large, cross-sectional, high-quality studies that reported common carotid artery CIMT values by age, sex, and race or ethnicity and were conducted in North America.[8,9,41,93] The 50th percentile mean far-wall common carotid artery CIMT values for white and black men and women between 45 and 64 years of age in ARIC and MESA were quite similar, given the differences between the studies.[9,41] For older patients, the 50th percentile maximum common carotid artery CIMT values in the CHS tended to be higher than in MESA, probably because individuals with known CVD were excluded from MESA but not from CHS.[8,9] Several large, high-quality studies from Europe also reported common carotid artery CIMT values.[9,19,22,94] These studies did not provide information about race or ethnicity but were conducted mostly in white individuals. In general, CIMT values in studies such as CAPS and the Malmö Diet and Cancer Study (MDCS) tended to be higher than in the North American studies.[9,19,22] Reasons for the thicker CIMT values observed in these studies include different population characteristics, instrumentation, imaging and recording standards, and measurement techniques, such as whether segments with plaque were included or excluded from the measurement protocol. The relative risks associated with increasing CIMT were similar across all of the studies in Table 30-1.

The ASE Consensus Statement recommends that CIMT of the distal 1 cm of the far wall of each common carotid artery be imaged and compared with a normative data set.[9] The distal common carotid artery is easy to image, and far-wall common carotid artery CIMT measurements predict future cardiovascular events (see Table 30-1). Although near-wall measurements and those from other segments also have been used in some studies, they are more challenging technically, less reproducible, and do not appreciably improve risk prediction.[54] In one study, the ultrasound measurement of the near-wall CIMT was 20% lower than the corresponding histologic measurement.[95] Although CIMT imaging is limited to the common carotid artery, a thorough scan of the extracranial carotid arteries for the presence of carotid plaque should be performed to increase sensitivity for identification of subclinical vascular disease. A circumferential plaque scan of both carotid arteries can compensate for reduced sensitivity that may result from measurement of only common carotid artery CIMT.[54,96]

A scanning protocol based on that used in the ARIC study was recommended by the ASE Consensus Statement because in ARIC, prevalent common carotid artery CIMT and carotid plaques predicted future cardiovascular events (see Tables 30-1 and 30-2), and the scanning methods are reproducible in most clinical laboratories.[7,9,18,41,46,97] Furthermore, ARIC was a very large study, and normative values based on age, sex, and race or ethnicity have been published in the age range that is considered most appropriate for screening.[41] The

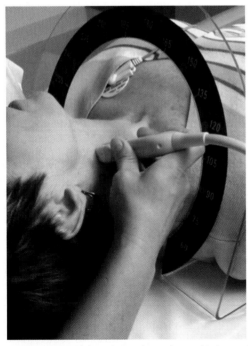

FIGURE 30-3 Position of the patient and setup for carotid ultrasound study.

recommended protocol includes a plaque scan and imaging of the common carotid artery from multiple angles for measurement of CIMT. The ARIC scanning protocol, limited to the common carotid artery, is summarized in the ASE Consensus Statement.[9] Additional information about frequently observed pitfalls and possible solutions to CIMT acquisition problems are provided in that document.[9] Other scanning protocols may be used if they are more germane to the clinical population being investigated. Which segments of the carotid artery are interrogated and at which angles, as well as which measurements are obtained, must match those in the normative data set of the representative epidemiologic study. The age, sex, and race or ethnicity of the patient should be considered in choosing the scanning and measuring protocols. For example, the CIMT measurements in the Bogalusa Heart Study have not yet been related to future CVD events; however, they are the only normative values for CIMT in young adults from North America.[93] The MESA study has the only normative values for CIMT in Chinese and Hispanic Americans. On the basis of the relatively similar relative risk associated with increasing CIMT across the age ranges described in Table 30-1, it can be inferred that increased CIMT in these patient groups (as determined by comparison with these data sets) is associated with increased cardiovascular risk. The use of values from clinically referred populations is discouraged because of the likelihood of referral bias and inaccurate risk estimates.

CAROTID INTIMA-MEDIA THICKNESS MEASUREMENT

The ASE Consensus Statement recommends use of digital images that are acquired and stored directly from the ultrasound system, rather than digitized video captures, as well as minimal compression and use of the DICOM standard.[9] The reader reviews overall image quality, thickness, presence or absence of plaque, and presence or absence of incidental findings such as possible obstructive carotid artery disease, carotid dissection, carotid tumors, thyroid abnormalities, and lymphadenopathy. Cine loops and R wave–gated still-frame images of the distal 1-cm segment of the far walls of the right and left common carotid artery, each from three different angles of incidence, are measured in triplicate. Measurement of each image involves tracing of the blood-intima and media-adventitia interfaces of the far wall by a leading edge–to–leading edge method (see Fig. 30-2).[9] Only clearly visualized images should be measured. If plaques are detected in the segment being measured, they are traced as part of the CIMT because they appear to have been included in CIMT measurements in most of the epidemiologic studies in Table 30-1.[27] Most studies that provided reference values were obtained by manual reading techniques; however, semiautomated border detection programs were used by some.[9] Semiautomated border detection programs are widely available, and when they are used, they tend to improve reproducibility and to shorten reading time, especially among newer readers.[9,98-101] The ASE Consensus Statement recommends use of a semiautomated border detection program with validated accuracy.[9] These programs tend to produce somewhat thicker CIMT values than are seen with manual tracing, especially if the generated borders are left unedited. Simple point-to-point measurement of CIMT should be avoided.

Depending on the protocol, the triplicate measurements are averaged or the highest value is taken. Most reading software will report the mean-mean (average of segmental mean CIMT values) and mean-maximum (average of segmental maximum CIMT values) thickness values. Mean-mean values are more reproducible because multiple points along the traced segment are averaged, but they are less sensitive to change. Mean-maximum values are more sensitive to change but less reproducible because they are derived from a single-point measurement along the 1-cm region. It is recommended that mean CIMT values from the far walls of the right and left common carotid arteries (mean-mean) be used for clinical studies.[9]

STUDY INTERPRETATION

The study report (1) provides the referring health care provider with data about the mean (or maximum) CIMT of the segments analyzed, depending on the scanning protocol and reference data base; (2) briefly summarizes the scanning protocol and reference data base used; (3) states whether the CIMT values are means or maxima; (4) compares the CIMT data with the reference population of individuals of similar age, sex, and race or ethnicity; (5) describes the presence or absence of carotid plaques; and (6) describes any other clinically relevant findings, such as the presence of obstructive carotid atherosclerosis. Each of these points is discussed in detail in the ASE Consensus Statement.[9] To avoid confusion with a duplex carotid ultrasound examination, the report should clearly identify the type of study being performed (i.e., "carotid ultrasound study for cardiovascular risk assessment") and explicitly state that the study measures the thickness of the walls of the carotid artery and that the results are not a "percent stenosis" and do not indicate the presence or absence of clinically significant obstruction, unless noted otherwise.[9] Reports also should include a clinically relevant percentile range for the CIMT value by stating a range of percentiles (such as quartile or quintile) for the measured value.[9] The communication of CIMT results can be facilitated by qualitatively describing broad ranges of percentiles to avoid the appearance of greater precision that is achievable when CIMT values are mapped to a reference population. This is because the percentile estimates in the population studies have confidence intervals surrounding them and because the instrumentation, scanning, and measurement techniques in a clinical laboratory will not be exactly the same as those used in these studies.[9] Values ≥75th percentile are considered high and indicative of increased risk. Values in the >25th percentile but <75th percentile are considered average and indicative of unchanged risk.[9] Values ≤25th percentile are considered low, but whether they are indicative of reduced risk is unclear.

CONCLUSION

Evaluation of CIMT and carotid plaque by B-mode ultrasound is a validated tool for CVD risk assessment that can be integrated into clinical practice. This noninvasive approach can detect subclinical vascular disease and refine CVD risk assessment in some asymptomatic patients. Strict attention to quality control in image acquisition, measurement, interpretation, and reporting is necessary for implementation of this technique in clinical practice.

REFERENCES

1. Lloyd-Jones D, Adams R, Carnethon M, et al: Heart disease and stroke statistics—2009 update: a report from the American Heart Association Statistics Committee and Stroke Statistics Subcommittee. *Circulation* 119:e21, 2009.
2. Virmani R, Burke AP, Farb A, Kolodgie FD: Pathology of the vulnerable plaque. *J Am Coll Cardiol* 47:C13, 2006.
3. McGill HC, Jr, McMahan CA, Herderick EE, et al: Effects of coronary heart disease risk factors on atherosclerosis of selected regions of the aorta and right coronary artery. PDAY Research Group. Pathobiological Determinants of Atherosclerosis in Youth. *Arterioscler Thromb Vasc Biol* 20:836, 2000.

4. Greenland P, Abrams J, Aurigemma GP, et al: Prevention Conference V: Beyond secondary prevention: identifying the high-risk patient for primary prevention: noninvasive tests of atherosclerotic burden: Writing Group III. *Circulation* 101:E16, 2000.

5. Taylor AJ, Merz CN, Udelson JE: 34th Bethesda Conference: Executive summary—can atherosclerosis imaging techniques improve the detection of patients at risk for ischemic heart disease? *J Am Coll Cardiol* 41:1860, 2003.

6. Baldassarre D, Amato M, Pustina L, et al: Measurement of carotid artery intima-media thickness in dyslipidemic patients increases the power of traditional risk factors to predict cardiovascular events. *Atherosclerosis* 191:403, 2007.

7. Chambless LE, Heiss G, Folsom AR, et al: Association of coronary heart disease incidence with carotid arterial wall thickness and major risk factors: the Atherosclerosis Risk in Communities (ARIC) Study, 1987-1993. *Am J Epidemiol* 146:483, 1997.

8. O'Leary DH, Polak JF, Kronmal RA, et al: Carotid-artery intima and media thickness as a risk factor for myocardial infarction and stroke in older adults. Cardiovascular Health Study Collaborative Research Group. *N Engl J Med* 340:14, 1999.

9. Stein JH, Korcarz CE, Hurst RT, et al: Use of carotid ultrasound to identify subclinical vascular disease and evaluate cardiovascular disease risk: a consensus statement from the American Society of Echocardiography Carotid Intima-Media Thickness Task Force. *J Am Soc Echocardiogr* 91:93, 2008.

10. Stein JH, Fraizer MC, Aeschlimann SE, et al: Individualizing coronary risk assessment using carotid intima media thickness measurements to estimate vascular age. *Clin Cardiol* 27:388, 2004.

11. Gepner AD, Keevil JG, Wyman RA, et al: Use of carotid intima-media thickness and vascular age to modify cardiovascular risk prediction. *J Am Soc Echocardiogr* 19:1170, 2006.

12. Bard RL, Kalsi H, Rubenfire M, et al: Effect of carotid atherosclerosis screening on risk stratification during primary cardiovascular disease prevention. *Am J Cardiol* 93:1030-1032, 2004.

13. Rembold KE, Ayers CR, Wills MB, Rembold CM: Usefulness of carotid intimal medial thickness and flow-mediated dilation in a preventive cardiovascular practice. *Am J Cardiol* 91:1475, 2003.

14. Ali YS, Rembold KE, Weaver B, et al: Prediction of major adverse cardiovascular events by age-normalized carotid intimal medial thickness. *Atherosclerosis* 187:186, 2006.

15. Barth JD: An update on carotid ultrasound measurement of intima-media thickness. *Am J Cardiol* 89:32B, 2002.

16. Young W, Gofman J, Tandy R, et al: The quantitation of atherosclerosis III. The extent of correlation of degrees of atherosclerosis with and between the coronary and cerebral vascular beds. *Am J Cardiol* 8:300, 1960.

17. Sharma K, Blaha MJ, Blumenthal RS, Musunuru K: Clinical and research applications of carotid intima-media thickness. *Am J Cardiol* 103:1316, 2009.

18. Chambless LE, Folsom AR, Clegg LX, et al: Carotid wall thickness is predictive of incident clinical stroke: the Atherosclerosis Risk in Communities (ARIC) study. *Am J Epidemiol* 151:478, 2000.

19. Lorenz MW, von Kegler S, Steinmetz H, et al: Carotid intima-media thickening indicates a higher vascular risk across a wide age range: prospective data from the Carotid Atherosclerosis Progression Study (CAPS). *Stroke* 37:87, 2006.

20. Salonen JT, Salonen R: Ultrasound B-mode imaging in observational studies of atherosclerotic progression. *Circulation* 87:II56, 1993.

21. Kitamura A, Iso H, Imano H, et al: Carotid intima-media thickness and plaque characteristics as a risk factor for stroke in Japanese elderly men. *Stroke* 35:2788, 2004.

22. Rosvall M, Janzon L, Berglund G, et al: Incident coronary events and case fatality in relation to common carotid intima-media thickness. *J Intern Med* 257:430, 2005.

23. van der Meer I, Bots ML, Hofman A, et al: Predictive value of noninvasive measures of atherosclerosis for incident myocardial infarction: the Rotterdam Study. *Circulation* 109:1089, 2004.

24. Johnsen SH, Mathiesen EB, Joakimsen O, et al: Carotid atherosclerosis is a stronger predictor of myocardial infarction in women than in men: a 6-year follow-up study of 6226 persons: the Tromsø Study. *Stroke* 38:2873, 2007.

25. Folsom AR, Kronmal RA, Detrano RC, et al: Coronary artery calcification compared with carotid intima-media thickness in the prediction of cardiovascular disease incidence: the Multi-Ethnic Study of Atherosclerosis (MESA). *Arch Intern Med* 168:1333, 2008.

26. Prati P, Tosetto A, Vanuzzo D, et al: Carotid intima media thickness and plaques can predict the occurrence of ischemic cerebrovascular events. *Stroke* 39:2470, 2008.

27. Lorenz MW, Markus HS, Bots ML, et al: Prediction of clinical cardiovascular events with carotid intima-media thickness: a systematic review and meta-analysis. *Circulation* 115:459, 2007.

28. Baldassarre D, Amato M, Bondioli A, et al: Carotid artery intima-media thickness measured by ultrasonography in normal clinical practice correlates well with atherosclerosis risk factors. *Stroke* 31:2426, 2000.

29. Belcaro G, Nicolaides AN, Ramaswami G, et al: Carotid and femoral ultrasound morphology screening and cardiovascular events in low risk subjects: a 10-year follow-up study (the CAFES-CAVE study). *Atherosclerosis* 156:379, 2001.

30. Craven TE, Ryu JE, Espeland MA, et al: Evaluation of the associations between carotid artery atherosclerosis and coronary artery stenosis. A case-control study. *Circulation* 82:1230, 1990.

31. Wattanakit K, Folsom AR, Chambless LE, Nieto FJ: Risk factors for cardiovascular event recurrence in the Atherosclerosis Risk in Communities (ARIC) study. *Am Heart J* 149:606, 2005.

32. Chambless LE, Folsom AR, Sharrett AR, et al: Coronary heart disease risk prediction in the Atherosclerosis Risk in Communities (ARIC) study. *J Clin Epidemiol* 56:880, 2003.

33. Urbina EM, Srinivasan SR, Tang R, et al: Impact of multiple coronary risk factors on the intima-media thickness of different segments of carotid artery in healthy young adults (The Bogalusa Heart Study). *Am J Cardiol* 90:953, 2002.

34. Li S, Chen W, Srinivasan SR, et al: Childhood cardiovascular risk factors and carotid vascular changes in adulthood: the Bogalusa Heart Study. *JAMA* 290:2271, 2003.

35. Tzou WS, Douglas PS, Srinivasan SR, et al: Increased subclinical atherosclerosis in young adults with metabolic syndrome: the Bogalusa Heart Study. *J Am Coll Cardiol* 46:457, 2005.

36. Davis PH, Dawson JD, Mahoney LT, Lauer RM: Increased carotid intimal-medial thickness and coronary calcification are related in young and middle-aged adults. The Muscatine study. *Circulation* 100:838, 1999.

37. Davis PH, Dawson JD, Riley WA, Lauer RM: Carotid intimal-medial thickness is related to cardiovascular risk factors measured from childhood through middle age: the Muscatine Study. *Circulation* 104:2815, 2001.

38. Oren A, Vos LE, Uiterwaal CS, et al: Cardiovascular risk factors and increased carotid intima-media thickness in healthy young adults: the Atherosclerosis Risk in Young Adults (ARYA) Study. *Arch Intern Med* 163:1787, 2003.

39. Knoflach M, Kiechl S, Kind M, et al: Cardiovascular risk factors and atherosclerosis in young males: ARMY study (Atherosclerosis Risk-Factors in Male Youngsters). *Circulation* 108:1064, 2003.

40. Raitakari OT, Juonala M, Kahonen M, et al: Cardiovascular risk factors in childhood and carotid artery intima-media thickness in adulthood: the Cardiovascular Risk in Young Finns Study. *JAMA* 290:2277, 2003.

41. Howard G, Sharrett A, Heiss G, et al; ARIC Investigators: Carotid artery intimal-medial thickness distribution in general populations as evaluated by B-mode ultrasound. *Stroke* 24:1297-1304, 1993.

42. Stein JH, Douglas PS, Srinivasan SR, et al: Distribution and cross-sectional age-related increases of carotid artery intima-media thickness in young adults: the Bogalusa Heart Study [correction *Stroke* 36:414, 2005]. *Stroke* 35:2782, 2004.

43. Espeland MA, Tang R, Terry JG, et al: Associations of risk factors with segment-specific intimal-medial thickness of the extracranial carotid artery. *Stroke* 30:1047, 1999.

44. Schott LL, Wildman RP, Brockwell S, et al: Segment-specific effects of cardiovascular risk factors on carotid artery intima-medial thickness in women at midlife. *Arterioscler Thromb Vasc Biol* 24:1951, 2004.

45. Spence DJ: The importance of distinguishing between diffuse carotid intima-media thickening and focal plaque. *Can J Cardiol* 24:61c, 2008.

46. Hunt KJ, Sharrett AR, Chambless LE, et al: Acoustic shadowing on B-mode ultrasound of the carotid artery predicts CHD. *Ultrasound Med Biol* 27:357, 2001.

47. Salonen JT, Salonen R: Ultrasonographically assessed carotid morphology and the risk of coronary heart disease. *Arterioscler Thromb* 11:1245, 1991.

48. Prabhakaran S, Rundek T, Ramas R, et al: Carotid plaque surface irregularity predicts ischemic stroke: the northern Manhattan study. *Stroke* 37:2696, 2006.

49. Stork S, van den Beld AW, von Schacky C, et al: Carotid artery plaque burden, stiffness, and mortality risk in elderly men: a prospective, population-based cohort study. *Circulation* 110:344, 2004.

50. Spence JD, Eliasziw M, DiCicco M, et al: Carotid plaque area: a tool for targeting and evaluating vascular preventive therapy. *Stroke* 33:2916, 2002.

51. Wyman RA, Gimelli G, McBride PE, et al: Does detection of carotid plaque affect physician behavior or motivate patients? *Am Heart J* 154:1072, 2007.

52. Touboul PJ, Hennerici MG, Meairs S, et al: Mannheim intima-media thickness consensus. *Cerebrovasc Dis* 18:346, 2004.

53. Touboul PJ, Hennerici MG, Meairs S, et al: Mannheim carotid intima-media thickness consensus (2004-2006). An update on behalf of the Advisory Board of the 3rd and 4th Watching the Risk Symposium, 13th and 15th European Stroke Conferences, Mannheim, Germany, 2004, and Brussels, Belgium, 2006. *Cerebrovasc Dis* 23:75, 2007.

54. Roman MJ, Naqvi TZ, Gardin JM, et al: Clinical application of noninvasive vascular ultrasound in cardiovascular risk stratification: a report from the American Society of Echocardiography and the Society of Vascular Medicine and Biology. *J Am Soc Echocardiogr* 19:943, 2006.

55. Spence JD: Technology Insight: ultrasound measurement of carotid plaque—patient management, genetic research, and therapy evaluation. *Nat Clin Pract Neurol* 2:611, 2006.

56. Spence JD: Ultrasound measurement of carotid plaque as a surrogate outcome for coronary artery disease. *Am J Cardiol* 89:10B, 2002.

57. Joakimsen O, Bonaa KH, Stensland-Bugge E: Reproducibility of ultrasound assessment of carotid plaque occurrence, thickness, and morphology. The Tromsø Study. *Stroke* 28:2201, 1997.

58. Ainsworth CD, Blake CC, Tamayo A, et al: 3D ultrasound measurement of change in carotid plaque volume: a tool for rapid evaluation of new therapies. *Stroke* 36:1904, 2005.

59. National Cholesterol Education Program (NCEP) Expert Panel (ATP III): Third Report of the National Cholesterol Education Program (NCEP) Expert Panel on Detection, Evaluation, and Treatment of High Blood Cholesterol in Adults (Adult Treatment Panel III) final report. *Circulation* 106:3143, 2002.

60. Graham I, Atar D, Borch-Johnsen K, et al: European guidelines on cardiovascular disease prevention in clinical practice: executive summary. *Eur Heart J* 28:2375, 2007.

61. Grundy SM, Pasternak R, Greenland P, et al: Assessment of cardiovascular risk by use of multiple-risk-factor assessment equations: a statement for healthcare professionals from the American Heart Association and the American College of Cardiology. *Circulation* 100:1481, 1999.

62. Greenland P, Smith SC, Jr, Grundy SM: Improving coronary heart disease risk assessment in asymptomatic people: role of traditional risk factors and noninvasive cardiovascular test. *Circulation* 104:1863, 2001.

63. Greenland P, Knoll MD, Stamler J, et al: Major risk factors as antecedents of fatal and nonfatal coronary heart disease events. *JAMA* 290:891, 2003.

64. Lloyd-Jones DM, Leip EP, Larson MG, et al: Prediction of lifetime risk for cardiovascular disease by risk factor burden at 50 years of age. *Circulation* 113:791, 2006.

65. Lloyd-Jones DM: Short-term versus long-term risk for coronary artery disease: implications for lipid guidelines. *Curr Opin Lipidol* 17:619, 2006.

66. Michos ED, Vasamreddy CR, Becker DM, et al: Women with a low Framingham risk score and a family history of premature coronary heart disease have a high prevalence of subclinical coronary atherosclerosis. *Am Heart J* 150:1276, 2005.

67. Michos ED, Nasir K, Braunstein JB, et al: Framingham risk equation underestimates subclinical atherosclerosis risk in asymptomatic women. *Atherosclerosis* 184:201, 2006.

68. Nasir K, Michos ED, Blumenthal RS, Raggi P: Detection of high-risk young adults and women by coronary calcium and National Cholesterol Education Program Panel III guidelines. *J Am Coll Cardiol* 46:1931, 2005.

69. Berry JD, Liu K, Folsom AR, et al: Prevalence and progression of subclinical atherosclerosis in younger adults with low short-term but high lifetime estimated risk for cardiovascular disease: the coronary artery risk development in young adults study and multi-ethnic study of atherosclerosis. *Circulation* 119:382, 2009.

70. Nambi V, Chambless L, Folsom AR, et al: Are all patients considered "low risk" for coronary heart disease really low risk? An analysis from the Atherosclerosis Risk in Communities (ARIC) Study [abstract 4985]. *Circulation* 118, S_1125. 2008.

71. Greenland P, LaBree L, Azen SP, et al: Coronary artery calcium score combined with Framingham score for risk prediction in asymptomatic individuals. *JAMA* 291:210, 2004.

72. Budoff MJ, Achenbach S, Blumenthal RS, et al: Assessment of coronary artery disease by cardiac computed tomography: a scientific statement from the American Heart Association Committee on Cardiovascular Imaging and Intervention, Council on Cardiovascular Radiology and Intervention, and Committee on Cardiac Imaging, Council on Clinical Cardiology. *Circulation* 114:1761, 2006.

73. Greenland P, Bonow RO, Brundage BH, et al: ACCF/AHA 2007 clinical expert consensus document on coronary artery calcium scoring by computed tomography in global cardiovascular risk assessment and in evaluation of patients with chest pain: a report of the American College of Cardiology Foundation Clinical Expert Consensus Task Force (ACCF/AHA Writing Committee to Update the 2000 Expert Consensus Document on Electron Beam Computed Tomography). *Circulation* 115:402, 2007.

74. Bild DE, Bluemke DA, Burke GL, et al: Multi-ethnic study of atherosclerosis: objectives and design. *Am J Epidemiol* 156:871, 2002.

75. Newman AB, Naydeck BL, Ives DG, et al: Coronary artery calcium, carotid artery wall thickness, and cardiovascular disease outcomes in adults 70 to 99 years old. *Am J Cardiol* 101:186, 2008.

76. McClelland RL, Chung H, Detrano R, et al: Distribution of coronary artery calcium by race, gender, and age: results from the Multi-Ethnic Study of Atherosclerosis (MESA). *Circulation* 113:30, 2006.

77. Budoff MJ, McClelland RL, Nasir K, et al: Characteristics of persons who have cardiovascular events with absent or minimal coronary calcification: the Multi-Ethnic Study of Atherosclerosis (MESA) [abstract 812-3]. *J Am Coll Cardiol* March 11:A160, 2008.

78. Coles DR, Smail MA, Negus IS, et al: Comparison of radiation doses from multislice computed tomography coronary angiography and conventional diagnostic angiography. *J Am Coll Cardiol* 47:1840, 2006.

79. Korcarz CE, DeCara JM, Hirsch AT, et al: Ultrasound detection of increased carotid intima-media thickness and carotid plaque in an office practice setting: does it affect physician behavior or patient motivation? *J Am Soc Echocardiogr* 21:1156, 2008.

80. Wyman RA, Fraizer MC, Keevil JG, et al: Ultrasound-detected carotid plaque as a screening tool for advanced subclinical atherosclerosis. *Am Heart J* 150:1081, 2005.

81. Crouse JR, III, Raichlen JS, Riley WA, et al: Effect of rosuvastatin on progression of carotid intima-media thickness in low-risk individuals with subclinical atherosclerosis: the METEOR Trial. *JAMA* 297:1344, 2007.

82. Espeland MA, O'Leary DH, Terry JG, et al: Carotid intimal-media thickness as a surrogate for cardiovascular disease events in trials of HMG-CoA reductase inhibitors. *Curr Control Trials Cardiovasc Med* 6:3, 2005.

83. Bovet P, Perret F, Cornuz J, et al: Improved smoking cessation in smokers given ultrasound photographs of their own atherosclerotic plaques. *Prev Med* 34:215, 2002.

84. Shahab L, Hall S, Marteau T: Showing smokers with vascular disease images of their arteries to motivate cessation: a pilot study. *Br J Health Psychol* 12:275, 2007.

85. Barth JD: Which tools are in your cardiac workshop? Carotid ultrasound, endothelial function, and magnetic resonance imaging. *Am J Cardiol* 87:8A, 2001.

86. Wyman RA, Gimelli G, McBride PE, et al: Does detection of carotid plaque affect physician behavior or motivate patients? *Am Heart J* 154:1072, 2007.

87. Taylor AJ, Bindeman J, Feuerstein I, et al: Community-based provision of statin and aspirin after the detection of coronary artery calcium within a community-based screening cohort. *J Am Coll Cardiol* 51:1337, 2008.

88. Orakzai RH, Nasir K, Orakzai SH, et al: Effect of patient visualization of coronary calcium by electron beam computed tomography on changes in beneficial lifestyle behaviors. *Am J Cardiol* 101:999, 2008.

89. Kalia NK, Miller LG, Nasir K, et al: Visualizing coronary calcium is associated with improvements in adherence to statin therapy. *Atherosclerosis* 185:394, 2006.

90. O'Malley PG, Feuerstein IM, Taylor AJ: Impact of electron beam tomography, with or without case management, on motivation, behavioral change, and cardiovascular risk profile: a randomized controlled trial. *JAMA* 289:2215, 2003.

91. Lederman J, Ballard J, Njike VY, et al: Information given to postmenopausal women on coronary computed tomography may influence cardiac risk reduction efforts. *J Clin Epidemiol* 60:389, 2007.

92. Mitchell CK, Aeschlimann SE, Korcarz CE: Carotid intima-media thickness testing: technical considerations. *J Am Soc Echocardiogr* 17:690, 2004.

93. Tzou WS, Douglas PS, Srinivasan SR, et al: Distribution and predictors of carotid artery intima-media thickness in young adults: THE Bogalusa Heart Study. *Prev Cardiol* 10:181, 2007.

94. Allan PL, Mowbray PI, Lee AJ, Fowkes FG: Relationship between carotid intima-media thickness and symptomatic and asymptomatic peripheral arterial disease. The Edinburgh Artery Study. *Stroke* 28:348, 1997.

95. Wong M, Edelstein J, Wollman J, Bond MG: Ultrasonic-pathological comparison of the human arterial wall. Verification of intima-media thickness. *Arterioscler Thromb* 13:482, 1993.

96. Gepner AD, Wyman RA, Korcarz CE, et al: An abbreviated carotid intima-media thickness scanning protocol to facilitate clinical screening for subclinical atherosclerosis. *J Am Soc Echocardiogr* 20:1269, 2007.

97. Bond M, Barnes R, Riley W, et al; ARIC Study Group: High-resolution B-mode ultrasound scanning methods in the Atherosclerosis Risk in Communities Study (ARIC). *J Neuroimaging* 1:68, 1991.

98. Gepner AD, Korcarz CE, Aeschlimann SE, et al: Validation of a carotid intima-media thickness border detection program for use in an office setting. *J Am Soc Echocardiogr* 19:223, 2006.

99. Stein JH, Korcarz CE, Mays ME, et al: A semi-automated border detection program that facilitates clinical use of ultrasound carotid intima-media thickness measurements. *J Am Soc Echocardiogr* 18:244, 2005.

100. Kanters SD, Algra A, van Leeuwen MS, Banga JD: Reproducibility of in vivo carotid intima-media thickness measurements: a review. *Stroke* 28:665, 1997.

101. Tang R, Hennig M, Bond MG, et al: Quality control of B-mode ultrasonic measurement of carotid artery intima-media thickness: the European Lacidipine Study on Atherosclerosis. *J Hypertens* 23:1047, 2005.

CHAPTER 31

Peripheral Arterial Disease Assessment and Management

Jeffrey S. Berger and Emile R. Mohler III

Peripheral arterial disease (PAD) is a disease that obstructs blood supply to the extremities. The most common pathologic process is atherosclerotic disease, but it may also result from connective tissue diseases, vasculitis, hematologic disorders, thrombosis, embolism, fibromuscular dysplasia, mechanical obstruction, and occupation-related diseases. This serious and highly prevalent disorder is associated with significant morbidity and mortality, commonly with impaired function and quality of life.

EPIDEMIOLOGY

Lower extremity PAD, a highly prevalent condition in the United States with an estimated general population prevalence of 12%, is estimated to affect approximately 8 to 12 million Americans.[1] In primary care office practices, PAD is present in 29% of patients older than 70 years or older than 50 years with a history of smoking or diabetes.[2] The prevalence of PAD and intermittent claudication increases progressively with age. Data from the 1999-2000 National Health and Nutrition Examination Survey (NHANES) demonstrated the prevalence of PAD (defined as an ankle-brachial index <0.90 in either leg) was 0.9% between the ages of 40 and 49 years, 2.5% between the ages of 50 and 59 years, 4.7% between the ages of 60 and 69 years, and 14.5% at the age of 70 years and older.[3] NHANES data from 1999 to 2004 demonstrated a 44% increase in the odds of PAD for every 10-year increase in age.[4] There are data to suggest that race or ethnicity plays a role in PAD.[3,5-7] The prevalence among non-Hispanic blacks was 7.9%, the highest among other racial and ethnic groups (4.4% in non-Hispanic whites and 3% in Mexican Americans). Consistently, the Atherosclerosis Risk in Communities (ARIC) study demonstrated a significantly higher prevalence of PAD in African Americans than in whites.[8] Collaborative data from seven community-based studies noted a higher rate of PAD in African Americans than in American Indians, Asian Americans, Hispanics, and non-Hispanic whites.[9]

Despite the high prevalence of PAD, detection and awareness are lower than for arterial disease in other locations.[2] A population-based telephone survey of a nationally representative sample of adults older than 50 years demonstrated that only 26% of respondents expressed familiarity with PAD.[10]

RISK FACTORS FOR PERIPHERAL ARTERIAL DISEASE

The risk factors for PAD are similar to those for arterial disease in the coronary and cerebrovascular territories.[5,11] Increasing age, hypertension, dyslipidemia, cigarette smoking, and diabetes mellitus are well-established risk factors for all arterial disease. Data derived from several observational studies demonstrate that cigarette smoking and diabetes are particularly strong risk factors for PAD. Data from the 1999-2000 NHANES survey found that in age- and sex-adjusted logistic regression analysis, current smoking had a greater than fourfold increased odds and diabetes almost a three-fold increased odds of prevalent PAD. In a longitudinal cohort study, data from the Framingham Heart Study of 381 men and women who were observed for 38 years revealed that the odds ratio for development of intermittent claudication was 2.6 for the presence of diabetes mellitus and 1.4 for each 10 cigarettes smoked per day.[12]

Dyslipidemia is also associated with an increased prevalence of PAD.[5] In comparison of a panel of lipid risk factors for PAD, total cholesterol, high-density lipoprotein cholesterol (HDL-C), low-density lipoprotein cholesterol (LDL-C), triglycerides, and apolipoprotein B were all significant predictors of increased risk of PAD, although the ratio of total cholesterol to HDL-C was the single strongest predictor (highest quartile versus lowest quartile relative risk, 3.9; 95% confidence interval, 1.7 to 8.6).[13]

There is growing evidence that several nontraditional risk factors, including inflammation, endothelial dysfunction, thrombotic and hemostatic markers, and platelet activity, may also be associated with increased PAD risk.[5] Multiple studies have shown elevated levels of inflammatory biomarkers in men and women with PAD.[13,14] In a community-based sample from the Framingham Offspring Study,[15] the group of inflammatory biomarkers was related to both ankle-brachial index and clinical PAD.

In the Edinburgh Artery Study,[16] a population-based cohort study, several markers of endothelial function and inflammation were compared. C-reactive protein, interleukin-6, and intercellular adhesion molecule 1 were significant predictors of lower extremity atherosclerotic progression measured by ankle-brachial index during 12 years of follow-up independently of cardiovascular risk factors. Elevated levels of inflammatory biomarkers are also associated with greater functional impairment and faster functional decline in people with PAD.[17,18] A study of proteomic profiling identified the protein β_2-thromboglobulin as being elevated in subjects with PAD, and a significant correlation was observed between β_2-microglobulin and the severity of disease.[19] The association of β_2-microglobulin with PAD may be related to vascular inflammation.

Abnormalities in hemostasis also associate with an increased prevalence of PAD. Data derived from the ARIC study found elevated levels of hemostatic markers in subjects with PAD. Specifically, higher levels of fibrinogen, von Willebrand factor, factor VIII, D-dimer, and thromboglobulin were associated with greater PAD prevalence. In a population of Scottish men and women aged 55 to 74 years, mean levels of fibrinogen, fibrin D-dimer, and plasma viscosity remained significantly higher among the diabetes/impaired glucose tolerant group with PAD compared with those with no PAD.[20]

In contrast, fibrinogen and homocysteine were not associated with development of PAD in the Women's Health Study. Considerable evidence links platelets, a major culprit in atherothrombosis, and the development of PAD. With use of data from NHANES, levels of mean platelet volume in peripheral blood independently associate with PAD (tertile 1, 4.4%; tertile 2, 6.1%; tertile 3, 7.0%; P for trend = 0.003), independent of traditional cardiovascular risk factors.[21] Ongoing studies will determine the usefulness of markers of inflammation, endothelial function, hemostasis, and platelet activity in the risk prediction of PAD.

PATHOPHYSIOLOGY

Although it is poorly understood, the pathophysiologic process leading to development of claudication and decline in functional status is thought to be progression of atherothrombosis,[22,23] the combination of atherosclerosis and thrombosis. The proatherogenic state can be classified into increased vasoconstriction, inflammation, and platelet activation and endothelial dysfunction. The natural history of atherosclerosis in the extremities involves progressive occlusion of the vessel, typically in susceptible regions where turbulent blood flow occurs, such as the proximal superficial femoral artery and the popliteal artery at Hunter canal.[24]

Vasodilator capability is severely decreased in subjects with PAD.[25,26] Normal arteries dilate in response to several different stimuli, such as acetylcholine, serotonin, thrombin, and bradykinin, as well as shear stress induced by increases in blood flow that increase nitric oxide production.[27-30] Endothelium from a subject with PAD is impaired; the production and bioavailability of nitric oxide in the artery wall are decreased.[31,32] There is increasing evidence for the participation of inflammatory cells as mediators in atherogenesis and plaque rupture in arterial disease of all vascular beds.[33]

Inflammatory mediators play an essential role in the pathogenesis of cardiovascular disease, being involved at all stages of plaque development and eventual rupture.[34]

Several studies have noted increased levels of inflammatory markers in subjects with PAD.[13,35] Subjects with PAD have increased platelet activity, platelet hyperactivity (as assessed by platelet aggregation), mean platelet volume, platelet factor 4, β-thromboglobulin, and P-selectin expression receptors on platelets.[21,36,37] Nevertheless, there is a lack of data comparing the association between platelet markers with different pathophysiologic mechanisms and PAD.

Other pathologic considerations for PAD include altered muscle structure and function. Repeated episodes of ischemia during exercise and reperfusion during recovery may promote oxidant injury to endothelial cells, muscle mitochondria, muscle fibers, and distal motor axons. Muscle denervation and alterations in muscle metabolism contribute to performance limitations.[38]

PAD has two distinct manifestations, claudication and critical limb ischemia. Patients with claudication infrequently progress to chronic limb ischemia and have a combined annual amputation mortality rate of 2% to 4% per patient per year, whereas patients with chronic limb ischemia have a 6-month amputation risk of 25% to 40% and an annual mortality rate as high as 20% (Fig. 31-1).[5]

Others have noted differences between large-vessel PAD and small-vessel PAD. In a longitudinal study of 403 subjects with a mean follow-up of 4.6 years, current cigarette smoking, the ratio of total cholesterol to HDL-C, high-sensitivity C-reactive protein, and lipoprotein(a) were independent predictors of large-vessel PAD progression. This was in contrast to progression of small-vessel PAD, for which diabetes was the only significant predictor.[39]

DIAGNOSIS OF PERIPHERAL ARTERIAL DISEASE

After a complete history and physical examination, the diagnosis of PAD should be confirmed with a vascular study. There are multiple modalities from which to choose for assessment of PAD. A simple, inexpensive, noninvasive tool that correlates well with angiographic disease severity and functional symptoms is the ankle-brachial index (ABI).[40-43] In the supine position, the ankle and arm systolic pressures are approximately the same, and on standing, the ankle systolic pressure is somewhat higher than that of the arm.[44] Thus, in the supine position, the measured ankle systolic blood pressure divided by the brachial systolic blood pressure is normally between 1.0 and 1.3.[45] However, if a fixed obstruction of the arterial lumen is present, as is the case with atherosclerotic disease, a pressure gradient occurs, resulting in a reduced downstream pressure and concomitant reduction in the ABI.[44]

An ABI < 0.9 is considered abnormal and diagnostic of PAD.[40,45,46] ABI values between 0.90 and 0.99 are considered borderline and equivocal for PAD. Of note, recent data indicate that even borderline ABI values have significant increased risk for a cardiovascular event (Fig. 31-2).[47] An ABI ranging from 0.70 to less than 0.90 indicates mild disease; moderate disease correlates with an ABI ranging from 0.40 to less than 0.70; and severe disease is associated with an ABI of no more than 0.40.[40] Studies evaluating the diagnostic accuracy of the ABI have demonstrated that it can differentiate between normal and angiographically diseased limbs with a sensitivity of 97% and a specificity of 100%[48] and that the resting ABI is a significant predictive variable for the severity of angiographic disease.[49]

Approximately one third of patients with PAD have typical claudication, defined as pain in one or both legs on walking,

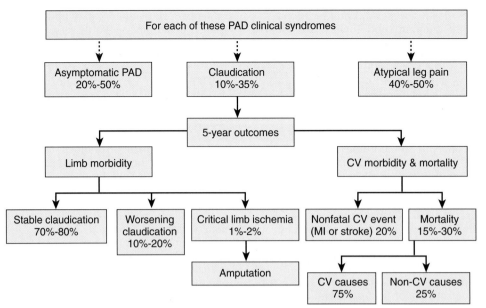

FIGURE 31-1 The natural history of atherosclerotic lower extremity peripheral arterial disease (PAD). Individuals with atherosclerotic lower extremity PAD may be asymptomatic (without identified ischemic leg symptoms, albeit with a functional impairment), present with leg symptoms (classic claudication or atypical leg symptoms), or present with critical limb ischemia. All individuals with PAD face a risk of progressive limb ischemic symptoms as well as a high short-term cardiovascular ischemic event rate and increased mortality. These event rates are most clearly defined for individuals with claudication or critical limb ischemia and less well defined for individuals with asymptomatic PAD. CV, cardiovascular; MI, myocardial infarction. *(Modified from Weitz JI, Byrne J, Clagett GP, et al: Diagnosis and treatment of chronic arterial insufficiency of the lower extremities: a critical review.* Circulation *94:3026, 1996.)*

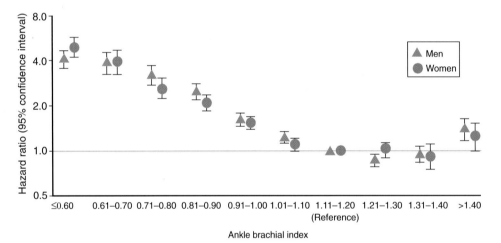

FIGURE 31-2 Hazard ratios for total mortality in men and women by ankle-brachial index in the ABI Collaboration.

primarily affecting the calves, that does not go away with continued walking and is relieved by rest.[45]

Ankle-Brachial Index Technique

The ABI can be measured in the office or hospital setting because the equipment required is inexpensive and portable[40,45,50] (Fig. 31-3). The study is done with the patient in the supine position after resting for at least 5 minutes. The "traditional" method for conduction of the ABI test is to use an ordinary blood pressure cuff and to measure the systolic blood pressure with a Doppler ultrasonic velocity signal probe. The blood pressure is measured in both arms, and if a discrepancy exists, the higher of the two systolic blood pressure values is used. The Doppler probe is then moved over the posterior tibial artery and then over the dorsalis pedis artery to measure the respective ankle pressures. The

higher of the two ankle pressures is typically used to calculate the leg ABI. However, recent information indicates that use of the lower of the two may identify more individuals with PAD.[51] The process should be repeated for the other leg. The lowest ABI between both legs is the ABI that stratifies the patient's risk for functional impairment and adverse cardiovascular event.[52,53]

Limitations of Ankle-Brachial Index

As with most tests, measurement of the ABI has some limitations. The pressures in the leg may be supranormal (ABI > 1.4) because of inability to compress the artery, especially in patients with diabetes.[44] A supranormal pressure does not allow determination of whether an obstructive plaque is present, and thus the information is considered not diagnostic. If an incompressible artery is found, the patient should be referred to an accredited vascular laboratory for

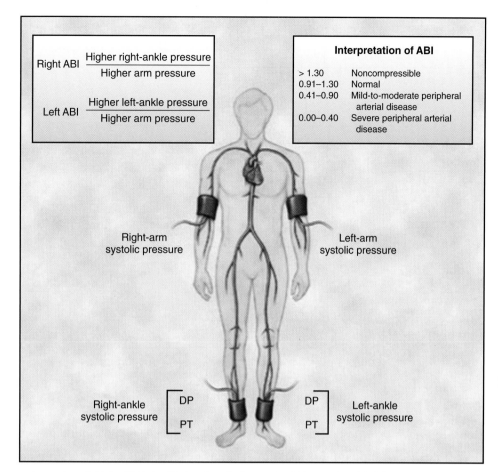

FIGURE 31-3 Ankle-brachial index. DP, dorsalis pedis; PT, posterior tibial artery. *(Modified from Hiatt WR: Medical treatment of peripheral arterial disease and claudication. N Engl J Med 344:1608, 2001.)*

measurement of a toe-brachial index or other noninvasive testing.[40,46]

Another problem that may preclude accurate analysis with the ABI is the presence of bilateral subclavian artery stenosis. The result of this hemodynamic occlusion is a false reduction in the "true" systemic circulation systolic pressure and inaccurate denominator in calculation of the ABI.[46] Other limitations of the ABI that should be recognized in considering surgery include its inability to localize arterial lesions accurately[54] and the lack of an association between ABI and the predicted potential for wound healing.[55]

Ankle-Brachial Index in Asymptomatic Peripheral Arterial Disease

Up to two thirds of patients who have a reduced ABI do not have classic symptoms of intermittent claudication.[45,56,57] Individuals with PAD who do not have classic intermittent claudication symptoms have significant functional impairment, functional decline, and cardiovascular events compared with those without PAD.[58] The collaboration of 16 international cohorts including more than 48,000 individuals demonstrated that the ABI provided independent risk information over and above the Framingham risk score, and a low ABI significantly increased the risk of total and cardiovascular mortality and major coronary events across all Framingham risk categories.[47] In fact, the ABI resulted in reclassification of the Framingham risk estimate in approximately 20% of men and one third of women. An analysis of 102 subjects with a recent stroke or transient ischemic attack found that 26% had asymptomatic PAD as detected by ABI measurement.[59] Subjects with asymptomatic PAD had a fivefold

greater adjusted increase in cardiovascular events than did subjects without PAD.

Recommendations for Screening for Ankle-Brachial Index

Given the wealth of information obtained from this simple hemodynamic test, current American College of Cardiology/ American Heart Association (ACC/AHA) and Inter-Society Consensus for the Management of Peripheral Arterial Disease (TASC II)[38,60] guidelines have provided Class IA recommendation for measurement of the ABI in "at-risk" populations. We recommend the following protocol for measurement of the ABI in at-risk populations (Fig. 31-4).

Vascular Exercise Testing

The measurement of the ABI before and after exercise provides additional diagnostic information about the presence and severity of claudication.[40,44,48] The normal response of the ankle systolic pressure is an increase with exercise. However, if significant lower extremity arterial obstruction is present, the ankle systolic pressure may decrease because of a pressure gradient across the blockage while the arm pressure may increase, resulting in reduced ABI.

The ABI typically will return to pre-exercise level within 5 minutes after cessation of exercise. Thus, if clinical suspicion is high that leg discomfort is due to claudication, an exercise test will provide confirmatory information in a patient with "normal" or borderline ABI. Alternatively, if the

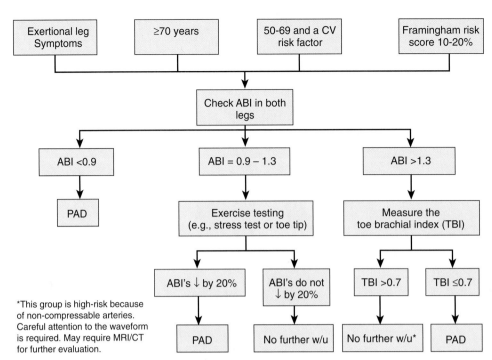

FIGURE 31-4 Flow diagram for measurement of ankle-brachial index.

ABI does not change with exercise, leg discomfort with exercise may be due to another cause, such as spinal stenosis.

The clinical protocol for vascular stress testing may use a standard exercise treadmill or pedal plantar flexion (heel raises).[61,62] One common regimen is for the patient to walk at a standard speed and grade for a predetermined period (i.e., 2 mph at 12% incline for 5 minutes) or until claudication develops.[44,46] Immediately after cessation of exercise, the patient is asked to lie in a supine position, and the ankle systolic blood pressure is measured.[44] The pedal plantar flexion exercise test involves the patient's standing facing a wall while using light fingertip support for balance. The patient raises the heels as high as possible while keeping the knees straight and then immediately lowers them; the cycle is repeated 30 to 50 times or until claudication symptoms occur. As with treadmill testing, the ABI is calculated with the patient in a supine position immediately after completion of the exercise sequence.[61,62] Postexercise measurement of the ABI may identify an additional 30% of patients with PAD.[63]

Segmental Pressures and Pulse Volume Recordings

The ABI, although useful for diagnosis of the presence of PAD, does not provide for the level of disease, an important factor in determining how to treat claudication. A common procedure in many vascular laboratories is measurement of multiple or segmental pressures in the lower extremities along with pulse volume recordings that measure the magnitude and contour of the blood pulse volume.[44,46] This combination of segmental pressures and pulse volume recordings has demonstrated 95% accuracy compared with angiography.[46]

An alternative to pulse volume recording measurement is blood velocity waveform analysis,[44,46] in which a continuous-wave Doppler probe is used over multiple arterial segments to detect the blood flow velocity and the velocity patterns.[44,46] The normal blood flow pattern is triphasic (forward, reverse, and late forward flow), and a change in this pattern to biphasic or monophasic indicates a flow-reducing lesion.[44] One major disadvantage of segmental pressure, pulse volume recording, and Doppler velocity waveform analysis is the inability to visualize the anatomy and to pinpoint the

artery being studied.[44,46] However, the pulse volume recording and Doppler velocity waveform analysis are particularly useful in assessing patients with supranormal pressures, such as may occur in diabetic patients, due to medial artery calcification.[44,46]

Ultrasonic Duplex Scanning

Duplex ultrasound B-mode imaging combined with spectral Doppler analysis is used to localize occlusions more precisely than arterial segments or to more fully characterize the severity and morphology of occlusions.[46] The artery characteristics provided from duplex ultrasound imaging include artery wall thickness, degree of flow turbulence, vessel morphology, and changes in blood flow velocity in areas of stenosis.[42]

Compared with x-ray contrast angiography, the accuracy (specificity) of duplex ultrasound is very high (92% to 98%), although its sensitivity for assessment of stenosis is variable, depending on the size of the vessel.[42]

Some data indicate that the sensitivity for stenosis measurement with duplex ultrasound is lower for smaller arteries than for larger arteries in the limb. The appropriate applications for duplex ultrasound include preparation for planned angioplasty or surgical procedure, detection of restenosis after an endovascular procedure, and surveillance of femoropopliteal or distal saphenous vein grafts for detection of myointimal lesions before graft failure.[40,44]

If the specific anatomic location and further assessment of stenosis are warranted, then other noninvasive imaging techniques such as spiral computed tomography angiography and magnetic resonance angiography may be used in addition to or instead of duplex ultrasonography.[46] Although noninvasive imaging studies are becoming more commonly used preoperatively, catheter-based angiography is still considered the "gold standard."

PROGNOSIS

Symptomatic and asymptomatic PAD is associated with an increased risk for morbidity and mortality. Pooled data from 11 studies in six countries found that PAD, defined by a low

ABI (<0.9), was associated with an increased risk of subsequent all-cause mortality (RR, 1.60), cardiovascular mortality (RR, 1.96), coronary heart disease (RR, 1.45), and stroke (RR, 1.35) after adjustment for age, sex, conventional cardiovascular risk factors, and prevalent cardiovascular disease. An analysis from the Reduction of Atherothrombosis for Continued Health (REACH) registry[64] spanning 44 countries demonstrated that patients with established atherosclerosis in more than one vascular bed had substantially higher event rates than did patients with atherosclerotic disease in only one vascular bed. In this cohort of approximately 68,000 patients, the annual rate of myocardial infarction, stroke, or death from cardiovascular causes for patients with PAD was 5%.[64]

A recent prospective cohort demonstrated a similar high risk of mortality in symptomatic and asymptomatic patients with PAD, and it was significantly higher than in those without PAD.[65] Data from the Clopidogrel for High Atherothrombotic Risk and Ischemic Stabilization, Management, and Avoidance (CHARISMA) trial showed an increased risk of all-cause death, cardiovascular death, myocardial infarction, and stroke in subjects with PAD versus no PAD and found no difference between symptomatic and asymptomatic PAD.[66] In a longitudinal study of older men with diabetes without symptomatic PAD, 14-year mortality was significantly higher in subjects with asymptomatic PAD versus no PAD. In the multivariate analysis of the 14-year follow-up, PAD and diabetes were both associated with an increased risk of death, whereas PAD but not diabetes was associated with increased cardiac events and cardiovascular mortality.[67] Data from the ARIC study between 1987 and 2001 found that for every 0.10 decrease in the ABI, the hazard for coronary heart disease increased by 25% in white men, by 20% in white women, by 34% in African American men, and by 32% in African American women.[68]

In a recent collaboration of 16 international cohorts,[47] the ABI provided independent risk information over and above the Framingham risk score. The hazard ratios for all-cause mortality at different levels of ABI compared with a reference ABI of 1.11 to 1.20 in all studies combined formed a reverse J-shaped curve for both men and women (see Fig. 31-2). For levels of ABI < 1.1, the hazard of death increased in a stepwise manner with decreasing ABI. An ABI > 1.40 was associated with an increased risk of death for men and women. Similar results were noted for cardiovascular mortality and major coronary events.[47]

TREATMENT

The treatment of PAD has evolved during the past decade to include a broad approach, focusing on reduction of the risk of the major factors associated with the development and progression of PAD.[45,69] Furthermore, because PAD subjects are at high risk for coronary and cardiovascular events and mortality,[70] much emphasis is placed on the reduction of cardiovascular risk. In fact, the National Cholesterol Education Program (NCEP) Expert Panel on Detection, Evaluation, and Treatment of High Blood Cholesterol in Adults (Adult Treatment Panel III) considered PAD a coronary heart disease risk equivalent, thereby elevating it to the highest risk category.[71] Nevertheless, patients with PAD are undertreated with regard to the use of lipid-lowering and antiplatelet drugs compared with patients with coronary artery disease.[72,73]

Smoking Cessation

A plethora of evidence exists that smoking is a very significant risk factor for the incidence of PAD and its consequences.[5,74] Cessation of cigarette smoking is associated with a lower amputation rate, a lower incidence of rest ischemia,

and an improvement in maximal treadmill walking distance.[75] Among subjects with PAD who are not smokers, there is a lower rate of myocardial infarction and mortality than among PAD subjects who do smoke. Furthermore, PAD subjects who discontinue smoking have an improved 5-year survival versus that of those who continue to smoke.[75] Physician advice must be the cornerstone of this strategy but should be in conjunction with other proven remedies, including group counseling sessions and pharmacologic interventions (nicotine replacement therapy, bupropion, and varenicline).

Lipid-Lowering Therapy

Although dietary modification is often the initial treatment for lowering of cholesterol concentration, the addition of pharmacotherapies may be necessary to achieve target total cholesterol, HDL-C, and LDL-C levels. All patients with PAD of any severity should achieve an LDL-C concentration of less than 100 mg/dL, whereas a target of less than 70 mg/dL is reasonable in subjects with PAD and atherosclerosis in other arterial beds.

In the Scandinavian Simvastatin Survival Study (4S), simvastatin (20 to 40 mg/day) significantly reduced the incidence of intermittent claudication from 3.6% to 2.3% during a median period of 5.4 years in 4444 patients with prior myocardial infarction or angina and a baseline plasma total cholesterol concentration between 212 and 309 mg/dL (relative risk reduction, 0.62%; 95% CI, 0.44%-0.88%).[76] In subjects with established PAD, statin therapy may reduce the incidence of cardiovascular events. In a subgroup analysis of 6748 subjects with PAD from the Heart Protection Study, simvastatin 40 mg daily was associated with a reduction in cardiovascular events, regardless of the presenting cholesterol levels.[77] Statin therapy also improves pain-free walking time.[78] Although statin drugs have the strongest data supporting use, cholesterol lowering by other means is effective in decreasing cardiovascular events as well.[79]

Blood Pressure Control

Antihypertensive therapy is effective at reducing cardiovascular events in subjects with PAD.[45,80] Concern has been raised about the use of beta blockers in the treatment of hypertension among patients with intermittent claudication, but data do not elicit such fears. In fact, a meta-analysis of 11 studies of beta blocker therapy in patients with intermittent claudication found no significant impairment on walking capacity.[81] As a result, these drugs are not contraindicated in patients with PAD. There is some evidence that angiotensin-converting enzyme inhibitor therapy may improve cardiovascular events and increase walking distance in selected patients with PAD. In the Heart Outcomes Prevention Evaluation (HOPE) trial, ramipril (5 to 10 mg/day) decreased cardiovascular events in subjects with PAD.[82]

Regarding drug choice, all drugs that lower blood pressure are effective at reducing the risk of cardiovascular events. According to the TASC II guidelines, thiazide diuretics and angiotensin-converting enzyme inhibitors should be considered as initial blood pressure–lowering drugs in PAD to reduce the risk of cardiovascular events.[60]

Antiplatelet Therapy

The Antithrombotic Trialists' Collaboration, a systematic overview of 135,000 high-risk patients from 287 trials, demonstrated a reduction in myocardial infarction, stroke, and death with antiplatelet therapy in patients at risk for cardiovascular events.[83] Among 42 PAD trials that included 9214 patients and used a variety of antiplatelet agents, compared with placebo, antiplatelet therapy (combining all agents)

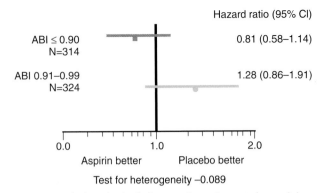

Hazard ratio (95% CI)

ABI ≤ 0.90
N=314   0.81 (0.58–1.14)

ABI 0.91–0.99
N=324   1.28 (0.86–1.91)

0.0   1.0   2.0

Aspirin better   Placebo better

Test for heterogeneity –0.089

31

FIGURE 31-5 The hazard ratio of adverse cardiovascular events (myocardial infarction, stroke, cardiovascular death, or amputation for chronic limb ischemia) in subjects with an ABI of 0.9 and an ABI between 0.91 and 0.99 according to treatment with aspirin 100 mg/day versus placebo in the POPADAD trial.

demonstrated a significant 23% reduction in the odds of cardiovascular events. However, nearly two thirds evaluated nonaspirin antiplatelet agents, questioning whether the overall benefit of antiplatelet therapy in PAD may have been driven by therapeutic regimens other than aspirin.

Subsequently, the prevention of progression of arterial disease and diabetes (POPADAD) trial found no benefit of aspirin 100 mg/day in diabetic subjects with asymptomatic PAD (ABI < 1.0).[84] However, a subgroup analysis from the POPADAD trial demonstrated a borderline interaction, suggesting a greater benefit in those with an ABI ≤ 0.9 (Fig. 31-5). A recent meta-analysis of randomized trials of aspirin versus placebo in participants with PAD did not show a significant reduction in cardiovascular events with aspirin.[85] However, aspirin was associated with a 35% reduction in the incidence of nonfatal stroke.[85]

Several hypotheses have emerged as to why aspirin was not found to significantly decrease cardiovascular events in subjects with PAD, including insufficient power, wrong dose, the variation in patient phenotype studied, and perhaps that PAD represents a diffuse form of atherosclerosis with a high inflammatory burden and platelet activity, which may be less responsive to aspirin. The overall benefit of antiplatelet therapies in the Antithrombotic Trialists' Collaboration was driven by data from trials using picotamide, dipyridamole, and ticlopidine. Importantly, aspirin has been shown to have other benefits, including delay in the rate of progression, reduction of the need for intervention, and reduction of graft failure in patients who have undergone revascularization procedures.[86,87]

The Clopidogrel versus Aspirin in Patients at Risk of Ischaemic Events (CAPRIE) trial demonstrated that clopidogrel (75 mg/day) had a modest although significant advantage over aspirin (325 mg/day) for the prevention of cardiovascular events in 19,185 patients with a recent stroke, myocardial infarction, or PAD.[88] Overall, there was a 9% relative risk reduction for cardiovascular events, yet among the subset of patients with PAD, clopidogrel resulted in 23% fewer cardiovascular events compared with aspirin. However, the CHARISMA trial found no significant benefit of dual antiplatelet therapy with aspirin plus clopidogrel versus aspirin alone in patients with established coronary artery disease, cerebrovascular disease, or PAD as well as in patients with multiple atherosclerotic risk factors.[89]

Although a benefit of dual antiplatelet therapy versus aspirin alone was noted in subjects with prior myocardial infarction, ischemic stroke, or symptomatic PAD,[90] no reduction in cardiovascular events was noted in the subgroup of subjects with PAD.[66] In a prospective randomized trial, picotamide significantly reduced mortality in diabetic patients

with PAD compared with aspirin.[91] This may reflect its greater potency, given a dual mechanism of action through inhibition of platelet thromboxane A$_2$ synthase and antagonism of thromboxane A$_2$ receptors. Future studies of this compound are warranted.

Current guidelines[5,60] recommend an antiplatelet agent in subjects with PAD, such as aspirin or clopidogrel. On the basis of the limitations of data available, recommendations for aspirin as an important therapeutic tool for secondary prevention in patients with PAD should not be modified. To best inform evidence-based clinical practice guidelines, more high-quality clinical trials are needed.

Anticoagulation Therapy

Oral anticoagulation with warfarin has not been established to reduce cardiovascular events in patients with PAD because it is no more effective than antiplatelet therapy and confers a higher risk of bleeding.[92] The Department of Veterans Affairs Cooperative Study tested combined oral anticoagulation and antiplatelet therapy in patients with PAD.[93] No significant difference was found between groups, and there were 133 deaths in the combined treatment group and 95 deaths in the group receiving aspirin alone.

More recently, the Warfarin and Antiplatelet Vascular Evaluation (WAVE) trial randomized PAD patients to combination therapy with an antiplatelet agent and an oral anticoagulant agent (target international normalized ratio, 2.0 to 3.0) or to antiplatelet therapy alone.[94] In this trial, the combination treatment arm was not more effective than antiplatelet therapy alone in preventing major cardiovascular complications and was associated with a more than threefold increase in life-threatening bleeding.[94]

Other Pharmacotherapy

In addition to treatment of cardiovascular risk factors and coexisting diseases to prevent cardiovascular events (myocardial infarction, stroke, and death) associated with atherosclerosis, therapies exist to provide a significant reduction or elimination of PAD symptoms. Claudication drug therapy for relief of symptoms may involve drugs different from those that would be used for risk reduction (an exception may be lipid-lowering therapy).[78]

Cilostazol is a phosphodiesterase type 3 inhibitor with properties that inhibit platelet aggregation and vascular smooth muscle proliferation and improve the lipid profile and vasodilation. A meta-analysis of six randomized trials demonstrated that cilostazol improved maximum walking distance and pain-free walking distance.[95] An advisory from the U.S. Food and Drug Administration stated that cilostazol should not be used in patients with congestive heart failure because other phosphodiesterase type 3 inhibitors have been demonstrated to worsen survival in this cohort. The effect of cilostazol on cardiovascular morbidity and mortality remains unknown.

Pentoxifylline is a xanthine derivative used to treat patients with intermittent claudication. Its mechanism of action is thought to be a rheologic modifier—increase in red blood cell deformity and decreases in fibrinogen concentration, platelet adhesiveness, and whole-blood viscosity. A meta-analysis demonstrated a modestly improved walking distance, substantially less effective than either cilostazol or a supervised exercise program.[96]

Exercise

For patients with symptomatic PAD, exercise therapy is a key component of reducing symptoms. A supervised program of treadmill-based walking exercise can induce a training response characterized by large improvements in treadmill exercise performance, peak oxygen consumption, endothelial function, and quality of life.[5,60] Exercise is more effective than angioplasty for improvement of walking time and is also more effective than antiplatelet therapy, but it does not differ significantly from surgical treatment.[97] Possible mechanisms underlying the exercise response in PAD include improvements in endothelial function, skeletal muscle metabolism, and blood viscosity and a reduction in systemic inflammation. Although it is less well studied, exercise may also improve survival.[98] In a prospective observational study of 225 men and women with PAD in whom physical activity was measured with a vertical accelerometer, individuals in the highest quartile of measured activity had a significantly lower mortality than those in the lowest quartile (hazard ratio, 0.29; 95% CI, 0.10-0.83).

Dietary Intervention

The dietary approach for treatment of PAD is the same as for patients with coronary artery and carotid artery atherosclerotic disease. Patients are advised to balance calorie intake and physical activity to achieve and to maintain a healthy body weight; to consume a diet rich in vegetables and fruits; to choose whole-grain, high-fiber foods; to consume fish, especially oily fish, at least twice a week; and to limit intake of saturated fat to <7% of energy, *trans*-fat to <1% of energy, and cholesterol to <300 mg/day.[99]

REVASCULARIZATION FOR PERIPHERAL ARTERIAL DISEASE

The treatment approach with revascularization for PAD involves two distinct populations, those with stable claudication and those with critical limb ischemia. According to the ACC/AHA guidelines, for patients with stable claudication, endovascular or surgical revascularization is "indicated for individuals with a vocational or lifestyle-limiting disability due to claudication when clinical features suggest a reasonable likelihood of symptomatic improvement with endovascular intervention and (a) there has been an inadequate response to exercise or pharmacological therapy and/or (b) there is a very favorable risk-benefit ratio (e.g., focal aortoiliac occlusive disease)" (Fig. 31-6). In contrast, those patients with critical limb ischemia deserve consideration for immediate revascularization.

The Inter-Society Consensus for the Management of PAD (TASC) was produced to assess the evidence for PAD diagnosis and treatment and to help guide clinicians in their care of patients with PAD.[60] The TASC recommendation regarding determination of the best method of revascularization for treatment of claudication is based on the balance between the risk of a specific intervention and the degree and durability of the improvement that can be expected from the intervention. The outcome of the revascularization procedure depends on the anatomic and clinical features of the lesion.

The anatomic features that have an impact on vessel patency after procedures are the severity of disease in run-off arteries (those distal to the treated lesion), the length of the stenosis or occlusion, and the number of lesions treated. The major clinical factors that affect the outcome of revascularization procedures include diabetes mellitus, smoking, renal disease, and severity of ischemia. The TASC classification of arterial lesions includes A lesions, which should be treated with endovascular approach; B lesions, which also should be treated with endovascular approach unless an open revascularization is required for other associated lesions in the same anatomic area; C lesions, for which open revascularization

produces superior results and endovascular treatment should be reserved for high-risk patients for surgery; and D lesions, for which the open surgical approach is preferred (Tables 31-1 and 31-2).

A detailed approach to revascularization is provided in the ACC/AHA and TASC II guidelines.[5,60] In brief, the endovascular treatment of iliac lesions results in the most durable outcome, whereas infrainguinal disease is much more problematic. There are only small clinical studies available directly comparing endovascular treatments with best medical management. The CLEVER (Claudication: Exercise Versus Endoluminal Revascularization) study, funded by the National Institutes of Health's Heart, Lung, and Blood Institute, is a prospective, multicenter, randomized, controlled clinical trial evaluating the relative efficacy, safety, and health economic impact of endovascular and noninvasive treatment strategies for people with aortoiliac PAD and claudication. The results of the CLEVER trial are anticipated to provide needed comparative evidence for revascularization and noninvasive medical approaches. Future studies comparing an invasive versus medical therapy approach are warranted in other anatomic areas, including the femoral and more distal arteries.

ABDOMINAL AORTIC ANEURYSM

An abdominal aortic aneurysm (AAA) is considered to be present when the minimum anteroposterior diameter of the aorta reaches 3.0 cm.[5] However, this primary definition does not account for the wide variation in body size, so other definitions have emerged, including a 50% increase in size relative to the proximal normal segment.[100,101]

During the last decade, AAA has increasingly been recognized as an important cause of mortality in older persons. In 2006, for example, AAA was noted to be the 13th and 14th leading cause of mortality in the United States among subjects 60 to 69 years and 70 to 79 years, respectively.[102]

Epidemiology

The most important risk factors for AAA are increasing age, smoking, and male sex.[103-105] Other factors share many of the same coronary risk factors, including race, atherosclerosis, hypertension, and family history.[103,106-111] A recent analysis from the Women's Health Initiative confirmed the importance of smoking and age as robust risk factors in women.[112] As in men, a negative association between diabetes and AAA was reported, suggesting a common pathophysiologic mechanism of AAA in men and women.[113]

A series of 46,000 autopsies done in Sweden found an age-standardized AAA prevalence rate of approximately 4.7% among men and 3.0% among women. The prevalence among men increased rapidly after the age of 55 years and reached a peak of 5.9% at the age of 80 years; the prevalence among women increased after the age of 70 years and reached a peak of 4.5% above the age of 90 years.[114] Because AAAs are easily detectable with ultrasonography, more recent studies have evaluated the prevalence of AAA in the community.

In the final result of the Aneurysm Detection and Management (ADAM) study screening program of the Department of Veterans Affairs, which screened more than 126,196 veterans aged 50 to 79 years, investigators reported a prevalence of 4.2% for aneurysms 3.0 cm or larger and 1.3% for aneurysms 4.0 cm or larger.[109] In general, the prevalence of AAAs 2.9 to 4.9 cm in diameter ranges from 1.3% for men aged 45 to 54 years up to 12.5% for men 75 to 84 years of age. Comparable prevalence figures for women are 0% and 5.2%, respectively.[5]

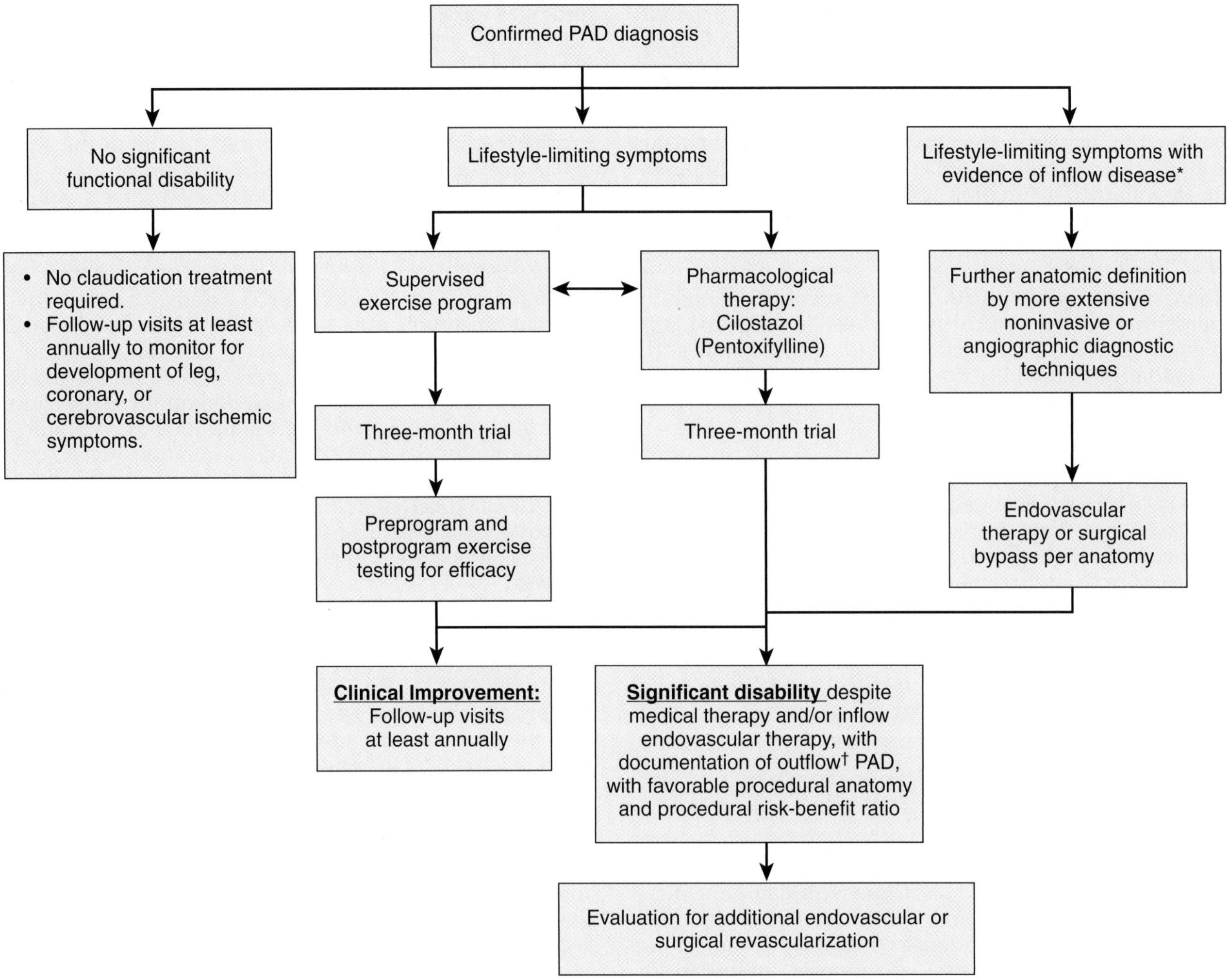

FIGURE 31-6 Treatment of claudication. *Inflow disease should be suspected in individuals with gluteal or thigh claudication and femoral pulse diminution or bruit and should be confirmed by noninvasive vascular laboratory diagnostic evidence of aortoiliac stenoses. †Outflow disease represents femoropopliteal and infrapopliteal stenoses (the presence of occlusive lesions in the lower extremity arterial tree below the inguinal ligament from the common femoral artery to the pedal vessels). *(Reproduced with permission from Hirsch AT, Haskal ZJ, Hertzer NR, et al: ACC/AHA 2005 Practice Guidelines for the management of patients with peripheral arterial disease [lower extremity, renal, mesenteric, and abdominal aortic]: a collaborative report from the American Association for Vascular Surgery/Society for Vascular Surgery, Society for Cardiovascular Angiography and Interventions, Society for Vascular Medicine and Biology, Society of Interventional Radiology, and the ACC/AHA Task Force on Practice Guidelines [Writing Committee to Develop Guidelines for the Management of Patients With Peripheral Arterial Disease]: endorsed by the American Association of Cardiovascular and Pulmonary Rehabilitation; National Heart, Lung, and Blood Institute; Society for Vascular Nursing; Trans-Atlantic Inter-Society Consensus; and Vascular Disease Foundation. J Am Coll Cardiol 47:1239, 2006.)*

Abdominal Aortic Aneurysm Screening

The evaluation for an AAA involves physical examination and abdominal ultrasonography. The bifurcation of the aorta occurs at the level of the umbilicus, and palpation may detect a pulsatile mass in the abdomen. Palpation of AAA appears to be safe and has not been reported to precipitate rupture.[115] The physical detection of AAA is significantly hampered by obesity but nonetheless should be included on all vascular examinations. Abdominal palpation will detect most AAAs large enough to warrant surgery, but it cannot be relied on to exclude the diagnosis.[115] The most reliable screening method for AAA is ultrasonography because of high sensitivity (95% to 100%) and specificity (nearly 100%) as well as safety and relatively low cost.[116] Other imaging modalities on which AAA may be seen are plain abdominal radiography, abdominal computed tomography, and magnetic resonance imaging, but they are not considered first-line evaluation for AAA.

The Multicenter Aneurysm Screening Study (MASS) evaluated a population-based sample of 67,800 men between the ages of 65 and 74 years.[117] Subjects were randomly assigned to receive an invitation to undergo ultrasound screening or no correspondence. Of the 33,839 men invited to undergo screening, 1333 aneurysms were detected (prevalence of 4.9%). Ultrasound examination was repeated yearly in those with an aortic diameter of 3.0 to 4.4 cm and every 3 months in those with an aortic diameter of 4.5 to 5.4 cm. Those patients with an aortic diameter ≥5.5 cm, an increase in aortic diameter by more than 1 cm in a year, or symptoms attributed to the aneurysm were referred to surgery. Surgical repair was performed significantly more often in the screened group (354 patients) versus the control group (146 patients). Overall, a substantial reduction in aneurysm-related mortality could be

TABLE 31–1	TASC Classification of Aortoiliac Lesions
Type A lesions	Unilateral or bilateral stenoses of CIA Unilateral or bilateral single short (≤3 cm) stenosis of EIA
Type B lesions	Short (≤3 cm) stenosis of infrarenal aorta Unilateral CIA occlusion Single or multiple stenosis totaling 3-10 cm involving the EIA not extending into the CFA Unilateral EIA occlusion not involving the origins of internal iliac or CFA
Type C lesions	Bilateral CIA occlusions Bilateral EIA stenoses 3-10 cm long not extending into the CFA Unilateral EIA stenosis extending into the CFA Unilateral EIA occlusion that involves the origins of internal iliac and/or CFA Heavily calcified unilateral EIA occlusion with or without involvement of origins of internal iliac and/or CFA
Type D lesions	Infrarenal aortoiliac occlusion Diffuse disease involving the aorta and both iliac arteries requiring treatment Diffuse multiple stenoses involving the unilateral CIA, EIA, and CFA Unilateral occlusions of both CIA and EIA Bilateral occlusions of EIA Iliac stenoses in patients with AAA requiring treatment and not amenable to endograft placement or other lesions requiring open aortic or iliac surgery

AAA, abdominal aortic aneurysm; CFA, common femoral artery; CIA, common iliac artery; EIA, external iliac artery.
Modified from Norgren L, Hiatt WR, Dormandy JA, et al: Inter-Society Consensus for the Management of Peripheral Arterial Disease (TASC II). *J Vasc Surg* 45(Suppl S):S5, 2007.

TABLE 31–2	TASC Classification of Femoral Popliteal Lesions
Type A lesions	Single stenosis ≤10 cm in length Single occlusion ≤5 cm in length
Type B lesions	Multiple lesions (stenoses or occlusions), each ≤5 cm Single stenosis or occlusion ≤15 cm not involving the infrageniculate popliteal artery Single or multiple lesions in the absence of continuous tibial vessels to improve inflow for a distal bypass Heavily calcified occlusion ≤5 cm in length Single popliteal stenosis
Type C lesions	Multiple stenoses or occlusions totaling >15 cm with or without heavy calcification Recurrent stenoses or occlusions that need treatment after two endovascular interventions
Type D lesions	Chronic total occlusions of CFA or SFA (>20 cm, involving the popliteal artery) Chronic total occlusion of popliteal artery and proximal trifurcation vessels

CFA, common femoral artery; SFA, superficial femoral artery.
Modified from Norgren L, Hiatt WR, Dormandy JA, et al: Inter-Society Consensus for the Management of Peripheral Arterial Disease (TASC II). *J Vasc Surg* 45(Suppl S):S5, 2007.

achieved by the implementation of a population screening program. The risk for dying of an AAA during 4.1 years was reduced from 3.3 per 1000 to 1.9 per 1000.[117]

For AAA ultrasound screening, the ACC/AHA guidelines recommend the following:

- Men 60 years of age or older who are either siblings or offspring of patients with AAAs should undergo physical examination and ultrasound screening for the detection of aortic aneurysms.
- Men who are 65 to 75 years of age who have ever smoked should undergo a physical examination and one-time ultrasound screening for detection of AAAs.

In January 2007, Medicare coverage for a one-time ultrasound study was made available for Medicare recipients who meet the following criteria:

- Referral from an initial "Welcome to Medicare" physical examination within 6 months of Medicare eligibility.
- Male between 65 and 75 years of age who smoked at least 100 cigarettes.
- Male or female with a family history of AAA.

A study that included 17,540 patients (10,012 women and 7528 men) from 100 hospitals and clinics across the United States reported that AAA occurred in 3.9% of the men and 0.7% of the women.[118] However, certain subgroups of women were at higher risk; women older than 65 years had a fourfold increased odds of having an AAA; women with a history of smoking or a history of heart disease had triple the risk of AAA. These data raise the question of whether certain high-risk groups of women should undergo AAA screening. Only adequately powered outcome studies will help provide therapeutic decisions.

Treatment of Abdominal Aortic Aneurysm

The treatment of AAA involves watchful waiting, open surgical repair, or endovascular stent graft placement. A systematic review of how to manage asymptomatic medium-sized (4.0 to 5.5 cm) aneurysms reported no improvement in survival with early surgical repair.[119] An elective repair is considered for AAA of 5.5 cm in diameter, for those that increase in diameter by more than 0.5 cm within a 6-month interval, or for those that are symptomatic (tenderness or abdominal or back pain).[5] However, the risk of intervention must be weighed against the potential benefit. The perioperative mortality rate for surgical aortic aneurysm repair ranges from 2.7% to 5.8%. The factors that increase risk include emergent operation due to rupture, advanced age, chronic kidney disease, cirrhosis, and cardiopulmonary disease.[120-122]

Endovascular repair of AAA is a potential alternative to open surgical repair, but the precise role of endografts in clinical practice has yet to be completely defined. The short-term morbidity and mortality of endografts compare favorably with surgical resection. The complications from stent graft placement include endovascular leaks (persistent blood flow into the aneurysmal sac after device placement), device migration, device failure (e.g., stent frame fracture), and postimplantation syndrome. Because of these potential complications, patients who have undergone endovascular repair of AAA require diligent follow-up with imaging studies annually to evaluate the status of the graft.

A recent randomized, multicenter clinical trial of 881 veterans with eligible AAA who were candidates for both elective endovascular repair and open repair demonstrated a lower 30-day mortality rate in the endovascular repair group (0.5% versus 3.0%; $P = 0.004$) without any significant difference in mortality at 2 years (7.0% versus 9.8%; $P = 0.13$).[123] Longer term outcome data are needed to determine whether endovascular repair is preferable to open surgical repair.[124]

Prognosis

The rupture of AAA has a mortality rate as high as 90%,[125-127] yet most AAAs never rupture. For that reason, considerable attention has been given to the decision of when and for whom to intervene for elective repair of an AAA and by what

TABLE 31–3	Mortality in Subjects with Abdominal Aortic Aneurysms				
Study	Type	Patient Population	Number	Follow-up	Death
Veterans Affairs Cooperative Study (2002)	Cohort	VA setting; AAA ≥5.5 cm for which repair was not planned (contraindication or refusal)	198	1.5 years	57% overall 1 year: 29.8% 2 year: 55.5% 3 year: 75.4%
DREAM (2004)	Randomized controlled trial	Netherlands and Belgium; AAA ≥5 cm eligible for both endovascular and open repair	Endovascular (n = 171) Open (n = 174)	30 days 2 years	Endovascular vs open Perioperative: 1.2% vs 4.6% (P = 0.10) 2-year: 10.3% vs 10.4% (P = 0.86)
EVAR 1 (2004)	Randomized controlled trial	United Kingdom; men and women ≥60 years with AAA ≥5.5 cm eligible for both endovascular and open repair	Endovascular (n = 543) Open (n = 539)	30 days 4 years	Endovascular vs open 30-day: 1.7% vs 4.7% (P <0.05) 4-year: 18.4% vs 20.2% (P = 0.46)
EVAR 2	Randomized controlled trial	United Kingdom; men and women ≥60 years with AAA ≥5.5 cm and unfit for open repair	Endovascular (n = 166) No intervention (n = 172)	3.3 years	Endovascular vs open Long term: 44.6 vs 39.5% (P = 0.10)
Medicare (2008)	Cohort	Medicare patients ≥67 years with a discharge diagnosis of AAA without rupture and a procedural code for open surgical repair or endovascular repair	Endovascular (n = 22,830) Open (n = 22,830)	4 years	Endovascular vs open Perioperative: 1.2% vs 4.8% (P <0.001) (Benefit from endovascular repair persisted for more than 3 years, after which the survival rates associated with the two procedures were similar)
OVER (2009)	Randomized controlled trial	VA setting; eligible for both endovascular and open repair for AAA ≥5 cm, or associated iliac aneurysm ≥3 cm, or AAA ≥4.5 cm with rapid enlargement or saccular morphology	Endovascular (n = 444) Open (n = 437)	1.8 years	Endovascular vs open 30 day: 0.5% vs 3.0% (P = 0.004) 2-year: 7.0% vs 9.8% (P = 0.13)

method.[128] In a surgical cohort of elective and acute infrarenal AAA surgery, mortality within 30 days was approximately fivefold higher for acute AAA surgery, yet no difference was observed during long-term follow-up.[128]

The natural history of clinically apparent AAAs of 5.5 cm or more is difficult to determine because most large aneurysms are repaired (Table 31-3). In an observational study from the Veterans Affairs Cooperative Study among 198 patients with AAA of at least 5.5 cm for whom elective repair was not planned because of medical contraindications or patient refusal, investigators reported a 57% mortality rate after a mean follow-up of 1.5 years.[129] Probable AAA rupture occurred in 23% of the population; the 1-year incidence rates of probable AAA rupture were 9% for AAAs of 5.5 to 5.9 cm, 10% for AAAs of 6.0 to 6.9 cm (19% in the subgroup of 6.5 to 6.9 cm), and 33% for AAAs of 7.0 cm or more.[129]

The strongest risk factor for the rupture of an AAA is maximal aortic diameter, and for that reason, it is the dominating indication for repair. A statement from the Joint Council of the American Association for Vascular Surgery and Society for Vascular Surgery estimated the annual rupture risk according to AAA diameter[130]:

- 0% for aneurysms <4.0 cm in diameter
- 0.5% to 5% for those 4.0 to 4.9 cm in diameter
- 3% to 15% for those 5.0 to 5.9 cm in diameter
- 10% to 20% for those 6.0 to 6.9 cm in diameter
- 20% to 40% for those 7.0 to 7.9 cm in diameter
- 30% to 50% for those ≥8.0 cm in diameter

Although several biomarkers have been proposed to help identify AAA rupture or expansion, most have weak or no correlation with the clinical course of AAA.[131,132] There are

some data that sex may dictate the risk of rupture[133]; the rate of rupture of aneurysms that were 4.0 to 5.5 cm in diameter was four times higher in women compared with men. A meta-analysis showed that the annual risk of rupture of large AAA (5 cm in diameter) was 18% (95% CI, 8% to 26%) in women versus 12% (95% CI, 5% to 20%) in men.[130,134] Other factors increase the risk of rupture, such as rate of expansion, continued smoking, uncontrolled hypertension, and increased wall stress.[130]

Importantly, morbidity and mortality from AAA have improved after elective repair.[135] Analysis of Medicare and Nationwide Inpatient Sample data bases has demonstrated an improvement in 30-day mortality and overall short-term outcomes with endovascular aneurysm repair.[136,137] A recent report from the Swedish aneurysm registry demonstrated an improvement in long-term survival of Swedish citizens treated for AAA with endovascular repair.[138] Data from the United States found similar results—endovascular repair of AAA is associated with a decrease in rupture of AAA and overall patient survival.[137] Long-term randomized data are essential to properly evaluate current therapy for AAA.

CONCLUSION

PAD, a highly prevalent condition, is most commonly caused by atherosclerotic occlusion of the arteries to the lower extremities, and it is an important manifestation of systemic atherosclerosis. The risk factors for PAD are similar to those for coronary disease, including increasing age, hypertension, dyslipidemia, cigarette smoking, and diabetes mellitus.

Symptomatic and asymptomatic PAD is associated with an increased risk for cardiovascular morbidity and mortality. A simple, inexpensive, noninvasive tool that correlates well with angiographic disease severity and functional symptoms is the ankle-brachial index, and the lower the ankle-brachial index, the greater the risk of adverse events.

The treatment of PAD has evolved during the past decade to include a broad approach, focusing on reduction of the risk of the major factors associated with the development and progression of atherosclerosis. This risk, along with severity of claudication in symptomatic patients, can be substantially reduced by targeting the prevalence and level of risk factors by means of lifestyle modification and effective medical therapies. Revascularization for treatment of PAD is based on the balance between the risk of a specific intervention and the degree and durability of the improvement that can be expected from the intervention.

REFERENCES

1. Lloyd-Jones D, Adams R, Carnethon M, et al: Heart disease and stroke statistics—2009 update: a report from the American Heart Association Statistics Committee and Stroke Statistics Subcommittee. *Circulation* 119:e21, 2009.
2. Hirsch AT, Criqui MH, Treat-Jacobson D, et al: Peripheral arterial disease detection, awareness, and treatment in primary care. *JAMA* 286:1317, 2001.
3. Selvin E, Erlinger TP: Prevalence of and risk factors for peripheral arterial disease in the United States: results from the National Health and Nutrition Examination Survey, 1999-2000. *Circulation* 110:738, 2004.
4. Selvin E, Hirsch AT: Contemporary risk factor control and walking dysfunction in individuals with peripheral arterial disease: NHANES 1999-2004. *Atherosclerosis* 201:425, 2008.
5. Hirsch AT, Haskal ZJ, Hertzer NR, et al: ACC/AHA 2005 guidelines for the management of patients with peripheral arterial disease (lower extremity, renal, mesenteric, and abdominal aortic): executive summary a collaborative report from the American Association for Vascular Surgery/Society for Vascular Surgery, Society for Cardiovascular Angiography and Interventions, Society for Vascular Medicine and Biology, Society of Interventional Radiology, and the ACC/AHA Task Force on Practice Guidelines (Writing Committee to Develop Guidelines for the Management of Patients With Peripheral Arterial Disease) endorsed by the American Association of Cardiovascular and Pulmonary Rehabilitation; National Heart, Lung, and Blood Institute; Society for Vascular Nursing; TransAtlantic Inter-Society Consensus; and Vascular Disease Foundation. *J Am Coll Cardiol* 47:1239, 2006.
6. Bennett PC, Silverman S, Gill PS, Lip GY: Ethnicity and peripheral artery disease. *QJM* 102:3, 2009.
7. Criqui MH, Vargas V, Denenberg JO, et al: Ethnicity and peripheral arterial disease: the San Diego Population Study. *Circulation* 112:2703, 2005.
8. Zheng ZJ, Rosamond WD, Chambless LE, et al: Lower extremity arterial disease assessed by ankle-brachial index in a middle-aged population of African Americans and whites: the Atherosclerosis Risk in Communities (ARIC) Study. *Am J Prev Med* 29(Suppl 1):42, 2005.
9. Allison MA, Ho E, Denenberg JO, et al: Ethnic-specific prevalence of peripheral arterial disease in the United States. *Am J Prev Med* 32:328, 2007.
10. Hirsch AT, Murphy TP, Lovell MB, et al: Gaps in public knowledge of peripheral arterial disease: the first national PAD public awareness survey. *Circulation* 116:2086, 2007.
11. Criqui MH: Peripheral arterial disease—epidemiological aspects. *Vasc Med* 6(Suppl):3, 2001.
12. Murabito JM, D'Agostino RB, Silbershatz H, Wilson WF: Intermittent claudication. A risk profile from The Framingham Heart Study. *Circulation* 96:44, 1997.
13. Ridker PM, Stampfer MJ, Rifai N: Novel risk factors for systemic atherosclerosis: a comparison of C-reactive protein, fibrinogen, homocysteine, lipoprotein(a), and standard cholesterol screening as predictors of peripheral arterial disease. *JAMA* 285:2481, 2001.
14. McDermott MM, Lloyd-Jones DM: The role of biomarkers and genetics in peripheral arterial disease. *J Am Coll Cardiol* 54:1228, 2009.
15. Murabito JM, Keyes MJ, Guo CY, et al: Cross-sectional relations of multiple inflammatory biomarkers to peripheral arterial disease: the Framingham Offspring Study. *Atherosclerosis* 203:509, 2009.
16. Tzoulaki I, Murray GD, Lee AJ, et al: C-reactive protein, interleukin-6, and soluble adhesion molecules as predictors of progressive peripheral atherosclerosis in the general population: Edinburgh Artery Study. *Circulation* 112:976, 2005.
17. McDermott MM, Ferrucci L, Liu K, et al: D-dimer and inflammatory markers as predictors of functional decline in men and women with and without peripheral arterial disease. *J Am Geriatr Soc* 53:1688, 2005.
18. McDermott MM, Liu K, Ferrucci L, et al: Circulating blood markers and functional impairment in peripheral arterial disease. *J Am Geriatr Soc* 56:1504, 2008.
19. Wilson AM, Kimura E, Harada RK, et al: β_2-Microglobulin as a biomarker in peripheral arterial disease: proteomic profiling and clinical studies. *Circulation* 116:1396, 2007.
20. Lee AJ, MacGregor AS, Hau CM, et al: The role of haematological factors in diabetic peripheral arterial disease: the Edinburgh artery study. *Br J Haematol* 105:648, 1999.
21. Berger JS, Eraso LH, Xie D, et al: Mean platelet volume and prevalence of peripheral artery disease, the National Health and Nutrition Examination Survey, 1999-2004. *Atherosclerosis* 2010 Sep 18, 2010. [Epub ahead of print]
22. Lip GY, Blann AD: Thrombogenesis, atherogenesis and angiogenesis in vascular disease: a new "vascular triad," *Ann Med* 36:1195, 2004.
23. Faxon DP, Fuster V, Libby P, et al: Atherosclerotic Vascular Disease Conference: Writing Group III: pathophysiology. *Circulation* 109:2617, 2004.
24. Levy PJ: Epidemiology and pathophysiology of peripheral arterial disease. *Clin Cornerstone* 4:1, 2002.
25. Yataco AR, Corretti MC, Gardner AW, et al: Endothelial reactivity and cardiac risk factors in older patients with peripheral arterial disease. *Am J Cardiol* 83:754, 1999.
26. Brevetti G, Silvestro A, Schiano V, Chiariello M: Endothelial dysfunction and cardiovascular risk prediction in peripheral arterial disease: additive value of flow-mediated dilation to ankle-brachial pressure index. *Circulation* 108:2093, 2003.
27. Toutouzas PC, Tousoulis D, Davies GJ: Nitric oxide synthesis in atherosclerosis. *Eur Heart J* 19:1504, 1998.
28. Furchgott RF, Zawadzki JV: The obligatory role of endothelial cells in the relaxation of arterial smooth muscle by acetylcholine. *Nature* 288:373, 1980.
29. Anderson TJ, Uehata A, Gerhard MD, et al: Close relation of endothelial function in the human coronary and peripheral circulations. *J Am Coll Cardiol* 26:1235, 1995.
30. Napoli C, de Nigris F, Williams-Ignarro S, et al: Nitric oxide and atherosclerosis: an update. *Nitric Oxide* 15:265, 2006.
31. Boger RH, Bode-Boger SM, Thiele W, et al: Biochemical evidence for impaired nitric oxide synthesis in patients with peripheral arterial occlusive disease. *Circulation* 95:2068, 1997.
32. Sydow K, Hornig B, Arakawa N, et al: Endothelial dysfunction in patients with peripheral arterial disease and chronic hyperhomocysteinemia: potential role of ADMA. *Vasc Med* 9:93, 2004.
33. Ross R: Atherosclerosis—an inflammatory disease. *N Engl J Med* 340:115, 1999.
34. Steinhubl SR, Newby L, Sabatine M, et al: Platelets and atherothrombosis: an essential role for inflammation in vascular disease—a review. *Int J Angiol* 14:211, 2005.
35. Shankar A, Li J, Nieto FJ, et al: Association between C-reactive protein level and peripheral arterial disease among US adults without cardiovascular disease, diabetes, or hypertension. *Am Heart J* 154:495, 2007.
36. Rajagopalan S, McKay I, Ford I, et al: Platelet activation increases with the severity of peripheral arterial disease: implications for clinical management. *J Vasc Surg* 46:485, 2007.
37. Blann AD, Tan KT, Tayebjee MH, et al: Soluble CD40L in peripheral artery disease. Relationship with disease severity, platelet markers and the effects of angioplasty. *Thromb Haemost* 93:578, 2005.
38. Hiatt WR, Brass EP: Pathology of intermittent claudication. In Creager MA, Dzau VJ, Loscalzo J, editors: *Vascular medicine: a companion to Braunwald's heart disease*, Philadelphia, 2006, Elsevier, pp 239-347.
39. Aboyans V, Criqui MH, Denenberg JO, et al: Risk factors for progression of peripheral arterial disease in large and small vessels. *Circulation* 113:2623, 2006.
40. Olin JW: Clinical evaluation and office-based detection of peripheral arterial disease. Available at: www.svmb.org/medpro/cme/p1/cme_part1.html. Accessed November 2, 2000.
41. McDermott MM: Ankle brachial index as a predictor of outcomes in peripheral arterial disease. *J Lab Clin Med* 133:33, 1999.
42. Hiatt WR, Jones DN: The role of hemodynamics and duplex ultrasound in the diagnosis of peripheral arterial disease. *Curr Opin Cardiol* 7:805, 1992.
43. Papamichael CM, Lekakis JP, Stamatelopoulos KS, et al: Ankle-brachial index as a predictor of the extent of coronary atherosclerosis and cardiovascular events in patients with coronary artery disease. *Am J Cardiol* 86:615, 2000.
44. Weitz JI, Byrne J, Clagett GP, et al: Diagnosis and treatment of chronic arterial insufficiency of the lower extremities: a critical review. *Circulation* 94:3026, 1996.
45. Hiatt WR: Medical treatment of peripheral arterial disease and claudication. *N Engl J Med* 344:1608, 2001.
46. Dormandy JA, Rutherford RB: Management of peripheral arterial disease (PAD). TASC Working Group. TransAtlantic Inter-Society Consensus (TASC). *J Vasc Surg* 31(pt 2):S1, 2000.
47. Fowkes FG, Murray GD, Butcher I, et al: Ankle brachial index combined with Framingham Risk Score to predict cardiovascular events and mortality: a meta-analysis. *JAMA* 300:197, 2008.
48. Ouriel K, McDonnell AE, Metz CE, Zarins CK: Critical evaluation of stress testing in the diagnosis of peripheral vascular disease. *Surgery* 91:686, 1982.
49. Muller-Buhl U, Wiesemann A, Oser B, et al: Correlation of hemodynamic and functional variables with the angiographic extent of peripheral arterial occlusive disease. *Vascr Med* 4:247, 1999.
50. Yao ST, Hobbs JT, Irvine WT: Ankle systolic pressure measurements in arterial disease affecting the lower extremities. *Br J Surg* 56:676, 1969.
51. Reed JF, 3rd, Eid S, Edris B, Sumner AD: Prevalence of peripheral artery disease varies significantly depending upon the method of calculating ankle brachial index. *Eur J Cardiovasc Prev Rehabil* 16:377, 2009.
52. Espinola-Klein C, Rupprecht HJ, Bickel C, et al: Different calculations of ankle-brachial index and their impact on cardiovascular risk prediction. *Circulation* 118:961, 2008.
53. McDermott MM, Fried L, Simonsick E, et al: Asymptomatic peripheral arterial disease is independently associated with impaired lower extremity functioning: the women's health and aging study. *Circulation* 101:1007, 2000.
54. Baxter GM, Polak JF: Lower limb colour flow imaging: a comparison with ankle:brachial measurements and angiography. *Clin Radiol* 47:91, 1993.
55. Treiman GS, Oderich GS, Ashrafi A, Schneider PA: Management of ischemic heel ulceration and gangrene: an evaluation of factors associated with successful healing. *J Vasc Surg* 31:1110, 2000.
56. McDermott MM, Greenland P, Liu K, et al: Leg symptoms in peripheral arterial disease: associated clinical characteristics and functional impairment. *JAMA* 286:1599, 2001.
57. McDermott MM, Greenland P, Liu K, et al: The ankle brachial index is associated with leg function and physical activity: the Walking and Leg Circulation Study. *Ann Intern Med* 136:873, 2002.

58. McDermott MM, Ades P, Guralnik JM, et al: Treadmill exercise and resistance training in patients with peripheral arterial disease with and without intermittent claudication: a randomized controlled trial. *JAMA* 301:165, 2009.
59. Sen S, Lynch DR, Jr, Kaltsas E, et al: Association of asymptomatic peripheral arterial disease with vascular events in patients with stroke or transient ischemic attack. *Stroke* 40:3472, 2009.
60. Norgren L, Hiatt WR, Dormandy JA, et al: Inter-Society Consensus for the Management of Peripheral Arterial Disease (TASC II). *J Vasc Surg* 45(Suppl S):S5, 2007.
61. McPhail IR, Spittell PC, Weston SA, Bailey KR: Intermittent claudication: an objective office-based assessment. *J Am Coll Cardiol* 37:1381, 2001.
62. Amirhamzeh MM, Chant HJ, Rees JL, et al: A comparative study of treadmill tests and heel raising exercise for peripheral arterial disease. *Eur J Vasc Endovasc Surg* 13:301, 1997.
63. Stein R, Hriljac I, Halperin JL, et al: Limitation of the resting ankle-brachial index in symptomatic patients with peripheral arterial disease. *Vasc Med* 11:29, 2006.
64. Steg PG, Bhatt DL, Wilson PW, et al: One-year cardiovascular event rates in outpatients with atherothrombosis. *JAMA* 297:1197, 2007.
65. Diehm C, Allenberg JR, Pittrow D, et al: Mortality and vascular morbidity in older adults with asymptomatic versus symptomatic peripheral artery disease. *Circulation* 120:2053, 2009.
66. Cacoub PP, Bhatt DL, Steg PG, et al: Patients with peripheral arterial disease in the CHARISMA trial. *Eur Heart J* 30:192, 2009.
67. Ogren M, Hedblad B, Engstrom G, Janzon L: Prevalence and prognostic significance of asymptomatic peripheral arterial disease in 68-year-old men with diabetes. Results from the population study "Men born in 1914" from Malmö, Sweden. *Eur J Vasc Endovasc Surg* 29:182, 2005.
68. Weatherley BD, Nelson JJ, Heiss G, et al: The association of the ankle-brachial index with incident coronary heart disease: the Atherosclerosis Risk In Communities (ARIC) study, 1987-2001. *BMC Cardiovasc Disord* 7:3, 2007.
69. Hankey GJ, Norman PE, Eikelboom JW: Medical treatment of peripheral arterial disease. *JAMA* 295:547, 2006.
70. Golomb BA, Dang TT, Criqui MH: Peripheral arterial disease: morbidity and mortality implications. *Circulation* 114:688, 2006.
71. Executive Summary of The Third Report of The National Cholesterol Education Program (NCEP) Expert Panel on Detection, Evaluation, And Treatment of High Blood Cholesterol In Adults (Adult Treatment Panel III). *JAMA* 285:2486, 2001.
72. McDermott MM, Mehta S, Ahn H, Greenland P: Atherosclerotic risk factors are less intensively treated in patients with peripheral arterial disease than in patients with coronary artery disease. *J Gen Intern Med* 12:209, 1997.
73. Clark AL, Byrne JC, Nasser A, et al: Cholesterol in peripheral vascular disease—a suitable case for treatment? *QJM* 92:219, 1999.
74. Agarwal S: The association of active and passive smoking with peripheral arterial disease: results from NHANES 1999-2004. *Angiology* 60:335, 2009.
75. Lu JT, Creager MA: The relationship of cigarette smoking to peripheral arterial disease. *Revs Cardiovasc Med* 5:189, 2004.
76. Pedersen TR, Kjekshus J, Pyorala K, et al: Effect of simvastatin on ischemic signs and symptoms in the Scandinavian simvastatin survival study (4S). *Am J Cardiol* 81:333, 1998.
77. Randomized trial of the effects of cholesterol-lowering with simvastatin on peripheral vascular and other major vascular outcomes in 20,536 people with peripheral arterial disease and other high-risk conditions. *J Vasc Surg* 45:645; discussion 653, 2007.
78. Mohler ER, 3rd, Hiatt WR, Creager MA: Cholesterol reduction with atorvastatin improves walking distance in patients with peripheral arterial disease. *Circulation* 108:1481, 2003.
79. Aung PP, Maxwell HG, Jepson RG, et al: Lipid-lowering for peripheral arterial disease of the lower limb. *Cochrane Database Syst Rev* (4):CD000123, 2007.
80. Mehler PS, Coll JR, Estacio R, et al: Intensive blood pressure control reduces the risk of cardiovascular events in patients with peripheral arterial disease and type 2 diabetes. *Circulation* 107:753, 2003.
81. Radack K, Deck C: Beta-adrenergic blocker therapy does not worsen intermittent claudication in subjects with peripheral arterial disease. A meta-analysis of randomized controlled trials. *Arch Intern Med* 151:1769, 1991.
82. Yusuf S, Sleight P, Pogue J, et al: Effects of an angiotensin-converting-enzyme inhibitor, ramipril, on cardiovascular events in high-risk patients. The Heart Outcomes Prevention Evaluation Study Investigators. *N Engl J Med* 342:145, 2000.
83. Collaborative meta-analysis of randomised trials of antiplatelet therapy for prevention of death, myocardial infarction, and stroke in high risk patients. *BMJ* 324:71, 2002.
84. Belch J, MacCuish A, Campbell I, et al: The prevention of progression of arterial disease and diabetes (POPADAD) trial: factorial randomised placebo controlled trial of aspirin and antioxidants in patients with diabetes and asymptomatic peripheral arterial disease. *BMJ* 337:a1840, 2008.
85. Berger JS, Krantz MJ, Kittelson JM, Hiatt WR: Aspirin for the prevention of cardiovascular events in patients with peripheral artery disease: a meta-analysis of randomized trials. *JAMA* 301:1909, 2009.
86. Goldhaber SZ, Manson JE, Stampfer MJ, et al: Low-dose aspirin and subsequent peripheral arterial surgery in the Physicians' Health Study. *Lancet* 340:143, 1992.
87. Hess H, Mietaschk A, Deichsel G: Drug-induced inhibition of platelet function delays progression of peripheral occlusive arterial disease. A prospective double-blind arteriographically controlled trial. *Lancet* 1:415, 1985.
88. A randomised, blinded, trial of clopidogrel versus aspirin in patients at risk of ischaemic events (CAPRIE). CAPRIE Steering Committee. *Lancet* 348:1329, 1996.
89. Bhatt DL, Fox KA, Hacke W, et al: Clopidogrel and aspirin versus aspirin alone for the prevention of atherothrombotic events. *N Engl J Med* 354:1706, 2006.
90. Bhatt DL, Flather MD, Hacke W, et al: Patients with prior myocardial infarction, stroke, or symptomatic peripheral arterial disease in the CHARISMA trial. *J Am Coll Cardiol* 49:1982, 2007.
91. Neri Serneri GG, Coccheri S, Marubini E, Violi F: Picotamide, a combined inhibitor of thromboxane A_2 synthase and receptor, reduces 2-year mortality in diabetics with peripheral arterial disease: the DAVID study. *Eur Heart J* 25:1845, 2004.
92. Mohler ER, 3rd: Atherothrombosis—wave goodbye to combined anticoagulation and antiplatelet therapy? *N Engl J Med* 357:293, 2007.
93. Johnson WC, Williford WO: Benefits, morbidity, and mortality associated with long-term administration of oral anticoagulant therapy to patients with peripheral arterial bypass procedures: a prospective randomized study. *J Vasc Surg* 35:413, 2002.
94. Anand S, Yusuf S, Xie C, et al: Oral anticoagulant and antiplatelet therapy and peripheral arterial disease. *N Engl J Med* 357:217, 2007.
95. Thompson PD, Zimet R, Forbes WP, Zhang P: Meta-analysis of results from eight randomized, placebo-controlled trials on the effect of cilostazol on patients with intermittent claudication. *Am J Cardiol* 90:1314, 2002.
96. Hood SC, Moher D, Barber GG: Management of intermittent claudication with pentoxifylline: meta-analysis of randomized controlled trials. *CMAJ* 155:1053, 1996.
97. Gardner AW, Poehlman ET: Exercise rehabilitation programs for the treatment of claudication pain. A meta-analysis. *JAMA* 274:975, 1995.
98. Garg PK, Tian L, Criqui MH, et al: Physical activity during daily life and mortality in patients with peripheral arterial disease. *Circulation* 114:242, 2006.
99. Lichtenstein AH, Appel LJ, Brands M, et al: Diet and lifestyle recommendations revision 2006: a scientific statement from the American Heart Association Nutrition Committee. *Circulation* 114:82, 2006.
100. Johnston KW, Rutherford RB, Tilson MD, et al: Suggested standards for reporting on arterial aneurysms. Subcommittee on Reporting Standards for Arterial Aneurysms, Ad Hoc Committee on Reporting Standards, Society for Vascular Surgery and North American Chapter, International Society for Cardiovascular Surgery. *J Vasc Surg* 13:452, 1991.
101. Ebaugh JL, Garcia ND, Matsumura JS: Screening and surveillance for abdominal aortic aneurysms: who needs it and when. *Semin Vasc Surg* 14:193, 2001.
102. Heron M: Deaths: leading causes for 2004. National vital statistics reports; vol 56, no 5. Hyattsville, Md, National Center for Health Statistics. Available at: http://www.cdc.gov/nchs/data/dvs/LCWK1_2006.pdf. Accessed October 29, 2009.
103. Lederle FA, Johnson GR, Wilson SE, et al: Prevalence and associations of abdominal aortic aneurysm detected through screening. Aneurysm Detection and Management (ADAM) Veterans Affairs Cooperative Study Group. *Ann Intern Med* 126:441, 1997.
104. Wilmink TB, Quick CR, Day NE: The association between cigarette smoking and abdominal aortic aneurysms. *J Vasc Surg* 30:1099, 1999.
105. Powell JT, Greenhalgh RM: Clinical practice. Small abdominal aortic aneurysms. *N Engl J Med* 348:1895, 2003.
106. Verloes A, Sakalihasan N, Koulischer L, Limet R: Aneurysms of the abdominal aorta: familial and genetic aspects in three hundred thirteen pedigrees. *J Vasc Surg* 21:646, 1995.
107. Darling RC, 3rd, Brewster DC, Darling RC, et al: Are familial abdominal aortic aneurysms different? *J Vasc Surg* 10:39, 1989.
108. Webster MW, Ferrell RE, St Jean PL, et al: Ultrasound screening of first-degree relatives of patients with an abdominal aortic aneurysm. *J Vasc Surg* 13:9; discussion 13, 1991.
109. Lederle FA, Johnson GR, Wilson SE, et al: The aneurysm detection and management study screening program: validation cohort and final results. Aneurysm Detection and Management Veterans Affairs Cooperative Study Investigators. *Arch Internal Med* 160:1425, 2000.
110. Allardice JT, Allwright GJ, Wafula JM, Wyatt AP: High prevalence of abdominal aortic aneurysm in men with peripheral vascular disease: screening by ultrasonography. *Br J Surg* 75:240, 1988.
111. Cabellon S, Jr, Moncrief CL, Pierre DR, Cavanaugh DG: Incidence of abdominal aortic aneurysms in patients with atheromatous arterial disease. *Am J Surg* 146:575, 1983.
112. Lederle FA, Larson JC, Margolis KL, et al: Abdominal aortic aneurysm events in the women's health initiative: cohort study. *BMJ* 337:a1724, 2008.
113. Lederle FA: Ultrasonographic screening for abdominal aortic aneurysms. *Ann Intern Med* 139:516, 2003.
114. Bengtsson H, Bergqvist D, Sternby NH: Increasing prevalence of abdominal aortic aneurysms. A necropsy study. *Eur J Surg* 158:19, 1992.
115. Lederle FA, Simel DL: The rational clinical examination. Does this patient have abdominal aortic aneurysm? *JAMA* 281:77, 1999.
116. Screening for abdominal aortic aneurysm: recommendation statement. *Ann Intern Med* 142:198, 2005.
117. Ashton HA, Buxton MJ, Day NE, et al: The Multicentre Aneurysm Screening Study (MASS) into the effect of abdominal aortic aneurysm screening on mortality in men: a randomised controlled trial. *Lancet* 360:1531, 2002.
118. Derubertis BG, Trocciola SM, Ryer EJ, et al: Abdominal aortic aneurysm in women: prevalence, risk factors, and implications for screening. *J Vasc Surg* 46:630, 2007.
119. Lederle FA, MacDonald R, Wilt TJ: Anticoagulant prophylaxis for hospitalized medical patients. *Ann Intern Med* 147:523; author reply 524, 2007.
120. Steyerberg EW, Kievit J, de Mol Van Otterloo JC, et al: Perioperative mortality of elective abdominal aortic aneurysm surgery. A clinical prediction rule based on literature and individual patient data. *Arch Intern Med* 155:1998, 1995.
121. Heller JA, Weinberg A, Arons R, et al: Two decades of abdominal aortic aneurysm repair: have we made any progress? *J Vasc Surg* 32:1091, 2000.
122. Huber TS, Wang JG, Derrow AE, et al: Experience in the United States with intact abdominal aortic aneurysm repair. *J Vasc Surg* 33:304; discussion 310, 2001.
123. Lederle FA, Freischlag JA, Kyriakides TC, et al: Outcomes following endovascular vs open repair of abdominal aortic aneurysm: a randomized trial. *JAMA* 302:1535, 2009.
124. Cao P, Verzini F, Parlani G, et al: Clinical effect of abdominal aortic aneurysm endografting: 7-year concurrent comparison with open repair. *J Vasc Surg* 40:841, 2004.
125. Mealy K, Salman A: The true incidence of ruptured abdominal aortic aneurysms. *Eur J Vasc Surg* 2:405, 1988.
126. Johansen K, Kohler TR, Nicholls SC, et al: Ruptured abdominal aortic aneurysm: the Harborview experience. *J Vasc Surg* 13:240, 1991.

127. Heikkinen M, Salenius J, Zeitlin R, et al: The fate of AAA patients referred electively to vascular surgical unit. *Scand J Surg* 91:345, 2002.

128. Welten GM, Schouten O, Hoeks SE, et al: Long-term prognosis of patients with peripheral arterial disease: a comparison in patients with coronary artery disease. *J Am Coll Cardiol* 51:1588, 2008.

129. Lederle FA, Johnson GR, Wilson SE, et al: Rupture rate of large abdominal aortic aneurysms in patients refusing or unfit for elective repair. *JAMA* 287:2968, 2002.

130. Brewster DC, Cronenwett JL, Hallett JW Jr, et al: Guidelines for the treatment of abdominal aortic aneurysms. Report of a subcommittee of the Joint Council of the American Association for Vascular Surgery and Society for Vascular Surgery. *J Vasc Surg* 37:1106, 2003.

131. Urbonavicius S, Urbonaviciene G, Honore B, et al: Potential circulating biomarkers for abdominal aortic aneurysm expansion and rupture—a systematic review. *Eur J Vasc Endovasc Surg* 36:273; discussion 281, 2008.

132. Golledge J, Tsao PS, Dalman RL, Norman PE: Circulating markers of abdominal aortic aneurysm presence and progression. *Circulation* 118:2382, 2008.

133. Norman PE, Powell JT: Abdominal aortic aneurysm: the prognosis in women is worse than in men. *Circulation* 115:2865, 2007.

134. Wong F, Brown LC, Powell JT: Can we predict aneurysm rupture? In Becquemin J-P, Alimi Y, editors: *Controversies and updates in vascular surgery*, Torino, Italy, 2006, Medica Italy, pp 35-43.

135. Sicard GA: The impact of a well structured vascular registry in assessing the long-term survival after repair of abdominal aortic aneurysms. *Circulation* 120:188, 2009.

136. Anderson PL, Arons RR, Moskowitz AJ, et al: A statewide experience with endovascular abdominal aortic aneurysm repair: rapid diffusion with excellent early results. *J Vasc Surg* 39:10, 2004.

137. Giles KA, Pomposelli F, Hamdan A, et al: Decrease in total aneurysm-related deaths in the era of endovascular aneurysm repair. *J Vasc Surg* 49:543; discussion 550, 2009.

138. Mani K, Bjorck M, Lundkvist J, Wanhainen A: Improved long-term survival after abdominal aortic aneurysm repair. *Circulation* 120:201, 2009.

31

Peripheral Arterial Disease Assessment and Management

Endothelial Function and Dysfunction

Mary C. Corretti, Gurusher S. Panjrath, and Steven R. Jones

KEY POINTS

- Advances in vascular biology and imaging technology have greatly contributed to further elucidation of the complexities of vascular structure and function and the significance of the endothelium in the development of atherosclerosis.

- Vascular endothelium is a vast dynamic paracrine system that regulates several key biologic and molecular functions serving to maintain vascular health and homeostasis.

- The endothelium functions primarily to modulate vascular tone/vasomotion, to maintain an anticoagulant/profibrinolytic state, to inhibit platelet aggregation and adhesion, to inhibit vascular smooth muscle cell proliferation and migration, and to maintain an anti-inflammatory milieu.

- Endothelial activation refers to the biologic response to impairment in vascular homeostasis that engenders a new molecular or functional homeostasis.

- Environmental and genetic factors, such as cardiovascular risk factors, impose an oxidative stress on the vasculature through mechanisms such as the nitric oxide pathway.

- Translational research from experimental discoveries in vascular biology to the clinical arena has spawned applications of new and emerging invasive and noninvasive techniques to measure endothelial function and dysfunction.

- Ongoing research in the development and application of primarily noninvasive imaging techniques to measure endothelial function

and dysfunction continues in the pursuit of tests for subclinical disease states, targeting therapeutic strategies and prognosis.

More commonly the arterio-sclerosis results from the bad use of good vessels.
William Osler (*The Principles and Practice of Medicine,* 1892)

Cardiovascular disease incurs a major burden to the public health and health care system. In the past several decades, advances in vascular biology have greatly contributed to our understanding of the complexities of vascular structure and function and the significance of the endothelium in the development of atherosclerosis. Atherosclerosis is a ubiquitous, complex disease process that is dynamic and multifactorial. Genetic and various environmental factors, with their complex interactions, lead to the initiation and progression of atherosclerosis during decades. The vascular endothelium, the largest paracrine organ, vastly forms the inner lining of all blood vessels in the vasculature to maintain vascular homeostasis through myriad complex biologic properties and physiologic processes. Strategically located between the vessel lumen and smooth muscle layer, the endothelium serves to modulate vascular tone, cell growth, platelet and leukocyte interactions, inflammation, and thrombogenicity.

Physical and chemical stimuli in the vascular milieu initiate and propagate diverse physiologic and molecular processes through signal transduction mechanisms not yet fully understood and through the elaboration and secretion of various substances. The magnitude and duration of exposure to cardiovascular risk factors impose injury on the vasculature, primarily through oxidative stress mechanisms that promote procoagulation, inflammation, vasoconstriction, and proliferation of cell growth. The complexity of atherosclerosis translates into a continuum of cardiovascular disease processes that manifest derangements in endothelial functions, which begin early in the pathogenesis of disease. The study of endothelium from cell to organ system poses the challenge for development and application of various genetic and chemical biomarkers and imaging

modalities for diagnosis, therapeutics, and prognosis.

Various invasive and noninvasive imaging modalities have evolved in the last several decades to clinically evaluate structure and function of various vascular beds in health and disease states. Advances in experimental and clinical research underscore the complexity of vascular homeostasis. Perturbations in vascular homeostasis induced by environmental factors or the local biologic milieu are manifestations of endothelial dysfunction that require further definition of the specific vascular property involved. The term *endothelial activation* refers to the biologic response to impairment in vascular homeostasis that engenders a new molecular functional homeostasis.[1]

Imaging techniques to assess endothelial function, particularly vascular vasomotion, emerged concurrently with the advances in vascular biology, coupled with a keen interest in the use of biomarkers and imaging modalities and techniques to detect subclinical disease while targeting preventive and therapeutic interventions. Investigation continues in the clinical applications to enhance early detection and to guide therapy and prognosis.

ENDOTHELIUM AND ENDOTHELIAL PHYSIOLOGY: GENERAL OVERVIEW

Malpighi's discovery in the 17th century of the endothelium as a physical separation between blood and tissue with no substantial functionality persisted through the 19th and mid-20th centuries. The endothelium is a 0.2- to 4-μm-thick monolayer of squamous endothelial cells lining the entire surface of the vasculature, including endocardium, arteries, arterioles, capillaries, venules,

TABLE 32–1	Role of Endothelium in Vascular Homeostasis

Vascular tone
Vascular permeability
Vascular remodeling
Anticoagulant, profibrinolytic, and procoagulant activities
Inflammatory and immunopathologic responses
Interactions with blood components

Healthy endothelium

Vasodilatory: endothelium dependent
Antihypertrophic: inhibits vascular smooth muscle cell proliferation and migration
Anticoagulant and profibrinolytic
Antithrombotic: inhibits platelet adhesion and aggregation
Anti-inflammatory: inhibits leukocyte adhesion and migration

veins, adventitial vasa vasorum, and other microcirculation.[1] Once thought to be a passive, semipermeable membrane between blood flow and vascular wall, the endothelium is essentially a vast autocrine, paracrine, and endocrine organ that spans a surface area of approximately 700 m^2.

The endothelium is strategically located at the interface of the blood circulation, blood components, and vascular smooth muscle and adventitia. As such, the endothelium is the major regulator of vascular homeostasis, which occurs through myriad diverse and interrelated physiologic functions. These include the regulation of vasomotion, smooth muscle cell proliferation, inflammation, thrombolysis, homeostasis, platelet aggregation, immune responses, cell proliferation, and free radical production. Normal healthy endothelium exerts a variety of effects to maintain vascular homeostasis of these various biologic functions (Table 32-1). It performs these functions through an elaborate array of secretable substances and signal transduction mechanisms in response to a number of different physiologic, chemical, and mechanical stimuli within and around its surrounding milieu and external environmental factors.[1-3]

One of the pivotal roles of the endothelium is the modulation of vascular tone, caliber, and blood flow in response to neural, humoral, and mechanical stimuli by synthesis and release of various vasoactive substances.[2-4] Specifically, the endothelium plays a key role in regulation of hemostasis and thrombosis, vascular tone, inflammation, and vascular growth and remodeling under normal conditions. Laminar stress is among the most important stimuli that help maintain the normal physiologic state of the endothelium. This is attained by reduction of biologic activity of proteins by S-nitrosylation of cysteine residues and oxidative phosphorylation in mitochondria.[5,6] However, during exposure to risk factors such as hypertension, diabetes mellitus, and tobacco smoking, dysfunction of endothelium ensues, thus disturbing the fine balance and subsequently resulting in atherosclerosis.

Vasomotion

Regulation of vascular tone by endothelium is achieved by generation and secretion of vasoactive substances. The endothelium exerts a significant effect on both vasodilation and vasoconstriction. Endothelium-mediated vasodilation is predominantly achieved by nitric oxide (NO) and prostacyclins (PGI$_2$). Endothelium-mediated vasoconstriction is regulated by secretion of angiotensin II, platelet-derived growth factors, platelet-activating factor, and endothelin 1, all of which have vasoconstrictive effects.[7] NO serves as an important vasodilator and forms a major basis for endothelial function and dysfunction.

Prostacyclin, another vasodilator synthesized in the endothelium, is a product of arachidonic acid, which is released from membrane phospholipids in response to shear stress.[1,8] Vasodilator effects of prostacyclins are dependent on expression of receptors in vascular smooth muscles. This limits the role of endothelium-mediated vasodilation in vascular beds where receptors are not expressed. Prostacyclins do not contribute to the maintenance of basal vascular tone of large conduit arteries. Prostacyclins mediate their effect through receptors coupled to adenylate cyclase and elevation of cyclic adenosine monophosphate (cAMP) levels in vascular smooth muscles, stimulation of ATP-sensitive potassium channels, hyperpolarization of cell membrane, and thus inhibition of the development of contraction. Inhibition of the contractile mechanism is also mediated by the expelling of calcium from the cytosol of vascular smooth muscles. In addition, prostacyclins contribute to release of NO by endothelial cells and have a synergistic effect with NO on antiplatelet activity.

Endothelin 1

Endothelin 1 (ET-1) is a potent vasoconstrictor generated in the endothelial cells along with other cell lines. It belongs to a family of structurally related peptides including ET-1, ET-2, and ET-3.[9,10] Mature human ET-1 is derived from a precursor, preproendothelin 1, through an intermediate molecule and requires a peptidase named ET-converting enzyme. This peptidase serves as a critical physiologic regulator of ET-1 activity. Shear stress and cyclic stress, along with other factors such as hypoxia, stimulate generation of ET-1 from endothelial cells. The vasoconstrictor effect of ET-1 is mediated by binding to ET$_A$ on vascular smooth muscle cells. The effect on NO and PGI$_2$ generation is mediated by binding to ET$_B$ receptors on the endothelium.

Vascular beds exhibit heterogeneity in vasoconstrictor response to ET-1. Whereas the renal endothelium and the coronary endothelium are extremely sensitive to ET-1, the pulmonary circulation exhibits a less sensitive response. In addition to vasoconstriction, ET-1 exhibits a wide range of activities. It has a positive inotropic effect on cardiomyocytes and stimulates release of atrial natriuretic peptide from atrial myocytes. In addition, it aids in release of aldosterone and catecholamines from the adrenal cortex and medulla. ET-1 augments the vascular actions of other vasoactive peptides (such as angiotensin II, norepinephrine, and serotonin), participates in leukocyte and platelet activation, and thus facilitates a prothrombotic state.[11,12] It also has an inhibitory effect on renin release from juxtaglomerular cells. Finally, it enhances release of endothelium-derived relaxing factor and PGI$_2$ and modulates vascular remodeling.[13]

Inflammation

The endothelium, as a result of its location, serves as a potent anti-inflammatory tissue. It is constantly exposed to various pathogens, anti-inflammatory cells, and immunoreactive substances. Disease states or exposures such as hypertension and atherosclerosis constitute inflammatory changes in the vascular wall. Inflammatory changes include altered expression of adhesion molecules. Under shear stress, endothelial cells exhibit a number of anti-inflammatory properties. This response includes prevention of adhesion of circulating inflammatory cells to endothelial cells and release of immunoreactive substances. NO released from endothelial cells aids in limiting leukocyte adhesion. Furthermore, NO has an inhibitory effect on release of prothrombotic substances, such as von Willebrand factor and P-selection.

NO limits activation of nuclear factor-κB (NF-κB) and thus inhibits adhesion molecule expression and subsequent attachment of immune cells to endothelium. Endothelial dysfunction, as a result of oxidative stress in the endothelial cells, results in activation of NF-κB, a redox-sensitive transcription factor. Subsequent steps include release of chemoattractant proteins such as monocyte chemotactic protein 1 and expression of adhesion molecules (E-selectin, P-selectin, intercellular adhesion molecule 1 [ICAM-1], and vascular cell adhesion molecule 1 [VCAM-1]). This results in monocyte attachment and rolling through the selectins, activation through selectins and chemokines (CCL2, CXCL8, and platelet-activating factor), arrest and adherence through the immunoglobulin G family (ICAM-1, VCAM-1) and integrins ($\alpha_V\beta_3$), and finally extravasation through platelet/endothelial cell adhesion molecule 1. Other molecules involved in extravasation of leukocytes include cadherins.[14,15]

Hemostasis and Thrombosis

The endothelium serves as a lining of a compartment that maintains blood flow while permitting delivery of important nutrients to other organs in the body. It serves this purpose by inhibiting platelet aggregation and clotting cascade activation. It achieves the antithrombotic properties by generating anticoagulants (antithrombin III, thrombomodulin, tissue factor pathway inhibitor, protein C, and heparan sulfate proteoglycans), fibrinolytics (tissue-type plasminogen activators and urokinase-type plasminogen activators), and platelet inhibitors (NO, prostacyclins, and ADPase [CD39]). On the opposite end of the spectrum, the endothelium maintains hemostasis by production and release of procoagulants (thrombin receptor, protein C receptor, tissue factor, and coagulation factor binding sites) and antifibrinolytics (plasminogen activator inhibitor 1) and by promotion of platelet activation (von Willebrand factor and platelet-activating factor).

Whereas normal endothelial cells do not express procoagulants such as tissue factor, activated endothelial cells rapidly express the same on their cell surface. Similarly, von Willebrand factor is stored in endothelial cells in granules called Weibel-Palade bodies, which are exposed on the endothelial surface in response to injury and other soluble mediators, resulting in formation of a hemostatic plug and platelet adhesion.[1]

Vascular Growth and Remodeling

With better understanding of developmental biology, it is now evident that a close relationship exists between endothelial cells and the hematopoietic cell lineage. It is now known that hemangioblasts may be the common precursor for both cell lineages. The hemangioblasts differentiate into either blood cell precursors or angioblasts, which are endothelial cell precursors.[16] Vessel growth or angiogenesis after the initial process of development of blood vessels involves formation of capillary sprouts by endothelial cells.[17] This process subsequently leads to remodeling and formation of a mature vessel.

Endothelial cells play an important role in the remodeling process during development by secretion of substances that recruit undifferentiated mesenchymal cells and cause their maturation into pericytes or smooth cells.[18] During endothelial dysfunction, in adult cells, vascular smooth muscle proliferation takes place in the presence of oxidative stress and as a result of decrease in endothelium-derived NO, which has an inhibitor effect on vascular smooth muscle growth.

It is now known that the endothelium along with the vasa vasorum contributes to angiogenesis and neovessel formation in atheromas. These neovessels are instrumental in atherosclerotic plaque progression, instability, and rupture. The microvascular channels formed by invagination of endothelial lumen may also serve for the transport of inflammatory cells, such as leukocytes. This is supported by selectively increased VCAM expression on microvascular endothelial cells.[19] In addition to leukocyte migration, microvessels cause intraplaque neovascularization, thus leading to hyperpermeability, and result in microhemorrhage and thrombosis.[19,20] Evidence of hemosiderin deposits in the neovascular plexus and their colocalization with thrombotic factors such as von Willebrand factor suggest hemorrhage and thrombosis within the atheroma. Hyperpermeable neovessels allow extravasation of red blood cells.[21] Lysis of red blood cells contributes to plaque progression by lipid expansion as their membranes are rich in cholesterol and generation of reactive oxygen species and macrophage activation.[20] As discussed elsewhere, reactive oxygen species deplete endothelium-derived NO and thus limit its inhibitory effect on vascular smooth muscle growth.

Nitric Oxide Pathway

In the early 1980s, Furchgott and Zawadski[22] first demonstrated the obligatory role of the endothelium for vascular relaxation in response to vasoactive substances such as acetylcholine and postulated the existence of an endothelium-derived relaxing factor, later discovered to be NO.[1,23,24] Of all substances secreted or controlled by the endothelium, NO is the most recognized molecule; it is pivotal in maintaining vascular tone and mediates inhibition of coagulation, platelet activation, smooth muscle cell proliferation, and inflammation. Inadequate or lack of NO is implicated in endothelial dysfunction.

NO is produced by the endothelial cells from l-arginine (Fig. 32-1). It is a heterodiatomic lipophilic free radical that is synthesized by endothelial nitric oxide synthase, a heme-containing NAD(P)H-dependent oxygenase that requires cofactors tetrahydrobiopterin and nicotinamide adenine dinucleotide phosphate.[25] Three distinct isoforms of nitric oxide synthase (NOS) are known to exist: endothelial NOS (eNOS), inducible NOS (iNOS), and neuronal NOS (nNOS). All three isoforms belong to a family of arginine hydroxylases.[26] Most of the NO production takes place in invaginations of the cell membrane (caveolae) of endothelial cells. It is made from the amino acid l-arginine, which is converted to l-citrulline by means of eNOS. Caveolin 1 regulates the activity of eNOS by binding to calmodulin, with the resultant inhibition of eNOS. However, eNOS activation and NO production are achieved by binding of calcium to calmodulin, causing a displacement of caveolin.[27,28]

Activity and synthesis of eNOS are modulated by physiologic inhibitors, such as asymmetric dimethylarginine and geranylgeranyl pyrophosphate (intermediate of cholesterol biosynthesis), or pharmacologic inhibitors, such as N^G-monomethyl-l-arginine (l-NMMA) and l-nitroarginine methyl ester. NO, a potent endogenous vasodilator, is basally secreted in response to various physiologic agonists, physical stimuli, and pharmacologic agents. It exerts its effect on vascular tone in multiple ways. The basal secretion of NO maintains the vessel in a vasodilatory state and assists in maintaining vascular health through its various antiatherogenic properties.

Once it is secreted, NO diffuses into the subendothelium and exerts a vasodilator effect on vascular smooth muscle cells. It activates the soluble guanylate cyclase, followed by an increase of the intracellular concentration of cyclic guanosine monophosphate. This results in a reduction in the intracellular calcium concentration, followed by a relaxation of vascular smooth muscle cells.[29] In addition, it decreases the expression and activity of the potent vasoconstrictor ET-1. NO has an inhibitory effect on vascular smooth muscle proliferation and migration and extracellular matrix production.[29] NO exerts this effect by inhibiting the activation of NF-κB. This particular attribute contributes to

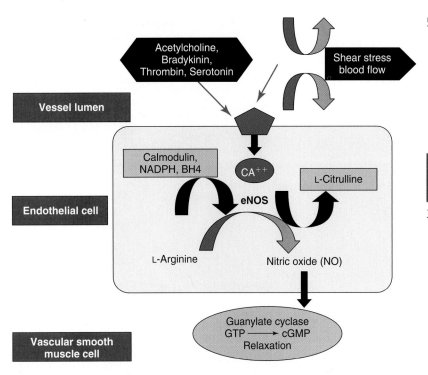

FIGURE 32-1 Production and release of nitric oxide leading to vasodilation. BH4, tetrahydrobiopterin; Ca^{2+}, calcium ion; cGMP, cyclic guanosine monophosphate; eNOS, endothelial nitric oxide synthase; GC, guanylate cyclase; GTP, guanosine triphosphate; NADPH, reduced nicotinamide adenine dinucleotide phosphate. *(Modified from Behrendt D, Ganz P: Endothelial function. From vascular biology to clinical applications. Am J Cardiol 90:40, 2002.)*

anti-inflammatory as well as to antiproliferative properties.[30,31] NO exerts its inhibitory effect on platelet activation and aggregation by stimulation of the cAMP pathway. Its effect on the fibrinolysis system is mediated by stimulation of tissue plasminogen activator release.[32] However, the effect on mobilization of progenitor cells and stem cell modulation of their survival and function are areas of immense interest.[33]

Diminished NO activity may be due to four distinct causes: decreased expression of eNOS enzyme, eNOS uncoupling, increased scavenging of NO, and impaired transmission of NO-mediated signaling.[34,35] Both physical and humoral stimuli can activate the transcription of eNOS gene. Activation of eNOS by physical stimuli such as shear stress is mediated by Raf, Ras, and ERK1/2 and NF-κB binding to shear stress response element.[36] Humoral factors influencing eNOS transcription include growth factors (vascular endothelial growth factor, basic fibroblast growth factor, epidermal growth factor, and transforming growth factor-β), cytokines, and oxygen radicals.

Uncoupling of eNOS refers to the process by which eNOS switches its predominant function of NO generation to reactive oxygen species formation. When this switch occurs as a result of tetrahydrobiopterin deficiency, generation of oxidants such as superoxide is dominant. However, deficiency of l-arginine also leads to production of hydrogen peroxide.[11] Superoxide anions rapidly interact with NO to form peroxynitrite. Peroxynitrite in turn decreases tetrahydrobiopterin and results in increased consumption and reduced production of NO.[35,36] Figure 32-2 summarizes the mechanism of decreased NO bioavailability mediated by reactive oxygen species. In addition, various factors known to regulate eNOS gene expression mediate endothelial function and dysfunction (Table 32-2).

ENDOTHELIAL DYSFUNCTION

No single definition of endothelial dysfunction exists, given the complex and ubiquitous nature of endothelial biology.

Endothelial dysfunction was first described as structural changes or loss of anatomic integrity in the context of atherosclerosis.[37] Endothelial dysfunction includes broad regulatory changes leading to abnormal vasomotion and the expression of a prothrombotic and proinflammatory phenotype of the vascular endothelium. This poses a challenge to define endothelial dysfunction in terms that include all the possible alterations in vascular homeostasis and at various time points in various disease states.

Endothelial dysfunction encompasses any alterations in the diverse vascular biology and function, particularly vasomotor function as well as the prothrombotic, proinflammatory, proatherogenic properties. Endothelial activation refers to the biologic response to alterations or impairment in vascular homeostasis that would elicit new molecular or functional homeostasis, including gene activation[1] and the repair response to damaged endothelium.[38,39]

Chronic exposure to injury stimuli and reactive oxygen species may surpass the inherent capacity of the endothelium to mount a suitable defense. This may subsequently lead to aging and senescence of the endothelial cells. Finally, the senescent endothelial cells may detach and be released in the circulation.

Activated endothelial cells, apoptotic cells, and their components in the circulation thus may serve as markers for endothelial dysfunction.[40] The levels of these cell types and their components have been shown to be increased in several inflammatory states, such as coronary artery disease, rheumatoid arthritis, and systemic lupus erythematosus.[41,42] Endothelial repair may be due to repopulation of the denuded endothelium by replication of adjacent mature endothelial cells or from circulating endothelial progenitor cells.[43]

Endothelial progenitor cells are circulating precursors recruited from the bone marrow, partly by NO-dependent mechanisms. These cells may transform into mature endothelial cells and contribute to maintenance of endothelial integrity and health. The extent to which this mechanism may be successful depends on the exposure to cardiovascular risk factors and inflammatory stimuli. Under certain circumstances, these cells may transform into macrophages and thus

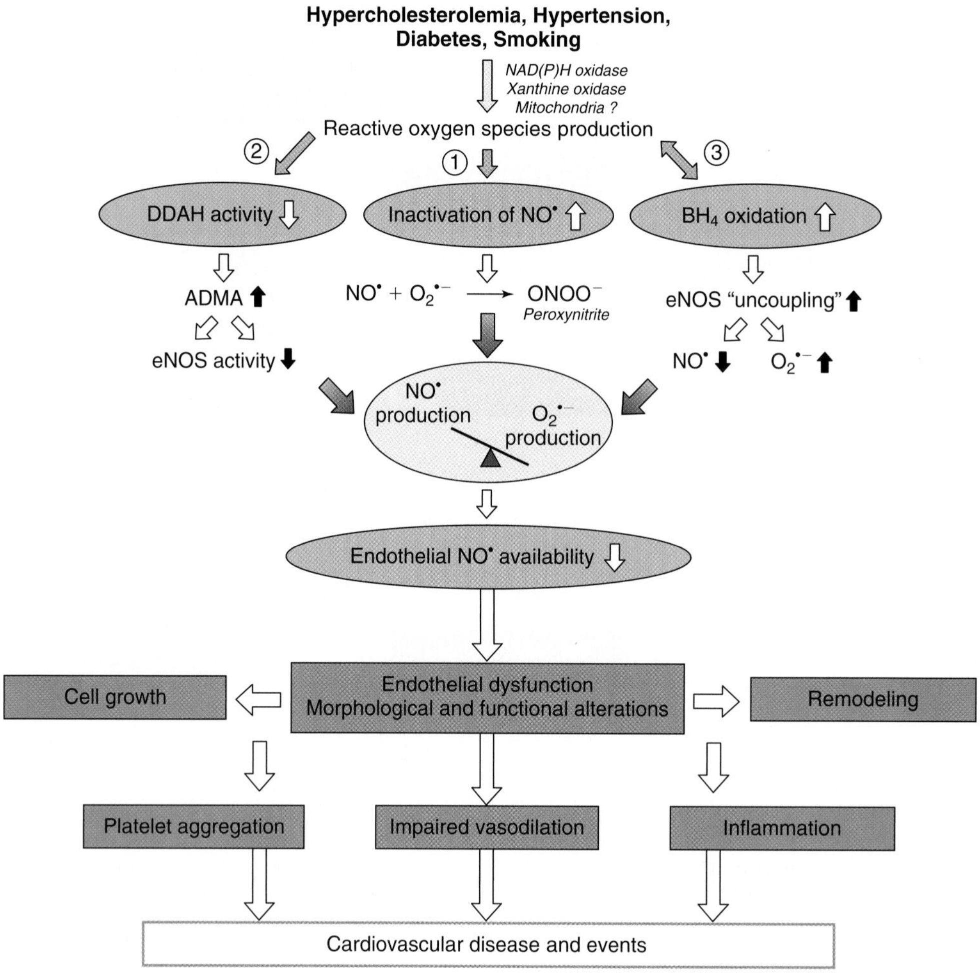

FIGURE 32-2 Schematic representation of mechanisms of decreased NO bioavailability resulting in endothelial dysfunction. Reactive oxygen species decrease the bioavailability of NO in endothelium by three different mechanisms: (1) superoxide reacts with NO to form peroxynitrite anions, causing a diminished bioavailability of NO; (2) reactive oxygen species cause an increased concentration of ADMA, an endogenous inhibitor of eNOS; and (3) uncoupling of eNOS enzyme due to degradation of BH$_4$. ADMA, asymmetric dimethylarginine; BH$_4$, tetrahydrobiopterin; DDAH, dimethylarginine dimethylaminohydrolase; eNOS, endothelial NO synthase; NO, nitric oxide. *(From Landmesser U, Hornig B, Drexler H: Endothelial function: a critical determinant in atherosclerosis?* Circulation *109[Suppl 1]:II27, 2004.)*

may contribute to endothelial dysfunction. Modification of risk factors by interventions such as exercise and statins, as discussed later, may help in mobilization of endothelial progenitor cells and aid in repair.[44,45] Any imbalance between injury and repair may result in endothelial dysfunction. Whereas levels of endothelial progenitor cells may be increased on exposure to acute insult, chronic inflammatory states result in reduced levels. Reduced levels of endothelial progenitor cells may be a result of overconsumption, inhibited mobilization, or accelerated senescence. Risk factors, by modulating the levels of oxidative stress or NO activity, may influence the levels of circulating progenitor cells. The precise underlying mechanism needs to be understood better.

Oxidative Stress and Endothelial Dysfunction

Oxidative stress refers to a state whereby the rate of formation of reactive oxygen species exceeds the capacity of physiologic antioxidant defense mechanisms. Chronic exposure to reactive oxidative species may overwhelm the inherent antioxidative mechanism and thus contribute to endothelial dysfunction or prolonged endothelial activation. Several enzyme systems are sources of free radical production (reactive oxygen

species), including NAD(P)H oxidases, nitric oxide synthases, lipoxygenases, cyclooxygenases, oxidoreductases, and mitochondrial oxidases.[46] Balance between production of reactive oxygen species and activity of superoxide dismutase during oxidative phosphorylation is maintained in normal physiologic conditions.[47]

An abundance of reactive oxidant species alters several important physiologic functions, including regulation of blood flow, vasodilation, coagulation, inflammation, and cellular growth, and activates multiple signaling pathways in vascular wall cells that also contribute to the impairments of vascular function and repair. On exposure to risk factors such as obesity and diabetes mellitus, there is an alteration in this balance due to increased substrate delivery, such as circulating free fatty acids.[13,45] In coronary artery disease, increased oxidative stress is a result of increased nicotinamide adenine dinucleotide phosphate oxidases and xanthine oxidase.[34,35,46,47] As depicted in Figure 32-2, diverse risk factors result in increased oxidative stress and contribute to decreased NO bioavailability by three distinct mechanisms. Production of superoxide is increased in the diseased vessels of patients with coronary vascular disease.[48] Superoxide interacts with NO, forming peroxynitrite anions, resulting in consumption of NO and loss of its activity.[48,49]

TABLE 32–2	Factors Regulating Endothelial Nitric Oxide Synthase Gene Expression	
Factors		**Effect**
Physical factors		
Shear stress		Stimulation
Hydrostatic pressure		Stimulation
Humoral factors		
Reactive oxygen species		
Nitric oxide		Inhibition
Oxidized low-density lipoprotein		Inhibition
H_2O_2		Stimulation
Inflammatory factors		
Tumor necrosis factor-α		Inhibition
Growth factors		
Vascular endothelial growth factor		Stimulation
Basic fibroblast growth factor		Stimulation
Epidermal growth factor		Stimulation
Transforming growth factor-β		Stimulation
Peptide hormones		
Angiotensin II		Stimulation
Endothelin 1		Stimulation
Erythropoietin		Stimulation or inhibition

NO is a key mediator in vascular homeostasis as it serves as an antiatherogenic molecule, promotes vasodilation, and counteracts inflammation, platelet aggregation, and vascular smooth muscle proliferation. A large body of evidence supports the tenet that endothelial dysfunction is caused to some degree by accelerated inactivation of NO by reactive oxygen species, although exact mechanisms are not entirely elucidated and strategies for targeted therapy are still under investigation. Another mechanism is the redox-dependent inhibition of the enzyme dimethylarginine dimethylaminohydrolase. This results in increased concentration of the endogenous eNOS inhibitor asymmetric dimethylarginine (ADMA). Levels of ADMA are elevated in a large number of conditions, including several associated with risk of endothelial dysfunction.[50,51] ADMA concentration may be increased because of impaired excretion or increased synthesis, as in the case of vascular shear stress.[50,51] Accumulation of ADMA acts as a competitive antagonist to the eNOS substrate L-arginine.

Role of Endothelial Dysfunction in the Presence of Specific Risk Factors and Atherosclerotic Disease

Several risk factors may play a critical role in contributing to endothelial dysfunction and thus atherosclerosis. Traditional and novel cardiovascular risk factors, including smoking, aging, hyperlipidemia, hypertension, diabetes, and family history of premature atherosclerosis, among others, are associated with a loss or attenuation of endothelium-dependent vasodilation in both children and adults.[52,53] Elevated C-reactive protein, chronic systemic infection, obesity, and several immune-mediated diseases are also associated with impaired endothelial function.[54,55] Given its complex biology, the term *endothelial dysfunction* applies broadly to the various perturbations that contribute over time to the development and clinical expression of atherosclerosis.

The underlying mechanism through which risk factors impart vascular injury initiating endothelial dysfunction is indeed multifactorial, yet it is generally accepted that the predominant mechanism is oxidative stress and redox injury resulting in decreased synthesis or increased degradation of NO. Given the diverse vasculoprotective properties of NO and related pathways, there is increasing evidence to support the notion that endothelial dysfunction begins with impairment of oxidative stress, with subsequent unavailability of NO. Factors that help stimulate the production and release of NO have also been an area of active research.

An important mechanical stimulus that evokes vasodilator release of vasoactive substances, particularly NO, from the vascular endothelium is pulsatile flow and shear stress induced from movement of blood along the endothelial cells.[2-4] Varying degrees of shear stimulus have been shown to have an impact on the degree of vasodilation, which points to the complexity of the underlying vasomotor function, the impact of vascular risk factors and disease states, and the ability to decipher specific mechanisms underlying impaired endothelial vasomotor function. Reactive hyperemia is a transient increase in blood flow, physiologically or mechanically invoked, that immediately follows a designated period of vessel occlusion or flow disturbance. High shear stress on the endothelium provides the stimulus for NO release. In addition, a variety of vasodilators, such as adenosine and hydrogen ions, among others, are released and act locally on the microvessel milieu.[56,57]

ENDOTHELIAL VASOMOTOR FUNCTION TESTING

The initial observations and discoveries in vascular biology since the 1980s stimulated intense basic research in vascular biology in the ensuing decades to further delineate the various components and mechanisms of vascular diseases. A vast body of work emerged emphasizing the importance of endothelium-derived NO as a potent endogenous vasodilator that contributes to vascular health in optimal conditions. Moreover, these observations formed the basis for translational research to study the characteristics and clinical significance of endothelium-dependent properties, such as vasodilation, in various vascular beds and in various vascular disease states.

Experimental and clinical techniques using physiologic agents and various imaging techniques were developed and applied to study vascular structure and functions of both conduit and resistance vessels in the normal state and within the context of cardiovascular risk factors, such as dyslipidemia, hypertension, diabetes, and early atherosclerosis. Such techniques also spurred further investigations of the impact of therapeutic and lifestyle modifications on endothelial dysfunction and its prognosis.[57]

Invasive Measures of Coronary Vasoactivity

With the discoveries in endothelial biology in the 1980s, there was growing interest in the potential to clinically examine perturbations in vascular function before the advent of detectable atherosclerosis and clinical events. Numerous studies and methods using various physiologic agents and techniques to study endothelium-dependent vasomotor function in conduit and resistance vessels in the normal state and in the presence of cardiovascular risk factors and atherosclerosis ensued. Ludmer and colleagues,[58] in the 1980s, first described impaired endothelium-dependent vasomotor function with intracoronary injection of acetylcholine and quantitative coronary angiography in humans with various degrees of atherosclerosis noted by angiography. They demonstrated that like isolated vascular rings used in basic experimentation, human coronaries that appeared angiographically normal or with mild stenosis paradoxically vasoconstricted to acetylcholine but not to nitroglycerin.[58] Subsequently, endothelium-dependent, NO-mediated vasomotor function testing gained notoriety as a useful tool to assess the functional integrity of vascular endothelium in vivo.

The endothelium-dependent vasodilator response may serve as a surrogate marker for the bioavailability of NO. Endothelial function is most commonly measured as the vasomotor response to pharmacologic stimuli, such as acetylcholine, methacholine, bradykinin, serotonin, papaverine, and substance P, or to a physical stimulus, such as shear stress (increased blood flow velocity), exercise, cold pressor test, and mental stress. During cardiac catheterization, alterations in arterial lumen diameter in response to such stimuli can be measured by computerized edge detection software to provide reproducible measurements of the angiographic lumen diameter compared with baseline diameters. Lumen diameter and coronary flow by quantitative coronary angiography and intracoronary Doppler study, respectively, can be used to assess changes in vessel diameter and coronary flow reserve.

Endothelial function in resistance vessels (microcirculation) is also critical in the assessment of endothelial vasomotor function. Resistance vessels regulate blood flow in response to changes in perfusion pressure (autoregulation) and metabolic needs (metabolic regulation). The vascular tone of resistance vessels determines blood flow; therefore, altered blood flow detected by techniques without considerable changes in mean blood pressure indicates changes in resistance vessel tone. Endothelial function of forearm resistance vessels can be assessed by measurement of coronary blood flow with intravascular Doppler study in response to intracoronary adenosine or by forearm blood flow responses to intra-arterial agonists with strain-gauge plethysmography.[59]

Angiography is invasive and carries some risk, and it is not conducive to repeated studies in the same individual over time or for the study of relatively low risk populations. Insights from these invasive studies of endothelial vasomotor function and flow reserve provoked a keen interest in the pursuit of similar studies in the peripheral circulation with both invasive and noninvasive techniques. This was motivated by the notion that endothelial dysfunction is both a local and systemic physiologic state, along with an interest in detecting the impact of cardiovascular risk factors and the presence of preclinical atherosclerotic disease.

Invasive Assessment of Forearm Microcirculation (Venous Occlusion Plethysmography)

The limitations inherent in coronary artery circulation studies of vasomotion led researchers to pursue the peripheral circulation for further investigation. There was also keen interest to determine whether there were methods to more broadly assess the systemic nature of atherosclerosis and the broader impact of cardiovascular risk factors and the potential role to evaluate the impact of interventions and risk factor modifications. Moreover, further study led to an interest in the relationship of conduit and resistance vessels in vascular health and disease.

Venous occlusion plethysmography is an invasive technique that indirectly measures microvessel function as forearm blood flow in response to an intra-arterial infusion of a vasoactive substance such as acetylcholine, substance P, or adenosine into either the brachial artery or radial artery or to reactive hyperemia (increased shear stress). The standard testing technique is well described, reliable, and highly reproducible and typically used in research protocols.[59] The invasive aspect of this technique with cannulation of peripheral arteries poses the potential for injury to the artery and

nerves, which makes it less desirable for routine clinical use and examination of larger populations. It is a valuable research tool to evaluate the pathologic mechanisms underlying endothelial dysfunction and the impact of various therapeutic interventions.

Noninvasive Assessment of Peripheral Conduit Vascular Reactivity: Brachial Artery Ultrasound

Ultrasound techniques have long been used to study vessel physiology. Ultrasound assessment of brachial artery vasoreactivity with high-resolution B-mode ultrasound emerged as a clinical research tool in the early 1990s to noninvasively study endothelium-dependent vasomotor function. In 1992, Celemajer and colleagues used B-mode ultrasound to study the brachial artery's vasoactive response to increased shear stress induced by hyperemia in adults with coronary artery disease or smoking exposure.[52,53] The key observation, termed flow-mediated vasodilation (FMD), expressed as a percentage (FMD%), was impaired vasoactivity detectable noninvasively with ultrasound in individuals with risk factors, coronary artery disease, or both. Concurrent with observations from basic studies and invasive coronary studies, flow-mediated vasodilation in the brachial artery is abolished by the NO synthase inhibitor l-NMMA.[60,61]

Since its inception, flow-mediated vasodilation has been applied widely as a research tool to evaluate the impact of cardiovascular risk factors and preclinical disease states and to improve endothelial function with targeted specific interventions and risk factor modifications. Further exploration of the technique led to studies of underlying mechanisms for the time course after the hyperemic response, the effect of blood pressure cuff occlusion duration, the effect of upper arm occlusion versus lower arm occlusion for technical ease of imaging and targeted NO stimulation, and the effect of other stimuli such as cold pressor and mental stress.[62-69]

Advances in vascular biology and the role of oxidative stress in enhancing lipid oxidation and promoting a proinflammatory state spearheaded further investigations with this technique. Basic studies of vascular rings exposed to chylomicron remnants[70] and the effect of fat meals with and without antioxidant vitamins on flow-mediated vasodilation[71,72] contributed to the notion that healthy vascular beds exposed to oxidative stressors manifest acute alterations in endothelial function. Studies that demonstrated significant improvement in flow-mediated brachial artery vasodilation inspired enthusiasm to study the impact of various risk factors and targeted therapies for cardiovascular disease. Correlative studies of brachial artery vasoactivity with intracoronary vasoactive substances and carotid intima-media thickness provided support for brachial artery vasoactivity as an index or marker of endothelial function.[73,74] Large clinical trials and epidemiologic longitudinal studies now incorporate FMD% as a marker of impaired vasomotor endothelial dysfunction.

Technique

The technique and examination protocol for brachial artery vasoactivity testing are well described in the literature. Seemingly simple, it is technically challenging, with a significant learning curve to achieve high-quality, consistent performance and reproducibility in both technique and interpretation.[63-65,74,75]

Standard ultrasound systems equipped with vascular software with B-mode two-dimensional imaging, color and spectral Doppler display, internal electrocardiographic monitor, and high-frequency vascular linear array transducer (range, 8 to 12 MHz) are required. Higher frequency transducers of 8 to 12 MHz compared with 7 to 7.5 MHz enable visualization

32

of the intima as opposed to the vessel wall alone, which has implications for the application of measurement techniques. Before brachial artery vasoactivity testing, the individual should avoid vasoactive substances or stimuli and rest quietly supine for 10 minutes.

The technical preparation involves positioning of the subject's arm extended and supinated to allow optimal imaging of the brachial artery antecubitally. Blood pressure occlusion for 5 minutes and release create the shear stress to induce flow-mediated vasodilation.

Application of an upper versus a lower arm cuff for occlusion has been studied, and the placement provides different stimuli. Upper arm occlusion provides a more robust shear stimulus for vasodilation and probably invokes other vasoactive mechanisms besides release of NO. Upper arm occlusion typically elicits an increase in hyperemic flow of four to five times from baseline and greater change in vasodilation compared with lower arm cuff occlusion. Furthermore, vasodilator response to upper arm occlusion hyperemia has been shown to be largely NO mediated. In addition, arteries smaller than 2.5 mm in diameter are difficult to measure, and vasodilation is difficult to perceive in vessels larger than 5.0 mm in diameter.

Flow-mediated vasodilation typically occurs 60 to 90 seconds after cuff release while accurately acquiring the image at the same position compared with baseline. Brachial artery flow returns to baseline by 1 minute after hyperemia, but dilation may ensue beyond 1 minute.[62,63] The physiologic characteristics of this response may be individually dependent as well as indicative of impaired vascular health in the setting of risk factors or genetic predisposition to disease states such as atherosclerosis. Brachial artery diameter is measured perpendicular to the longitudinal axis in which the lumen-intima interface is visualized on the near (anterior) and far (posterior) walls. The lumen-intima interface or media-adventitia interface is identified with electronic calipers from the ultrasound system analysis software or determined through edge detection computer software typically performed off-line. Edge detection programs that can account for skew by elliptical modeling have less variance in their measurements of brachial artery diameter.[76] Maximal vasodilation after hyperemia may be variable within an individual or in certain disease states, although most individuals dilate maximally at approximately 60 to 90 seconds after cuff release. Consequently, it is recommended that B-mode acquisition of the brachial artery be acquired from 30 seconds up to at least 2 minutes after hyperemia for off-line analysis (Fig. 32-3).

Flow-Mediated Vasodilation. FMD% is expressed as the change in post-stimulus diameter as a percentage of the baseline diameter.

$$FMD\% = post\text{-}hyperemic\ diameter - baseline\ diameter \div$$
$$baseline\ diameter \times 100$$

Doppler: Baseline and Hyperemic Flow. Baseline and hyperemic blood flow are calculated from the time-averaged pulsed Doppler spectral trace (TVI, time-velocity integral) from the onset of one waveform to the beginning of the next waveform.

$$Blood\ flow\ velocity\ (TVI) \times vessel\ diameter\ (\pi r^2)$$
$$\times heart\ rate = blood\ flow$$

Endothelium-Independent Vasodilation with Nitroglycerin

In most studies to date, an exogenous NO donor, such as a single high dose (0.4 mg) of nitroglycerin spray or sublingual tablet, has been given to determine the maximum obtainable vasodilator response and to serve as a measure of endothelium-independent vasodilation reflecting vascular smooth muscle function.[67,68] Peak vasodilation occurs 3 to 4 minutes after nitroglycerin administration, on the order of 15% to 20% maximum dilation increase from baseline diameter. Brachial artery images and Doppler velocity signal are continuously recorded during this time. The effect of nitroglycerin on the vessel diameter persists up to 20 to 30 minutes.

TIME COURSE OF FLOW-MEDIATED DILATION (FMD) EXAM PROTOCOL

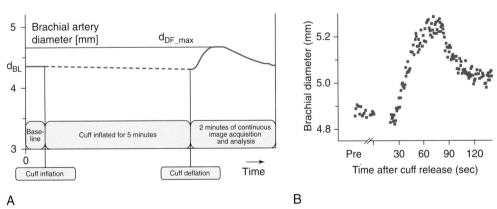

FIGURE 32-3 A, Schematic diagram of the brachial artery B-mode ultrasound imaging protocol for brachial artery vasoactivity testing. B-mode longitudinal images of the brachial artery segment of interest are recorded during baseline and after cuff deflation. Baseline and deflation image sequences are analyzed to assess vessel diameter function. Diameter *d* is the averaged arterial diameter at baseline; duration of baseline acquisition typically ranges between 10 and 20 seconds; *d* is the maximum diameter during the 2 minutes after cuff release. **B,** Time course of brachial artery flow-mediated vasodilation by upper arm occlusion shear stress stimulus in a healthy individual. (**A** from Sonka M, Liang W, Lauer RM: Automated analysis of brachial ultrasound image sequences: early detection of cardiovascular disease via surrogates of endothelial function. IEEE Trans Med Imaging 21:1271, 2002. **B** from Corretti MC, Anderson TJ, Benjamin EJ, et al: Guidelines for the ultrasound assessment of endothelial-dependent flow-mediated vasodilation of the brachial artery. J Am Coll Cardiol 39:257, 2002.)

534	Nitroglycerin should not be administered to individuals with clinically significant bradycardia or hypotension. Determination of the vasodilator responses to increasing doses of nitroglycerin (an NO donor), rather than to a single dose, may further elucidate changes in smooth muscle function or arterial compliance that might be playing a role in any observed changes in flow-mediated vasodilation.[67,68] This may further the understanding of impaired vasodilator responses in the presence of cardiovascular risk factors or disease states.

Quality Control Metrics and Reproducibility

Quality control of measures of flow-mediated vasodilation requires optimal hands-on training to ensure the highest quality and consistency in data acquisition and measurement techniques.[63] Intraobserver and interobserver variability for technical and interpretive expertise is highly dependent on the mastery of this technique. This requires a learning curve founded on appropriate instruction, consistent application, and quality control. The image analysis and measurement of the vasodilator response from repeated studies should be done by an individual who is blinded as to sequence. Investigator-initiated studies, large-cohort epidemiologic studies, and core laboratories should adhere to a standardized protocol for training, implementation of technique and analysis, and reproducibility. Experienced laboratories with excellent reproducibility maintain a coefficient of variation <2% and a 2% to 4% improvement in FMD% in small crossover trials (N = 20 to 30 subjects) and parallel group trials (N = 25 to 50) per intervention arm.[63,69,77,78]

Interpretation

To date, there are no specific nomograms for flow-mediated vasodilation other than data from ongoing data bases such as the Framingham study or other individual institutions. Consistency in technical approach and data acquisition is necessary, along with consideration of physiologic factors that mediate basal vasomotor tone and diameter. A larger baseline diameter yields a smaller measure of percentage change for any given absolute change in post-stimulus diameter. Inversely, smaller arteries dilate relatively more than larger arteries do. In sum, this merits consideration in attempting to compare vasodilator responses between individuals and groups with different baseline diameters. For studies in which multiple measures are made within the same individual over time or comparisons are made before and after an intervention in the same individuals, percentage change may be the easiest metric, provided baseline diameter remains stable over time. The baseline diameter, absolute change, and percentage change in diameter are therefore typically reported in publications.

Flow-mediated vasodilation is also affected by a change in the hyperemic stimulus. The flow stimulus should be consistent; otherwise, any change in FMD% of the conduit artery may be related to changes in flow (even indirectly mediated by changes in the microcirculation) rather than to improvement of endothelial function of the conduit vessel. Further studies with noninvasive techniques of vasomotion and of hyperemic flows as shear stimulus and its physiologic significance are currently under way.[79-83]

EMERGING TECHNIQUES OF VASCULAR FUNCTION

Assessment of the pulse characteristics is one of the earliest recorded medical skills, replaced with the objective recordings with sphygmography, later replaced by the sphygmomanometer. Pulse characteristics and arterial hemodynamics have always been an important focus of the study of vessel function and ventriculoarterial coupling. Advances in vascular biology coupled with computer technology and techniques to measure arterial waveforms, pressures, and flows generated a greater interest in noninvasive study of vascular structure and function with age, other cardiovascular risk factors, and more recently the impact of disease and risk factor modification. The association of arterial stiffening and aging is well described.

Elastin and collagen, major components of the vasculature, largely regulate vascular tone or stiffness and undergo significant degenerative changes with age and other cardiovascular risk factors or disease processes, as in hypertension, diabetes, end-stage renal disease, and smokers. Arterial stiffness has been extensively studied and accepted as a surrogate marker of atherosclerosis and the effects of advancing age and as a prognostic indicator for cardiovascular events.

Arterial stiffness is structurally determined by the components of the blood vessel, but it is in part under the functional control of the endothelium through its release of vasoactive mediators. The emerging data that arterial stiffness may be involved in the pathogenesis of cardiovascular disease underscore the interest in and importance of physiologic mechanisms that may be targeted for risk assessment and therapeutics. Various techniques to noninvasively study vascular properties and function through assessment of arterial waveforms, pulse velocity, and measures of arterial stiffness, along with flow-mediated vasoactive surrogates of endothelial function, may be used selectively and comprehensively to fully evaluate the status of vascular function in an individual and the impact of risk factors and interventions. These include Doppler-based techniques and applanation tonometry to assess velocities or flow and arterial waveforms including pulse wave analysis, pulse wave velocity measurement, and pulse amplitude tonometry (also known as pulse volume amplitude).

Given the challenges in mastering ultrasound assessment of brachial artery vasodilation in response to reactive hyperemia, interest has shifted to the utility of measuring digital pulse amplitude tonometry at rest and in response to reactive hyperemia to assess cardiovascular risk in individual subjects.[84]

Pulse amplitude tonometry (commercially available as Endo-PAT2000, Itamar Medical) is a relatively new noninvasive technique that records pulse amplitude in the fingertip at baseline and during reactive hyperemia. Hyperemia flow-mediated dilation in the fingertip increases the pulse amplitude. With use of proprietary software, the net response is expressed as the reactive hyperemia pulse amplitude tonometry index. Preliminary studies with this technique have demonstrated that an intra-arterial infusion of L-NMMA into the brachial artery blocks hyperemia-induced increase in pulse amplitude. This indicates that the reactive hyperemia pulse amplitude is at least partially dependent on an NO synthesis process.[84-87] Other investigations have shown a correlation between reactive hyperemia–induced pulse amplitude tonometry index and brachial artery flow-mediated vasodilation and the coronary circulation[85] and that it too is inversely related to cardiovascular risk factors,[85,86] as previously shown with brachial artery flow-mediated vasodilation and other invasive techniques.

The technique can be simultaneously employed with ultrasound assessment of brachial artery flow-mediated vasodilation to provide further insights into hyperemia-induced vasomotor function. Pulse amplitude tonometry appears to be a promising technique, particularly given its ease of application; however, more studies are needed to confirm its correlation with other well-established techniques and protocols.

Laser Doppler Flowmetry: Measure for Cutaneous Microvessels

An emerging noninvasive technique to study the microvasculature is laser Doppler flowmetry, which provides a semi-quantitative measure of blood flow in the small blood vessels of the microvasculature. These vessels have low-velocity flows associated with nutrient blood flow delivery, regulation of skin temperature, and vascular resistance in the capillaries, arterioles, and venules. A low-intensity laser beam scans across the skin surface, allowing measurements with good temporal and spatial resolution of rapid blood flow changes. Application of this technique to the study of endothelium-dependent and endothelium-independent vasomotor function with use of substances that change skin perfusion, such as acetylcholine, is under study; therefore, its exact role remains uncertain.

Arterial Compliance and Arterial Stiffness

Each pulsation of the heart generates a velocity of the pressure wave (pulse wave velocity) that is transmitted centrifugally throughout the peripheral vascular system. The waveform is related to the biomechanical properties of the arterial system, including arterial wall stiffness. The ascending aortic pressure waveform can be measured from the carotid artery, femoral artery, or radial artery by noninvasive techniques such as applanation tonometry and Doppler ultrasound. Arterial stiffness can be examined with a variety of approaches. These include measurement of the arterial pulse pressure from blood pressure readings, applanation tonometry assessment and analysis of the pulse wave contour, and ultrasound assessment of the arterial distensibility and pulse wave velocity.[88,89]

Pulse wave analysis is a technique that provides accurate recording of peripheral pressure waveforms with assessment of the corresponding central waveform. From this, the augmentation index and central pressure can be derived, providing information about arterial stiffness and altered pulse dynamics. Pulse wave analysis is a stable, easy to perform,

and highly reproducible technique that relates arterial structure to vascular tone. Implementation of the technique is not dependent on a flow stimulus or infusion of a vasodilator agent. Pulse wave analysis is typically applied to the aorta and carotid, brachial, or femoral arteries.

Applanation tonometry (SphygmoCor CPV, AtCor Medical, Sydney, Australia) is a method used for pulse wave analysis to derive the central aortic pressure waveform and pulse wave velocity. There are two main methods of applanation tonometry to assess the pulse pressure waveform. It can be analyzed by applying a valid transfer function based on Fourier analysis, which allows derivation of an aortic pressure waveform, the augmentation index, and time to reflected wave. The other method involves use of a modified windkessel model of the circulation. This model allows calculation of large- and small-vessel compliance but does not include the effects of wave reflections. The tonometer is positioned over the maximal arterial pulsation of an accessible superficial artery (e.g., radial, brachial, and femoral) to minimally flatten or applanate the arterial wall. This results in normalization of the circumferential stress in the arterial wall. Changes in the electrical resistance of a piezoelectric crystal within the tonometer allow recording of the pressure waveform. This pressure waveform is then digitalized for application of a "generalized transfer function," derived from simultaneous recording of peripheral arterial and the invasively recorded central ascending aortic pressures, allowing automated calculation of the central aortic pressure waveform from the peripheral pressure and tonometry data. Reflection of pressure waves in the arterial tree leads to augmentation of the central aortic pressure wave. Peripheral vessels with higher impedance reflect the incident wave to the aorta, resulting in augmentation of the central aortic pressure. Thus, the resulting central aortic pressure represents the sum of the incident and the reflected waveforms.[90]

The obtained pulse waveform shape provides information about arterial compliance and serves as the basis for the calculation of the augmentation index as illustrated in Figure 32-4. Augmentation index is commonly used as a measure of arterial stiffness. Applanation tonometry–based assessment of peripheral pressure waveforms and calculation of augmentation index have been studied as a tool for assessment of endothelial function. However, in a comparison between flow-mediated vasodilation and pulse wave analysis as a

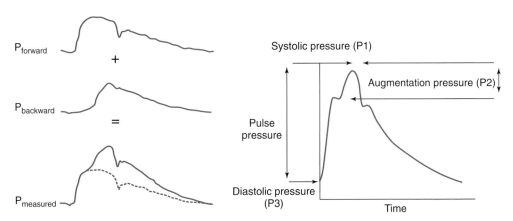

FIGURE 32-4 **Left,** Diagram of aortic pressure wave. Invasive hemodynamic measure of aortic pressure waveforms: forward, backward, and summated to yield measured pressure and flow waveforms. **Right,** Applanation tonometry: pulse wave analysis and augmentation index assessment of arterial stiffness. Augmentation index = augmentation pressure/pulse pressure. The peak systolic pressure is represented by P1. P3 is the minimum diastolic pressure. An inflection point, P2, in the waveform identifies the merging point of the beginning upstroke of the reflected pressure wave. (**Left** from Murgo JP, Westerhof N, Giolma JP, Altobelli SA: Manipulation of ascending aortic pressure and flow wave reflections with the Valsalva maneuver: relationship to input impedance, Circulation 63:122, 1981. **Right** from Laurent S, Cockcroft J, Van Bortel L, et al: Expert consensus document on arterial stiffness: methodological issues and clinical applications, Eur Heart J 27:2588, 2006.)

536 function of endothelial function in response to inflammation, flow-mediated vasodilation was found to be more reproducible. Multiple variables (age, height, and heart rate) may influence calculations. In addition, standardization of arteries used for calculations needs to be determined. Paucity of long-term longitudinal studies assessing the predictive value of these tests on mortality and the effect of interventions is a limitation in wide-scale adoption of this tool.

Augmentation index and pulse wave velocity are dependent on arterial stiffness and ventricular-arterial coupling and wave reflections that include effects of the mechanical properties of the arterial wall in addition to the effects of atherosclerosis and dysfunctional endothelium. This is particularly notable in renal failure, hypertension, presence of advanced glycation end products in diabetes mellitus, and advanced age. There may be discordance with FMD% and some of these other techniques, which speaks to the additive value of the two methods.[87-93]

32

LIFESTYLE MODIFICATIONS AND THERAPEUTICS

There is a growing body of evidence that endothelial dysfunction can be both a consequence of and a major contributor to cardiovascular disease and events. Experimental and clinical techniques have demonstrated various manifestations of endothelial dysfunction in the presence of traditional and novel cardiovascular risk factors and in diseases such as diabetes, dysmetabolic syndrome, hypertension, and coronary artery disease. Endothelial dysfunction also invokes the inability to optimally repair in the setting of vascular injury. The presence of endothelial dysfunction represents in itself a risk factor burden that seeks to be assessed and quantified; however, the complexity and multifactorial nature of endothelial dysfunction elude simple diagnostic tests. It is the final common pathway through which vascular risk factors initiate the pathogenesis of atherosclerosis. Current evidence supports the fact that endothelial function is an integrative indicator of the net effects of the magnitude and duration of arterial injury and repair over time. The focus on specific perturbations of endothelial dysfunction allows the application of noninvasive imaging and hemodynamic techniques with or without concurrent biomarkers. Numerous studies employing flow-mediated vasodilation as a marker of endothelial vasomotor dysfunction have demonstrated impairment (less vasodilation in response to shear stress) in various conditions and improvement with such interventions as lifestyle modifications and therapeutics.

PROGNOSIS

Numerous studies have emerged in the last decade that employed several techniques to measure endothelial dysfunction as a potential surrogate marker for clinical events. Table 32-3 summarizes a variety of retrospective and prospective studies of endothelial function testing by invasive and noninvasive modalities with cardiovascular events.[94-103] These studies lend further support to other experimental and clinical evidence that endothelium plays an active critical role in atherosclerosis. This small group of studies

TABLE 32–3	Prognosis and Endothelial Function					
Author	Design and Patient Cohort	Vascular Bed	Technique	Stimulus	Follow-up	Cardiovascular Events
Suwaidi (2000)	Retrospective 157 mild CAD	Coronary	IVUS, QCA/CBF	Acetylcholine adenosine, nitroglycerin	28 months	14%, 10 events Events with lowest acetylcholine response
Schachinger (2000)	Retrospective 147 CAD	Coronary	IVUS, QCA/CBF	Acetylcholine, cold	7.7 years	11%, 28 events Acetylcholine independent predictor of events
Neunteufl (2000)	Retrospective 73 CAD	Brachial	FMD%	Hyperemia	5 years	FMD% independent predictor of events
Heitzer (2001)	Prospective 281 CAD	Brachial	Venous plethysmography	Acetylcholine	4.5 years	Acetylcholine independent predictor of events
Perticone (2001)	Prospective 225 HTN	Brachial	Venous plethysmography	Acetylcholine	32 months	Acetylcholine independent predictor of events
Gokce (2002)	Prospective 187 preoperative vascular	Brachial	FMD%	Hyperemia	30 days	15% (FMD% < 8%) FMD% independent predictor of postoperative events
Halcox (2002)	Retrospective 308 diagnostic catheterization	Coronary	QCA/CBF	Acetylcholine, adenosine	46 months	11.4% Acetylcholine independent predictor of events
Modena (2002)	Prospective 400 postmenopausal women with HTN	Brachial	FMD%	Hyperemia	67 months	21.3% with persistent impaired FMD%; no improvement with therapy
Schindler (2003)	Prospective 130 normal coronary angiograms	Coronary	Vasoactivity	Cold pressor	45 months	26 with events Cold pressor independent predictor of events
Gokce (2003)	Prospective 199 vascular surgery	Brachial	FMD%	Hyperemia	14 months	Cardiovascular death, unstable angina, stroke

CAD, coronary artery disease; CBF, coronary blood flow; FMD, flow-mediated vasodilation; HTN, hypertension; IVUS, intravascular ultrasound; QCA, quantitative coronary angiography.

demonstrates prognostic insight into selected high-risk groups with multiple risk factors for atherosclerosis that have an impact on endothelial function; data to support the prognostic value in low- and intermediate-risk groups are currently lacking. Nevertheless, these prognostic studies suggest that endothelial function testing may provide insight into an individual's risk burden, the response to therapy, and perhaps the need for more aggressive management. All biologic systems, individuals with cardiovascular risk factors, and disease demonstrate a wide range of responses to endothelium-dependent techniques and heterogeneity in the magnitude of dysfunction in individuals with similar risk factor profiles. With advances in development and application, such techniques will serve as useful diagnostic and prognostic clinical and research tools.

CLINICAL TRIALS

The study of endothelial function in clinical research has had a universal interest as an important functional barometer of cardiovascular risk as well as a marker of endothelial injury coupled with other circulating biomarkers and emerging imaging techniques. Throughout the 1990s, pharmacologic and lifestyle modifications known to decrease cardiovascular risk were studied with endothelial function testing as a clinical endpoint. Numerous clinical studies reported the effect of pharmacologic or physiologic interventions on endothelial function by brachial artery flow-mediated vasodilation and other endothelial function testing as a surrogate marker for altered endothelial vasomotor function in healthy individuals and in those with risk factors or known coronary disease. Acute and chronic studies, both parallel group and crossover designs, were successfully conducted on the effects of angiotensin-converting enzyme inhibitors,[52,53,57] antioxidant vitamins,[52,57] statins,[52,57,69] diet changes,[69,71] and hormone replacement therapy[52,69] on endothelial function, putatively through improvement in NO-mediated mechanisms. Although several intervention therapies demonstrate improvement in endothelial function and also reduce cardiovascular risk, the literature is variable in this regard.

Implications of the approach for standardization of techniques and sample size determinations have been reported. Subsequently, assessment of flow-mediated brachial artery vasodilation has been incorporated into clinical studies and larger longitudinal studies such as the Framingham study and other similar epidemiologic-genetic studies. There are technical and interpretive challenges that must be mastered to ensure consistency and reproducibility in data acquisition owing to the variable nature of vascular reactivity. Several important considerations are optimal technical training, study design, and sample size along with uniform technique in scanning protocol and analysis and validation of reproducibility in controlled research settings. Most studies have been of cohorts of individuals with risk factors or disease states that undergo assessment of endothelial function testing for diagnostic or therapeutic assessment from single centers and less so from multicenter studies. Multicenter studies optimally require one site serving as the core laboratory to ensure uniform methodology and analysis.

To date, there is no direct evidence that therapeutic improvement in endothelial function translates into lower cardiovascular morbidity and mortality because large prospective clinical trials with improved endothelial function as a primary therapeutic endpoint have not been conducted. This is in part due to the technical and physiologic challenges in optimizing standardization and reproducibility consistently to study the dynamic nature of the endothelium. Further development and investigation of various noninvasive techniques to clinically assess the functional properties

of normal and activated endothelium are essential as no one technique can be used exclusively to assess and to monitor the dynamic nature of vascular biology. Currently, endothelial function testing is not used clinically to routinely assess risk or to guide management of risk factor modification or therapeutics. At this time, these methods have yet to emerge as powerful diagnostic tools alone or in addition to traditional clinical tools, particularly for subclinical atherosclerosis and vascular disease. Ongoing studies with these techniques continue to address their full potential. This requires endothelial function testing to be sensitive, specific, and accurate. It should be standardized and reproducible along with validated population norms to help provide insight into the status of vascular health and possibly guide therapy. It should provide prognostic information to current clinical information and parameters and assist in the identification of individuals who might benefit from various therapies. An improvement displayed by endothelial function testing should predict a measurable reduction in risk of clinical cardiovascular events. Genetic susceptibility as well as complex multiple risk factor interactions throughout the continuum of vascular health and disease will likely determine any one individual's response to testing. The complex causal mechanisms of atherosclerosis, the diverse effects of various interventions imposed along the continuum of vascular health, and the genetic-environmental response to such interventions make it unlikely that any single surrogate of endothelial function can optimally stratify risk or predict clinical outcomes. Nevertheless, endothelial function testing methods hold significant promise in providing added beneficial information. The enormous body of studies to date in this field underscores an interest in and a potential for endothelial function testing to be a useful tool for diagnostics, therapeutics, and prognostication.

CONCLUSION

Understanding of the pathophysiology of endothelial dysfunction due to underlying injury and repair has made significant progress. Whereas risk factors associated with endothelial dysfunction are increasingly recognized, detection of endothelial dysfunction is still primarily a research tool. With advances in biomarkers and imaging technology, it may be possible to detect injury early in the process before expression of the cardiovascular phenotype. In addition, with recent advances in the repair process, it will be imperative to identify and to track circulating endothelial progenitor cells to document repair and re-endothelialization.

Various invasive and noninvasive techniques have been applied to further study the endothelial vasomotor dysfunction in the wake of the discoveries made in NO biology and oxidative injury. Ultrasound assessment of brachial artery flow-mediated vasodilation has yielded important information about vascular function in health and disease, yet several new technologic advances and techniques have emerged to expand the scope in the detection of mechanisms of and impairments in vascular structure and function. The ongoing discoveries from basic experimentation to translational clinical studies remain essential to the study of mechanisms of impaired vascular homeostasis and to determine the incremental value of the presence of endothelial dysfunction beyond known and established risk factors and clinical predictors. Whether treatment strategies aimed at modifying risk factors suffice or a need for endothelium-directed therapy is required is an exciting area of investigation and needs to be proven.

Diagnostic and prognostic studies of endothelial dysfunctions—be they imaging modalities of structure and function along with circulating biomarkers—will provide

538 insight and guidance into an individual's overall cardiovascular risk burden, the treatment plan, and the response to therapy. These goals for brachial artery vasoactivity testing and other related noninvasive vascular techniques require rigorous standardization and correlations, data from large-scale population and randomized studies, and correlation studies with other imaging modalities coupled with genomics and environmental research. Prospective studies comparing vascular function testing with modalities such as intravascular ultrasound, carotid intima-media thickness, multidetector computed tomography, and computed tomographic angiography in the context of interventions and prognosis will further define the potential clinical role for ultrasound measures of brachial artery vasoactivity testing with other emerging techniques and biomarkers to assess cardiovascular health and disease.

REFERENCES

1. De Caterina R, Massaro M, Libby P: Endothelial functions and dysfunctions. In DeCaterina R, Libby P, editors: *Endothelial dysfunctions and vascular disease,* Malden, 2007, Blackwell Futura Publishing, pp 3-25.
2. Vane JR, Anggard EE, Botting RM: Mechanisms of disease—regulatory functions of the vascular endothelium. *N Engl J Med* 323:27, 1990.
3. Vanhoutte PM: Other endothelium-derived vasoactive factors. *Circulation* (Suppl V):V9, 1993.
4. Davies PF: Flow-mediated endothelial mechanotransduction. *Physiol Rev* 75:519, 1995.
5. Gimbrone MA, Jr: Vascular endothelium, hemodynamic forces, and atherogenesis. *Am J Pathol* 155:1, 1999
6. Ghosh S, Karin M: Missing pieces in the NF-κB puzzle. *Cell* 109(Suppl):S81, 2002.
7. Kinlay S, Behrendt D, Wainstein M, et al: Role of endothelin-1 in the active constriction of human atherosclerotic coronary arteries. *Circulation* 104:1114, 2001.
8. Moncada S, Higgs EA, Vane JR: Human arterial and venous tissues generate prostacyclin (prostaglandin x), a potent inhibitor of platelet aggregation. *Lancet* 1:18, 1977.
9. Campia U, Panza JA: Endothelial vasodilator dysfunction in hypertension. In DeCaterina R, Libby P, editors: *Endothelial dysfunctions and vascular disease,* Malden, 2007, Blackwell Futura Publishing, pp 212-231.
10. Inoue A, Yanagisawa M, Kimura S, et al: The human endothelin family: three structurally and pharmacologically distinct isopeptides predicted by three separate genes. *Proc Natl Acad Sci U S A* 86:2863, 1989.
11. Forstermann U, Munzel T: Endothelial nitric oxide synthase in vascular disease: from marvel to menace. *Circulation* 113:1708, 2006.
12. Halcox JP, Narayanan S, Cramer-Joyce L, et al: Characterization of endothelium-derived hyperpolarizing factor in the human forearm microcirculation. *Am J Physiol Heart Circ Physiol* 280:H2470, 2001.
13. Creager MA, Beckman JA: Vascular function and diabetes mellitus. In DeCaterina R, Libby P, editors: *Endothelial dysfunctions and vascular disease,* Malden, 2007, Blackwell Futura Publishing, pp 232-244.
14. Szmitko PE, Wang CH, Weisel RD,, et al: New markers of inflammation and endothelial cell activation. Part I. *Circulation* 108:1917, 2003.
15. Szmitko PE, Wang CH, Weisel RD, et al: Biomarkers of vascular disease linking inflammation to endothelial activation. Part II. *Circulation* 108:2141, 2003.
16. Folkman J, Shing Y: Angiogenesis. *J Biol Chem* 267:10931, 1992.
17. Beck L, Jr, D'Amore PA: Vascular development: cellular and molecular regulation. *FASEB J* 11:365, 1997.
18. O'Brien KD, Allen MD, McDonald TO, et al: Vascular cell adhesion molecule-1 is expressed in human coronary atherosclerotic plaques. Implications for the mode of progression of advanced atherosclerosis. *J Clin Invest* 92:945, 1993.
19. Brogi E, Winkles JA, Underwood R, et al: Distinct patterns of expression of fibroblast growth factors and their receptors in human atheroma and nonatherosclerotic arteries. Association of acidic FGF with plaque microvessels and macrophages. *J Clin Invest* 92:2408, 1993.
20. Kolodgie FD, Gold HK, Burke AP, et al: Intraplaque hemorrhage and progression of coronary atheroma. *N Engl J Med* 349:2316, 2003.
21. Moreno PR, Purushothaman KR, Sirol M, et al: Neovascularization in human atherosclerosis. *Circulation* 113:2245, 2006.
22. Furchgott RF, Zawadzki JV: The obligatory role of endothelial cells in the relaxation of arterial smooth muscle by acetylcholine. *Nature* 288:373, 1980.
23. Ignarro LJ, Buga GM, Wood KS, et al: Endothelium-derived relaxing factor produced and released from artery and vein is nitric oxide. *Proc Natl Acad Sci U S A* 184:9265, 1987.
24. Palmer RM, Ferrige AC, Moncada S: Nitric oxide release accounts for the biological activity of endothelium-derived relaxing factor. *Nature* 327:524, 1987.
25. Moens AL, Kass DA: Tetrahydrobiopterin and cardiovascular disease. *Arterioscler Thromb Vasc Biol* 26:2439, 2006.
26. Govers R, Rabelink TJ: Cellular regulation of endothelial nitric oxide synthase. *Am J Physiol Renal Physiol* 280:F193, 2001.
27. Vasquez-Vivar J, Kalyanaraman B, Martasek P, et al: Superoxide generation by endothelial nitric oxide synthase: the influence of cofactors. *Proc Natl Acad Sci U S A* 95:9220, 1998.
28. Dudzinski DM, Igarashi J, Greif D, et al: The regulation and pharmacology of endothelial nitric oxide synthase. *Annu Rev Pharmacol Toxicol* 46:235, 2006.
29. Kolpakov V, Gordon D, Kulik TJ: Nitric oxide–generating compounds inhibit total protein and collagen synthesis in cultured vascular smooth muscle cells. *Circ Res* 76:305, 1995.
30. Zuckerbraun BS, Stoyanovsky DA, Sengupta R, et al: Nitric oxide–induced inhibition of smooth muscle cell proliferation involves *S*-nitrosation and inactivation of RhoA. *Am J Physiol Cell Physiol* 292:C824, 2007.
31. Ohkita M, Takaoka M, Shiota Y, et al: Nitric oxide inhibits endothelin-1 production through the suppression of nuclear factor kappa B. *Clin Sci (Lond)* 103(Suppl 48):68S, 2002.
32. Giannarelli C, De Negri F, Virdis A, et al: Nitric oxide modulates tissue plasminogen activator release in normotensive subjects and hypertensive patients. *Hypertension* 49:878, 2007.
33. Aicher A, Heeschen C, Mildner-Rihm C, et al: Essential role of endothelial nitric oxide synthase for mobilization of stem and progenitor cells. *Nat Med* 9:1370, 2003.
34. Cai H, Harrison DG: Endothelial dysfunction in cardiovascular diseases: the role of oxidant stress. *Circ Res* 87:840, 2000.
35. Harrison DG: Cellular and molecular mechanisms of endothelial cell dysfunction. *J Clin Invest* 100:2153, 1997.
36. Corson MA, James NL, Latta SE, et al. Phosphorylation of endothelial nitric oxide synthase in response to fluid shear stress. *Circ Res* 79:984, 1996.
37. Gimbrone MA, Jr, editor: *Endothelial dysfunction and the pathogenesis of atherosclerosis,* New York, 1980, Springer-Verlag.
38. Mel LG, Pachori AS, Kong D, et al: Endothelium-targeted gene and cell-based therapy for cardiovascular disease. In DeCaterina R, Libby P, editors: *Endothelial dysfunctions and vascular disease,* Malden, 2007, Blackwell Futura Publishing, pp 365-399.
39. Hill JM, Zalos G, Halcox JP, et al: Circulating endothelial progenitor cells, vascular function and cardiovascular risk. *N Engl J Med* 348:593, 2003.
40. Mallat Z, Benamer H, Hugel B, et al: Elevated levels of shed membrane microparticles with procoagulant potential in the peripheral circulating blood of patients with acute coronary syndromes. *Circulation* 101:841, 2000.
41. Rajagopalan S, Somers EC, Brook RD, et al: Endothelial cell apoptosis in systemic lupus erythematosus: a common pathway for abnormal vascular function and thrombosis propensity. *Blood* 103:3677, 2004.
42. Werner N, Wassmann S, Ahlers P, et al: Circulating CD31+/annexin V+ apoptotic microparticles correlate with coronary endothelial function in patients with coronary artery disease. *Arterioscler Thromb Vasc Biol* 26:112, 2006.
43. Laufs U, Werner N, Link A, et al: Physical training increases endothelial progenitor cells, inhibits neointima formation, and enhances angiogenesis. *Circulation* 109:220, 2004.
44. Walter DH, Rittig K, Bahlmann FH, et al: Statin therapy accelerates reendothelialization: a novel effect involving mobilization and incorporation of bone marrow–derived endothelial progenitor cells. *Circulation* 105:3017, 2002.
45. Siekmeier R, Grammer T, Marz W: Roles of oxidants, nitric oxide, and asymmetric dimethylarginine in endothelial function. *J Cardiovasc Pharmacol Ther* 13:279, 2008.
46. Landmesser U, Merten R, Spiekermann S, et al: Vascular extracellular superoxide dismutase activity in patients with coronary artery disease: relation to endothelium-dependent vasodilation. *Circulation* 101:2264, 2000.
47. Spiekermann S, Landmesser U, Dikalov S, et al: Electron spin resonance characterization of vascular xanthine and NAD(P)H oxidase activity in patients with coronary artery disease: relation to endothelium-dependent vasodilation. *Circulation* 107:1383, 2003.
48. Sorescu D, Weiss D, Lassegue B, et al: Superoxide production and expression of nox family proteins in human atherosclerosis. *Circulation* 105:1429, 2002.
49. Gryglewski RJ, Palmer RM, Moncada S: Superoxide anion is involved in the breakdown of endothelium-derived vascular relaxing factor. *Nature* 320:454, 1986.
50. Vallance P, Leiper J: Cardiovascular biology of the asymmetric dimethylarginine:dimethylarginine dimethylaminohydrolase pathway. *Arterioscler Thromb Vasc Biol* 24:1023, 2004.
51. Osanai T, Saitoh M, Sasaki S, et al: Effect of shear stress on asymmetric dimethylarginine release from vascular endothelial cells. *Hypertension* 42:985, 2003.
52. Adams Mark R, Celermajer DS: Endothelial vasodilatory dysfunction and risk factors in adults. In DeCaterina R, Libby P, editors: *Endothelial dysfunctions and vascular disease,* Malden, 2007, Blackwell Futura Publishing, pp 189-198.
53. Halcox JPJ, Deanfield JE: Endothelial vasodilatory dysfunction in early life. In DeCaterina R, Libby P, editors: *Endothelial dysfunctions and vascular disease,* Malden, 2007, Blackwell Futura Publishing, pp 199-212.
54. Yeh ETH: CRP as a mediator of disease. *Circulation* 109(Suppl 1):II11, 2004.
55. Zampolli A, Falk E, DeCaterina F: Anti-atherogenic effects of omega-3 fatty acids. In DeCaterina R, Libby P, editors: *Endothelial dysfunctions and vascular disease,* Malden, 2007, Blackwell Futura Publishing, pp 286-299.
56. Pyke KA, Dwyer EM, Tschakovsky ME: Impact of controlling shear rate on flow-mediated dilation responses in the brachial artery of humans. *J Appl Physiol* 97:499, 2004.
57. Frick M, Weidinger F: Endothelial function: a surrogate endpoint in cardiovascular studies. *Curr Pharm Des* 13:1741, 2007.
58. Ludmer PL, Selwyn AP, Shook TL, et al: Paradoxical vasoconstriction induced by acetylcholine in atherosclerotic coronary arteries. *N Engl J Med* 315:1046, 1986.
59. Wilkinson IB, Webb DJ: Venous occlusion plethysmography in cardiovascular research: methodology and clinical applications [review]. *Br J Clin Pharmacol* 52:631, 2001.
60. Joannides R, Haefeli WE, Linder L, et al: Nitric oxide is responsible for flow-dependent dilatation of human peripheral conduit arteries in vivo. *Circulation* 91:1314, 1995.
61. Doshi SN, Naka KK, Payn N, et al: Flow-mediated dilatation following wrist and upper arm occlusion in humans: the contribution of nitric oxide. *Clin Sci* 101:629, 2001.
62. Corretti MC, Plotnick GD, Vogel RA: Technical aspects of evaluating brachial artery vasodilatation using high-frequency ultrasound. *Am J Physiol* 268:H1397, 1995.

32

63. Corretti MC, Anderson TJ, Benjamin EJ, et al: Guidelines for the ultrasound assessment of endothelial-dependent flow-mediated vasodilation of the brachial artery. *J Am Coll Cardiol* 39:257, 2002.

64. Deanfield J, Donald A, Ferri C, et al: Endothelial function and dysfunction. Part I: methodological issues for assessment in the different vascular beds: a statement by the Working Group on Endothelin and Endothelial Factors of the European Society of Hypertension. *J Hypertens* 23:7, 2005.

65. Vogel RA, Corretti MD, Plotnick GD: A comparison of the assessment of flow-mediated brachial artery vasodilation using upper versus lower arm arterial occlusion in subjects with and without coronary risk factors. *Clin Cardiol* 23:571, 2000.

66. Mannion TC, Vita JA, Keaney JF, Jr, et al: Non-invasive assessment of brachial artery endothelial vasomotor function: the effect of cuff position on level of discomfort and vasomotor responses. *Vasc Med* 3:263, 1998.

67. Leeson P, Thorne S, Donald A, et al: Non-invasive measurement of endothelial function: effect on brachial artery dilatation of graded endothelial dependent and independent stimuli. *Heart* 78:22, 1997.

68. Ducharme A, Dupuis J, McNicoll S, et al: Comparison of nitroglycerin lingual spray and sublingual tablet on time of onset and duration of brachial artery vasodilation in normal subjects. *Am J Cardiol* 84:952, A8, 1999.

69. Widlansky ME, Gokce N, Keaney JF, et al: The clinical implications of endothelial dysfunction. *J Am Coll Cardiol* 42:1149, 2003.

70. Doi H, Kugiyama K, Ohta Y, et al: Remnants of chylomicron and VLDL impair endothelium-dependent vasorelaxation. *Circulation* 92(Suppl I):1, 1995.

71. Plotnick GD, Corretti MC, Vogel RA: Effect of antioxidant vitamins on the transient impairment of endothelium-dependent brachial artery vasoactivity following a single high-fat meal. *JAMA* 278:1682, 1997.

72. Leeson CP, Hingorani AD, Mullen MJ, et al: Glu298Asp endothelial nitric oxide synthase gene polymorphism interacts with environmental and dietary factors to influence endothelial function. *Circ Res* 90:1153, 2002.

73. Anderson TJ, Uehata A, Gerhard MD, et al: Close relation of endothelial function in the human coronary and peripheral circulation. *J Am Coll Cardiol* 26:1235, 1995.

74. Corretti MC: Endothelial dysfunction: ultrasound measurement of endothelium-dependent flow-mediated brachial artery vasodilation. In Bianco JA, editor: *Subclinical atherosclerosis—assessing the risks*, New York, 2006, Taylor & Francis, pp 3-12.

75. Bots ML, Westerink J, Rabelink TJ, de Koning EJP: Assessment of flow-mediated vasodilatation (FMD) of the brachial artery: effects of technical aspects of the FMD measurement of the FMD response. *Eur Heart J* 26:363, 2005.

76. Haluska B, Sutherland A, Case C, et al: Automated edge-detection technique for measurement of brachial artery reactivity: a comparison of concordance with manual measurements. *Ultrasound Med Biol* 27:1285, 2001.

77. Sorensen KE, Celermajer DS, Spiegelhalter DJ, et al: Non-invasive detection of human endothelium dependent arterial responses: accuracy and reproducibility. *Br Heart J* 74:247, 1995.

78. Herrington DM, Fan L, Drum M, et al: Brachial flow-mediated vasodilator responses in population-based research: methods, reproducibility and effects of age, gender and baseline diameter. *J Cardiovasc Risk* 8:319, 2001.

79. Slyper AH: What vascular ultrasound testing has revealed about pediatric atherogenesis, and a potential clinical role for ultrasound in pediatric risk assessment. *J Clin Endocrinol Metab* 89:3089, 2004.

80. Philpott A, Anderson TJ: Reactive hyperemia and cardiovascular risk. *Arterioscler Thromb Vasc Biol* 27:2065, 2007.

81. Palínkás A, Tóth E, Venneri L, et al: Temporal heterogeneity of endothelium-dependent and -independent dilatation of brachial artery in patients with coronary artery disease. *Int J Cardiovasc Imaging* 18:3372, 2002.

82. Berk BC: Atheroprotective signaling mechanisms activated by steady laminar flow in endothelial cells. *Circulation* 117:1082, 2008.

83. Nohria A, Herhard-Herman M, Creager MA, et al: Role of nitric oxide in the regulation of digital pulse volume in humans. *J Appl Physiol* 101:545, 2006.

84. Hamburg NM, Keyes MJ, Larson MG, et al: Cross-sectional relations of digital vascular function to cardiovascular risk factors in the Framingham Heart Study. *Circulation* 117:2467, 2008.

85. Gerhard-Herman M, Hurley S, Mitra D, et al: Assessment of endothelial function (nitric oxide) at the tip of a finger [abstract]. *Circulation* 106:II170, 2002.

86. Kuvin JT, Patel AR, Sliney KA, et al: Assessment of peripheral vascular endothelial function with finger arterial pulse wave amplitude. *Am Heart J* 78:1210, 2003.

87. Safar ME, Levy BI, Struijker-Boudier H: Current perspectives on arterial stiffness and pulse pressure in hypertension and cardiovascular disease. *Circulation* 107:2864, 2003.

88. Davies JA, Struthers AD: Pulse wave analysis and pulse wave velocity: a critical review of their strengths and weaknesses. *J Hypertens* 21:463, 2003.

89. O'Rourke MF, Adji A: An updated clinical primer on large artery mechanics: implications of pulse waveform analysis and arterial tonometry. *Curr Opin Cardiol* 20:275, 2005.

90. Murgo JP, Westerhof N, Giolma JP, Altobelli SA: Manipulation of ascending aortic pressure and flow wave reflections with the Valsalva maneuver: relationship to input impedance. *Circulation* 63:122, 1981.

91. McEniery MC, Wallace S, Mackenzie IS, et al: Endothelial function is associated with pulse pressure, pulse wave velocity, and augmentation index in healthy humans. *Hypertension* 48:602, 2006.

92. Nigam A, Mitchell GF, Lambert J, Tardiff JC: Relation between conduit vessel stiffness (assessed by tonometry) and endothelial function (assessed by flow-mediated dilatation) in patients with and without coronary heart disease. *Am J Cardiol* 92:395, 2003.

93. Barac A, Campia U, Panza JA: Methods for evaluating endothelial function in humans. *Hypertension* 49:748, 2007.

94. Suwaidi JA, Hamasaki S, Higano ST, et al: Long-term follow-up of patients with mild coronary artery disease and endothelial dysfunction. *Circulation* 101:948, 2000.

95. Schachinger V, Britten MB, Zeiher AM: Prognostic impact of coronary vasodilator dysfunction on adverse long-term outcome of coronary heart disease. *Circulation* 101:1899, 2000.

96. Neunteufl T, Heher S, Katzenschlager R, et al: Late prognostic value of flow-mediated dilation in the brachial artery of patients with chest pain. *Am J Cardiol* 86:207, 2000.

97. Heitzer T, Schlinzig T, Krohn K, et al: Endothelial dysfunction, oxidative stress, and risk of cardiovascular events in patients with coronary artery disease. *Circulation* 104:2673, 2001.

98. Perticone F, Ceravolo R, Pujia A, et al: Prognostic significance of endothelial dysfunction in hypertensive patients. *Circulation* 104:191, 2001.

99. Gokce N, Keaney JF, Jr, Hunter LM, et al: Risk stratification for postoperative cardiovascular events via noninvasive assessment of endothelial function: a prospective study. *Circulation* 105:1567, 2002.

100. Halcox JP, Schenke WH, Zalos G, et al: Prognostic value of coronary vascular endothelial dysfunction. *Circulation* 106:653, 2002.

101. Modena MG, Bonetti L, Coppi F, et al: Prognostic role of reversible endothelial dysfunction in hypertensive postmenopausal women. *J Am Coll Cardiol* 40:505, 2002.

102. Schindler TH, Hornig B, Buser PT, et al: Prognostic value of abnormal vasoreactivity of epicardial coronary arteries to sympathetic stimulation in patients with normal coronary angiograms. *Arterioscler Thromb Vasc Biol* 23:495, 2003.

103. Gokce N, Keaney JF, Jr, Hunter LM, et al: Predictive value of noninvasively determined endothelial dysfunction for long-term cardiovascular events in patients with peripheral vascular disease. *J Am Coll Cardiol* 41:1769, 2003.

Endothelial Function and Dysfunction

Exercise/Emotional Aspects of Preventive Cardiology

CHAPTER 33

Exercise for Restoring Health and Preventing Vascular Disease

Kerry J. Stewart, Elizabeth V. Ratchford, and Mark A. Williams

KEY POINTS

- Increased levels of physical activity and exercise are associated with increased longevity and a decrease in cardiovascular disease risk factors, metabolic syndrome, and diabetes.

- By adding a sedentary lifestyle to its list of controllable risk factors for coronary artery disease, the American Heart Association has made regular exercise a major focus for preventive medicine.

- Exercise regimens should include aerobic, muscle strengthening, and flexibility exercises.

- Cardiac rehabilitation is recognized as integral to the comprehensive care of patients with cardiovascular disease and is recommended as useful and effective (Class I) by the American Heart Association and the American College of Cardiology in patients with coronary artery disease and chronic heart failure.

- The efficacy and effectiveness of cardiac rehabilitation on improvements in health outcomes are beyond the improvements in morbidity and mortality already available through revascularization and optimal pharmacotherapy.

- Elderly individuals with heart disease can benefit greatly from exercise training and other aspects of cardiac rehabilitation and secondary prevention programs.

- Exercise training plays a critical role as a primary treatment of patients with peripheral arterial disease, with the goal of improving quality of life and functional capacity.

This chapter describes the cardiovascular health benefits of regular exercise, the benefits and risks of exercise training and cardiac rehabilitation for individuals with established cardiovascular disease including peripheral arterial disease, and the major types of exercise recommended for cardiovascular health. Exercise prescription guidelines are provided to ensure maximal efficacy and safety of the exercise program.

ROLE OF INCREASED PHYSICAL ACTIVITY IN PRIMARY PREVENTION OF CARDIOVASCULAR DISEASE

The cardiovascular health benefits of regular exercise are well established.[1-3] According to the U.S. Department of Health and Human Services,[3] strong evidence demonstrates that compared with less active persons, more active men and women have lower rates of all-cause mortality, coronary heart disease, hypertension, stroke, type 2 diabetes, metabolic syndrome, colon cancer, breast cancer, and depression. The risk of dying prematurely declines as people become physically active, as evidenced by data shown in Table 33-1.[1-3]

Strong evidence also supports the conclusion that compared with less active people, physically active adults and older adults exhibit a higher level of cardiorespiratory and muscular fitness, have a healthier body mass and composition, and have a metabolic profile that is more favorable for prevention of cardiovascular disease and type 2 diabetes. Modest evidence indicates that physically active adults and older adults have better quality sleep, health-related quality of life, and enhanced bone health.

A recent meta-analysis[4] of 26 studies, incorporating 513,472 individuals (20,666 coronary heart disease events) followed up for 4 to 25 years, showed that individuals who reported performing a high level of leisure-time physical activity had significant protection against coronary heart disease (relative risk, 0.73; P <0.00001), whereas those individuals who practiced a moderate level of physical activity also had a reduced risk of coronary heart disease (relative risk, 0.88; P <0.0001). Data from the Physicians' Health Study[5] showed that adherence to healthy lifestyle factors (normal body weight, never smoking, regular exercise, moderate alcohol intake, and consumption of breakfast cereal and fruits and vegetables) is independently

TABLE 33–1	Risk of Premature Death According to Duration of Leisure-Time Physical Activity
Minutes per Week of Moderate- or Vigorous-Intensity Physical Activity	**Relative Risk**
30	1
90	0.8
180	0.73
330	0.64
420	0.615

33

associated with an 11% lifetime risk of heart failure with exercising ≥5 times per week versus a 14% risk for exercising <5 times per week. Thus, there is substantial protection against the occurrence of cardiovascular disease from moderate to high levels of physical activity, thereby strengthening the recommendations of guidelines.[6]

Increased levels of physical activity and exercise are also associated with increased longevity and a decrease in cardiovascular disease risk factors, metabolic syndrome, and diabetes. In 2009, the American College of Sports Medicine's position statement "Exercise and Physical Activity for Older Adults"[7] reported that although no amount of physical activity can stop the biologic aging process, there is evidence that regular exercise can minimize the physiologic effects of an otherwise sedentary lifestyle and increase active life expectancy by limiting the development and progression of chronic disease and disabling conditions. There is also emerging evidence for significant psychological and cognitive benefits accruing from regular exercise participation by older adults.

Ideally, exercise prescriptions for older adults should include aerobic exercise, muscle strengthening exercises, and flexibility exercises. Although this chapter focuses on cardiovascular disease, adults with chronic conditions such as type 2 diabetes, cancer, osteoarthritis, cognitive disorders, and renal disease are also likely to derive significant therapeutic benefit from prescribed exercise and increased physical activity.[3] In many cases, persons with cardiovascular disease also suffer from these comorbidities, thereby enhancing the importance of exercise training as part of their overall treatment plan.

Despite numerous epidemiologic and experimental studies supporting the beneficial effects of being physically active, this scientific knowledge has not resulted in a more active population. According to the Centers for Disease Control and Prevention,[8] the prevalence of leisure-time physical inactivity throughout the United States ranged from 16% to 49%, whereas the prevalence of adults who engaged in at least moderate physical activity ranged from 33% to 62%, and the prevalence of vigorous physical activity ranged from 15% to 42%. Among adults aged 60 years or older, more than half reported no leisure-time physical activity at all.[9] Thus, a substantial number of adults do not engage in levels of activity sufficient to produce health benefits.

People with chronic disease are more likely to report a sedentary lifestyle, as are minorities and individuals in lower socioeconomic classes.[10] Unfortunately, less than 30% of individuals at high risk for cardiovascular disease receive physical activity counseling during ambulatory care visits.[11] By adding a sedentary lifestyle to its list of controllable risk factors for coronary artery disease, the American Heart Association has made regular exercise a major focus for preventive medicine.[6]

The physical activity goal in the *Healthy People 2010* report by the Centers for Disease Control and Prevention is to increase the proportion of adults who engage in regular exercise and moderate activity for at least 30 minutes each day. This goal matches the Surgeon General's recommendation that all Americans should accumulate at least 30 minutes of activity throughout the day on most days of the week.[12] These guidelines establish the minimal effort needed to derive health benefits from physical activity, although individuals exceeding these recommendations in terms of frequency or intensity are likely to derive additional health and fitness benefits.

Several studies have established an inverse dose-response relationship between the amount of physical activity performed and health risk. Thus, the most fit and active individuals generally have the best risk profiles and reduced levels of early mortality and morbidity from a variety of diseases, including cardiovascular disease. For example, men and women who were generally healthy but less fit by exercise testing had a higher risk of all-cause mortality during an 8-year follow-up compared with those who were moderately or highly fit. Data from the Nurses' Health Study[13] found that physical activity of less than 3.5 hours per week and excess body weight (defined as a body mass index of 25 or higher) accounted for 31% of all premature deaths, 59% of cardiovascular deaths, and 21% of cancer deaths.

In another study, Puerto Rican men in the middle of the physical activity distribution had a 32% to 37% reduction in risk for all-cause mortality.[14] Moreover, compared with the most sedentary quartile of participants, the next most active quartile had an accumulated survival that was approximately 3 years longer. We previously showed that exercise-induced reductions in total and abdominal obesity after 6 months of training were associated with favorable changes in risk factors for cardiovascular disease, including those that constitute metabolic syndrome.[15]

EXERCISE TRAINING EFFECT

The underlying principles for enhanced cardiovascular and musculoskeletal function are similar for those with and without cardiovascular disease and also apply to most other chronic health conditions, such as type 2 diabetes.[16] A brief summary of these principles is provided.

The body adapts to the kind and amount of physical demands placed on it. The response is specific, with the most change generally occurring in those parts of the body on which demands are placed. For exercise to improve fitness, it must overload the muscles or organ system involved in the exercise. In this context, overload is defined as performing exercise at a greater intensity than the intensity to which one is accustomed. Because the effects of exercise are specific to the type of activity engaged, an optimal exercise program should include a variety of activities designed to improve each of the major components of fitness. These are cardiovascular endurance, muscle strength, muscle endurance, and flexibility.

Cardiovascular endurance depends on the ability of the muscles to use oxygen during exercise; hence, it is also known as aerobic endurance. Cardiovascular endurance is dependent on cardiac output providing sufficient oxygen-carrying blood, distribution of the blood to the working muscles, and capacity of the muscles to extract oxygen from a given blood flow.

The principal hemodynamic adaptation to aerobic exercise in individuals with and without heart disease takes place in the peripheral vascular and muscular systems. With regular exercise, the skeletal muscles can extract more oxygen from a given blood flow, and there is a better distribution of the cardiac output. Heart rate and blood pressure are also lower at rest and at a given submaximal workload. As a result, the individual can do more work with less cardiac effort. This adaptation is especially beneficial to cardiac patients who may have limited coronary artery blood supply or poor left ventricular function. Angina may occur at the same threshold, that is, the same double product (heart rate × systolic blood pressure), but this threshold is reached at a higher level of body work.

RISKS OF INCREASED PHYSICAL ACTIVITY

Although habitual physical activity reduces coronary heart disease events, vigorous activity can also acutely and transiently increase the risk of sudden cardiac death and acute myocardial infarction in susceptible persons, as discussed in detail in an American Heart Association Scientific Statement.[17] Exercise-associated acute cardiac events generally occur in individuals with structural cardiac disease. Hereditary or congenital cardiovascular abnormalities are predominantly responsible for cardiac events among young individuals, whereas atherosclerotic disease is primarily responsible for these events in adults.

The absolute rate of exercise-related sudden cardiac death varies with the prevalence of disease in the study population. The incidence of acute myocardial infarction and sudden death is greatest in the habitually least physically active individuals. Although no specific strategies have been widely studied to reduce exercise-related acute cardiovascular events, maintaining regular physical activity may help reduce events because a disproportionate number of events occur in the least physically active subjects performing unaccustomed physical activity. Other strategies, such as screening patients before participation in exercise, excluding high-risk patients from certain activities, promptly evaluating possible prodromal symptoms, training fitness personnel for emergencies, and encouraging patients to avoid high-risk activities, appear prudent but have not been systematically evaluated.

CARDIAC REHABILITATION

Cardiac rehabilitation and secondary prevention programs are recognized as integral to the comprehensive care of patients with cardiovascular disease and as such are recommended as useful and effective (Class I) by the American Heart Association and the American College of Cardiology in the treatment of patients with coronary artery disease and chronic heart failure.[18] In 2009,[19] an estimated 785,000 Americans had a new coronary event, and about 470,000 had a recurrent event. It is estimated that an additional 195,000 silent first myocardial infarctions occur each year. At the same time, the death rate from cardiovascular disease declined by 26% from 1995 to 2005. Thus, the burden of chronic cardiovascular disease remains high, and a growing number of patients will be candidates for cardiac rehabilitation.

In 2007,[18] the American Heart Association and the American Association of Cardiovascular and Pulmonary Rehabilitation recommended that cardiac rehabilitation programs provide several important core components consisting of baseline patient assessment, nutritional counseling, risk factor management (lipids, hypertension, weight, diabetes, and smoking), psychosocial management, physical activity counseling, and exercise training. The American Heart Association also recommends these cardiac rehabilitation components for the elderly.[20] Whereas secondary prevention therapies, such as pharmacologic management of atherosclerosis risk factors and depression, are provided by clinicians in their offices, cardiac rehabilitation is often the most advantageous setting for bringing many of these core components

together in a comprehensive approach to provide exercise training, patient education, behavioral counseling, and psychosocial support.

Studies of efficacy and effectiveness of cardiac rehabilitation document reductions in mortality and improvements in clinical and behavioral outcomes beyond the improvements in morbidity and mortality already available through revascularization and optimal pharmacotherapy. Yet cardiac rehabilitation, like many preventive measures, is underused.[21]

Unfortunately, it is estimated that only 10% to 40% of eligible patients participate in cardiac rehabilitation programs.[22,23] These rates of participation are even less for older patients, a group with the highest prevalence of cardiovascular disease.[24,25] Although Medicare provides payment for cardiac rehabilitation for the diagnoses of myocardial infarction, coronary artery bypass surgery, stable angina, and, more recently, percutaneous revascularization, heart transplantation, and heart valve surgery, there is no such payment for patients who have heart failure or peripheral arterial disease. Insurance coverage by other third-party payers varies considerably throughout the United States.

There are also numerous disparities in cardiac rehabilitation program participation; women with lower incomes are less likely to be referred and less likely to enroll in cardiac rehabilitation, and there is a strong trend for African American women to be less likely to be referred and to enroll.[26] Among 1933 cardiac patients who met the selection criteria of the American College of Cardiology guidelines of eligibility for cardiac rehabilitation, whites were more likely to be referred for cardiac rehabilitation than were blacks.[27] Because almost all patients who have had an acute coronary event, with or without revascularization procedures, will benefit from cardiac rehabilitation, automatic referral systems should be considered to increase use and to reduce disparities.[26]

To compound the problem of access to cardiac rehabilitation based on race, blacks are more likely to have a greater number of adverse risk factors compared with whites.[28] Although both groups gained secondary prevention benefits, the degree of improvement was less for blacks than for whites, and this was especially evident among black women.

A review of all components of cardiac rehabilitation and secondary prevention (such as smoking cessation, behavioral counseling, and pharmacotherapy) is beyond the scope of this chapter. To some extent, the scope is also limited by the nature of the studies on cardiac rehabilitation, which used supervised exercise training as the primary treatment modality. Although not fully evaluated in large-scale trials, a comprehensive approach to cardiac rehabilitation would be more than just exercise training and presumably would produce greater improvements in health and functional status for patients than is evident in the literature.[29] Nevertheless, there is considerable evidence that exercise training by itself produces substantial physiologic benefits, improves risk factors, reduces mortality, and increases aerobic capacity, muscle strength, and functional performance.

Regular exercise training, with the goal of attaining a training effect, is beneficial for almost all patients after myocardial infarction.[30] Contemporary cardiac rehabilitation programs are also experienced in addressing the educational deficiencies of patients, including the special needs of those with cardiac pacemakers and implanted defibrillators, chronic heart failure, diabetes, peripheral arterial disease, and other comorbidities.

In recent years, there is also increased recognition of the importance of resistance training for individuals with and without cardiovascular disease. The American Heart Association recently updated its Scientific Advisory "Resistance Exercise in Individuals With and Without Cardiovascular Disease."[31] It notes that after appropriate screening, resistance training is an effective method to improve muscle strength

544 and endurance, to prevent and manage a variety of chronic medical conditions, to modify cardiac risk factors, and to enhance psychosocial well-being. Although weight machines are most commonly used in formal cardiac rehabilitation programs, alternative modes of resistance training are calisthenics, isometrics, and use of elastic stretch bands.

Most activities requiring lifting and straining, such as weight training, have a large static component. In such activities, there is increased peripheral vascular resistance, with an expected increase in blood pressure but much less of an increase in heart rate or cardiac output compared with aerobic exercise. Nevertheless, brief periods of moderate resistive exercise appear safe and may pose less of a cardiac burden than aerobic exercises of similar effort. In fact, studies show that cardiac patients who were required to carry or lift weights or to perform isometric exercise after a myocardial infarction had fewer ischemic electrocardiographic changes and arrhythmias during resistance exercise than during aerobic exercises. Gradual involvement in resistance training may therefore be beneficial and desirable, especially for patients whose jobs or recreational activities require static efforts.

33

KEY BENEFITS OF EXERCISE TRAINING IN PATIENTS WITH CARDIOVASCULAR DISEASE

Coronary Artery Disease

Candidates for cardiac rehabilitation services historically were patients who recently had a myocardial infarction or had undergone coronary artery bypass graft surgery but now include patients who have undergone percutaneous coronary interventions, are heart transplantation candidates or recipients, or have stable heart failure, peripheral arterial disease with claudication, or other forms of cardiovascular disease.[30] In addition, patients who have undergone other cardiac surgical procedures, such as those with valvular heart disease, also benefit from such programs.[32]

Patients who exercise regularly increase their physical working capacity and are therefore able to perform at higher levels of effort with less fatigue. Among those patients who experience exertional angina pectoris, regular exercise leads to cardiovascular adaptations as described earlier that result in the occurrence of angina at higher exercise levels. This increased anginal threshold allows the patient to do more work, and at any given level of work, the patient feels more comfortable because the work represents a lower percentage of a higher maximal capacity.

As summarized in the American Heart Association Scientific Statement "Cardiac Rehabilitation and Secondary Prevention of Coronary Heart Disease,"[30] exercise training, as part of a comprehensive rehabilitation program, has been shown to slow the progression or partially reduce the severity of coronary atherosclerosis. Multiple factors directly or indirectly appear to contribute to this effect. For example, increased flow-mediated shear stress on artery walls during exercise results in improved endothelial function, which is associated with enhanced synthesis, release, and duration of action of nitric oxide. Nitric oxide is responsible for endothelium-dependent vasodilation and inhibits multiple processes involved in atherogenesis and thrombosis.

Hambrecht and colleagues[33] demonstrated a significant improvement in endothelium-dependent arterial dilation in patients with coronary heart disease and abnormal endothelial function after only 4 weeks of vigorous endurance exercise training. Arterial inflammation probably plays a key role in the development and progression of atherosclerosis, as evidenced by the fact that acute myocardial infarctions often

evolve from mild to moderate coronary artery stenoses and that patients who experience a fatal coronary event invariably had antecedent exposure to one or more major coronary risk factors.[34] Thus, another potential mechanism by which exercise training and increased cardiorespiratory fitness improve prognostic markers in persons with and without heart disease is through reductions in systemic inflammation.[35]

Percutaneous coronary interventions are effective for interruption of the process of acute coronary stenosis. Although it is of great benefit that myocardial tissue damage can be avoided or minimized if the patient is treated in a timely manner, the need to treat the underlying disease that precipitated the stenosis is not changed after a revascularization procedure.[32] Despite the revascularization, some patients are anxious about resuming physical activity after percutaneous coronary intervention and need supervised cardiac rehabilitation to enhance their confidence to undertake physical activity and other favorable lifestyle changes. Supervised cardiac rehabilitation also promotes early identification of new signs and symptoms indicating possible restenosis, leading to prompt medical evaluation and treatment.

Despite the expanded use of percutaneous coronary interventions, there are few controlled studies of cardiac rehabilitation after these procedures. In one study,[36] patients who had undergone percutaneous coronary interventions were randomly assigned to a behaviorally oriented intervention or a control group. After 12 months, the intervention patients, compared with controls, improved significantly on self-rated measures of smoking, exercise, and diet habits. Patients also lost weight, improved their exercise capacity, and experienced less chest pain during exertion. Although the mechanisms for decreased mortality with exercise have not been fully explained, exercise training improves the lipid profile,[37,38] reduces blood pressure,[38,39] lowers fasting glucose concentration,[38,40] and reduces body fat and increases lean body mass.[15,37,41]

Exercise training has been shown to reduce mortality in patients after myocardial infarction. In one meta-analysis on the combined results of 10 randomized clinical trials that included 4347 patients (control, 2145 patients; rehabilitation, 2202 patients), the pooled odds ratios of 0.76 for all-cause death and of 0.75 for cardiovascular death were significantly lower in the rehabilitation group than in the control group, with no significant difference for nonfatal recurrent myocardial infarction.[42]

In a later meta-analysis of the combined results of 48 clinical trials with 8940 patients, there was a similar 25% reduction in cardiovascular mortality but no significant difference in the rates of nonfatal myocardial infarction and revascularization.[43] This beneficial effect of cardiac rehabilitation on mortality was independent of coronary heart disease diagnosis, type of cardiac rehabilitation, dose of exercise intervention, length of follow-up, trial quality, and trial publication date, which was through March 2003.

Heart Failure

Patients with heart failure often experience fatigue and dyspnea with exertion. Although the primary pathology of heart failure results from cardiovascular dysfunction, abnormalities in peripheral blood flow, skeletal muscle morphology, metabolism, strength, and endurance all contribute to the heart failure syndrome.[32] Rest was frequently recommended for patients with heart failure in the past,[44] but it is now established that exercise training produces substantial physiologic benefits, attenuation of symptoms, and improved quality of life for patients with left ventricular dysfunction and chronic heart failure.[32,45-49]

Several mechanisms contribute to improved functional capacity in patients with heart failure who participate in exercise training and cardiac rehabilitation.[32] Central hemodynamic mechanisms include increases in peak cardiac output, heart rate, and stroke volume. Peripheral vascular and metabolic mechanisms include improved endothelial vasodilator function, increased cellular oxidative enzyme activity, greater oxygen extraction from the blood, and improved neurohumoral axis. These adaptations result in increased oxygen delivery or use in the metabolically more active skeletal muscle, thus delaying reliance on anaerobic metabolism. Exercise training has beneficial effects on skeletal muscle by improving functional, histologic, and biochemical characteristics and by reducing the activation of the muscle neural afferents known as ergoreceptors.

Adverse events related to exercise training in heart failure in published studies have been few. A limitation in the existing literature is that most studies have been relatively small and have not been adequately powered to evaluate mortality and morbidity. To examine the issue of exercise safety and effectiveness in a large sample of patients with heart failure, Heart Failure: A Controlled Trial Investigating Outcomes of Exercise Training (HF-ACTION) was undertaken to determine whether aerobic-type exercise training reduces all-cause mortality or all-cause hospitalization and improves quality of life.[44,50]

Participants in HF-ACTION were randomized from April 2003 through February 2007 at 82 centers within the United States, Canada, and France, and the median follow-up was 30 months. The 2331 participants were medically stable patients with heart failure and reduced ejection fraction. The interventions were usual care plus aerobic exercise training (n = 1172), consisting of 36 supervised sessions followed by home-based training, and usual care alone (n = 1159). Overall, the performance of exercise training was well tolerated and safe, with only 37 patients in the exercise training group having at least one hospitalization due to an event that occurred during or within 3 hours of exercise, whereas 22 patients had such a hospitalization despite not undergoing exercise training.

Among patients in the exercise group, 759 (65%) experienced a primary clinical event compared with 796 (68%) in the usual care group. In the primary analysis adjusted for heart failure etiology, exercise training resulted in a nonsignificant reduction in all-cause mortality or hospitalization by an absolute reduction of 4%. However, after adjustment for key baseline characteristics that are prognostic for these clinical endpoints (exercise test duration, left ventricular ejection fraction, depression, and history of atrial fibrillation or flutter), exercise training reduced the incidence of all-cause mortality or hospitalization by 11% ($P = 0.03$). Participants in exercise training also achieved significant improvements in cardiopulmonary exercise test parameters and distance in the 6-minute walk test.

Exercise training also conferred modest but statistically significant improvements in self-reported health status compared with usual care without training.[50] Improvements occurred early and persisted over time. Based on the safety of exercise, improvements in quality of life and functional work capacity, and modest reductions in clinical events, HF-ACTION supports a prescribed exercise training program for patients with chronic heart failure above and beyond usual medical care.

CARDIAC REHABILITATION IN THE ELDERLY

Increasing evidence has accumulated during the past 3 decades that elderly individuals with coronary heart disease can benefit greatly from exercise training and other aspects of cardiac rehabilitation and secondary prevention

programs.[23] This is especially important given that those ≥65 years of age represent the greatest number of individuals with heart disease.[19] Traditionally, components of secondary prevention programming (exercise; smoking cessation; management of dyslipidemia, hypertension, diabetes, and weight; and interventions directed at return to work and psychosocial issues) are provided by the clinician through the office setting or through cardiac rehabilitation programs. Cardiac rehabilitation programs are particularly well suited to the provision of secondary prevention services, but unfortunately, many older patients who would derive benefit from these interventions do not participate because of lack of referral or a variety of societal and other barriers.[51,52]

A structured exercise program may be novel to older individuals or, in some instances, an activity in which they have not participated for many years. Furthermore, for older persons with coronary heart disease, the clinical manifestations represent the effects of the disease superimposed on the physiologic effects of age, which too often lead to decreases in exercise capacity and overall physical activity.

Whereas exertional angina pectoris remains common in this age group, an increased percentage of older patients have atypical manifestations of myocardial ischemia, including dyspnea on exertion and poor functional capacity, often exacerbated by comorbidities such as chronic lung disease, peripheral arterial disease, arthritis, and neuromuscular disorders that may limit ambulation. Thus, the absence of exercise-related anginal symptoms in older patients with suspected coronary heart disease may merely reflect the lack of physical activity.[53,54]

As a means of increasing physical activity and fitness for older persons with heart disease, the prescription of exercise is an essential component of secondary prevention.[20,55] The basis for the exercise intervention in these patients includes improved functional capacity with reduced activity-related abnormal signs or symptoms, including fatigue.[52,56-61] Expected outcomes are similar to those for younger patients, although absolute levels of functional capacity in the elderly are less, and results may require longer program participation in this age group.[52,56] As with younger patients, a multidisciplinary approach to secondary prevention that includes exercise may have a positive impact on other heart disease risk factors.[23,60,62]

Whether exercise as a part of secondary prevention is associated with a reduction in morbidity or mortality as in younger patients has yet to be established. However, studies of older patients with and without heart disease have suggested a positive impact of physical activity on mortality.[63-65] Findings have suggested that light to moderate activity is associated with a significantly lower risk of all-cause mortality in persons with established coronary heart disease and an inverse association between physical activity and all-cause mortality in both older men and women.

ROLE OF EXERCISE TRAINING IN PATIENTS WITH PERIPHERAL ARTERIAL DISEASE

Exercise training plays a critical role as a primary treatment of patients with peripheral arterial disease (PAD), with the goal of improving quality of life and functional capacity. According to the practice guidelines of the American College of Cardiology and the American Heart Association (ACC/AHA) for the management of PAD, supervised exercise training is rated as Class I, Level of Evidence A, for the initial treatment of claudication.[66] The first randomized controlled trial was published in 1966; a marked improvement in walking ability was seen in patients with claudication assigned to daily exercise.[67]

Several prospective randomized trials have demonstrated that exercise training improves claudication symptoms.[68-70] Studies differ in terms of the magnitude of the reported response to exercise, a finding likely explained by variability both in the exercise intervention itself (duration, frequency, and intensity) and in outcome measures.[71] A meta-analysis of 21 nonrandomized and randomized studies reported a 179% increase in pain-free walking distance and a 122% increase in maximum walking distance.[68] A more recent Cochrane review of 22 randomized controlled trials for claudication reported an overall improvement in walking ability of approximately 50% to 200%.[70]

Overall, patients can expect approximately a doubling of their pain-free and maximum walking distances with exercise training, with the best results occurring in supervised programs compared with unsupervised home-based training. Another Cochrane review of eight small trials including a total of 319 subjects found a significant improvement in maximum treadmill walking distance in supervised compared with unsupervised programs, with a difference of approximately 150 meters.[72] The magnitude and durability of the benefits of home-based exercise for treatment of claudication, however, remain controversial.

Surprisingly, only a small number of studies have compared exercise training with lower extremity revascularization for the treatment of claudication. One such prospective randomized trial compared supervised exercise with angioplasty and found that mean maximum walking distances progressively increased in the supervised exercise group at 6, 9, and 12 months but did not increase in the angioplasty group even though the ankle-brachial indices improved with angioplasty.[73] Subsequently, the same group reported that after a median follow-up of 70 months, the functional outcome was the same between the exercise and angioplasty groups.[74] Among 62 patients randomized to angioplasty or medical treatment,[75] there were no significant group differences at 2 years in treadmill walking distances or quality of life; the medical group was not in a supervised program but was given "exercise advice" to walk at home.

A trial from the Netherlands randomized 151 patients with claudication to either endovascular revascularization (angioplasty with conditional stenting) or 24 weeks of twice-weekly 30-minute hospital-based treadmill exercise sessions.[76] Endovascular revascularization provided more immediate clinical success, but after 6 and 12 months, the treatment groups were equivalent in terms of functional capacity and quality of life scores. The CLEVER (Claudication: Exercise Versus Endoluminal Revascularization) trial is a similar ongoing National Institutes of Health/National Heart, Lung, and Blood Institute–funded multicenter randomized clinical trial comparing supervised exercise with endovascular revascularization for the treatment of claudication due to aortoiliac disease.[77] The results of the CLEVER trial are hoped to provide more definitive data on the optimal approach to treatment of aortoiliac disease.

The exact mechanism to explain why exercise training improves claudication symptoms is not known but is likely multifactorial. Initial theories proposed that exercise increases collateral vessels through angiogenesis or leads to increased blood flow, but subsequent data on these hypotheses are inconsistent.[71,78] More likely, mechanisms for the benefit of exercise training include metabolic adaptations with improved oxygen extraction by the muscle, better walking efficiency from a biomechanical standpoint, and enhanced endothelial function.[79,80] Calf skeletal muscle may increase its oxidative capacity; improvements in exercise have correlated with changes in carnitine metabolism.[78]

In addition, the benefits of exercise may not be fully explained by local effects on the lower extremities, as evidenced by a randomized trial in which 104 patients with PAD were assigned to upper limb aerobic exercise, lower limb aerobic exercise, or no exercise for 24 weeks.[81] Similar improvements in claudication distance and maximum walking distance were observed in both exercise groups but not in the control group, suggesting a systemic benefit of exercise; an increase in exercise pain tolerance was also noted in the exercise groups.

Exercise may attenuate the inflammatory response in the long term[71] and has well-established beneficial effects on cardiovascular risk factors such as hypertension, diabetes, dyslipidemia, and obesity. Further rigorous prospective investigation is needed to ascertain whether this global improvement in vascular health may translate into reduced morbidity or mortality in patients with PAD. A retrospective cohort study from Japan showed that completion of a 12-week supervised exercise training program reduced both cardiovascular morbidity and mortality in patients with PAD.[82] The long-term impact of supervised exercise training on outcomes in PAD patients remains unknown.

Whereas the efficacy of exercise training for the treatment of *symptomatic* PAD has been well established, recent evidence now suggests that exercise training may also play an important role in the treatment of *asymptomatic* PAD. McDermott and coworkers[79] found that supervised treadmill training improved walking and quality of life outcomes in patients with PAD with and without claudication. Lower extremity resistance training was also beneficial for improving functional performance but not to the same degree as supervised treadmill training. Given that the large majority of patients with PAD are either asymptomatic or have atypical symptoms, these findings are particularly important and may herald a significant change in the clinical approach to treatment of PAD; further research in this area is warranted.

In spite of the numerous studies demonstrating the efficacy of exercise training, several barriers prevent its widespread use. Perhaps most notably, supervised exercise is not generally a covered benefit under most health insurance plans including Medicare, although PAD rehabilitation has had a Current Procedural Terminology code (CPT 93668) since 2001. Other barriers to participation include a time commitment and lack of broad availability of PAD rehabilitation centers.

Barriers also exist at the provider level, as many clinicians may hesitate to refer a high-risk patient with multiple comorbidities to an exercise program. However, that same patient may in fact derive the greatest benefit from exercise. Because of the systemic nature of obstructive atherosclerotic vascular disease and the high prevalence of coronary artery disease in this population, patients with PAD in many cases may qualify for cardiac rehabilitation from an insurance standpoint by meeting one of the other criteria as noted elsewhere in this chapter (e.g., recent myocardial infarction, coronary revascularization, or angina).[29] The decision to enroll a patient with PAD in an exercise training program should be individualized and may be affected by medical comorbidities that limit walking ability, such as pulmonary or degenerative joint disease. Treadmill exercise is not recommended in patients with foot ulcers or critical limb ischemia.

A meta-analysis found that the best results were seen with walking programs lasting more than 30 minutes per session, at least three times per week, for at least 6 months.[68] Studies suggest that the benefits of the supervised program may extend beyond the duration of the program. For example, among patients who attended supervised training twice weekly for 10 weeks, the improvements in claudication distance and maximum walking distance were sustained at 3 years[83]; there was no difference between the results at 3 months and at 1, 2, or 3 years.

EXERCISE TESTING FOR PERIPHERAL ARTERIAL DISEASE

Per the ACC/AHA guidelines, standardized treadmill testing should ideally be performed before initiation of exercise training to establish the magnitude of the functional limitation due to claudication and to provide a baseline for measurement of the response to therapy.[66] The treadmill test may reveal nonvascular factors contributing to the impaired walking ability (such as degenerative joint disease) and assist in individualizing the exercise prescription. Continuous electrocardiographic monitoring is useful, particularly given the high prevalence of concomitant coronary artery disease.

A graded treadmill test is preferable to a constant-load test because it is more reproducible and shows less variability.[84] For example, the Gardner protocol starts at 2 mph at a 0% grade; the grade is then increased by 2% every 2 minutes.[85] Data including the time at onset of claudication symptoms and the maximum walking time should be recorded. A 6-minute walk test may be used as an alternative to treadmill testing.[66,86]

The need for formal cardiac testing before initiation of a PAD exercise program should be individualized. Exercise centers differ in terms of enrollment requirements. At present, a limited though growing number of clinical exercise centers in the United States offer PAD rehabilitation programs. At minimum at most centers, the patient will need a referral from a physician and a baseline electrocardiogram. Preferably, the referral should also include a recent clinic note and the results of a graded exercise test to establish the cardiovascular response to exercise. Sessions are supervised with monitoring of heart rate and blood pressure; electrocardiographic telemetry is recommended for at least the first session and may be used throughout each session if necessary. Patients with diabetes require blood glucose monitoring to avoid hypoglycemia as exercise increases insulin sensitivity. In addition, proper footwear and routine self-examination of the feet are important, particularly in patients with diabetic neuropathy.

GUIDELINES FOR EXERCISE PRESCRIPTION INCLUDING THE ROLE OF AEROBIC AND RESISTANCE TRAINING

Healthy Adults

Most epidemiologic studies confirm significant risk reduction for those achieving at least moderate-intensity physical activity on most days of the week compared with those who are sedentary.[3] Further increases in fitness produce relatively modest additional benefits. Thus, individuals do not need to attain high levels of fitness to accrue substantial health benefits from exercise.

In 2007, the American College of Sports Medicine and the American Heart Association updated their physical activity guidelines for adults.[1] To promote and to maintain health, all healthy adults aged 18 to 65 years old need moderate-intensity aerobic physical activity for a minimum of 30 minutes on 5 days each week or vigorous-intensity aerobic physical activity for a minimum of 20 minutes on 3 days each week. Combinations of moderate- and vigorous-intensity activity can be performed to meet this recommendation. For example, a person can meet the recommendation by walking briskly for 30 minutes twice during the week and then jogging for 20 minutes on two other days.

Moderate-intensity aerobic activity, which is equivalent to a brisk walk and noticeably accelerates the heart rate, can be accumulated toward the 30-minute minimum by performing bouts each lasting 10 minutes or more. Vigorous-intensity activity is exemplified by jogging and causes rapid breathing and a substantial increase in heart rate. In addition, every adult should perform activities that maintain or increase muscle strength and endurance a minimum of 2 days each week. Because of the dose-response relationship between physical activity and health, persons who wish to further improve their personal fitness, reduce their risk for chronic diseases and disabilities, or prevent unhealthy weight gain may benefit by exceeding the minimum recommended amounts of physical activity.

Exercise Prescription Guidelines for Patients with Cardiovascular Disease Including the Older Patient

Methods for prescribing exercise for cardiac patients generally do not require significant modification for older patients. The exercise prescription should define individual patient guidelines for activity while promoting variety in the exercise regimen. The exercise prescription should encourage the participant to engage in all aspects of physical fitness, including aerobic capacity and muscle endurance, range of motion and flexibility, and muscle strength. Modification of the components of the exercise prescription should be routinely considered, particularly for those persons with comorbidities that limit mobility (e.g., musculoskeletal limitations, arthritis, pulmonary disease, and peripheral arterial disease). Increase in energy expenditure and enhancement of functional independence should be emphasized, as well as participation in activities that increase socialization, which should affect feelings of isolation and depression, not uncommon in this age group. Increasing frequency and duration of activity should supersede increases in intensity, thereby reducing the likelihood for overuse injuries.

Recommendations for increasing participation in programs of physical activity should include a broader interpretation of exercise programming, including vocational and recreational activities as well as activities of daily living. Recommendations should also be sensitive to considerations of differences in needs between women and men and ethnic and racial diversity. Because likelihood of participation is increased with physician referral and support, it is incumbent on clinicians to strongly and repeatedly encourage participation in a supervised exercise program.

The use of strength training and flexibility activities for all patients as integral components of the overall exercise prescription should also assist in improving neuromuscular function, muscle strength, and endurance. Such training is essential to improvement of responses to the various physical demands of daily living as well as occupational and recreational activities and improvement of functional independence, self-esteem, and health-related quality of life. In men and women, strength training improves through neuromuscular adaptation, muscle fiber hypertrophy (although limited), and increased muscle oxidative capacity due to the combination of aerobic exercise and strength development, which is a feature of resistance-type circuit training.[87] Even in the oldest persons, resistance training significantly increases strength, gait velocity, balance and coordination, walking endurance, and stair-climbing power.[88-90]

Aerobic Training

Aerobic forms of exercise training are designed to increase functional capacity and endurance and to increase overall energy expenditure while enhancing quality of life. The primary components of the aerobic exercise prescription are

TABLE 33–2 | Recommended Components of the Aerobic Exercise Prescription

Frequency
3 to 5 session/week initially, progressing to every day when appropriate

Intensity
Heart rate reserve: Define a target heart rate based on peak exercise heart rate, resting heart rate, and a selected percentage based on fitness level (50% to 60% initially, progressing to ≥70% as indicated).
Percentage of peak heart rate: Select a target percentage of peak exercise heart rate (60% to 70% initially, progressing to 85% as indicated).
Percentage of peak MET level: Select a target percentage of peak functional capacity in METs (50% to 60% initially, progressing to ≥70% as indicated).
Perception of exertion: On the Borg Scale of Perceived Exertion (rating of 6 to 20), patients should attempt to achieve a perceived exertion level of 11 to 16. It is particularly useful for patients who have difficulty measuring heart rate or as an adjunct to heart rate measurement.

Duration
5 to 20 minutes initially, dependent on intensity of effort and the patient's tolerance, progressing to 30 to 40 minutes as indicated

Modality
Exercise activities should use large muscle groups, that is, legs and arms alone or in combination (e.g., outdoor or treadmill walking, cycling, arm ergometry, rowing, swimming).
Avoid high-impact activities (e.g., jogging), particularly early in the exercise program, to reduce the potential for injury.
Exercise may be continuous (few, if any, short rest periods during the exercise session) or discontinuous (periodic rest periods during the exercise session).

Progression
Changes in the exercise prescription should be based on the patient's tolerance to activity.
Signs or symptoms of intolerance (e.g., angina, significant cardiac arrhythmias, abnormal blood pressure response, unusual shortness of breath, or muscle/orthopedic distress) require evaluation and possible reduction in intensity or duration of exercise.
Conversely, patients may periodically receive increases in exercise intensity or duration of activity as exercise training responses improve (e.g., reduced exercise heart rate and systolic blood pressure, as well as perception of effort to standardized exercise workloads).

From American College of Sports Medicine; Thompson WR, Gordon NF, Pescatello LS: *ACSM's guidelines for exercise testing and prescription,* ed 8, Philadelphia, 2010, Lippincott Williams & Wilkins.

TABLE 33–3 | Examples of Estimated MET Levels for Various Activities

Specific Activity	Estimated MET Level
Bicycling for leisure (light to moderate effort)	4-8
Conditioning exercises (light to moderate effort)	3-7
Home activities (light to moderate effort)	2-6
Lawn/garden activities (light to moderate effort)	2-6
Fishing and hunting	2-6
Jogging/running (light to moderate effort)	7-8
Self-care	2-4
Sexual activity	1-2
Various sport activities	2-10
Walking 2.0 mph	2-3
Walking 3.0 mph	3-4
Walking 4.0 mph	4-5
Swimming for leisure (light to moderate effort)	6-8

From Ainsworth BE, Haskell WL, Whitt MC, et al: Compendium of physical activities: an update of activity codes and MET intensities. *Med Sci Sports Exerc* 32(Suppl):S498, 2000.

interrelated and include frequency, intensity, and duration. As an example, when intensity of the activity is limited, as is often the case with older patients with cardiovascular disease who have reduced functional capacity or various comorbid conditions, frequency or duration of the activity might be increased. Table 33-2 provides a general schematic for the prescription of aerobic exercise in older cardiac patients.

Increasing overall levels of physical activity may also be accomplished by less specific programming, which might include any number of daily vocational and recreation activities. Estimates of various levels of energy expenditure are available that can assist both patients and physicians in making decisions about which activities are appropriate. An example is found in Table 33-3, in which estimated metabolic equivalent (MET) levels are described in multiples of resting oxygen uptake. However, these estimations of energy expenditure can be highly disparate from actual values, dependent on the individual's level of vigor.

Resistance Training

Aging skeletal muscle responds to progressive overload through resistance training. However, emphasis must be placed on providing older persons with adequate time for musculoskeletal adaptation and the development of appropriate training technique, particularly at the initiation of a resistance training program; this practice will reduce the likelihood of muscle overuse, soreness, and injury.[31] This is important in older patients with cardiovascular disease and is also essential for those with hypertension, arthritis, pulmonary disease, or other physically limiting conditions.[91]

The initial workload intensity and frequency of training should be modest, providing for the use of proper body mechanics and avoidance of breath-holding and straining during exercise. The initial exercise prescription and subsequent progression of resistance should be undertaken with caution. Alternatives to traditional resistance can be considered, including aquatic resistance exercise and modification of the exercise components, such as variation of exercises, more gradual progression, and increased rest periods within each session.

Table 33-4 describes recommendations for the prescription of resistance training. In general, the methods and considerations for prescribing resistance in older adults are not different from those in younger persons. However, as mentioned previously, modifications may be needed to accommodate health conditions and other individual limitations.[31] Because the effects of any exercise program including resistance are specific to the muscle groups being trained, training regimens should involve all major muscle groups.[92]

Although few data identifying the appropriate timing for initiation of resistance training after a cardiac event are available, conventional guidelines suggest a restrictive maximal weight limit (of 10 to 20 pounds) for up to 12 to 16 weeks, particularly in unsupervised activities. However, Stewart and colleagues[93] initiated resistance training as part of a combined resistance and aerobic program as soon as 6 weeks after myocardial infarction, demonstrating significantly improved functional capacity and arm and leg strength with no adverse clinical or exercise-related events. As the resistance participant progresses in the training program, resistance intensity may be increased to provide for further improvement. In

TABLE 33–4	Prescription of Resistance Training for Older Adults (>50 years)

Select 6-8 Different Exercises That Involve Major Muscle Groups (Examples)

Upper body: chest press, shoulder press, triceps extension, biceps curl, and pull-down (upper back)

Midsection of the body: lower back extension and abdominal crunch/curl-up

Lower body: quadriceps extension or leg press, leg curls (hamstrings), and calf raise

Exercise Prescription Components

Initially, use single sets of 6-8 varied exercises, 2 days per week.

Each set should include 10-15 repetitions of an exercise at <40% of 1-repetition maximum (1-RM).*

Provide 1-2 minutes rest between exercises.

Alternate between upper and lower body work.

Exercise Technique

Perform each exercise through a full range of motion, in a controlled rhythmic manner, at a slow to moderate speed.

Avoid breath-holding and straining (Valsalva maneuver) by exhaling during the contraction or exertion phase of the exercise and inhaling during the relaxation or rest phase of the exercise.

Emphasize proper body mechanics throughout each exercise.

Progression of Exercise

As 12-15 repetitions of a given exercise become easily accomplished, consider updating the prescription in the following order:

Vary type of exercises.

Increase level of resistance: increasing by 5% of 1-RM, up to 40% 1-RM for arm exercises and up to 60% 1-RM for leg exercises.

Add a second set of exercises without increasing level of resistance.

Add a third day of resistance training during the week.

*1-RM is the greatest amount of resistance (i.e., weight) that can be lifted or pushed with a single effort. As an alternative approach, a method of trial and error to determine a level of resistance for which the participant can perform 10 repetitions can be used. The participant can thus work toward comfortably progressing to 15 repetitions before increasing resistance.

older persons, this increase can be achieved by increasing the resistance (or weight) or adding a second set per exercise. Increasing the number of repetitions within a set or decreasing the duration of rest periods between sets or exercises is generally not recommended for this age group.[31]

Cardiovascular responses to resistance training should be measured, including heart rate, blood pressure, and perception of exertion. Because of the short duration of individual resistance exercises, heart rate response is generally lower than during aerobic exercise. However, blood pressure response can be greater, and thus heart rate alone may not accurately reflect overall cardiovascular response.[94]

In patients who have a history of hypertension, blood pressure response to resistance training should be evaluated, especially in those who have known heart disease. However, blood pressure measured immediately after rather than during the actual resistance exercise is likely to underestimate the pressure response.[95] Consequently, blood pressure ideally should be assessed during the last couple of repetitions during resistance training, along with a rating of perceived exertion; a rating of 11 to 14 ("fairly light" to "somewhat hard") on the Borg category scale is recommended.[31,96] Participants should be frequently reminded of potential adverse signs and symptoms, such as dizziness, excessive shortness of breath, chest discomfort, heart rhythm irregularities, or acute pain in the muscles or joints; resistance training should be immediately discontinued with these occurrences.[31,96]

EXERCISE PRESCRIPTION FOR PERIPHERAL ARTERIAL DISEASE

A standardized program consists of three sessions per week for 12 weeks, although more recent studies have employed a 24-week program.[76,79] The participant starts with 5 minutes of warm-up, followed by 50 minutes of intermittent exercise and 5 minutes of cool-down. The treadmill typically starts at 0% grade at 2 mph; the grade is kept constant during the course of each session. A graded pain scale of 1 to 5 is used to rate the claudication symptoms to allow the exercise physiologist to monitor the progress.[97]

The participant walks on the treadmill until the claudication discomfort reaches a moderate level (4), preferably within the first 5 minutes on the treadmill. He or she then gets off the treadmill and rests in a chair until the discomfort completely subsides. Treadmill walking then commences again, with repeated bouts of exercise and rest, ideally for a total of 50 minutes.

To maximize the benefit of the exercise training sessions, the grade and speed are increased as walking ability improves. When the patient is able to walk for 5 to 8 minutes at the current speed and grade without stopping, the settings should be changed for the next session. For example, the grade may be increased by 2% per session up to 10%; the speed may then be progressively increased as tolerated. Patients should also be instructed to walk at home for 30 to 60 minutes at least twice per week in addition to the three supervised sessions.

Progress in an exercise program should be objectively measured with subsequent treadmill testing, recording variables such as pain-free walking time or distance, maximum walking time or distance, or the work performed in metabolic equivalents calculated from the speed and grade of the treadmill. Questionnaires such as the Walking Impairment Questionnaire are not typically used in clinical practice but may be employed as time permits to assess functional status.[84]

Repeated testing with ankle-brachial indices is not generally necessary as the results typically do not change in spite of the expected improvement in functional capacity.[71] As claudication symptoms improve and exercise tolerance increases, patients should be monitored closely for any signs or symptoms of cardiac ischemia, which may have initially been masked by a limited walking ability.

After the completion of a supervised program, patients should be given an exercise prescription for a home-based maintenance program with the use of claudication symptoms as a guide. Home-based exercise should be similar to the supervised program with intermittent periods of exercise to moderate levels of pain followed by rest until the pain completely subsides.

Several tools may improve compliance at home, such as follow-up phone calls, using a pedometer, joining a gym, setting goals, keeping a walking diary or logbook, finding an exercise "buddy," and putting daily exercise on a "to-do list." Websites such as http://startwalkingnow.org/ sponsored by the American Heart Association may be used to plot walking routes and to log walking times and distances. Throughout the supervised exercise training and beyond, regular medical follow-up should be encouraged to optimize medical management focused on cardiovascular risk reduction.

LONG-TERM MAINTENANCE OF EXERCISE TRAINING

Unfortunately, long-term adherence to formal exercise programs remains a continuing challenge. Because regular exercise training and participation in physical activity are

33

Exercise for Restoring Health and Preventing Vascular Disease necessary to maintain the physiologic benefits described throughout this chapter, many of these benefits are lost in a few weeks when adherence fails. Asking and advising the patient about exercise and physical activity patterns should be a routine part of each visit.

To further emphasize its importance, health care providers may refer to specific advice about activity as an "exercise prescription," underscoring that it is just as important as medicines that might also be prescribed. Both patients and health care providers should adopt the understanding that "exercise is medicine" in terms of its importance to restoration of health and prevention of disease.

REFERENCES

1. Haskell WL, Lee IM, Pate RR, et al: Physical activity and public health: updated recommendation for adults from the American College of Sports Medicine and the American Heart Association. *Circulation* 116:1081, 2007.
2. Nelson ME, Rejeski WJ, Blair SN, et al: Physical activity and public health in older adults: recommendation from the American College of Sports Medicine and the American Heart Association. *Circulation* 116:1094, 2007.
3. Physical Activity Guidelines Advisory Committee report, 2008, Washington, DC, 2008, U.S. Department of Health and Human Services.
4. Sofi F, Capalbo A, Cesari F, et al: Physical activity during leisure time and primary prevention of coronary heart disease: an updated meta-analysis of cohort studies. *Eur J Cardiovasc Prev Rehabil* 15:247, 2008.
5. Djousse L, Driver JA, Gaziano JM: Relation between modifiable lifestyle factors and lifetime risk of heart failure. *JAMA* 302:394, 2009.
6. Thompson PD, Buchner D, Pina IL, et al: Exercise and physical activity in the prevention and treatment of atherosclerotic cardiovascular disease: a statement from the Council on Clinical Cardiology (Subcommittee on Exercise, Rehabilitation, and Prevention) and the Council on Nutrition, Physical Activity, and Metabolism (Subcommittee on Physical Activity). *Circulation* 107:3109, 2003.
7. Chodzko-Zajko WJ, Proctor DN, Fiatarone Singh MA, et al: American College of Sports Medicine position stand. Exercise and physical activity for older adults. *Med Sci Sports Exerc* 41:1510, 2009.
8. Chowdhury PP, Balluz L, Murphy W, et al: Surveillance of certain health behaviors among states and selected local areas—United States, 2005. *MMWR Surveill Summ* 56:1, 2007.
9. Hughes JP, McDowell MA, Brody DJ: Leisure-time physical activity among US adults 60 or more years of age: results from NHANES 1999-2004. *J Phys Act Health* 5:347, 2008.
10. Crespo CJ, Smit E, Andersen RE, et al: Race/ethnicity, social class and their relation to physical inactivity during leisure time: results from the Third National Health and Nutrition Examination Survey, 1988-1994. *Am J Prev Med* 18:46, 2000.
11. Ma J, Urizar GG, Jr, Alehegn T, Stafford RS: Diet and physical activity counseling during ambulatory care visits in the United States. *Prev Med* 39:815, 2004.
12. Physical activity and health: a report of the Surgeon General, Atlanta, Georgia, 1996, U.S. Department of Health and Human Services, Centers for Disease Control and Prevention, National Center for Chronic Disease Prevention and Health Promotion.
13. Hu FB, Willett WC, Li T, et al: Adiposity as compared with physical activity in predicting mortality among women. *N Engl J Med* 351:2694, 2004.
14. Crespo CJ, Palmieri MR, Perdomo RP, et al: The relationship of physical activity and body weight with all-cause mortality: results from the Puerto Rico Heart Health Program. *Ann Epidemiol* 12:543, 2002.
15. Stewart KJ, Bacher AC, Turner KL, et al: Effect of exercise on blood pressure in older persons: a randomized controlled trial. *Arch Intern Med* 165:756, 2005.
16. Marwick TH, Hordern MD, Miller T, et al: Exercise training for type 2 diabetes mellitus: impact on cardiovascular risk: a scientific statement from the American Heart Association. *Circulation* 119:3244, 2009.
17. Thompson PD, Franklin BA, Balady GJ, et al: Exercise and acute cardiovascular events placing the risks into perspective: a scientific statement from the American Heart Association Council on Nutrition, Physical Activity, and Metabolism and the Council on Clinical Cardiology. *Circulation* 115:2358, 2007.
18. Balady GJ, Williams MA, Ades PA, et al: Core components of cardiac rehabilitation/secondary prevention programs: 2007 update: a scientific statement from the American Heart Association Exercise, Cardiac Rehabilitation, and Prevention Committee, the Council on Clinical Cardiology; the Councils on Cardiovascular Nursing, Epidemiology and Prevention, and Nutrition, Physical Activity, and Metabolism; and the American Association of Cardiovascular and Pulmonary Rehabilitation. *Circulation* 115:2675, 2007.
19. Lloyd-Jones D, Adams R, Carnethon M, et al: Heart disease and stroke statistics—2009 update: a report from the American Heart Association Statistics Committee and Stroke Statistics Subcommittee. *Circulation* 119:e21, 2009.
20. Williams MA, Fleg JL, Ades PA, et al: Secondary prevention of coronary heart disease in the elderly (with emphasis on patients > or = 75 years of age): an American Heart Association scientific statement from the Council on Clinical Cardiology Subcommittee on Exercise, Cardiac Rehabilitation, and Prevention. *Circulation* 105:1735, 2002.
21. Bittner V, Sanderson B: Cardiac rehabilitation as secondary prevention center. *Coron Artery Dis* 17:211, 2006.
22. Thomas RJ, Miller NH, Lamendola C, et al: National Survey on Gender Differences in Cardiac Rehabilitation Programs. Patient characteristics and enrollment patterns. *J Cardiopulm Rehabil* 16:402, 1996.
23. Wenger NK, Froelicher ES, Smith LK, et al: Cardiac rehabilitation as secondary prevention. Agency for Health Care Policy and Research and National Heart, Lung, and Blood Institute. *Clin Pract Guidel Quick Ref Guide Clin* 17:1, 1995.
24. Lavie CJ, Milani RV: Cardiac rehabilitation and preventive cardiology in the elderly. *Cardiol Clin* 17:233, 1999.
25. Ades PA: Cardiac rehabilitation in older coronary patients. *J Am Geriatr Soc* 47:98, 1999.
26. Allen JK, Scott LB, Stewart KJ, Young DR: Disparities in women's referral to and enrollment in outpatient cardiac rehabilitation. *J Gen Intern Med* 19:747, 2004.
27. Gregory PC, LaVeist TA, Simpson C: Racial disparities in access to cardiac rehabilitation. *Am J Phys Med Rehabil* 85:705, 2006.
28. Sanderson BK, Mirza S, Fry R, et al: Secondary prevention outcomes among black and white cardiac rehabilitation patients. *Am Heart J* 153:980, 2007.
29. Thomas RJ, King M, Lui K, et al: AACVPR/ACC/AHA 2007 performance measures on cardiac rehabilitation for referral to and delivery of cardiac rehabilitation/secondary prevention services endorsed by the American College of Chest Physicians, American College of Sports Medicine, American Physical Therapy Association, Canadian Association of Cardiac Rehabilitation, European Association for Cardiovascular Prevention and Rehabilitation, Inter-American Heart Foundation, National Association of Clinical Nurse Specialists, Preventive Cardiovascular Nurses Association, and the Society of Thoracic Surgeons. *J Am Coll Cardiol* 50:1400, 2007.
30. Leon AS, Franklin BA, Costa F, et al: Cardiac rehabilitation and secondary prevention of coronary heart disease: an American Heart Association scientific statement from the Council on Clinical Cardiology (Subcommittee on Exercise, Cardiac Rehabilitation, and Prevention) and the Council on Nutrition, Physical Activity, and Metabolism (Subcommittee on Physical Activity), in collaboration with the American association of Cardiovascular and Pulmonary Rehabilitation. *Circulation* 111:369, 2005.
31. Williams MA, Haskell WL, Ades PA, et al: Resistance exercise in individuals with and without cardiovascular disease: 2007 update: a scientific statement from the American Heart Association Council on Clinical Cardiology and Council on Nutrition, Physical Activity, and Metabolism. *Circulation* 116:572, 2007.
32. Stewart KJ, Badenhop D, Brubaker PH, et al: Cardiac rehabilitation following percutaneous revascularization, heart transplant, heart valve surgery, and for chronic heart failure. *Chest* 123:2104, 2003.
33. Hambrecht R, Wolf A, Gielen S, et al: Effect of exercise on coronary endothelial function in patients with coronary artery disease. *N Engl J Med* 342:454, 2000.
34. Franklin BA, Trivax JE, Vanhecke TE: New insights in preventive cardiology and cardiac rehabilitation. *Curr Opin Cardiol* 23:477, 2008.
35. Pedersen BK: The anti-inflammatory effect of exercise: its role in diabetes and cardiovascular disease control. *Essays Biochem* 42:105, 2006.
36. Lisspers J, Sundin O, Hofman-Bang C, et al: Behavioral effects of a comprehensive, multifactorial program for lifestyle change after percutaneous transluminal coronary angioplasty: a prospective, randomized controlled study. *J Psychosom Res* 46:143, 1999.
37. Brubaker PH, Warner JG, Jr, Rejeski WJ, et al: Comparison of standard- and extended-length participation in cardiac rehabilitation on body composition, functional capacity, and blood lipids. *Am J Cardiol* 78:769, 1996.
38. LaMonte MJ, Eisenman PA, Adams TD, et al: Cardiorespiratory fitness and coronary heart disease risk factors: the LDS Hospital Fitness Institute cohort. *Circulation* 102:1623, 2000.
39. Kelemen MH, Effron MB, Valenti SA, Stewart KJ: Exercise training combined with antihypertensive drug therapy. Effects on lipids, blood pressure, and left ventricular mass. *JAMA* 263:2766, 1990.
40. Wei M, Gibbons LW, Mitchell TL, et al: The association between cardiorespiratory fitness and impaired fasting glucose and type 2 diabetes mellitus in men. *Ann Intern Med* 130:89, 1999.
41. Stewart KJ, Bacher AC, Turner K, et al: Exercise and risk factors associated with metabolic syndrome in older adults. *Am J Prev Med* 28:9, 2005.
42. Oldridge NB, Guyatt GH, Fischer ME, Rimm AA: Cardiac rehabilitation after myocardial infarction. Combined experience of randomized clinical trials. *JAMA* 260:945, 1988.
43. Taylor RS, Brown A, Ebrahim S, et al: Exercise-based rehabilitation for patients with coronary heart disease: systematic review and meta-analysis of randomized controlled trials. *Am J Med* 116:682, 2004.
44. O'Connor CM, Whellan DJ, Lee KL, et al: Efficacy and safety of exercise training in patients with chronic heart failure: HF-ACTION randomized controlled trial. *JAMA* 301:1439, 2009.
45. Coats AJ: Exercise rehabilitation in chronic heart failure. *J Am Coll Cardiol* 22(Suppl A):172A, 1993.
46. Coats AJ, Adamopoulos S, Radaelli A, et al: Controlled trial of physical training in chronic heart failure. Exercise performance, hemodynamics, ventilation, and autonomic function. *Circulation* 85:2119, 1992.
47. Keteyian SJ, Brawner CA: Chronic heart failure and cardiac rehabilitation for the elderly: is it beneficial? *Am J Geriatr Cardiol* 8:80, 1999.
48. Keteyian SJ, Levine AB, Brawner CA, et al: Exercise training in patients with heart failure. A randomized, controlled trial. *Ann Intern Med* 124:1051, 1996.
49. Sullivan MJ, Higginbotham MB, Cobb FR: Exercise training in patients with severe left ventricular dysfunction. Hemodynamic and metabolic effects. *Circulation* 78:506, 1988.
50. Flynn KE, Pina IL, Whellan DJ, et al: Effects of exercise training on health status in patients with chronic heart failure: HF-ACTION randomized controlled trial. *JAMA* 301:1451, 2009.
51. Ades PA, Waldmann ML, McCann WJ, Weaver SO: Predictors of cardiac rehabilitation participation in older coronary patients. *Arch Intern Med* 152:1033, 1992.
52. Maniar S, Sanderson BK, Bittner V: Comparison of baseline characteristics and outcomes in younger and older patients completing cardiac rehabilitation. *J Cardiopulm Rehabil Prev* 29:220, 2009.
53. Gurwitz JH, McLaughlin TJ, Willison DJ, et al: Delayed hospital presentation in patients who have had acute myocardial infarction. *Ann Intern Med* 126:593, 1997.
54. Paul SD, O'Gara PT, Mahjoub ZA, et al: Geriatric patients with acute myocardial infarction: cardiac risk factor profiles, presentation, thrombolysis, coronary interventions, and prognosis. *Am Heart J* 131:710, 1996.
55. Williams MA, Maresh CM, Esterbrooks DJ, et al: Early exercise training in patients older than age 65 years compared with that in younger patients after acute myocardial infarction or coronary artery bypass grafting. *Am J Cardiol* 55:263, 1985.

56. Ades PA, Hanson JS, Gunther PG, Tonino RP: Exercise conditioning in the elderly coronary patient. *J Am Geriatr Soc* 35:121, 1987.

57. Ades PA, Waldmann ML, Poehlman ET, et al: Exercise conditioning in older coronary patients. Submaximal lactate response and endurance capacity. *Circulation* 88:572, 1993.

58. Lavie CJ, Milani RV: Effects of cardiac rehabilitation and exercise training on exercise capacity, coronary risk factors, behavioral characteristics, and quality of life in women. *Am J Cardiol* 75:340, 1995.

59. Lavie CJ, Milani RV: Benefits of cardiac rehabilitation and exercise training programs in elderly coronary patients. *Am J Geriatr Cardiol* 10:323, 2001.

60. Lavie CJ, Milani RV, Littman AB: Benefits of cardiac rehabilitation and exercise training in secondary coronary prevention in the elderly. *J Am Coll Cardiol* 22:678, 1993.

61. Williams MA, Maresh CM, Aronow WS, et al: The value of early out-patient cardiac exercise programmes for the elderly in comparison with other selected age groups. *Eur Heart J* 5(Suppl E):113, 1984.

62. Lavie CJ, Milani RV: Effects of cardiac rehabilitation programs on exercise capacity, coronary risk factors, behavioral characteristics, and quality of life in a large elderly cohort. *Am J Cardiol* 76:177, 1995.

63. Hakim AA, Petrovitch H, Burchfiel CM, et al: Effects of walking on mortality among nonsmoking retired men. *N Engl J Med* 338:94, 1998.

64. Kushi LH, Fee RM, Folsom AR, et al: Physical activity and mortality in postmenopausal women. *JAMA* 277:1287, 1997.

65. Fried LP, Kronmal RA, Newman AB, et al: Risk factors for 5-year mortality in older adults: the Cardiovascular Health Study. *JAMA* 279:585, 1998.

66. Hirsch AT, Haskal ZJ, Hertzer NR, et al: ACC/AHA 2005 Practice Guidelines for the management of patients with peripheral arterial disease (lower extremity, renal, mesenteric, and abdominal aortic): a collaborative report from the American Association for Vascular Surgery/Society for Vascular Surgery, Society for Cardiovascular Angiography and Interventions, Society for Vascular Medicine and Biology, Society of Interventional Radiology, and the ACC/AHA Task Force on Practice Guidelines (Writing Committee to Develop Guidelines for the Management of Patients With Peripheral Arterial Disease): endorsed by the American Association of Cardiovascular and Pulmonary Rehabilitation; National Heart, Lung, and Blood Institute; Society for Vascular Nursing; TransAtlantic Inter-Society Consensus; and Vascular Disease Foundation. *Circulation* 113:e463, 2006.

67. Larsen OA, Lassen NA: Effect of daily muscular exercise in patients with intermittent claudication. *Lancet* 2:1093, 1966.

68. Gardner AW, Poehlman ET: Exercise rehabilitation programs for the treatment of claudication pain. A meta-analysis. *JAMA* 274:975, 1995.

69. Robeer GG, Brandsma JW, van den Heuvel SP, et al: Exercise therapy for intermittent claudication: a review of the quality of randomised clinical trials and evaluation of predictive factors. *Eur J Vasc Endovasc Surg* 15:36, 1998.

70. Watson L, Ellis B, Leng GC: Exercise for intermittent claudication. *Cochrane Database Syst Rev* (4):CD000990, 2008.

71. Stewart KJ, Hiatt WR, Regensteiner JG, Hirsch AT: Exercise training for claudication. *N Engl J Med* 347:1941, 2002.

72. Bendermacher BL, Willigendael EM, Teijink JA, Prins MH: Supervised exercise therapy versus non-supervised exercise therapy for intermittent claudication. *Cochrane Database Syst Rev* (2):CD005263, 2006.

73. Creasy TS, McMillan PJ, Fletcher EW, et al: Is percutaneous transluminal angioplasty better than exercise for claudication? Preliminary results from a prospective randomised trial. *Eur J Vasc Surg* 4:135, 1990.

74. Perkins JM, Collin J, Creasy TS, et al: Exercise training versus angioplasty for stable claudication. Long and medium term results of a prospective, randomised trial. *Eur J Vasc Endovasc Surg* 11:409, 1996.

75. Whyman MR, Fowkes FG, Kerracher EM, et al: Is intermittent claudication improved by percutaneous transluminal angioplasty? A randomized controlled trial. *J Vasc Surg* 26:551, 1997.

76. Spronk S, Bosch JL, den Hoed PT, et al: Intermittent claudication: clinical effectiveness of endovascular revascularization versus supervised hospital-based exercise training—randomized controlled trial. *Radiology* 250:586, 2009.

77. Murphy TP, Hirsch AT, Ricotta JJ, et al: The Claudication: Exercise Vs. Endoluminal Revascularization (CLEVER) study: rationale and methods. *J Vasc Surg* 47:1356, 2008.

78. Hiatt WR, Regensteiner JG, Hargarten ME, et al: Benefit of exercise conditioning for patients with peripheral arterial disease. *Circulation* 81:602, 1990.

79. McDermott MM, Ades P, Guralnik JM, et al: Treadmill exercise and resistance training in patients with peripheral arterial disease with and without intermittent claudication: a randomized controlled trial. *JAMA* 301:165, 2009.

80. Stewart KJ: Exercise training and the cardiovascular consequences of type 2 diabetes and hypertension: plausible mechanisms for improving cardiovascular health. *JAMA* 288:1622, 2002.

81. Zwierska I, Walker RD, Choksy SA, et al: Upper- vs lower-limb aerobic exercise rehabilitation in patients with symptomatic peripheral arterial disease: a randomized controlled trial. *J Vasc Surg* 42:1122, 2005.

82. Sakamoto S, Yokoyama N, Tamori Y, et al: Patients with peripheral artery disease who complete 12-week supervised exercise training program show reduced cardiovascular mortality and morbidity. *Circ J* 73:167, 2009.

83. Ratliff DA, Puttick M, Libertiny G, et al: Supervised exercise training for intermittent claudication: lasting benefit at three years. *Eur J Vasc Endovasc Surg* 34:322, 2007.

84. Hiatt WR, Hirsch AT, Regensteiner JG, Brass EP: Clinical trials for claudication. Assessment of exercise performance, functional status, and clinical end points. Vascular Clinical Trialists. *Circulation* 92:614, 1995.

85. Gardner AW, Skinner JS, Cantwell BW, Smith LK: Progressive vs single-stage treadmill tests for evaluation of claudication. *Med Sci Sports Exerc* 23:402, 1991.

86. McDermott MM, Ades PA, Dyer A, et al: Corridor-based functional performance measures correlate better with physical activity during daily life than treadmill measures in persons with peripheral arterial disease. *J Vasc Surg* 48:1231, 2008.

87. American College of Sports Medicine; Thompson WR, Gordon NF, Pescatello LS: *ACSM's guidelines for exercise testing and prescription*, ed 8, Philadelphia, 2010, Lippincott Williams & Wilkins.

88. Jette AM, Lachman M, Giorgetti MM, et al: Exercise—it's never too late: the strong-for-life program. *Am J Public Health* 89:66, 1999.

89. Fiatarone MA, O'Neill EF, Ryan ND, et al: Exercise training and nutritional supplementation for physical frailty in very elderly people. *N Engl J Med* 330:1769, 1994.

90. Brochu M, Savage P, Lee M, et al: Effects of resistance training on physical function in older disabled women with coronary heart disease. *J Appl Physiol* 92:672, 2002.

91. American College of Sports Medicine position stand: Progression models in resistance training for healthy adults. *Med Sci Sports Exerc* 41:687, 2009.

92. Anderson K, Behm DG: Trunk muscle activity increases with unstable squat movements. *Can J Appl Physiol* 30:33, 2005.

93. Stewart KJ, McFarland LD, Weinhofer JJ, et al: Safety and efficacy of weight training soon after acute myocardial infarction. *J Cardiopulm Rehabil* 18:37, 1998.

94. Graves JE, Franklin BA: *Resistance training for health and rehabilitation*, Champaign, Ill, 2001, Human Kinetics.

95. MacDougall JD, Tuxen D, Sale DG, et al: Arterial blood pressure response to heavy resistance exercise. *J Appl Physiol* 58:785, 1985.

96. American Association of Cardiovascular & Pulmonary Rehabilitation: *Guidelines for cardiac rehabilitation and secondary prevention programs*, ed 4, Champaign, Ill, 2004, Human Kinetics.

97. Regensteiner JG, Steiner JF, Hiatt WR: Exercise training improves functional status in patients with peripheral arterial disease. *J Vasc Surg* 23:104, 1996.

33

Exercise for Restoring Health and Preventing Vascular Disease

Psychological Risk Factors and Coronary Artery Disease: Epidemiology, Pathophysiology, and Management

Alan Rozanski

KEY POINTS

- During the last three decades, epidemiologic studies have demonstrated a consistent relationship between psychosocial variables and coronary artery disease.

- Psychosocial risk factors for coronary artery disease include depression; various anxiety syndromes, such as phobias, panic, and post-traumatic stress syndrome; anger/hostility; negative cognitive patterns such as pessimism; and chronic stress, including work stress, marital stress, social isolation, and low socioeconomic status.

- Important new data indicate that positive psychological factors, including positive emotions and having a sense of purpose, improve physiology and increase longevity.

- The pathophysiology governing these relationships stems from chronic activation of the autonomic nervous system and the hypothalamic-pituitary-adrenal axis.

- Both the brain itself, which is remodeled by chronic stress, and the heart are end-target organs of chronic psychosocial stress.

- Psychosocial factors such as depression and chronic stress lead to widespread peripheral effects that promote coronary artery disease, such as inflammation, hypercoagulability, metabolic syndrome and diabetes, hypertension, endothelial dysfunction, and enhanced physiologic reactivity to environmental stimuli.

- Acute psychological stress can increase the risk for cardiac events among patients with coronary disease through widespread pathophysiologic effects.

- Mixed results among sparse large-scale studies have inhibited the adoption of formal guidelines for management of psychosocial stress in clinical practice.

- New developments within medical psychology hold promise for optimizing behavioral interventions in the future.

Since antiquity, there has been a strong lay notion concerning the relationship between psychological stress and the development of heart disease. However, it was not until the late 1970s that a significant scientific evidence base began to coalesce in this arena. By the early 1960s, the Framingham study had already identified key clinical risk factors for coronary artery disease (CAD), including smoking, hypertension, hyperlipidemia, diabetes, and a family history of premature CAD. At that time and into the following decade, interest in potential psychosocial risk factors for CAD was principally dominated by a construct proposed by Friedman and Rosenman.[1] They conceived of a coronary-prone type A personality pattern, characterized as hard driving, time impatient, and prone to hostility. Initial research linked type A personality to a higher risk of cardiac disease compared with type B. Whereas this concept proved popular and became part of the cultural vernacular for many years, ultimately the construct was largely abandoned because of the lack of sufficient confirmatory evidence during prospective study.

Subsequent research, however, began to define strong links between various psychosocial risk factors and CAD. For instance, in 1979, the landmark Alameda County study was published, noting a stepwise gradient between the size of individuals' social network and all-cause mortality.[2] New and more sophisticated epidemiologic studies, which for the first time corrected for concurrent risk factors such as smoking and involving increasing, more representative sample sizes, began to demonstrate a similar stepwise gradient between the magnitude of depressive symptoms and adverse cardiac outcomes.[3] At the same time, important animal work began to define pathophysiologic links between chronic stress and atherosclerosis.[4] With respect to acute stress, newly available imaging techniques were able to show for the first time a relationship between acute stress and myocardial perfusion, ischemic wall motion abnormalities, and coronary vasoconstriction.[3] Since then, a markedly vast literature has developed to link a large variety of psychosocial risk factors to CAD.

This chapter reviews current understanding of the epidemiologic link between psychosocial risk factors and CAD. Both negative factors that cause CAD and more recently defined positive factors that help buffer against the development of CAD are reviewed. The pathophysiologic basis for these links is broadly examined, and treatment considerations that are relevant to cardiologists are considered.

THE EPIDEMIOLOGY LINKING PSYCHOSOCIAL RISK FACTORS TO CARDIOVASCULAR DISEASE

During the last few decades, a number of negative psychosocial factors have been linked to the development of cardiovascular disease (CVD). More recently, various positive psychological factors, such as the

BOX 34-1 Psychosocial Factors That Have Been Linked to the Progression or Prevention of Cardiovascular Disease

Negative Thought Patterns and Emotions
Depressive syndromes
  Mild to moderate depressive symptoms
  Major depression
  Hopelessness
Anxiety syndromes
  Generalized anxiety disorder
  Phobic anxiety
  Panic disorder
  Post-traumatic stress disorder
Hostility and anger
Worry
Pessimism

Chronic Stress
Work stress
Marital stress and dissatisfaction
Social isolation and lack of social support
Low socioeconomic status
Caregiver strain
Adverse childhood experience
Perceived injustice

Positive Psychological Factors
Positive emotions
Optimism
Social support
Sense of purpose

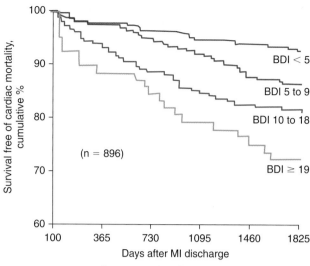

FIGURE 34-1 Grouping of post–myocardial infarction (MI) patients according to their Beck Depression Inventory (BDI) scores, ranging from those with no depressive symptoms (BDI < 5) to those with moderately severe depression (BDI ≥ 19). A gradient relationship was observed for frequency of death according to the magnitude of depressive symptoms. Notably, increased events occurred even among patients with mild depressive symptoms (BDI scores of 5 to 9).

presence of positive emotions and having a sense of purpose, have been demonstrated to protect against CVD and to promote longevity. The psychological factors that have been shown to be epidemiologically linked to CVD are listed in Box 34-1. These factors can be divided into three broad categories: (1) chronic negative thought patterns and emotions; (2) chronic stress; and (3) positive psychosocial factors that promote health and buffer against CAD. Each of these categories is reviewed.

Thought Patterns and Emotions

Thought patterns and emotions are logically linked because they are bidirectionally related. Thoughts commonly generate concomitant emotional responses, but our moods and emotional states can also affect the quality of our thinking. Depression, anxiety, and anger/hostility have been most commonly studied; but in recent years, other thought patterns, such as pessimism/optimism, have also emerged as an important area of study.

Depression

Depression has been particularly studied as a risk factor for CAD, for a variety of clinical reasons. First, depressive symptoms are common in society; major depression, alone, affects approximately 5% of the U.S. population at any time, with an increased frequency in cardiac cohorts. Second, depression is painful and debilitating, leading to loss of productivity and high economic costs.[5] Third, various effective quantifiable tools exist to measure depressive symptoms, and epidemiologic studies that use these tools have consistently demonstrated that depression is associated with a heightened frequency of atherosclerotic heart disease and adverse clinical events.

Validated standardized scales, such as the Beck Depression Inventory and the Center for Epidemiologic Studies

Depression Scale (CES-D), allow depressive symptoms to be characterized along a full spectrum, ranging from mild to severe depressive symptoms. At the severe end of this spectrum is major depression, which is a specific clinical psychiatric disorder that is established by formal diagnostic interview according to the following *Diagnostic and Statistical Manual of Mental Disorders,* fourth edition (DSM-IV) criteria: the presence of severely depressed mood and/or inability to take pleasure in all or most things that were previously considered enjoyable, lasting ≥2 weeks and accompanied by functional impairment and somatic complaints, such as fatigue or loss of energy nearly every day, insomnia or hypersomnia, change in appetite, diminished ability to concentrate, feelings of worthlessness or inappropriate guilt, and recurrent thoughts of death or suicidal ideation.

Studies have consistently demonstrated that the prevalence of major depression is increased by at least threefold in cardiac populations, occurring in at least 15% to 20% of patients who are status post–myocardial infarction, unstable angina, angioplasty, bypass surgery, or valve surgery or who have congestive heart failure.[3] In addition, at least another 15% of cardiac patients can be expected to manifest minor to moderate depressive symptoms that do not meet the criteria for major depression according to DSM-IV criteria. This high prevalence of depressive symptoms in cardiac populations is believed to be due to a bidirectional relationship between depression and CAD.

This high frequency of depressive symptoms in cardiac patients is of particular concern given repeated evidence of a strong gradient relationship between the frequency of depressive symptoms and the occurrence of adverse cardiac events both among community cohorts who are observed prospectively and among cardiac disease cohorts. Evidence indicates that even mild depressive symptoms are associated with an increased frequency of cardiac events compared with patients who have no depressive symptoms[6] (Fig. 34-1).

Various meta-analyses have been performed, and each has found a prognostic association between depression and adverse outcomes.[7-11] For example, meta-analyses of community-based cohorts conducted by Rugulies[7] and by Wulsin and Singal[9] found depression to be associated with a relative risk ratio of 1.64 for the development of CAD. Similarly, Van Melle and coworkers[10] and Barth and colleagues[11]

Study, Year	No. of Subjects	Follow-up	Scale	Endpoints	Adjusted Risk Ratios
McCarron et al,[13] 2003	9,239	20 years	Physician impression	ACM	1.36 (1.07-1.72)
Eaker et al,[14] 2005	3,682	10 years	Framingham anxiety scale	ACM, male ACM, female	1.22 (1.08-1.38) 1.27 (1.05-1.55)
Ringbäck Weitoft and Rosén,[15] 2005 (3 different cohorts)	10,733 10,035 9,100	5 years	Hospital ICD codes	ACM ACM ACM	1.71 (1.1-2.5) 2.3 (1.6-3.3) 1.8 (1.1-1.3)
Ostir and Goodwin,[16] 2006	506	5 years	Zung	ACM	1.52 (1.02-2.28)
Mykletun et al,[17] 2007	61,349	4.4 years	HADS	ACM CD	0.90 (0.83-0.98) 0.89 (0.67-3.38)
Fan et al,[18] 2008	129,499	N/A	History of anxiety on PHQ-8	Self-reported CVD	1.46 (1.37-1.54)
Shen et al,[19] 2008	735	12.4 years	MMPI anxiety subscales	MI	1.43 (1.17-1.75)
Phillips et al,[20] 2009	4,256	15 years	DSM-III (interview)	ACM CD	1.80 (1.16-2.80) 1.84 (0.98-3.45)

TABLE 34–1 Outcomes by Anxiety in General Population Samples

ACM, all-cause mortality; CD, cardiac death; CVD, cardiovascular disease; HADS, Hospital Anxiety and Depression Scale; MI, myocardial infarction; MMPI, Minnesota Multiphasic Personality Inventory; PHQ, Patient Health Questionnaire.

found depression to be associated with at least a twofold increase in event risk for cardiac populations among meta-analyses involving 22 studies and 20 studies, respectively.

Anxiety Syndromes

Like depression, feelings of anxiety vary across a wide spectrum, but anxiety disorders are more common than depression. For instance, within the National Comorbidity Survey, the 12-month prevalence of diagnosed anxiety disorders within a representative national survey was approximately 20%.[12] Transient experience of anxiety is a universal phenomenon that is often an adaptive warning of threat or danger. When anxiety is chronic or cannot be controlled, however, it becomes maladaptive. Many studies have now assessed the epidemiologic significance of both self-reported anxious symptoms and various pathologic forms of anxiety, as characterized in the DSM-IV.

In early study, conflicting results were obtained regarding anxiety as a CVD risk factor, but in recent years, increasing study has clarified the status of anxiety syndromes relative to cardiac risk. Table 34-1 lists the outcomes associated with measurements of anxiety in community samples for studies reported since 2003.[13-20] In general, these studies found anxiety to be associated with significant risk ratios for adverse clinical events, although in some studies, anxiety was not a significant predictor after full adjustment for covariates of risk.[13,20] This sensitivity to covariate adjustment may help explain some of the conflicting data concerning anxiety among earlier epidemiologic studies.

There have also been many studies concerning anxiety within cardiac populations, but most of these have involved small sample sizes. Among three studies with cardiac populations >500 individuals, each demonstrated an increased risk for adverse clinical events in the presence of anxiety.[21-23] In an interesting study in this arena, Frasure-Smith and Lesperance[23] compared self-reported anxiety symptoms versus the identification of generalized anxiety disorder (GAD) according to use of the Structured Clinical Interview for DSM-IV. The diagnostic criteria for GAD include excessive anxiety or worry for more days than not for >6 months, with difficulty in controlling the worry and symptoms of functional impairment and distress (e.g., fatigue, insomnia). The study assessed 804 patients with stable CAD observed for a composite index of major adverse cardiac events. Whereas both self-reports of

anxiety and GAD were associated with increased events before covariate adjustment, only GAD remained a significant predictor of risk after covariate adjustment. These results are indicative of a gradient relationship, whereby more pathologic anxiety exerts greater pathophysiologic effects.

In addition to GAD, most of the other DSM-IV anxiety syndromes have been assessed relative to their clinical sequelae. Among the anxiety disorders that will be encountered by cardiologists is panic disorder, because the symptoms associated with panic attacks, including chest pain, palpitations, and dyspnea, can lead to frequent emergency department presentations. Panic disorder involves the presence of recurrent and unexpected panic attacks, with the occurrence of anticipatory anxiety or worry and a significant change in behavior related to the attacks. Among studies concerning panic attack, Smoller and coworkers[24] observed 3369 women for 5.3 years and found panic attacks to be associated with a substantial hazard ratio for the development of CVD and stroke as well as all-cause mortality. Panic disorder was also found to be associated with an increased frequency of acute myocardial infarction in the follow-up of 9641 patients with panic disorder who were matched to 28,923 controls,[25] and similar findings were noted in other large studies.[26,27]

The most common of the DSM-IV forms of anxiety disorders is presence of phobic disorders. The 12-month prevalence of simple phobias was approximately 9% among the individuals within the National Comorbidity Survey, and social phobias were found within approximately 8%.[20] The DSM-IV criteria for phobia include the presence of excessive and persistent fear that is cued by the presence or anticipation of exposure to a specific object or situation, with the exposure usually invoking an immediate anxiety response. Notably, phobic anxiety, as assessed by the Crown-Crisp Index, has also been linked to cardiac death in large cohorts, including the follow-up of 33,999 men from the Health Professionals Follow-up Study[28] and 72,359 women from the Nurses' Health Study.[29]

Another anxiety disorder that has recently been strongly linked to cardiovascular sequelae is post-traumatic stress disorder (PTSD). PTSD is considered present if, after the exposure of an inciting traumatic event, subjects report re-experiencing of the traumatic event, hyperarousal, and avoidance of traumatic reminders and emotional numbing. In a prospective study of men who had served in the military, a stepwise relationship was noted between increasing symptoms of PTSD and both cardiac death and nonfatal myocardial infarction,[30] and a second study found a relationship between PTSD and incident CAD among a community cohort of 1059 women who were observed for 14 years.[31] In a third study, Boscarino[32] evaluated 4328 men who had served in the Vietnam War. The presence of PTSD was associated with a more than twofold increase in the frequency of subsequent cardiac mortality, with the effect being independent of the presence of depression. PTSD patients are more prone to depression, but evidence indicates that pathophysiologic effects from PTSD, such as hypertension, may occur independently of depressive symptoms.[33]

Anger and Hostility

Anger and hostility are often grouped together in studies of psychological risk factors because of overlapping characteristics. Hostility refers to an entrenched cognitive trait of easily precipitated resentfulness, cynicism, or suspicious negative thoughts about others. This cognitive style leads to frequent expressions of anger and negative social exchanges. Anger is an acute negative emotion, but individuals may by temperament or due to life experience be predisposed to a cognitive style of angry thoughts that may result in either expressed or suppressed feelings of anger. Hostile individuals are frequently angry, but anger can be experienced without hostility.

Unlike for depression or anxiety, no psychiatric system of classification has been developed for patients manifesting syndromal hostility or anger. Also, research in this arena has been characterized by the use of widely varying scales, which may have contributed to disparate findings over the years. Moreover, whereas anxiety and depression can be assessed both by self-report and by independent structured interview, the use of a standard structured interview approach has not been commonly applied for the study of anger and hostility. This represents a potential limitation in this arena because lack of self-awareness or self-denial may potentially limit the accuracy of self-reports concerning anger and hostility. Nevertheless, despite such limitations, an increasing literature regarding anger and hostility has emerged.

Chida and Steptoe[34] recently conducted a meta-analysis of published prospective cohort studies concerning anger and hostility. Among 25 studies involving community samples, the hazard ratio for CVD events in initially healthy populations in association with anger and hostility was 1.19 (95% CI, 1.05-1.35). Similarly, the hazard ratio was increased to 1.24 (95% CI, 1.08-1.42) among 19 studies involving patients with known CVD. Further support for the link between hostility or anger and CVD comes from a number of studies that have found these psychological variables to be associated with greater presence or progression of objectively measured atherosclerosis.[3]

Pessimism Versus Optimism

The tendency that people have toward thinking in pessimistic versus optimistic patterns has been closely linked to health outcomes. Optimism and pessimism have most commonly been measured in medical research in two ways. One characterization, developed by Seligman and colleagues, defines optimism versus pessimism in terms of the way individuals attribute the *causes* to life events.[35] Optimists tend to see negative events as temporary and positive events as more permanent; they tend to attribute specific causes to negative events while viewing positive events in more global terms; and they tend to attribute external causes to negative events rather than employing self-condemnation. Pessimists have the opposite "explanatory style." Another characterization of optimism versus pessimism, as developed by Scheier and

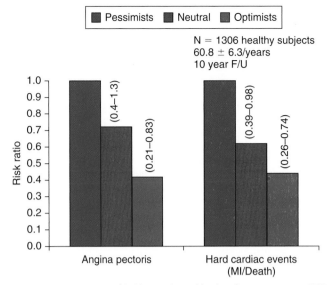

FIGURE 34-2 Occurrence of incident angina and hard cardiac events among 1306 healthy subjects in the Normative Aging Study, followed up for 10 years.[37] A gradient relationship was noted for outcomes for subjects classified as having a pessimistic, neutral, or optimistic explanatory speaking style.

34

Carver,[36] defines optimism versus pessimism in terms of individuals' disposition toward expecting positive or negative future outcomes. This disposition toward optimism or pessimism is seen as influencing peoples' behaviors, how they pursue goals, and their resilience to life stress.

Both approaches toward measurement of pessimism and optimism have been linked to adverse clinical events. A 10-year follow-up of 1306 men from the Normative Aging Study found that those with a pessimistic explanatory speaking style had the highest frequency and those with an optimistic speaking style had the lowest frequency of incident angina and coronary events (myocardial infarction or cardiac death) during follow-up, whereas those who had a neutral speaking style had an event rate that was intermediate (Fig. 34-2).[37]

In a study of 7216 subjects who were observed during four decades, those who tested pessimistic on a personality inventory showed a significant linear trend toward greater all-cause mortality with increasing pessimism.[38] Among elderly subjects observed for approximately 9 years, those subjects who tested high for optimism, compared with high scores for pessimism, had a substantially reduced hazard ratio for all-cause mortality (0.55; 95% CI, 0.42-0.74) and cardiac mortality (0.23; 95% CI, 0.10-0.55).[39] In another elderly cohort, the degree of measured dispositional optimism was found to be inversely associated with the frequency of cardiovascular death in a cohort of 545 men observed for 15 years.[40]

Most recently, Tindle and associates[41] assessed the relationship between optimism and CVD in the largest cohort yet studied, 97,253 women from the Women's Health Initiative. Optimistic women, compared with pessimistic women, again manifested a reduced adjusted risk ratio for cardiac mortality (0.70; 95% CI, 0.55-0.90) in this study. Together, these studies provide consistent evidence for a strong relationship between pessimism and optimism and adverse clinical events.

Worry, Rumination, and Other Negative Thought Patterns

A variety of other negative thought patterns, which may relate to anxiety or depression or serve as precursors to these psychological states, have received attention in the cardiovascular literature but not with a sufficient breadth of epidemiologic study to date. One of these cognitive states is chronic worry, which represents a cognitive component or precursor of anxiety. Among 1757 men in the Normative Aging Study, worry was associated with an increased risk ratio for nonfatal myocardial infarction (RR, 2.41; 95% CI, 1.40-4.13), with a dose-response relationship noted for both nonfatal myocardial infarction and total cardiac events.[42]

Rumination is another negative cognitive state involving the tendency to repetitively think about negative events. Whereas epidemiologic study is lacking, ruminators have been shown to have heightened heart and blood pressure reactivity to acute stress and delayed recovery of these responses.[43] Perfectionism also represents a negative cognitive state. Perfectionism is characterized as the tendency to set excessively high standards for performance, accompanied by a highly critical style of self-examination. Preliminarily, perfectionism has been linked both to mortality in one study[44] and to excessive cortisol secretion during psychological stress in a second study.[45] The cognitive tendency to be forgiving or unforgiving is another cognitive pattern that was found to influence the degree of cardiovascular reactivity to stress in one study.[46] Clearly, much more study is needed in this arena, but combined, these studies are suggestive of a broad link between chronic negative cognitive states and cardiovascular sequelae.

Chronic Stress

The study of chronic stress is unique within the context of psychological risk factors for CVD because chronic stress can be readily studied in controlled animal models of stress, complementing the epidemiologic study in humans. A set of investigations performed in cynomolgus monkeys (*Macaca fascicularis*) has been particularly insightful for elucidating the relationship between chronic stress and atherosclerosis.[4,47-49]

Cynomolgus monkeys are an apt model for correlative study because they develop coronary atherosclerosis when under stress or when fed fatty diets, with similarities to humans in terms of coronary pathology and pathophysiology. Cynomolgus monkeys also have definable and quantifiable social characteristics, and their social environment can easily be modified to create conditions of chronic stress. One approach to inducing chronic stress in these monkeys is to take advantage of the fact that they form well-defined social status hierarchies, with the most dominant monkeys reliably defeating more subordinate monkeys during competitive interactions. Once dominance rank is established, these monkeys form stable hierarchical societies. However, if monkeys are constantly placed into new social groups, a chronically stressful environment is created as the monkeys continually reinitiate their attempt to establish dominance within their new social groups. When male monkeys within stable versus unstable groups were kept on a low-cholesterol diet, the dominant male monkeys within the unstable social groups developed endothelial injury.[4] When both the stable and unstable social groups of monkeys were fed a high-cholesterol diet, both groups developed atherosclerosis, but the magnitude of disease was greater in the dominant male monkeys that were in the unstable environments.[47]

Chronic stress has been well studied within the epidemiologic literature. The most commonly studied chronic stress in this regard has been work stress. Estimates as to the frequency of chronic work stress vary widely, but it is a common stressor. The leading models of work stress are the model of job strain as developed by Karasek and associates[50] and the effort-reward imbalance model as developed by Siegrist[51] (Fig. 34-3). The job strain model posits that individuals experience job strain when experiencing work that is highly demanding but associated with low job latitude. Lack of control, however, appears to be a more toxic factor than high job demand.[52] In the effort-reward imbalance model, stress

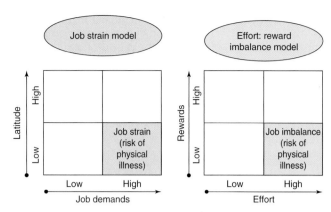

FIGURE 34-3 Two common conceptual models of job stress. The job strain model **(left)** is based on assessment of the amount of job demand and decision latitude at work. The presence of high demand but low decision latitude is characteristic of job stress. The effort-reward imbalance model **(right)** is based on assessment of job demand versus "reward" at work, whether financial or in terms of nonfinancial factors such as recognition, advancement, and prestige at work. High effort with low reward is characteristic of job imbalance. *(From Rozanski A, Blumenthal JA, Davidson KW, et al: The epidemiology, pathophysiology, and management of psychosocial risk factors in cardiac practice: the emerging field of behavioral cardiology.* J Am Coll Cardiol 45:637, 2005.)

occurs when high demand is associated with low "reward," either in terms of financial or professional reward (e.g., opportunities for promotion) or in terms of psychological reward (e.g., sense of security or self-esteem). Notably, both models have been linked to adverse CAD outcomes, as summarized in a review of 13 prospective cohort studies.[53] Compared with each other, the job strain and effort-reward imbalance models were comparable predictors for adverse outcome.[54]

Other studies have also linked work stress to the presence of accelerated atherosclerosis during serial carotid ultrasound study.[55] The effects of work stress tend to be accentuated in individuals with lower socioeconomic status and those with lower social support. However, work stress may also affect white-collar and higher socioeconomic status workers with seemingly more autonomous jobs as high work demand or low latitude commonly occurs because of internal psychodynamic factors, such as the need for recognition or perfectionistic tendencies.

Although marital stress or dissatisfaction is common in society, for years it was less studied than work stress relative to its association with CVD. Many studies over the years have studied clinical outcomes relative to marital status (e.g., remaining married, single, divorced, or widowed), but only recently have investigators begun to focus on outcomes as a function of marital quality. Among community cohorts, the quality of marital communications and marital conflict were found to strongly influence the frequency of adverse cardiac outcomes during a 10-year follow-up of 3682 subjects in the Framingham Offspring Study.[56] For example, women who self-silenced themselves during marital conflicts were noted to have a fourfold increase in mortality during follow-up. Similarly, an increased frequency of cardiac events was noted among those reporting more negative marital interactions during a 12.2-year follow-up of 9011 British civil servants.[57] Among patients with CAD, Orth-Gomer and coworkers[58] found marital stress to be associated with a 2.9-fold increased risk of recurrent events during a 5-year follow-up of women who were status post–myocardial infarction, and Coyne and associates[59] found that marital quality influences mortality rates among patients with congestive heart failure. Marital quality has also been found to influence the rate of progression of atherosclerosis as measured during both serial carotid ultrasound and coronary artery calcium scanning.[60]

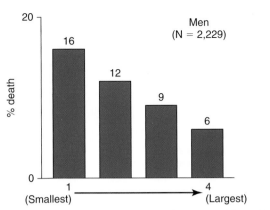

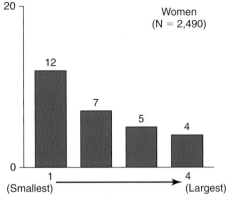

FIGURE 34-4 Mortality in the Alameda County study[2] according to the size of subjects' reported social network for men and for women, ranging from smallest to largest network size. An inverse gradient was observed in both men and women.

34

Data garnered during three decades provide strong epidemiologic proof for the health damaging of poor social support and social isolation. Social support in epidemiologic study is commonly divided into the amount of tangible or instrumental support (e.g., the size of one's social network) and the amount of emotional social support. Inadequacy in both types of support is linked to a heightened incidence of CVD and reduced longevity, both among community-based cohorts and among patients with known CAD.[3] Within these studies, an inverse gradient has consistently been noted between the amount of social support and the development of CAD or cardiac events[3] (Fig. 34-4).

Two other common stressors are low socioeconomic status and caregiver stress. Low socioeconomic status is associated with such psychosocial factors as higher anxiety resulting from hardship and environmental threat, poorer social support, demoralized feelings, and lower self-esteem. There is strong evidence to suggest that the impact of socioeconomic status on outcomes is due not only to material disadvantage and poorer health habits but also to psychological and stress-related mechanisms.[61-63] By contrast, whereas caregiver strain is commonplace in today's society, it has been much less studied, especially in terms of cardiac outcomes. In the Nurses' Health Study, caregiving for >9 hours per week was found to be associated with significantly increased risk of fatal CAD or nonfatal myocardial infarction.[64] More study in this arena is required. Recently, other forms of chronic stress have begun to receive attention as potential risk factors for CVD, including the long-lasting influence of adverse childhood experiences[65,66] and the experience of organizational injustice.[67]

Positive Psychological Factors

Until recently, most investigation regarding psychosocial factors and CVD has focused on just the negative relationships associated with factors such as depression and anxiety. However, two psychosocial factors have been persistently associated with a full spectrum of both negative and positive effects: optimism and social support, as reviewed before. More recently, new research has focused on the buffering and health-promoting effects of other positive factors, including positive emotions and the satisfaction of basic psychological needs that can induce a state of relative flourishing.[68-73] Positive emotions in the context of this research have been defined broadly to include both emotions such as happiness and states of being that reflect a positive engagement with the environment, such as the presence of curiosity and interest.[68]

In important work, Fredrickson[68] developed the broaden-and-build model concerning emotions. This work has demonstrated an important directional relationship between the quality of emotions and cognitive functions, such as a broader scope of attention, more flexibility, and better problem-solving and creativity skills. In positive emotional states, individuals are seen as more likely to be friendly and optimistic. Thus, positive emotion is seen as increasing individuals' personal resources and providing them with increased resilience to cope with stress. A recent meta-analysis has assessed the relationship between positive well-being and longevity among 35 studies involving initially healthy populations and 35 other studies involving patients.[74] In both cohorts, the presence of positive well-being was associated with reduced mortality. To date, however, there has been little study regarding the effect of positive emotions on cardiac outcomes. Certain attitudinal states have also received recent attention as to their impact on overall well-being. These include the practice of gratitude[75] and social altruism.[76] These parameters, however, have not yet been well assessed in terms of cardiac epidemiology.

In addition to positive emotions, various theorists have postulated that individuals have psychological needs that must be met for optimal satisfaction and that the absence of these needs leads to psychological tension.[69,73] Whereas these theorists differ in what constitutes these needs, there is general agreement among virtually all theorists that social connection is a basic psychological need. This may help explain why measured levels of social support have consistently been a very strong disease predictor. In addition, some theorists also posit that individuals have a basic need for meaning or sense of purpose,[69,72] which when unmet leads to chronic tension.

Recent data support this assertion. For example, in a study of 1238 elderly individuals, purpose in life was assessed according to a 10-item scale, and the subjects were then observed for a mean of 2.7 years.[77] Those who were identified as having a higher level of purpose in life had a substantially adjusted reduced risk of mortality (0.60; 95% CI, 0.42-0.87) (Fig. 34-5). Similarly, in the MacArthur Study of Successful Aging, older adults in the age range of 70 to 79 years who reported being more useful to friends and family during a baseline interview had reduced mortality and disability during a 7-year follow-up compared with those who reported never or rarely feeling useful.[78] Similar findings were also noted in a third study involving a 6-year follow-up of elderly subjects in Japan.[79] More study is needed to assess the epidemiologic effects of having a sense of purpose in younger subjects and its specific relationship to cardiovascular disease.

Psychological Risk Factors and Coronary Artery Disease: Epidemiology, Pathophysiology, and Management

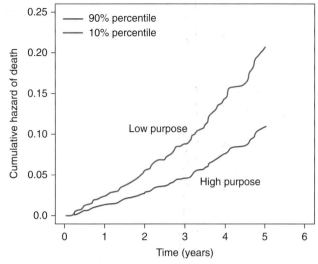

FIGURE 34-5 Cumulative hazard among 1238 older community-dwelling individuals observed for 5 years, according to the presence of a low versus high sense of purpose. The hazard rate for mortality in persons with high scores for purpose in life was about 57% of that for persons with low scores. *(From Boyle PA, Barnes LL, Buchman AS, et al: Purpose in life is associated with mortality among community-dwelling older persons. Psychosom Med 71:575, 2009.)*

34

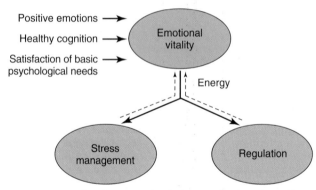

FIGURE 34-6 Paradigm for emotional vitality. Emotional vitality is fostered by positive emotions, healthy thought patterns such as optimism, and satisfaction of basic psychological needs, such as social connectedness. High emotional vitality provides energy and resilience for dealing with stress and negative emotions. In turn, successful stress management and resilience in the face of negative emotions build self-esteem and preserve emotional vitality. *(From Rozanski A, Blumenthal JA, Davidson KW, et al: The epidemiology, pathophysiology, and management of psychosocial risk factors in cardiac practice: the emerging field of behavioral cardiology. J Am Coll Cardiol 45:637, 2005.)*

The influence of positive and negative psychological factors as well as the influence of biologic and behavioral factors has been postulated to be contained within a composite variable, one's sense of emotional vitality,[80] as conceptualized in Figure 34-6. The emotional aspect of vitality is augmented by positive emotions, positive thought patterns like optimism, and the satisfaction of basic psychological needs like social support and a sense of purpose. By contrast, chronic negative emotions, negative thought patterns like rumination and worry, dissatisfaction of basic psychological needs, and chronic stress are all seen as depleting vitality.

Support for this concept comes from a study by Kubzansky and Thurston,[81] who assessed the link between the emotional aspects of vitality and incident CAD among 6025 subjects in the National Health and Nutrition Examination Survey (NHANES) I. During a mean follow-up of 15 years, those who

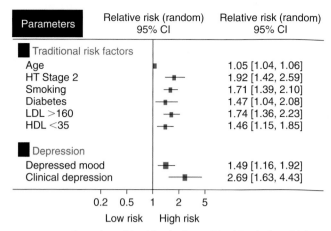

FIGURE 34-7 Comparison of the risk ratios for traditional Framingham risk factors in men versus the risk ratios for depressive symptoms and clinical depression as reported by Rugulies.[7] The risk ratios for traditional risk factors are for death due to cardiac causes (death, myocardial infarction, coronary artery insufficiency, development of angina). For depressive symptoms and clinical depression, the risk ratios are for death due to cardiac disease and myocardial infarction. CI, confidence interval; HT, hypertension; HDL, high-density lipoprotein; LDL, low-density lipoprotein. *(From Rozanski A, Blumenthal JA, Davidson KW, et al: The epidemiology, pathophysiology, and management of psychosocial risk factors in cardiac practice: the emerging field of behavioral cardiology. J Am Coll Cardiol 45:637, 2005.)*

manifested higher levels of emotional vitality manifested less CAD.

Comparison of Cardiovascular Disease Risk Factors

In summary, epidemiologic studies have identified an increasing number of psychosocial risk factors associated with CAD. Although these risk factors have been studied in isolation, very frequently they cluster together. For example, the frequency of depression has been found to be increased *threefold* among individuals experiencing high job stress.[82] The risk for CAD and cardiac events associated with many psychological risk factors for CAD generally demonstrates a gradient relationship and a level of risk that is comparable to conventionally studied CAD risk factors (Fig. 34-7).

A unique study that compared psychosocial risk with other CAD risk factors was the INTERHEART case-control study.[83] This study examined a variety of CAD risk factors among an international population of 12,461 acute post–myocardial infarction patients, matched to 14,637 control subjects. A simple psychological index in this study was comparable to other CAD risk factors in terms of myocardial infarction risk (Fig. 34-8). This psychosocial index remained a robust predictor of myocardial infarction independent of geographic or ethnic context.[84]

Of note, within epidemiologic study, the risk associated with psychological risk factors is adjusted for other CAD risk factors. However, because behavioral and metabolic CAD risk factors tend to aggregate disproportionately among individuals with psychosocial stress, in causative fashion, the true cardiovascular risk posed by psychosocial risk factors may be even greater than that reported within the literature.

PATHOPHYSIOLOGY

For many years, the pathophysiologic mechanisms responsible for the morbidity and mortality associated with

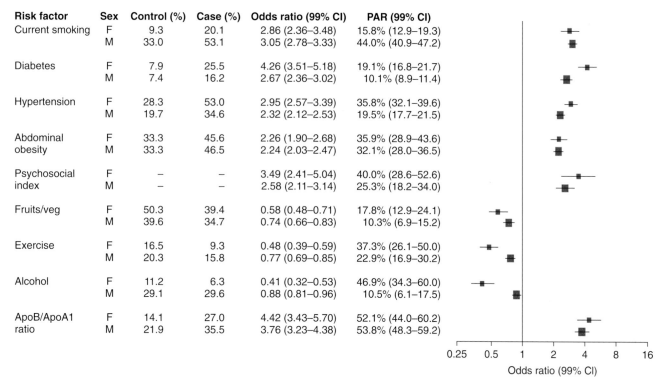

Risk factor	Sex	Control (%)	Case (%)	Odds ratio (99% CI)	PAR (99% CI)
Current smoking	F	9.3	20.1	2.86 (2.36–3.48)	15.8% (12.9–19.3)
	M	33.0	53.1	3.05 (2.78–3.33)	44.0% (40.9–47.2)
Diabetes	F	7.9	25.5	4.26 (3.51–5.18)	19.1% (16.8–21.7)
	M	7.4	16.2	2.67 (2.36–3.02)	10.1% (8.9–11.4)
Hypertension	F	28.3	53.0	2.95 (2.57–3.39)	35.8% (32.1–39.6)
	M	19.7	34.6	2.32 (2.12–2.53)	19.5% (17.7–21.5)
Abdominal obesity	F	33.3	45.6	2.26 (1.90–2.68)	35.9% (28.9–43.6)
	M	33.3	46.5	2.24 (2.03–2.47)	32.1% (28.0–36.5)
Psychosocial index	F	–	–	3.49 (2.41–5.04)	40.0% (28.6–52.6)
	M	–	–	2.58 (2.11–3.14)	25.3% (18.2–34.0)
Fruits/veg	F	50.3	39.4	0.58 (0.48–0.71)	17.8% (12.9–24.1)
	M	39.6	34.7	0.74 (0.66–0.83)	10.3% (6.9–15.2)
Exercise	F	16.5	9.3	0.48 (0.39–0.59)	37.3% (26.1–50.0)
	M	20.3	15.8	0.77 (0.69–0.85)	22.9% (16.9–30.2)
Alcohol	F	11.2	6.3	0.41 (0.32–0.53)	46.9% (34.3–60.0)
	M	29.1	29.6	0.88 (0.81–0.96)	10.5% (6.1–17.5)
ApoB/ApoA1 ratio	F	14.1	27.0	4.42 (3.43–5.70)	52.1% (44.0–60.2)
	M	21.9	35.5	3.76 (3.23–4.38)	53.8% (48.3–59.2)

Odds ratio (99% CI)
0.25 0.5 1 2 4 8 16

FIGURE 34-8 The risk of acute myocardial infarction results from the international INTERHEART case-control study for each of nine CAD risk factors were evaluated, adjusted for age, gender, and geographic location. The prevalence of each CAD risk factor is presented for controls and cases in the third and fourth columns. The prevalence rates for the psychosocial index were not calculated as it was derived from a statistical odds ratio. PAR, population attributable risk. *(From Yusuf S, Hawken S, Ounpuu S, et al: Effect of potentially modifiable risk factors associated with myocardial infarction in 52 countries (the INTERHEART study): case-control study. Lancet 364:937, 2004.)*

psychosocial risk factors for CVD were obscure. However, this is no longer the case. Both animal study and sophisticated research in humans have elucidated a complex pathophysiology that is unleashed by negative psychosocial factors, resulting in widespread systemic effects. The pathophysiology associated with depression and chronic stress is summarized in Figure 34-9. These two psychosocial conditions have been most studied relative to pathophysiology and are thus reviewed herein. However, there is also ample research into the pathophysiologic effects associated with other common psychosocial risk factors for CVD, such as poor social support, anxiety, and anger/hostility, as well as increasing study of the beneficial effects associated with positive factors such as positive emotions and optimism that are not reviewed in this chapter but are well documented in the literature.

Effects of Chronic Stress

The brain serves as a constant sentinel for all stimuli that are perceived as physically or psychologically threatening in our environment. Perceived threat induces an acute stress response that involves activation of both the autonomic nervous system and the hypothalamic-pituitary-adrenal (HPA) axis.[85] When perceived or real threat remains persistent, a chronic stress response ensues, involving profound dysregulation of both systems.

Under conditions of acute stress, the secretion of cortisol serves as a negative feedback system, helping to terminate the physiologic response to acute stress. By contrast, chronic stress results in turn-off of this negative feedback loop, with resultant high cortisol secretion.[86] In addition, there is elevated sympathetic nervous system stimulation during chronic stress. The chronic stimulation of the HPA and sympathetic nervous systems within the brain during chronic stress leads to the cascade of peripheral pathophysiologic effects that are outlined in Figure 34-9, including increased inflammation,[87] hypercoagulability,[88] metabolic syndrome,[89] central obesity,[90] and hypertension.[91,92]

In addition, an important and consistent effect of chronic stress is that it leads to impaired and exaggerated physiologic reactivity, as characterized by augmented heart rate and blood pressure responses to physiologic stimuli. A variety of clinical data indicate that such enhanced physiologic reactivity leads to accelerated atherosclerosis. For example, in experimental study, cynomolgus monkeys manifesting higher heart rate responses to a threatening experimental stimulus demonstrated atherosclerotic lesions in coronary and carotid arteries that were twice as large as those of less reactive monkeys.[49] Pretreatment with beta blockade abolished the excess atherosclerosis that is observed in dominant males housed in unstable social environments, indicating that sympathetic activation is an important mediator of this stress-induced atherosclerosis.[48] In parallel to this animal work, individuals with greater physiologic reactivity have been found to manifest accelerated atherosclerosis during serial carotid ultrasound study.[3]

An area of recent interest is an apparent relationship between chronic stress and premature aging, as assessed by the effect of stress on the length of leukocyte telomeres. Telomeres are repetitive DNA sequences complexed with proteins that cap and protect chromosome ends. They decline in length with age, but limited study has found shortened telomere length among those with more perceived stress[93] (Fig. 34-10) and in caregivers,[94] and a study suggests an association between pessimism and shorter telomeres as well.[95]

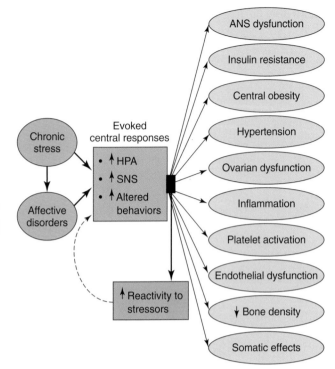

FIGURE 34-9 Schematic representation of the principal pathways by which chronic stress and affective disorders promote disease. The primary effect of perceived stress on chronic negative emotions is chronic activation of the hypothalamic-pituitary-adrenal (HPA) axis and the sympathetic nervous system (SNS). Widespread peripheral effects derive from this central nervous system activation (see text). In addition, there are direct effects on central nervous system remodeling that may help drive altered behaviors. Another consequence is a heightened physiologic responsivity to acute environmental stimuli. ANS, autonomic nervous system. *(From Rozanski A, Blumenthal JA, Davidson KW, et al: The epidemiology, pathophysiology, and management of psychosocial risk factors in cardiac practice: the emerging field of behavioral cardiology.* J Am Coll Cardiol *45:637, 2005.)*

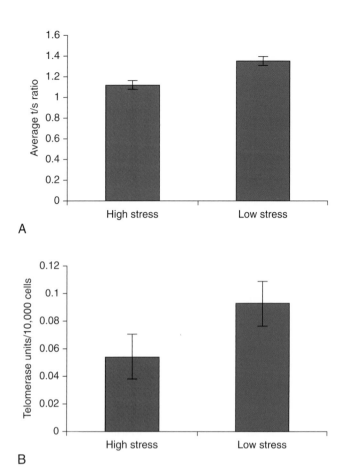

FIGURE 34-10 Comparison of mean telomerase length and telomerase enzyme activity in subjects with high versus low perceived stress. *(From Epel ES, Blackburn EH, Lin J, et al: Accelerated telomere shortening in response to life stress.* Proc Natl Acad Sci U S A *101:17312, 2004.)*

Finally, extensive research by McEwen and others has established that the brain, itself, is an important end-organ target of chronic stress. Specifically, chronic stress leads to profound primary alterations in brain chemistry and circuitry, including functional remodeling of the amygdala and hippocampus within the brain's limbic system and in the prefrontal cortex.[96] Under conditions of chronic stress, the hippocampus, an essential structure for memory and spatial navigation, manifests functional atrophy of its neural dendrites; concomitantly, the amygdala, a region that regulates fear responses and is involved in hormonal, autonomic, and behavioral responses to stress, manifests growth and expansion in its neuronal dendrites (Fig. 34-11). The prefrontal cortex, the master region for executive decision making and regulation of neurohumoral and autonomic responses during stress, also manifests shrinkage of its dendrites during chronic stress. The functional consequences of these central nervous system effects may include impairment in judgment, attention, and memory and an increased vulnerability toward anxiety. Importantly, both the shrinkage in the hippocampus and prefrontal cortex and the hypertrophy of the amygdala are reversible in animal models of stress, and limited human imaging data suggest that this may also be the case in humans.[96]

Effects of Depression

Like chronic stress, depression is also associated with widespread systemic effects resulting from activation of the

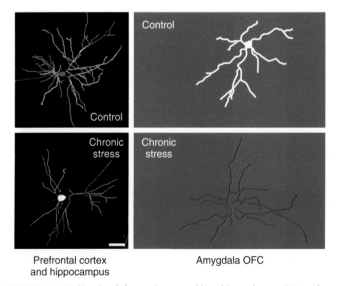

FIGURE 34-11 Directional changes in neuronal branching and connectivity under conditions of chronic stress. Chronic stress causes functional atrophy of neuronal dendrites in the medial prefrontal cortex and CA3 region of the hippocampus and hypertrophy (i.e., growth and expansion) in the basolateral amygdala and orbitofrontal cortex. Within animal models, these changes are reversible. *(Courtesy of Dr. Bruce McEwen.)*

autonomic nervous system and HPA axis. Hypercortisolemia is characteristic in chronic depression, as is heightened stimulation of the sympathetic nervous system, resulting in higher concentrations of circulating plasma norepinephrine and an increase in total body sympathetic activity. As a consequence of the latter, depressed patients commonly manifest autonomic nervous system dysfunction, with diminished heart rate variability, baroreflex dysfunction, increased rest heart rate, and increased QT variability.[97,98] Metabolic abnormalities are also common in depressed patients, including increase in insulin resistance,[99] metabolic syndrome,[100] visceral fat,[101] and diabetes mellitus, which is increased three-fold in depressed patients compared with nondepressed counterparts.[102] The concomitant increase in cortisol and decrease in growth and sex hormone concentrations associated with depression, and possibly induced local inflammatory protein interactions, result in an increased frequency of bone demineralization and osteoporosis.[103] Enhanced platelet activation is also characteristic, apparently resulting from multiple pathophysiologic effects of depression. These include elevations in β-thromboglobulin, platelet factor 4, and functional glycoprotein IIb/IIIa receptors; increased responsiveness of platelets to serotonin; and hyperactivity of the 5-hydroxytryptamine transporter 2A receptor signal transduction system.[97]

Substantial data now indicate that depression is also pro-inflammatory, a result of chronic stimulation of the HPA axis and the sympathetic nervous system, probably acting in concert with various peripheral effects of depression, such as hyperglycemia. Depression is associated with increases in C-reactive protein, fibrinogen, interleukin-6, and tumor necrosis factor and other inflammatory proteins, occurring independently of other CVD risk factors and body mass index.[104] Evidence suggests that the elevation of proinflammatory cytokines contributes to many of the typical somatic symptoms associated with depression, such as fatigue, decreased appetite and weight loss, and sleep and mood disturbances. Another pathophysiologic consequence of depression is endothelial dysfunction (Fig. 34-12).[105] This pathophysiologic effect may be aided by abnormalities in vascular cell adhesion and proliferation, as manifested by increased levels of intercellular adhesion molecules among depressed subjects. Together, these changes produce a strongly proatherosclerotic environment.

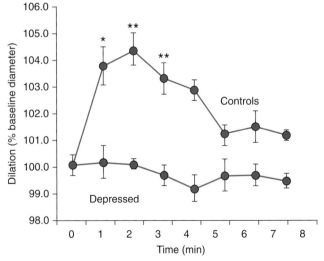

FIGURE 34-12 Comparison of degree of flow-mediated artery dilation after cuff release in 12 depressed patients and 10 healthy controls. Arterial endothelial function is significantly impaired in the depressed patients. *(From Broadley AJ, Korszun A, Jones CJ, Frenneaux MP: Arterial endothelial function is impaired in treated depression. Heart 88:521, 2002.)*

Behavioral Mechanisms

Besides their direct pathophysiologic effects, common to all psychosocial factors is strong evidence linking these factors to adverse health behaviors, such as poor diet and overeating, smoking, lack of exercise, poor sleep hygiene, social isolation, and decreased adherence to recommended health habit change. For instance, meta-analyses indicate substantially increased noncompliance with medical treatment regimens among patients with depression[106] and poor social support.[107] In the long term, these negative health behaviors both increase the risk for CAD and lead to a vicious circle of a decreased sense of physical and psychological well-being and worsening psychosocial status.

Acute Psychological Stress

An acute increase in cardiac events has been noted during the presence of natural or man-made real-life stressors, including earthquakes, missile attacks, and sporting events such as soccer matches and the Super Bowl.[108-111] Moreover, prospective epidemiologic study using a unique case-crossover design has permitted comparison of potential triggers surrounding the occurrence of cardiac events to control periods in a corresponding earlier period (e.g., 24 hours earlier).[112,113] This design helps eliminate some bias because if a patient is chronically stressed, the presence of stress before the clinical event will not add to the assessed risk ratio for the population under study. Using this design, investigators have found that the relative risk of acute myocardial infarction is increased more than twofold in the face of acute anger,[113-115] with work stress (e.g., high-pressured deadlines),[116] and during acute depression.[117] Patients of lower socioeconomic status may be more prone to the effects of these acute stressors.[113,117]

The pathophysiologic mechanisms that may place cardiac patients at increased risk for myocardial ischemia and cardiac events appear to be multifactorial. Acute psychological stress causes sudden increase in heart rate and often substantial blood pressure elevations,[118] thus increasing myocardial oxygen demand. Simultaneously, among patients with coronary disease, acute psychological stress can cause coronary vasoconstriction, through an endothelium-dependent mechanism, at the sites of coronary stenoses, thus resulting in a concomitant decrease in myocardial oxygen supply.[119] In the laboratory setting, mild psychological stressors can cause transient myocardial perfusion defects[120] and the induction of transient wall motion abnormalities[3]; the transient wall motion abnormalities are inducible in approximately half of patients with exercise-inducible myocardial ischemia. Patients who manifest ischemia during mental stress testing are at increased risk of mortality.[121,122] In one study, three different types of mental stressors were compared for their ability to induce regional wall motion abnormalities among CAD patients. Notably, a stressor involving speaking on issues of personal stress was substantially more potent than other mental tasks (the Stroop Word Task and math stress) in inducing myocardial ischemia. When CAD patients are monitored for ischemia with ambulatory electrocardiographic monitoring, ischemia is also often noted during nonexercise stressors, including those of an emotional nature.[123,124] Interestingly, mental stress–induced ischemia is most commonly clinically "silent" (i.e., it occurs in the absence of chest pain), and it occurs at a substantially lower double product compared with exercise-induced ischemia. Overall, mental stress–induced ischemia is not common among patients who do not have exercise-induced myocardial ischemia.

Besides these pathophysiologic effects, acute mental stress may cause a worsening of endothelial function that may last for hours.[125] Pretreatment with metapyrone, a competitive inhibitor of the conversion of 11-deoxycortisol to cortisol, can ablate this effect of acute mental stress.[126] Other work has demonstrated that acute mental stress has the ability to induce platelet activation,[127] to augment indices of arterial wall stiffness,[128] and to promote inflammation.[129-131] In one unique study that was designed to examine the prospective effects of a real-life stressor on inflammatory and vasoconstrictive mediators, investigators compared the serum from subjects watching World Cup soccer with that from reference groups of patients with acute coronary syndrome and healthy volunteers.[131] Various inflammatory and vasoconstrictor mediators, such as monocyte chemoattractant protein 1 and endothelin 1, were substantially elevated among the subjects who were watching the soccer matches. In addition, an extensive literature has demonstrated the ability of acute mental stress to produce a more proarrhythmic environment and to stimulate cardiac arrhythmias, both in the laboratory and in real-life settings.[3,132]

Paralleling the general increased interest in positive psychological factors that may buffer against illness, there has also been recent study in the potential acute beneficial effects of positive moods on physiology. For example, Frederickson and Levenson[133] have demonstrated that whereas negative moods that are induced in the laboratory setting can lengthen the time of hemodynamic recovery from an acute mental stressor, the preinduction of a positive mood can shorten hemodynamic recovery. In other work, films designed to produce laughter and mental stress produced divergent effects on indices of arterial wall stiffness.[134] Using a similar design, other investigators have demonstrated divergent effects of viewing laughter versus mental stress–related films on subsequent endothelial function[135] (Fig. 34-13). The clinical significance of such findings awaits further study.

Stress Cardiomyopathy

Acute stress also has the ability to produce an uncommon but increasingly recognized form of acute reversible heart failure, associated with a distinct pattern of acute left ventricular hypocontraction, involving prominent apical akinesis with relative sparing of the base of the left ventricle.[136-138] This syndrome has been referred to by different names, including takotsubo cardiomyopathy and apical ballooning syndrome. A study has characterized a relatively large group of 130 such patients.[139] Predominantly, these patients, as in most series, were women, with stress cardiomyopathy induced by either intensely emotional or physical stress in the majority of these patients. However, some patients had no identifiable trigger, and in a very small number, there was either delayed return of ventricular function or evidence of left ventricular thrombi, raising the issue of screening some patients for anticoagulation.[139]

THE CLINICAL MANAGEMENT OF PSYCHOLOGICAL RISK FACTORS IN CARDIOLOGY PRACTICE

Psychosocial problems such as depression are highly distressing and severely damage quality of life. Moreover, the convincing epidemiology and pathophysiology associated with psychosocial risk factors for CAD form a further compelling reason for development of behavioral interventions to protect against their adverse effects. Because psychosocial problems are commonly concentrated in cardiac patients, screening will provide cardiologists with the opportunity to identify and manage or refer patients with such problems in clinical practice. To date, however, there are no accepted practice guidelines to steer management of psychosocial problems in clinical practice. Issues to be solved include a lack of evidence base to suggest optimal therapies; the lack of organized health care systems to aid physicians in such management, particularly as it relates to time constraints that physicians commonly face; and the lack of reimbursement for practicing behavioral interventions. These issues are addressed in this section.

Evidence Base Concerning Behavioral Interventions

To date, there have been only sparse large studies that specifically evaluated the clinical efficacy of stand-alone behavioral interventions in cardiac populations (Table 34-2). The first of these was the Recurrent Coronary Prevention Project study.[140] In this study, 862 individuals were randomized into two groups; 270 received group counseling, and 592 received both group counseling and type A behavioral modification counseling. Another 151 patients served as a nontreated comparison group. During a 4.5-year follow-up, the occurrence of subsequent cardiovascular mortality or nonfatal myocardial infarction was significantly lower in the group that received type A behavioral counseling compared with the other two groups. Subsequently, the Ischemic Heart Disease study demonstrated a reduction in cardiac events among a group of patients who underwent a home-based stress reduction program.[141] Two other large-scale stress management studies were negative, but in neither study did the intervention actually reduce psychological distress.[142,143] In a secondary analysis of one of these two studies, a significant reduction in cardiac mortality was noted for the subgroup with reduction in distress within the psychological intervention arm of the study.[144]

The fifth and most recent large-scale behavioral intervention study was the Enhancing Recovery in Coronary Heart Disease Patients (ENRICHD) trial.[145] This differed from the prior studies in that it focused on alleviating depression or low perceived social support. This trial randomized 2841 acute post–myocardial infarction patients who had evidence of either depression or low perceived social support into

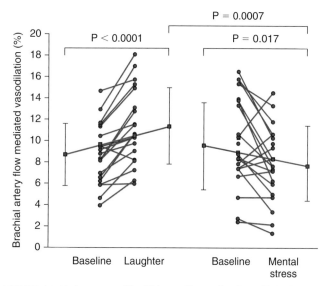

FIGURE 34-13 Assessment of brachial artery flow-mediated vasodilation in 20 healthy volunteers at baseline and during viewing of a cinematic film designed to induce laughter (left) and at baseline and during viewing of a film designed to induce mental stress (right). The mean flow-mediated dilation was increased by 22% ± 15% in testing that was performed after inducing laughter and decreased by 35% ± 47% after viewing of the mental stress film clips. *(From Miller M, Mangano C, Park Y, et al: Impact on cinematic viewing on endothelial function. Heart 92:261, 2006.)*

	No. of Patients					
Investigations	Control Group	Intervention Group	Follow-up	Type of Intervention	Reduced Psychosocial Stress?	Reduced Cardiac Events?
Friedman et al,[140] 1986	270	592	4.5 years	Type A behavior pattern modification/group counseling	Yes	Yes
Frasure-Smith and Prince,[141] 1985	229	232	5 years	Home-based nursing intervention	Yes	Yes
Jones and West,[142] 1996	1155	1159	1 year	Group stress management sessions	No	No
Frasure-Smith et al,[143] 1997	684	692	1 year	Home-based nursing intervention	No	No*
ENRICHD investigators,[145] 2003	1243	1238	2.4 years	Cognitive-behavior therapy for depression	Yes†	No*

TABLE 34–2 | Large-Scale Psychosocial Intervention Trials Among Patients with Known Coronary Artery Disease

*Secondary analysis with the intervention groups revealed decreased cardiac events among those patients with reduced stress.
†Substantial decreases in depression scores were noted in both the control and intervention groups.

34

Psychological Risk Factors and Coronary Artery Disease: Epidemiology, Pathophysiology, and Management

either usual medical care or a treatment arm that employed cognitive-behavioral therapy, supplemented by the use of a selective serotonin reuptake inhibitor (SSRI) for severe or unremitting depression. Physicians were permitted to also use SSRIs within the usual care group. A similar frequency of the composite endpoint of all-cause mortality and nonfatal myocardial infarction was observed in both treatment arms after 29 months of follow-up. The results of this trial may have been influenced by a greater than expected reduction in depression and improvement in social support in the usual care group, resulting in only modest difference in psychosocial functioning between both treatment arms by the end of the trial. Also, potential differences may have been obscured by a relatively high use of antidepressants in both treatment arms and a high rate of referral of recruits to myocardial revascularization, occurring in approximately 40% of the patients within 12 weeks of acute myocardial infarction. A later secondary analysis of the ENRICHD trial found that within the intervention arm, those who responded with a reduction in depression had a lower risk for late mortality compared with patients whose depression persisted or worsened.[146]

The combined efficacy of psychosocial interventions that involved smaller sample sizes has been assessed in a meta-analysis of 36 psychological intervention trials involving 12,851 patients.[147] Overall, these interventions were found to result in only a small reduction in the frequency of nonfatal myocardial reinfarction and no reduction in cardiac mortality or the frequency of subsequent myocardial revascularization procedures. Among the findings emphasized in this meta-analysis was the observation that these trials frequently yielded negligible improvement in depression or anxiety levels. In the absence of such effect, the utility of such studies must be interpreted with caution.

A variety of investigators have attempted to address the paucity of clinical trial evidence on cardiovascular outcomes by examining the effect of psychosocial interventions on intermediary processes that are connected to atherosclerosis or risk for cardiac events. As an example, Blumenthal and colleagues compared the beneficial effects of three management approaches—exercise, stress management, and usual care—among three intermediate endpoints in 134 randomized patients (changes in flow-mediated dilation, left ventricular ejection fraction, and wall motion during radionuclide ventriculography) and in variables reflecting cardiac autonomic control.[148] Both among patients assigned to exercise and stress management, favorable findings in these indices were observed compared with patients assigned to usual medical care. A review of studies that have examined the effects of psychological interventions on such intermediary endpoints is beyond the purview of this chapter, but a practical problem posed by these smaller trials is that they often involve considerably more intense caregiver interactions than is possible in everyday practice.

The end result of the evidence base to date is a lack of certainty as to best practical approaches for management of psychosocial distress in cardiac practice. Nevertheless, in the absence of formal data, there are many insights, practical experiences, and new work in the arena of medical psychology that may guide physicians regarding the management of psychosocial issues in cardiac patients, as discussed here.

Screening for Psychological Distress in Cardiac Populations

A recent American Heart Association Science Advisory calls for the routine screening for depression in cardiac practice and suggests that at a minimum, a two-question survey from the Patient Health Questionnaire (PHQ) be applied.[148] The two-item questionnaire includes the following:
Over the past 2 weeks, how often have you been bothered by any of the following problems?
 1. Little interest or pleasure in doing things.
 2. Feeling down, depressed, or hopeless.
If the answer to either question is yes, the Advisory suggests that the full nine items of the PHQ be assessed (the PHQ-9; Box 34-2). Patients with high PHQ scores (≥10) should be referred for qualified professional evaluation according to this Advisory.

A number of issues are pertinent relative to this new recommendation. First, to-date, there is insufficient study to determine whether the screening for depression, per se, without additional structured follow-up care sufficiently impacts on clinical care. Notably, a meta-analysis suggests that the stand-alone use of a depression-screening questionnaire has little impact on depression management.[149] In primary care settings, the utility of screening for depression is improved if such screening is tied to some form of collaborative care intervention following screening.[150,151] Second, the American Heart Association Science Advisory did not deal with recommendations for screening for anxiety, which, although substantially comorbid with depression, may occur in its absence and exert significant effect on morbidity, mortality, health cost, and quality of life. Third, and significantly, despite the widespread emphasis on DSM-IV diagnoses, they largely cover depression, anxiety, and substance abuse disorders; but as reviewed in this chapter, there are a large variety of other psychosocial problems that can exert significant clinical and pathophysiologic effects, including chronic stress and social isolation. Whereas there are also short-version questionnaires that can be used to screen for these psychosocial factors, the use of questionnaires is probably

BOX 34-2 Patient Health Questionnaire-9 (PHQ-9) for Screening for Depression

Over the past 2 weeks, how often have you been bothered by any of the following problems?
1. Little interest or pleasure in doing things.
2. Feeling down, depressed, or hopeless.
3. Trouble falling asleep, staying asleep, or sleeping too much.
4. Feeling tired or having little energy.
5. Poor appetite or overeating.
6. Feeling bad about yourself, feeling that you are a failure, or feeling that you have let yourself or your family down.
7. Trouble concentrating on things such as reading the newspaper or watching television.
8. Moving or speaking so slowly that other people could have noticed.
9. Thinking that you would be better off dead or that you want to hurt yourself in some way.
   Questions are scored: not at all = 0; several days = 1; more than half the days = 2; and nearly every day = 3. Add together the item scores to get a total score for depression severity.

From Lichtman JH, Bigger JT, Blumenthal JA, et al: Depression and coronary heart disease recommendations for screening, referral, and treatment. *Circulation* 118:1768, 2008. Reproduced with permission.

BOX 34-3 Suggested Open-Ended Questions to Screen for Psychosocial Risk Factors

How would you describe your energy level?
How have you been sleeping?
How has your mood been recently?
Do you feel anxious or unduly worried?
Are you under undue pressure at work or at home?
Do you have difficulty unwinding after work or at the end of the day?
Who do you turn to for support?

Modified from Rozanski A, Blumenthal JA, Davidson KW, et al: The epidemiology, pathophysiology, and management of psychosocial risk factors in cardiac practice: the emerging field of behavioral cardiology. *J Am Coll Cardiol* 45:637, 2005.

unnecessary in daily practice. Rather, just as physicians are accustomed to performing a quick oral review of all organ systems in daily practice, a very short series of questions, such as those proposed in Box 34-3, can be used to screen for chronic negative emotions, chronic stress, and somatic complaints that may be stress or emotion related. There is a conception that such investigation is necessarily lengthy and thus impractical, but to the contrary, a practiced clinician can often obtain relevant screening information in a matter of minutes by using simple questions such as those listed in Box 34-3.

Synergy of Managing "Behavioral" and Psychological Risk Factors

There is a common division made between the management of behavioral lifestyle factors associated with CAD, such as smoking, poor diet, and sedentary behavior, and the management of psychological risk factors, but these factors commonly cluster together. There are reasons that grouping the consideration of these factors is beneficial. Psychological risk factors, such as depression, anxiety, and chronic stress, are

causative factors with respect to poor health behaviors, and they constitute a strong barrier to the successful adherence of recommended health behavior change.[106,107] Equally important, poor health behavior is one of the mechanisms by which psychological risk factors cause or worsen CAD, and favorable behavioral change is one means of ameliorating some aspects of psychological distress.

As an example, exercise represents a behavioral intervention that can be used to ameliorate psychological distress, as shown by cross-sectional and randomized controlled trials demonstrating lower depression among those who exercise.[152,153] In other work, Blumenthal and coworkers randomized 156 depressed subjects to exercise, antidepressant medication, or both.[154] Exercise was just as effective as sertraline hydrochloride in reducing depressive symptoms in this cohort, but the study did not contain a control group.

A subsequent randomized controlled trial compared four therapies: supervised group exercise, home-based exercise, antidepressant medication, and placebo groups.[155] Comparable reductions in depression were again observed with exercise and antidepressant medication, with a lesser but beneficial effect associated with placebo medication. Further, examination of the effects of exercise within the ENRICHD study found that it was associated with both a significant reduction in depression and a 30% reduction in mortality.[156] A cardiac rehabilitation program is a common clinical setting in which psychosocial interventions have been combined with exercise training and standard behavioral risk factor modification.

In a recent meta-analysis of 23 randomized controlled trials that involved cardiac rehabilitation, Linden and colleagues[157] observed a reduction in all-cause mortality at 2-year follow-up for those studies incorporating psychosocial interventions compared with those that did not (odds ratio of 0.72; 95% CI, 0.56-0.94). Notably, paralleling results seen among studies involving stand-alone psychosocial interventions, reduction in mortality was significant only among patients in whom there was successful reduction of psychological distress within this meta-analysis.

New Potential Paradigms for Psychosocial Interventions

Potential advances in the psychosocial management of cardiac patients can be inhibited when strict boundaries are maintained between what cardiologists and behavioral specialists manage. New insights into the determinants and means of augmenting human motivation, the bidirectional relationship between thoughts and emotions, and the potential application of positive psychology practices represent new opportunities to develop more optimal and potentially efficient interventions in cardiac practice.

An example of how cardiologists might think about stress, moods, emotions, and health behaviors in an integrative way stems from work conducted by Thayer and colleagues.[158] In a series of experimental subjects, they assessed the relationship between four parameters: feelings of tension, energy levels, moods, and behaviors. The paradigm that evolved from their work revolves around four energy-tension states, as illustrated in Figure 34-14. These investigators noted that when subjects reported low tension, whether in association with high energy (i.e., "calm energy") or low energy (i.e., "calm tiredness"), corresponding mood states were generally positive. By contrast, when subjects reported high tension, moods varied according to subjects' corresponding energy levels; "tense tiredness" was associated with a high frequency of negative moods, but "tense energy" was not.

These findings offer insights into a potential management paradigm, involving four categories of intervention, for the amelioration of psychosocial risk factors in cardiac practice.

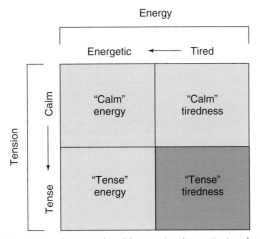

FIGURE 34-14 Thayer's proposed model concerning characterization of subjects' momentary states according to energy and tension levels. The majority of negative moods in this experimental work occurred in subjects when they reported both high tension and low energy (i.e., "tense tiredness"). *(From Thayer RE, Newman R, McClain TM: Self-regulation of mood: strategies for changing a bad mood, raising energy and reducing tension.* J Pers Soc Psychol 67:910, 1994.)

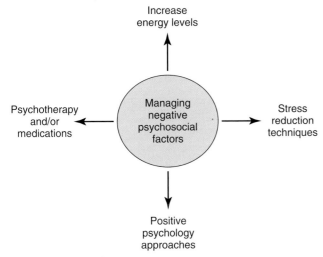

FIGURE 34-15 Potential methods for management of negative psychosocial interventions in clinical practice (see text).

Whereas these categories are listed as separate approaches in Figure 34-15, in fact there is considerable overlap and potential synergy among these approaches. One approach is to focus subjects on managing their energy. This can be beneficial because when patients are under prolonged stress, there is often a tendency to become more self-centered and to feel greater urgency to manage stress, even though at such times patients may not be at their best for problem solving.[68] The work of Thayer implies that when patients lift their energy, their mood may also lift, thus providing them with greater self-efficacy for problem solving afterward. Patients may benefit from advice on how to increase their energy effectively. A common quick fix for patients when they are feeling tense-tired is the ingestion of unhealthy energy-dense foods.[158,159] Rather, physicians can suggest such energy-boosting activities as short bursts of exercise activity, switching from draining work to inspiring work, taking naps, or listening to inspiring music.

Alternatively, methods that are designed to physically and emotionally unwind or reduce stress may be useful, including such practices as simple breathing exercises and the application of mindful meditation. Practices such as yoga and Tai Chi represent approaches that may both increase energy and reduce stress when they are employed over time. There is increasing evidence that such techniques have beneficial physiologic effects.[160-162]

When patients are tense-tired or moody, there is a tendency to become more cognitively inflexible, impatient, and less creative.[68] A behavioral approach that teaches patients to take their negative thoughts, moods, and problems less seriously or to turn away from these thoughts to positive pursuits that generate positive emotions is becoming commonplace among practitioners of positive psychology and might be helpful to cardiac patients as well. As an example of this approach, a couple under marital stress may choose to focus on their specific complaints under standard marital therapy. In this alternative approach, a positive psychology practitioner may have the couple focus and dwell on the positive aspects of their relationship during counseling sessions, with the intention of raising emotional well-being, with enhanced problem solving evolving as a secondary outcome of that effort. To date, there is a dearth of study regarding the potential effects of positive psychological interventions on clinical outcomes, but the beneficial effects of positive interventions on some mediators of physiology and central nervous system function have been noteworthy.[163,164]

When stress, anxiety, or mood disorders become more severe, referral of patients to trained mental health professionals for formal psychotherapy should be considered. Some sources of stress and the health behaviors they induce, such as overeating and sedentary behavior, poor social support, loneliness, overwork, and life imbalance (sometimes leading to unduly severe voluntary sleep restriction), may be amenable to physician advice or referral to community or Internet resources. Notably, many of these psychosocial problems do not necessarily fall within the traditional division of what physicians versus mental health care specialists manage.

The Use of Psychopharmacologic Medications

When depression or anxiety is sufficiently severe, patients are candidates for the use of pharmacologic agents or some form of professional psychotherapeutic counseling, such as cognitive-behavioral therapy or problem-solving therapy. Cardiologists do not commonly manage depression, but they may either refer patients directly to psychiatrists for psychiatric evaluation or work with general practitioners who are accustomed to treating depression or collaborating with psychiatrists for mental health care. In either case, it behooves cardiologists to be well acquainted with the medical side effects of psychopharmacologic agents and potential drug interactions. In recent years, SSRIs have become the preferred medication for treatment of depression in cardiac patients, and they are also used as a first-line medication for treatment of significant anxiety. SSRI medication (sertraline) was found to have a very good safety profile for use in post–myocardial infarction patients in the SADHART study,[165] but recent study has suggested that the use of SSRIs is not necessarily benign. A 5.9-year follow-up of 136,293 women from the Women's Health Initiative found that SSRIs were not associated with an increased risk of cardiac events, but there was an increased risk for all-cause mortality and hemorrhagic and fatal stroke.[166] However, the increase in absolute event rate with SSRI use during this follow-up was still low. In another large follow-up of 63,469 women from the Women's Health Study, Whang and associates[167] found that major depression and antidepressant use were associated with an increased cardiac event rate, and antidepressant use alone was associated with an increased event rate for sudden cardiac arrest. It is not clear whether this effect merely signaled the presence of greater underlying

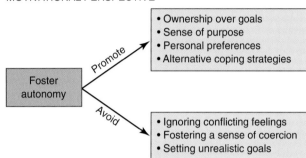

MOTIVATIONAL PERSPECTIVE

FIGURE 34-16 Attempts to promote treatment adherence commonly make use of techniques that involve external regulation. Alternatively, attempts to promote patients' personal autonomy can foster intrinsic motivation. Examples of this approach include attempts to promote patient ownership over recommended behavioral changes (i.e., getting patients to voice their own reasons for initiating change) and helping patients to find meaningful purpose for suggested change. *(From Rozanski A, Blumenthal JA, Davidson KW, et al: The epidemiology, pathophysiology, and management of psychosocial risk factors in cardiac practice: the emerging field of behavioral cardiology. J Am Coll Cardiol 45:637, 2005.)*

BOX 34-4 Steps to Promote Effective Adherence to Behavioral Suggestions

1. Use clear and effective communication and make recommendations as specific and simple as possible.
2. Schedule follow-up visits to check adherence, especially during the early practice phase, as opposed to the later, more ingrained habit phase.
3. Provide a motivating rationale for the patient's treatment regimen, with consideration of explanations that befit the patient's level of "health literacy."
4. Follow key oral suggestions with written ones to reinforce the cardiologist's message.
5. Begin with "micro" goals for patients who are resistant to behavior change or who have fewer available personal resources.
6. Help patients establish realistic goals and expectations.
7. Involve patients in tailoring behavioral suggestions that reflect their autonomous desires and tendencies rather than just dictating change.
8. Provide positive feedback.
9. Openly and candidly explore potential patient barriers to adherence (such as lack of personal motivation, time, family support, facilities, or knowledge; fears; job, home, or other pressures; and cultural issues) and assist patients with problem solving and developing strategies (e.g., self-monitoring approaches, written agreements, and relapse prevention) at the time of recommendations.
10. Make use of "implementation intentions."
11. Help patients to become cognizant of environmental stimuli that may inadvertently prime negative health behaviors nonconsciously.
12. Refer patients with poor structural or functional social support to programs or activities that will enhance adherence by providing social support.

Modified from Rozanski A, Blumenthal JA, Davidson KW, et al: The epidemiology, pathophysiology, and management of psychosocial risk factors in cardiac practice: the emerging field of behavioral cardiology. *J Am Coll Cardiol* 45:637, 2005.

---

depression among those taking antidepressant medication or represented an important side effect of SSRI use. Such recent observations point out the need for further prospective study regarding the use of SSRIs in cardiac patients, both to study their potential benefits in promoting survival, which to date has been poorly studied, and to better assess potential medical side effects of SSRI use in cardiac patients. Still, these medications enjoy a substantially improved patient profile compared with various prior generations of antidepressant agents, such as tricyclic depressants.

The Psychological Management of Patient Adherence

Behavioral risk factors for CAD are well established, including sedentary behavior, smoking, overeating, and poor nutritional diets. Depression, anxiety, poor social support, and other psychosocial risk factors offer a powerful barrier to patients' attempts to modify these adverse health behaviors as well as to medication adherence. Research indicates that understanding of psychological principles can increase patients' internal motivation and help them plan and maintain adherence to health behaviors. For instance, patients become more motivated and they relapse less often when they formulate health goals that are more consonant with their own autonomously endorsed values or patterns of behavior, rather than just being told by their physicians what to do[97] (Fig. 34-16). Increasingly, it is also recognized that patients are nonconsciously or "mindlessly" cued into behaviors by their external environment.[168,169] Along these lines, physicians can advise patients about environmental factors that induce "mindless eating"[170] or promote stress. The

tendency to behave nonconsciously can also be positively manipulated to promote healthful behaviors through the formation of "implementation intentions," as developed by Gollwitzer.[171] Implementation intentions involve patients' declaration that when it is X, I will do Y. For instance, "when I finish work at 6 PM at night, I will drive to the gym before coming home." Although this formulation seems simplistic, meta-analysis indicates that it can be effective in fostering behavioral change.[172] Approaches to augment patients' adherence to recommended health behaviors are listed in Box 34-4.

Potential Practice Model for Psychosocial Interventions in Cardiac Practice

The management of both behavioral and psychological problems varies widely in complexity and in terms of time and resource demands. A potential stepped care model for integration of psychosocial interventions into medical care is shown in Figure 34-17. Patients with milder forms of psychosocial distress and with a tendency to be highly adherent to medical suggestions can be readily managed within routine physician practice.[173] Physicians can enhance their management of patients by being cognizant of principles designed to promote the adherence of patients to suggested behavioral change.[97] Whereas physician time is limited, physicians can complement their management of patients by suggesting to them community-based exercise and social programs and

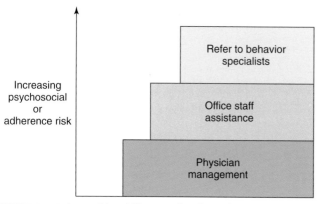

STEPPED CARE BEHAVIORAL
MANAGEMENT FOR CLINICAL PRACTICE

Increasing
psychosocial
or
adherence risk

Refer to behavior
specialists

Office staff
assistance

Physician
management

FIGURE 34-17 A potential model for stepped psychosocial interventions in clinical cardiac practice. Routine counseling and psychosocial interventions may be addressed at the physician level. Somewhat increased difficulty in adherence to medical regimens or psychosocial stress may benefit from adjunctive care, monitoring, or feedback from office staff (see text). Patients with significant psychosocial distress (e.g., depression) or poor adherence difficulty may benefit from additional referral to behavioral health specialists or programs.[3]

Internet-based programs that can support dietary and other behavioral changes. The range of such programs varies widely within local communities. For patients with somewhat increased psychosocial distress or with greater difficulty in adhering to behavioral change, added instruction, support, monitoring, or feedback might be accomplished by use of ancillary office staff.

Added support is often quite helpful in the early stages of requested behavioral changes because unlike habits, which are automatic and noneffortful, new behavioral practices are intentional and effortful. Patients who are poorly adherent or resistant to recommended behavioral change or manifest a high level of psychological distress can be referred to appropriate health care professionals, according to the nature of the patient's problems. Prospective work is needed to test the potential of this stepped care model.

CONCLUSION

Epidemiologic studies have been consistent in demonstrating a strong relationship between various psychosocial risk factors and heart disease. These factors include chronic negative emotions, such as depression and various forms of anxiety; negative cognitive patterns, such as pessimism; chronic stress; and the lack of certain basic psychological needs, such as poor social support. In general, a strong dose-response association exists among many psychosocial risk factors and CAD outcomes. Importantly, new evidence indicates that positive psychological factors and life experiences can benefit physiology and improve longevity. Great strides have been made into understanding of the pathophysiology linking psychosocial risk factors to CAD, involving chronic activation of the autonomic nervous system and the hypothalamic-pituitary axis, leading to remodeling of central nervous system structures, physiologic hyperreactivity, apparent accelerated aging, and negative metabolic, coagulation, and immune effects that serve to promote accelerated atherosclerosis and increase the risk for cardiac events. Results of psychosocial intervention trials have resulted in mixed data, but new paradigms and developments within medical psychology offer new potential means to improve the efficacy of psychosocial interventions in cardiac patients.

Acknowledgment

I would like to thank Elana Feinerman for her expert technical assistance in the preparation of this manuscript and Dr. Bruce McEwen for providing Figure 34-11.

REFERENCES

1. Friedman M, Rosenman RH: Association of specific overt behavior with blood and cardiovascular findings. *JAMA* 169:1286, 1959.
2. Berkman LF, Syme SL: Social networks, host resistance, and mortality: a nine-year follow-up study of Alameda county residents. *Am J Epidemiol* 109:186, 1979.
3. Rozanski A, Blumenthal JA, Kaplan J: Impact of psychological factors on the pathogenesis of cardiovascular disease and implications for therapy. *Circulation* 99:2192, 1999.
4. Kaplan JR, Manuck SS, Clarkson TB, et al: Social stress and atherosclerosis in normocholesterolemic monkeys. *Science* 220:733, 1983.
5. Rutledge T, Vaccarino V, Johnson BD, et al: Depression and cardiovascular health care costs among women with suspected myocardial ischemia: prospective results from the WISE (Women's Ischemia Syndrome Evaluation Study). *J Am Coll Cardiol* 53:176, 2009.
6. Lesperance F, Frasure-Smith N, Talajiv M, et al: Five-year risk of cardiac mortality in relation to initial severity and one-year changes in depression symptoms after myocardial infarction. *Circulation* 105:1049, 2002.
7. Rugulies R: Depression as a predictor for coronary heart disease. A review and meta-analysis. *Am J Prev Med* 23:51, 2002.
8. Cuijpers P, Smit F: Excess mortality in depression: a meta-analysis of community studies. *J Affect Disord* 72:227, 2002.
9. Wulsin LR, Singal BM: Do depressive symptoms increase the risk for the onset of coronary disease? A systematic quantitative review. *Psychosom Med* 65:201, 2003.
10. Van Melle JP, den Jonge P, Spijkerman TA, et al: Prognostic association of depression following myocardial infarction with mortality and cardiovascular events: a meta-analysis. *Psychosom Med* 66:814, 2004.
11. Barth J, Schumacher M, Hermann-Lingen C: Depression as a risk factor for mortality in patients with coronary heart disease: a meta-analysis. *Psychosom Med* 66:802, 2004.
12. Kessler RC, Chiu WT, Demler O, Walters EE: Prevalence, severity, and comorbidity of 12-month DSM-IV disorders in the National Comorbidity Survey Replication. *Arch Gen Psychiatry* 62:617, 2005.
13. McCarron P, Gunnell D, Harrison GL, et al: Temperament in young adulthood and later mortality: prospective observational study. *J Epidemiol Community Health* 57:888, 2003.
14. Eaker ED, Sullivan LM, Kelly-Hayes M, et al: Tension and anxiety and the prediction of the 10-year incidence of coronary heart disease, atrial fibrillation, and total mortality: the Framingham Offspring Study. *Psychosom Med* 67:692, 2005.
15. Ringbäck Weitoft G, Rosén M: Is perceived nervousness and anxiety a predictor of premature mortality and severe morbidity? A longitudinal follow up of the Swedish survey of living conditions. *J Epidemiol Community Health* 58:794, 2005.
16. Ostir GV, Goodwin JS: High anxiety is associated with an increased risk of death in an older tri-ethnic population. *J Clin Epidemiol* 59:534, 2006.
17. Mykletun A, Bjerkeset O, Dewey M: Anxiety, depression, and cause-specific mortality: the HUNT Study. *Psychosom Med* 69:323, 2007.
18. Fan AZ, Strine TW, Jiles R, et al: Depression and anxiety associated with cardiovascular disease among persons aged 45 years and older in 28 states of the Unites States, 2006. *Prev Med* 46:445, 2008.
19. Shen BJ, Avivi YE, Todaro JF, et al: Anxiety characteristics independently and prospectively predict myocardial infarction in men. *J Am Coll Cardiol* 51:113, 2008.
20. Phillips AC, Batty GD, Gale CR: Generalized anxiety disorder, major depressive disorder, and their comorbidity as predictors of all-cause and cardiovascular mortality: the Vietnam experience study. *Psychosom Study* 71:395, 2009.
21. Shibeshi WA, Young-Xu Y, Blatt CM: Anxiety worsens prognosis in patients with coronary artery disease. *J Am Coll Cardiol* 49:2021, 2007.
22. Rothenbacher D, Hahmann H, Wusten B, et al: Symptoms of anxiety and depression in patients with stable coronary heart disease: prognostic value and consideration of pathogenetic links, 2009. *Eur J Cardiovasc Prev Rehabil* 14:547, 2007.
23. Frasure-Smith N, Lesperance F: Depression and anxiety as predictors of 2-year cardiac events in patients with stable coronary artery disease. *Arch Gen Psychiatry* 65:62, 2008.
24. Smoller JW, Pollack MG, Wassertheil-Smoller S, et al: Panic attacks and risk of incident cardiovascular events among postmenopausal women in the Women's Health Initiative Observational Study. *Arch Gen Psychiatry* 64:1153, 2007.
25. Chen YH, Tsai SY, Lee HS, et al: Increased risk of acute myocardial infarction for patients with panic disorder: a nationwide population-based study. *Psychosom Med* 71:798, 2009.
26. Caminero AG, Blumentals WA, Russo LJ, et al: Does panic disorder increase the risk of coronary heart disease? A cohort study of a national managed care database. *Psychosom Med* 67:688, 2005.
27. Walters K, Rait G, Petersen I, et al: Panic disorder and risk of new onset coronary heart disease, acute myocardial infarction, and cardiac mortality: cohort study using the general practice research database. *Eur Heart J* 29:2981, 2008.
28. Kawachi I, Colditz GA, Ascherio A, et al: Prospective study of phobic anxiety and risk of coronary heart disease in men. *Circulation* 89:1992, 1994.
29. Albert CM, Chae CU, Rexrode KM, et al: Phobic anxiety and risk of coronary heart disease and sudden cardiac death among women. *Circulation* 111:480, 2005.
30. Kubzansky LD, Koenen KC, Spiro A, et al: Prospective study of posttraumatic stress disorder symptoms and coronary heart disease in the Normative Aging Study. *Arch Gen Psychiatry* 64:109, 2007.

34

Psychological Risk Factors and Coronary Artery Disease: Epidemiology, Pathophysiology, and Management

31. Kubzansky LD, Koenen KC, Jones C, et al: A prospective study of posttraumatic stress disorder symptoms and coronary heart disease in women. *Health Psychol* 28:125, 2009.

32. Boscarino JA: A prospective study of PTSD and early-age heart disease mortality among Vietnam veterans: implications for surveillance and prevention. *Psychosom Med* 70:668, 2008.

33. Kibler JL, Joshi K, Ma M: Hypertension in relation to posttraumatic stress disorder and depression in the US National Comorbidity Survey. *Behav Med* 34:125, 2008.

34. Chida Y, Steptoe A: The association of anger and hostility with future coronary heart disease. *J Am Coll Cardiol* 59:936, 2009.

35. Peterson C, Seligman MEP, Vaillant GE: Pessimistic explanatory style is a risk factor for physical illness: a thirty-five-year longitudinal study. *J Pers Soc Psychol* 55:23, 1988.

36. Scheier MG, Carver CS: Optimism, coping, and health: assessment and implications of generalized outcome expectancies. *Health Psychol* 4:219, 1985.

37. Kubzansky LD, Sparrow D, Vokonas P, et al: Is the glass half empty or half full? A prospective study of optimism and coronary heart disease in the normative aging study. *Psychosom Med* 63:910, 2001.

38. Grodbardt BR, Bower JH, Geda YE, et al: Pessimistic, anxious, and depressive personality traits predict all-cause mortality: the Mayo Clinic Cohort Study of Personality and Aging. *Psychosom Med* 71:491, 2009.

39. Giltay EJ, Geleijnse JM, Zitman FG, et al: Dispositional optimism and all-cause and cardiovascular mortality in a prospective cohort of elderly Dutch men and women. *Arch Gen Psychiatry* 61:1126, 2004.

40. Giltay EJ, Kamphuis MH, Kalmijn S, et al: Dispositional optimism and the risk of cardiovascular death. *Arch Intern Med* 166:431, 2006.

41. Tindle HA, Chang YF, Kuller LH, et al: Optimism, cynical hostility, and incident coronary heart disease and mortality in the Women's Health Initiative. *Circulation* 120:656, 2009.

42. Kubzansky LD, Kawachi I, Spiro A, III, et al: Is worrying bad for your heart? A prospective study of worry and coronary heart disease in the Normative Aging Study. *Circulation* 95:818, 1997.

43. Glynn LM, Christenfeld N, Gerin W: The role of rumination in recovery from reactivity: cardiovascular consequences of emotional states. *Psychosom Med* 64:714, 2002.

44. Fry PS, Debats DL: Perfectionism and the five-factor personality traits as predictors of mortality in older adults. *J Health Psychol* 14:513, 2009.

45. Wirtz PH, Elsenbruch S, Emini L, et al: Perfectionism and the cortisol response to psychosocial stress in men. *Psychosom Med* 69:249, 2007.

46. Lawler KA, Younger JW, Piferi RL, et al: A change of heart: cardiovascular correlates of forgiveness in response to interpersonal conflict. *J Behav Med* 26:373, 2003.

47. Kaplan JR, Manuck SB, Clarkson TB, et al: Social status, environment and atherosclerosis in cynomolgus monkeys. *Arteriosclerosis* 2:359, 1982.

48. Kaplan JR, Manuck SB, Adams MR, et al: Inhibition of coronary atherosclerosis by propranolol in behaviorally predisposed monkeys fed an atherogenic diet. *Circulation* 76:1365, 1987.

49. Manuck SB, Kaplan JR, Adams MR: Effects of stress and the sympathetic nervous system on coronary artery atherosclerosis in the cynomolgus macaque. *Am Heart J* 116:328, 1988.

50. Karasek R, Baker D, Marxer F, et al: Job decision latitude, job demands, and cardiovascular disease: a prospective study of Swedish men. *Am J Public Health* 71:694, 1981.

51. Siegrist J: Adverse health effects of high-effort/low-reward conditions. *J Occup Health Psychol* 71:694, 1996.

52. Bosma A, Marmot MG, Hemingway H, et al: Low job control and risk of coronary heart disease in Whitehall II (prospective cohort) study. *BMJ* 314:558, 1997.

53. Kuper H, Marmot M, Hemingway H: Systematic review of prospective cohort studies of psychosocial factors in the etiology and prognosis of coronary heart disease. *Semin Vasc Med* 2:267, 2002.

54. Peter R, Siegrist J, Hallqvist J, et al: Psychosocial work environment and myocardial infarction: improving risk estimation by combining two complementary job stress models in the SHEEP study. *J Epidemiol Community Health* 56:294, 2002.

55. Lynch J, Krause N, Kaplan, GA, et al: Workplace demands, economic reward, and progression of carotid atherosclerosis. *Circulation* 96:302, 1997.

56. Eaker ED, Sullivan LM, Kelly-Hayes M, et al: Marital status, marital strain, and risk of coronary heart disease or total mortality: the Framingham Offspring Study. *Psychosom Med* 69:509, 2007.

57. De Vogli R, Chandola T, Marmot MG: Negative aspects of close relationships and heart disease. *Arch Intern Med* 167:1951, 2007.

58. Orth-Gomer K, Wamala SP, Horsten M, et al: Marital stress worsens prognosis in women with coronary heart disease: the Stockholm Female Coronary Risk Study. *JAMA* 248:3008, 2000.

59. Coyne JC, Rohrbaugh MJ, Shoham V, et al: Prognostic importance of marital quality for survival of congestive heart failure. *Am J Cardiol* 88:526, 2001.

60. Gallo LC, Troxel WM, Kuller LH, et al: Marital status, marital quality, and atherosclerotic burden in postmenopausal women. *Psychosom Med* 65:952, 2003.

61. Adler NE, Boyce T, Chesney MA, et al: Socioeconomic status and health: the challenge of the gradient. *Am Psychol* 49:15, 1994.

62. Marmot M: *The status syndrome: how social standing affects our health and longevity*, New York, 2004, Henry Holt and Company.

63. Dohrenwend BP: The role of adversity and stress in psychopathology: some evidence and its implications for theory and research. *J Health Soc Behav* 41:1, 2000.

64. Lee S, Colditz GA, Berkman LF, et al: Caregiving and risk of coronary heart disease in U.S. women: a prospective study. *Am J Prev Med* 24:113, 2003.

65. Batten S, Aslan M, Maciejewski PK, et al: Childhood maltreatment as a risk factor for adult cardiovascular disease and depression. *J Clin Psychiatry* 65:249, 2004.

66. Dong M, Giles WH, Felitti VJ, et al: Insights into causal pathways for ischemic heart disease: adverse childhood experiences study. *Circulation* 100:1761, 2004.

67. Kivimaki M, Ferrie JE, Brunner E, et al: Justice at work and reduced risk of coronary heart disease among employees: the Whitehall II Study. *Arch Intern Med* 165:2245, 2005.

68. Fredrickson BL: The role of positive emotions in positive psychology: the broaden-and-build theory of positive emotions. *Am Psychol* 56:218, 2001.

69. Ryff CD, Singer B: The contours of positive human health. *Psychol Inquiry* 9:1, 1998.

70. Pressman SD, Cohen S: Does positive affect influence health? *Psychol Bull* 131:925, 2005.

71. Maslow A: *Motivation and personality*, New York, 1954, Harper.

72. Frankl VE: *Man's search for meaning: an introduction to logotherapy*, New York, 1959, Simon & Schuster.

73. Ryan RM, Deci EL: Self-determination theory and the facilitation of intrinsic motivation, social development, and well-being. *Am Psychol* 55:68, 2000.

74. Chida Y, Steptoe A: Positive psychological well-being and mortality: a quantitative review of prospective observational studies. *Psychosom Med* 70:741, 2008.

75. Emmons RA, McCullough ME: Counting blessings versus burdens: experimental studies of gratitude and subjective well-being. *J Pers Soc Psychol* 84:377, 2003.

76. Schwartz C, Meisenhelder JB, Ma Y: Altruistic social interest behaviors are associated with better mental health. *Psychosom Med* 65:778, 2003.

77. Boyle PA, Barnes LL, Buchman AS, et al: Purpose in life is associated with mortality among community-dwelling older persons. *Psychosom Med* 71:575, 2009.

78. Gruenewald TL, Karlamangla AS, Greendale GA, et al: Feelings of usefulness to others, disability, and mortality in older adults: the MacArthur Study of Successful Aging. *J Gerontol B Psychol Sci Soc Sci* 62:P28, 2007.

79. Okamoto K, Tanaka Y: Subjective usefulness and 6-year mortality risks among elderly persons in Japan. *J Gerontol B Psychol Sci Soc Sci* 59:P246, 2004.

80. Rozanski A, Kubzansky LD: Psychological functioning and physical health: a paradigm of flexibility. *Psychosom Med* 67:S47, 2005.

81. Kubzansky LD, Thurston RC: Emotional vitality and incident coronary heart disease: Benefits of healthy psychological functioning. *Arch Gen Psychiatry* 64:1393, 2007.

82. Mausner-Dorsch H, Easton WW: Psychosocial work environment and depression: epidemiologic assessment of the demand-control mode. *Am J Public Health* 90:1765, 2000.

83. Yusuf S, Hawken S, Ounpuu S, et al: Effect of potentially modifiable risk factors associated with myocardial infarction in 52 countries (the INTERHEART study): case-control study. *Lancet* 364:937, 2004.

84. Rosengren A, Hawken S, Ounpuu S, et al: Association of psychosocial risk factors with risk of acute myocardial infarction in 11,119 cases and 13,648 controls from 52 countries (the INTERHEART study): case-control study. *Lancet* 364:953, 2004.

85. McEwen BS: Protective and damaging effects of stress mediators. *N Engl J Med* 338:171, 1998.

86. Dallman MG, La Fleur S, Pecoraro NC, et al: Minireview: glucocorticoids—food intake, abdominal obesity, and wealthy nations in 2004. *Endocrinology* 145:2633, 2004.

87. Kiecolt-Glaser JK, Preacher KJ, MacCallum RC, et al: Chronic stress and age-related increases in the proinflammatory cytokine IL-6. *Proc Natl Acad Sci U S A* 100:9090, 2003.

88. Jain S, Mills PH, Kanel RV: Effects of perceived stress and uplifts on inflammation and coagulability. *Psychophysiology* 44:154, 2007.

89. Brunner EJ, Hemmingway H, Walker BR: Adrenocortical, autonomic, and inflammatory causes of the metabolic syndrome: nested case-control study. *Circulation* 106:2659, 2002.

90. Brunner EJ, Chandola T, Marmot MG: Prospective effect of job strain on general and central obesity in the Whitehall II Study. *Am J Epidemiol* 165:828, 2007.

91. Schnall PL, Schwartz JE, Landsbergis PA, et al: A longitudinal study of job strain and ambulatory blood pressure: results from a three-year follow-up. *Psychosom Med* 60:697, 1998.

92. Vrijkotte TGM, van Doornen LJP, de Geus EJC: Effects of work stress on ambulatory blood pressure, heart rate, and heart rate variability. *Hypertension* 35:880, 2000.

93. Epel ES, Blackburn EH, Lin J, et al: Accelerated telomere shortening in response to life stress. *Proc Natl Acad Sci U S A* 101:17312, 2004.

94. Damjanovic AK, Yang Y, Glaser R, et al: Accelerated telomere erosion is associated with a declining immune function of caregivers of Alzheimer's disease patients. *J Immunol* 179:4249, 2007.

95. O'Donovan A, Lin J, Wolkowitz O, et al: Pessimism correlates with leukocyte telomere shortness and elevated interleukin-6 in post-menopausal women. *Brain Behav Immun* 23:446, 2009.

96. McEwen BS: Physiology and neurobiology of stress and adaptation: central role of the brain. *Physiol Rev* 87:873, 2007.

97. Rozanski A, Blumenthal JA, Davidson KW, et al: The epidemiology, pathophysiology, and management of psychosocial risk factors in cardiac practice: the emerging field of behavioral cardiology. *J Am Coll Cardiol* 45:637, 2005.

98. Koschke M, Boettger MK, Schulz S, et al: Autonomy of autonomic dysfunction in major depression. *Psychosom Med* 71:852, 2009.

99. Timonen M, Salmenkaita I, Jokelainen J, et al: Insulin resistance and depressive symptoms in young adult males: findings from Finnish Military Conscripts. *Psychosom Med* 69:723, 2007.

100. Vaccarino V, McClure C, Johnson D, et al: Depression, the metabolic syndrome and cardiovascular risk. *Psychosom Med* 70:40, 2008.

101. Everson-Rose SA, Lewis TT, Karavolus K, et al: Depressive symptoms and increased visceral fat in middle-aged women. *Psychosom Med* 71:410, 2009.

102. De Groot M, Anderson R, Freedland KE, et al: Association of depression and diabetes complications: a meta-analysis. *Psychosom Med* 63:619, 2001.

103. Michelson D, Stratakis C, Hill L, et al: Bone mineral density in women with depression. *N Engl J Med* 335:1176, 1996.

104. Howren MB, Lamkin DM, Suls J: Associations of depression with C-reactive protein, IL-1, and IL-6: a meta-analysis. *Psychosom Med* 71:171, 2009.

105. Broadley AJ, Korszun A, Jones CJ, Frenneaux MP: Arterial endothelial function is impaired in treated depression. *Heart* 88:521, 2002.

106. DiMatteo MR, Lepper HS, Croghan TW: Depression is a risk factor for noncompliance with medical treatment. Meta-analysis of the effects of anxiety and depression on patient adherence. *Arch Intern Med* 160:2101, 2000.

107. DiMatteo MR: Social support and patient adherence to medical treatment: a meta-analysis. *Health Psychol* 23:207, 2004.

108. Meisel SR, Kutz I, Dayan K, et al: Effects of Iraqi missile war on incidence of acute myocardial infarction and sudden death in Israeli civilians. *Lancet* 338:660, 1991.

109. Kario K, Matsuo T, Kobayashi H, et al: Earthquake-induced potentiation of acute risk factors in hypertensive elderly patients: possible triggering of cardiovascular events after a major earthquake. *Am Coll Cardiol* 29:926, 1997.

110. Wilbert-Lampen U, Leistner D, Greven S, et al: Cardiovascular events during World Cup soccer. *N Engl J Med* 385:475, 2008.

111. Kloner RA, McDonald S, Leeka J, Poole K: Comparison of total and cardiovascular death rates in the same city during a losing versus winning super bowl championship. *Am J Cardiol* 103:1647, 2009.

112. Tofler GH, Muller JE: Triggering of acute cardiovascular disease and potential preventive strategies. *Circulation* 114:1863, 2006.

113. Mottleman MA, Maclure M, Sherwood JB, et al: Triggering of acute myocardial infarction onset by episodes of anger. *Circulation* 92:1720, 1995.

114. Moller J, Hallqvist J, Diderichsen F, et al: Do episodes of anger trigger myocardial infarction? A case-crossover analysis in the Stockholm Heart Epidemiology Program (SHEEP). *Psychosom Med* 61:842, 1999.

115. Lipovetzky N, Hod H, Roth A, et al: Emotional events and anger at the workplace as triggers for a first event of the acute coronary syndrome: A case-crossover study. *Isr Med Assoc J* 9:310, 2007.

116. Moller J, Theorell T, de Faire U, et al: Work related stressful life events and the risk of myocardial infarction. Case-control and case-crossover analyses within Stockholm heart epidemiology programme (SHEEP). *J Epidemiol Community Health* 59:23, 2005.

117. Steptoe A, Strike PC, Perkins-Porras L, et al: Acute depressed mood as a trigger of acute coronary syndromes. *Biol Psychiatry* 60:837, 2006.

118. Rozanski A, Bairey CN, Krantz DS, et al: Mental stress and the induction of silent myocardial ischemia in patients with coronary artery disease. *N Engl J Med* 318:1005, 1983.

119. Yeung AC, Vekshtein VI, Krantz DS, et al: The effect of atherosclerosis on the vasomotor response of the coronary arteries to mental stress. *N Engl J Med* 325:1551, 1991.

120. Deanfield JE, Shea M, Kensett M, et al: Silent myocardial ischemia due to mental stress. *Lancet* 2:1001, 1984.

121. Sheps DS, McMahon RP, Becker L, et al: Mental stress–induced ischemia and all-cause mortality in patients with coronary artery disease: results from the psychophysiological investigations of myocardial ischemia study. *Circulation* 105:1780, 2002.

122. Babyak MA, Blumenthal JA, Hinderliter A, et al: Prognosis after change in left ventricular ejection fraction during mental stress testing in patients with stable coronary artery disease. *Am J Cardiol* 105:25, 2010.

123. Gabbay RH, Krantz DS, Kop WJ, et al: Triggers of myocardial ischemia during daily life in patients with coronary artery disease: physical and mental activities, anger and smoking. *J Am Coll Cardiol* 27:585, 1996.

124. Gullette ECD, Blumenthal JA, Babyak M, et al: Effects of mental stress on myocardial ischemia during daily life. *JAMA* 277:1521, 1997.

125. Ghiadoni L, Donald AE, Cropley M, et al: Mental stress induces transient endothelial dysfunction in humans. *Circulation* 102:2473, 2000.

126. Broadley AJM, Korszun A, Abdelaal E, et al: Inhibition of cortisol production with metyrapone prevents mental stress–induced endothelial dysfunction and baroreflex impairment. *J Am Coll Cardiol* 46:344, 2005.

127. Reid GJ, Seidelin PH, Kop WJ, et al: Mental stress–induced platelet activation among patients with coronary artery disease. *Psychosom Med* 71:438, 2009.

128. Vlachopoulos C, Kosmopoulou F, Alexopoulos N, et al: Acute mental stress has a prolonged unfavorable effect on arterial stiffness and wave reflections. *Psychosom Med* 68:231, 2006.

129. Kop WJ, Weissman NJ, Zhu J, et al: Effects of acute mental stress and exercise on inflammatory markers in patients with coronary artery disease and healthy controls. *Am J Cardiol* 101:767, 2008.

130. Cankaya B, Chapman BP, Talbot NL, et al: History of sudden unexpected loss is associated with elevated interleukin-6 and decreased insulin-like growth factor-1 in women in an Urban primary care setting. *Psychosom Med* 71:914, 2009.

131. Wilbert-Lampen U, Nickel T, Leistner D, et al: Modified serum profiles of inflammatory and vasoconstrictive factors in patients with emotional stress–induced acute coronary syndrome during World Cup soccer 2006. *J Am Coll Cardiol* 55:637, 2010.

132. Ziegelstein RC: Acute emotional stress and cardiac arrhythmias. *JAMA* 298:324, 2007.

133. Frederickson BL, Levenson RW: Positive emotions speed recovery from the cardiovascular sequelae of negative emotions. *Cognition Emotion* 12:191, 1998.

134. Vlachopoulos C, Xaplanteris P, Alexopoulos N, et al: Divergent effects of laughter and mental stress on arterial stiffness and central hemodynamics. *Psychosom Med* 71:1, 2009.

135. Miller M, Mangano C, Park Y, et al: Impact on cinematic viewing on endothelial function. *Heart* 92:261, 2006.

136. Wittstein IS, Thiemann DR, Lima JAC, et al: Neurohumoral features of myocardial stunning due to sudden emotional stress. *N Engl J Med* 352:539, 2005.

137. Sharkey SW, Lesser JR, Zenovich AG, et al: Acute and reversible cardiomyopathy provoked by stress in women from the United States. *Circulation* 111:472, 2005.

138. Wittstein IS: Apical-ballooning syndrome. *Lancet* 370:545, 2007.

139. Sharkey SW, Windenburg DC, Lesser JR, et al: Natural history and expansive clinical profile of stress (tako-tsubo) cardiomyopathy. *J Am Coll Cardiol* 55:333, 2010.

140. Friedman M, Thoresen CE, Gill J, et al: Alteration of type A behavior and its effect on cardiac recurrences in post myocardial infarction patients: summary results of the Recurrent Coronary Prevention Project. *Am Heart J* 112:653, 1986.

141. Frasure-Smith N, Prince R: The ischemic heart disease life stress monitoring program: impact on mortality. *Psychosom Med* 47:431, 1985.

142. Jones DA, West RR: Psychological rehabilitation after myocardial infarction: multicenter randomized control trial. *Br Med J* 313:1517, 1996.

143. Frasure-Smith N, Lesperance F, Prince RH, et al: Randomized trial of home-based psychosocial nursing intervention for patients recovering from myocardial infarction. *Lancet* 350:473, 1997.

144. Cossette S, Frasure-Smith N, Lesperance F: Clinical implications of a reduction in psychological distress on cardiac prognosis in patients participating in a psychosocial intervention program. *Psychosom Med* 63:257, 2001.

145. The ENRICHD Investigators: Effects on treating depression and low perceived social support on clinical events after a myocardial infarction: the Enhancing Recovery in Coronary Heart Disease Patients (ENRICHD) randomized trial. *JAMA* 289:3106, 2003.

146. Carney RM, Blumenthal JA, Freedland KE, et al: Depression and late mortality after myocardial infarction in the Enhancing Recovery in Coronary Heart Disease (ENRICHD) Study. *Psychosom Med* 66:466, 2004.

147. Rees K, Bennett P, West R, et al: Psychological interventions for coronary heart disease. *Cochrane Database Syst Rev* 3:1, 2009.

148. Blumenthal JA, Sherwood A, Babyak MA: Effects of exercise and stress management training on markers of cardiovascular risk in patients with ischemic heart disease. A randomized controlled trial. *JAMA* 293:1626, 2005.

149. Gilboy S, Sheldon T, House A: Screening and case-finding instruments for depression: a meta-analysis. *CMAJ* 178:997, 2008.

150. Thombs BD, De Jonge P, Coyne JC, et al: Depression screening and patient outcomes in cardiovascular care. A systematic review. *JAMA* 300:2161, 2008.

151. Whooley MA: To screen or not to screen? Depression in patients with cardiovascular disease. *J Am Coll Cardiol* 54:891, 2009.

152. Blumenthal JA, Jiang W, Babyak MA, et al: Stress management and exercise training in cardiac patients with myocardial ischemia. *Arch Intern Med* 157:2213, 1997.

153. Barbour KA, Edenfield TM, Blumenthal JA: Exercise as a treatment for depression and other psychiatric disorders. *J Cardiopulm Rehabil Prev* 27:359, 2007.

154. Blumenthal JA, Babyak MA, Moore KA, et al: Effects of exercise training on older patients with major depression. *Arch Intern Med* 159:2349, 1999.

155. Blumenthal JA, Babyak MA, Doraiswamy M, et al: Exercise and pharmacotherapy in the treatment of major depressive disorder. *Psychosom Med* 69:587, 2007.

156. Blumenthal JA, Babyak MA, Carney RM, et al: Exercise, depression, and mortality after myocardial infarction in the ENRICHD trial. *Med Sci Sports Exerc* 36:746, 2004.

157. Linden W, Phillips MJ, Leclerc J: Psychological treatment of cardiac patients: a meta-analysis. *Eur Heart J* 28:2972, 2007.

158. Thayer RE, Newman R, McClain TM: Self-regulation of mood: strategies for changing a bad mood, raising energy and reducing tension. *J Pers Soc Psychol* 67:910, 1994.

159. Thayer RE: Energy, tiredness, and tension effects of a sugar snack vs moderate exercise. *J Pers Soc Psychol* 52:119, 1987.

160. Kiecolt-Glaser JK, Christian L, Preston H, et al: Stress, inflammation, and yoga practice. *Psychosom Med* 72:113, 2010.

161. Motivala SJ, Sollers J, Thayer J, Irwin MR: Tai Chi Chih acutely decreases sympathetic nervous system activity in older adults. *J Gerontol A Biol Sci Med Sci* 61:1177, 2006.

162. Pace TWW, Negi LT, Adame DD, et al: Effect of compassion meditation on neuroendocrine, innate immune and behavioral responses to psychosocial stress. *Psychoneuroendocrinology* 34:87, 2009.

163. Gordon BA, Rykhlevskaia EI, Brumback CR, et al: Neuroanatomical correlates of aging, cardiopulmonary fitness level, and education. *Psychophysiology* 45:825, 2008.

164. Carlson MC, Erickson KI, Kramer AF: Evidence for neurocognitive plasticity in at-risk older adults: the experience corps program. *J Gerontol A Biol Sci Med Sci* 64:1275, 2009.

165. Glassman AH, O'Connor CM, Califf RM, et al: Sertraline treatment of major depression in patients with acute MI or unstable angina. *JAMA* 258:701, 2002.

166. Smoller JW, Allison M, Cochrane BB, et al: Antidepressant use and risk of incident cardiovascular morbidity and mortality among postmenopausal women in the Women's Health Initiative study. *Arch Intern Med* 169:2128, 2010.

167. Whang W, Kubzansky LD, Kawachi I, et al: Depression and risk of sudden cardiac death and coronary heart disease in women. *J Am Coll Cardiol* 53:950, 2009.

168. Bargh JA, Gollwitzer PM, Lee-Chai AT, et al: The automated will: nonconscious activation and pursuit of behavioral goals. *J Pers Soc Psychol* 81:1014, 2004.

169. Harris JL, Bargh JA, Brownell KD: Priming effects of television food advertising on eating behavior. *Health Psychol* 28:404, 2009.

170. Wansink B: *Mindless eating: why we eat more than we think*, New York, 2006, Bantam Books.

171. Gollwitzer PM, Schaal B: Metacognitoon in action: the importance of implementation intentions. *Pers Soc Psychol Rev* 2:124, 1998.

172. Gollwitzer PM, Sheeran P: Implementation intentions and goal achievement: a meta-analysis of effects of processes. *Adv Exp Soc Psychol* 38:69, 2006.

173. Rozanski A: Integrating psychologic approaches into the behavioral management of cardiac patients. *Psychosom Med* 67:S67, 2005.

CHAPTER 35

The Role of Treatment Adherence in Cardiac Risk Factor Modification

Thomas M. Maddox and P. Michael Ho

KEY POINTS

- Treatment adherence is essential for the optimal control of cardiac risk factors.

- Poor adherence, with subsequent adverse cardiac outcomes, is evident in hypertension, hyperlipidemia, diabetes, smoking cessation, and weight loss.

- Elements associated with poor adherence include social and economic factors, health care system and team-related factors, condition-related factors, therapy-related factors, and patient-related factors.

- Medication simplification and team-based approaches to identification and treatment of cardiac risk factors have shown promise in improving treatment adherence.

- Future approaches to improvement of treatment adherence may include moving to a home-based model of care, activating patients to participate in their care, and employing information technology to identify nonadherence and to initiate interventions.

Drugs don't work in patients who don't take them.

C. Everett Koop

For patients with coronary artery disease (CAD) or at risk for CAD, optimal control of cardiac risk factors, such as hypertension, hyperlipidemia, and smoking, is one of the most effective methods to reduce subsequent cardiac morbidity and mortality. For this control to be achieved, a variety of therapeutic options, both pharmacologic and nonpharmacologic, are available to patients and their health care providers. However, none of these therapeutic options can provide optimal cardiac risk factor control without diligent adherence to their use. Indeed, treatment adherence serves as the "final common pathway" for risk factor treatment and has been characterized as the "key mediator between medical practice and patient outcomes."[1] Despite this essential and somewhat obvious role in risk factor optimization, treatment adherence has been a relatively neglected area of research because of difficulties in both characterizing the factors that drive adherence and designing effective interventions for improvement. Thus, a critical step in optimizing cardiac risk factors in patients with CAD is understanding and improving treatment adherence.

Adherence to treatments of cardiac risk factors is difficult for a variety of reasons. Many risk factors, such as hypertension and hyperlipidemia, are chronic, life-long conditions that require daily administration of treatments, including both pharmacologic agents and lifestyle choices. Furthermore, these conditions are largely asymptomatic. Thus, an important motivator for treatment—relief from bothersome symptoms—is largely absent in the management of cardiac risk factors. In fact, the treatments themselves may cause symptoms via side effects, thus adding another disincentive for adherence among affected patients. Finally, adherence is also influenced by a variety of patient, provider, and health care system characteristics.

This chapter reviews the current definitions of treatment adherence, methods of its measurement, and current gaps in the treatment of cardiac risk factors. Although both lifestyle and pharmacologic treatments are important for optimal risk factor control, the bulk of the research has focused on adherence patterns to pharmacologic therapies and thus comprises the majority of the review. Barriers to treatment adherence, including those at the patient, provider, and health care system levels, are reviewed. Interventions to improve adherence are also reviewed for both their relative effectiveness and potential dissemination. Finally, future directions for adherence research and interventions are presented.

ADHERENCE DEFINED

Treatment adherence is defined as the extent to which patients take treatments (medications or lifestyle modifications) as prescribed by their health care providers.[2] A variety of terms have been used to describe treatment adherence in the past, such as compliance, concordance, and fidelity, but these terms have been largely abandoned because of the pejorative nature underlying their use.[3,4] Adherence is usually measured on a continuous scale as a percentage calculated by the number of treatments actually taken relative to the number of treatments prescribed.[5] For example, a patient who is prescribed 30 pills of an anti-hypertensive medication and actually takes only 20 pills is 67% adherent to the prescribed regimen. The adherence scale can range from 0% to >100% (because some patients can take more than their prescribed treatments).[5] Truly perfect adherence, with fidelity to precise timing of each dose of treatment, is rare, occurring in only one sixth of patients in one survey.[6,7] Furthermore, many of the treatments for cardiac risk factors (e.g., statin therapy for hyperlipidemia) may not require such precision for optimal control to be achieved. Accordingly, most studies on adherence have used a dichotomous cutoff of ≥80% to define good versus poor treatment adherence.[5]

A related but separate concept to treatment adherence is treatment persistence.

Persistence is the duration of time that a patient remains on treatment from the initiation to discontinuation of a prescribed therapy.[3] Unlike adherence, persistence patterns not only can describe patient adherence actions but also can identify other reasons for therapy discontinuation, such as intolerance of therapy due to side effects or provider-initiated discontinuation.

Treatment adherence and persistence can be measured in a variety of ways. In general, measurement can be direct or indirect, with tradeoffs made between precision and ease of measurement for each type of method. Direct methods of adherence measurement include directly observed therapy and measurement of the blood concentration of a medication or its metabolite. Both of these techniques, although accurate, require substantial time and expense and are thus rarely employed. Indirect methods of adherence measurement include patient self-report of treatment adherence, pill counting, assessment of medication refill rates, assessment of a clinical response to a prescribed therapy, and medication electronic monitoring systems (MEMS) that track the frequency and timing of opening of the pill containers. In general, self-report and pill counts are not considered reliable methods of assessment, in part because of the social desirability bias that occurs when patients exaggerate their behavior in an effort to please their health care providers. This bias also affects the ascertainment of patients' adherence to prescribed lifestyle modifications. On the other hand, medication refill rate assessment is a reliable method of adherence assessment, especially in closed health care systems in which patients receive their medications from a single pharmacy source. MEMS assessments are also considered reliable, although their use is expensive and logistically complex. Finally, use of a combination of adherence measurement methods can also be a valuable and reliable way to determine adherence patterns.[2]

PATTERNS OF NONADHERENCE AND ASSOCIATED OUTCOMES

Research into adherence patterns for cardiac risk factor treatments has uncovered significant gaps. As previously noted, adherence is generally worse among those patients who have chronic asymptomatic conditions, such as hypertension and hyperlipidemia, than among those with acute symptomatic illnesses. Even among those patients participating in clinical trials, which are optimized for medication provision and follow-up and generally have high adherence rates, adherence rates for chronic conditions average only 43% to 78%.[8-10] In addition, several studies have documented that both adherence to and persistence with chronic treatments drop precipitously after the first 6 months of therapy.[9,11,12]

Most deviations from adherent behavior are omissions of or delays in medication administration, rather than outright discontinuation of treatments. Urquhart and colleagues characterized specific patterns of medication-taking behavior, using MEMS, among patients initiated on chronic preventive therapies. They found that patients exhibited six types of medication-taking behavior, with roughly even allocation of patients to each group. One sixth of patients exhibited nearly perfect medication-taking behavior, taking almost all of their doses at their prescribed frequency. One sixth took all of the prescribed doses but had some timing irregularity. One sixth had an occasional missed dose, along with some timing irregularity. One sixth of patients took "drug holidays," or several consecutive missed doses, three or four times a year. One sixth took drug holidays monthly or more often, and the final group of patients took few or no doses, although they would often report good medication adherence.[6,7,13] Consistent with this desire by patients to exhibit good adherence behavior,

Feinstein and colleagues[14] demonstrated that many patients improve adherence in the 5 days preceding a visit to the physician, a phenomenon dubbed "white coat adherence" by the investigators.

Predictably, these gaps in treatment adherence lead to worse health outcomes and increased health care costs. A variety of studies have demonstrated that patients with poor adherence have higher all-cause mortality and cardiovascular event rates compared with those with good adherence.[15-18] In addition, two studies have demonstrated that among medication-related hospitalizations in the United States, between 39% and 69% are due to nonadherence.[19,20] Specific studies examining patients with chronic medical conditions such as hypertension and hyperlipidemia have found associations between nonadherence and worse treatment outcomes, higher hospitalization rates, and increased health care costs.[21,22] McCombs and colleagues demonstrated that patients with hypertension who interrupted or terminated their blood pressure treatment accumulated an additional $873 in health care costs (primarily hospitalization related) during the following year.[23] This finding was supported by an analysis of the U.K.-based MediPlus data base that demonstrated an association between the discontinuation of antihypertensive treatments and increased hospital and general physician costs.[24]

NONADHERENCE IN HYPERTENSION

Hypertension is a principal risk factor for the development of both CAD and cerebrovascular disease and a major contributor to worldwide cardiovascular mortality.[25] Uncontrolled hypertension among CAD patients is associated with recurrent cardiovascular events, including death, myocardial infarction, and stroke.[26] Fortunately, a wide variety of treatments exist to achieve blood pressure control and to minimize the risk of these adverse events. Currently, more than 10 classes of antihypertension medications are available, and achieving a sustained decrease in blood pressure of 12 mm Hg with one or more of these treatments can prevent one death for every 11 patients treated.[27]

Despite this availability of treatment and evidence of its benefit, blood pressure control for a large number of hypertensive patients remains suboptimal, and nonadherence to treatment is a major factor. Several studies have demonstrated that less than 50% of CAD patients with hypertension have their blood pressure at recommended levels.[28,29] Nonadherence is a major contributor to this lack of control and, in one study, appeared to contribute to uncontrolled blood pressure more than the lack of adequate prescription of hypertension treatments.[30,31] Furthermore, patients with greater than 80% adherence rates demonstrated improved blood pressure control relative to those patients with less than 50% adherence rates. Treatment adherence to hypertension medications is especially problematic given the asymptomatic nature of the condition, the common occurrence of side effects associated with hypertension treatments, and the daily commitment required for proper medication adherence.[2] These factors all lead to difficulty with adherence. Haynes and colleagues[32] illustrated these difficulties by finding that more than 50% of newly diagnosed hypertensive patients with poor blood pressure control had problems with treatment adherence.

Nonadherence to hypertension treatments with its accompanying uncontrolled blood pressure leads to adverse outcomes. Maronde and colleagues[33] found that Medicare patients who were rehospitalized had significantly higher rates of antihypertension medication nonadherence than a comparable group of nonhospitalized Medicare patients. Similarly, Psaty and colleagues[34] found that patients who were recently nonadherent to beta blocker therapy for their hypertension demonstrated a 4.5-fold increased risk for coronary heart disease complications.

NONADHERENCE IN HYPERLIPIDEMIA

Among CAD patients, lipid-lowering therapies, especially statin medications, can significantly decrease the risk of recurrent cardiac events and mortality. For example, the Heart Protection Study evaluated the effects of simvastatin among CAD, diabetic, or treated hypertensive patients and found an 18% reduction in cardiac-related deaths and a 24% reduction in major cardiovascular events.[35] Similarly, the PROVE-IT TIMI 22 trial compared differing intensities of statin therapies (pravastatin versus atorvastatin) among acute coronary syndrome patients. After 2 years, the atorvastatin patients had lower low-density lipoprotein levels and a 16% reduction in the primary endpoint (death from any cause, myocardial infarction, unstable angina requiring rehospitalization, revascularization, or stroke).[36] Meta-analyses of statin therapy echo these benefits. One involving approximately 25,000 subjects from 34 trials found that 4 years of cholesterol-lowering therapy would prevent one death, one coronary heart disease death, and one cardiovascular death for every 110, 96, and 117 patients treated, respectively.[37] In addition, a survival benefit was seen in studies in which more than 50% of patients were myocardial infarction survivors, had a total cholesterol reduction of more than 10%, and were treated for at least 4 years. In addition, statins produced a greater reduction in the odds of death than other lipid-lowering therapies.

Despite these clear benefits of statin use, nonadherence is a significant problem. Benner and colleagues[38] found that more than half of patients started on statin medications will discontinue the medication within 6 months. Jackevicius and colleagues[12] noted a similar gap in a study of statin adherence patterns among elderly patients. They found that the 2-year rate of statin adherence among this cohort was less than 50%. Furthermore, they demonstrated differential rates of adherence based on the presence of known CAD (Fig. 35-1).

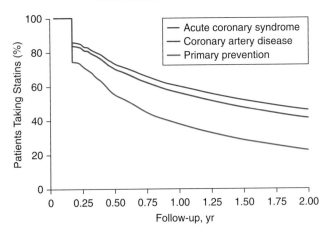

SURVIVAL CURVES FOR ADHERENCE
WITH STATINS IN 3 COHORTS

— Acute coronary syndrome
— Coronary artery disease
— Primary prevention

No. at Risk					
Acute coronary syndrome	22379	16312	12901	10662	8977
Coronary artery disease	36106	25416	19558	15823	13094
Primary prevention	85020	47685	33564	26401	21602

FIGURE 35-1 Survival curves for adherence with statins in three cohorts. All curves are based on a Cox proportional hazards model adjusted for covariates. The median follow-up was 494 days for acute coronary syndrome, 430 days for coronary artery disease, 235 days for primary prevention, and 303 days overall. (*From Jackevicius CA, Mamdani M, Tu JV: Adherence with statin therapy in elderly patients with and without acute coronary syndromes. JAMA 288:462, 2002.*)

Although patients who had experienced acute coronary syndrome had higher 2-year adherence rates than those with chronic CAD or receiving statins for primary prevention (40% for acute coronary syndrome, 36% for chronic CAD, and 25% for primary prevention), all patient groups demonstrated significant adherence gaps.

Nonadherence to statins is significantly associated with adverse outcomes. Wei and colleagues[39] found that post–myocardial infarction patients who had at least 80% adherence rates to statin therapy experienced relative risk reductions of 81% for recurrent myocardial infarction and 53% for all-cause mortality, but those patients who had adherence rates <80% had no significant risk reduction in either recurrent cardiac events or mortality. The Lescol Intervention Prevention Study supported these findings by demonstrating that post–myocardial infarction patients who discontinued their statin medications experienced a twofold increase in major adverse cardiovascular events.[40] These benefits of adherence appear to be medication specific, as demonstrated in an elegant study by Rasmussen and colleagues.[41] They found that adherence to statins exhibited a "dose-response" relationship with mortality, with higher adherence corresponding to decreased mortality. A similar relationship between calcium channel blockers and mortality among the same cohort was not seen, suggesting that the adherence-mortality relationship was statin specific.

NONADHERENCE IN DIABETES

Diabetes is another major cardiac risk factor among CAD patients. Diabetic patients are at higher risk for development of CAD and dying of it.[42] In addition, concurrent cardiac risk factors (e.g., hypertension, smoking) are more prevalent among diabetic patients and appear to exert worse effects in the setting of poor glycemic control. Diabetes is a complex disorder that requires constant attention to diet, exercise, glucose monitoring, and medication to achieve good glycemic control.[3] Glycemic control in diabetes plays an important role in reducing microvascular disease, such as nephropathy, retinopathy, and neuropathy.[43-45] In addition, a 17-year study of type 1 diabetics indicated that tight glycemic control reduces the risk of cardiac events by 42%.[46] In contrast, tight glycemic control among type 2 diabetics has not demonstrated conclusive benefits for reduction of cardiac events and may be associated with harm in some cases.[47] Despite this uncertainty, multifactorial cardiac risk factor control, including glycemic control, is an important element of effective prevention of cardiac events. For example, the Steno-1 trial demonstrated the benefit in achieving multiple risk factor control among diabetics.[48] Patients were randomized to usual care or an intensive treatment regimen that included both behavioral and pharmacologic treatments targeting hypertension, hyperglycemia, dyslipidemia, microalbuminuria, and secondary prevention of CAD events with aspirin. After 7.8 years of follow-up, patients receiving the intensive treatment experienced 53% reduction in cardiovascular disease. Furthermore, these benefits were sustained, with the patients receiving intensive treatment experiencing a 57% reduction in cardiovascular deaths during the following 4 years after the cessation of the trial.

As with the other cardiac risk factors requiring prolonged chronic treatments, treatment adherence is a substantial problem among diabetics. Among patients receiving oral hypoglycemic therapies, adherence rates range widely from 36% to 93%.[3] Boccuzzi and colleagues[49] profiled adherence rates among patients taking oral antidiabetic medications and found that 12 months after initiation of these therapies, adherence to metformin was 60%; to sulfonylureas, 56%; to repaglinide, 48%; and to α-glucosidase, 31%. Adherence rates with insulin therapy were not much better; one study demonstrated that only 63% of insulin doses were taken as prescribed.[3]

Nonadherence to diabetic treatments is further complicated by the common occurrence of other cardiac risk factors and comorbidities, many of which require multiple additional medications. Piette and colleagues[50] demonstrated that 50% of U.S. diabetic patients were receiving at least seven medications, including at least two glucose-lowering medications. Adherence rates are adversely affected by this increased number of medications. Rubin[51] found that rates of adherence to polytherapy versus monotherapy are 10% to 20% lower among diabetic patients. In addition, treatments that require multiple administrations during the day also adversely affect adherence. Paes and colleagues[52] found that the adherence rates were 79% for once-daily dosing of medications, 66% for twice-daily dosing, and 38% for three-times-daily dosing.

Predictably, nonadherence to antidiabetic medications is linked to adverse outcomes. Pladevall and colleagues[53] illustrated that 10% increases in nonadherence to antidiabetic treatments were associated with 0.14% increases in hemoglobin A1c. Lau and Nau[54] demonstrated that patients who were nonadherent to their diabetic regimen were more likely to be hospitalized. In contrast, increased medication adherence to antidiabetic medications (at a threshold rate of 60%+) resulted in decreased medical care costs, although overall costs were not reduced because medication costs offset these savings.[55] Similarly, Balkrishnan and colleagues[56] demonstrated that 10% increases in medication possession ratios were associated with 8.6% to 28.9% decreases in annual health care costs.

NONADHERENCE IN SMOKING

Smoking is a major cardiac risk factor and remains a significant public health issue. In 2007, 19.8% of U.S. adults were active smokers.[57] Smoking increases all-cause and cardiovascular mortality, and among patients with CAD, it increases the risk of reinfarction and mortality.[58,59] Quitting smoking, in turn, reduces all-cause mortality by 36% in CAD patients, even in long-term smokers.[60] In addition, there is some evidence that public health policies such as smoking bans can have salutary effects. A small study in Colorado demonstrated a 27% reduction in myocardial infarction hospitalizations after institution of a smoking ban.[61] A similar study in Scotland demonstrated a 14% to 21% reduction in acute coronary syndrome admissions during the 10 months after a smoking ban.[62]

Quitting smoking is a difficult process, with high recidivism rates. For example, in a study of long-term abstinence rates among smokers who tried to quit without any behavioral or pharmacologic assistance, only 5% to 7% were abstinent at 1 year.[63] Accordingly, a variety of both behavioral and pharmacologic interventions have been developed to assist with smoking cessation. Behavioral interventions include in-person counseling, remote (phone, Web) counseling, group counseling, and financial incentives. Pharmacologic treatments for quitting smoking include nicotine replacement therapies in a variety of formulations (e.g., patch, gum, lozenge, inhaler, nasal spray), bupropion, and varenicline.

Despite the wide variety of treatments, the rates of adherence to these programs, measured as abstinence from smoking after completion of the treatment, remain remarkably low. For example, quit rates for in-person clinical counseling are 12.3% at 3 months and 6.5% at 12 months[64]; for group programs, 20% at 1 year[65]; and for remote counseling, 10% at 1 year.[66] Financial incentive programs resulted in quit rates of 14.7% at 9 to 12 months and 9.4% at 15 to 18 months.[67] Quit rates with pharmacologic therapies are better than with behavioral therapies, but the absolute rates of adherence and

smoking abstinence remain low. Among nicotine replacement therapies, the highest adherence rates were with the patch, but 12-week abstinence rates were similar for all nicotine replacement modalities (gum, 20%; patch, 21%; spray, 24%; inhaler, 24%).[68] Bupropion resulted in quit rates of 44% (compared with 19% with placebo) at 7 weeks and 23% (compared with 12% with placebo) at 1 year.[69] Longer term bupropion (administered for 52 weeks versus 7 weeks) had better short-term abstinence rates (47% versus 37%) at 16 weeks after cessation of therapy but similar rates of abstinence to short-term bupropion at 2 years (41% versus 40%). Varenicline demonstrated abstinence rates of 44% 4 weeks after medication cessation, compared with 30% with bupropion and 18% with placebo. At 1 year, abstinence rates were 23% with varenicline, 16% with bupropion, and 9% with placebo.[70,71]

NONADHERENCE IN OBESITY

Obesity is a growing problem in the United States and worldwide and serves as a risk factor for cardiac disease. The NHANES survey from 1988 to 1991 demonstrated that 36% of surveyed patients were obese.[72] Obesity is associated with coronary disease; Bogers and colleagues[73] showed a 29% increase in CAD with each 5-unit increase in body mass index. Although the direct cardiac risk due to obesity is confounded by the common presence of concurrent cardiac risk factors, obesity appears to be an independent risk factor for CAD, probably by contributing to insulin resistance, hypertension, lipid abnormalities, left ventricular hypertrophy, endothelial dysfunction, and obstructive sleep apnea.[74] Most if not all of these risk factors can be better controlled or even eliminated with weight loss. Although no randomized controlled clinical trials have linked weight loss to decreased mortality or CAD, a large observational study found that overweight women who lost more than 20 pounds had a 25% decrease in mortality, CAD, and cancer mortality. Among the subset of women with CAD or heart failure, any weight loss was associated with a 10% reduction in CAD and a 20% reduction in all-cause mortality.[75]

Similar to smoking cessation, weight loss is difficult to achieve. A variety of weight loss strategies exist and include behavioral modification, dietary therapy, exercise, drug therapy, liposuction, and bariatric surgery. Despite these options, though, adherence to weight loss programs, measured by achievement and maintenance of weight loss, is low.

Behavioral modification strategies include self-monitoring, control of the stimuli that activate eating, slowing down eating, goal setting, behavioral contracting and reinforcement, nutrition education, modification of physical activity, social support, and cognitive restructuring. These techniques are usually paired with dietary weight loss programs, and the combination has been demonstrated to increase weight loss by 7.7 kg at 12 months.[76] In addition, ongoing behavioral modification strategies may be useful in maintaining weight loss. Wing and colleagues[77] showed that those patients who achieved a mean weight loss of 19 kg in the prior year had a lower amount of weight re-gain with in-person support (face-to-face support resulted in weight gain of 2.9 kg; Internet-based support, 4.7 kg; and newsletter only, 4.9 kg).

Commercial diet programs, which rely primarily on calorie restriction, have demonstrated efficacy in weight loss. Both Weight Watchers and the Jenny Craig programs have been studied. Weight Watchers resulted in the loss of 5.3% of baseline weight compared with 1.5% in the placebo group at 1 year.[78] At 2 years, both groups had regained weight, but the Weight Watchers participants gained back less. Similarly, Jenny Craig participants lost 7.1% of their baseline weight versus 0.7% in the placebo group at 1 year.[79] In addition to overall calorie restriction, a variety of diets with differing

35

macronutrient composition have been promoted, but data have been conflicting about the superiority of one over the other. For example, a comparison of the Atkins, Ornish, Weight Watchers, and Zone diets showed similar modest reductions in weight and cardiac risk factors at 1 year. Importantly, all diets had adherence rates of only 50% to 65%, and adherence, more than macronutrient composition of the diets, had a significant correlation with weight loss.[80]

Pharmacologic therapies for weight loss include sympathomimetic drugs (e.g., sibutramine), drugs that alter fat digestion (e.g., orlistat), antidepressants, antiepileptics, and diabetes drugs (e.g., metformin). Many of these have shown modest efficacy for weight loss over placebo. A meta-analysis of sibutramine demonstrated additional mean weight loss of 4.5 kg over placebo.[81] Similarly, a meta-analysis of orlistat showed an additional mean weight loss of 2.89 kg.[82] As with all medications, adherence is essential for maximum efficacy of therapy, and these weight loss medications require at least 1 year if not 2 years of therapy. Tellingly, only 67% of the participants in the Kelley orlistat trial completed therapy.

A final, invasive option for weight loss is bariatric surgery. The procedure is generally successful; a meta-analysis demonstrated that mean weight loss is 61% of baseline weight.[83] In addition, cardiac risk factors such as hypertension and diabetes were greatly improved in the majority of patients. Despite these encouraging results, the surgery has 30-day mortalities ranging from 0.1% to 1%. In addition, the salutatory effects on weight loss and cardiac risk factor control are primarily seen only in morbidly obese patients, making this therapy less attractive for less obese patients.

FACTORS ASSOCIATED WITH NONADHERENCE

Treatment adherence is a multidimensional construct that is determined by the interplay of a variety of factors. However, many providers believe that patients are solely responsible for their adherence behavior and thus fail to account for other factors outside a patient's locus of control that can facilitate or impede the ability to adhere to a prescribed treatment (i.e., therapy or system factors).[84] Understanding of these factors and their impact on adherence behavior is essential to the proper design of interventions to improve adherence rates.

The 2003 World Health Organization report *Adherence to Long-Term Therapies: Evidence for Action* organized the factors affecting adherence into five dimensions: social/economic factors, health care system and team-related factors, condition-related factors, therapy-related factors, and patient-related factors (Fig. 35-2).[84] The bulk of prior research on adherence factors has focused primarily on patient-related factors, but there is increasing recognition, with accompanying research, that factors in the other four dimensions are equally important in characterizing and improving adherence.

Socioeconomic factors are major determinants of a patient's ability to adhere to treatment plans. Several studies have documented that low socioeconomic status, financial difficulty, high cost of medications, low health literacy, and unemployment are correlated with poor treatment adherence.[85,86] These factors are especially onerous in the treatment of chronic cardiac risk factors, for which multiple medications are required to be administered for years.

Health care system and team-related factors are another important component in treatment adherence. The currently fragmented health care system in the United States presents multiple challenges in maintaining good treatment adherence. Imposed limits on access to care, restricted medication formularies, switching of formularies, and high costs of

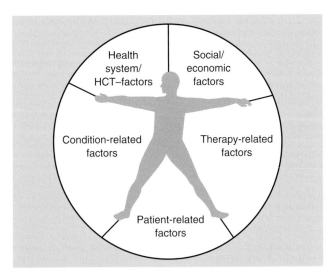

FIGURE 35-2 The five dimensions of adherence. HCT, health care team. *(From Adherence to long-term therapies: evidence for action, Geneva, 2003, World Health Organization.)*

medications have all been demonstrated to have a negative impact on adherence.[2]

Multiple components of the individual patient-provider relationship can positively or negatively affect adherence. Bodenheimer,[87] in a recent review, described the difficulties that health care providers have in making sure their patients understand the care they receive and assisting patients in self-management of their treatments. Both of these areas require attention to optimize adherence. In a review, Osterberg and Blaschke[2] outlined provider actions that have a negative impact on subsequent treatment adherence, including the prescription of complex dosing regimens, the failure of the provider to explain the benefits and potential side effects of treatments, the failure of the provider to consider the patient's lifestyle or the affordability of medications in prescription decisions, and merely the presence of a poor provider-patient therapeutic relationship. A series of studies looking at patient comprehension of treatment plans underscores these points. Roter and Hall[88] found that 50% of patients leave an office not understanding what they were told by the provider. Schillinger and colleagues,[89] on asking patients to restate the provider's instructions, found that 47% responded incorrectly. Finally, in another study by Schillinger and colleagues,[90] 50% of patients, when asked to state how they were supposed to take a prescribed medication, did not understand how the provider had prescribed the medication. Clearly, these factors will adversely affect treatment adherence.

Condition-related factors are another component affecting treatment adherence. Cardiac risk factors, as previously noted, are often asymptomatic conditions, a characteristic that obviates some of the immediate positive feedback that symptomatic conditions provide for treatment adherence (e.g., analgesics for pain). In addition, the chronic nature of the conditions, often requiring daily, life-long therapy, often results in poorer adherence patterns, as the commitment to administer daily treatments (both pharmacologic and lifestyle modification) wanes.

Therapy-related factors are a major contributor to treatment adherence. Factors such as drug tolerability, regimen complexity, frequency of dosing, number of concurrent medications, and changes in medications can affect a patient's willingness and ability to adhere to treatments.[84] A variety of studies have demonstrated an inverse correlation between treatment adherence and number of daily doses of a

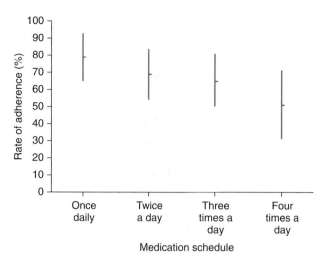

FIGURE 35-3 Adherence to medication according to frequency of doses. Vertical lines represent 1 SD on either side of the mean rate of adherence (horizontal bars). *(From Osterberg L, Blaschke T: Adherence to medication. N Engl J Med 353:487, 2005.)*

medication prescribed (Fig. 35-3).[91-94] Although some studies have found a positive correlation between number of medications and treatment adherence,[95] the bulk of the evidence demonstrates that simplifying medication regimens as much as possible increases the likelihood of adherence.[96]

Finally, patient factors are an important aspect of treatment adherence. Interestingly, basic demographic categories—age, sex, race, and educational level—are not strong predictors of treatment adherence.[97] A study by Steiner and associates[98] underscored this point by demonstrating that prediction models for treatment adherence using only patient factors were poor. In two different health systems, the C-statistics, which measure the ability of factors to distinguish between adherers and nonadherers, were only 0.58 and 0.61. On the other hand, mental health status, including depression, cognitive impairment, anxiety, stress, and substance abuse, is strongly linked to nonadherence.[2,99-101]

In contrast to basic demographic patient factors, patients' knowledge about their cardiac risk factors, health beliefs, health attitudes, self-management skills, and active participation in their care appear to be strong predictors of adherence.[100,102-104] Several studies have documented that patient beliefs and attitudes, such as low perceived risk of a condition, low perceived need for treatment, perceived ineffectiveness of a treatment, or perceived harm from a treatment, negatively affect adherence.[100,105,106] These beliefs are especially prevalent in asymptomatic conditions such as cardiac risk factors, underlining the challenge to treatment adherence for these conditions. Other patient characteristics that negatively affect adherence include a lack of self-efficacy, negative or avoidant coping strategies, and different degrees of readiness to change.[100,105,106] Patients' misperceptions or lack of insight into their particular condition or conditions can also negatively affect adherence.[107-109] For example, a common patient belief about hypertension is that it is an intermittent but acutely symptomatic condition that can be treated solely with nonpharmacologic therapies—beliefs that would seemingly invalidate the need for life-long adherence to hypertension treatments.[110-112]

INTERVENTIONS TO IMPROVE ADHERENCE

Once gaps in adherence and the factors underlying them are understood, interventions can be designed to improve them.

However, successful interventions to improve adherence are rare and point to the difficulty in overcoming the multiple barriers to adherence in the treatment of cardiac risk factors. Because the factors that result in nonadherence are multiple and involve patient, provider, and health care system factors, interventions that are successful and sustainable will need to be multimodal, to account for the particular barriers to adherence in their targeted population, and to integrate well into practice patterns.

Several Cochrane reviews have been conducted to assess the overall effectiveness of interventions to improve treatment adherence for chronic cardiac risk factor conditions.[113,114] In general, synthesis of common elements of effective interventions was difficult because of the multifaceted nature of many of the interventions. Nonetheless, behavioral interventions, such as reducing dosing demands or incorporating monitoring and feedback to patients and providers, had the most successful, albeit modest, effects.[115]

In general, elements of successful interventions can be divided into patient, provider, and health care system factors. In a review of patient-focused interventions, the most effective strategy was simplifying the treatment regimen.[114] In contrast, motivational strategies, such as home monitoring, small group sessions, or reminder calls, were only moderately effective, and patient education alone was least effective. Claxton and colleagues[8] demonstrated that simplifying medication dosing by reducing the frequency of daily medication administration was associated with improved adherence. Additional studies supported this conclusion and found that minimizing the total number of daily doses of medication was more effective at improving adherence than minimizing the total number of medications.[93,116] In addition to minimizing daily doses, selection of medications with longer half-lives, and thus "more forgiving" of occasional nonadherence, may improve overall cardiac risk factor control, such as with hypertension.[6,7] Monitoring and feedback, although less effective than medication simplification, can nonetheless be valuable in improving adherence.[117,118] For example, a trial using MEMS caps to inform adherence behavior and to provide feedback to both patients and providers among patients with refractory hypertension demonstrated improved adherence.[119] Among these patients, 30% had improvement in adherence and blood pressure control with monitoring; 20% had treatment nonadherence identified; and a subgroup of patients achieved blood pressure control with audit, feedback, and medication adjustment with use of the MEMS information.

In contrast to patient-focused interventions, provider-focused interventions have been largely disappointing. Continuing medical education efforts, audit and feedback programs, academic detailing, and computerized decision support have all been ineffective at improving adherence.[120] Interestingly, one of the few successful provider-focused interventions targeted the specific interaction between provider and patients. Rosen and colleagues[121] demonstrated improved adherence among diabetic patients by use of feedback from MEMS caps data as the basis for a conversation between providers and patients on barriers to adherence and potential solutions (e.g., establishing cues to trigger timely medication administration).

Health care system interventions have had success in improving adherence when team management approaches for risk factor management were employed.[122,123] In Cooper's review of successful cardiac risk factor interventions, seven of the eight successful programs used either nurse- or pharmacist-directed programs or collaborative care of the patient with a pharmacist.[120] In addition, employment of communication with patients between clinic visits, by modalities such as the telephone or the Internet, also has demonstrated promise. Piette and colleagues[124] showed improved adherence to diabetic treatments with a nurse-directed program and telephonic interactive voice recognition technology.

FUTURE DIRECTIONS IN ADHERENCE

To date, most of the research into cardiac risk factor treatment nonadherence has focused on the patient, provider, health care system, condition, and treatment factors associated with nonadherence. The next step, then, is to translate these insights to effective interventions to improve adherence. Research into both the barriers to adherence and successful adherence interventions suggests that fruitful paths for improvement may involve team-based approaches to risk factor management; movement from episodic, office-based management of cardiac risk factors to more continual, home-based management; activation of patients in their care; and alignment of health care systems to facilitate these changes in care.

35

The majority of successful adherence interventions remove the locus of risk factor management from physicians and assign responsibility to a team of other health care providers, usually composed of nurses and pharmacists. This redesign overcomes the multiple barriers that physicians face in attempting to manage chronic conditions in the compressed setting of a short office visit—competing demands, "tyranny of the urgent," and clinical inertia. In addition, nurses and pharmacists who are charged with risk factor management, by virtue of having a more single-minded focus to their efforts, can achieve an efficiency and experience in identifying nonadherence among the cardiac population and methods to overcome it.

Movement of risk factor management and adherence efforts from the office to the home setting can potentially improve adherence. Both blood pressure and lipid measurements can occur more frequently between episodic office visits, and information can be relayed to both providers and patients by telephone, mail, and Internet. In addition, information about medication refill patterns and other adherence data can also be fed back to providers and patients in a "real-time" format. This iterative audit and feedback mechanism for both risk factor control and adherence can allow positive reinforcement of treatment, which is an especially important feature for chronic, asymptomatic conditions. In addition, this process can identify problems earlier and allow corrective measures to occur sooner, thus minimizing the total amount of time of nonadherence and suboptimal control of risk factors.

Patient activation is another potentially important area for adherence improvement. Improving a patient's understanding of the condition, the need for treatment, and the efficacy of controlling risk factors can lead to improved "buy-in" of treatment and subsequent adherence. In addition, these targeted patient education efforts could be combined with a personalized assessment of each patient's lifestyle to identify potential barriers to adherence, to direct inquiry to patients about their adherence behavior, and to identify solutions before significant nonadherence occurs.

Finally, health care systems will need to provide incentives and to remove disincentives for measures to improve adherence. Improved access to medical care and medications will need to allow efficient management of medication and visit costs. In addition, improved delivery of medications, such as automating refills and allowing mail delivery of medications, may also facilitate adherence. For more continual, home-based care to be feasible, improvements in communication between patients and health care teams will be necessary. Although privacy issues will need consideration, tools such as automated telephone calls and Internet-based communication could be employed to assist with this process.

Another potential system feature that could positively affect medication adherence is automated screens of patient populations for both treatment adherence (e.g., automatic detection and notification of missed medication refills) and cardiac risk factor control. Such screens necessitate electronic medical records with good data quality but could potentially result in early identification of and intervention for patients with suboptimal adherence and control. Finally, any system redesign will require alignment of reimbursement to facilitate its success. Because most medical care is currently reimbursed in fee-for-service, office- or procedure-based model, changes that move care to a team-based and home-based model will need accompanying changes to ensure fair reimbursement for these efforts.

CONCLUSION

Treatment adherence is an essential component to optimization of cardiac risk factors, and significant gaps currently exist in its provision. Causes of these gaps are a complex interplay of patient, provider, health care system, condition, and treatment factors. Accordingly, simple interventions have been elusive. Nonetheless, promising elements to improve adherence, such as medication simplification, team-based management, and patient activation, have been identified and can serve as a foundation for larger, multimodal interventions that can improve adherence and realize the ultimate goal of optimal risk factor control and minimization of adverse cardiac outcomes among the CAD population.

REFERENCES

1. Peterson AM, Takiya L, Finley R: Meta-analysis of trials of interventions to improve medication adherence. *Am J Health Syst Pharm* 60:657, 2003.
2. Osterberg L, Blaschke T: Adherence to medication. *N Engl J Med* 353:487, 2005.
3. Cramer JA: A systematic review of adherence with medications for diabetes. *Diabetes Care* 27:1218, 2004.
4. Steiner JF, Earnest MA: The language of medication-taking. *Ann Intern Med* 132:926, 2000.
5. Rudd P, Byyny RL, Zachary V, et al: Pill count measures of compliance in a drug trial: variability and suitability. *Am J Hypertens* 1:309, 1988.
6. Urquhart J: The electronic medication event monitor. Lessons for pharmacotherapy. *Clin Pharmacokinet* 32:345, 1997.
7. Urquhart J: The odds of the three nons when an aptly prescribed medicine isn't working: non-compliance, non-absorption, non-response. *Br J Clin Pharmacol* 54:212, 2002.
8. Claxton AJ, Cramer J, Pierce C: A systematic review of the associations between dose regimens and medication compliance. *Clin Ther* 23:1296, 2001.
9. Cramer J, Rosenheck R, Kirk G, et al: Medication compliance feedback and monitoring in a clinical trial: predictors and outcomes. *Value Health* 6:566, 2003.
10. Waeber B, Leonetti G, Kolloch R, McInnes GT: Compliance with aspirin or placebo in the Hypertension Optimal Treatment (HOT) study. *J Hypertens* 17:1041, 1999.
11. Haynes RB, McDonald HP, Garg AX: Helping patients follow prescribed treatment: clinical applications. *JAMA* 288:2880, 2002.
12. Jackevicius CA, Mamdani M, Tu JV: Adherence with statin therapy in elderly patients with and without acute coronary syndromes. *JAMA* 288:462, 2002.
13. Cramer JA, Scheyer RD, Mattson RH: Compliance declines between clinic visits. *Arch Intern Med* 150:1509, 1990.
14. Feinstein AR: On white-coat effects and the electronic monitoring of compliance. *Arch Intern Med* 150:1377, 1990.
15. Influence of adherence to treatment and response of cholesterol on mortality in the coronary drug project. *N Engl J Med* 303:1038, 1980.
16. Ho PM, Magid DJ, Shetterly SM, et al: Medication nonadherence is associated with a broad range of adverse outcomes in patients with coronary artery disease. *Am Heart J* 155:772, 2008.
17. Horwitz RI, Horwitz SM: Adherence to treatment and health outcomes. *Arch Intern Med* 153:1863, 1993.
18. LaRosa JC: Poor compliance: the hidden risk factor. *Curr Atheroscler Rep* 2:1, 2000.
19. McDonnell PJ, Jacobs MR: Hospital admissions resulting from preventable adverse drug reactions. *Ann Pharmacother* 36:1331, 2002.
20. Schiff GD, Fung S, Speroff T, McNutt RA: Decompensated heart failure: symptoms, patterns of onset, and contributing factors. *Am J Med* 114:625, 2003.
21. DiMatteo MR, Giordani PJ, Lepper HS, Croghan TW: Patient adherence and medical treatment outcomes: a meta-analysis. *Med Care* 40:794, 2002.
22. Sokol MC, McGuigan KA, Verbrugge RR, Epstein RS: Impact of medication adherence on hospitalization risk and healthcare cost. *Med Care* 43:521, 2005.
23. McCombs JS, Nichol MB, Newman CM, Sclar DA: The costs of interrupting antihypertensive drug therapy in a Medicaid population. *Med Care* 32:214, 1994.

24. Hughes D, McGuire A: The direct costs to the NHS of discontinuing and switching prescriptions for hypertension. *J Hum Hypertens* 12:533, 1998.
25. Lloyd-Jones D, Adams R, Carnethon M, et al: Heart disease and stroke statistics—2009 update: a report from the American Heart Association Statistics Committee and Stroke Statistics Subcommittee. *Circulation* 119:e21, 2009.
26. Pepine CJ, Kowey PR, Kupfer S, et al: Predictors of adverse outcome among patients with hypertension and coronary artery disease. *J Am Coll Cardiol* 47:547, 2006.
27. Ho PM, Rumsfeld JS: Beyond inpatient and outpatient care: alternative model for hypertension management. *BMC Public Health* 6:257, 2006.
28. Cooper-DeHoff RM, Handberg EM, Cohen J, et al: Characteristics of contemporary patients with hypertension and coronary artery disease. *Clin Cardiol* 27:571, 2004.
29. Ho PM, Masoudi FA, Peterson ED, et al: Cardiology management improves secondary prevention measures among patients with coronary artery disease. *J Am Coll Cardiol* 43:1517, 2004.
30. Ho PM, Magid DJ, Shetterly SM, et al: Importance of therapy intensification and medication nonadherence for blood pressure control in patients with coronary disease. *Arch Intern Med* 168:271, 2008.
31. Weir MR, Maibach EW, Bakris GL, et al: Implications of a health lifestyle and medication analysis for improving hypertension control. *Arch Intern Med* 160:481, 2000.
32. Haynes RB, Taylor DW, Sackett DL, et al: Can simple clinical measurements detect patient noncompliance? *Hypertension* 2:757, 1980.
33. Maronde RF, Chan LS, Larsen FJ, et al: Underutilization of antihypertensive drugs and associated hospitalization. *Med Care* 27:1159, 1989.
34. Psaty BM, Koepsell TD, Wagner EH, et al: The relative risk of incident coronary heart disease associated with recently stopping the use of beta-blockers. *JAMA* 263:1653, 1990.
35. MRC/BHF Heart Protection Study of cholesterol lowering with simvastatin in 20,536 high-risk individuals: a randomised placebo-controlled trial. *Lancet* 360:7, 2002.
36. Cannon CP, Braunwald E, McCabe CH, et al: Intensive versus moderate lipid lowering with statins after acute coronary syndromes. *N Engl J Med* 350:1495, 2004.
37. Marchioli R, Marfisi RM, Carinci F, Tognoni G: Meta-analysis, clinical trials, and transferability of research results into practice. The case of cholesterol-lowering interventions in the secondary prevention of coronary heart disease. *Arch Intern Med* 156:1158, 1996.
38. Benner JS, Glynn RJ, Mogun H, et al: Long-term persistence in use of statin therapy in elderly patients. *JAMA* 288:455, 2002.
39. Wei L, Wang J, Thompson P, et al: Adherence to statin treatment and readmission of patients after myocardial infarction: a six year follow up study. *Heart* 88:229, 2002.
40. Lesaffre E, Kocmanova D, Lemos PA, et al: A retrospective analysis of the effect of noncompliance on time to first major adverse cardiac event in LIPS. *Clin Ther* 25:2431, 2003.
41. Rasmussen JN, Chong A, Alter DA: Relationship between adherence to evidence-based pharmacotherapy and long-term mortality after acute myocardial infarction. *JAMA* 297:177, 2007.
42. Franco OH, Steyerberg EW, Hu FB, et al: Associations of diabetes mellitus with total life expectancy and life expectancy with and without cardiovascular disease. *Arch Intern Med* 167:1145, 2007.
43. Intensive blood-glucose control with sulphonylureas or insulin compared with conventional treatment and risk of complications in patients with type 2 diabetes (UKPDS 33). UK Prospective Diabetes Study (UKPDS) Group. *Lancet* 352:837, 1998.
44. United Kingdom Prospective Diabetes Study (UKPDS). 13: Relative efficacy of randomly allocated diet, sulphonylurea, insulin, or metformin in patients with newly diagnosed non–insulin dependent diabetes followed for three years. *BMJ* 310:83, 1995.
45. The effect of intensive treatment of diabetes on the development and progression of long-term complications in insulin-dependent diabetes mellitus. The Diabetes Control and Complications Trial Research Group. *N Engl J Med* 329:977, 1993.
46. Nathan DM, Cleary PA, Backlund JY, et al: Intensive diabetes treatment and cardiovascular disease in patients with type 1 diabetes. *N Engl J Med* 353:2643, 2005.
47. Gerstein HC, Miller ME, Byington RP, et al: Effects of intensive glucose lowering in type 2 diabetes. *N Engl J Med* 358:2545, 2008.
48. Gaede P, Vedel P, Larsen N, et al: Multifactorial intervention and cardiovascular disease in patients with type 2 diabetes. *N Engl J Med* 348:383, 2003.
49. Boccuzzi SJ, Wogen J, Fox J, et al: Utilization of oral hypoglycemic agents in a drug-insured U.S. population. *Diabetes Care* 24:1411, 2001.
50. Piette JD, Heisler M, Wagner TH: Problems paying out-of-pocket medication costs among older adults with diabetes. *Diabetes Care* 27:384, 2004.
51. Rubin RR: Adherence to pharmacologic therapy in patients with type 2 diabetes mellitus. *Am J Med* 118(Suppl 5A):27S, 2005.
52. Paes AH, Bakker A, Soe-Agnie CJ: Impact of dosage frequency on patient compliance. *Diabetes Care* 20:1512, 1997.
53. Pladevall M, Williams LK, Potts LA, et al: Clinical outcomes and adherence to medications measured by claims data in patients with diabetes. *Diabetes Care* 27:2800, 2004.
54. Lau DT, Nau DP: Oral antihyperglycemic medication nonadherence and subsequent hospitalization among individuals with type 2 diabetes. *Diabetes Care* 27:2149, 2004.
55. Hepke KL, Martus MT, Share DA: Costs and utilization associated with pharmaceutical adherence in a diabetic population. *Am J Manag Care* 10:144, 2004.
56. Balkrishnan R, Rajagopalan R, Camacho FT, et al: Predictors of medication adherence and associated health care costs in an older population with type 2 diabetes mellitus: a longitudinal cohort study. *Clin Ther* 25:2958, 2003.
57. Cigarette smoking among adults—United States, 2007. *MMWR Morb Mortal Wkly Rep* 57:1221, 2008.
58. Goldenberg I, Jonas M, Tenenbaum A, et al: Current smoking, smoking cessation, and the risk of sudden cardiac death in patients with coronary artery disease. *Arch Intern Med* 163:2301, 2003.
59. Qiao Q, Tervahauta M, Nissinen A, Tuomilehto J: Mortality from all causes and from coronary heart disease related to smoking and changes in smoking during a 35-year follow-up of middle-aged Finnish men. *Eur Heart J* 21:1621, 2000.
60. Critchley J, Capewell S: Smoking cessation for the secondary prevention of coronary heart disease. *Cochrane Database Syst Rev* (1):CD003041, 2004.
61. Reduced hospitalizations for acute myocardial infarction after implementation of a smoke-free ordinance—City of Pueblo, Colorado, 2002-2006. *MMWR Morb Mortal Wkly Rep* 57:1373, 2009.
62. Pell JP, Haw S, Cobbe S, et al: Smoke-free legislation and hospitalizations for acute coronary syndrome. *N Engl J Med* 359:482, 2008.
63. Rigotti NA: Clinical practice. Treatment of tobacco use and dependence. *N Engl J Med* 346:506, 2002.
64. Borland R, Balmford J, Bishop N, et al: In-practice management versus quitline referral for enhancing smoking cessation in general practice: a cluster randomized trial. *Fam Pract* 25:382, 2008.
65. Jamrozik K: Population strategies to prevent smoking. *BMJ* 328:759, 2004.
66. Myung SK, McDonnell DD, Kazinets G, et al: Effects of Web- and computer-based smoking cessation programs: meta-analysis of randomized controlled trials. *Arch Intern Med* 169:929, 2009.
67. Volpp KG, Troxel AB, Pauly MV, et al: A randomized, controlled trial of financial incentives for smoking cessation. *N Engl J Med* 360:699, 2009.
68. Hajek P, West R, Foulds J, et al: Randomized comparative trial of nicotine polacrilex, a transdermal patch, nasal spray, and an inhaler. *Arch Intern Med* 159:2033, 1999.
69. Hurt RD, Sachs DP, Glover ED, et al: A comparison of sustained-release bupropion and placebo for smoking cessation. *N Engl J Med* 337:1195, 1997.
70. Gonzales D, Rennard SI, Nides M, et al: Varenicline, an $\alpha_4\beta_2$ nicotinic acetylcholine receptor partial agonist, vs sustained-release bupropion and placebo for smoking cessation: a randomized controlled trial. *JAMA* 296:47, 2006.
71. Jorenby DE, Hays JT, Rigotti NA, et al: Efficacy of varenicline, an $\alpha_4\beta_2$ nicotinic acetylcholine receptor partial agonist, vs placebo or sustained-release bupropion for smoking cessation: a randomized controlled trial. *JAMA* 296:56, 2006.
72. Kuczmarski RJ, Flegal KM, Campbell SM, Johnson CL: Increasing prevalence of overweight among US adults. The National Health and Nutrition Examination Surveys, 1960 to 1991. *JAMA* 272:205, 1994.
73. Bogers RP, Bemelmans WJ, Hoogenveen RT, et al: Association of overweight with increased risk of coronary heart disease partly independent of blood pressure and cholesterol levels: a meta-analysis of 21 cohort studies including more than 300 000 persons. *Arch Intern Med* 167:1720, 2007.
74. Poirier P, Giles TD, Bray GA, et al: Obesity and cardiovascular disease: pathophysiology, evaluation, and effect of weight loss: an update of the 1997 American Heart Association Scientific Statement on Obesity and Heart Disease from the Obesity Committee of the Council on Nutrition, Physical Activity, and Metabolism. *Circulation* 113:898, 2006.
75. Williamson DF, Pamuk E, Thun M, et al: Prospective study of intentional weight loss and mortality in never-smoking overweight US white women aged 40-64 years. *Am J Epidemiol* 141:1128, 1995.
76. Avenell A, Broom J, Brown TJ, et al: Systematic review of the long-term effects and economic consequences of treatments for obesity and implications for health improvement. *Health Technol Assess* 8:(iii) 1, 2004.
77. Wing RR, Tate DF, Gorin AA, et al: A self-regulation program for maintenance of weight loss. *N Engl J Med* 355:1563, 2006.
78. Heshka S, Anderson JW, Atkinson RL, et al: Weight loss with self-help compared with a structured commercial program: a randomized trial. *JAMA* 289:1792, 2003.
79. Rock CL, Pakiz B, Flatt SW, Quintana EL: Randomized trial of a multifaceted commercial weight loss program. *Obesity (Silver Spring)* 15:939, 2007.
80. Dansinger ML, Gleason JA, Griffith JL, et al: Comparison of the Atkins, Ornish, Weight Watchers, and Zone diets for weight loss and heart disease risk reduction: a randomized trial. *JAMA* 293:43, 2005.
81. Li Z, Maglione M, Tu W, et al: Meta-analysis: pharmacologic treatment of obesity. *Ann Intern Med* 142:532, 2005.
82. Kelley DE, Bray GA, Pi-Sunyer FX, et al: Clinical efficacy of orlistat therapy in overweight and obese patients with insulin-treated type 2 diabetes: a 1-year randomized controlled trial. *Diabetes Care* 25:1033, 2002.
83. Buchwald H, Avidor Y, Braunwald E, et al: Bariatric surgery: a systematic review and meta-analysis. *JAMA* 292:1724, 2004.
84. Adherence to long-term therapies: evidence for action, Geneva, 2003, World Health Organization.
85. Briesacher BA, Gurwitz JH, Soumerai SB: Patients at-risk for cost-related medication nonadherence: a review of the literature. *J Gen Intern Med* 22:864, 2007.
86. Piette JD: Perceived access problems among patients with diabetes in two public systems of care. *J Gen Intern Med* 15:797, 2000.
87. Bodenheimer T: A 63-year-old man with multiple cardiovascular risk factors and poor adherence to treatment plans. *JAMA* 298:2048, 2007.
88. Roter DL, Hall JA: Studies of doctor-patient interaction. *Annu Rev Public Health* 10:163, 1989.
89. Schillinger D, Piette J, Grumbach K, et al: Closing the loop: physician communication with diabetic patients who have low health literacy. *Arch Intern Med* 163:83, 2003.
90 Schillinger D, Machtinger E, Wang F, et al: *Preventing medication errors in ambulatory care: the importance of establishing regimen concordance*, vol 1, Rockville, Md, 2005, Agency for Healthcare Research and Quality.
91. Chapman RH, Benner JS, Petrilla AA, et al: Predictors of adherence with antihypertensive and lipid-lowering therapy. *Arch Intern Med* 165:1147, 2005.
92. Dunbar-Jacob J, Bohachick P, Mortimer MK, et al: Medication adherence in persons with cardiovascular disease. *J Cardiovasc Nurs* 18:209, 2003.
93. Eisen SA, Miller DK, Woodward RS, et al: The effect of prescribed daily dose frequency on patient medication compliance. *Arch Intern Med* 150:1881, 1990.
94. Yiannakopoulou EC, Papadopulos JS, Cokkinos DV, Mountokalakis TD: Adherence to antihypertensive treatment: a critical factor for blood pressure control. *Eur J Cardiovasc Prev Rehabil* 12:243, 2005.

578

95. George JP, Shalansky SJ: Predictors of refill non-adherence in patients with heart failure. *Br J Clin Pharmacol* 63:488–493, 2007.
96. Iskedjian M, Einarson TR, MacKeigan LD, et al: Relationship between daily dose frequency and adherence to antihypertensive pharmacotherapy: evidence from a meta-analysis. *Clin Ther* 24:302, 2002.
97. DiMatteo MR: Variations in patients' adherence to medical recommendations: a quantitative review of 50 years of research. *Med Care* 42:200, 2004.
98. Steiner JF, Ho PM, Beaty B, et al: Sociodemographic and clinical characteristics are not clinically useful predictors of refill adherence in patients with hypertension. *Circ Cardiovasc Qual Outcomes* 2:451, 2009.
99. DiMatteo MR, Lepper HS, Croghan TW: Depression is a risk factor for noncompliance with medical treatment: meta-analysis of the effects of anxiety and depression on patient adherence. *Arch Intern Med* 160:2101, 2000.
100. Dunbar-Jacob J, Schlenk EA, Burke LE, Matthews JT: Predictors of patient adherence: patient characteristics. In Shumaker SA, Schron EB, Ockene JK, McBee WL, editors: *The handbook of health behavior change*, ed 2, New York, 1998, Springer, pp 491–511.
101. Ziegelstein RC, Fauerbach JA, Stevens SS, et al: Patients with depression are less likely to follow recommendations to reduce cardiac risk during recovery from a myocardial infarction. *Arch Intern Med* 160:1818, 2000.
102. Joosten EA, Fuentes-Merillas L, de Weert GH, et al: Systematic review of the effects of shared decision-making on patient satisfaction, treatment adherence and health status. *Psychother Psychosom* 77:219, 2008.

103. Rand C, Weeks K: Measuring adherence with medication regimens in clinical care and research. In Shumaker SA, Schron EB, Ockene JK, McBee WL, editors: *The handbook of health behavior change*, ed 2, New York, 1998, Springer, pp 114–132.
104. Vermeire E, Hearnshaw H, Van Royen P, Denekens J: Patient adherence to treatment: three decades of research. A comprehensive review. *J Clin Pharm Ther* 26:331, 2001.
105. DiMatteo MR, Haskard KB, Williams SL: Health beliefs, disease severity, and patient adherence: a meta-analysis. *Med Care* 45:521, 2007.
106. Glanz K, Lewis FM, Rimer BK: Models of individual health behavior. *Health behavior and health education: theory, research, and practice*, San Francisco, 1997, Jossey-Bass, p. 41.
107. Lacro JP, Dunn LB, Dolder CR, et al: Prevalence of and risk factors for medication nonadherence in patients with schizophrenia: a comprehensive review of recent literature. *J Clin Psychiatry* 63:892, 2002.
108. Okuno J, Yanagi H, Tomura S: Is cognitive impairment a risk factor for poor compliance among Japanese elderly in the community? *Eur J Clin Pharmacol* 57:589, 2001.

109. Perkins DO: Predictors of noncompliance in patients with schizophrenia. *J Clin Psychiatry* 63:1121, 2002.
110. Meyer D, Leventhal H, Gutmann M: Common-sense models of illness: the example of hypertension. *Health Psychol* 4:115, 1985.
111. Schlomann P, Schmitke J: Lay beliefs about hypertension: an interpretive synthesis of the qualitative research. *J Am Acad Nurse Pract* 19:358, 2007.
112. Sharkness CM, Snow DA: The patient's view of hypertension and compliance. *Am J Prev Med* 8:141, 1992.
113. Haynes RB, Yao X, Degani A, et al: Interventions to enhance medication adherence. *Cochrane Database Syst Rev* (4):CD000011, 2005.
114. Schroeder K, Fahey T, Ebrahim S: Interventions for improving adherence to treatment in patients with high blood pressure in ambulatory settings. *Cochrane Database Syst Rev* (2):CD004804, 2004.
115. Kripalani S, Yao X, Haynes RB: Interventions to enhance medication adherence in chronic medical conditions: a systematic review. *Arch Intern Med* 167:540, 2007.
116. Schroeder K, Fahey T, Ebrahim S: How can we improve adherence to blood pressure–lowering medication in ambulatory care? Systematic review of randomized controlled trials. *Arch Intern Med* 164:722, 2004.
117. Feldman R, Bacher M, Campbell N, et al: Adherence to pharmacologic management of hypertension. *Can J Public Health* 89:I16, 1998.
118. Vrijens B, Goetghebeur E: Comparing compliance patterns between randomized treatments. *Control Clin Trials* 18:187, 1997.
119. Burnier M, Schneider MP, Chiolero A, et al: Electronic compliance monitoring in resistant hypertension: the basis for rational therapeutic decisions. *J Hypertens* 19:335, 2001.
120. Cooper LA: A 41-year-old African American man with poorly controlled hypertension: review of patient and physician factors related to hypertension treatment adherence. *JAMA* 301:1260, 2009.
121. Rosen MI, Rigsby MO, Salahi JT, et al: Electronic monitoring and counseling to improve medication adherence. *Behav Res Ther* 42:409, 2004.
122. Fahey T, Schroeder K, Ebrahim S: Interventions used to improve control of blood pressure in patients with hypertension. *Cochrane Database Syst Rev* (4):CD005182, 2006.
123. Walsh JM, McDonald KM, Shojania KG, et al: Quality improvement strategies for hypertension management: a systematic review. *Med Care* 44:646, 2006.
124. Piette JD, Weinberger M, McPhee SJ, et al: Do automated calls with nurse follow-up improve self-care and glycemic control among vulnerable patients with diabetes? *Am J Med* 108:20, 2000.

35

CHAPTER **36**

Clinical Practice Guidelines and Performance Measures in the Treatment of Cardiovascular Disease

Sidney C. Smith, Jr.

KEY POINTS

- Therapeutic options for treatment of patients to prevent cardiovascular disease events have increased at an exponential rate during the past quarter century.

- The Institute of Medicine has emphasized that treatment strategies and recommendations must be founded on a strong evidence base.

- Comprehensive scientific guidelines, performance measures, and policies supporting preventive therapies will rely on this foundation of scientific information.

- Evolving data confirm the efficacy of evidence-based medicine to improve patient outcomes.

- It is imperative that health care providers shape their practices to keep abreast of the concepts put forth in the cardiovascular disease guidelines and performance measures.

The therapeutic options for treatment of patients to prevent cardiovascular disease (CVD) events have increased at an exponential rate during the past quarter century. This increase in medical therapies, procedures, and tests coupled with growing numbers of patients at risk for CVD events or surviving after an event has resulted in a wide array of treatment strategies, often leaving the health care provider uncertain about the appropriate course of action. Mounting evidence during the past decade has documented significant variation in the performance of recommended tests and therapies and patient outcomes.[1,2] On the basis of these trends and observations, the Institute of Medicine recommended in its 2001 report *Crossing the Quality Chasm: A New Health System for the 21st Century,*[3] "Patients should receive care based on the best available scientific knowledge. Care should not vary illogically from clinician to clinician or from place to place." The cardiovascular community has responded by the development of evidence-based practice guidelines and performance measures with the intent of providing consistent high-quality care and outcomes for patients with CVD.

CLINICAL PRACTICE GUIDELINES: BACKGROUND

Current strategies for prevention or treatment of CVD are increasingly based on guideline recommendations. Among such guideline statements, those issued by the American College of Cardiology (ACC) and the American Heart Association (AHA) have gained widespread recognition and use.[4,5] The origins of the ACC/AHA practice guidelines date to the early 1980s, when the federal government requested the recommendations of the ACC and AHA on the indications for cardiac pacemakers. In the early years of the guideline efforts, several statements were developed for a variety of procedures and diagnostic tests, including coronary bypass graft surgery, exercise treadmill testing, percutaneous coronary interventions, and radionuclide testing. Understanding that physicians providing patient care need information on the treatment and management of a complete disease state rather than isolated advice about when to perform a procedure or diagnostic test, the ACC/AHA practice guidelines have evolved to a focus on disease states such as ST-segment elevation myocardial infarction (STEMI), valvular heart disease, chronic stable angina, and heart failure. This has resulted in an increasing number of recommendations supported by varying levels of evidence and expert consensus opinion.

GUIDELINE RECOMMENDATIONS AND EVIDENCE

The definitions used by the ACC/AHA guideline statements for the classification of recommendations and supporting level of evidence are shown in Figure 36-1. The recommendations range from Class I, for which the benefit of a test, treatment, or procedure greatly exceeds the risk and it is recommended that the test, treatment, or procedure be done, to Class III, for which the benefit of a test, treatment, or procedure is less than or equivalent to the risk and therefore should not be done. Situated between these strong recommendations in favor for or against performing a test, procedure, or treatment are Class IIa and IIb recommendations, for which benefit exceeds risk such that the performance of the test, procedure, or treatment is deemed reasonable (IIa) or might be considered (IIb). For each class of recommendation, the guidelines must further state the level of evidence on which the recommendation is based. Level A represents multiple randomized clinical trials or meta-analyses obtained in multiple subgroups including age, gender, and ethnicity;

SIZE OF TREATMENT EFFECT →

	CLASS I *Benefit >>>Risk* Procedure/Treatment **SHOULD** be performed/administered	CLASS IIa *Benefit >>Risk* *Additional studies with focused objectives needed* **IT IS REASONABLE** to perform procedure/administer treatment	CLASS IIb *Benefit ≥ Risk* *Additional studies with broad objectives needed; additional registry data would be helpful* Procedure/Treatment **MAY BE CONSIDERED**	CLASS III *Risk ≥ Benefit* Procedure/Treatment should NOT be performed/administered **SINCE IT IS NOT HELPFUL AND MAY BE HARMFUL**
LEVEL A Multiple populations evaluated* Data derived from multiple randomized clinical trials or meta-analyses	■ Recommendation that procedure or treatment is useful/effective ■ Sufficient evidence from multiple randomized trials or meta-analyses	■ Recommendation in favor of treatment or procedure being useful/effective ■ Some conflicting evidence from multiple randomized trials or meta-analyses	■ Recommendation's usefulness/efficacy less well established ■ Greater conflicting evidence from multiple randomized trials or meta-analyses	■ Recommendation that procedure or treatment is not useful/effective and may be harmful ■ Sufficient evidence from multiple randomized trials or meta-analyses
LEVEL B Limited populations evaluated* Data derived from a single randomized trial or nonrandomized studies	■ Recommendation that procedure or treatment is useful/effective ■ Evidence from single randomized trial or nonrandomized studies	■ Recommendation in favor of treatment or procedure being useful/effective ■ Some conflicting evidence from single randomized trial or nonrandomized studies	■ Recommendation's usefulness/efficacy less well established ■ Greater conflicting evidence from single randomized trial or nonrandomized studies	■ Recommendation that procedure or treatment is not useful/effective and may be harmful ■ Evidence from single randomized trial or nonrandomized studies
LEVEL C Very limited populations evaluated* Only consensus opinion of experts, case studies, or standard of care	■ Recommendation that procedure or treatment is useful/effective ■ Only expert opinion, case studies, or standard of care	■ Recommendation in favor of treatment or procedure being useful/effective ■ Only diverging expert opinion, case studies, or standard of care	■ Recommendation's usefulness/efficacy less well established ■ Only diverging expert opinion, case studies, or standard of care	■ Recommendation that procedure or treatment is not useful/effective and may be harmful ■ Only expert opinion, case studies, or standard of care
Suggested phrases for writing recommendations †	should is recommended is indicated is useful/effective/beneficial	is reasonable can be useful/effective/beneficial is probably recommended or indicated	may/might be considered may/might be reasonable usefulness/effectiveness is unknown/unclear/uncertain or not well established	is not recommended is not indicated should not is not useful/effective/beneficial may be harmful

ESTIMATE OF CERTAINTY (PRECISION) OF TREATMENT EFFECT

36

FIGURE 36-1 ACC/AHA guideline classification of recommendations and level of evidence.
*Data available from clinical trials or registries about the usefulness/efficacy in different subpopulations, such as gender, age, history of diabetes, history of prior myocardial infarction, history of heart failure, and prior aspirin use. A recommendation with Level of Evidence B or C does not imply that the recommendation is weak. Many important clinical questions addressed in the guidelines do not lend themselves to clinical trials. Even though randomized trials are not available, there may be a very clear clinical consensus that a particular test or therapy is useful or effective.
†In 2003, the ACC/AHA Task Force on Practice Guidelines developed a list of suggested phrases to use when writing recommendations. All recommendations in this guideline have been written in full sentences that express a complete thought, such that a recommendation, even if separated and presented apart from the rest of the document (including headings above sets of recommendations), would still convey the full intent of the recommendation. It is hoped that this will increase readers' comprehension of the guidelines and will allow queries at the individual recommendation level.
(From Smith SC, Allen J, Blair SN, et al: AHA/ACC guidelines for secondary prevention for patients with coronary and other atherosclerotic vascular disease: 2006 update: endorsed by the National Heart, Lung, and Blood Institute. Circulation 113:2363, 2006.)

level B represents data from single randomized trials or non-randomized studies in which limited populations have been evaluated; and level C is based on consensus opinion of experts, case studies, or standards of care. A level of evidence of B or C does not necessarily imply a weak recommendation. There are many important clinical questions for which the number of patients available for a randomized controlled trial is too small to provide significant results or the clinical circumstances are such that there is a clear and strong consensus regarding the indication for a test, procedure, or treatment. However, the guidelines are written with the objective of having the strongest evidence base possible.

During recent years, considerable efforts have been directed toward avoiding conflicts of interest and relationships with industry that might potentially bias the

recommendations in guideline statements. The ACC and AHA have instituted strong policies to see that such interests are avoided in the development of guideline statements. Members of guideline writing committees must recuse themselves from voting when such conflicts or relationships are present, and their recusal is noted in the guideline statement. Membership of the guideline writing groups is being structured with a goal that no more than 30% of the writing group may have conflicts of interest or relationships with industry for the tests, procedures, and treatments being discussed. Further review and recommendations for approval of all ACC/AHA guidelines are provided by additional individuals, including members of the Science Advisory Committee of the AHA, Board of Trustees of the ACC, expert content reviewers, and representatives from other societies participating in the development or endorsement of the guideline. These measures help ensure that the guidelines are strongly based on evidence or objective expert consensus.

STATUS OF CURRENT GUIDELINE EVIDENCE BASE

The largest continuous experience with the development of cardiovascular guidelines is found in the joint efforts of the ACC and AHA.[4,5] These guidelines have provided critical information to assist with the establishment of standards of care and benchmarks to assess quality of care. The evolution of recommendations in these guidelines and the development of evidence base for these recommendations have been analyzed and provide insight into challenges facing development of current guideline statements.[6] Since the first ACC/AHA clinical practice guideline was released in 1984 on the indications for cardiac pacemakers to September 2008, the ACC/AHA Task Force on practice guidelines has published 53 guidelines on 22 topics resulting in a total of 7196 recommendations. Among these 53 guidelines, there were 22 that were diseased based, 15 that were interventional procedure based, and 14 that were diagnostic procedure based. The use of level of evidence for guideline recommendations was first introduced in 1998, and analysis of the 16 guidelines current at the time of the report[6] comprising a total of 2711 recommendations revealed a high proportion of recommendations (48%) to be based on expert consensus, standard of care, or case studies (level of evidence C), whereas a small number (11%) were derived from a high evidence base of multiple randomized controlled trials or meta-analyses (level of evidence A). Moreover, among those guidelines that had undergone one revision or update, there was a 48% increase in recommendations, with the greatest number occurring in Class II, indicating a level of uncertainty in the recommendation. Importantly, the secondary prevention guideline recommendations had the highest evidence base, with more than 90% being level of evidence A or B, attesting to the strong evidence available to support recommendations for preventive therapies.

FUTURE CONSIDERATIONS FOR GUIDELINE DEVELOPMENT

The observations from the review of ACC/AHA guidelines support the need for more evidence to assist with the clinical decisions faced by physicians who treat patients with CVD. The current system of clinical research that generates evidence from randomized controlled trials is largely supported by the pharmaceutical industry and in most instances is understandably directed toward gaining approval of new medical therapies. There is limited sponsorship of trials that focus on questions relating to clinical practice combining or comparing existing tests, procedures, and treatments. Broader support and funding are necessary if we are to advance the knowledge base for guideline development.

The purpose of the ACC/AHA practice guidelines is to assist health care providers in clinical decision making by describing a range of reasonably acceptable approaches to assist in the diagnosis, management, and prevention of cardiovascular diseases or conditions. Guideline recommendations attempt to define practices that will meet the needs of most patients in most circumstances. However, the ultimate judgment regarding care of a particular patient should be made by the health care provider and patient, with all of the circumstances presented by that patient taken into consideration. Thus, there are circumstances in which deviations from these guidelines may be appropriate, especially when a recommendation is of lower certainty, such as Class IIb, and supported primarily by expert opinion level C. Clinical decision making should also consider the quality and availability of expertise in the area where care is provided. On occasion, the ACC/AHA guidelines may be used as the basis for regulatory or payer decisions, but their ultimate goal is to improve quality of care and to serve the patient's best interests.

GUIDELINES FOR SECONDARY PREVENTION

The AHA/ACC Guidelines for Secondary Prevention, endorsed by the National Heart, Lung, and Blood Institute (NHLBI), provide concise evidence-based recommendations for the prevention of cardiovascular events in patients with established CVD.[7] The goal for controlling each risk factor is listed in conjunction with recommended therapeutic interventions to achieve that goal (Table 36-1). The class of recommendation and evidence base for each intervention are concisely summarized, and the references and supplemental search criteria are provided. As noted earlier in this chapter, these guidelines have a high evidence base, with more than 90% being level A or B. They are widely used and quoted and provide the basis for the AHA and ACC quality improvement programs reviewed later in this chapter.

The recommendations are closely coordinated with statements from the National Institutes of Health/NHLBI and the Centers for Disease Control and Prevention (CDC) and updated on the basis of the evolving evidence base for each risk factor. For example, recommendations on target goals for lipids and hypertension are consistent with those put forth by the NHLBI National Cholesterol Adult Treatment Panel[8,9] and the Joint National Committee on Prevention, Detection, Evaluation, and Treatment of High Blood Pressure,[10] and the recommendations for influenza vaccine in all patients with atherosclerotic vascular disease are consistent with those of the CDC Advisory Committee on Immunization Practices.[11] These guideline recommendations are also integrated into other relevant guideline statements from the ACC/AHA, such as those for ST-segment myocardial infarction, unstable angina/non–ST-segment myocardial infarction, chronic stable angina, and percutaneous coronary interventions, and updated as dictated by new evidence from randomized controlled trials and other sources.

A consistent focus of these guidelines has been the assessment of the evidence base according to gender, age, and ethnicity. Many randomized controlled trials have cut points for study inclusion at 75 or 80 years of age or have underrepresentation of women or minority ethnic groups. Thus, the evidence base for recommendations may not be universally consistent across age, gender, and ethnic groups. Recognizing the differences that do exist in the evidence base for women and the elderly, the AHA has developed guideline statements[12,13] focusing specifically on the evidence base for those groups that serve as valuable additions to the general guideline statements.

PERFORMANCE MEASURES: BACKGROUND

Numerous studies have demonstrated a gap between guideline recommendations and the quality of care rendered to patients. The Institute of Medicine has outlined deficiencies that exist in delivery of effective, timely, safe, and equitable care to patients. Recognizing the importance of these concerns, the ACC and AHA have taken a leadership role in the development of performance measures[14] for several cardiovascular conditions (Table 36-2). These performance

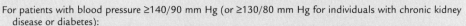

| **TABLE 36–1** | **AHA/ACC Secondary Prevention for Patients with Coronary and Other Vascular Disease*: 2006 Update** |

Intervention Recommendations with Class of Recommendation and Level of Evidence

Smoking

Goal
Complete cessation. No exposure to environmental tobacco smoke.

- Ask about tobacco use status at every visit. **I (B)**
- Advise every tobacco user to quit. **I (B)**
- Assess the tobacco user's willingness to quit. **I (B)**
- Assist by counseling and developing a plan for quitting. **I (B)**
- Arrange follow-up, referral to special programs, or pharmacotherapy (including nicotine replacement and bupropion). **I (B)**
- Urge avoidance of exposure to environmental tobacco smoke at work and home. **I (B)**

Blood Pressure Control

Goal
<140/90 mm Hg
or
<130/80 mm Hg if patient has diabetes or chronic kidney disease

For all patients:
- Initiate or maintain lifestyle modification—weight control; increased physical activity; alcohol moderation; sodium reduction; and emphasis on increased consumption of fresh fruits, vegetables, and low-fat dairy products. **I (B)**

For patients with blood pressure ≥140/90 mm Hg (or ≥130/80 mm Hg for individuals with chronic kidney disease or diabetes):
- As tolerated, add blood pressure medication, treating initially with beta blockers and/or ACE inhibitors, with addition of other drugs such as thiazides as needed to achieve goal blood pressure. **I (A)**
[For compelling indications for individual drug classes in specific vascular diseases, see Seventh Report of the Joint National Committee on Prevention, Detection, Evaluation, and Treatment of High Blood Pressure (JNC 7).][10]

Lipid Management

Goal
LDL-C <100 mg/dL
If triglycerides are ≥200 mg/dL, non–HDL-C should be <130 mg/dL[†]

For all patients:
- Start dietary therapy. Reduce intake of saturated fats (to <7% of total calories), *trans*–fatty acids, and cholesterol (to <200 mg/d). **I (B)**
- Adding plant stanol/sterols (2 g/d) and viscous fiber (>10 g/d) will further lower LDL-C.
- Promote daily physical activity and weight management. **I (B)**
- Encourage increased consumption of omega-3 fatty acids in the form of fish[‡] or in capsule form (1 g/d) for risk reduction. For treatment of elevated triglycerides, higher doses are usually necessary for risk reduction. **IIb (B)**

For lipid management:
Assess fasting lipid profile in all patients, and within 24 hours of hospitalization for those with an acute cardiovascular or coronary event. For hospitalized patients, initiate lipid-lowering medication as recommended below before discharge according to the following schedule:
- LDL-C should be <100 mg/dL **I (A)**, **and**
- Further reduction of LDL-C to <70 mg/dL is reasonable. **IIa (A)**
- If baseline LDL-C is ≥100 mg/dL, initiate LDL-lowering drug therapy.[§] **I (A)**
- If on-treatment LDL-C is ≥100 mg/dL, intensify LDL-lowering drug therapy (may require LDL-lowering drug combination[||]). **I (A)**
- If baseline LDL-C is 70 to 100 mg/dL, it is reasonable to treat to LDL-C <70 mg/dL. **IIa (B)**
- If triglycerides are 200 to 499 mg/dL, non–HDL-C should be <130 mg/dL. **I (B)**, **and**
- Further reduction of non–HDL-C to <100 mg/dL is reasonable. **IIa (B)**
- Therapeutic options to reduce non–HDL-C are:
  - More intense LDL-C–lowering therapy **I (B)**, or
  - Niacin[¶] (after LDL-C–lowering therapy) **IIa (B)**, or
  - Fibrate therapy[#] (after LDL-C–lowering therapy) **IIa (B)**
- If triglycerides are ≥500 mg/dL,[#] therapeutic options to prevent pancreatitis are fibrate[¶] or niacin[¶] before LDL-lowering therapy; and treat LDL-C to goal after triglyceride-lowering therapy. Achieve non–HDL-C <130 mg/dL if possible. **I (C)**

Physical Activity

Goal
30 minutes, 7 days per week (minimum 5 days per week)

- For all patients, assess risk with a physical activity history and/or an exercise test, to guide prescription. **I (B)**
- For all patients, encourage 30 to 60 minutes of moderate-intensity aerobic activity, such as brisk walking, on most, preferably all, days of the week, supplemented by an increase in daily lifestyle activities (e.g., walking breaks at work, gardening, household work). **I (B)**
- Encourage resistance training 2 days per week. **IIb (C)**
- Advise medically supervised programs for high-risk patients (e.g., recent acute coronary syndrome or revascularization, heart failure). **I (B)**

Weight Management

Goal
Body mass index: 18.5 to 24.9 kg/m^2

Waist circumference: men <40 inches, women <35 inches

- Assess body mass index and/or waist circumference on each visit and consistently encourage weight maintenance/reduction through an appropriate balance of physical activity, caloric intake, and formal behavioral programs when indicated to maintain/achieve a body mass index between 18.5 and 24.9 kg/m^2. **I (B)**
- If waist circumference (measured horizontally at the iliac crest) is ≥35 inches in women and ≥40 inches in men, initiate lifestyle changes and consider treatment strategies for metabolic syndrome as indicated. **I (B)**
- The initial goal of weight loss therapy should be to reduce body weight by approximately 10% from baseline. With success, further weight loss can be attempted if indicated through further assessment. **I (B)**

TABLE 36–1 | **AHA/ACC Secondary Prevention for Patients with Coronary and Other Vascular Disease*: 2006 Update—cont'd**

583

	Intervention Recommendations with Class of Recommendation and Level of Evidence
Diabetes Management *Goal* HbA1c <7%	• Initiate lifestyle and pharmacotherapy to achieve near-normal HbA1c. **I (B)** • Begin vigorous modification of other risk factors (e.g., physical activity, weight management, blood pressure control, and cholesterol management as recommended above). **I (B)** • Coordinate diabetic care with patient's primary care physician or endocrinologist. **I (C)**

Antiplatelet Agents/Anticoagulants	• Start aspirin 75 to 162 mg/d and continue indefinitely in all patients unless contraindicated. **I (A)**
	  • For patients undergoing coronary artery bypass grafting, aspirin should be started within 48 hours after surgery to reduce saphenous vein graft closure. Dosing regimens ranging from 100 to 325 mg/d appear to be efficacious. Doses higher than 162 mg/d can be continued for up to 1 year. **I (B)**
	• Start and continue clopidogrel 75 mg/d in combination with aspirin for up to 12 months in patients after acute coronary syndrome or percutaneous coronary intervention with stent placement (≥1 month for bare metal stent, ≥3 months for sirolimus-eluting stent, and ≥6 months for paclitaxel-eluting stent). **I (B)**
	  • Patients who have undergone percutaneous coronary intervention with stent placement should initially receive higher-dose aspirin at 325 mg/d for 1 month for bare metal stent, 3 months for sirolimus-eluting stent, and 6 months for paclitaxel-eluting stent. **I (B)**
	• Manage warfarin to international normalized ratio = 2.0 to 3.0 for paroxysmal or chronic atrial fibrillation or flutter, and in post–myocardial infarction patients when clinically indicated (e.g., atrial fibrillation, left ventricular thrombus). **I (A)**
	• Use of warfarin in conjunction with aspirin and/or clopidogrel is associated with increased risk of bleeding and should be monitored closely. **I (B)**

Renin-Angiotensin-Aldosterone System Blockers	ACE inhibitors: • Start and continue indefinitely in all patients with left ventricular ejection fraction ≤40% and in those with hypertension, diabetes, or chronic kidney disease, unless contraindicated. **I (A)** • Consider for all other patients. **I (B)** • Among lower-risk patients with normal left ventricular ejection fraction in whom cardiovascular risk factors are well controlled and revascularization has been performed, use of ACE inhibitors may be considered optional. **IIa (B)**
	Angiotensin receptor blockers: • Use in patients who are intolerant of ACE inhibitors and have heart failure or have had a myocardial infarction with left ventricular ejection fraction ≤40%. **I (A)** • Consider in other patients who are ACE inhibitor intolerant. **I (B)** • Consider use in combination with ACE inhibitors in systolic-dysfunction heart failure. **IIb (B)**
	Aldosterone blockade: • Use in post–myocardial infarction patients, without significant renal dysfunction** or hyperkalemia,^{††} who are already receiving therapeutic doses of an ACE inhibitor and beta blocker, have a left ventricular ejection fraction ≤40%, and have either diabetes or heart failure. **I (A)**
Beta Blockers	• Start and continue indefinitely in all patients who have had myocardial infarction, acute coronary syndrome, or left ventricular dysfunction with or without heart failure symptoms, unless contraindicated. **I (A)** Consider chronic therapy for all other patients with coronary or other vascular disease or diabetes unless contraindicated. **IIa (C)**
Influenza Vaccination	Patients with cardiovascular disease should have an influenza vaccination. **I (B)**

*Patients covered by these guidelines include those with established coronary and other atherosclerotic vascular disease, including peripheral arterial disease, atherosclerotic aortic disease, and carotid artery disease. Treatment of patients whose only manifestation of cardiovascular risk is diabetes will be the topic of a separate AHA scientific statement. ACE indicates angiotensin-converting enzyme.

†Non-HDL-C, total cholesterol minus HDL-C.

‡Pregnant and lactating women should limit their intake of fish to minimize exposure to methylmercury.

§When LDL-lowering medications are used, obtain at least a 30% to 40% reduction in LDL-C levels. If LDL-C <70 mg/dL is the chosen target, consider drug titration to achieve this level to minimize side effects and cost. When LDL-C <70 mg/dL is not achievable because of high baseline LDL-C levels, it generally is possible to achieve reductions of >50% in LDL-C levels by either statins or LDL-C–lowering drug combinations.

‖Standard dose of statin with ezetimibe, bile acid sequestrant, or niacin.

¶The combination of high-dose statin + fibrate can increase risk for severe myopathy. Statin doses should be kept relatively low with this combination. Dietary supplement niacin must not be used as a substitute for prescription niacin.

#Patients with very high triglycerides should not consume alcohol. The use of bile acid sequestrant is relatively contraindicated when triglycerides are >200 mg/dL.

**Creatinine should be <2.5 mg/dL in men and <2.0 mg/dL in women.

††Potassium should be <5.0 mEq/L.

From Smith SC, Allen J, Blair SN, et al: AHA/ACC guidelines for secondary prevention for patients with coronary and other atherosclerotic vascular disease: 2006 update: endorsed by the National Heart, Lung, and Blood Institute. *Circulation* 113:2363, 2006.

TABLE 36–2	ACCF/AHA Performance Measure Sets		
Topic	**Original Publication Date**	**Partnering Organizations**	**Status**
Chronic heart failure	2005	ACC/AHA—inpatient measures ACC/AHA/PCPI—outpatient measures	Currently undergoing update Currently undergoing update
Chronic stable coronary artery disease	2005	ACC/AHA/PCPI	Currently undergoing update
Hypertension	2005	ACC/AHA/PCPI	Currently undergoing update
ST elevation and non-ST elevation myocardial infarction	2006	ACC/AHA	Updated 2008
Cardiac rehabilitation	2007	AACVPR/ACC/AHA	
Atrial fibrillation	2008	ACC/AHA/PCPI	
Primary prevention of cardiovascular disease	2009	ACCF/AHA	
Peripheral arterial disease	2010*	ACCF/AHA/ACR/SCAI/SIR/SVM/SVN/SVS	

*Planned publication date.

AACVPR, American Association of Cardiovascular and Pulmonary Rehabilitation; ACC, American College of Cardiology; ACCF, American College of Cardiology Foundation; ACR, American College of Radiology; AHA, American Heart Association; PCPI, American Medical Association–Physician Consortium for Performance Improvement; SCAI, Society for Cardiac Angiography and Interventions; SIR, Society for Interventional Radiology; SVM, Society for Vascular Medicine; SVN, Society for Vascular Nursing; SVS, Society for Vascular Surgery.

From Redberg RF, Benjamin E, Bittner V, et al: ACCF/AHA 2009 performance measures for primary prevention of cardiovascular disease in adults. *J Am Coll Cardiol* 54:1364, 2009.

measures can be used for quality improvement programs directed toward improving patient outcomes. The basis for performance measures has generally been Class I or Class III recommendations from the ACC/AHA guidelines, which identify procedures or treatments that should or should not be given to patients. These processes of care measures are now combined with recommendations regarding structure of care that deal with the environment in which patients are treated and outcomes of care that assess health care systems on the basis of improved outcomes for patient care. The initial purpose of the ACC/AHA performance measures was for use in quality improvement efforts; however, their application has been expanded by other organizations for public reporting or external review. This development has led the performance measure writing groups to characterize their recommendations as either performance measures or test measures. The distinction between the two is that performance measures are those recommendations that are deemed appropriate for use in both quality improvement programs and external reporting, whereas test measures are those thought to be appropriate for quality improvement but not for external reporting until their efficacy has been validated. Thus, field testing of performance measures is strongly recommended if they are considered for use beyond quality improvement.

DEVELOPMENT AND SELECTION OF PERFORMANCE MEASURES

Performance measures generally target a specific patient population that is observed during a particular time period. For example, the performance measures for primary prevention outlined later in this chapter define the population as those patients older than 18 years to avoid conflict with recommendations for children. In addition, certain measures are given an upper age limit of 80 years because of the absence of evidence to support the recommendation in patients older than 80 years. Criteria for final selection of performance measures include (1) those Class I or III guideline recommendations with the strongest class of recommendation and level

of evidence, (2) the ease or complexity of the measurement, and (3) coverage in other performance measurement sets. The phrasing of performance measures is given careful consideration. For example, many patients are unable to achieve recommended blood pressure control because of medication noncompliance, costs, side effects, or other reasons. To avoid penalizing the physician for these issues that are beyond the physician's control, the measure is written to accept documentation of the use of at least two medications in patients whose blood pressures are greater than the target of 140/90 mm Hg or the achievement of the recommended target outcome.

Potential performance measures are developed with use of criteria that carefully define measurement parameters and evidence for or against the recommended measure as well as their applicability, interpretability, and feasibility. Specific attributes of highly desirable performance measures have been carefully defined by the ACC/AHA Task Force on Performance Measures (Table 36-3). Not all performance measures are based on level A evidence. For example, in dealing with a recommendation to counsel regarding cessation of tobacco use, the absence of multiple large randomized controlled studies does not preclude consideration of this important measure. By contrast, in the case of pharmaceutical agents that lend themselves to large randomized controlled trials, the need for level A evidence base is greater.

PERFORMANCE MEASURES FOR PRIMARY PREVENTION OF CARDIOVASCULAR DISEASE IN ADULTS

The 2009 ACC/AHA performance measures for primary prevention in adults[15] list 13 measures including recommendations involving lifestyle, blood pressure, lipids, global risk, and aspirin (Table 36-4). These 13 measures apply to all adults without CVD, including those without diabetes. They support practices expected to reduce the long-term risk of cardiovascular events. Because any single visit may not provide full opportunity for the full range of the performance

TABLE 36–3	Summary of ACCF/AHA Attributes of Performance Measures
Consideration	**Attribute**
Useful in improving patient outcomes	Evidence based Interpretable Actionable
Measure design	Denominator precisely defined Numerator precisely defined Validity type • Face* • Content† • Construct‡ Reliability
Measure implementation	Feasibility • Reasonable effort • Reasonable cost • Reasonable time period for collection
Overall assessment	Overall assessment of measure for inclusion in measurement set

*The measure intuitively appears to capture what it is intended to capture.
†The extent to which the items comprehensively capture the domain they are intended to measure.
‡The extent to which the measures correlate with other methods of quantifying the underlying construct.
From Redberg RF, Benjamin E, Bittner V, et al: ACCF/AHA 2009 performance measures for primary prevention of cardiovascular disease in adults. *J Am Coll Cardiol* 54:1364, 2009.

measures to be addressed, at least two encounters during a period of 1 year are recommended before the physician is expected to have responsibility for primary CVD prevention. Two of the measures, aspirin use and global risk estimation, are considered appropriate for internal quality improvement only. Statins are recognized as the mainstay of lipid-lowering therapy; however, given the variable response to lipid-lowering agents and their side effects, the writing group chose to accept either the attainment of a target goal for lipid lowering or the documented use of more than one lipid-lowering agent.

VALIDATION THAT GUIDELINES AND PERFORMANCE MEASURES IMPROVE CARDIOVASCULAR DISEASE OUTCOMES

The AHA and ACC have both developed programs aimed toward improving the use of guideline-recommended therapies by physicians. The ACC Guidelines Applied in Practice (GAP) program studied the potential benefits of guideline-recommended evidenced-based therapies among 2857 Medicare patients admitted to 38 hospitals in southeastern Michigan.[16] For GAP patients receiving guideline-recommended therapies, a significant reduction was observed in the in-hospital, 30-day, and 1-year mortality. After multivariate analysis, GAP accounted for a 21% to 26% reduction in mortality.

The AHA Get With The Guidelines (GWTG) program uses local physician champions, multidisciplinary teams, and preprinted orders along with a web-based Patient Management Tool to improve the use of evidence-based guideline-recommended therapies. Early results from GWTG[17] from 45,988 patients in 92 hospitals revealed improvement in the use of 10 of 11 guideline-recommended measures. This

TABLE 36–4	ACC/AHA Primary Prevention of Cardiovascular Disease Performance Measurement Set	
Performance Measure Name	**Measure Description**	**Designation**
1. Lifestyle/risk factor screening	Assessment of lifestyles and risk factors for development of CVD	A/PR IQI
2. Dietary intake counseling	Counseling to eat a healthy diet	A/PR
3. Physical activity counseling	Counseling to engage in regular physical activity	A/PR
4. Smoking/tobacco use	Risk assessment for smoking and tobacco use behaviors	A/PR IQI
5. Smoking/tobacco cessation	Cessation intervention for active smoking (tobacco use)	A/PR
6. Weight/adiposity assessment	Measurement of weight and body mass index and/or waist circumference	A/PR
7. Weight management	Counseling to achieve and maintain ideal body weight	A/PR IQI
8. Blood pressure measurement	Measurement of blood pressure in all patients	A/PR
9. Blood pressure control	Effective blood pressure control or combination therapy for patients with hypertension	A/PR IQI
10. Blood lipid measurement	Fasting lipid profile performed	A/PR IQI
11. Blood lipid therapy and control	Proportion of patients who meet current LDL-C treatment targets *or* who are prescribed ≥1 lipid-lowering medications at maximum tolerated dose	A/PR
12. Global risk estimation	Use of a multivariable risk score to estimate a patient's absolute risk for development of coronary heart disease	IQI
13. Aspirin use	Aspirin in patients without clinical evidence of atherosclerotic disease who are at higher CVD risk	IQI

A/PR, accountability/public reporting measures (appropriate for all uses, including internal quality improvement, pay for performance, physician ranking, and public reporting); CVD, cardiovascular disease; IQI, internal quality improvement measures (recommended for use in internal quality improvement programs only; not appropriate for any other use, e.g., pay for performance, physician ranking, or public reporting); LDL-C, low-density lipoprotein cholesterol.
From Redberg RF, Benjamin E, Bittner V, et al: ACCF/AHA 2009 performance measures for primary prevention of cardiovascular disease in adults. *J Am Coll Cardiol* 54:1364, 2009.

improvement in the use of recommended therapies occurred during a 1-year period, much faster than would have been expected from traditional quality improvement programs. Subsequent studies[18] comparing use of guideline-recommended measures in 233 GWTG hospitals with 3407 non-GWTG hospitals also observed better results for the GWTG hospitals. Results from the GWTG data base have also provided important information about differences in therapy.

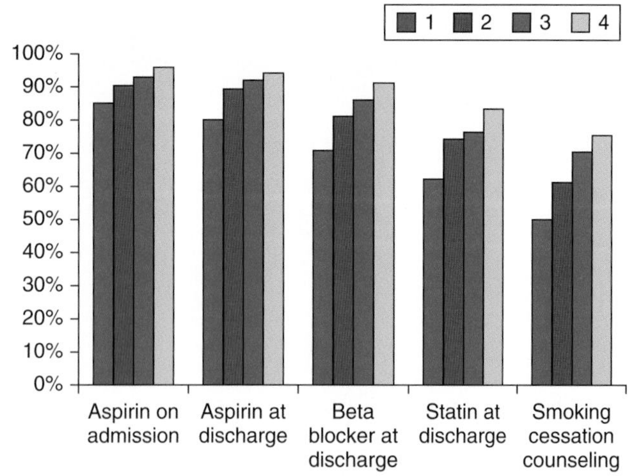

FIGURE 36-2 Compliance by quartile with guidelines of acute myocardial infarction. Bars show percentage compliance for quartiles of hospitals grouped by performance. *(From Braunwald's heart disease,* ed 8; *after Peterson ED, Roe MT, Mulgund J, et al: Association between hospital process performance and outcomes among patients with acute coronary syndromes.* JAMA 295:1912, 2006.)

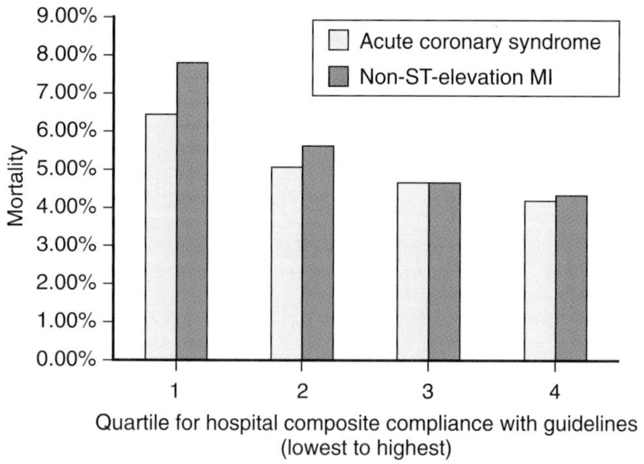

FIGURE 36-3 In-hospital mortality for patients with acute coronary syndrome and non–ST elevation myocardial infarction correlated with hospital compliance with guidelines. Bars show percentage compliance for quartiles of hospitals grouped by performance. *(From Braunwald's heart disease,* ed 8; *after Peterson ED, Roe MT, Mulgund J, et al: Association between hospital process performance and outcomes among patients with acute coronary syndromes.* JAMA 295:1912, 2006.)

36

In 78,254 patients with acute myocardial infarction admitted to 420 GWTG hospitals, women were shown to be less likely to receive aspirin and beta blockers on admission and less likely to undergo cardiac catheterization and revascularization.[19]

Important observational data indicate that broader use of guideline-based therapies is associated with improved outcomes.[20] Analysis of hospital care in 350 academic and nonacademic hospitals involving 64,775 patients presenting with findings consistent with non–ST elevation myocardial infarction revealed wide variation in adherence (63% to 82%) to nine ACC/AHA guideline-recommended therapies (Fig. 36-2). Further, the guideline adherence rate was significantly associated with in-hospital mortality, with mortality rates significantly decreasing from 6.31% for the lowest adherence quartile to 4.15% for the highest adherence quartile. After risk adjustment, every 10% increase in composite adherence to guidelines at a hospital was associated with a 10% decrease in patients' likelihood of in-hospital mortality (Fig. 36-3). These findings strongly support the use of guideline-based treatments at the system-wide level for the management of patients with CVD.

ADHERENCE TO PREVENTIVE THERAPIES

The success of evidence-based guideline implementation is founded on adherence by patients and physicians to the recommended therapies. As aptly put by Surgeon General C. Everett Koop, "Drugs don't work in patients who don't take them." Effective adherence to recommended medical therapies involves an active partnership between patients and physicians within a health care system to implement and to continue appropriate treatments and behaviors. Unfortunately, there is mounting evidence that nonadherence is widely present and results in worsened outcomes and increased cost of care.[21] Nearly one of four patients with myocardial infarction does not fill medications after discharge from the hospital by day 7.[22] Lack of adherence to medications has been shown to result in adverse outcomes.[23] Among patients with chronic coronary heart disease, nonadherence to medications such as beta blockers, statins, and

TABLE 36–5	Reasons for Medical Nonadherence	
Categories of Nonadherence	**Examples**
Health system	Poor quality of provider-patient relationship; poor communication; lack of access to health care; lack of continuity of care
Condition	Asymptomatic chronic disease (lack of physical cues); mental health disorders (e.g., depression)
Patient	Physical impairments (e.g., vision problems or impaired dexterity); cognitive impairment; psychological/behavioral; younger age; nonwhite race
Therapy	Complexity of regimen; side effects
Socioeconomic	Low literacy; higher medication costs; poor social support

From Ho PM, Bryson CL, Rumsfeld JS: Medication adherence. *Circulation* 119:3028, 2009.

angiotensin-converting enzyme inhibitors has been associated with a 10% to 40% increase in hospitalizations for cardiovascular causes and a 50% to 80% relative increase in risk of mortality.[24]

There are many reasons for nonadherence that have been summarized by the World Health Organization into five major categories (Table 36-5).[25] Younger patients, especially those who are depressed or nonwhite, are less likely to adhere to recommended therapies. Chronic conditions requiring ongoing therapy are associated with nonadherence. Low literacy, higher medication costs, and poor social support are important considerations. Successful implementation of medical therapies requires a combined effort involving health care providers, patients, and organizations delivering or paying for health care. The AHA GWTG program has demonstrated success in improving health care provider adherence to recommended guideline therapies. Patient education is the first step to improvement of patient adherence and must be repeated on subsequent outpatient visits. Telephone follow-up and other reminders can also be an effective tool to improve adherence. Finally, hospitals and payers are increasingly recognizing that cost of medical care is adversely associated with nonadherence and are therefore becoming involved in programs that assist health care providers and patients to implement and to sustain recommended therapies.

Whereas great progress has been recognized in the development of guidelines and performance measures for patient care, the success of these efforts resides with effective programs directed toward ensuring adherence by providers and patients with recommended therapies. This will be a growing area of research and emphasis for our health care system.

CONCLUSION

Health care is currently undergoing major changes. The Institute of Medicine has emphasized that treatment strategies and recommendations must be founded on a strong evidence base. Comprehensive policies supporting preventive therapies will rely on this foundation of scientific information. Evolving data confirm the efficacy of evidence-based medicine to improve patient outcomes. It is imperative that health care providers shape their practices to keep abreast of the concepts put forth in the CVD guidelines and performance measures and enable patients to adhere to the recommended therapies.

REFERENCES

1. McGlynn EA, Asch SM, Adams J, et al: The quality of health care delivered to adults in the United States. *N Engl J Med* 348:2635, 2003.
2. Lee TH, Meyer GS, Brennan TA: A middle ground on public accountability. *N Engl J Med* 350:2409, 2004.
3. National Academies Committee on Quality of Health Care in America, Institute of Medicine: *Crossing the quality chasm: a new health system for the 21st century*, Washington, DC, 2001, National Academies Press.
4. Gibbons RJ, Smith S, Antman E: American College of Cardiology/American Heart Association clinical practice guidelines: part I: where do they come from? *Circulation* 107:2979, 2003.
5. Gibbons RJ, Smith S, Antman E: American College of Cardiology/American Heart Association clinical practice guidelines: part II: evolutionary changes in a continuous quality improvement project. *Circulation* 107:3101, 2003.
6. Tricoci P, Allen JM, Kramer JM, et al: Scientific evidence underlying the ACC/AHA clinical practice guidelines. *JAMA* 301:831, 2009.
7. Smith SC, Allen J, Blair SN, et al: AHA/ACC guidelines for secondary prevention for patients with coronary and other atherosclerotic vascular disease: 2006 update: endorsed by the National Heart, Lung, and Blood Institute. *Circulation* 113:2363, 2006.
8. Expert Panel on Detection, Evaluation, and Treatment of High Blood Cholesterol in Adults: Executive Summary of the Third Report of The National Cholesterol Education Program (NCEP) Expert Panel on Detection, Evaluation, And Treatment of High Blood Cholesterol In Adults (Adult Treatment Panel III). *JAMA* 285:2486, 2001.
9. Grundy SM, Cleeman JI, Merz CN, et al: National Heart, Lung, and Blood Institute; American College of Cardiology Foundation; American Heart Association: Implications of recent clinical trials for the National Cholesterol Education Program Adult Treatment Panel III guidelines [erratum in *Circulation* 110:763, 2004]. *Circulation* 110:227, 2004.
10. Chobanian AV, Bakris GL, Black HR, et al: Joint National Committee on Prevention, Detection, Evaluation, and Treatment of High Blood Pressure. National Heart, Lung, and Blood Institute; National High Blood Pressure Education Program Coordinating Committee: Seventh report of the Joint National Committee on Prevention, Detection, Evaluation, and Treatment of High Blood Pressure. *Hypertension* 42:1206, 2003.
11. Harper SA, Fukuda K, Uyeki TM, et al: Advisory Committee on Immunization Practices (ACIP), Centers for Disease Control and Prevention (CDC): Prevention and control of influenza. Recommendations of the Advisory Committee on Immunization Practices (ACIP) [erratum in *MMWR Morb Mortal Wkly Rep* 54:750, 2005]. *MMWR Recomm Rep* 54:1, 2005.
12. Williams MA, Fleg JL, Ades PA, et al: Secondary prevention of coronary heart disease in the elderly (with emphasis on patients ≥75 years of age). *Circulation* 105:1735, 2002.
13. Mosca L, Banka CL, Benjamin EJ, et al: Evidence-based guidelines for cardiovascular disease prevention in women: 2007 update. *Circulation* 115:1481, 2007.
14. Spertus JA, Eagle KA, Krumholz HM, et al: American College of Cardiology and American Heart Association methodology for the selection and creation of performance measures for quantifying the quality of cardiovascular care. *J Am Coll Cardiol* 45:1147, 2005.
15. Redberg RF, Benjamin E, Bittner V, et al: ACCF/AHA 2009 performance measures for primary prevention of cardiovascular disease in adults. *J Am Coll Cardiol* 54:1364, 2009.
16. Eagle KA, Montoye CK, Riba AL, et al: Guideline-based standardized care is associated with substantially lower mortality in Medicare patients with acute myocardial infarction. *J Am Coll Cardiol* 46:1242, 2005.
17. LaBresh KA, Fonarow GC, Smith SC, et al: Improved treatment of hospitalized coronary artery disease patients with the get with the guidelines program. *Crit Pathw Cardiol* 6:98, 2007.
18. Lewis WR, Peterson ED, Cannon CP, et al: An organized approach to improvement in guideline adherence for acute myocardial infarction. *Arch Intern Med* 168:1813, 2008.
19. Jneid H, Fonarow GC, Cannon CP, et al: Sex differences in medical care and early mortality after acute myocardial infarction. *Circulation* 118:2803, 2008. DOI: 10.1161/ CIRCULATIONAHA. 108.789800.
20. Peterson ED, Roe MT, Mulgund J, et al: Association between hospital process performance and outcomes among patients with acute coronary syndromes. *JAMA* 295:1912, 2006.
21. Osterberg L, Blaschke T: Adherence to medication. *N Engl J Med* 353:487, 2005.
22. JackeviciusCA, Li P, Tu JV: Prevalence, predictors, and outcomes of primary nonadherence after acute myocardial infarction. *Circulation* 117:1028, 2008.
23. Ho PM, Spertus JA, Masoudi FA, et al: Impact of medication therapy discontinuation on mortality after myocardial infarction. *Arch Intern Med* 166:1842, 2006.
24. Ho PM, Magid DJ, Shetterly SM, et al: Medication nonadherence is associated with a broad range of adverse outcomes in patients with coronary artery disease. *Am Heart J* 155:772, 2008.
25. Ho PM, Bryson CL, Rumsfeld JS: Medication adherence. *Circulation* 119:3028, 2009.

A